Transforming Social Determinants to Promote Global Health

Jill B. Hamilton · Charles E. Moore
Editors

Transforming Social Determinants to Promote Global Health

Achieving Health Equity through Lived Experiences

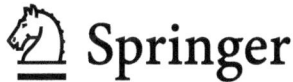 Springer

Editors
Jill B. Hamilton
Nell Hodgson Woodruff
School of Nursing
Emory University
Atlanta, GA, USA

Charles E. Moore
Department of Otolaryngology
Grady Health System
Emory University
Atlanta, GA, USA

ISBN 978-3-031-61159-9   ISBN 978-3-031-61160-5   (eBook)
https://doi.org/10.1007/978-3-031-61160-5

This Springer imprint is published by the registered company Springer Nature Switzerland AG
The registered company address is: Gewerbestrasse 11, 6330 Cham, Switzerland

If disposing of this product, please recycle the paper.

Foreword

As health professionals strive to be more knowledgeable about the impact of social determinants of health (SDOH), stories are needed to illustrate the multiple ways that these factors have influenced the huge variations in health outcomes that we see across communities nationally and globally. This book addresses this need and includes the voices of researchers, clinicians, community stakeholders, and leaders of faith-based institutions in their efforts to integrate knowledge of SDOH into their community-based work. The authors of this book represent communities from the global north (rural, urban-inner city, southern, northeastern, and western geographical regions of the USA) and the global south (Botswana, Ethiopia, Ghana, the Grenadines, Kenya, Malawi, Nigeria, Peru, and Tanzania). The various chapters capture these authors' experiences with the integration of SDOH into communities using a storytelling approach that will hopefully capture the interest of readers in the academy as well as individuals from the communities they represent. We anticipate that this book can be used as an illustrative guide to understanding diverse approaches to the integration of SDOH in community initiatives. The stories also provide examples of how transdisciplinary teams of faculty and students from schools of nursing, public health, medicine, clinicians in healthcare settings, and community leaders address SDOH in their communities. Readers may also find that content of the book useful for students beginning to explore practical approaches to the integration of SDOH into interventions or programs designed to alleviate health disparities and health inequities that exist among populations located in historically underserved and low resource communities globally. I wish to thank all the authors for the rich contributions they made to this work and especially acknowledge Dr. Jill Hamilton's vision and knowledge in bringing these authors together for a book that will have impact in advancing our knowledge of SDOH.

Nell Hodgson Woodruff School of Nursing   Linda A. McCauley
Emory University,
Atlanta, GA, USA

Acknowledgments

This book features stories that illustrate the ways in which SDOH is integrated into communities to address health inequities and promote global health. We are grateful for the researchers, clinicians, community partners, and students who either contributed to the chapters presented in this book or provided administrative support that enabled the completion of this project.

We would like to acknowledge with gratitude, the support from Nell Hodgson Woodruff School of Nursing administrative staff Margie Hutson, Kayla Vivian Slack, and colleague Lalita Kaligotla for their editorial assistance. We are also extremely grateful to Charlyne Anne Nicolas, Nakia C. Best, and Autherine Abiri for their continual support throughout this project.

Contents

About the Editors

Jill B. Hamilton, PhD, MRPL, RN, FAAN is Professor (tenured) and Senior Faculty Fellow of SDOH and Health Disparities at the Nell Hodgson Woodruff School of Nursing and Affiliate Professor at Candler School of Theology at Emory University in Atlanta, Georgia. Dr. Hamilton earned her BSN, MSN, and PhD in nursing from the University of North Carolina at Chapel Hill, a BS in Accounting from North Carolina Central University, postdoctoral training in the nursing care of older adults at the Oregon Health and Science University, and a Master's in Religion and Public Life at the Candler School of Theology. She previously held faculty positions at Johns Hopkins University and the University of North Carolina at Chapel Hill where she was a tenured Associate Professor. Dr. Hamilton's research interests include social determinants of health, health disparities, and the mental health promoting strategies used among older African American their families in response to life-threatening illness. Dr. Hamilton is Leading Editor of a text with Springer Nature titled *Integrating a Social Determinants of Health Framework into Nursing Education* published in 2023. She has done original research on the effects of storytelling that incorporates Black Sacred Music and scripture on psychological distress among older and younger African Americans. She was a Georgia Cancer Coalition Distinguished Cancer Scholar from 2003 to 2007 and a member of the 2014 Class of the UNC Thorp Faculty Engaged Scholars. Dr. Hamilton is currently a Fellow in the American Academy of Nursing and a Faculty Scholar of the Center for Spirituality, Theology and Health at Duke University. She was the recipient of the 2019 Distinguished Alumni Award from the School of Nursing at the University of North Carolina, the 2011 Oncology Nursing Society (ONS) Publishing's Division Award for Excellence in Writing Qualitative Research and the ONS 2023 Award for Excellence in Cancer Education. Dr. Hamilton was born and raised in the Southern Appalachian region of North Carolina.

Charles E. Moore, MD received a Bachelor of Science from Union College and his medical degree from Harvard Medical School. He subsequently completed residency training in Otolaryngology-Head and Neck Surgery and fellowship training in Craniomaxillofacial—Cranial Base, Facial Plastic, and Reconstructive Surgery at the University of Michigan. Dr. Moore is a Professor at Emory University and the Chief of Service in the Department of Otolaryngology—Head and Neck Surgery at Grady Health System. Dr. Moore has a longstanding and profound commitment to the training and development of learners from all backgrounds. His research focus has been in the investigation of factors involved in healthcare disparity with a particular focus on head and neck cancer incidence in medically underserved communities. He is the President and Founder of Health Education, Assessment and Leadership (HEAL), Inc. Through this organization, he strives to educate the community on health issues, assess its needs, and in the process, build leaders from within the community to address those issues. This traveling resource has grown into the Healing Community Center (HCC), one of Atlanta's newest Federally Qualified Healthcare Centers. This center is a free and affordable medical facility with four separate locations, which provide general adult medical care, pediatric medical care, specialty medical care, dental services, as well as mental health services for the uninsured and disadvantaged. The HCC is focused on those who fall in the gap between public funded health care and the privately insured. A primary emphasis is on preventative health, nutrition, and wellness. This center incorporates all of the major Atlanta academic institutions and community organizations in an integrated fashion to provide service-learning experiences while also providing the necessary care to those in need.

Introduction with Overview of Significance of the Community and Faith-Based Institutions in Transforming Social Determinants to Promote Health

Jill B. Hamilton and Charles E. Moore

The idea for this book came from conversations about the role of social determinants of health (SDOH) in the alleviation of health disparities and health inequities in marginalized communities in the U.S and internationally. In this chapter, Dr. Moore and I will share the origins of our passion for understanding and addressing SDOH conditions and the ways in which this passion has shaped the contents of this book. We also describe the diversity of authors and coauthors and their insights into SDOH and conclude with our vision that this book will be the catalyst for change in the health outcomes in the communities that we are so passionate about.

Dr. Moore and I became acquainted with each other's passion for giving back to the communities from which we came in 2006. Prior to meeting Dr. Moore in 2003, I had accepted a faculty position in the Nell Hodgson Woodruff School of Nursing after having completed a two-year postdoctoral fellowship at the Oregon Health and Science University School of Nursing with a focus on the care of older adults. As a postdoctoral fellow, and even during my predoctoral studies, I was committed to understanding the ways in which social support and spirituality (as SDOH conditions) were positive rather than negative influences on health outcomes of older African Americans. The evidence on this topic available to me during those years suggested that African Americans were lacking social support. The few studies that considered spirituality concluded that when African Americans did rely on their faith in God during illness, they were reluctant to seek medical treatment. It was as if African Americans chose one over the other, leading many healthcare professionals to assume that religion and spirituality were in opposition to medical care. This assumption had not been my experience. To change that narrative, I began conducting a series of descriptive studies that led to the development of the Ways of Helping Questionnaire, a measure of social support that was relevant and culturally sensitive to the African American experience. In 2006, I was awarded my first R01 award through the National Institutes of Health/National Institute of Nursing Research (1R01NR009271) to develop a culturally sensitive questionnaire to measure social support among older African American cancer survivors.

The findings from this funded study supported what I had known all along and what I had witnessed in the social interactions of the elders in the community where I was raised, attended school, worked, and worshipped. I saw these

J. B. Hamilton (✉)
Nell Hodgson Woodruff School of Nursing,
Emory University, Atlanta, GA, USA
e-mail: jbhamil@emory.edu

C. E. Moore
Emory University School of Medicine,
Emory University, Atlanta, GA, USA
e-mail: cemoore@emory.edu

relationships through a different lens, one of strength and resilience and not pathology and deviance. I was now equipped to contribute to the evidence and change the narrative about the social support experiences of African Americans. However, more importantly, I could now use this information to adapt intervention studies to support cancer patients in meaningful ways.

In the early years of my research, I was grateful to the African American cancer patients in Portland, Oregon and in the Cancer Center at Grady Health System for sharing their stories to teach me about their support needs [1, 2]. These patient participants taught me what was working and what was not working in their social relationships. These patients also taught me about the conditions that led to whether support was or was not available to them during the diagnosis and treatment for cancer. However, the more valuable lesson from these patients was how to communicate and how to listen so you could learn from them. Twenty years later, I continue to be grateful to this population for the lessons, the stories, the relationships, and even their prayers for my success.

Shortly after receiving this award, I heard about this African American MD who was seeing head and neck cancer patients in his clinic. I introduced myself and asked for his help with my research. At the time, Dr. Moore and I were both Assistant Professors and beginning our respective careers. I was passionate about learning more about the social support experiences of African Americans and, although Charles was an Otolaryngologist, he was passionate about using his knowledge and skills as an MD to help underserved communities in Atlanta.

Dr. Moore's story is another illustration of the passion we have to improve outcomes among this patient population. Dr. Moore had moved to Atlanta to take a position at Emory after medical school at Harvard followed by residency and fellowship training at the University of Michigan. The position was as Chief of Service at Grady Health System, a safety net hospital in Atlanta, GA. From the initial days of starting this position, he would regularly see patients in his clinic that would come in only after their disease progress had progressed to such an extent that there was very little that could be done except to race up to the operating room to place a surgical airway that would allow the patient to continue to breathe. Once the airway was controlled, the only option left for the patient was to be set up for hospice care. Seeing this day after day and week after week, he decided that something needed to be done. Not knowing what could be done, if anything, he began by identifying the top three zip codes where his patients lived. These three zip codes were all medically underserved areas. At that point, he tells the story of getting into his car and driving to those areas to meet with people to see how he might help. He describes his feelings and desire to do more than to treat patients when their illness was in the advanced stages. He thought that since he was a head and neck cancer surgeon, he might begin by giving head and neck cancer prevention talks in the community, and he focused his cancer prevention efforts on those communities with the poorest outcomes. He saw firsthand all of the issues caused by SDOH in addition to a myriad of unaddressed medical issues. This realization demanded that he relearn primary care skills in order to deliver primary care and cancer screening services in those communities. He started this community outreach from his car. Dr. Moore targeted churches and health fairs in those three zip codes for his head and neck cancer talks and cancer screenings and also focused his efforts on individuals in places like under bridges, crack houses, anyplace he could draw a listening audience. Initially, he didn't tell many people about what he was doing because early feedback was so negative and discouraging. For example, he talked to one person about his community outreach activities and the response was, "if those people wanted help they would come to you." Dr. Moore gradually realized that he could have greater impact in these communities if there were more people involved. Ignoring the naysayers, he started asking colleagues to join him in cancer screening events in more traditional places. He initially reached out to interested ENT residents from his clinic. Then, over the years, the interest in and participation from other healthcare providers grew for his community outreach. He now delivers his community outreach in a building that is now widely known as the HEALing Community Center.

The HEALing Community is a federally qualified healthcare center with five locations providing healthcare (medical, dental, behavioral health, supportive services, specialty care) in an integrated fashion. Two of these locations are school-based healthcare centers, which permit children to receive much needed health care without missing school. Offering easily accessible care to children in low resourced communities reduces school absenteeism rates and facilitates the child being successful in school. These services are of benefit to parents as well as they don't miss work when their child is sick. Ultimately, issues contributing to childhood illnesses might be prevented and sick childcare can be delivered in a neutral and familiar environment (school).

Over the years, Dr. Moore and I have shared stories of our shared passion to help individuals from marginalized communities. What has become apparent is our drive to use our knowledge and skills to help others that "look like" those individuals that made it possible for us to occupy our respective roles in a major, private predominately white institution. In the beginning of our journey, our colleagues were not supportive, they didn't see the value and importance of our work to marginalized communities. The support of our colleagues might have made our journey easier, but we persevered the negative and discouraging comments. Our desire to help overcome the wrongs done to us and former generations was important; the impetus that motivated our work and this book focused on SDOH and Community engagement.

1   Getting Started

Writing an edited book is never easy. However, we were surprised and elated at the interest from our colleagues, mentees, and students to contribute to this project. Similar to recruiting for a qualitative research study, we reached out to individuals we knew that were engaged in SDOH and community engagement. We wanted to include faculty in the academy but since true community engagement work includes the community, we encouraged our colleagues to include them as coauthors. One group of individuals from the community for which we are extremely honored to have contribute to this project are Black ministers. In Chap. 26, these individuals share the work they do in communities in collaboration with and apart from predominantly white institutions.

The final book includes chapters from a diverse group of faculty, students, and community members that span four continents and 20 countries. This diverse group of authors transcends racial/ethnic groups, geographic regions, levels of rankings and disciplines in the academy, and community members.

Racial/ethnic groups represented in this book include U.S. populations that identify as American Indian, Black or African American, Filipino American, Hispanic or Latino, and White. Geographic regions represented in the U.S. consist of authors from the Northeast, South, Midwest, and West Coast. U.S. academic Institutions represented include Brown University, Duke University, Emory University, Harvard University, Iowa State University, Johns Hopkins University, Michigan State University, Spellman College, University of Michigan, University of Minnesota, University of California (Irvin and San Francisco Campuses), University of North Carolina at Chapel Hill, University of Rhode Island, University of Pennsylvania, University of Texas (San Antonio), and Vanderbilt University.

International authors represent countries of Botswana, El Salvador, Ethiopia, Ghana, Haiti, India, Jamaica, Kenya, Malawi, Mexico, Nepal, Nigeria, Peru, South Korea, St. Vincent and the Grenadines, Uganda, Vietnam, and Venezuela. International Academic Institutions include Addis Ababa University, Addis Ababa, in Ethiopia, Dedan Kimathi University of Technology in Kenya, Kamuzu University of Health Sciences in Malawi, Kwame Nkrumah University of Science and Technology in Ghana, PAN Africa University Ibadan in Nigeria, St.

Vincent and the Grenadines School of Continuing Education, and the University of Botswana in Botswana.

Diversity of faculty from academic institutions includes those with associate degrees, bachelor's degrees, master's degrees, and doctoral degrees. Faculty authors are from Environmental and Health Sciences, NCI-Designated Cancer Centers, and Schools of Medicine, Nursing, and Public Health. Student authors who have contributed to this book as corresponding or coauthors are at the level of undergraduate, master's, and doctoral levels from Biology, nursing, photojournalism, and public health.

We are especially excited to have community leaders from the global south and U.S. faith-based institutions as authors and coauthors. These individuals are from communities that work to alleviate SDOH among marginalized populations residing in more urban heavily populated areas to those more rural, remote areas. Although Dr. Moore and I have led the collection of works in this book, we are genuinely grateful for the opportunity to learn about community engagement from these incredible authors.

The chapters in this book are organized according to the Nell Hodgson Woodruff School of Nursing Four Pillars of SDOH [3]. This Four Pillar approach categorizes SDOH into social, cultural, environmental (physical and social), and policy conditions. Chapters in Part 1 emphasize the Social Pillar—those factors that occur in society due to systemic (structural) racism and imbalances in power, financial resources, education, and occupation that influence wellness or lack thereof. Chapters in Part 2 emphasize the Cultural Pillar— those customary beliefs, social norms, attitudes, values, and practices shared by a group of people (community or society) in a place and time with regards to health and healthcare. Chapters in Part 3a emphasize the Physical Environment—the part of the human environment that includes purely physical factors that contribute to health inequities and health disparities. Chapters in Part 3b emphasize the Social Environment and might be further defined as the social surroundings (social settings, institutions, and relationships) that contribute to health inequ-

uities and health disparities. Finally, the Chapters in Part 4 emphasize Policy—those guidelines, principles, legislation, and political activities that affect the living conditions conducive to the welfare of individuals, communities, and societies quality of life.

2   Our Instructions to Authors

In our initial discussions, we desired an end product that would be read by academic individuals but also would be read by individuals in communities where we ultimately want to address SDOH and alleviate health disparities and inequities. We were clear, that we absolutely did not want a collection of research reports or documents generally submitted to peer reviewed journals. We wanted authors to tell the story behind the research, how they worked with communities to identify issues, design studies, develop trusting collaborative relationships and of course disseminate findings in ways that were relevant and meaningful. In the section below are the instructions provided authors as a guide to writing their stories. The emphasis was that these instructions were a guide as we wanted authors in collaboration with community members to be creative in telling their story.

3   SDOH Book Guideline for Chapters

1. The problem as it relates to some social determinants of health/why your work is important/significant to the reduction of some health disparity.
2. Who/what informed the problem (the literature, the community)/what are goals. In this second section, authors were instructed to consider writing about how or why a particular SDOH was selected—a personal experience, the literature, an experience with a patient or family, or the community.
3. Describe the community where you are doing the work (the setting, the people)—insert pictures if you have them. What are community

resources? Authors were encouraged to talk about the community (s) where their work was conducted. To write about the setting of these communities, the people living in these communities, and the resources generally available to people living in these communities as related to the issue being presented.

4. What are some of the programs (or just one program) you are developing, implementing, evaluating in the community/describe any outcomes. We became aware that many authors were in the beginning phases of their community work while others were more advanced in the delivery of interventions. Therefore, authors would be writing their chapters solo and describing their initial efforts to begin community-engaged work, while others had developed extensive collaborative networks in their communities and able to describe in greater detail their relationships, program implementation, and evaluative efforts. This diversity was important to the book and potential readers.

5. How has the community been involved in project. What were strategies to engage trust? Maintain trust. Describe collaborators what were strategies to develop or maintain collaborations. In this section, authors were encouraged to write about their experience with their community, their community members, how community members were identified, how community members were involved in the work, and ways in which faculty and community members collaborated in dissemination of the research in academic setting and to the community.

6. A concluding reflections piece of what were challenges/barriers, what have been successes, what are future plans. Are demographics changing in communities, how do future efforts address these changes.

A final guiding instruction was to encourage authors to be creative in telling the story, to use pictures, case studies, and community member's stories.

4   Final Thoughts on this Book

The overarching goal of this book is to showcase the true work of community engagement. In our experience and over the last nearly 20 years, there appears to be a disconnect between academia and the work related to SDOH in the community. For example, scholars in the academy have traditionally determined the issues, designed the research, and wrote proposals to conduct research in the community with little or no community input. Community has generally only been consulted and brought into these funded projects for the purpose of recruitment of eligible participants and data collection. Once data has been collected, there is a disconnect again and the findings are analyzed and interpreted again with little or no input from community. The perspective from academic scholars is the research is being conducted for the benefit of the community but in reality, the programs and interventions are not necessarily what the community needs or even wants. Oftentimes, academic scholars may not be willing to adapt or compromise that which they desire to bring to the community.

Our hope is that this book will accomplish a few things. The first is that scholars in academic institutions will pay greater attention to the community-based work and realize the need to reshape and refocus the ways in which research is conducted in community. Secondly, we hope to bring attention to academic scholars that collaborations with community members should be approached from the position of being equal partners and that the voice of the community is important. The third desire and outcome of this book is that readers of this text will realize that the issues being addressed should be guided by community members and even though funds may be awarded based on a specific need, there should be flexibility to adapt the goals of the funder to match the needs of the community. Finally, it is our hope that academic scholars will read chapters in this book and be inspired to include community partners in the dissemination of their work and that community partners will see their value in the participation in efforts to disseminate findings that directly affect their well-being. That their experiences are accurately captured and disseminated in ways that are accessible to the community.

Probably our most desired outcome from this book is a greater appreciation for the work that truly goes into community collaborations. Building trusting community collaborations and obtaining funding to do the work is an extremely time-intensive effort. Historically, the time to develop relationships and do the work that addresses the issues of marginalized communities has not been recognized as scholarly in the academy. The time-intensive nature of developing community partnerships, recruitment, and data collection while simultaneously meeting the metrics for success in academic institutions has been a challenge. Frequently, the conduct of research to meet the needs of communities is not consistent with priority topics funded at the National Institutes of Health, the gold standard of funding in the academy. It has also been a challenge to meet the metric for the publications in high impact, peer reviewed journals since community research is not on the level of randomized controlled trials or epidemiological studies with larger sample sizes.

In spite of these challenges, we have found community-engaged work to be especially.

rewarding. This work reminds us of how we were raised, that it is not about the survival of the individual but about the family; the community that you're part of. It's about people that you are associated with and have a genuine concern for their well-being. And I think before the language of social determinates of health became a catchphrase, those of us who grew up in communities where you relied on each other for survival were already familiar with this concept. We inherently knew that if our neighbor wasn't doing well, we checked on them. If our neighbor needed food or clothes, we gave them food and clothes. If the elderly or children needed a place to stay, you opened your home to them because you knew that if they're better off, then you're better off.

And so, for us, social determinants of health and community really aren't separated but, they're really one in the same. But we don't really like the focus on deficits because it makes it seems like folks in certain communities don't have resources. However, the strengths of communities should also be emphasized. For example, the informal networks in communities are frequently the community's biggest resource because they'll make it work with whatever they've got. So, when we reflect on our passion for social determinants of health, we think about the communities from which we came, we remember our families, our extended families of aunts and uncles who modeled ways to address the needs of communities. We remember the values taught in our respective churches and through interactions with the elders in our Sunday School classes and youth groups. We remember and honor them through the work we do in the community and through this edited book on Social Determinants of Health.

References

1. Hamilton JB, Moore CE, Powe BD, Agarwal M, Martin P. Perceptions of support among older African American cancer survivors. Oncol Nurs Forum. 2010;37(4):484–93. https://doi.org/10.1188/10.onf.484-493.
2. Hamilton JB, Stewart BJ, Crandell JL, Lynn MR. Development of the ways of helping questionnaire: a measure of preferred coping strategies for older African American cancer survivors. Res Nurs Health. 2009;32(3):243–59. https://doi.org/10.1002/nur.20321.
3. Hamilton JB. Integrating a social determinants of health framework into nursing education. In: Hamilton JB, Swan BA, McCauley L, editors. Integrating a social determinants of health framework into nursing education. Cham: Springer International Publishing; 2023. p. 9–53.

Jill B. Hamilton PhD, MRPL, RN, FAAN, is Professor (tenured) and Senior Faculty Fellow of SDOH and Health Disparities at the Nell Hodgson Woodruff School of Nursing and Affiliate Professor at Candler School of Theology at Emory University in Atlanta, Georgia. Dr. Hamilton earned her BSN, MSN, and PhD in nursing from the University of North Carolina at Chapel Hill, a BS in Accounting from North Carolina Central University, postdoctoral training in the nursing care of older adults at the Oregon Health and Science University, and a Master's in Religion and Public Life at the Candler School of Theology. She previously held faculty positions at Johns Hopkins University and the University of North Carolina at Chapel Hill where she was a tenured Associate Professor. Dr. Hamilton's research interests include social determinants of health, health disparities, and the mental health promoting strategies used among older African American their families in response to life-threatening illness. Dr. Hamilton is Leading Editor of a text with Springer Nature titled *Integrating a Social Determinants of Health Framework into Nursing Education* published in 2023. She has done original research on the effects of storytelling that incorporates Black Sacred Music and scripture on psychological distress among older and younger African Americans. She was a Georgia Cancer Coalition Distinguished Cancer Scholar from 2003 to 2007 and a member of the 2014 Class of the UNC Thorp Faculty Engaged Scholars. Dr. Hamilton is currently a Fellow in the American Academy of Nursing and a Faculty Scholar of the Center for Spirituality, Theology and Health at Duke University. She was the recipient of the 2019 Distinguished Alumni Award from the School of Nursing at the University of North Carolina, the 2011 Oncology Nursing Society (ONS) Publishing's Division Award for Excellence in Writing Qualitative Research and the ONS 2023 Award for Excellence in Cancer Education. Dr. Hamilton was born and raised in the Southern Appalachian region of North Carolina.

Charles E. Moore received a Bachelor of Science from Union College and his medical degree from Harvard Medical School. He subsequently completed residency training in Otolaryngology- Head and Neck Surgery and fellowship training in Craniomaxillofacial—Cranial Base, Facial Plastic, and Reconstructive Surgery at the University of Michigan. Dr. Moore is a Professor at Emory University and the Chief of Service in the Department of Otolaryngology—Head and Neck Surgery at Grady Health System. Dr. Moore has a longstanding and profound commitment to the training and development of learners from all backgrounds. His research focus has been in the investigation of factors involved in healthcare disparity with a particular focus on head and neck cancer incidence in medically underserved communities. He is the President and Founder of Health Education, Assessment and Leadership (HEAL), Inc. Through this organization, he strives to educate the community on health issues, assess its needs, and in the process, build leaders from within the community to address those issues. This traveling resource has grown into the Healing Community Center (HCC), one of Atlanta's newest Federally Qualified Healthcare Centers. This center is a free and affordable medical facility with four separate locations, which provide general adult medical care, pediatric medical care, specialty medical care, dental services, as well as mental health services for the uninsured and disadvantaged. The HCC is focused on those who fall in the gap between public funded health care and the privately insured. A primary emphasis is on preventative health, nutrition, and wellness. This center incorporates all of the major Atlanta academic institutions and community organizations in an integrated fashion to provide service-learning experiences while also providing the necessary care to those in need.

The Influence of Racism on Social Determinants of Health and Health Disparities

Jill B. Hamilton

1 The Nell Hodgson Woodruff School of Nursing Social Determinants of Health Framework

The Emory School of Nursing Framework is a Four-Pillar approach to integration of SDOH content into the curriculum (see Fig. 1). This framework pulls content from those SDOH frameworks frequently cited with a consideration for the many social-cultural determinants not easily measured. Our SDOH framework consists of four pillars of social determinants—*Social, Cultural, Environment (physical and social), and Policy* and is illustrated using interwoven puzzle pieces (see Fig. 1). This illustration depicts the real-life experiences of individuals that at any given time, these four determinants impact health outcomes. Although one pillar may emerge and be prominent in the promotion of health or alleviation of disease, an imbalance in one is likely to influence the other three SDOH pillars. It is important to consider that at any given time, any one or more of these four pillars can be protective or place individuals at risk for illness and health inequities. In the next sections we describe each of the four SDOH pillars with exemplars drawn

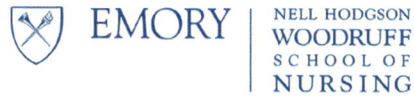

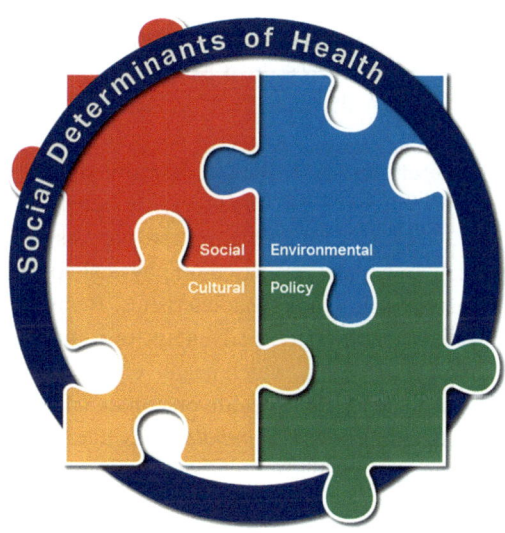

Fig. 1 SDOH framework

from research on Americans of African descent. This population is used for exemplars of each SDOH pillar given the persistent disparities in morbidity and mortality rates experienced among this population.

J. B. Hamilton (✉)
Nell Hodgson Woodruff School of Nursing,
Emory University, Atlanta, GA, USA
e-mail: jbhamil@emory.edu

2   Social Conditions (Part I)

Social Conditions are those factors that occur in society due to systemic (structural) racism and imbalances in power, financial resources, education, and occupation that influence wellness or lack thereof (see Fig. 2). Social conditions shaped by power imbalances and systemic racism for consideration include:

- Access to financial resources, education, type occupation.
- Health literacy.
- Access to health care.
- Social support as a social resource.

2.1   Systemic Racism, Power Imbalance, and Social Conditions

The experience of racism can be from structural and/or interpersonal practices, policies, and social norms that marginalize and oppress individuals or populations based on physical appearances or other visible characteristics. Racism in health care results in the advantage of some populations over others, which negatively affects the physical and mental health outcomes of those less advantaged. *Power imbalance* is interwoven with racism and occurs when one group asserts power or dominates another group in ways that disadvantages or is not in the best interest of the other group. *Systemic (structural) racism* and *the*

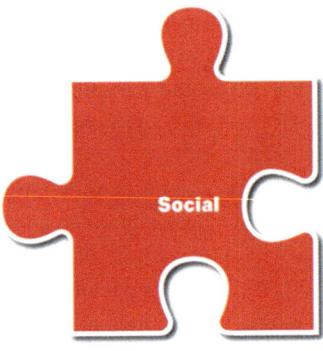

Fig. 2 Social conditions

imbalance of power in society is the current focus of educators and health care practitioners in their attempts to understand and dismantle SDOH and health inequities among people of color. Referred to as a major driver of health inequities, systemic racism generally refers to a system of ideas and policies that operate to oppress or marginalize subgroups of its population; a system of beliefs that one group is inherently inferior to another [1, 2]. This type of far-reaching determinant is a widely known and recognized determinant that continues to limit minority groups' access to opportunities and movement from lower stratifications of social classes. Systemic racism has historically limited the ability of people of color to obtain *(1) financial resources— high paying jobs with private insurance, (2) a quality education, and (3) access to quality health care.*

2.2   Historical Context of Systemic Racism and Social Conditions

Perhaps the greater illustration of the impact of systemic racism on the interrelatedness of *financial resources (insurance and high paying jobs), education, and access to health care* can be learned from the history of the enslaved African in the U.S. Historical records dating back to the nineteenth century documents the poor health outcomes among African Americans that resulted from a system of laws and policies (widely known as Jim Crow Laws) that supported a legal segregation system and also restricted access to health care [3, 4]. During the nineteenth century, systemic racist policies and practices contributed to disproportionately high rates of preventable illnesses such as pneumonia, pellagra, tuberculosis, and syphilis that led to some of the highest rates of premature mortality in the U.S. [5]. In fact, at the turn of the twentieth century, the life expectancy for these former enslaved Americans was 32 years in comparison to 49 years for white Americans [6]. This racial disparity in mortality rates has been largely attributed to the levels of poverty prevalent among unskilled and skilled occupations and the lack of access to quality education during that time [4, 7].

Employment in low-paying occupations on poor health outcomes among formerly enslaved Americans was especially apparent during the Civil Rights Era [8]. As a result of occupying the lowest income strata, premature mortality rates among this subgroup of Americans continued to be especially high. Even with the integration that occurred during this historical era, access to health care continued to be dismal. In addition to the excessive morbidity rates from deadly illness such as cancer, heart disease, and stroke, over one-half of the nations' maternal deaths were African American women, and the highest infant mortality rates were among African Americans. Persistent racism in the health care system resulted in access to health care that was determined by a persons' race but also social class. Even with more advanced cases of cancer and coronary artery disease, African Americans continued to have less accessibility to health care compared to white Americans.

Access to a Quality Education has historically been out of reach for a majority of Americans of African descent. During segregation for example, African Americans were discouraged from continuing their education beyond what was necessary for employment in service sectors such as a domestics or laborers [9]. Reportedly, while white employers were encouraging their descendants and white employees to attend college, they would communicate to their African American employees that they did not need a college education. Inequities in obtaining a quality education were also apparent from the quality of textbooks available to schools in low-income African American communities. Textbooks in schools in communities of color were reportedly discarded from white schools and with pages missing [10]. During the early and mid-twentieth century years, African Americans for example, grew up attending racially segregated schools and were transported to segregated high schools in a different city (if at all), even when a white school might have been in closer proximity [10]. Although a few participants managed to complete high school during this time, their ability to attend college was hampered by work obligations necessary to assist the family with finances. The experience of African Americans in these segregated schools may have been characterized by an education with less experienced or less qualified teachers, high levels of teacher turnover, less successful peer groups, and inadequate facilities and learning materials than that available to students in majority white schools.

Access to health care facilities expanded during the twentieth century but was still out of reach for many Americans, especially low-income and African Americans. For example, although child health programs were increasingly being established, these programs still were not accessible to the many African Americans in dire need of their services. This increase in access to health care programs during this time was likely a major influence in the improvements in the life-expectancy of African American males and females (47 and 49 years respectively) but was still substantially less than that for white Americans (59 years for males and 62 years for females) [5]. For example, while the average life expectancy had increased for both populations since the turn of the century, the gap between the groups had widened from a previous estimate of 5–7 years to 12–13 years [5]. The availability of government-sponsored insurance plans (e.g., Medicaid and Medicare) at least provided payment for some services as these participants became eligible which was believed to increase access to care. However, given the life expectancy of individuals born in the 1920s and 1930s, it is unlikely that many African Americans lived to the age of 65 when they would be eligible.

2.3   Current and Persistent Social Influences on Health Inequities

Financial resources continue to be a risk factor for disease and mortality rates. The lack of financial resources is often associated with a lack of information and knowledge and timely access to health care when diagnosed with life-threatening illness [11]. For example, persistent white-black disparities among cancer patients has been attributed to lower rates of timely follow-up care after abnormal mammograms and scheduling follow-up appointments which subsequently leads to delays in treatment [11]. And, despite advances in cancer diagnosing and treatment, individuals of a lower SES status (most often identified as racial minorities) are among those with the highest cancer mortality rates [12, 13]. When there is heart disease, the low SES individual is also at risk for higher levels of morbidity and mortality. In at least one national survey, patients with congenital heart disease who identified as Black, of a lower SES (including income and educational levels) had a greater likelihood of death [14]. Similarly, education and income are also determinants of poor hospital outcomes in research among stroke patients [15]. That is, stroke patients with a higher SES (income and educational level) had low mortality rates while those patients with a low SES (income and education) had high mortality rates [15].

A *quality education* is more accessible today, however, low educational attainment continues to be a marker for socioeconomic status and resulting higher mortality rates [16]. African Americans are still confronted with the harsh realities of structural racism and the racial segregation that persists among our educational and health care institutions. Older African Americans that lived prior to the Civil Rights Era would likely be disappointed—that, in spite of the change in laws prohibiting segregation, school segregation is on the rise in the United States [17]. Even in diverse schools, within-school segregation exists where Black, Indigenous, and Latinx adolescents are likely tracked into less rigorous courses and long-term outcomes are likely detrimental on mental health that persist through adulthood [18].

Health literacy is associated with low levels of education and SES status [19]. When patients are not able to understand written information related to their illness, they are less likely to ask questions or to be engaged in their care. For example, in a study examining the association of health literacy on health outcomes among patients with Type 2 diabetes, low levels of health literacy was associated with limitations with medication adherence, depressed moods, and self-management [20]. However, this finding is not

consistent. In another study, African American patients with low incomes and health literacy levels were less engaged in behaviors known to lead to better health outcomes [21].

Racial inequities in health care access have persisted into the twenty-first century [22]. Disparate health outcomes have been attributed to poor health behaviors such as lack of exercise, eating fatty foods, and cigarette smoking. However, public health experts and health care practitioners are now acknowledging the powerful influence of structural racism or those influences beyond the control of the individual [23]. Structural inequities such as poverty, the scarcity of health care providers in rural townships, and low paying jobs without insurance continues to contribute to the limited access to care among low income and African Americans today [24].

2.4 Social Support as a Resource from Family and Friends

Social support from family and friends is generally perceived as a social or financial resource for achieving and maintaining levels of wellness. The most widely known form of social support is emotional support which is the expression of love, liking, or both, and listening to worries and concerns. As a social resource, emotional support might also be in the form of expressions from others that result in feelings of being valued, esteemed, and positive feedback about one's self-worth. Instrumental support is the social resource of material aid or assistance with finances, household tasks, goods, and services. The third type of social support, and less frequently studied, is the support from information or advice about some problem or illness.

As a social resource, or SDOH, the availability of social support can be protective or place an individual at risk for poor health outcome. For many years, the assumption was that social support available to individuals with chronic and life-threatening illness was only available among white middle class and college-educated women; a type of social support not available to lower income persons and women of color. Scholars have concluded that white and married women were generally among those with higher levels of social support. That is, the support of having someone to confide in about personal and illness concerns among family and friends and to subsequently have an improved outlook on life, better physical functioning, and less likely to have premature mortality rates [25]. The perception that low income and persons of color lack social support is likely influenced by a pattern of research that was conducted primarily among the white middle class and by scientists of similar racial/ethnic backgrounds.

Systemic racism and social support. In response to harsh and oppressive living conditions, former enslaved Americans adapted their previous knowledge of family. Family was a system whereby individuals cared for one another and shared available social and financial resources in spite of blood kinship. Even among the lowest of paid workers where there was little or no money, historical accounts of former enslaved Americans document ways in which they shared material resources that enabled their survival—albeit a poor one [7].

Exemplars of the ways in which social support was a resource for low income and persons of color can be examined from narrative accounts during the Great Depression [26]. The Great Depression was difficult for all races/ethnicities; but was particularly devastating for African Americans. Poverty for African Americans was so severe in some situations that there was often little or no money for physical necessities [7, 27]. In situations where there was a lack of money, the support from family and close friends was extremely important to the survival of the African American family; a source of mutual assistance as members shared or bartered services for food, shelter, and clothing [7].

Recent evidence that suggests that a lack of social support among African Americans is likely the result of differences in types of social resources available and utilized among African Americans in comparison to whites. For example, in spite of having very similar health problems, African Americans are less likely to utilize confiding support or be willing to express feelings to others about their problems [28]. The reluctance to confide in others about illness-related problems is related to a fear that one's illness will be a direct burden on family and friends [25]. In fact, the value of not asking for help during times of crisis might be the norm for many members of this population as they are likely to value being perceived as being strong during adverse sitations [29]. Emotional support among this population might be expressed through material forms of social support or an emotional presence such as "sitting with the sick" [30], assistance to maintain important social roles at home, church, and work, and sharing stories of hope [28, 31, 32].

Current Influences of Social Support on health inequities. A culmination of risk factors among African Americans places them among populations most likely to encounter challenges with family support during illness. In comparison to other racial/ethnic groups, African Americans continue to rank lowest with home ownership and least likely to receive inheritances, gifts, and other financial family support, types of generational wealth that has contributed to better health outcomes among other populations for generations [33]. Additionally, in comparison to white Americans, African Americans are least likely to have recovered from generations of inequities in the job market or even the most recent financial devastation of the Great Recession [33]. The lack of financial resources coupled with generations of limited access to health care services has shaped patterns of giving and receiving social support such that patients are reluctant to ask for help when sick for fear of being a burden to family and friends. Indeed, this perception of being a burden is likely accurate given the harsh realities of limited financial resources in addition to a greater severity of illness and mortality rates experienced.

Inequities in the receipt of social support during illness is especially apparent among African Americans when there is a cancer diagnosis. African Americans continue to experience the highest overall mortality rates, more advanced staged cancers [34, 35] and higher levels of psychological distress from cancer than non-

Hispanic Whites [36]. High levels of psychological distress have been linked to unmet needs for support from family and friends and information from health care providers [37]. Root causes of this high level of psychological distress are from a history of past experiences of suffering, death, and isolation witnessed among cancer patients who likely did not survive treatment [32, 34, 35, 38, 39]. African American cancer patients and family members frequently recall images and horror stories of African American cancer patients who "suffered and died," after a period of "wasting away" and in excruciating pain [32]. The stories available to patients and family members are often replete with memories of other cancer patients diagnosed at a late stage and subsequently died from a disease that had spread to the point where treatment would not be effective [32, 38]. Despite high levels of psychological distress, African American patients and family members are not likely to seek mental health services [40] or to participate in hospital-based support groups [41]. African Americans are however, more likely to participate in community or faith-based support groups as these groups are sensitive to the values and need to remain hopeful and optimistic in the context of life-threatening illness.

2.5 Summary of Social Conditions Pillar

In this Social Conditions Pillar, we have covered, at least to some extent, the ways in which the social conditions of financial resources, quality education, type occupation, health literacy and access to care as SDOH influences to health outcomes. The influence of social conditions on health disparities is especially evident among African Americans, a U. S. population that continues to experience the greater health inequities within the context of systemic racism. Other related social factors will be discussed in other SDOH Pillars, i.e. physical environment (safe neighborhoods, access to healthy foods, parks and recreation areas), and social environment (social integration, support from faith-based institutions).

3 Cultural Conditions (Part II)

Cultural conditions are those customary beliefs, social norms, attitudes, values, and practices shared by a group of people (community or society) in a place and time (see Fig. 3). Cultural conditions shaped by power imbalances and systemic racism for consideration include:

- Interpersonal racism/discrimination.
- Religion/spirituality (individual/family values, beliefs).
- Racial Memories.
- Social norms.

Interpersonal racism/discrimination occurs among one-on-one social interactions, can be negative treatment based on an individual's characteristics, is more identifiable, and likely based on personal beliefs of one group toward another group. In a survey conducted by the Pew Research Center, a majority of African American adults (71%) reported having experienced racial discrimination at some point in their lives from interactions that occurred at the individual level [42]. It has been estimated that during the course of a year, 50% of African American adults report being suspected of wrongdoing (47%), considered as not smart (45%), experiencing unfair treatment in hiring or promotion opportunities (21%), or encountering racial profiling by police (18%) [42]. Although experiences with racism are likely common among African Americans, individuals at greatest risk include men, young

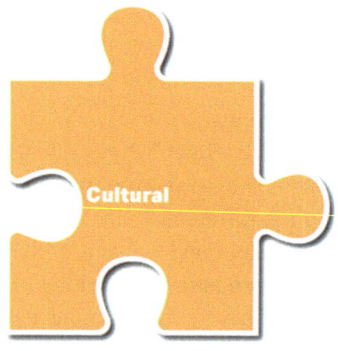

Fig. 3 Cultural conditions

adults, and those with some college education. Americans of African descent have consistently reported harsh treatment from the very health care providers in charge of their care when they are most vulnerable [43]. Health care practitioners have a long history of interpersonal racism with former enslaved individuals. The medical mistreatment of African Americans is well known, including the racism encountered with the Tuskegee Study, medical experimentation on the vulnerable, and the nonverbal communication that low income and folk of color were to blame for their poor health [44, 45]. When seeking care from physicians, African Americans have reported an insensitive nature in their communications and this has included spending less time with this population, and lack of respect and warmth during clinic visits [45].

Religion and spirituality have emerged as powerful determinants of health among U.S. and global populations. Religion is conceptualized as an adherence to a set of beliefs, values, and rituals, and symbols and participation in practices supported by organized faith-based institutions. Religiosity or religious involvement is another concept used among scholars to refer to beliefs and practices related to organized religious institutions [46]. The evidence to support the relationship of religious attendance to higher mortality rates is established. For example, in national surveys, respondents who attend church frequently have a lower hazard of mortality [47].

Spirituality, on the other hand, occurs on a more personal level and apart from affiliations with organized religious institutions. Conceptualizations of spirituality may include a search for answers to questions about life, a relationship to God, and making meaning of individual human experience through dimensions of connectedness: within oneself; to others and the environment; or, to God or other higher power [48]. Conceptualized as the religious practice of praying, spirituality is associated with cognitive functioning and depression [49].

Again, we look to the African American experience to illuminate the ways in which religion/spirituality might be protective and/or place the individual at risk for poor health. African Americans are the most religious group in the United States (U.S.) as evidenced by their religious affiliations, engagement in religious practices, and the frequency with which they believe that God exists [50]. Historically, a strong religious culture has been a widely recognized protective factor in illness situations and has enabled African Americans to survive generations of oppression and racism [51]. In comparison to other racial/ethnic groups, African Americans are more likely to rely on religious beliefs and practices in response to daily life challenges [50]. These religious beliefs and practices have been transmitted through African American oral history and subsequently are closely intermingled with everyday life [51]. As such, they are an important part of African American culture and sources of strength and comfort when confronted with social, personal, and mental health issues.

The practice of using faith-based strategies in response to experienced racial discrimination among African Americans is consistent with a strong religious culture that is generationally influenced [52]. Faith-based strategies may include finding meaning and purpose in the experience or turning to God for support and guidance [53]. Faith-based strategies promote a sense of resilience that buffers the impact of experienced racism on psychological and emotional well-being [54, 55]. A strong religious culture has historically existed among formerly enslaved Americans, which has provided individuals with a sense of order and control over their illness. This strong religious culture also promotes self-management of side effects from medical treatments and illness. For example, the survival of the African slave in in the U.S largely depended the use of religious songs or memorized scripture passages to communicate their struggles and fears to God and used to encourage one another in during adverse and life-threatening situations [56]. Scholars who have studied the content and purpose of religious songs have determined that these songs consist of Bible-based stories of God delivering oppressed or enslaved persons [57], expressions of the hopes of being delivered from a lifetime of evil and suffering to a lifetime of joy and happiness in this world or the next [57–60].

Religion and spirituality continue to be social determinants among individuals with life-threatening illness, particularly among low income and folk of color [61]. The evidence suggests that in comparison to whites, African Americans pray more, and this practice has promoted a more positive attitude toward their cancer experience [62, 63]. In my own research with African Americans, religious beliefs and practices have been used to cope with the loneliness and fears that frequently accompany the cancer experience but to also positively influence the utilization of cancer care services [61]. For example, African American cancer patients have reported praying to God and trusting Him to intercede on their behalf with their worries and providing guidance with treatment-related decisions [64, 65]. A faith in God has been used among recently diagnosed African American cancer survivors to overcome their fears and fatalistic attitudes of cancer being a death sentence and undergo prescribed cancer treatment [66]. A higher level of faith in God and use of religious practices among African American cancer survivors also minimizes treatment side effects, which likely also promotes adherence to treatment [67].

Negative aspects of religion and spirituality are certainly a possibility and associated with poor health outcomes. Fatalism, a pessimistic perspective, might also occur when patients are blamed and told that their illness is the result of a weakened or lack of faith in God [68]. Rather than religion/spirituality being perceived as a source of comfort, individuals may become distressed with thoughts that they need to pray more or are somehow being tested to see if their faith is strong. These negative and fatalistic attitudes and nonadherence to preventative care may occur when patients believe their illness is the result of a punishment for some sinful behavior. A fatalistic attitude might also be associated with a lack of engagement in cancer screenings [69] and depression [70].

Racial memories are those experiences, beliefs, and general recollections transmitted from one generation to another. Scholars tend to agree that the intergenerational transmission of stories with racial overtones occur as early as childhood, and persist well into adulthood [71]. Racial memories of the harmful effects of racism might be from structural and/or interpersonal practices, policies, and social norms that marginalized and oppressed individuals or populations based on physical appearances or other visible characteristic. Both historical and even recent scholarship highlights the centuries old negative impact of racism on the lives of African Americans. For example, in their formative years and much of their adulthood years, older African Americans were exposed to racial violence, segregation, and Jim Crow laws that restricted access to public accommodations, educational institutions, stores, and even access to health care [10]. In rural areas of the Southern U.S., many African Americans supported themselves through work as sharecroppers which was a form of labor exploitation that resulted in families working for little or no pay [7]. Opportunities for work included employment for men as skilled and unskilled laborers and for women in low paying jobs as domestics and seamstresses [7]. However, these types of employment were without the benefit of private health insurance and therefore a significant contributor to the burden of illness and mortality rates among this population.

In the context of life-threatening illnesses such as cancer, African Americans' racial memories include past recollections of times when cancer was an automatic death sentence. Overall cancer mortality rates for African Americans have also exceeded those of other racial/ethnic groups [34, 35]. In the 1960s, the overall 5-year survival rate for African Americans was a mere 27% which likely fueled the racial memory an African American cancer experience replete with "suffering and death" after a period of "wasting away" and in excruciating pain [72]. And, among a population that values social connectedness, the fear of death and change in appearance as a result of treatment further fuels the worry and fear among African Americans that too will die or, even worse, be isolated and "pitied" when there is a cancer diagnosis [72]. Racial memories may not lead to a reduction in seeking health care when needed but certainly increase the fear of a negative outcome [72].

Social norms are those accepted behaviors or ways of thinking that are culturally influenced among groups and can be expected responses to adverse situations such as illness. For example, one possible social norm that influences health outcomes among African American populations can be linked to an internalized value of needing to be strong [29]. Self-reliance or the value of needing to be strong in the face of adversity, occurs when individuals have a preference of relying on their own inner resources. Therefore, help from others is not needed or accepted. The value of self-reliance among an African American population could be attributed to a cultural attitude about asking for help. In a study with older persons of African ancestry (African Americans, Afro-Barbadians, and Afro-Haitians), participants believed they should give help but not ask for help in return [73]. In a study of low-income African American women, 15% said they never call on friends or relatives for help with health problems, rather they tend to rely only on themselves [74].

Another social norm that occurs among African Americans is to not openly discuss certain illnesses. Mental illness, for example, is associated with a stigma that results in a significant problem among African American populations [75–77]. African Americans are 20% more likely than whites to report serious psychological distress [78], fear public prejudice and discrimination [77, 79], and to be misdiagnosed by health care providers [77]. African Americans also report being fearful of being labeled "crazy" within their families and communities when there is mental illness [80]. Although the precise origins of this mental illness stigma is less clear, there is general agreement that stigma results in a higher illness burden among African Americans [79, 81]. High levels of psychological distress requires appropriate health care; however, mental health care providers skilled at delivering culturally competent care are limited and Americans of African descent are also more likely to turn to forms of religious coping such as prayer and a belief in God [77, 82].

3.1 Summary of Cultural Conditions Pillar

In this Cultural Conditions Pillar, we have covered, at least to some extent, the ways in which the cultural conditions of interpersonal racism/discrimination, religious beliefs, spirituality, racial memories as SDOH influence health outcomes and health equities among a former enslaved U. S. population. Depending on the population, other cultural conditions important for consideration might include societal values and nursing values. Although these cultural conditions have been discussed somewhat in this chapter among African Americans of a protestant religious tradition, further consideraton might include the ways in which social norms or informal rules exist among patients from varied cultures and other religious traditions.

4 Environmental (Physical) Conditions (Part IIIa)

Physical— the part of the human environment that includes purely physical factors (see Fig. 4). Physical environmental conditions for consideration include:

- Natural resources/natural disasters.
- Climate change/extremes in heat and cold temperatures.
- Exposure to toxic substances.
- Recreational resources—Safe play spaces.

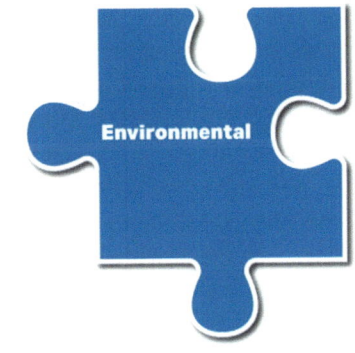

Fig. 4 Environmental conditions (physical)

Historical Overview of Nursing and Environmental Health Threats. Nursing has a long history of responding to threats to health from disruptions in the environment. Dating back to Florence Nightingale, nurses have stepped into global or national leadership roles in response to environmental hazards that have threatened the lives of families and the communities in which they lived [83]. In the nineteenth and early twentieth century, housing and labor protections were in their infancy and primarily focused on shoddy construction sites, substandard sanitation systems, abusive landlords, and poor urban planning [83]. Around the mid-twentieth century, patient care transitioned from community to hospital settings, where the focus of care on sick patient care was emphasized [83]. Care in hospital settings encouraged nurses to focus on sick patient care among patients with specific illness; a shift from a holistic approach to care [83]. This shift to sick patient care also fostered a perspective of care that is now largely focused on optimizing care rather than optimizing an environment that is healthy.

Several other historical events in the twentieth century shifted the perception of environmental issues being isolated events to those more widespread social issues. These social issues have included military troops' exposure to Agent Orange abroad and devastating community exposures to pollutants on the homeland. For example, the 1956 "Smog Complex" caused more than 2000 traffic accidents in the city of Los Angeles, California, in just 1 day [83]. Another environmental threat of great magnitude was from the devastation from wastewater and industrial runoff that contaminated farm soil and water supplies that disproportionately affected low income and minority communities [83]. Environmental threats have been from rivers and lakes that have been so riddled with sewage, oil, and industrial runoff, like Cuyahoga River in 1969, that the pollutants caught fire and resulted in the deaths of countless wildlife [83].

In the next sections, we highlight a few determinants related to physical and social environmental conditions. As with the social and cultural determinants, we illustrate environmental conditions using the evidence from populations most affected; low income and African Americans.

Natural Resources/Natural Disasters. Poverty and/or racism has influenced the severity of impact of natural disasters on individuals, communities, and societies. Natural disasters can affect anyone at any given time, the long-term impact of flooding from hurricanes and extremes in temperature disproportionately affects residents of low-income communities globally. In the U.S., systemic racism has led to an inadequate infrastructure in some cities that fails to protect its low-income citizens. Poverty guarantees that the financial resources of some individuals will only get worse during natural disasters. Perhaps one of the most devastating encounters from a natural disaster occurred over a decade ago that disproportionately affected low-income African Americans in Louisiana during the aftermath of Hurricane Katrina [84]. Hurricane Katrina was a destructive and deadly Category 5 tropical storm that made landfall in Louisiana and Mississippi on August 29, 2005. The flooding in the city of New Orleans in Louisiana has been largely attributed to engineering flaws in the levees (flood protection system constructed by the U. S. government) around the city [84]. Residents of this city with financial resources were able to evacuate before the hurricane made landfall. However, low-income and African Americans were not so fortunate. Those residents without the financial resources to evacuate endured days without water, food, or shelter. Many residents died from thirst, fatigue, and the violence that occurred in shelters. Katrina victims were either displaced from their homes, relocated and separated from family. Those that did return found homes in shambles and uninhabitable.

Climate Change/Extremes in Heat and Cold Temps. The earth's climate has experienced a change in the atmosphere which has raised the global temperature and extremes in weather patterns [85]. Threats to society from warmer temperatures have been the focus of the Environmental Protection Agency (EPA) for several years. Extremes in the weather have resulted in wildfires, air pollution, and floods. Extreme heat has been linked to illness and deaths, especially among the poor, pregnant women, children, elderly, and migrant farm workers [85–87]. Climate change is a global issue and known contributor to a rise in cardiovascular disease [88], complications of diabetes [89], asthma mortality rates [90], and increased mortality risk among the elderly [90]. In North America, however, low income and communities of color are especially impacted given the inequitable distribution of resources and social status [87, 91].

Increases to morbidity and mortality rates from environmental threats is predicted for the next several decades. The burden of extremes in weather is expected to be especially high among non-Hispanic Black infants and Australian indigenous infants who are much more likely to be born preterm than other racial/ethnic groups [92]. The increase in premature births among these populations is attributed to racism and classism (lack of access to high quality care) and community and environmental health (exposure to air pollution, lack of green space, and exposure to violence) [92]. The elderly is another population more likely to be negatively impacted by extremes in heat. Among the elderly and elderly African Americans, extremes in heat is a known contributor to increased Emergency Room (ER) visits for mental health issues [93]. Extremes in heat also contributes to increases in hospitalizations from myocardial infarctions particularly during summer months [94].

Exposure to Toxic Substances. Toxic substances are harmful to individual, family, and community health. These include exposure to fumes from cleaning agents, harmful chemicals present in drinking water or foods, air pollutants, and even pesticides used in the production of the foods we eat [85, 86]. Probably one of the more well-known toxins that had widespread harmful health effects was from asbestos exposure. Exposure to asbestos is known to increase the incidence of lung disease so much so that major national initiatives were implemented to ban the use of this substance and mandate its removal from public buildings [85, 86]. Another more recent example of an environmental threat was from toxic substances found in drinking water exposed during the Flint water crisis. The Flint

water crisis began when elevated levels of lead were found in children who had been drinking the city's water. Scholars have suggested that this lead contaminated water disproportionately affected a city that is largely low income and African American. This contaiminated drinking water resulted in excessive fetal deaths and other harmful health effects from ingesting lead from a water supply to numerous children during their formative years [95, 96]. Although the state of Michigan installed water filters, replaced pipes, and provided health care, educational and food resources to those affected, residents remain distrustful that the water is truly safe [97]. Moreover, research conducted years later suggest long-term effects leading to depression and posttraumatic distress disorder among adults living in the aftermath of this disaster [97].

Recreational Resources—Safe Play Spaces. Access to recreational resources including safe play spaces that permit children and adults to engage in outdoor activities has many benefits. In a community–academic partnership, renovated safe play spaces in schoolyards increased physical activity and social interactions in a low-income, urban neighborhood [98]. Green schoolyards may buffer against the effects of urbanization through increasing access to nature. A renovated green schoolyard has been shown to increase physical activity, school yard safety, school–community relationships, and less bullying behaviors [98]. Green schoolyards also offer a safe space for children and adults to engage in social, outdoor activities, particularly in low-income, urban neighborhoods [98]. Additonally, safe and green spaces that incorporate strategies to lower the traffic flow in urban areas decrease unhealthy weight trajectories in children [99].

Although safe green spaces generally encourage outdoor play and social activities, these healthy behaviors were reduced for some populations during the COVID pandemic when youth and adults were physically restrained to their homes [100]. For example, while youths with higher incomes and access to a safe built environment were more active and played more outdoors, low-income and Hispanic minority youth felt less safe [100]. Low income residents who were older, female, and black engaged in outdoor physical activity even though their neighborhoods were not safe [101].

4.1 Summary of Physical Environment

In this section we discussed some of the prevailing physical environmental threats to human health. Nursing has a long history of identifying and addressing physical environmental threats beginning with a focus on holistic care in communities to sick patient care in hospital settings. This shift to sick patient care with specific illness may have contributed to a lack of focus on holistic care, an emphasis of nursing care in previous years. In this section on physical environmental conditions we have focused our discussion on natural resources/natural disasters, climate change, exposure to toxic substances, and safe play spaces, conditions prevalent in our communities. Although we recognize there are many other threats from the physical environment, we are hopeful that the ones discussed will inspire your thinking on ways to incorporate those of interest to your faculty and students.

5 Environmental (Social) Conditions (Part IIIb)

Social environment is defined as a social setting in which people live (see Fig. 5).

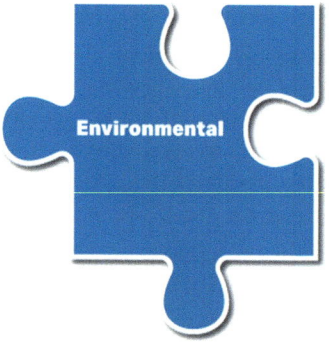

Fig. 5 Environmental conditions (social)

Social environment might be further defined as the surroundings (social settings) that are influenced by humans. In this section we detail a few social settings important to health equity to include quality of schools/academic settings, housing, access to affordable transportation, faith-based institutions, quality of schools, and composition of families. Other aspects of social settings important to consider as SDOH would be transportation, safety of neighborhoods, and community design. We have previously discussed access to health care and education. In this section, we consider:

- Quality of schools/academic settings.
- Workforce diversity in health care.
- Housing (safe and quality housing),
- Faith-based institutions.
- Composition of families.

Quality of Schools, Academic Settings. Historically, former enslaved Americans fought to obtain higher educational levels believing this to be the path to equality, independence, and respect [102]. A major triumph with the struggle for a quality education for this population was the passage of the Civil Rights Act of 1964. In the years leading up to the Civil Rights Act, older African Americans recalled attending racially segregated schools and being transported to segregated high schools in a different city, even when a white school might have been in closer proximity [10]. In rural areas especially, this transportation issue prevented many older African Americans from graduating from high school or even attending college. In addition to transportation issues, poverty contributed to the unequal access to educational resources. For example, in rural areas and among low-income families, the ability to complete high school and attend college was hampered by work obligations [10]. Poverty often dictated that everyone in the family contribute financially to keep the family housed and fed. Not unheard of are stories of children missing school days for work or teens dropping out of school altogether to enter the workforce [10]. Even when schools were accessible, students in segregated schools in African

American communities could have received an inferior education with less experienced or less qualified teachers, high levels of teacher turnover, less successful peer groups, and inadequate facilities and learning materials than exist in majority white schools.

Although there have been gains made in accessing a quality education post-segregation for African Americans, the harsh realities of structural racism and racial segregation persists among our educational institutions. In spite of the change in laws prohibiting segregation, school segregation is on the rise in the United States [17]. Even in schools claiming a diverse student population, within-school segregation exists. Moreover, attaining a quality education continues to be linked to one's social status. Today, the overwhelming majority of African American students attend under sourced schools where a majority of them are also African American [103]. Low income and African American students in these schools are also likely tracked into less rigorous courses resulting in detrimental long-term outcomes that are detrimental to their health and wellness; outcomes that persist throughout adulthood [18]. Our sickest patients today with the highest mortality rates are those with a low educational level [104].

Health Care Workforce Diversity. A diverse health care workforce is critical to the delivery of care that is culturally sensitive. Health care is still lacking adequate numbers of providers with with the knowledge and skillset necessary for care that is respectful and equitable. Scholars believe this lack of diversity in health care is severe and not likely to change [105, 106]. Historically, a period of racial segregation (Jim Crow) contributed greatly to a lack of hospitals and health care providers within majority African American and rural communities [3, 107]. During segregation, black owned and run hospitals filled the void in health care, however, due to a lack of funding, hospitals and clinics in these areas were also of a lower quality than those of majority white communities and virtually nonexistent today [107]. Even among hospitals that were integrated, African American health care providers were not allowed to practice in these settings, further

alienating low-income African Americans from receiving optimal health care [107]. In the twenty-first century, hospitals with Magnet status, NCI-Designated Cancer Centers, and Designated Trauma Centers generally provide a higher level of care and likely to employ a more diverse workforce. However, these medical centers are not easily accessible to populations with limited financial resources and challenges with transportation.

Housing (safe and quality housing). Substandard housing as an SDOH among low-income, rural, and African American populations was especially brought to light during the COVID-19 pandemic. Substandard housing interwoven with limited access to health care, and prolonged occupational exposure from this virus was especially noticeable among low income and residents of rural communities [108]. The impact of substandard housing among these populations has been devastating and particularly noticeable with the excessive mortality rates experienced among rural populations [108]. Even among rural residents, African Americans have been more likely than whites to live in substandard housing, in poverty, and in households headed by women.

Substandard housing is important to health care for several reasons. First, families in communities with substandard housing are less likely to have access to financial resources, quality educational institutions, or even health care than residents living in more affluent neighborhoods. Secondly, residents of substandard housing are at higher risk for poor mental and physical health [109]. The findings of recent research suggests that an overwhelming majority of U.S. households reported one or more subpar housing domain associated with poor health [110]. Prevalent among these domains included household fuel combustion, dampness and mold, inadequate water and sanitation, and injury hazards. Pests and allergens, low indoor temperatures, and injury hazards were consistently associated with older homes, lower rent costs, and lower unit satisfaction [110].

A more troubling issue for impoverished communities of color comes from the persistent violence that occurs among residents in these communities [111]. Communities with substandard housing are also communities with high rates of violence. For example, homicide is the number one killer of young black males while intimate partner violence disproportionately kills black women [111]. These communities are also characterized by gang violence, excessive use of police force, and the rise in suicide rates [111].

Faith-Based Institutions. Historically, a primary social institution that promoted the well-being of African Americans has been the Black Church. This faith-based and social institution originated from gatherings of former enslaved Americans as a place where they could exercise their religious beliefs apart from the control of the white slave owners. Although the African slave came to America from many different African tribes and religious backgrounds, historians tend to agree that religion was very important to the survivorship of this population [56, 112, 113]. In fact, historical literature describes the Black Church as an "invisible institution" whereby the African slave in America secretly met to worship and express their sorrows to God and to believe in His ability to deliver them from the evils of this world [56]. These expressions were important mental health promoting strategies that permitted the African slave to express pent-up emotions about their slave experiences and to receive emotional support for their plight through socializing and visiting with family and friends [114].

The Black Church has maintained its role as a major faith-based institution for largely African American congregations. Over time and since slavery, the Black Church has expanded its' role from religious service to the promotion of services specifically designed to combat specific health and social problems that disproportionately affect the larger African American community [115, 116, 117]. For example, in response to increases in youth crime rates, poor educational systems, and the need for after school care for working parents, the Black Church has developed educational programs for children [117]. In response to the disproportionate rates of cancer among African Americans, churches have orga-

nized large-scale cancer screening programs [118, 119] and cancer support groups [120]. Other ongoing formal support services provided assistance with personal care services and housekeeping and transportation to church, stores, and physician appointments [121].

In recent years, health care providers have partnered with the Black Church to enhance the delivery of health care services in underserved communities. Since the Black Church is generally embedded in underserved communities with long-term trusting relationships, health care providers have effectively delivered the influenza vaccine [122], cancer control interventions [123], COVID information and vaccines [124–127], and cardiovascular mobile health interventions [124].

Compositions of Families/Naturally Occurring Social Interactions and Social Connectedness. Extended family generally refers to close familial relationships among people that otherwise would not be included in the traditional nuclear household [115, 128, 129]. McAdoo [117] described extended family members as close relationships that include persons related by blood or marriage but a unit that often extends to include friends and neighbors who are referred to as fictive kin [117]. The phrase fictive kin is used because these persons are not related by blood but relationships with these persons are so close they are considered to be "like family." The relationships of these persons are so close that they are often referred to as aunt, uncle, cousin, play sister or brother [129]. Extended family members may consist of family members who reside in the same household or throughout several households.

A dominant thought in American culture is that the traditional family structure consists of a married couple with children. However, the traditional family structure is less likely among African Americans and individuals living in poverty [130]. One prevalent family structure is the single-mother household. Single-mother households are less likely to have completed college and more likely to live in poverty than other family structures. This disparity is especially pronounced among African American women, who in recent years are much more likely to be never married or divorced [130]. African American children in these single-mother households are even more affected—with a majority living in poverty [130].

Scholars studying the African American family have noted that any deviation from the traditional two-parent nuclear family has been negatively criticized and labeled dysfunctional [115, 131]. A predominant stereotype that the African American female-headed household is largely dependent on the welfare system is an erroneous assumption not verified by research. In fact, data show that aid to African American female-headed households from welfare and food stamps accounts for only 28% of the income for these family groups [132]. Moreover, Census Bureau data reveal that, in the time period between 1979 and 1989, the percentage of African American families receiving welfare benefits decreased from 24% to 21% [116]. When researchers focus on negative elements of African American families, such as persons on welfare, they fail to see positive characteristics that exemplify the majority of African American families. For example, although 28% of African American female-headed households receives public welfare, the overwhelming majority, or 72% of these households, is not dependent on welfare as a source of income but self-sufficient, productive members of society [132].

5.1 Summary of Social Environmental Conditions

In this social environmental conditions section, we discussed the ways in which social settings were determinants of health inequities. The quality of schools/academic settings, workforce in health care diversity, safe and quality housing, faith-based institutions, and composition of families were discussed. Other social environmental conditions for consideration would be access to public transportation that is convenient and affordable and a discussion on the access to advanced education at quality educational institutions continues to be out of reach for low income

and persons of color. Not surprisingly, education that is affordable and of high quality continues to be less accessible to low income and persons of color. The lack of a diverse workforce in health care has been an issue for decades. Health care providers with the skillset to truly understand social and cultural issues of relevance to diverse patient populations is desperately needed, particularly as society becomes more diverse. It is no surprise that substandard housing is influenced by a lack of financial resources and places low income individuals in unsafe neighborhoods, leading to fears of safety and low levels of physical activity. On the other hand, when individuals have the resources to live in quality houses, safe neighborhood, health outcomes are improved. Finally, faith-based institutions and the composition of families especially among African Americans have been a protective influence, a strategy to alleviate situations where there is a lack of financial resources. The Black Church and system of extended family has historically responded to racism and oppression through community and sharing what resources were available to them.

6   Policies/Laws (Part IV)

Guidelines, principles, legislation and activities that affect the living conditions conducive to the welfare of individuals, communities, societies quality of life (see Fig. 6). Policies implemented on a national, regional, or even within institutions

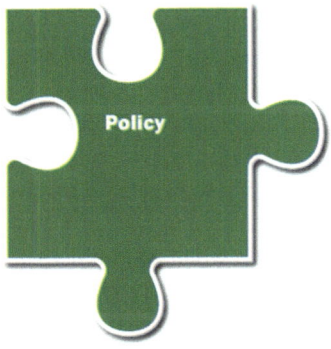

Fig. 6 Political conditions

at a local level have been protective for some populations and devastating for others. In this section we discuss a few policies/laws initiated at a national level that have contributed to health outcomes for individuals, families, and communities. In this section we reflect on the following:

- Jim Crow Laws/Civil Rights Act.
- Government-Sponsored insurance plans.
- Abortion (Roe vs. Wade).
- COVID-19 Vaccine Policies.

Black Codes and Jim Crow Laws. Perhaps the law with the greater influence on persistent racial disparities in health care originated from Jim Crow Laws that legalized racial segregation for nearly 100 years after the Civil War. Enforced until 1965, Jim Crow laws mandated racial segregation in public institutions in Southern U. S. States [133]. The intent of these laws was to marginalize African Americans through the denial of certain rights—the right to a quality education, high paying jobs, and health care [134]. Interwoven with Jim Crow Laws were Black codes that restricted the rights and freedoms of African Americans [134, 135, 136. Black codes were strict local and state laws that dictated when and where formerly enslaved Americans could work, where they could live, how they could travel, and whether they could vote [134, 136]. There were also laws that would permit authorities to seize formerly enslaved individuals, including children, for forced labor without pay [133]. Segregation was enforced in neighborhoods, recreation parks, public pools, hospitals, and residential homes for handicapped and disabled individuals [136].

Although *Jim Crow* laws ended in 1968, the effect of racial segregation persists and is an SDOH for descendants of the American slavery system [137]. Jim Crow laws dictated that African Americans attend segregated schools that provided an education that was of a lower quality than that of their white counterparts [134, 136]. In spite of the Brown vs. Board of Education ruling that racial segregation in public schools was unconstitutional, there are reports of continued segregation in public schools today [138]. An inferior education frequently translates into the inability to obtain higher paying jobs with the benefit of private insurance, to obtain housing in safe neighborhoods with better quality schools, financial resources to purchase fresh fruits and vegetables, and greater access to quality health care.

Jim Crow laws have not only had negative impact on education but is also apparent in the utilization of hospital services and the structure and functioning of minority communities. Moreover, these negative effects have persisted long after these laws ended in 1965 and influence racial disparities in health care today. For example, in comparison to whites, blacks under-utilize primary care and over-utilize emergency department services. Health care practitioners have long believed that the under-utilization of primary care was the result of distrust. However, recent research presented evidence to suggest that this pattern of health care services use is likely attributed to the ways in which non-Hispanic blacks were socialized during this extended period of racial segregation [139]. That is, the denial of access to health care during segregation contributes to a population's underuse of primary care and seeking care when the illness has advanced to a severe stage. In other research, social capital among residents in the Southern U.S was found to have persisted after Jim Crow laws were abolished. In comparison to non-Jim Crow states, the effects of racial segregation on lower levels of income, lower social connectedness, and the ability of communities to respond collectively to threats [137].

Government-Sponsored Insurance. Racism and racial inequities in the delivery of health care have persisted into the twenty-first century [22]. Although disparate health outcomes are attributed to poor health behaviors such as a lack of exercise, fatty foods, and cigarette smoking, public health experts and health care practitioners are now acknowledging the powerful influence of conditions beyond the control of the individual [23]. Poverty, the scarcity of health care providers in rural townships, and low paying jobs without insurance all contribute to a poor quality of care experienced among African Americans today [140]. The availability of government-sponsored insurance plans (e.g., Medicaid and Medicare) at least provided payment for some services as these participants became eligible. However, given the life expectancy of individuals born in the 1920s and 1930s, it is unlikely that many African Americans born during that time period lived to the age of eligibility. Without health insurance and no health care providers in some geographical areas, low income and African Americans were destined for high mortality rates.

Government-sponsored insurance plans such as Medicare and Medicaid that came after the Jim Crow years and is thought of as the most important Civil Rights Achievements in U.S. history [141]. The federal government literally threatened to withhold federal funding from hospitals that refused to desegregate [141]. This government-sponsored insurance forced the desegregation of hospitals benefited African Americans but low income persons as well [141]. In the next sections, we examine advantages and disadvantages of government-sponsored insurance plans particularly among low income and African Americans.

Medicare and Medicaid are the more well-known types of government-sponsored insurance programs [142, 143]. Medicare generally covers hospital care for people over the age of 65, younger disabled persons, and patients on dialysis [142, 143]. There are no premiums for medicare Part A (Hospital Insurance) for individuals age 65 who are permanent citizens or residents of the United States. Medicare Part A is also available to U. S. citizens under the age of 65 who, for example, are on dialysis or have had a kidney transplant [142, 143]. Medicare Part B (Medical Insurance) has a premium that is paid either monthly or quarterly. Medicare Part C, referred to as a Medicare Advantage Plan, is offered by private companies approved by Medicare. For an additional premium, Medicare Advantage Plans provide extra coverage for vision, hearing, dental, or health and wellness plans. Medicare Part D is another option that comes with a premium to help cover the cost of prescription medications. Out-of-pocket costs for these Medicare Advantage Plans can vary by company according

to their rules. These plans have rules that set fees for out-of-pocket costs that can change yearly. Medicaid is a health care coverage program for low income children, adults, pregnant women, seniors, and people with disabilities [142, 143]. For those individuals that are eligible, Medicaid covers emergency ambulance services, dental services.

The Affordable Care Act (ACA) is a health insurance coverage available to individuals, families, and small businesses [142, 143]. These insurance plans are operated by individual states and may be used to expand Medicaid coverage to their low income families and individuals. The ACA was signed into law on March 23, 2010 as the Patient Protection and Affordable Care Act and amended on March 30, 2010 by the Health Care and Education Reconciliation Act. The ACA addresses gaps in health insurance coverage, health care costs, and preventive care among U.S. citizens and residents. The benefit of being insured under the ACA is that health insurance companies cannot refuse to pay for care related to preexisting conditions like other individual insurance policies.

These government-sponsored insurance plans were designed to lessen the burden of cost to access to health care among low income individuals and to decrease health disparities. However, recent scholarship suggests that disparities in accessing health care persists among socioeconomically disadvantaged patients. For example, low income patients with Medicaid were more likely than private/Medicare patients to be diagnosed with later-staged cancers [144, 145]. Low income women with breast cancer are more likely to have longer travel times to a plastic surgeon and less likely to receive breast construction than other similarly staged women with Medicaid insurance coverage [146]. Still other research suggests that persons experiencing homelessness, a subpopulation of Medicaid patients, are underutilizing health care services that would be covered under this program [147]. The underutilization of health care services among low income persons with Medicaid coverage suggests that social factors other than one's ability to pay for services play a role in health outcomes.

Roe v. *Wade*. The original Roe v. Wade was a legal case decided by the U. S Supreme Court on January 22, 1973 that ruled that state regulation of restricting abortions was unconstitutional [148]. The Roe v. Wade opinion stated that in most instances the criminalization of abortion violated a woman's constitutional right of privacy. This was a constitutional right and consistent with a clause of the Fourteenth Amendment that no state shall deprive any person of life, liberty, or property, without due process of law. The 1973 Roe v. Wade decision was based on a federal action against the district attorney of Dallas county, Texas. At that time, the U.S. Supreme Court disagreed that women should have the right to terminate pregnancy in any way and at any time and supported the termination of a pregnancy at approximately the end of the first trimester of pregnancy. In 2022, after many years of discussions and disagreements about the constitutionality of abortions, Roe vs. Wade was reversed.

The decision to overturn Roe v. Wade has become extremely controversial and in this chapter we will not argue whether or not women's rights are being violated. Rather, we examine the influence of increased illegal and unsafe abortions on the morbidity and mortality of women that may result from this policy. Scholars have presented evidence that abortions are safe when conducted in a legal setting under safe condtions, however, the general consensus is that the majority of abortions are not conducted under safe conditions [149–151]. According to the World Health Organization (WHO), approximately 45% of all abortions are unsafe and 97% of those occur in developing countries [152]. The WHO has reported that abortions performed under unsafe conditions have contributed to injuries and deaths of women worldwide [152]. Unsafe abortions contribute to 4.7–13.2% of maternal deaths yearly and in 2012 alone, estimates are that seven million women per year were hospitalized for complications from unsafe abortions [152]. Currently, illegal abortions are reportedly much lower in the U.S. in comparison to women of lower resourced developing countries [150, 151].

Globally, low income women bear the greater financial burden of unsafe abortions. There may be costs associated with travel, mandatory waiting periods, or loss of income that limit access to safe abortion care for women with low resources [152]. Unsafe abortions are not only financially burdensome for the women but this burden extends to the family. WHO estimates from 2006 suggest that the cost of unsafe abortions to U.S. households was 922 million in loss of income as a result of long-term disability from unsafe abortions [152]. In comparison, unsafe abortions are significantly higher in countries with highly restrictive abortion laws than in those countries with less restrictive laws [152]. However, when abortions have been legalized and subsidized, the maternal morbidity rates have declined drastically [153].

Coronavirus Disease (COVID-19) and Vaccine Rollout. COVID-19 is an infectious disease caused by the SARS—CoV-2 virus which was initially discovered in December 2019 in Wuhan, China. Since that time COVID-19 rapidly spread throughout the world resulting in the deaths of millions. The contagiousness of the COVID-19 virus is due to its ability to replicate inside of a cell and quickly spread to other cells. It's ability to constantly mutate has resulted in a virus with variants that is deadly and must be continually monitored [1, 2].

According to the latest COVID-19 statistics, there have been 615 million recorded cases and 6.5 million deaths worldwide [154]. In the U.S alone, there have been 95.9 million cases and 1.05 million deaths. COVID-19 also resulted in what is now known as post-COVID (Long COVID) conditions that can occur after a COVID-19 infection and include a wide range of ongoing health problems that last weeks, months, and can lead to disability [1, 2]. Individuals at higher risk for post-COVID conditions include those not vaccinated [1, 2].

Information about the COVID-19 virus began to be disseminated in the U.S. in January 2020 which initially followed with guidelines for physical distancing and wearing masks. However, news was slow to reach some communites and information that was disseminated was not trusted particularly among those most vulnerable. COVID-19 was especially devastating for the African American community. African Americans have experienced a higher number of COVID-19 cases and hospitalizations than non-Hispanic whites [155]. In fact, COVID-19 mortality rates for African Americans are a third higher than for Latinos and more than double that for whites [156]. Although we are still in this pandemic, scholars have posited that the stark COVID-19 disparity among African Americans is a result of a long existing systemic racist policies. Policies that continue to have lasting effects on access to quality education, financial resources, housing, employment, and access to care [155]. The COVID-19 pandemic brought to light the determinants that prevented many African Americans from adhering to WHO and CDC guidelines for social distancing. Housing, community, and ecomonic status is a priviledge that permitted those with resources to adhere to protective guidelines, i.e., the priviledge to work from home, to shop online, to buy N95 masks and hand sanitizer. African Americans account for a larger percentage of Americans with low resources—jobs that are low paying and in the service sector and among those who use public transportation which increased their exposure to this community-acquired infection [155].

Despite the CDC's commitment to vaccine equity, access to this antiviral medication has been especially challenging for African American and Latino people and likely contributed to their higher incidence of illness and higher mortality rates from COVID-19 [157]. Scholars have concluded that the low rates of COVID-19 vaccines among African American and Latino populations have been the result of hesitancy or resistance behaviors [158–160]. Hesitancy behaviors have been linked back to mistreatment of African American and Latino communities, distrust of health care, and structural barriers to accessing the vaccine [158].

Although scholars have focused their attention to vaccine hesitancy and mistrust as the contributor to a lack of vaccine uptake, lack of access to the vaccine is likely the greater issue [161, 162]. When the focus of low rates of vaccine uptake

has been directed to vaccine hesitancy, scholars and practitioners have not recognized the burden imposed from factors not within the individual's control. Moreover, that latest trends in vaccine hesitancy suggests that in comparison to whites, there has been a recent shift from fewer Black adults with the "wait and see" attitude to higher numbers waiting to get vaccinated [161]. Reports from communities of color suggest that the initial vaccine rollout was not accessible due to structural barriers. One structural barrier included a lack of access to pharmacies or pharmacy services in rural areas or communities of color. Scheduling, computer literacy, transportation difficulties, and computer/internet access have also been reported as structural barriers that created challenges to persons of color wanting to be vaccinated [161].

The U.S. Census Bureau has reported that among all households in 2018, 92% had at a computer, laptop, tablet, or smartphone and 85% had a broadband internet subscription [163]. However, the creation of a vaccine scheduling system that was complex to navigate made it difficult to impossible even for persons with internet access to schedule an appointment. The initial phases of the vaccine rollout required that eligible persons make an appointment through a system where appointments were often closed out before they could be confirmed. Even when an appointment was confirmed, it was frequently with a government-sponsored vaccine center located in another town or city not easily accessible via car or public transportation. Additionally, while many households had internet connections, Black, Hispanic, and low-income households rely on smartphones and likely to incur costs should data usage exceed that allowed under specific plans with cell phone providers [163].

A vast majority of U.S. citizens travel by car or use public transportation. However, the American Public Transportation Association (APTA) reports that nearly 42% of Americans have only one car and 45% of Americans still do not have access to public transportation [164]. Initially, travel to government-sponsored vaccine centers required access to private or public transportation which limited access for the homebound, elderly, and disabled. Structural barriers from transportation challenges limited access to the vaccine for those at higher risk for contracting and dying from COVID-19.

Other challenges were related to the inconvenience of scheduling for essential employees and immigration status. Essential workers generally include those in health care, food service, transportation, and emergency services [165]. These individuals are among those least likely to have flexibility in their schedules that permits access to the vaccine. Since oftentimes appointments were only available during traditional 9–5 office or clinic hours, both essential workers and immigrants may have had scheduling issues. Immigrants may have also encountered language issues, fears related to immigration enforcement arrests, or fears related to residency status [161].

6.1   Summary of Policy Conditions

Although Policy Conditions have not generally been the focus of social determinants of health, this pillar is truly the foundation of the other three pillars (Social, Cultural, and Environmental) of the Nell Hodgson Woodruff SDOH Framework presented in this chapter. In this chapter on Policy Conditions, we discuss four policies that have shaped health outcomes particularly for low income and African American populations. Jim Crow laws that ended in 1968 legalized racial segregation in public spaces in the Southern U.S. However, these years of racial segregation have had long lasting effects on inequities in education, income, wealth, home ownership, and even the type occupation available to decendants of former enslaved Americans. In spite of widespread integration in public spaces, schools and neighborhoods remain segregated. We also discuss three other controversial policies implemented at the national level: Affordable Care Act, Roe v. Wade, and the rollout of the COVID-19 vaccine. Even though policies were intended to have equitable benefit to all persons, evidence suggests that low-income and persons of color with limited resources were disadvantaged most.

Medicaid for example, was designed to alleviate the burden of lack of access to care but in reality, the low income patient still has other challenges to overcome to access care. Roe v. Wade brought to light the challenges women have when access to safe abortions is limited. This is not just a U.S. problem but globally, where women with low resources are more likely to be hospitalized or even worse die from complications of an unsafe abortion. Finally, we have all learned about issues that originate from policies that are implemented based on resources available to the majority in the U.S. Precious time elapsed getting the vaccine to low income, disabled, and computer illiterate persons because of a policy that was implemented for the majority of persons known to have computers, cars, and access to public transportation.

References

1. CDC. Basics of COVID-19. 2021a. Retrieved September 27, 2022, from https://www.cdc.gov/coronavirus/2019-ncov/your-health/about-covid-19/basics-covid-19.html#:~:text=COVID%2D19%20(coronavirus%20disease%202019,%2C%20a%20flu%2C%20or%20pneumonia.
2. CDC. Racism and health. 2021b. Retrieved September 6, 2022, from https://www.cdc.gov/healthequity/racism-disparities/index.html.
3. Newkirk VRI. America's health segregation problem: has the country done enough to overcome its Jim crow health care system? The Atlantic Monthly Group. 2016. https://www.theatlantic.com/politics/archive/2016/05/americas-health-segregation-problem/483219/.
4. Rouse JA. Lugenia burns Hope: black southern reformer. Athens, GA: The University of Georgia Press; 1989.
5. Gamble VN. Germs have no color line: blacks and American medicine, 1900–1940. New York, NY: Garland Publishing, Inc; 1989.
6. Byrd WM, Clayton LA. Race, medicine, and health care in the United States: a historical survey. J Natl Med Assoc. 2001;93(3 Suppl):11S–34S.
7. Jones J. Labor of love, labor of sorrow. New York, NY: Vintage Books; 1995.
8. Giddings P. When and where I enter: the impact of black women on race and sex in America. New York, NY: William Morrow; 1984.
9. Lovett BL. America's historically black colleges and universities: a narrative history, 1837–2009. Macon, GA: Mercer University Press; 2015.

10. Hamilton JB. Black Appalachia's oldest: untold stories of racism, religion and mental health. 2022.
11. Gerend MA, Pai M. Social determinants of black-white disparities in breast cancer mortality: a review. Cancer Epidemiol Biomarkers Prev. 2008;17(11):2913–23.
12. Bhambhvani HP, Peterson DJ, Sheth KR. Sociodemographic factors associated with Wilms tumor treatment and survival: a population-based study. Int Urol Nephrol. 2022;54:3055–62.
13. Moubadder L, Collin LJ, Nash R, Switchenko JM, Miller-Kleinhenz JM, Gogineni K, Ward KC, McCullough LE. Drivers of racial, regional, and socioeconomic disparities in late-stage breast cancer mortality. Cancer. 2022;128(18):3370–82.
14. Tran R, Forman R, Mossialos E, Nasir K, Kulkarni A. Social determinants of disparities in mortality outcomes in congenital heart disease: a systematic review and meta-analysis. Front Cardiovasc Med. 2022;9:829902.
15. Yadav RS, Chaudhary D, Avula V, Shahjouei S, Azarpazhooh MR, Abedi V, Li J, Zand R. Social determinants of stroke hospitalization and mortality in United States' counties. J Clin Med. 2022;11(14):4101.
16. Jemal A, Thun MJ, Ward EE, Henley SJ, Cokkinides VE, Murray TE. Mortality from leading causes by education and race in the United States, 2001. Am J Prev Med. 2008;34(1):1–8.
17. Facing History and Ourselves. The persistence of racial segregation. 2021. https://www.facinghistory.org/educator-resources/current-events/persistence-racial-segregation-american-schools.
18. Walsemann KM, Bell BA. Integrated schools, segregated curriculum: effects of within-school segregation on adolescent health behaviors and educational aspirations. Am J Public Health. 2010;100(9):1687–95.
19. Lincoln AK, Eyllon M, Prener C, Garverich S, Griffith J, Adams W, Arford T, Rosenfeld L, Nykiel S, Johnson P, Guyer M, Leung YJ, Paasche-Orlow M. Prevalence and predictors of limited literacy in public mental health care. Community Ment Health J. 2021;57(6):1175–86.
20. Ajuwon AM, Insel K. Health literacy, illness perception, depression, and self-management among African Americans with type 2 diabetes. J Am Assoc Nurse Pract. 2022;34(9):1066–74.
21. Thomson MD, Williams AR, Sutton AL, Tossas KY, Garrett C, Sheppard VB. Engaging rural communities in cancer prevention and control research: development and preliminary insights from a community-based research registry. Cancer Med. 2021;10(21):7726–34.
22. Largent EA. Public health, racism, and the lasting impact of hospital segregation. Public Health Rep. 2018;133(6):715–20.
23. Gillispie-Bell V. The contrast of color: why the black community continues to suffer health disparities. Obstet Gynecol. 2021;137(2):220–4.
24. Kaufman HW, Niles JK, Nash DB. Disparities in SARS-CoV-2 positivity rates: associations with race and ethnicity. Popul Health Manag. 2021;24(1):20–6.
25. Hamilton JB, Stewart BJ, Crandell JL, Lynn MR. Development of the ways of helping questionnaire: a measure of preferred coping strategies for older African American cancer survivors. Res Nurs Health. 2009;32(3):243–59.
26. Hermence B. Before freedom: 48 oral histories of former North and South Carolina slaves. Winston-Salem, NC: John F. Blair; 1990.
27. Powdermaker H. After freedom: a cultural study in the deep south. Madison, WS: University of Wisconsin Press; 1937.
28. Hamilton JB, Sandelowski M. Types of social Suppport among African American cancer patients. Oncol Nurs Forum. 2004;31(4):792–800.
29. Poussaint AF, Alexander A. Lay my burden down: unraveling suicide and the mental health crisis among African Americans. Boston, MA: MA, Beacon Press Books; 2000.
30. Carlton-LaNey I, Hamilton J, Ruiz D, Alexander S. Sitting with the sick: African American women's philanthropy. Affilia J Women Soc Work. 2001;16(4):447–66.
31. Haas KB. Forgotten veterinarians, 4. John Boyd Dunlop and his pneumatic tire. Vet Herit. 2005;28(1):10–2.
32. Hamilton JB, Worthy VC, Moore AD, Best NC, Stewart JM, Song MK. Messages of Hope: helping family members to overcome fears and fatalistic attitudes toward cancer. J Cancer Educ. 2015b;32(1):190–7.
33. Bhutta N, Chang AC, Dettling LJ, Hsu JW. Disparities in wealth by race and ethnicity in the 2019 survey of consumer finances. 2020. Retrieved September 16, 2022, from https://www.federalreserve.gov/econres/notes/feds-notes/disparities-in-wealth-by-race-and-ethnicity-in-the-2019-survey-of-consumer-finances-20200928.html.
34. American Cancer Society. Cancer facts and figures for African Americans 2019–2021. Atlanta, GA: American Cancer Society; 2019a.
35. American Cancer Society. Cancer facts and figures. Atlanta, GA: American Cancer Society; 2019b.
36. Alcala HE. Differential mental health impact of cancer across racial/ethnic groups: findings from a population-based study in California. BMC Public Health. 2014;14:930.
37. Sklenarova H, Krumpelmann A, Haun MW, Friederich HC, Huber J, Thomas M, Winkler EC, Herzog W, Hartmann M. When do we need to care about the caregiver? Supportive care needs, anxiety, and depression among informal caregivers of patients with cancer and cancer survivors. Cancer. 2015;121(9):1513–9.
38. Rositch AF, Atnafou R, Krakow M, D'Souza G. A community-based qualitative assessment of knowledge, barriers, and pro-

moters of communicating about family cancer history among African-Americans. Health Commun. 2018;34(10):1192–201.

39. Schoenfeld ER, Francis LE. Word on the street: engaging local leaders in a dialogue about prostate cancer among African Americans. Am J Mens Health. 2016;10(5):377–88.

40. Traeger L, Cannon S, Keating NL, Pirl WF, Lathan C, Martin MY, He Y, Park ER. Race by sex differences in depression symptoms and psychosocial service use among non-Hispanic black and white patients with lung cancer. J Clin Oncol. 2014;32(2):107–13.

41. Somayaji D, Cloyes KG. Cancer fear and fatalism: how African American participants construct the role of research subject in relation to clinical cancer research. Cancer Nurs. 2015;38(2):133–44.

42. PewForum. On views of race and inequality. Black and Whites are Worlds Apart; 2016.

43. Blair IV, Havranek EP, Price DW, Hanratty R, Fairclough DL, Farley T, Hirsh HK, Steiner JF. Assessment of biases against Latinos and African Americans among primary care providers and community members. Am J Public Health. 2013;103(1):92–8.

44. Moore AD, Hamilton JB, Knafl GJ, Godley PA, Carpenter WR, Bensen JT, Mohler JL, Mishel M. Patient satisfaction influenced by interpersonal treatment and communication for African American men: the North Carolina-Louisiana prostate cancer project (PCaP). Am J Mens Health. 2012;6(5):409–19.

45. Moore AD, Hamilton JB, Knafl GJ, Godley PA, Carpenter WR, Bensen JT, Mohler JL, Mishel M. The influence of mistrust, racism, religious participation, and access to care on patient satisfaction for African American men: the North Carolina-Louisiana prostate cancer project. J Natl Med Assoc. 2013;105(1):59–68.

46. Koenig HG, King DE, Carson VB. Handbook of religion and health. New York, NY: Oxford University Press; 2012.

47. Idler E, Blevins J, Kiser M, Hogue C. Religion, a social determinant of mortality? A 10-year follow-up of the health and retirement study. PLoS One. 2017;12(12):e0189134.

48. Reed PG. An emerging paradigm for the investigation of spirituality in nursing. Res Nurs Health. 1992;15(5):349–57.

49. Britt KC, Kwak J, Acton G, Richards KC, Hamilton J, Radhakrishnan K. Measures of religion and spirituality in dementia: an integrative review. Alzheimers Dement (N Y). 2022;8(1):e12352.

50. PewForum. A religious portrait of African-Americans. Pew Forum on Religion & Public Life; 2007.

51. Raboteau AJ. A fire in the bones: reflections on African-American religious history. Boston, MA: Beacon Press; 1995.

52. Miller TN, Matthie N, Best NC, Price MA, Hamilton JB. Intergenerational influences on faith-based strategies used in response to racial discrimination among Young African American adults. J Natl Med Assoc. 2020;112(2):176–85.

53. Hamilton JB, Fluker WE. An exploration of suffering and spirituality among older African American cancer patients as guided by howard thurman's theological perspective on spirituality. J Relig Health. 2021;60:2810–29.

54. Chung B, Meldrum M, Jones F, Brown A, Jones L. Perceived sources of stress and resilience in men in an African American community. Prog Community Health Partnersh. 2014;8(4):441–51.

55. Teti M, Martin AE, Ranade R, Massie J, Malebranche DJ, Tschann JM, Bowleg L. "I'm a keep rising. I'm a keep going forward, regardless": exploring Black men's resilience amid sociostructural challenges and stressors. Qual Health Res. 2012;22(4):524–33.

56. Raboteau AJ. Slave Religion. In: The "invisible institution" in the antebellum south. New York, NY: Oxford University Press; 1978.

57. Walker WT. Somebody's calling my name. Black sacred music and social change. Valley Forge, PA: Judson Press; 1979.

58. Cone JH. The spirituals and the blues. Maryknoll, NY: Orbis Books; 2008.

59. Pinn AB. Why lord? Suffering and evil in Black theology. New York, NY: Continuum; 1999.

60. Reagon BJ. If you don't go don't hinder me. The African American Sacred Song Tradition. University of Nebraska Press, Bison Books; 2001.

61. Hamilton JB, Galbraith KV, Best NC, Worthy VC, Moore LT. African-American cancer survivors' use of religious beliefs to positively influence the utilization of cancer care. J Relig Health. 2015a;54(5):1856–69.

62. Lambe CE. Complementary and alternative therapy use in breast cancer: notable findings. J Christ Nurs. 2013;30(4):218–25.

63. Sterba KR, Burris JL, Heiney SP, Ruppel MB, Ford ME, Zapka J. "We both just trusted and leaned on the Lord": a qualitative study of religiousness and spirituality among African American breast cancer survivors and their caregivers. Qual Life Res. 2014;23:1909–20.

64. Hamilton J, Powe B, Pollard A, Lee K, Felton A. Spirituality among African American cancer survivors. Cancer Nurs. 2007;30(3):309–16.

65. Henderson P, Gore SV, Davis BL, Condon EH. African American women coping with breast cancer: a qualitative analysis. Oncol Nurs Forum. 2003;30(4):641–7.

66. Maliski SL, Connor SE, Williams L, Litwin MS. Faith among low-income, African American/black men treated for prostate cancer. Cancer Nurs. 2010;33(6):470–8.

67. DiIorio C, Steenland K, Goodman M, Butler S, Liff J, Roberts P. Differences in treatment-based beliefs and coping between African American and white men with prostate cancer. J Community Health. 2011;36(4):505–12.

68. Hamilton JB, Worthy VC, Moore AD, Best NC, Stewart JM, Song MK. Messages of Hope: Helping Family Members to Overcome Fears and Fatalistic Attitudes Toward Cancer. Journal of cancer education : the official journal of the American Association for Cancer Education, 2017;32(1):190–97. https://doi.org/10.1007/s13187-015-0895-z.

69. Colón-López V, Valencia-Torres IM, Ríos EI, Llavona J, Vélez-Álamo C, Fernández ME. Knowledge, attitudes, and beliefs about colorectal cancer screening in Puerto Rico. J Cancer Educ. 2023;38(2):552–61.

70. Guariglia L, Ieraci S, Villani V, Tanzilli A, Benincasa D, Sperati F, Terrenato I, Pace A. Coping style in glioma patients and their caregiver: evaluation during disease trajectory. Front Neurol. 2021;12:709132.

71. Bengtson VL, Copen CE, Putney NM, Silverstein M. A longitudinal study of the intergenerational transmission of religion. Int Sociol. 2009;24(3):325–45.

72. Hamilton JB, Best NC, Galbraith KV, Worthy VC, Moore LA. Strategies African-American cancer survivors use to overcome fears and fatalistic attitudes. J Cancer Educ. 2015;30(4):629–35.

73. Degazon CE. Ethnic identification, social support and coping strategies among three groups of ethnic African elders. J Cult Divers. 1994;1(4):79–85.

74. Tessaro I, Eng E, Smith J. Breast cancer screening in older African-American women: qualitative research findings. Am J Health Promot. 1994;8(4):286–92.

75. Abdullah T, Brown TL. Mental illness stigma and ethnocultural beliefs, values, and norms: an integrative review. Clin Psychol Rev. 2011;31(6):934–48.

76. Haynes TF, Cheney AM, Sullivan JG, Bryant K, Curran GM, Olson M, Cottoms N, Reaves C. Addressing mental health needs: perspectives of African Americans living in the rural south. Psychiatr Serv. 2017;68(6):573–8.

77. Vance TA. Addressing mental health in the black community. 2019. Retrieved October 1, 2022, from https://www.columbiapsychiatry.org/news/addressing-mental-health-black-community.

78. Dworak-Peck S. Why mental health care is stigmatized in Black Communities. 2019. Retrieved October 1, 2022, from https://dworakpeck.usc.edu/news/why-mental-health-care-stigmatized-black-communities.

79. Gary FA. Stigma: barrier to mental health care among ethnic minorities. Issues Ment Health Nurs. 2005;26(10):979–99.

80. Conner KO, Lee B, Mayers V, Robinson D, Reynolds CF, Albert S, Brown C. Attitudes and beliefs about mental health among African American older adults suffering from depression. J Aging Stud. 2010;24(4):266–77.

81. Rivera KJ, Zhang JY, Mohr DC, Wescott AB, Pederson AB. A narrative review of mental illness stigma reduction interventions among African Americans in the United States. J Ment Health Clin Psychol. 2021;5(2):20–31.

82. Taylor RJ, Chatters L, Woodward AT, Boddie S, Peterson GL. African Americans' and black Caribbeans' religious coping for psychiatric disorders. Soc Work Public Health. 2021;36(1):68–83.

83. McCauley L, Hayes R. From Florence to fossil fuels: nursing has always been about environmental health. Nurs Outlook. 2021;69(5):720–31.

84. Greenberg M. Hurricane Katrina: A signature cascading risk event and a warning. Am J Public Health. 2020;110(10):1493–4.

85. EPA, United States Environmental Protetion Agency. Climate change indicators: weather and climate. 2022a. Retrieved September 21, 2022, from https://www.epa.gov/climate-indicators/weather-climate.

86. EPA, United States Environmental Protection Agency. Chemicals and toxics topics. 2022b. Retrieved September 23, 2022, from https://www.epa.gov/environmental-topics/chemicals-and-toxics-topics.

87. Giudice LC, Llamas-Clark EF, DeNicola N, Pandipati S, Zlatnik MG, Decena DCD, Woodruff TJ, Conry JA. Climate change, women's health, and the role of obstetricians and gynecologists in leadership. Int J Gynaecol Obstet. 2021;155(3):345–56.

88. Du J, Cui L, Ma Y, Zhang X, Wei J, Chu N, Ruan S, Zhou C. Extreme cold weather and circulatory diseases of older adults: A time-stratified case-crossover study in jinan, China. Environ Res. 2022;214(Pt 3):114073.

89. Kim KN, Lim YH, Bae S, Kim JH, Hwang SS, Kim MJ, Oh J, Lim H, Choi J, Kwon HJ. Associations between cold spells and hospital admission and mortality due to diabetes: a nationwide multi-region time-series study in Korea. Sci Total Environ. 2022b;838(Pt 3):156464.

90. Zhou Y, Pan J, Xu R, Lu W, Wang Y, Liu T, Fan Z, Li Y, Shi C, Zhang L, Liu Y, Sun H. Asthma mortality attributable to ambient temperatures: a case-crossover study in China. Environ Res. 2022;214(Pt 4):114116.

91. Berberian AG, Gonzalez DJX, Cushing LJ. Racial disparities in climate change-related health effects in the United States. Curr Environ Health Rep. 2022;9(3):451–64.

92. Clougherty JE, Burris HH. Rising global temperatures is likely to exacerbate persistent disparities in preterm birth. Paediatr Perinat Epidemiol. 2022;36(1):23–5.

93. Yoo EH, Eum Y, Gao Q, Chen K. Effect of extreme temperatures on daily emergency room visits for mental disorders. Environ Sci Pollut Res Int. 2021;28(29):39243–56.

94. Fisher JA, Jiang C, Soneja SI, Mitchell C, Puett RC, Sapkota A. Summertime extreme heat events and increased risk of acute myocardial infarction hospitalizations. J Expo Sci Environ Epidemiol. 2017;27(3):276–80.

95. Allgood KL, Mack JA, Novak NL, Abdou CM, Fleischer NL, Needham BL. Vicarious structural rac-

ism and infant health disparities in Michigan: the flint water crisis. Front Public Health. 2022;10:954896.

96. Roy S, Edwards MA. Are there excess fetal deaths attributable to waterborne lead exposure during the Flint water crisis? Evidence from bio-kinetic model predictions and vital records. J Expo Sci Environ Epidemiol. 2022;32(1):17–26.

97. Reuben A, Moreland A, Abdalla SM, Cohen GH, Friedman MJ, Galea S, Rothbaum AO, Schmidt MG, Vena JE, Kilpatrick DG. Prevalence of depression and posttraumatic stress disorder in Flint, Michigan, 5 years after the onset of the water crisis. JAMA Netw Open. 2022;5(9):e2232556.

98. Bohnert AM, Nicholson LM, Mertz L, Bates CR, Gerstein DE. Green schoolyard renovations in low-income urban neighborhoods: benefits to students, schools, and the surrounding community. Am J Community Psychol. 2022;69(3–4):463–73.

99. Putra I, Astell-Burt T, Feng X. Association between built environments and weight status: evidence from longitudinal data of 9589 Australian children. Int J Obes. 2022;46(8):1534–43.

100. Gu X, Keller J, Zhang T, Dempsey DR, Roberts H, Jeans KA, Stevens W, Borchard J, VanPelt J, Tulchin-Francis K. Disparity in built environment and its impacts on Youths' physical activity behaviors during COVID-19 pandemic restrictions. J Racial Ethn Health Disparities. 2022:1–11.

101. Child ST, Kaczynski AT, Fair ML, Stowe EW, Hughey SM, Boeckermann L, Wills S, Reeder Y. 'We need a safe, walkable way to connect our sisters and brothers': a qualitative study of opportunities and challenges for neighborhood-based physical activity among residents of low-income African-American communities. Ethn Health. 2019;24(4):353–64.

102. Darling-Hammond L. Unequal opportunity: race and education. 1998. Retrieved September 18, 2022, from https://www.brookings.edu/articles/unequal-opportunity-race-and-education/.

103. Garcia E. Schools are still segregated, and black children are paying a price. ." 2020. Retrieved September, 18, 2022, from https://www.epi.org/publication/schools-are-still-segregated-and-black-children-are-paying-a-price/.

104. Jackson H, Engelman M. Deaths, disparities, and cumulative (dis)advantage: how social inequities produce an impairment paradox in later life. J Gerontol A Biol Sci Med Sci. 2022;77(2):392–401.

105. GWToday. New study finds severe lack of diversity in the health care workforce. 2021. https://gwtoday.gwu.edu/new-study-finds-severe-lack-diversity-health-care-workforce.

106. Hynson E, Bloomer J, Samson Z, Price K, Tran D, Muench U. Workforce trends of underrepresented minority nurses in the united states over the last decade: progress towards equal representation? Policy Polit Nurs Pract. 2022;23(4):215–27. https://doi.org/10.1177/15271544221118319.

107. Taylor J. Racism, inequality, and health care for African Americans. 2019. Retrieved September 16, 2022, from https://tcf.org/content/report/racism-inequality-health-care-african-americans/?session=1.

108. CDC. COVID-19 cases, hospitalization, and death by race/ethnicity. 2020.

109. Sonik RA, Herrera AL. Associations between inspections for unsafe housing conditions and evictions in New York City public housing buildings. J Community Health. 2022;47(5):849–52.

110. Chu MT, Fenelon A, Rodriguez J, Zota AR, Adamkiewicz G. Development of a multidimensional housing and environmental quality index (HEQI): application to the American housing survey. Environ Health. 2022;21(1):56.

111. Frazer E, Mitchell RA Jr, Nesbitt LS, Williams M, Mitchell EP, Williams RA, Browne D. The violence epidemic in the African American community: a call by the national medical association for comprehensive reform. J Natl Med Assoc. 2018;110(1):4–15.

112. Blassingame JW. The slave community. Plantation life in the ante-bellum south. New York, NY: Oxford University Press; 1972.

113. Lincoln CE, Mamiya LH. The black church in the African American experience. Durham, NC: Duke University Press; 1995.

114. Boles JB. Black southerners, 1619–1869. Lexington, KY: The University Press of Kentucky; 1984.

115. Billingsley A. Black families in white America. Englewood Cliffs, NJ: Prentice-Hall; 1968.

116. Hill RB. The strengths of African-American families: twenty-five years later. Baltimore, MD: R & B Publishers; 1997.

117. McAdoo HP, Crawford V. The black church and family support programs. Prev Hum Serv. 1991;9(1):193–203.

118. Leone LA, Allicock M, Pignone MP, Walsh JF, Johnson LS, Armstrong-Brown J, Carr CC, Langford A, Ni A, Resnicow K, Campbell MK. Cluster randomized trial of a church-based peer counselor and tailored newsletter intervention to promote colorectal cancer screening and physical activity among older African Americans. Health Educ Behav. 2016;43(5):568–76.

119. Maxwell AE, Lucas-Wright A, Santifer RE, Vargas C, Gatson J, Chang LC. Promoting cancer screening in partnership with health ministries in 9 African American churches in South Los Angeles: an implementation pilot study. Prev Chronic Dis. 2019;16:E128.

120. Barg FK, Gullatte MM. Cancer support groups: meeting the needs of African Americans with cancer. Semin Oncol Nurs. 2001;17(3):171–8.

121. Chatters LM, Taylor RJ, Woodward AT, Nicklett EJ. Social support from church and family members and depressive symptoms among older African Americans. Am J Geriatr Psychiatry. 2015;23(6):559–67.

122. Corley AMS, Gomes SM, Crosby LE, Hopkins M, Cranley D, Lynch B, Mitchell M. Partnering with faith-based organizations to offer flu vacci-

nation and other preventive services. Pediatrics. 2022;150(3):e2022056193.

123. Knott CL, Chen C, Bowie JV, Mullins CD, Slade JL, Woodard N, Robinson-Shaneman BR, Okwara L, Huq MR, Williams R, He X. Cluster-randomized trial comparing organizationally tailored versus standard approach for integrating an evidence-based cancer control intervention into African American churches. Transl Behav Med. 2022;12(5):673–82.

124. Brewer LC, Jenkins S, Hayes SN, Kumbamu A, Jones C, Burke LE, Cooper LA, Patten CA. Community-based, cluster-randomized pilot trial of a cardiovascular mobile health intervention: preliminary findings of the FAITH! Trial. Circulation. 2022;146(3):175–90.

125. Moore D, Mansfield LN, Onsomu EO, Caviness-Ashe N. The role of black pastors in disseminating COVID-19 vaccination information to black communities in South Carolina. Int J Environ Res Public Health. 2022;19(15):8926.

126. Nwaozuru U, Obiezu-Umeh C, Diallo H, Graham D, Whembolua GL, Bourgeau MJ, Ritchwood TD, Nelson LE, Shato T, Mathews A, Moise R, Ward MC, Raude J, Ahonkhai AA, Young DJ, Conserve DF. Perceptions of COVID-19 self-testing and recommendations for implementation and scale-up among black/African Americans: implications for the COVID-19 STEP project. BMC Public Health. 2022;22(1):1220.

127. Rogers CR, Rogers TN, Matthews P, Le Duc N, Zickmund S, Powell W, Thorpe RJ Jr, McKoy A, Davis FA, Okuyemi K, Paskett ED, Griffith DM. Psychosocial determinants of colorectal cancer screening uptake among African-American men: understanding the role of masculine role norms, medical mistrust, and normative support. Ethn Health. 2022;27(5):1103–22.

128. Azibo, D. A. (1992). Understanding the proper and improper usage of the comparative research framework. African American psychology: theory, research, and practice. A. K. H. Burlew, W. C. Banks, H. P. McAdoo and D. A. Azibo. Newbury Park, CA, Sage Publications, Inc.: 5–27.

129. Dilworth-Anderson P. Extended kin networks in black families. Generations. 1992;16(3):29–32.

130. Pew Research Center. On views of race and inequality, Blacks and Whites are worlds apart. 2016. Retrieved September 19, 2022, from https://www.pewresearch.org/social-trends/2016/06/27/1-demographic-trends-and-economic-well-being/.

131. Morton P. Disfigured images. Westport, CT: Praeger Publishers; 1991.

132. Taylor RJ, Chatters LM, Jackson JS. In: Taylor RJ, Chatters LM, Jackson JS, editors. Changes over time in support network involvement among Black Americans. Family life in Black America. Thousand Oaks, CA: Sage Publications; 1997. p. 295–318.

133. A & E Television Networks. Jim Crow Laws. History. 2022. https://www.history.com/topics/early-20th-century-us/jim-crow-laws.

134. Gates J, Louis H. Stony the road: reconstruction, white supremacy, and the rise of Jim crow. New York, NY: Penguin Press; 2019.

135. Valk A, Leslie B. Living with Jim crow: African American women and memories of the segregated south. New York, NY: Pelgrave-McMillan; 2010.

136. Woodward CV. The strange life of Jim crow. New York, NY: Oxford University Press; 2002.

137. Hswen Y, Qin Q, Williams DR, Viswanath K, Brownstein JS, Subramanian SV. The relationship between Jim crow laws and social capital from 1997-2014: A 3-level multilevel hierarchical analysis across time, county and state. Soc Sci Med. 2020;262:113142.

138. Smedley BD, Stith AY, Colburn L, Evans CH, Institute of Medicine. The right thing to do, the smart thing to do: Enhancing diversity in the health professions: summary of the symposium on diversity in health professions in honor of Herbert W. Nickens, M.D. Washington, DC: National Academies Press (US); 2001. Copyright 2001 by the National Academy of Sciences. All rights reserved

139. Hua CL, Bardo AR, Brown JS. Mistrust in physicians does not explain black-white disparities in primary care and emergency department utilization: the importance of socialization during the Jim crow era. J Natl Med Assoc. 2018;110(6):540–6.

140. Kaufman JC. The health consequences of black subordination and white domination: a relational and located approach to studying the health of US older adults born 1938–1948 dissertation. 2021.

141. Sternberg S. Desegregation: the hidden legacy of medicare. 2015. Retrieved October 1, 2022, from https://www.usnews.com/news/articles/2015/07/30/desegregation-the-hidden-legacy-of-medicare.

142. U.S. Department of Health and Human Services. Health insurance reform. Washington, DC: HHS; 2022a.

143. U.S. Department of Health and Human Services. Medicare and medicaid. Washington, DC: HHS; 2022b.

144. Kim G, Qin J, Hall CB, In H. Association between socioeconomic and insurance status and delayed diagnosis of gastrointestinal cancers. J Surg Res. 2022a;279:170–86.

145. Zaveri S, Nevid D, Ru M, Moshier E, Pisapati K, Reyes SA, Port E, Romanoff A. Racial disparities in time to treatment persist in the setting of a comprehensive breast center. Ann Surg Oncol. 2022;29(11):6692–703.

146. Stankowski TJ, Schumacher JR, Hanlon BM, Tucholka JL, Venkatesh M, Yang DY, Poore SO, Neuman HB. Barriers to breast reconstruction for socioeconomically disadvantaged women. Breast Cancer Res Treat. 2022;195(3):413–9.

147. Patel CG, Williams SP, Tao G. Access to healthcare and the utilization of sexually transmitted infections among homeless Medicaid patients 15 to 44 years of age. J Community Health. 2022;47(5):853–61.

148. Duignan B. Roe v. Wade. 2022. Retrieved October 1, 2022, from https://www.britannica.com/event/Roe-v-Wade.

149. Cameron S. Recent advances in improving the effectiveness and reducing the complications of abortion. F1000Res. 2018;7:F1000 Faculty Rev-1881.

150. Grimes DA, Benson J, Singh S, Romero M, Ganatra B, Okonofua FE, Shah IH. Unsafe abortion: the preventable pandemic. Lancet. 2006;368(9550):1908–19.

151. Rasch V. Unsafe abortion and postabortion care—an overview. Acta Obstet Gynecol Scand. 2011;90(7):692–700.

152. WHO. Abortion. 2021. Retrieved September 27, 2022, from https://www.who.int/news-room/fact-sheets/detail/abortion.

153. Clarke D, Mühlrad H. Abortion laws and women's health. J Health Econ. 2021;76:102413.

154. WHO. WHO coronavirus (COVID-19) dashboard. 2022. Retrieved September 27, 2022, from https://covid19.who.int/.

155. Maness SB, Merrell L, Thompson EL, Griner SB, Kline N, Wheldon C. Social determinants of health and health disparities: COVID-19 exposures and mortality among African American people in the United States. Public Health Rep. 2021;136(1):18–22.

156. Vasquez Reyes M. The disproportional impact of COVID-19 on African Americans. Health Hum Rights. 2020;22(2):299–307.

157. CDC. COVID-19 vaccine equity. 2022. Retrieved September 27, 2022, from https://www.cdc.gov/coronavirus/2019-ncov/community/health-equity/vaccine-equity.html.

158. Balasuriya L, Santilli A, Morone J, Ainooson J, Roy B, Njoku A, Mendiola-Iparraguirre A, O'Connor Duffany K, Macklin B, Higginbottom J, Fernández-Ayala C, Vicente G, Venkatesh A. COVID-19 vaccine acceptance and access among black and Latinx communities. JAMA Netw Open. 2021;4(10):e2128575.

159. Moore JX, Gilbert KL, Lively KL, Laurent C, Chawla R, Li C, Johnson R, Petcu R, Mehra M, Spooner A, Kolhe R, Ledford CJW. Correlates of COVID-19 vaccine hesitancy among a community sample of African Americans living in the southern United States. Vaccines (Basel). 2021;9(8):879.

160. Willis DE, Andersen JA, Bryant-Moore K, Selig JP, Long CR, Felix HC, Curran GM, McElfish PA. COVID-19 vaccine hesitancy: race/ethnicity, trust, and fear. Clin Transl Sci. 2021;14(6):2200–7.

161. Njoku A, Joseph M, Felix R. Changing the narrative: structural barriers and racial and ethnic inequities in COVID-19 vaccination. Int J Environ Res Public Health. 2021;18(18):9904.

162. Reverby SM. Racism, disease, and vaccine refusal: people of color are dying for access to COVID-19 vaccines. PLoS Biol. 2021;19(3):e3001167.

163. Bureau USC. Computer and internet use in the United States: 2018. 2021. Retrieved Press Release Number CB21-TPS.38, 2022, from https://www.census.gov/newsroom/press-releases/2021/computer-internet-use.html.

164. APTA. Public transportation facts. 2022. Retrieved September 29, 2022, from https://www.apta.com/news-publications/public-transportation-facts/.

165. McNicholas C, Poydock M. Who are essential workers? A comprehensive look at their wages, demographics, and unionization rates. 2020. Retrieved September 29, 2022, from https://www.epi.org/blog/who-are-essential-workers-a-comprehensive-look-at-their-wages-demographics-and-unionization-rates/.

Jill B. Hamilton PhD, MRPL, RN, FAAN, is Professor (tenured) and Senior Faculty Fellow of SDOH and Health Disparities at the Nell Hodgson Woodruff School of Nursing and Affiliate Professor at Candler School of Theology at Emory University in Atlanta, Georgia. Dr. Hamilton earned her BSN, MSN, and PhD in nursing from the University of North Carolina at Chapel Hill, a BS in Accounting from North Carolina Central University, postdoctoral training in the nursing care of older adults at the Oregon Health and Science University, and a Master's in Religion and Public Life at the Candler School of Theology. She previously held faculty positions at Johns Hopkins University and the University of North Carolina at Chapel Hill where she was a tenured Associate Professor. Dr. Hamilton's research interests include social determinants of health, health disparities, and the mental health promoting strategies used among older African American their families in response to life-threatening illness. Dr. Hamilton is Leading Editor of a text with Springer Nature titled *Integrating a Social Determinants of Health Framework into Nursing Education* published in 2023. She has done original research on the effects of storytelling that incorporates Black Sacred Music and scripture on psychological distress among older and younger African Americans. She was a Georgia Cancer Coalition Distinguished Cancer Scholar from 2003 to 2007 and a member of the 2014 Class of the UNC Thorp Faculty Engaged Scholars. Dr. Hamilton is currently a Fellow in the American Academy of Nursing and a Faculty Scholar of the Center for Spirituality, Theology and Health at Duke University. She was the recipient of the 2019 Distinguished Alumni Award from the School of Nursing at the University of North Carolina, the 2011 Oncology Nursing Society (ONS) Publishing's Division Award for Excellence in Writing Qualitative Research and the ONS 2023 Award for Excellence in Cancer Education. Dr. Hamilton was born and raised in the Southern Appalachian region of North Carolina.

Looking Back on a 16-Year Academic/Community Partnership

Valarie Worthy and Jill B. Hamilton

In this chapter the authors describe their experiences with an academic/community partnership. Their story focuses on when the partnership started and ways in which this collaboration has been maintained since 2007. The authors are both Registered Nurses, the first is a patient navigation manager at Duke Healthcare Systems and past president of Sisters Network Triangle, Inc., the second a tenured Professor at the Nell Hodgson Woodruff School of Nursing.

1 Starting with the Community: Our Early Experiences

Community Partner (Valarie). When I think about Sisters Network Triangle and the whole support group, I can't help but remember how totally frightened I was as a 40-year-old breast cancer survivor, with literally having nobody to talk to, because Black people don't talk openly about cancer. In fact, my fear of breast cancer came from a place—the church that should've brought me comfort. For example, when I attended funerals, people would say, "well, they had cancer," but you never saw the struggle or even if there was a struggle. The assumption, even for me as a 40-year-old nurse and before working in the field of oncology, is that when people have cancer, they die. Because I certainly didn't see the evidence of God being a healer through the witness of other cancer survivors. Among the cancer survivors visible to me, there was silence, so the only survivorship stories I had access to were from friends and families about those individuals who had died. The experience of only hearing stories about cancer as a death sentence was frightening. Even with my nursing background, hearing that I had a cancer diagnosis was devastating because no one had shared with me positive stories of breast cancer survivors.

So, when I was diagnosed, I didn't really have anyone to talk to except maybe one lady in a church that wasn't my home church. She said to me, "you know, I'm far out, things may have changed since I was diagnosed, but any way that I can help you and answer questions, I will." But that was it. This lady was at least 10–15 years older than me, she had a husband, children, and was established in her career. I was younger and just trying to define who I was and what my career would look like. I needed to find someplace where I could see and hear people that looked like me share their experiences of how they overcame their fears.

V. Worthy (✉)
Duke Cancer Institute, Duke University,
Durham, NC, USA
e-mail: Valarie.worthy@duke.edu

J. B. Hamilton
Nell Hodgson Woodruff School of Nursing,
Emory University, Atlanta, GA, USA

Academic Partner (Jill) I think the earliest experience that heavily influenced my program of research occurred in the 1980s when I was a graduate student in nursing. I was sitting in the classroom with a White professor and White classmates and remember feeling exhausted at listening to the weekly lectures that concluded that Black folk in published research studies were somehow pathologic or deficit. At that time and even now, researchers compare the behaviors of what is published about African Americans to that of Whites without any consideration of cultural influences on those behaviors and conclude that Black folk are lacking in some way. The prevailing research then as is now focuses on the weaknesses, rather than the strengths of the population. This prevailing assumption of cultural equivalence reflected in comparison studies with African Americans and Whites is also apparent in social support research, which was my topic of interest at the time.

In published research on social support, the presumption of cultural equivalence is evident when researchers compare social support resources known to be available to Whites with those available to and utilized by African Americans. While this pervasive assumption appears to be one of cultural equivalence, the interpretation of the findings is one of pathology or deviance. For instance, in health and illness literature, researchers who compare the social networks and social support resources of Whites to African Americans often interpret differences found in the African American sample negatively. In social support research, researchers acknowledge that African Americans are being compared to standards based on the perspectives of White and middle-class persons. However, in those studies where African Americans use types of social support not emphasized in research with White populations, they are assumed to be socially isolated or lacking social support. Although this negative view of social support may be widely accepted or unchallenged, it is not clear whether these lower amounts of social support are actually due to a lack of this resource or the researchers' failure to identify such because of insensitivity to cultural differences.

Research methodologies emphasizing that differences found among Black populations in comparison to White populations are culturally insensitive. Especially irritating was this White Professor's assertion that African Americans were socially isolated and lacking social support. I spoke up to say that as an African American, that had not been my experience and that possibly those stories emphasizing the strengths of the population were absent from published research. However, the professor at that time quickly dismissed my response and made the comment that if those stories that I was referring to were not published, they did not exist. I never spoke up in that class again but walked away determined to change that narrative. I enrolled in a PhD Program not long after that time and began my career of conducting research to elucidate the strengths of African Americans. I completed my PhD in Nursing in 2001 with beginning a program of research focused on the positive social support experiences among African American cancer survivors.

In another experience as an independent academic researcher, I was conducting a pilot study to evaluate a new and culturally relevant measure of social support that captured the strengths of African Americans. It was fall 2001, in my postdoctoral fellowship at OHSU in Portland, Oregon, when I was planning to recruit for this pilot study. I will always remember submitting my application to the University IRB and being initially denied since, based on previous attempts, the reviewer believed that I would never be able to recruit African American cancer survivors in Portland. Portland was the whitest city I had ever lived, and statistics supported my perception and likely that of this IRB Reviewer, since only 2.6% of the population was non-Hispanic, Black. I had traveled across country from Durham, North Carolina and didn't know anyone in Portland except for my two White mentors at Oregon Health and Science University (OHSU). I had joined a Black Church in Portland but had not been there long enough to establish a positive relationship with the Black community.

I pushed back with that IRB reviewer, and eventually received approval to conduct my research, but still had no idea where to start recruiting. I had placed flyers around town, but I doubted that would be a successful way to recruit older African Americans with cancer. However, God surely was looking out for me because I was standing in line one day at a Post Office in Northeast Portland (where a majority of African Americans lived) and saw this African American woman wearing a T shirt with a logo that read breast cancer survivor. I'm sure that I broke protocol, but I approached her, introduced myself, and asked if I might interview her for my study. She said yes, asked for my phone number, and said she would call me and also introduce me to other African American cancer survivors in the area. I remember leaving the Post Office thinking, I'll never hear from her again. To my surprise, she called me within 2 hours and by the end of the day, she had set me up for interviews with other African American cancer survivors in Northeast Portland. I had tapped into an informal support group of African American cancer survivors in Northeast Portland and by the month's end, I had interviewed the 30 participants I needed for my pilot study. I was repeatedly told by this group of cancer survivors that they would have participated in research at OHSU but they had never been asked.

2 Our Experiences with Cancer Support Groups

Community Partner (Valarie). Not long after my cancer diagnosis, I went to the support group that was offered at my cancer center. When I went in, I wasn't really shocked at the racial makeup of this support group because all my life I had been the only Black person, with the majority being White. So, that didn't really bother me that I was the only Black person. What was a problem for me was that most of the women in this cancer center-based support group were older, in their late fifties and sixties, and either retiring or near retirement. Whereas here I was in my early forties, in the prime of my life and my career. I wanted to be in a support group where I could talk with people in my age range, while they wanted to talk about life after retirement and grandchildren. So, even if they could've shared

information with me, which they would've openly done, the information they would have given me would not have been very relevant to what I was experiencing at the time. However, their willingness to share any information was better than what I had experienced in my church.

This cancer center support group was led by a nurse and a therapist, which is customary for academic cancer centers. In an academic environment, there are rules and regulations of how to proceed. Of course, there was not an opening or closing prayer or any conversations referencing God which was important to me. As a result, I didn't have the support from my peers in my age range with whom I would have had similar life challenges and the faith-based support was also missing. The cancer center support group lacked so much. Often, at the end of those support meetings, I left feeling worse than when I came in. I was thinking, "this is not… this is not for me."

Prior to joining the support group at the cancer center, I tried unsuccessfully to start my own support group. However, I couldn't get Black women to openly disclose that they were breast cancer survivors—not one—except for that one lady from the church I spoke about earlier. On occasion, one breast cancer survivor would whisper in my ear, "I had *that*" as if saying the words "breast cancer" were unspeakable or somehow shameful. *They wouldn't even say the word cancer.* I needed and wanted to hear people's positive stories, get encouragement, and support. I wanted to hear stories of other women that looked like me, women who were survivors, in my age bracket, with shared goals, values, and beliefs. The stories with mostly White and older breast cancer survivors were not encouraging and did not provide the support that I needed. I was discouraged and I only attended this support group for about 3 months.

After this experience, I began to realize that God had a plan for me. While receiving treatment for breast cancer, I began to share my story in the way that I wanted to hear it. I purchased a breast model and started doing impromptu breast cancer awareness sessions at my church or any venue that would permit me to do so. I would do little things to tell my story about breast cancer at my church and talk to my friends about the importance of getting a mammogram and conducting self-breast exams.

3 Starting an African American Breast Cancer Support Group

Community Partner (*Valarie*). About 10 years prior to my breast cancer diagnosis, I developed strong relationships with coworkers at my place of employment. One person was diagnosed with breast cancer about 2 or 3 years after I was diagnosed. After I had totally given up on the idea of being part of a support group with my peers, this friend and former co-worker called me while I was driving down the highway and she said, "Valarie, let's start a support group." When she said that, I thought I was going to run off the highway to think the support group I wanted was now going to be a possibility. My friend said, "do you know anybody?" I said, "no, not really, everybody I talk to, are not interested in being a part of a support group." She said, "Well, I got this patient that I've seen over the years. And she just called me to tell me she was diagnosed with breast cancer. Let's go visit her and see if she would be interested in being part of our support group."

This patient that my friend knew was also very interested in a different type of support group. When we met with her, she had recently had surgery and still had drains coming from her breast incision. Being a nurse, I asked her if she wanted me to empty her drain. As my friend was writing her information down for the application and interviewing her, I was providing nursing care. She was interested; however, we knew we had to get others interested in order to meet the requirement of five breast cancer survivors for an affiliate chapter of Sisters Network. As fate would have it, I crossed paths with my insurance agent in the parking lot of a bank and she said, "Val, you're a breast cancer survivor, aren't you?" I said, "Yes," and she said, "I just got diagnosed with breast cancer." I replied, "You're kidding me!" She said, "No, and I need somebody to talk to!" I told her, "we're trying to start a support group. would you be interested in being part of it?" She said, "absolutely," so we then we were four. Now we only needed one more survivor. My friend, the insurance agent, that I met in the bank parking lot then said, "I have another friend and

I'm sure that she would help us start this chapter." She talked to her friend who promised to join our group, and did all the paperwork, but then her house was destroyed by fire. After that we were not going to burden her with begging her to join the support group" On top of the cancer diagnosis, she was dealing with her the loss of her home; that was enough stress. Instead, for our fifth person, I approached a lady at church who was recently diagnosed. I said to her, "We need one more person to start this support group. If you are not interested in being an active member, that is fine. We just need your help to get it started". She gave us her paperwork, but to our surprise, the lady whose house burned down also submitted her paperwork. She told us "I made a promise." Now we had six "charter members" who started our new chapter of Sisters Network.

Academic Partner (Jill). Valarie's experience with the initial reluctance for African American women to join a support group is not surprising. During the early years of my career, when recruiting participants for my research, I visited groups designed to support cancer survivors. Rarely were these groups attended by African Americans. I since learned from my research that, generally. African Americans prefer the support from family and friends rather than the strangers at cancer center support groups. Ironically, while African Americans desire support from family and friends, those diagnosed with cancer are fearful that this disease will be a burden to family and friends. They are also reluctant to share a cancer diagnosis for fear of being ostracized and pitied among people in their social environments. In order to avoid these negative, isolating experiences, African American cancer survivors are likely to keep their diagnosis of cancer to themselves, only sharing the news with a few selected individuals. The social support available to African American cancer survivors sometimes will come from other survivors in their workplace or churches, individuals who may have kept their cancer diagnosis a secret for many years, who only disclosed their diagnosis when necessary to help someone else.

Beginning in 2007, I attended several support group meetings with Sister's Network, Triangle, and was impressed at the difference in mood, optimistic conversations, and caring shared among these African American breast cancer survivors. The meetings always began with meditation, welcoming new members, and getting updates on treatment of members still in treatment. I remember initially sitting in the back of the room as observer but quickly became member of the group—actually an Associate Member. And although I was never a breast cancer survivor, these women became a huge source of support for me and for the research that I was doing in the academy. They were there to listen to my research ideas, to encourage me, and cheered me on as I struggled as an African American scientist on tenure track in a research-intensive environment attempting to be successful with community engaged research.

3.1   Start Up of an African American Cancer Survivors Support Group

Community Partner (Valarie). A requirement from Sisters Network is that you must have five survivors to start your group. We ended up with six people that were interested.

My friend and co-founder, Dean Johnson, who knew a ton of people, just started calling people she knew, and they started calling people they knew, and I think at our very first meeting we had 15 to 20 people, a good number. Dean had a friend who had office space with a long table, enough for everyone to sit around it for our first meeting.

The National Office of Sisters Network gave us an agenda that we could follow, and we started from there. Honestly, I didn't want to be president. But my friend Dean said, "I'm not gonna be it." I said, "I thought you were, because you like to lead." She replied, "no." And then she said, "you really always wanted a support group." So, I started leading the group, but that wasn't my plan. I didn't necessarily want to *lead* it; I just wanted to be a *part* of it.

I was amazed at how quickly the membership of this support group grew. We started doing out-reach events where we were telling our stories. I was also amazed that these women were openly talking about breast cancer and others' responses to this openness, for example "oh, you don't look like you had cancer." I became acutely aware that the Black community had preconceived ideas about what cancer looked like. So, to address this need and provide culturally relevant support to women with breast cancer, we started our support group Sisters Network Triangle, Inc. in 2003.

Academic Partner (Jill). I became aware of Sister's Network in 2007 and invited to attend one of their monthly meetings through a childhood friend, also a breast cancer survivor. My initial goals for attending these meetings were to learn more about the social support experiences of African American cancer survivors. A secondary goal was to learn how, as nurse scientist, I might somehow use my knowledge to give back to this organization. I did not want to just come in and get what I needed and exit as many of my peers had done. I was a nurse scientist yes, but I identified with them as an African American woman and wanted to provide something in return, and in the back of my mind, given the stats on the incidence of breast cancer, thought it might very well be that 1 day I too might be a breast cancer survivor.

For several months, I attended these meetings, always sitting in the back of the room. However, it was not long before I felt like one of the group. I also attended the social activities they sponsored. One of the highlights of my experience with this group occurred a few short months after my first meeting when Valarie asked me to teach a few members of the group the language of research. They wanted to be better able to advocate for the group when approached by researchers, to understand their language. I was honored. I had taught research methods in the academy to undergraduate and graduate students and was very confident that I could give them research knowledge useful to their purpose. During that time, I had a 9-month faculty appointment with a lot of flexibility during the summer months to meet with them. They scheduled the time and place and more importantly showed up to learn from me. Again, I was honored.

4   Sister's Network and Community Outreach

Community Partner (Valarie). I think that calling our group a cancer survivors' organization instead of a support group, helped us to offer breast cancer survivors support and cancer education and as well as community outreach. When you think about a breast cancer support group, you are limited to the concept of women gathering to talk solely about their diagnosis which can be depressing. I have even heard from some women that attending traditional support groups with conversations focused on the cancer and its treatment were sad and depressing. And people didn't want to be a part of those type conversations. But when you said *survivorship*—that word had its own energy in and of itself.

The beauty of what we were offering in our survivorship group was, in addition to offering support to survivors of breast cancer, their family members, and caregivers, was our outreach services that really spoke to the heart of what we were all about. Our mission was to educate the community and show them that cancer was not automatically a death sentence. We tried as best as we could to show the Black community in the Triangle area that we were still very much alive and thriving and others could too with early screening and diagnosing. We wanted to change the narrative of cancer being a death sentence. Dean, as a Social Worker, and me, as a Registered Nurse, had worked in the community prior to being diagnosed and already had established a lot of relationships in the community. We both had done a lot of outreach in churches prior to becoming cancer survivors. Shortly after I was diagnosed with breast cancer, I discovered that the mother of the pastor's had been diagnosed with breast cancer and would advocate for breast cancer survivors. So, the pastor's wife was extremely involved in community outreach and engagement which also opened doors for us.

For me, my breast cancer diagnosis was the catalyst of starting my outreach and community engagement. My diagnosis was the key to unlocking the door for African Americans having a better understanding of cancer, of cancer screenings, and just understanding that there is a more excellent way for survivorship. That death was not the only outcome. This is when I began to see breast cancer survivors being transformed. Because, as a cancer survivor helping others, you not only receive the Gospel as it speaks to God's plan for your life or about healing scriptures, but also, in your role as a health professional, you can talk to others in your community about cancer, cancer prevention, and cancer screenings. It was like a hand in a glove.

Once Sisters Network started, we continued to build on the relationships and work we had already started in our community. As a home health nurse, I was already out there visiting people in the community, so people knew me. I was going to doctor's offices, clinics, all that kind of thing to get their support with our community outreach activities. I lived in the community where I received treatment, so I had access to cancer care and I could talk to my oncologist and his team. The benefit of this interaction led to their collaboration and engagement with me in community outreach activities. It really became a village to disseminate health information. And we did it without a struggle. Once we realized the source of people's fears, we knew how to attack the elephant (so to speak) before it really came out in the room. You knew how to address those fears in a way that wasn't confrontational, but educational.

Academic Partner (Jill). As an academic partner with a program of research focused on the social support experiences of cancer survivors, I did not directly participate in community outreach activities with Sister's Network Triangle, Inc. However, I did attempt to show my support for Sister's Network Triangle's community outreach activities when asked to be invited speaker at their events and attending the Annual Tea Events when I was in town. For example, I was invited speaker at the **"Spirituality and Cancer" Sisters Network tenth Annual Surviving and Thriving Symposium**, Durham, NC. At other times, I was able to contribute financially, for example purchasing extra tickets for the Annual Tea Event, to enable other members to attend. Over the years, I have also contributed Walmart cards to the Health and Wellness committee of Sister's Network Triangle. The Health and Wellness committee then used these gift cards to relieve the burden to members in treatment, assisting them to buy gas, medications, or food. I wish I would have done more but I did what I could at the time.

5   Developing a Trusting Relationship

Community Partner (Valarie). Jill is probably responsible for me being open to researchers. If it weren't for her, I probably wouldn't make the effort that I make when it comes to researchers I encounter in the community—like researchers wanting to hear the voice of the real people. And because of my collaboration with Jill, I knew how to set a standard. Jill was a nurse and scientist I was able to see her in a nontraditional position—because back then, nurses were primarily bedside folk, either in a clinic or still doing traditional nursing care to patients. That was my previous experience. But seeing a nurse as a researcher and Black? That was amazing!! When Jill came into our organization, and we finally did get to talk, I learned so much from her. And then Jill started the research about religious songs, and me being a Baptist girl who played the piano for Sunday school until I graduated high school, that topic really resonated with me. Listening to religious songs (gospel music) and hymns was like medicine to us.

I remember relying on songs when I was diagnosed. If I had to get an x-ray or radiation, I would always have some music playing. I would be listening to some Gospel music, or I'd be singing. It was always Gospel songs that would give me peace. So, when Jill started her research about Gospel songs, it really resonated with me, and it all came together. It's like what my grandmother taught me. What I learned at church, it just all came together. What Jill did really brought credibility to what many cancer survivors felt about the usefulness of gospel music to our cancer experience.

Listening to and singing gospel music was like you took chemo and all the other medicine that got you better. But we always knew—the secret sauce was the scripture-based songs that were in our heart. God takes chemo, the medicine, and everything else and blesses it, but the secret sauce was having that song, that scripture, in our heart. I felt as if God gave me a song that the angels can't sing. In your mind, you think about how *There is a bright side somewhere, don't rest until you find it.* Those songs that carried you through, they don't make you sad. God, like the speed of sound, that song transfers you from that place of remembering that thing that hurt you, and before you can even grab ahold of the bitterness of that hurt, that song has already lifted you up beyond it.

To be able to have a person like Jill now quantify what we all had felt, I thought, "Yes, this is how this thing is supposed to be." Jill was authentic and became my litmus test to how someone in academia should behave and respond to the community. Jill raised the standard of what to expect from others. If my interactions with others didn't feel right, if I didn't feel like this was something Jill Hamilton would do, then I wouldn't work with them. Really, that's how I felt. That wasn't Jill's intent to teach me that, but that's what I learned because that's where my level of comfort was. Jill never projected herself as *"her vs. us."* She was always part of the *we*, and that made a big difference for us. I never felt like, "we are schooling her on something." It was always an equal exchange. As it says in the Bible, we were equally yoked.

Academic Partner (Jill). I didn't initially realize the purpose for my collaboration with Valarie back in 2007. I initially only wanted to learn more from them about how I could ensure that the research I was conducting was relevant and useful. However, over the years, I believe I had become a voice for this group to the larger academic community. I had become a conduit to capture the stories of these African American women with breast cancer, to portray the strengths of these women. I had finally achieved my goal of contributing to the scientific literature that African American cancer survivors do indeed have social support from family and friends, that their belief in God lends to a faith and optimistic perspective needed during the diagnosis and treatment for cancer but also in their years of survivorship. They became the voice to support that interventions need to be adapted to be culturally relevant, that African American women can rely on God for support during cancer, but still be adherent to prescribed plans for treatment. That the positive survivorship experience for African American women depended on hospital prescribed surgery, chemotherapy, immunotherapy, and radiation therapy for cancer, but also their faith in God and those songs and scripture passages learned during their formative years. Ultimately, it was the story communicated through a song or scripture passage that enabled them to endure a prescribed cancer treatment and to overcome the fears of recurrence that may come during the years of survivorship.

6   Finding Meaningful Ways to Give Back to the Community

Community Partner (Valarie). We [breast cancer survivors of Sisters Network, Triangle] all must have known Jill was not the norm. But she could've been a wolf in sheep's clothing. We didn't know anything, but God had mercy on us. Jill was always so humble and willing to teach us. I think another member of the support group and cancer survivor said, "Can you believe this?" "She doesn't mind teaching us this stuff." And that was the beauty of it. A lot of people talk about community engagement, but Jill was walking the walk and talking the talk.

We had an event at one of my churches where Jill shared her research with faith-based cancer survivorship stories with people. It's the type of research that people have never been exposed to. It's like the testimonies that people talk about at church, the songs they sing at church, they sing them on the way home from church. They sing them in their homes, and they know what those songs mean to them and how they make them feel. But the fact that a researcher can take those

lines, and chorus, and frame it, and describe it in a way that is literally like medicine, an elixir was what we needed. Jill had captured how religious songs are used and was able to describe it to the world in a way that the world understands it.

For the African American experience, the use of religious songs during cancer now becomes comparable to yoga. Moreover, all the other research has said, "Oh, well, we have scientific data to suggest that yoga does XYZ and meditation does XYZ," but for us, for the African American experience we turn to our religious songs for strength and comfort. We've known this a long time, but nobody took the time to really look at it, to dissect it. And for cancer survivors that used it to give voice to this strategy, did help calm fears. But nobody said that outside of the four walls of their home and church. Jill put our thoughts, what we believe in our heart; and ways we describe our faith in actionable ways. We never could've described it.

We appreciate the therapists, psychiatrists, and chaplains, but it's the songs, the scriptures in the midnight hour that gets us through. The songs get us through when the chaplain, therapist, psychiatrist are not there. There's a song; there's a scripture; there's something that people are saying that is bringing them peace in the midst of this crazy storm. Just listening to that song, such as '*Joy Cometh in the Morning.*' People were so into the song that if someone that wasn't familiar with the meaning of the song, if they asked you, "Really? In the morning you're gonna feel better?" You say to them, "Not literally in the morning." We were so in tune with '*Joy Cometh in the Morning.*' We weren't talking about literally, "*Oh, it's light time, morning,*" but we all knew what it meant. You're at that point in your life where these words just take on a life of their own. You feel as if, "If I can just grab this song, grab these words and put them in my heart, then I know that I will feel better."

Jill explained this research about religious songs to us in a way that people otherwise would not have understood, now they began to understand. And not only did they understand how we dealt with cancer, but how we dealt with life in America. Because for some people, it's like, "If I can deal with the life and the hand that I've been dealt, and if those hymns carried me, surely it will carry me through a cancer diagnosis." Or the young person might say, "If it carried my grand-mamma and my granddaddy, my great-great and all they went through, surely it can carry me through this cancer diagnosis."

That's how religious songs work in our lives. That's why when you get in church, in anybody's church, you can sing those songs. I have nothing against these modern-day gospel singers or praise worshippers—beautiful songs. But when some-body, an older person that has known the meaning of those songs starts singing a hymn, it is some-thing about that song that breaks down all com-munication barriers. Folks that may not have ever heard a hymn—some of the young people, they haven't but they know there's something different about those hymns. Reminds me of the song "*It will never lose its power*." It's just like the song, *The blood, that Jesus shed for me*, that hymn, it will never, ever, ever, ever lose its power. *It reaches to the highest mountain and it flows to the lowest valley*. That hymn would take you above the clouds, but when you are down at your lower moment and you can't even get a sound out, just the thought of that song would lift you up. I'm not saying lift you up high, just that a lift is better than where you are.

That's what those songs do for the African American experience. For Jill to give it a tag and a title, beyond what it already was, like a hymn, it becomes a heart, a scab over a wound. It becomes the peacemaker, you know, the healer. That's what really spoke to the African American expe-rience. That's what makes the difference. I used to speak in front of people and I would tell my story, and then I would say to myself, "Well, how do I end this thing?" More times than I can count, I would end it by saying a couple of lines from a hymn. "This is my story. This is my song. *Praising my Savior All the Day Long*." And I would end my talk with those lines. "This is my story." And it was.

Academic Partner (Jill). I have previously described ways in which I as individual academic partner attempted to maintain a reciprocal rela-tionship with Valarie as community partner and

to the African American breast cancer survivors who have supported me and my program of research over the years. However, my greater purpose is to use my scholarship and knowledge to contribute to the larger population of Black/African American cancer patients/survivors throughout the globe. Through my academic appointment at a leading research university, I have the capability to retell the stories of cancer survivorship that I have collected over the years, to package those stories in a way that will be accessible to Black/African American cancer patients/survivors globally. This shift will call for a difference in how these stories made accessible to the population orally and through written lan-guage that may appear less rigorous and unac-ceptable in the health sciences. The style of writing that I am referring to is widely accepted in the humanities and theology, a form of creative nonfiction, a style accessible by the public.

During the next phase I will use my collabora-tion with Valarie, my community partner, to guide me in ways to best disseminate these sto-ries to the broader community of Black/African American cancer survivors. Valarie has the vision and knowledge of what survivors need and I have the skill to language the stories for accessibility and utility.

7 A Partnership with Dissemination of Findings in Academia and the Community

Community Partner (Valarie). If you really think about it, all the literature and evidence you read even in nursing school about African Americans, it really doesn't capture our truth. But I felt like what Jill wrote had a multifunctional purpose. One, it had to inform people that didn't know any-thing about our culture. Secondly, her writing was informative and gave voice to an experience that wasn't an imitation of anyone elses. For example, Jill's writing captured who we are as African Americans, so that a person could read it and understand and think, "Yes, that's exactly how I felt." Similarly, a researcher could understand through Jill's descriptions how religious songs impact the lives of African American cancer survivors.

When writing with Jill, I didn't always know what to say. I knew it was in my heart, but I didn't know how to put it in words. And Jill has always had a great way of pulling things out of me. Before I knew it, I was able to describe and write down my thoughts. For me, it was always that I couldn't give that thing a tag or title. But I knew when I felt it.

When writing for publication, sometimes the Lord would put something on my heart, and He was like, "You need to call Jill." And I would say, "Lord, we just talked." And he would say, "But you have to tell her this is what..." Just different things. So, I'd call Jill and say, "I don't know when we're gonna need this, but this is what the Lord said."

A final thought about learning to write with Jill was an experience I had with her while in graduate school. I would frequently call Jill for her advice and guidance on my class assignments. I was always amazed at how she was able to explain those concepts I was reading in those textbooks and hearing in classroom lectures. But one piece of advice Jill provided when beginning to write for academic audiences. Jill would say "when you come across a word or phrase when reading articles, write those words on a Post-it note and place it on your computer monitor so you will remember to use that word or phrase when writing." I still remember that advice and use it today.

Academic Partner (Jill). One of the metrics for success in the academy is the number of papers from your research in peer-reviewed publications. I can remember asking Valarie to write with me, having the expectation that she would write paragraphs that I could integrate into the manuscripts I was drafting. I remember sending Valarie drafts of manuscripts asking her feed-back. In my academic world, feedback was generally written and that was my expectation with Valarie. And my traditional thinking of publishing together meant, I write something, you write something; I write something, you write something. And I remember thinking 1 day, I said, "This ain't working with us." Valarie's feedback would come in a late-night phone call where we would spend an hour or two talking about the findings and my interpretation and conclusion of those findings. On one occasion, Valarie called me and said "I hate to mess you up but you didn't get it." After laughing at the way she said it, my response was "Valarie, tell me again. Just tell me again, because I'm going to get this thing right."

We revised that particular manuscript, which was the first manuscript that I had ever submitted and had accepted on the first attempt. I learned then that a true collaboration that includes dissemination of findings is more than putting words on paper, it is truly a process of conceptualization that occurs at the inception of the project through publication.

In addition to dissemination in academic journals, another metric for success in the academy is presentations at international, national, and regional conferences with a goal of informing and receiving feedback from our peers. However, because of my collaboration with Valarie and Sister's Network, I was invited to present my research to other cancer survivors during events in community settings as well as faith-based institutions. The benefit of sharing my research in community settings was that survivors could see the results of their participation in my research and also to know that their experiences were indeed helping other survivors and family members.

8 Reflection

The collaboration between Jill and myself has been a very rewarding one. We have learned from each other, supported each other to achieve our respective professional goals, and are planning for more years of a research/community partnership.

Valarie Worthy MSN, RN, is Patient Navigator Manager at Duke University Health System and Co-Founder of TOUCH, the Black Breast Cancer Alliance, to bolster Black women's breast cancer clinical trial participation by 2025—with the goal of reaching 350,000 Black women and motivating 25,000 into trial portals. Valarie is a two-decade-plus breast cancer survivor, has been a nurse for more than 41 years, and worked at Duke for the past 20 years. Her hometown is Ahoskie, in northeastern North Carolina.

Jill B. Hamilton PhD, MRPL, RN, FAAN, is Professor (tenured) and Senior Faculty Fellow of SDOH and Health Disparities at the Nell Hodgson Woodruff School of Nursing and Affiliate Professor at Candler School of Theology at Emory University in Atlanta, Georgia. Dr. Hamilton earned her BSN, MSN, and PhD in nursing from the University of North Carolina at Chapel Hill, a BS in Accounting from North Carolina Central University,

postdoctoral training in the nursing care of older adults at the Oregon Health and Science University, and a Master's in Religion and Public Life at the Candler School of Theology. She previously held faculty positions at Johns Hopkins University and the University of North Carolina at Chapel Hill where she was a tenured Associate Professor. Dr. Hamilton's research interests include social determinants of health, health disparities, and the mental health promoting strategies used among older African American their families in response to life-threatening illness. Dr. Hamilton is Leading Editor of a text with Springer Nature titled *Integrating a Social Determinants of Health Framework into Nursing Education* published in 2023. She has done original research on the effects of storytelling that incorporates Black Sacred Music and scripture on psychological distress among older and younger African Americans. She was a Georgia Cancer Coalition Distinguished Cancer Scholar from 2003 to 2007 and a member of the 2014 Class of the UNC Thorp Faculty Engaged Scholars. Dr. Hamilton is currently a Fellow in the American Academy of Nursing and a Faculty Scholar of the Center for Spirituality, Theology and Health at Duke University. She was the recipient of the 2019 Distinguished Alumni Award from the School of Nursing at the University of North Carolina, the 2011 Oncology Nursing Society (ONS) Publishing's Division Award for Excellence in Writing Qualitative Research and the ONS 2023 Award for Excellence in Cancer Education. Dr. Hamilton was born and raised in the Southern Appalachian region of North Carolina.

Those factors that occur in society due to systemic (structural) racism and imbalances in power, financialresources, education, and occupation that influence wellness or lack thereof.

Access to Quality Education and Technology: Examining Digital and Health Literacy

Diana Baptiste, Tamar Rodney,
Ruth-Alma Turkson-Ocran,
Oluwabunmi Ogungbe,
and Yvonne Commodore-Mensah

1 Introduction

Amid the COVID-19 pandemic, healthcare systems in the United States faced challenges in sustaining their healthcare delivery capacity, prompting a rapid adoption of technology to provide healthcare services. In this evolving "new normal," telehealth services have swiftly become an integral part of routine care practices. With the ongoing imperative of social distancing for high-risk patients, healthcare providers are increasingly adopting telehealth services and the use of health information technologies (HIT) to communicate with patients with diverse health needs such as management of chronic conditions, psy-

chiatric care, counseling, non-urgent medical visits, and healthcare educational sessions.

There is an intersection of digital literacy and health literacy within urban communities. Racial and ethnic disparities exist among individuals, especially in inner-city areas access and utilize technology, particularly in the context of health information and services [1–3]. This chapter aims to shed light on the challenges and opportunities related to digital and health literacy in urban settings, where disparities in education and technology access are often pronounced. This chapter provides valuable insights into the potential impact of these disparities on healthcare outcomes and suggests strategies for improving digital and health literacy in inner-city populations.

D. Baptiste (✉) · T. Rodney · Y. Commodore-Mensah
Johns Hopkins University School of Nursing,
Johns Hopkins University, Baltimore, MD, USA
e-mail: dbaptis1@jhu.edu; trodney1@jhu.edu;
Ycommod1@jhmi.edu

R.-A. Turkson-Ocran
Division of General Medicine, Harvard Medical
School, Beth Israel Deaconess Medical Center,
Boston, MA, USA
e-mail: rturkson@bidmc.harvard.edu

O. Ogungbe
Department of Epidemiology, Johns Hopkins
Bloomberg School of Public Health,
Johns Hopkins University, Baltimore, MD, USA
e-mail: Oogungb3@jhu.edu

2 Telehealth

Telehealth offers patients the opportunity to engage in remote healthcare visits, primarily aimed at addressing non-urgent concerns, promoting medication adherence, and reducing emergency department visits [4]. The utilization of telehealth services presents numerous advantages for both patients and healthcare providers. For patients, telehealth enhances access to high-quality healthcare, preventive services, patient education, and lifestyle counseling, ultimately resulting in fewer hospitalizations [4]. Additionally, it can eliminate obstacles to timely care for individuals facing challenges such as limited transportation and childcare access.

Telehealth is designed to facilitate a seamless transition from traditional in-person visits to healthcare encounters conducted via telephone, remote monitoring, wireless communication, or videoconferencing [5]. For healthcare providers, telehealth increases provider-to-patient interactions, facilitates the use of interpretation services for non-English speakers and enhances the utilization of healthcare services. However, despite the prevalence of advanced technology, it is important to recognize that not all patients have easy access to phones and computers due to various social, structural, and economic barriers. Low health and digital literacy, limited internet or computer access, and a lack of technological proficiency can pose significant challenges [1, 6]. Addressing these social barriers to telehealth and HIT adoption is essential to ensure equitable access to healthcare services and technology-driven health information. Strategies should focus on education, improving access, fostering trust, and considering the diverse needs of patients from different backgrounds and communities.

3 Health Information Technology (HIT)

The use of health information technology (HIT) has also created opportunities for individuals to access their electronic medical records and other important health information and education. There are numerous potential obstacles to the use of HIT, especially among older adults, including limited health literacy, challenges related to HIT's usability and accessibility, and difficulties in effectively utilizing HIT due to complications stemming from chronic illnesses, such as vision impairment, limited fine motor mobility, and cognitive impairment [7]. It has been demonstrated that HIT can enhance care management and health promotion among older adults. Consequently, it would be beneficial to develop strategies aimed at overcoming these barriers to

further boost its effectiveness. Younger family members and caregivers can also play a role in supporting older adults in effectively accessing and using HIT.

4 Social Barriers to Using Telehealth and Health Information Technology (HIT) Include

- **Digital Literacy:** Many individuals, particularly older adults or those from underserved communities, may not have the necessary digital literacy skills to effectively navigate and use telehealth platforms or HIT. This lack of familiarity with technology can be a significant barrier.

- **Access to Technology:** Not everyone has access to the required technology, such as smartphones, computers, or a reliable internet connection, which is essential for telehealth and HIT usage. Disparities in technology access can hinder people from benefiting from these services.

- **Language and Cultural Differences:** Language barriers and cultural differences can create challenges in using telehealth and HIT. If services are not available in multiple languages or don't consider cultural norms, it can deter some individuals from using them.

- **Privacy Concerns:** Some people may be concerned about the privacy of their health information when using telehealth or HIT. Worries about data breaches or unauthorized access can deter individuals from fully engaging with these technologies.

- **Lack of Trust:** Trust in healthcare providers and technology companies is crucial for the adoption of telehealth and HIT. Skepticism about the security of data or the quality of care provided remotely can discourage usage.

- **Socioeconomic Status:** Socioeconomic factors, such as income and education level, can influence access to telehealth and HIT. People with lower incomes or less education may be less likely to have the means or knowledge to use these technologies effectively.

- **Resistance to Change:** Resistance to change is a common social barrier. Some individuals and healthcare providers may prefer traditional in-person interactions and be reluctant to switch to telehealth or HIT solutions.
- **Geographic Barriers:** In rural or remote areas, access to reliable internet and telehealth services may be limited. Geographic barriers can significantly impact the feasibility of using these technologies.
- **Family and Caregiver Support:** An individual's ability to use telehealth and HIT can be influenced by the support they receive from family members or caregivers. Lack of support can hinder utilization.
- **Health Disparities:** Existing health disparities can exacerbate social barriers. Minority populations and those with chronic health conditions may face additional challenges in accessing and using telehealth and HIT, further widening healthcare inequalities.

Vulnerable populations, particularly those who are Black with lower incomes and unemployment, are at a higher risk of experiencing the "digital divide" [2, 3, 8]. Individuals who are employed and have higher incomes are more likely to communicate with healthcare providers through methods like text, phone apps, or email. Previous studies reaffirm there is a clear association between lower income and education levels with lower HIT usage [2, 3, 5]. Therefore, ensuring the affordability and accessibility of HIT is paramount in expanding access to potentially beneficial interventions that may currently be limited by financial constraints.

Strategies for improving telehealth and HIT usage should address these gaps associated with social determinants of health and health and digital literacy, as individuals with adequate health literacy are more likely to have internet access at home, use the internet for health-related information, use telehealth resources appropriately, engage in email correspondence with healthcare providers, and effectively communicate with them compared to patients with marginal to low health literacy [6]. Therefore, when considering the adoption of telehealth and the use of HIT, we must take into account not only the suitability and available support for telehealth but also the challenges related to access. These challenges may encompass issues such as technological literacy, environmental support, and socioeconomic factors.

5   Moving beyond Technology and Connecting Back to the Community

In addressing communities affected by the digital divide, it is crucial to acknowledge our ability to make a meaningful impact by directly engaging with these community members. It underscores the importance of creating a balance between technological advancements and maintaining meaningful connections within communities [9]. The central idea is that while technology has facilitated various aspects of modern life, it should not replace or diminish the essential bonds that exist within communities. Instead, we recommend that healthcare providers should make deliberate efforts to use technology as a tool to enhance and strengthen community connections. This approach acknowledges the value of face-to-face interactions, local engagement, and the social context that communities provide [9]. Ultimately, we advocate for a holistic perspective that embraces both technological progress and the preservation of genuine community ties. A significant opportunity exists to meet with patients and community members "right where they are." Here are some suggestions for enhancing community engagement:

1. **Collaborate with Community-Based Organizations:** Consider forming partnerships with local community-based organizations and grassroots groups. Together, you can craft messages that resonate with the community's specific context, increasing awareness of healthcare programs tailored to their needs.
2. **Conduct Community Screenings**: Organize community health screenings to improve healthcare accessibility within vulnerable populations. These screenings should take place in community gathering spots like

workplaces, barbershops, beauty salons, and churches, where community members frequently convene.

3. **Leverage Digital Platforms:** While addressing the digital divide, don't overlook the opportunities presented by digital platforms to facilitate health-related discussions and foster social support. Examples include virtual networks, webinars, social media groups, and online discussion forums, which can all play a significant role in promoting health awareness and engagement.

A Case Example

Background:

AG is a 47-year-old Haitian immigrant female. AG resides in a low-income neighborhood in a densely populated urban area. She has a high school diploma from her native country and speaks English as her second language. She lives alone in a small apartment and has a part-time job as a cleaner at a local elementary school. Due to her limited education and job opportunities, AG's income is modest, making her financially vulnerable. She has a history of managing chronic hypertension and type 2 diabetes, which require regular medical attention and monitoring.

Challenges with accessing telehealth services:

- *Limited access to technology:* AG does not own a personal computer or a smartphone with internet access. She cannot afford these devices due to her low income.
- *Lack of digital literacy:* While she understands the basics of using a cellphone for calls and texts, AG lacks the digital literacy required to navigate telehealth platforms or video conferencing apps effectively.
- *Language barrier:* AG's primary language is Haitian creole, and her proficiency in English is limited. She struggles with understanding complex medical instructions or discussing her health concerns in English, which is often the language used in telehealth services.
- *Unreliable internet connectivity*: Even if she had access to a smartphone, her neighborhood frequently experiences internet connectivity issues, making reliable telehealth consultations challenging.

Financial constraints: AG has no health insurance due to her low income and cannot afford the cost of telehealth consultations, which are often not covered by public health programs.

Impact on health:

AG's inability to access telehealth services has several significant consequences:

- *Missed appointments:* Without access to virtual healthcare, AG frequently misses medical appointments, leading to inadequate management of her chronic conditions.
- *Limited health education*: She misses out on essential health education and preventive care information, which could empower her to manage her conditions more effectively.
- *Health inequities:* The lack of access to telehealth exacerbates existing health inequities, as AG faces greater challenges in receiving timely and quality healthcare compared to individuals with better access.

Potential solutions:

- *Community outreach:* Local healthcare organizations can initiate community outreach programs to identify individuals like AG who lack access to technology and provide them with subsidized or donated devices, such as tablets or smartphones.
- *Digital literacy training:* Programs aimed at improving digital literacy can be offered within the community to help patients like AG become more comfortable with using technology for healthcare purposes.
- *Language access services:* Healthcare providers should ensure that they have interpreters or multilingual staff available to assist patients with limited English proficiency, bridging the language barrier during telehealth consultations.
- *Affordable internet services:* Advocacy for affordable internet access in underserved communities can help address connectivity issues.
- *Financial assistance*: Healthcare facilities can offer sliding-scale fees or financial assistance programs to make telehealth consultations more affordable for low-income patients.

AG's case highlights the complex challenges faced by individuals from low socioeconomic backgrounds when accessing telehealth services. Addressing these barriers requires a multifaceted approach involving technology provision, education, language support, and financial assistance to ensure equitable healthcare access for all.

The association between social determinants of health and education, as well as health and digital literacy, underscores the complex relationships between individual well-being and the broader socioeconomic context [1, 6, 9]. It is evident that education plays a pivotal role in shaping health outcomes, with higher educational attainment often correlating with improved health [2]. Moreover, education equips individuals with the skills necessary for digital literacy, enabling them to access and utilize technology for health-related purposes. Additionally, health and digital literacy can also be influenced by social determinants. Individuals from disadvantaged or underserved backgrounds may face barriers to accessing education and digital resources, perpetuating health inequalities [2, 6]. Bridging the gap in digital literacy can empower communities to harness technology for health improvement. Furthermore, reconnecting directly within communities is another way to lessen the digital divide [9–11].

Recognizing these scenarios highlights the need for comprehensive strategies that address social determinants, promote education, and enhance digital and health literacy. Such initiatives can help break down social barriers, reduce health disparities, and empower individuals to take charge of their health through informed decision-making and equitable access to healthcare resources. Ultimately, fostering a synergy between education, health, and digital literacy is a vital step toward achieving health equity and improving overall well-being for all.

References

1. McCall T, Asuzu K, Oladele CR, Leung TI, Wang KH. A socio-ecological approach to addressing digital redlining in the United States: a call to action for health equity. Front Digit Health. 2022;4:897250.
2. Nwokeji U, Spaulding EM, Shan R, Turkson-Ocran RA, Baptiste D, Koirala B, et al. Health information technology use among persons with self-reported atherosclerotic cardiovascular disease: analysis of the 2011-2018 National Health Interview Survey. J Med Internet Res. 2021;23(8):e23765.
3. Saeed SA, Masters RM. Disparities in health care and the digital divide. Curr Psychiatry Rep. 2021;23(9):61. https://doi.org/10.1007/s11920-021-01274-.
4. Smith S, Raskin S. Achieving health equity: examining telehealth in response to a pandemic. J Nurse Practitioners. 2020;17(2):214–7. https://doi.org/10.1016/j.nurpra.2020.10.001.
5. Pew Research Center. Internet/broadband fact sheet. 2019. https://www.pewresearch.org/internet/fact-sheet/internet-broadband/.
6. Zemlak JL, Wilson P, VanGraafeiland B, Rodney T. Telehealth and the psychiatric mental health nurse practitioner: beyond the COVID-19 pandemic. J Am Psychiatr Nurses Assoc. 2024;30(1):174–9. https://doi.org/10.1177/10783903211045119.
7. Bagchi A, Melamed B, Yeniyurt S, Holzemer W, Reyes D. Telemedicine delivery for urban seniors with low computer literacy: a pilot study citation. Online J Nurs Inform. 2018;22(2)
8. Connolly KK, Crosby ME. Examining e-health literacy and the digital divide in an underserved population in Hawai'i. Hawai'i J Med Public Health. 2014;73(2):44–8.
9. Gallegos-Rejas VM, Thomas EE, Kelly JT, Smith AC. A multi-stakeholder approach is needed to reduce the digital divide and encourage equitable access to telehealth. J Telemed Telecare. 2023;29(1):73–8. https://doi.org/10.1177/1357633X221107995.
10. Early J, Hernandez A. Digital disenfranchisement and COVID-19: broadband internet access as a social determinant of health. Health Promot Pract. 2021;22(5):605–10.
11. Fisher K, Magin P. The telehealth divide: health inequity during the COVID-19 pandemic. In Fam Pract. 2022;39:547–9. https://doi.org/10.1093/fampra/cmab173.

Diana Baptiste DNP, RN, FAAN, is an Associate Professor at the Johns Hopkins School of Nursing. She is a certified nurse educator whose teaching is grounded in cutting-edge, evidence-based instructional methods with a strong commitment to health equity in education, practice, and research. Her sustained scholarship focuses on cardiovascular health across the care continuum for underserved populations, grounded in responding to social justice issues influencing health outcomes.

Tamar Rodney PhD, RN, PMHNP-BC, CNE, FAAN, is an Assistant Professor at the Johns Hopkins School of Nursing. She is a board-certified psychiatric nurse practitioner who has worked in trauma and psychiatry. She is the track coordinator for the Psychiatric Mental Health Nurse Practitioner DNP and Certificate programs and maintains a clinical practice in Baltimore City serving families recovering from substance use. She has over 10 years of experience providing medication management and psychotherapy services to individuals with mental health needs. She continues to lead a strong program of research that includes identifying biomarkers for PTSD in individuals with a history of traumatic brain injury and addressing coping issues for students with mental health needs.

Ruth-Alma Turkson-Ocran PhD, MPH, APRN, FNP-BC, CNE, is a clinical investigator with the Division of General Medicine in the Research Section at Beth Israel Deaconess Medical Center and Harvard Medical School and a board-certified nurse practitioner. She is committed to ethical research that empowers underserved and marginalized populations. Her research interests are centered around social determinants of health, cardiometabolic and kidney disease, and wearable devices, particularly among persons of African descent.

Oluwabunmi Ogungbe DNP, FNP-BC, MPH, is an Assistant Professor at Johns Hopkins School of Nursing and Johns Hopkins Bloomberg School of Public Health. She is a cardiovascular epidemiologist dedicated to using her clinical, research, and public health expertise to implement several community-engaged interventions leveraging digital technologies to improve cardiovascular health. Dr. Ogungbe is an emerging leader in community-engaged research seeking to advance health equity, both locally in the USA and globally.

Yvonne Commodore-Mensah PhD, RN, FAAN, is a cardiovascular nurse epidemiologist whose current program of research seeks to reduce the burden of cardiovascular disease risk among Africans locally (United States) and globally (sub-Saharan Africa) through community-engaged research. Her research expertise includes immigrant health, global health, cardiovascular disease epidemiology, and social determinants of health.

A Community Partnership to Train Nursing Students as Advocates for Health and Social Justice among Marginalized Communities

Lalita Kaligotla, Heather Allstrom, Leah Bercovitch, and Guadalupe Castaneda

1 Introduction

Health disparities are differences among and between population groups affecting the attainment of optimal health. These disparities can be measured by differences in incidence, prevalence, mortality, burden of disease, and other adverse health conditions [1]. Disparities can exist across many dimensions, including race, gender, sexual orientation, age, disability status, socioeconomic status, and geographic location. According to Healthy People 2030, all of these factors shape an individual's ability to achieve optimal health [2]. Furthermore, existing evidence on health disparities reveals differential health outcomes across and within all of the identity groups mentioned above [3]. Health disparities can stem from health inequities—systematic differences in the health of groups and communities occupying unequal positions in society that are avoidable and unjust [4]. These disparities in health and access to healthcare translate to stark differences in life expectancy. In Atlanta, for instance, life expectancy can vary by as much as over a decade—dropping precipitously from 84 to 71 years in communities that are barely a few miles apart [5]. With regard to the health and well-being of children, child poverty is a persistent issue, and the poverty rate for children in Atlanta (24%) is well above state (20%) and national averages (17%). Lack of access to consistent and reliable healthcare among children is also a vexing problem in the city with the rate of uninsured children rising from 4% to 9% between the years 2019 and 2021 [6]. The status of women's health, particularly perinatal health, remains a concerning issue in the state, with maternal mortality rates that are amongst the worst in the nation, at 46.2 maternal deaths per 100,000 live births and are particularly alarming for Black mothers at 66.6 deaths per 100,000 live births [7].

In this context, Emory University and Emory Healthcare (EHC) have demonstrated a continuing commitment and passion toward serving the community. In order to provide medical care regardless of individuals' ability to pay, EHC provided more than $148 million in compassionate, cutting-edge care to the poor, underinsured, and uninsured. The three schools that comprise the Woodruff Health Sciences Center (WHSC) educate aspiring clinicians and scientists who go on to improve the health and lives of people in Atlanta, Georgia, and around the globe [8]. One of these schools, the Nell Hodgson Woodruff School of Nursing (NHWSN), is a global leader in nursing education with a strong commitment

L. Kaligotla (✉) · H. Allstrom · L. Bercovitch
G. Castaneda
Nell Hodgson Woodruff School of Nursing,
Emory University, Atlanta, GA, USA
e-mail: lalita.kaligotla@emory.edu;
heather.allstrom@emory.edu;
leah.bercovitch@emory.edu;
guadalupe.castaneda@emory.edu

© The Author(s), under exclusive license to Springer Nature Switzerland AG 2024
J. B. Hamilton, C. E. Moore (eds.), *Transforming Social Determinants to Promote Global Health*,
https://doi.org/10.1007/978-3-031-61160-5_5

to service and community engagement with students logging over 15,000 service-learning hours annually and serving over 7500 clients [9].

2   Fuld Fellowship for Social Responsibility

The Fuld Fellowship for Social Responsibility is one example of NHWSN's commitment to giving back to the broader community. This fellowship is awarded to outstanding future nurse leaders that have chosen nursing as a second career. As Fuld Fellows, these students are pursuing an educational track to first earn a Master of Science in Nursing and become credentialed as a registered nurse followed by graduate training as a nurse practitioner to earn an advanced practice graduate degree or a doctorate in nursing within a designated specialty area, such as family nurse practitioner, certified nurse midwife, or pediatric nurse practitioner. The fellowship program started in 2002 with a $5 million grant from the Helene Fuld Health Trust, the nation's largest private funder devoted exclusively to nursing education. Over the past two decades, this program has provided $8.1 million in tuition aid to 71 students.

The mission of Emory School of Nursing is to create visionary nurse leaders, and fulfilling social responsibility to local and global communities is a core value. Through this program, the School aims to build mutually beneficial partnerships with local organizations in support of healthy communities. Placing nursing students in community-based contexts expands students' capacities to understand the healthcare needs of underserved populations, aligns with the school's vision and core values, and builds on strategic national initiatives to create a culture of health across America. Students are selected based on their interests in community engagement and social responsibility, with the goal to enable them to play a broader role in providing healthcare to underserved populations.

This fellowship program enables students to provide service to our community while learning about the potential community impact through immersive engagement with local nonprofit organizations for approximately 12–18 months. As a culmination of their service activities, students work with a community partner on a project that is of strategic importance to the organization and is aligned with the students' professional aspirations, and interests.

3   Meet the Fuld Fellows

This article features the work of three Fuld Fellows for Social Responsibility doing community-based work to help address the heath care needs of three different groups of underserved populations in metro Atlanta.

Heather Allstrom works with Our House Health, a part of Our House, a community based organization serving families experiencing homelessness. The primary sites for this work are Restoration House and Our House.

Leah Bercovitch works with Strong4Life, which is an initiative of Children's Healthcare of Atlanta with the mission to help families raise healthy, safe, resilient kids by serving as wellness advocates in Metro Atlanta communities.

Guadalupe "Lupe" Castaneda works with the Latino Community Fund (LCF) Georgia, a Latino-serving and Latino-led nonprofit organization. In partnership with LCF Georgia, the NHWSN is engaged in providing health screening and health education to members of the Latinx community, particularly underserved members of the community through engagement and outreach.

The next sections provide an overview and descriptions of some of the impactful ways in which the Fuld Fellows are shaping the healthcare landscape in metro Atlanta and attempting to mitigate adverse impacts of social determinants of health.

4   Overview Community-Based Work Being Conducted by Fuld Fellows

4.1   Our House Health

Our House Health is part of Our House, an organization that serves the needs of families experiencing homelessness. Previously called Community Advanced Practice Nurses (CAPN), Inc. it was fully integrated with Our House and the name was changed to Our House Health. Our House's mission is to provide transformative care to end the cycle of homelessness for families. Our House achieves its mission through interrelated programs that address the root causes of homelessness and social determinants of health: housing, early childhood education, employment training, healthcare, and family advocacy. Our House cares for more than 4000 individuals and families every year and ensures every family served has the tools needed to achieve lasting self-sufficiency. Our House Health is a nurse practitioner led program that provides free low-barrier healthcare services to patients that are unhoused, uninsured, and low income. Our House's healthcare program was founded by Nurse Practitioners who believe that strengthening the lives of those who have been systematically excluded is essential to restoring communities. The organization has several clinics co-located at multiple shelters across Atlanta, where Nurse Practitioners provide compassionate whole person, family-centered care that is high quality, evidence based, and rooted in the Nursing model. Each clinic serves children and adults of all ages and specializes in preventive, reproductive, and mental health. The emphasis is on increasing access to care and remaining easily accessible for those who would otherwise not have received care. Thus, Our House Health functions as a transitional medical home that provides essential health services free of charge while working hard to transition clients to a trustworthy and compassionate permanent primary care medical home.

The population that Our House serves is amongst the most vulnerable in the city and faces a multitude of complex health disparities and social determinants of health [10]. Limited health literacy further compounds health inequities amongst this population. Therefore, and as identified by the Healthy People 2030 initiative, health communication is a crucial mechanism to mitigate these disparities [2].

Our House is an access to point to healthcare organization with compassionate and attentive nurse practitioners that use the nursing model to provide whole-person care that serves about 4000 families annually and is growing each year. Our House specializes in caring for families experiencing homelessness and compassionately meeting the needs of the entire family unit. When people think about those experiencing homelessness, they often envision adult individuals. However, families with young children are one of the largest populations that experience homelessness. Often, these families are sleeping in their cars, living in motels, or living at the largesse of friends and family members. According to Atlanta Mission there are about 10,000 unhoused people in Atlanta, with about 2000 people that sleep on the street every night [11]. Furthermore, Georgia has the third highest rate of uninsured individuals in the country at 13.7% [12]. Research shows that uninsured, unhoused, and/or low-income populations have lower rates of health literacy [13] and that "Patients who are unable to successfully interpret health information have increased hospitalization rates, develop more diseases, and experience higher mortality" ([13], p.51). In working alongside this population, it is vital to create tools that will increase their understanding of health, improve health outcomes, and increase their quality of life and life expectancy.

This work with Our House is guided by prior experience and informed by the literature. Therefore, the most appropriate tools to mitigate health inequities amongst this population are easily accessible health education brochures. The specific topics for the brochures were determined through a process of conversation and consensus with community members about their health-related concerns and questions. Through dissemination of up-to-date recommendations and evidence-based interventions from peer-reviewed literature to the community, the goal was to facilitate positive changes that will improve quality of life and health outcomes. However, given the alienation among healthcare professionals and vulnerable communities, it was imperative to first build trust.

Engaging clients and trusted nurse practitioners from the beginning stages of this project helped build this trust. Having conversations, listening, and making space for the client's voice to be an integral part of the decision-making process were all means to this end. By working with nurse practitioners and clients, and using evidence-based resources to gather information, this project resulted in the creation of health education brochures that the clients could use to improve their understanding of their health.

Health literacy is strongly associated with patients being able to engage in complex disease management and self-care. Patients who are unable to successfully interpret health information have increased hospitalization rates, develop more diseases, and experience higher mortality [13]. Through a process of conversation, consensus, trust, and relationship building, this project resulted in the development of evidence-based recommendations and translated them into digestible, health education brochures. Education about critical health topics increases health literacy amongst this underserved population and empowers them to have greater agency in advocating for themselves in the healthcare space [14].

This project served to bridge the gap between academic research and underserved communities, and in translating knowledge in an accessible manner. As healthcare professionals and those with the privilege of advanced academic training, we have an obligation to tailor interventions, and to disseminate the most up to date, evidence-based information to everyone in order to expand health equity and improve quality of life and health outcomes for all.

4.2   Strong4Life

The field of healthcare is increasingly recognizing the importance of integrating an understanding of social determinants of health into clinical care [15]. Social factors such as food and housing insecurity are well-documented contributors to poor health outcomes, and the risks of these factors can be mitigated through preventative screening in a primary care setting [16]. The American Academy of Pediatrics has endorsed primary care screening for risk factors within social determinants of health to provide a buffer against the epigenetic changes and behavioral challenges that toxic stress can create [17]. Screening for risk factors is effective to the extent that screening tools have proven specificity and sensitivity and that the screening is tied to specific interventions. Thus, although the need to integrate pediatric primary care screens has been almost unilaterally endorsed, it has proven challenging to implement screening tools that are accurate and seamlessly integrated with community services.

Strong4Life represents the preventative arm of Children's Healthcare of Atlanta (CHOA) with the mission to help families raise healthy, safe, resilient kids. Their approach addresses key influencers and environments where kids live, learn, and play with a goal of impacting healthy behaviors and creating thriving communities. Through projects such as promoting healthy habits in schools, and providing information about nutrition, coping skills, and emotional wellness, Strong4Life engages parents, healthcare providers, schools, early care and education centers, faith-based organizations, out of school time organizations, and community partners. They promote Stong4Life healthy habits and act as influencers among their pediatric care providers, patients, families, and communities. Strong4Life has had good positive momentum in impacting kids and families through programs and community partnerships designed to deliver consistent messages and support that bring about sustainable lifestyle change.

One of the social risk factors they have identified in the Atlanta area is food insecurity. In Fulton County, 16.4% of children are food insecure and rates are even higher in neighboring counties such as Clayton County, at 26.1%. As with all social issues, the issue of food insecurity cannot be tackled without acknowledging racial disparities. In Fulton County, the general rate of food insecurity among White Non-Hispanic individuals is 5%, whereas the rates among Hispanic and Black individuals are 14% and 20% respectively. Further complicating the issue, 34% of food-insecure children in Fulton County have a household income that renders them ineligible from receiving federal food assistance [18]. These statistics paint a picture of the problem that has driven Strong4Life to seek an effective system to integrate food insecurity screening and the provision of resources in the clinical pediatric setting.

This project started with a scoping literature review primarily looking at screening tools that are being used and published examples of pediatric clinics screening for food insecurity. One of the critical issues Strong4Life identified is that food insecurity screening tools are used to evaluate access to food without determining the quality of this food. The United States Department of Agriculture (USDA) is expanding on its long-standing efforts to combat food insecurity by taking action to address nutrition insecurity as well. The USDA defines nutrition insecurity as consistent access to safe and healthy food, and thus integrates a measure of diet quality, which a food insecurity screening tool may miss. This framework recognizes social determinants of health, as historically underserved populations are disproportionately impacted by diet-linked chronic diseases [19]. The Strong4Life project sought out examples of screening for nutrition insecurity in the literature as well as the use of standardized tools.

The literature review conducted revealed that the standardized tool most often used for identifying food insecurity is referred to as "the Hunger Vital Sign," and includes two questions that ask parents whether they have been worried about food running out or have run out of food in the past 12 months [20]. However, there is no consensus in the literature on how to best screen for nutrition insecurity [21], which is consistent with the relative recency of this concept. The absence of a universal nutrition insecurity screening tool presents an equity issue, as lack of access to

nutrient-dense foods is a structural barrier that contributes to disparities in chronic disease.

Published quality improvement projects examining food insecurity screening in pediatric clinics vastly outnumber those piloting nutrition insecurity screening. These projects and the research surveying pediatric providers on food insecurity, reveal consistent barriers to screening. Barriers on the provider side include uncertainty around handling a positive screen, discomfort in discussing food insecurity, and a lack of time [22, 23]. Caregivers may be reluctant to engage in conversations about food insecurity with providers due to fear of stigmatization, fear of negative repercussions following a positive screen, and the perception that food insecurity is not a medical issue [22].

Several pediatric clinics have successfully integrated food insecurity screening into their practice, such as the Kaiser clinic in Oakland, which uses the Hunger Vital Sign and also screens for other social determinants of health [24]. Other successful programs have been implemented at a pediatric cardiology clinic in Pittsburgh [25] and a pediatric nephrology clinic in Seattle [26]. As with screening, similar barriers to implementation were identified across studies. It was difficult for providers to integrate documentation of food insecurity into electronic medical records and families were often lost to follow-up after a positive screen. One clinic at the University of California, San Diego addressed the issue of follow-up by allowing same day onsite enrollment into Supplemental Assistance Nutrition Program (SNAP) benefits [27].

As food and nutrition are deeply intertwined with identity and culture, any successful nutrition intervention must engage the community it is serving in order to be successful. The next stage of this project involves reaching out to stakeholders in the Metro Atlanta community such as pediatric providers and caregivers to better assess the state of food and nutrition insecurity in the area. Using a socially conscious approach, this outreach addresses questions about the type of food caregivers feed their children and if the diet they provide their children is influenced by factors such as cost and access. This information will guide the creation of a nutrition screening tool, which will then be implemented throughout local pediatric clinics. The difficulties involved with following up on a positive screen are well documented in the research. Therefore, it is vital to address this prophylactically by building partnerships with organizations such as community food banks and gardens, who already have established relationships with Atlanta families. The information obtained from the Strong4Life project thus far has revealed the urgency of expanding food insecurity screening practices. As previously described, food insecurity impacts under-resourced populations, and disproportionately people of color, in Atlanta. Nutrition insecurity has only recently received attention as a factor that contributes to disparities in chronic disease and a standardized way of assessing this dimension has not yet been created. A successful intervention to combat nutrition insecurity will use community resources to construct a screening tool, and the findings of previous quality improvement projects to implement this tool. By integrating the community and an interdisciplinary team of healthcare providers that are invested in the intersection of nutrition with social determinants of health, Strong4Life aims to expand the scope and quality of equitable healthcare among children in Atlanta.

4.3   Latino Community Fund

Founded in 2017, the nonprofit LCF Georgia is run largely by people of Latinx descent. The organization's primary mission is strengthening the Latinx communities' rights, knowledge, education, and access to opportunities across three pillars—expanding economic opportunity, fostering community, and enhancing democratic capacity [28]. The Latinx community in Georgia encounters many obstacles to receiving high-quality healthcare, despite the state's diverse demographics.

With an estimated 54 million people making up 17% of the population, Latinos are one of the major minority groups in the United States [29]. The Latino American association projects that

the Hispanic population will roughly double from its current level of about 50 million to nearly 106 million in 2050 [30]. Georgia is one of the top ten states with the largest Hispanic populations, with approximately one million Latinos making up 9% of the state's total population, and with an increase of over 96% from 2000 to 2010. Over half of the state's Latinos (500,000) live in Cobb, Dekalb, Fulton, and Gwinnett counties, and make up 11% of the total population of metro Atlanta [30].

The Latino population makes numerous and significant contributions to the United States in a variety of areas, including the workforce participation, economic development, and being part of the entrepreneurship ecosystem. However, in comparison to their White counterparts, Latinos have higher rates of poverty, food insecurity, obesity, and the prevalence of serious chronic diseases such high blood pressure, cholesterol, and diabetes. For the underserved, undocumented, and low-income populations, many of whom are Hispanic, it is essential that they have access to quality, affordable healthcare. However, for many Hispanics trying to get healthcare services, financial factors continue to be a major obstacle [31].

LCF of Georgia engages in advocacy and outreach initiatives such as community health fairs and educational workshops to raise awareness about health issues affecting the Latinx community. The organization partners with Emory University's NHWSN and other healthcare providers to offer on-site cholesterol, blood pressure, and diabetes screenings. Building the bridge between the gap in healthcare access caused by financial hurdles and healthcare illiteracy is one of the primary initiatives led by the NHWSN student.

A key priority for collaboration between NHWSN and LCF is to build a database that lists all the available community services in the area. Among these community options are low-cost to free general or specialized health screenings, finding rental homes, assistance with utilities, emergency shelter, transportation services, and food access. There is continual involvement and follow through with community members from their initial screening to the recommendation and the follow-up to ensure that they seek healthcare services or treatment they need. NHWSN students in collaboration with LCF Georgia seek to empower the Latinx community by supplying crucial knowledge about the services that are accessible in healthcare and assisting them in successfully navigating the healthcare system through targeted campaigns, neighborhood activities, and educational workshops.

This work has a transformational effect on the student(s) and in their commitment to increase access to healthcare for the Latinx community through the engagement with the LCF of Georgia. The partnership between NHWSN and the LCF of Georgia is an ongoing and multipronged initiative with multiple collaborations with student and faculty involvement.

involving them in decision-making processes helps establish trust and ensures long-term success. Culturally and linguistically appropriate engagement, along with an asset-based approach, are also important for successful collaborations.

Communication: Open communication, humility, and coordination with those closest to the issues are vital—those most proximal to the issues being tackled are often best equipped to identify solutions. Students are encouraged to communicate frequently with community members for information sharing, feedback, and ongoing support. This fosters learning opportunities for students and helps build reciprocal networks between academic health centers, civil society organizations, and community members effected by the issues being addressed.

5 Best Practices in Community Engagement: Building Collaborations, Community, and Continuity

Building sustainable and mutually beneficial relationships with communities is crucial for addressing social determinants of health (SDOH). Collaborative relationships have the potential to foster meaningful partnerships, improve health outcomes, and promote health equity for underserved communities. In the interest of sharing best practices, we present below a few lessons we have drawn in working on these projects and in building relationships with community partners to tackle critical health challenges in metro Atlanta.

Shared Vision: Aligning with the vision and aspirations of communities is essential. Students working on these projects found success by learning from community members and partner organizations to find common purpose. Understanding the needs of the communities they serve and the differential impacts of SDOH contributes to seeking sustainable change.

Building Trust: Building trust and mutual understanding is crucial. Active and respectful engagement with community members, listening to their needs and perspectives with empathy, and

6 Looking Ahead

In summary, building collaborations, community, and continuity is crucial to addressing SDOH in community contexts. Best practices include building trust, finding shared vision, and maintaining open communication. By incorporating these practices, organizations and institutions can work towards achieving health equity and improving well-being for all.

Looking ahead, partnerships and projects like those described herein have the potential to demonstrate institutional commitment to the community. Through open dialog and by incorporating evidence-based approaches, and a justice-oriented focus, we believe that this work transforms students' experiences. In so doing, and paraphrasing the words of the Rev. Martin Luther King Jr., we also hope that it contributes to bending the arc of the moral universe closer to greater justice and good health for all [32].

References

1. National Institutes of Health. Health disparities 2014. 2016. https://www.nhlbi.nih.gov/health/educational/healthdisp/.
2. Office of Disease Prevention and Health Promotion. Health communication. Healthy People 2030.

U.S. Department of Health and Human Services. https://health.gov/healthypeople/objectives-and-data/browse-objectives/health-communication

3. Weinstein JN, Geller A, Negussie Y, Baciu A. The state of health disparities in the U.S. In: Weinstein JN, Geller A, Negussie Y, Baciu A, editors. Communities in action: pathways to health equity. National Academies Press; 2017. https://www.ncbi.nlm.nih.gov/books/NBK425844/.

4. Graham H. Social determinants and their unequal distribution: clarifying policy understandings. Milbank Q. 2004;82(1):101–24. https://doi.org/10.1111/j.0887-378X.2004.00303.x.

5. Lawler K, Fuller E, Wilson M, Henry E, Minyard K. Reducing health disparities in Atlanta. Stanf Soc Innov Rev. 2016;14(2):A22–3. https://doi.org/10.48558/Z5MQ-KK32.

6. Anne E. Casey Foundation. A profile of youth and young adults in Atlanta. 2023. https://www.aecf.org/blog/a-profile-of-youth-and-young-adults-in-atlanta.

7. Armstrong-Mensah E, Dada D, Bowers A, Muhammad A, Nnoli C. Geographic, health care access, racial discrimination, and socioeconomic determinants of maternal mortality in Georgia, United States. Int J MCH AIDS. 2021;10(2):278–86. https://doi.org/10.21106/ijma.524.

8. Nolan M. Woodruff Health Sciences Center Community Benefits Report: Improving Lives and Providing Hope. Emory News Center. 2023. https://news.emory.edu/stories/2023/06/hs_community_benefits_report_07-06-2023/story.html.

9. Emory Nursing. Atlanta based service learning. https://www.nursing.emory.edu/pages/atlanta-based-service-learning.

10. Our House. Our house health: healthcare programs. 2023. https://ourhousega.org/capn-clinics/

11. Atlanta Mission. The hidden homeless: what you're not seeing in the statistics. 2023. https://atlantamission.org/the-hidden-homeless-what-youre-not-seeing-in-the-statistics/.

12. Harker L. Fast facts on medicaid expansion. Georgia Budget and Policy Institute. 2020. https://gbpi.org/fast-facts-on-medicaid-expansion/.

13. Hickey KT, Masterson Creber RM, Reading M, Sciacca RR, Riga TC, Frulla AP, Casida JM. Low health literacy: implications for managing cardiac patients in practice. Nurse Pract. 2018;43(8):49–55. https://doi.org/10.1097/01.NPR.0000541468.54290.49. PMID: 30028773; PMCID: PMC6391993

14. Odoh C, Vidrine JI, Businelle MS, Kendzor DE, Agrawal P, Reitzel LR. Health literacy and self-rated health among homeless adults. Health Behav Res. 2019;2(4):13. https://doi.org/10.4148/2572-1836.1055.

15. Sandhu S, Sharma A, Cholera R, Bettger J. Integrated health and social care in the United States: a decade of policy progress. Int J Integr Care. 2021;21(4):9. https://doi.org/10.5334/ijic.5687.

16. Massar RE, Berry CA, Paul MM. Social needs screening and referral in pediatric primary care clinics: a multiple case study. BMC Health Serv Res. 2022;22(1):1369. https://doi.org/10.1186/s12913-022-08692-x.

17. Gitterman BA, Flanagan PJ, Cotton WH, Dilley KJ, Duffee JH, Green AE, Nelson JL. Poverty and child health in the United States. Pediatrics. 2016;137(4):e20160339. https://doi.org/10.1542/peds.2016-0339.

18. Feeding America Research Team. Map the meal gap data. United States of America. 2021. https://foundationfar.org/impact/insights/geographic-variation-in-food-insecurity-in-the-united-states-findings-from-feeding-americas-map-the-meal-gap/?gclid=Cj0KCQjwnMWkB-hDLARIsAHBOfto9pryRS3SiEBU-ajo6ikTA80fM_E9Ips2P6g54EHJUxJh4QLIPhbEaAkMOEALw_wcB.

19. United States Department of Agriculture. USDA announces actions on nutrition security. United States Department of Agriculture. 2022. Retrieved June 18, 2023, from https://www.usda.gov/media/press-releases/2022/03/17/usda-announces-actions-nutrition-security.

20. Hager ER, Quigg AM, Black MM, Coleman SM, Heeren T, Rose-Jacobs R, Cook J, Ettinger de Cuba S, Casey P, Chilton M, Cutts D, Meyers A, Frank DA. Development and validity of a 2-item screen to identify families at risk for food insecurity. Pediatrics. 2010;126(1):e26. https://doi.org/10.1542/peds.2009-3146.

21. Becker PJ, Bellini SG, Vega MW, Corkins MR, Spear BA, Spoede E, Hoy M, Piemonte T, Rozga M. Validity and reliability of pediatric nutrition screening tools for hospital, outpatient, and community settings: a 2018 evidence analysis center systematic review. J Acad Nutr Diet. 2020;120(2):288–318. https://doi.org/10.1016/j.jand.2019.06.257.

22. Barnidge E, Labarge G, Krupsky K, Arthur J. Screening for food insecurity in pediatric clinical settings: opportunities and barriers. J Community Health. 2017;42(1):51–7. https://doi.org/10.1007/s10900-016-0229-z.

23. Hoisington AT, Braverman MT, Hargunani DE, Adams EJ, Alto CL. Health care providers' attention to food insecurity in households with children. Prev Med. 2012;55(3):9–22. https://doi.org/10.1016/j.ypmed.2012.06.007. Epub 2012 Jun 16

24. Fort V, Weintraub MR, Conell C, Dandekar A, Hayes E. Food insecurity screening in a pediatric clinic: findings on documentation and multidimensional care needs. Perm J. 2022;26(4):62–8. https://doi.org/10.7812/TPP/21.198.

25. Black AK, Pantalone J, Marrone AC, Morell E, Telles R, DeBrunner M. Identifying food insecurity in cardiology clinic and connecting families to resources. Pediatrics. 2022;149(5) https://doi.org/10.1542/peds.2020-011718.

26. Starr MC, Fisher K, Thompson K, Thurber-Smith K, Hingorani S. A pilot investigation of food inse-

curity among children seen in an outpatient pediatric nephrology clinic. Prev Med Rep. 2018;10:113–6. https://doi.org/10.1016/j.pmedr.2018.02.019.

27. Smith S, Malinak D, Chang J, Perez M, Perez S, Settlecowski E, Rodriggs T, Hsu M, Abrew A, Aedo S. Implementation of a food insecurity screening and referral program in student-run free clinics in San Diego, California. Prev Med Rep. 2017;5:134–9. https://doi.org/10.1016/j.pmedr.2016.12.007.

28. Latino Community Fund Inc. About. 2023. https://lcfgeorgia.org/about/.

29. United States Census Bureau. Quick Facts: DeKalb County, Georgia; Georgia. 2023. https://www.census.gov/quickfacts/fact/table/dekalbcountygeorgia,GA,US/RHI225221.

30. Camilo M. About the Latino population in USA: the LAA. Latin American Association. 2021. https://the-laa.org/latino-population/#:~:text=Georgia%20is%20home%20to%20nearly,with%20the%20largest%20Hispanic%20populations.

31. Pérez-Escamilla R. Health care access among Latinos: implications for social and health care reforms. J Hisp High Educ. 2009;9(1):43–60. https://doi.org/10.1177/1538192709349917.

32. King MLK Jr. 1929–1968. A testament of hope: the essential writings of Martin Luther King, Jr. Harper. 1991.

Lalita Kaligotla PhD, is Professor of the Practice and Senior Director for Leadership and Community Engagement at Emory University's Nell Hodgson Woodruff School of Nursing. Her work is centered on values-based leadership, social innovation, human-centered design, and community-based research. She currently envisions and implements leadership development programming for faculty, staff, and students as well as experiential, and interprofessional, experiences for students. She has a keen interest in addressing inequities in access to healthcare and health outcomes. She also serves as the faculty director for the Fuld Fellowship for Social Responsibility, a scholarship program designed to support high achieving nursing students with a strong commitment to civic engagement and social responsibility.

Heather Allstrom MN, RN, is a 2024 Doctor of Nursing Practice candidate at Emory University, studying to become a women's health and gender-related nurse practitioner. She received her Master of Nursing, also from Emory, is a Sigma Alpha Epsilon inductee and a Fuld Service-Learning Fellow. She completed her undergraduate training at the University of Connecticut earning a Bachelor of Science in Molecular and Cellular Biology and a Bachelor of Arts in Human Development and Family Sciences in 2020. As a Fuld Service-Learning Fellow, Heather volunteers with Our House Health working on health literacy initiatives for low-income and unhoused clients of the organization.

Leah Bercovitch is a hematology/oncology nurse at Children's Healthcare of Atlanta. She is also a Fuld Fellow and pediatric primary care doctoral student at the Emory University School of Nursing.

Guadalupe Castaneda is a dedicated Registered Nurse who earned her Master of Nursing from Emory University in August 2023. She previously completed her Bachelor's in microbiology with a minor in chemistry at San Jose State University in 2021. Guadalupe is a published researcher with an article on the CRISPR/Cas9 system's efficiency in Science Direct. She currently serves as a Fuld Fellow, focusing on community outreach in the Latinx community with the Latino Community Fund of Georgia. Additionally, she is an active member of the National Association of Hispanic Nurses, working to promote healthcare equity and diversity.

The Blueprint to STEM Mentorship for Inner City Youth

Brittany Prince

People of color are inadequately represented in the United States Health Care System. Health disparities exist in part due to a lack of representation in healthcare fields. Emory School of Medicine's Health Careers Collaborative (HCC) mentorship program addresses health inequities by exposing high school students from inner city, underserved, low-socioeconomic status, minority communities to health topics and mentorship within the health professions.

Inner city youth face unique challenges due to socioeconomic and environmental factors. An inner city is defined as a highly populated city that is frequently deteriorating and inhabited mainly by poor, often minority groups of people [1]. Being an inner-city kid provides advantages but has disadvantages as well. Advantages include exposure to different cultures, lifestyles, and beliefs on a daily basis. Being part of a densely populated community allows youth to become more social and gain life skills at a very young age, learning to adjust to a complex environment where rural kids may struggle [2]. Children living in the inner city are exposed to a variety of food options. They often are confident and not afraid to try new things [2].

Disadvantages of living in the inner city include higher rates of poverty, crime, violence, and inequities in education. High poverty rates create financial insecurity, forcing youth to prioritize short-term survival over the creation of long-term goals. Children living in the inner city experience higher crime rates. Their safety is questioned on a daily basis, leading to increased stress levels [3]. This can affect their mental health and intensify trauma levels. Schools in the inner cities may have inadequate educational resources due to a lack of funding [3]. The result is a negative impact on academic performance. Poor-performing schools can lead to socioeconomic disparities.

Another challenge for inner city youth is limited role models in the community who are accomplished professionally or academically. A lack of role models can impede a child's ambition and restrict their insight into existing opportunities. Mentorship programs are essential in addressing disparities and improving opportunities. Mentoring is a way to create an atmosphere that develops youth regardless of their background [4].

1 STEM Mentorship Among High School Students

There is significant data supporting the long-term benefits of providing STEM mentorship programs for high school students in Title 1 schools. A study conducted by the National

B. Prince (✉)
Urban Health Initiative, Emory University,
Atlanta, GA, USA
e-mail: brittany.prince@emory.edu

© The Author(s), under exclusive license to Springer Nature Switzerland AG 2024
J. B. Hamilton, C. E. Moore (eds.), *Transforming Social Determinants to Promote Global Health*,
https://doi.org/10.1007/978-3-031-61160-5_6

Science Foundation found that students who participate in STEM mentoring programs are more likely to pursue STEM majors and careers than those who do not. Another study published in the Journal of STEM Education: Innovations and Research found that mentoring can help high school students develop STEM-related skills, such as problem-solving and critical thinking [5]. Problem-solving and critical thinking are essential in examining situations successfully.

The American Society for Engineering Education has reported that mentoring can be particularly beneficial for underrepresented groups in STEM, including students from low-income backgrounds. A report from the National Academies of Sciences, Engineering, and Medicine emphasizes the importance of providing STEM opportunities to students from diverse backgrounds, including those in Title 1 schools, in order to address the underrepresentation of certain groups in STEM fields [6].

Emory's High School STEM program, the Health Career Collaborative (HCC), is a rewarding and innovative association between high school students and teaching partners in health and medicine, public health, and other allied health fields. The HCC advances the possibilities of further studies and careers in medicine and allied health sciences for underrepresented, low-income high school students. The program centers on inspiration, cultivating a feeling of real potential, and awakening a sense of vision and purpose in students' educational journeys. It is an opportunity to build meaningful relationships between a cohort of high school students at an early stage in their development and a team of dedicated older students and healthcare professionals immersed in delivering medical care and health services [7].

HCC is staffed by faculty members from the Emory University School of Medicine and the Emory Urban Health Initiative who help shape the curriculum and facilitate the discussions around health care. The program relies on volunteers who are either healthcare practitioners or students from Emory University Schools of Medicine, Nursing, and Public Health, as well as Registered Dietitians from Open Hand Atlanta.

The Health Career Collaborative program consists of four overarching goals [7]:

1. Engage students in project-based learning focusing on science and healthcare-related issues.
2. Encourage students to graduate from high school (current graduation rates at partner high schools 50–60%).
3. Model a diverse range of health-related career pathways.
4. Empower students to identify the most pressing health needs in their community and engage students in community-based health promotion activities.

2 Emory Urban Health Initiative and Health Career Collaborative

Under the Emory Urban Health Initiative, faculty and students from Emory University School of Medicine launched the Health Career Collaborative (formerly known as the Health Careers Academy) program during the 2016–2017 school year with four area high schools: Benjamin E. Mays High School, Redan High School, Maynard Jackson High School, and Clarkston High School. At that time, Mays High School student enrollment was 1244; the graduation rate was 78%; 98% of enrolled students were Black or African American; 97% were eligible for free lunch; and 3% were eligible for reduced lunch. Mays High School ranks in the bottom 50% of all schools in Georgia for overall test scores, including math and reading proficiency [8]. The demographics of the other schools are similar: all are predominantly minorities, with high percentages of African Americans, and all are Title 1 schools with high levels of free/reduced lunch eligibility. Clarkston High School is unique due to being part of the City of Clarkston, the most diverse city in the nation, which has a very high refugee population and more than 50% of residents born outside the United States. 90% of Clarkston High School students are Asian or African American [8]. Partnering with these area high schools was consistent with HCC's program mission to provide mentorship, engaging health curriculum, and exposure to health careers to high school students from low-income, underrepresented minority communities [7].

Initial steps in the development of the program consisted of recruitment of mentors in the fall semester of the academic year. Potential mentors for the program were required to fill out a mentorship application to be considered. Individuals had to pass a background check, be in good standing with an academic institution, and major or work in a STEM-related field. Once selected, mentors were required to attend a mentor orientation to discuss roles, responsibilities, dress code, and proper etiquette with students. Email is the only acceptable form of communication a mentor can have with a student, with zero tolerance for sharing social media with students. The responsibilities of a mentor were the following:

- Committing to 1.5 h/week from February to April.
- Serving as a role model.
- Teaching medical/health case studies.
- Helping students create community-based health projects.
- Guiding students through the many health career opportunities available to them.

HCC strategically identified mentors with similar ethnic and geographic backgrounds. Mentors were recruited from student minority organizations and HBCUs. Our guest speakers for program sessions also typically reflected the background of our students.

3 Exemplars of Student Experiences/Curriculum

Once our first cohort of mentors were identified and recruited, HCC worked with the partner high schools to promote the program. Students partici-

pated in an intuitive surgical robot experience in the fall. Engineers from underrepresented groups donated equipment worth over $20,000 for the day. HCC provided a 30-min presentation followed by a 20-min hands-on demo. Not only did our partner teachers participate, but also the experience was opened to other science teachers at the schools.

Aside from the robot event to create engagement and interest before the initial launch of the program, the curriculum has remained fairly consistent over the years. The program kick-off is typically held 2–3 weeks before the mentors enter the schools. Students are invited to the host (Emory) University for approximately 3 h. Students are given an overview of the program and expectations. Students interact with various students from other schools and participate in health competitions. Students have the opportunity to participate in field trips throughout the program. All of the field trips are held at Emory University. The field trips include the kick-off event, medical lab, and our final event.

Grade 10 Curriculum. The tenth-grade program is a 12-session project-based learning curriculum that brings hospital and medical student volunteers into the high school's health classroom. The curriculum focuses on the following Hospital Emergency Room cases: open fracture, kidney stone, gunshot wound, peanut allergy, concussion, and pneumonia. Each lesson has suggested research goals [9].

Grade 11 Curriculum. The 11th-grade curriculum concentrates on public health issues: trauma and violence prevention, nutrition, diabetes, obesity, HIV, STIs, hypertension, and heart disease. Each session also includes a hands-on activity [10]. For the final project, students are encouraged to create an informative video highlighting prevention connected to adolescents.

Grade 12 Curriculum. The 12th-grade curriculum collaborates with health organizations to host a student health fair. Students learn how to establish community partnerships. The project aims to inspire the students to become advocates and Changemakers of health [11].

Final Project. Students are encouraged to create a final project similar to the 11th-grade final project, but with broader methods of expression. Students pick a public health topic associated with their age range to research and present. Instead of only having the option of creating a video, students can get as creative as they want. In the past, students have made songs, spoken words, plays, and PowerPoint presentations. Healthcare professionals serve as guest judges and provide feedback to the students.

3.1 Scheduling Format

We tried two different scheduling formats to deliver the HCC curriculum. The first approach paired HCC mentors with a high school science teacher to teach the Health Careers Collaborative curriculum during their allotted time period with the students. The teacher selected the class based on the grade levels and curriculum. We worked with chemistry, biology, and sport medicine courses.

The second approach was running the program for students as an after-school program. Both programs operated for 1-h sessions each week. Both approaches had positives and negatives.

4 Successes and Challenges

Running the program during the school day had a higher attendance rate. Students were automatically assigned to the Health Career Collaborative if they were enrolled in a particular class taught by our partner teacher. Our ability to garner the support of the principal and school board was essential for using classroom time for the program and field trip approvals.

Transportation was a major challenge to having the program after school. Because the students did not have access to bus transportation, attendance was low, and students could not attend sessions consistently. However, having the program after school allowed every student the opportunity to participate regardless of their class schedule.

5 Program Adaptations Due to COVID

The COVID Pandemic created unanticipated challenges requiring a shift from in person to virtual classes similar to that occurring in the rest of the world. Mentors transitioned from in person format to the platform Zoom for their weekly sessions. We utilized platform polls capabilities to engage students and to answer questions in real time during the sessions. To enhance continued participation in the program, students attending sessions were automatically entered into a drawing to win an Amazon gift card. Pear deck, flipgrid, jamboard, and google forms were engagement tools used to increase session involvement. Icebreakers were also used as a form of check-in. However, creativity was limited to utilization of PowerPoints for discussions of public health topics for their final reports.

While the pandemic created some challenges, it created opportunities to expand the program. During the pandemic, the program offered free virtual tutoring programs for all our students provided by college students using the zoom platform. This idea to incorporate college students came as the result of disruptions in classroom education due to the infectious nature of COVID-19 and potential for negative outcomes on state test scores. During the initial phases of this expansion, we met with teachers to identify the subjects for which students would need the most assistance. We then proceeded to recruit college students based on their tutoring skills. Mentors were recruited from Emory University, Morehouse College, Spelman College, Clark Atlanta University and Georgia Tech. The positions as college mentors were advertised on student listserves, social media outlets, and professional group chats. Once student and mentors were matched, tutoring sessions were held once a week for 1 h via Zoom. Breakout rooms in Zoom were created for individuals that required focused one-on-one attention. Typically, 2–3 mentors were assigned to each tutoring session with 3–5 students.

6 Challenges and Opportunities

In addition to the challenges imposed by the COVID Pandemic, other challenges to the programs included our ability to access funding. Due to limited funds from our partner schools, Health Careers Collaborative had to cover all expenses. We were responsible for paying for field trips, memberships for health organizations, food for events, staff time, and giveaways. Grants to Emory Urban Health Initiative made this support possible.

Despite funding challenges, Health Career Collaborative had the opportunity to support other STEM programs. For example, we were able to work with Health Occupations Students of America (HOSA) program. The mission of HOSA is to empower HOSA-Future Health Professionals to become leaders in the global health community through education, collaboration, and experience [12]. HOSA promotes careers in health and is recognized by the Department of Health and Human Services, the U.S. Department of Education, and other federal and state agencies. Created in 1974, HOSA is a global organization that provides intense training related to healthcare. Through this collaboration, we assisted students with their HOSA competition projects and sponsored membership and conference dues to compete in the HOSA competition at the state level. The competitive category events include health science, health professions, emergency preparedness, leadership, and teamwork. There are a total of 67 competitive events and 14 academic testing events [12]. Our staff and mentors also served as guest judges on district and state levels for the events.

7 Reflection

Since 2016, 10 cohorts of students have progressed through Emory School of Medicine's Health Care Collaborative program. We have had a 100% retention rate and very positive student evaluations. Additionally, the majority of our students have enrolled in higher education programs including PWI's, HBCU's, and technical schools. The HCC program has recently received grant funding from Health Resources and Services Administration (HRSA), United Healthcare, and Jesse Parker Williams Foundation. This will allow us to expand the program to more schools in inner city areas across Metro-Atlanta. We also will be able to provide additional field trips and more hands-on activities.

References

1. Dictionary.com. Inner city. In Dictionary.com dictionary. Retrieved November 15, 2023, from https://www.dictionary.com/browse/inner-city.
2. BKK Kids. The pros and cons of raising kids in a big city. 2022. Retrieved November 15, 2023 from https://www.bkkkids.com/blog/the-pros-cons-of-raising-kids-in-a-big-city/.
3. Johnson MR. Educational inequality in inner city schools: challenges and solutions. Urban Educ. 2019;25(2):167–83.
4. Mark A. The pros and cons of living inner city. Baltimore Post-Examiner. 2019. Retrieved November 16, 2023 from https://baltimorepostexaminer.com/the-pros-and-cons-of-living-inner-city/2019/08/13.
5. Bullough RV, Gitonga LM. Mentoring high school students in STEM: a longitudinal study. J STEM Educ. 2017;18(1):17–25.
6. National Academies of Sciences, Engineering, and Medicine. Minority serving institutions: America's underutilized resource for strengthening the STEM workforce. The National Academies Press. 2018. https://doi.org/10.17226/25257
7. Health Career Collaborative. Mission. 2019. Retrieved November 15, 2023 from https://healthcareercollaborative.com/mission/.
8. Public School Review. Benjamin E. Mays High School. Retrieved November 15, 2023 from https://www.publicschoolreview.com/benjamin-e-mays-high-school-profile.
9. Health Career Collaborative. 10th grade—A hands-on introduction. 2015. Retrieved November 15, 2023, from https://healthcareercollaborative.com/for-teaching-partners/10th-grade-program-title/.
10. Health Career Collaborative. 11th grade—Deepening understanding of health science. Retrieved November 16, 2023 from https://healthcareercollaborative.com/for-teaching-partners/11th-grade-program-title/.
11. Health Career Collaborative. 12th grade—Community health. 2016. Retrieved November 15, 2023 from https://healthcareercollaborative.com/for-teaching-partners/12th-grade-program-title/.

12. Hosa Inc. Future health professionals. About HOSA. 2021. https://hosa.org/about-hosa.

Brittany Prince received a BS from the University of South Carolina in Public Health and a Master of Health Administration from Clayton State University. Brittany, currently enrolled at Georgia Southern University, is pursuing a Doctorate in Public Health. Brittany is the Assistant Director at Emory University Urban Health Initiative and an Engagement Manager for Georgia Memory Net. She is the CEO and Founder of a nonprofit, WellStart Initiatives, and CEO of Brittany Monea Consulting Firm.

SDOH Influences on Chronic Stress: The Physiological Cost That Increases Risk of Heart Disease in Early Midlife African American Women

Telisa Spikes

As a former nursing manager of an advanced heart failure transplant/cardiovascular stepdown unit, exposure to many different patient populations with an array of chronic conditions was nothing new. Hypertension seemed to be the most common diagnosis shared by all patients, regardless of if they were young or old. Unbeknownst to me, I was about to experience and bear witness to a dire clinical situation that would set the trajectory for the research that I would be conducting in early midlife African American women. On this particular morning of our weekly heart failure-transplant multidisciplinary team meeting, there was a 29-year-old African American woman that had been admitted with a diagnosis of advanced heart failure due to peripartum cardiomyopathy. In a nutshell, the discussion went something like this, "Ms. Morrison[a] is a 29 y/o African American woman admitted with a diagnosis of advanced heart failure, current ejection fraction (EF) is 10%, and the patient is not a candidate for a heart transplant or a left ventricular assist device (LVAD)." To provide some context, an ejection fraction or EF, is an estimate of how well the heart is pumping blood with each contraction. A normal EF ranges between 50–75% [1]. The left ventricular assist device (LVAD) is a mechanical pump that is surgically inserted into the heart and assists the left ventricle in pumping blood throughout the entire body's circulatory system. Recommendation for this supportive therapy is reserved for those who have an extremely weak heart that is not responding to guideline-based pharmacological therapies, and when sudden cardiac death is imminent. Typically, patients that receive the LVAD fall within three categories, those with end-stage heart failure who may not be a candidate for heart transplantation, those that require what is known as bridge-to-transplant therapy, or bridge-to-recovery [2].

The initial reaction after hearing the clinical case of the 29-year-old Ms. Morrison was shock, followed by a moment of silence, then an internal sadness. The question now became, "how did this young woman get to this point?" The heart failure transplant team informed both the patient and her mother that there were no additional medical therapies that could be done to improve her heart condition and given the severity of her heart failure, their subsequent recommendations now involved end-of-life care planning for the coordination of hospice care. Then came the most grueling part of the conversation to which the patient's mother asked, "so what does this mean for my daughter?" and the heart failure physician responds, "your daughter may have at most, 4–6 weeks left to live, and the next steps would be hospice care where she will be kept comfortable". The room fell completely silent for what

T. Spikes (✉)
Nell Hodgson Woodruff School of Nursing,
Emory University, Atlanta, GA, USA
e-mail: tspikes@emory.edu

seemed like 10 min, then the mom looked at her daughter and said firmly, "do not receive what they are telling you, only God knows when your time is up." Ms. Morrison remained quiet, stoic in her appearance, and when asked if she had any additional questions, she responded softly, "no". After the heart failure team left the room, I learned the patient had four small children, with the youngest nearly a month-old, and no local familial support as her mother resided in another state.

Unfortunately, she was not the last young African American woman that was admitted with a diagnosis of heart failure. In fact, there was a slight influx of African American women between the ages of 30–35 years old that had been admitted with a new diagnoses of heart failure. Fortunately, most of the cases were not as severe as this 29-year-old if there was a silver lining to be found in the midst of these circumstances. However, the one common denominator these women shared was a diagnosis of hypertension. In order to understand why Black women have the highest burden of hypertension relative to other racial/ethnic groups in the United States, one must first understand the role that social determinants of health (SDOH) has on fostering disparate health conditions. SDOH are those conditions in which people are born, grow, live, work, and age and includes socioeconomic status, neighborhood and physical environment, education access and quality, food, community and social context, healthcare access, and racism [3]. Based on this definition, it is clear to understand why social conditions are considered the fundamental cause of disease since health outcomes do not occur independent of the social conditions which people live [4]. Past health research had mostly centered around the role of nonmodifiable (age, sex, race) and modifiable (health behaviors and weight) attributes of health; however, a significant limitation of this research scope failed to incorporate elements of the social environment or consider how they might potentially influence health and health outcomes [5]. As Dr. Donald Berwick was quoted, "No scientific doubt exists that, mostly circumstances outside of health care nurture or impair health. Except for a few clinical preventive

services, most hospitals and physician offices are repair shops, trying to correct the damage of causes collectively denoted social determinants of health" [6]. In view of this perspective, we now know that genetics accounts for a small proportion as it relates to who gets a disease and why, but rather one's social environment can determine if certain genes are expressed or suppressed [7], thus impacting the likelihood of developing a given disease(s). We also know that race is not a biological attribute, but rather socially constructed categories created to designate class, status, and power that have a significant impact on the lives of individuals by their perception and in turn how other's perceive them [8, 9]. We now know that many of the chronic comorbid conditions such as heart disease, diabetes, and certain types of cancers begin to clinically manifest in Black women as young as 20–30 years old [10], while many of these same conditions do not appear in White women until they are much older [11]. Additionally, African American populations begin to show signs of premature biological aging, the speed at which the biological systems age relative to their chronological age, much earlier than White populations which tend to demonstrate biological aging patterns that are consistent with their chronological age [11, 12]. These aging patterns are especially insightful as they are implicated in the premature onset for the development of most prevalent chronic diseases including hypertension and heart disease, which disproportionately impact African American women [13].

1 Health Equity and Systemic Racism's Influence on Black Women's Lives

The attainment of health equity is met with systemic racism, which has a robust influence on all dimensions of SDOH resulting in vast structural inequities that exist both internal and external to the healthcare system. Income inequality and the pay gap continue to remain significant burdens that impact the economic well-being and quality of life for African American women. African American women earn $0.64 for every dollar earned by a White male, while Asian and White women earn $0.80 and $0.73, respectively [14]. African American women are more likely to be the sole head-of-household income earners, which results in assuming more financial obligations with fewer financial resources. Of all racial groups, African American women are the most likely to be impacted by student loan debt. After completing a Bachelor's degree, African American women average an estimated $41,466 in debt contrast to the $33,851 or 22% less owed among White women [15]. Additionally, the historical impact of residential redlining, defined as the outlining of areas of maps where African American populations resided and were used to determine a neighborhoods' risk level based on property values and home ownership [16], has also severely impacted the attainment of wealth for African American families compared to White populations. In a recent analysis conducted by my colleagues and I, we investigated the impact of net worth and blood pressure phenotypes and found that African American women that reported a negative net worth, defined as debts greater than assets, had higher 48-h daytime and nighttime blood pressure levels and sustained hypertension [17]. The lack of wealth accumulation has also had a considerable impact on residential neighborhood contextual factors including poor or no access to health-promoting activities and resources (walkable communities, sidewalks, access to healthy foods), residence in moderate to high crime areas regardless of socioeconomic status, and reduced access to high quality medical care. These residential mediators have been linked to cardiovascular disease-related risk factors of obesity, hypertension, poor diet, diabetes, poor sleep, and undiagnosed sleep disorders [18]. Lastly, within the healthcare system, racial and gender bias among African American women such as being ignored and not heard has been linked to delays in diagnosis, and adverse health outcomes especially relating to Black women's maternal health [19]. These are just some of the examples, though not exhaustive, in which SDOH influences the quality of life and well-being of Black women.

2 SDOH and Persistent Physiological Stress and CVD in Black Women

The overall social context or lived experience of African American women that is associated with hardship and struggle is linked to constant, continuous, and long-lasting stressors. Based on societal norms, if one works hard, follow the rules, and live responsibly, then attainment of the American dream is possible for all regardless of your race or class status; however, the error with this perspective neglects to factor in the effects of systemic and institutional racism that produces societal inequities that does not benefit everyone equally. An often cited yet powerful quote from the late Fannie Lou Hamer's speech in 1964 where she states, *"For three hundred years, we've given them time. And I've been tired so long, now I am sick and tired of being sick and tired, and we want a change. We want a change in this society in America because, you see, we can no longer ignore the facts and getting our children to sing, Oh say can you see, by the dawn's early light, what so proudly we hailed"* [20], is a sentiment that African Americans still consider relevant in the present day society and demonstrates the hypocrisy and inequities in American society. Voting rights, effects of the law, income inequality, educational policy, and the financial/banking industry are all sectors through which social conditions operate to affect health.

Until recently, the role of psychosocial stress as a risk factor for hypertension and heart disease among African American women was underappreciated and considered less explicit of a risk factor relative to widely established tangible cardiovascular-related risk factors of obesity, hypertension, and health-behaviors [21]. Although stress is a universal phenomenon that affects all groups and classes of people, voluminous research suggests that differential exposure to certain stressors, individual differences in the magnitude of stressor-evoked physiological reactions, and vulnerability to those stressors are what distinguishes who becomes susceptible to illness [22]. Briefly, stressors fall within two broad categories, acute or chronic, with the former lasting a period of minutes to weeks and the latter persisting for hours per day for weeks, months, or years. Acute stressors are associated with an immunoprotective response that are health-promoting such as healing of a wound and heightened immune response to combat infections, while chronic stressors are associated with maladaptive responses that are associated with pathological changes due to overactivation of the physiological immune response [23]. The connection between chronic stress and CVD is highly complex and is believed to be the result of chronic and sustained activation of numerous biological systems that results in inflammation. To further complicate this process, chronic stress is also associated with the promotion of health-risk behaviors including smoking, consumption of high caloric foods, and alcohol use that are often deployed as coping mechanisms, further heightens inflammation, thereby magnifying CVD risk. Notably, these risk factors still do not fully account for the association between stress and CVD indicating that mechanisms beyond these health-risk behaviors, such as the social environment, may have an important role in the stress–health paradox, thus increasing vulnerability to adverse health outcomes.

To better understand how chronic stress induces CVD risk and CVD, key physiological mechanisms and processes must be understood. Imagine going on a walk and seeing a rattlesnake, the hypothalamus or the control center of the brain undergoes an adaptive response of protection which promotes active engagement of the sympathetic nervous system. Both the innate and adaptive immune responses become active causing the release of proinflammatory cytokines, which prepare the body to destroy and dispose of pathogens if attacked, and the release of various catecholamines, including epinephrine and nor-epinephrine, promotes vasoconstriction and peripheral vascular resistance [24]. These catecholamines cause an increase in blood pressure and heart rate allowing for successful escape from the threat. Additionally, the endocrine system also becomes engaged activating the hypothalamus pituitary (HPA) axis that involves the pituitary and adrenal glands. The HPA axis is responsible for the synthesis and release of corticotropin-releasing factor (CRF) and vasopressin [25]. CRF causes the anterior pituitary gland to release adrenocorticotropic hormone (ACTH) which signals the adrenal cortex to release cortisol which is also known as the stress hormone. The simultaneous production of glucocorticoids that are responsible for metabolic, anti-inflammatory, immune-suppression, and neurologic effects are also released [26]. Upregulation of glucocorticoid receptors, which are responsible for reducing the HPA activation via negative feedback mechanisms are also increased. Successful activation of this system is contingent upon the negative feedback mechanisms at the glucocorticoid receptor sites, thus inhibiting the release of pro-inflammatory cytokines to achieve allostasis [24]. But what happens when this system does not recede and the negative feedback mechanism no longer functions adequately as in the case with African American women that constantly live in a heightened stated of vigilance secondary to chronic stress? The overexposure to stress hormones over a prolonged period is associated with increased levels of systemic inflammation. The glucocorticoid negative feedback HPA axis is postulated to become diminished resulting in stress-induced epigenetic modifications causing dysregulation of this feedback mechanism, overactivation of the immune system, and a hyperinflammatory physiological state [27]. These stress-induced changes have been associated with major depressive disorder, malignancies involving the bone marrow and white blood cells, allergies, lupus, sleep disorders, and cardiovascular disease [24]. The heightened stress-response has also been related to maladaptive behavioral responses including adiposity, excessive eating, and decreased physical activity [24, 25]. Hyperactivity of the immune system in the presence of chronic stressors combined with cardiovascular risk factors are thought to exert a detrimental effect on the cardiovascular system via chronic low-grade inflammation resulting in impaired vascular function. Systemic low-grade chronic inflammation is closely related to many cardiovascular risk factors including hypertension, impaired arterial elasticity, arteriosclerosis, and atherosclerosis [28]. Evidence suggest hypertension is the result of stiff arteries and consequently, linked to the development of heart failure [29]. When the heart is pumping against increased resistance due to stiffer arteries over time, this will ultimately cause the heart to enlarge, which in turns affects the efficacy of its pumping ability by decreasing coronary and systemic perfusion thus culminating in adverse cardiovascular events of heart attack, stroke, heart failure, and even death. Regarding the young African American women that were admitted with heart failure, knowledge of their social lives and whether they were navigating various chronic stressors and, if so, how they were managing those stressors remains unknown, yet highlights the critical need to further understand the role that socio-contextual factors may have contributed to their diagnosis.

3   Next Steps for the development of multilevel Interventions

Academic clinicians and health researchers are poised to make substantial contributions to the health of populations that are disproportionately impacted by health disparities. The COVID-19 pandemic revealed the stark health inequities of African American populations as well as the unequal effects of the social landscape specifically among African American and Hispanic populations in the United States. Despite the inherent challenges of addressing the SDOH, these cannot and should not be a reason to circumvent how they interact to determine the health and well-being of populations. The knowledge to be gained in understanding how these factors impact health may offer insight that can be used for the guidance of multilevel strategies to develop and inform interventions that includes the individual, the community, and health/public policy sectors. Now that we better understand interconnectedness of the social and health context, it is important that we begin to move beyond individual level interventions broadening the

scope to include community as well as policy interventions. Research suggest that downstream interventions which primarily focuses on change at the individual level, may in fact increase health inequities as opposed to upstream interventions which focus on social and policy change [29].

Given the various mechanisms in which chronic stress is associated with the development of heart disease and the mounting evidence indicating the disproportionate burden of socially derived stressors (i.e., race, gender, economic, social networks) [30] that are linked to the excess physiological wear and tear of African American women [31, 32] very few studies have been conducted to investigate these connections in younger African American women. These stressors are also considered to have a greater impact on cardiovascular health than traditional CVD-related risk factors of obesity, and may override the biological protectiveness from heart disease that is unique to women [33]. To understand and disentangle these relationships, we will test multiple hypothesis to investigate the contributing role that chronic stress has on biological and vascular aging in early midlife Black women, 30–44 years old. Further, we will examine the independent and combined effects of these stressors to determine if or which are most harmful for health and whether psychosocial resources of resilience, which are suggested to mitigate vulnerability to environmental risk experiences [34], are in fact health promoting or deleterious to health. When positive psychosocial resources are deployed to successfully cope and manage external threats, the risk for adverse outcomes are postulated to diminish [35]; however, when constantly exposed to chronic stressors, this normal and dynamic process is suggested to enhance as opposed to buffer the negative effects of stress [36]. Although the social context of African American women is often characterized by hardship and struggle, many do succeed and overcome these social adversities to achieve optimal health and well-being.

Recognizing the strengths of African American women, my research team and I will incorporate a mixed methodology approach to understand why women who are exposed to very similar social contexts have better health outcomes than those who do not. These findings will be informative in formulating strategies to develop tailored and targeted interventions for testing earlier in the life course, a critical period before the development of hypertension and other chronic conditions.

4 Reflection

Socially derived stressors have a profound impact on the overall health and well-being of African American women. There is a growing urgency to incorporate appropriate health equity frameworks to investigate the many complexities that influence the health of African American women. Additionally, it is imperative that clinicians consider the roles of SDOH and incorporate these factors into care models that extend beyond the walls of healthcare facilities. Although African American women have made significant strides in society ranging from political achievements to educational attainment, this group continues to lag as it relates to indices of health. If we are serious about improving the health and well-being of all populations, then the attainment of health equity for African American women must be of heightened priority if we are to narrow the health disparities encountered by this subgroup of women.

References

1. Kosaraju A, Goyal A, Grigorova Y, Makaryus AN. StatPearls. Left Ventricular Ejection Fraction. 2023. https://www.ncbi.nlm.nih.gov/books/NBK459131/.
2. Vaidya Y, Riaz S, Dhamoon AS. StatPearls [Internet]. Left Ventricular Assist Devices. 2022. https://www.ncbi.nlm.nih.gov/books/NBK499841/.
3. U.S. Department of Health and Human Services. Social determinants of health. Washington, DC. 2022. https://health.gov/healthypeople/priority-areas/social-determinants-health.
4. Phelan J, Link B, Diez-Roux A, Kawachi I, Levin B. Fundamental causes of social inequalities in mortality: a test of the theory. J Health Soc Behav. 2004;45(September):265–85.
5. Geronimus A. Weathering the extraordinary stress of ordinary life in an unjust society. New York, NY: Little Brown Spark; 2023.
6. Berwick DM. The moral determinants of health. JAMA. 2020;324:225–6. https://doi.org/10.1001/jama.2020.11129.
7. Reiss D, Leve LD, Neiderhiser JM. How genes and the social environment moderate each other. Am J Public Health. 2013;103 Suppl 1(Suppl 1):S111–21. https://doi.org/10.2105/ajph.2013.301408.
8. Cole ER, Omari SR. Race, class and the dilemmas of upward mobility for African Americans. J Soc Issues. 2003;59:785–802. https://doi.org/10.1046/j.0022-4537.2003.00090.x.
9. Weinstein JN, Geller A, Negussie Y, Baciu A. Communities in action: pathways to health equity. In: National Academies of Sciences, Engineering, and Medicine; Health and Medicine Division; Board on Population Health and Public Health Practice; Committee on Community-Based Solutions to Promote Health Equity in the United States, editor. The State of Health Disparities in the United States. Washington, DC: National Academies Press (US); 2017. p. 58–9.
10. Chinn JJ, Martin IK, Redmond N. Health equity among black women in the United States. J Women's Health. 2021;30(2):212–9. https://doi.org/10.1089/jwh.2020.8868.
11. Geronimus AT, Hicken MT, Keene D, Bound J. "Weathering" and age patterns of allostatic load scores among blacks and whites in the United States. Am J Public Health. 2006;96(5):826–33.
12. Levine ME, Crimmins E. Evidence of accelerated aging among African Americans and its implications for mortality. Soc Sci Med. 2014;118(1):27–32. https://doi.org/10.1016/j.socscimed.2014.07.022.
13. Simons RL, Lei M-K, Klopack E, Zhang Y, Gibbons FX, Beach SRH. Racial discrimination, inflammation, and chronic illness among African American women at midlife: support for the weathering perspective. J Racial Ethnic Health Disparities. 2021;8(2):339–49. https://doi.org/10.1007/s40615-020-00786-8.
14. Carrazana C, Mithani J. Happy Equal Pay Day? Here are 6 charts showing why it's not much of a celebration. In: The 19th. 2023.
15. AAUW. Deeper in debt 2021 update [Press release]. 2021. https://www.aauw.org/app/uploads/2021/05/Deeper_In_Debt_2021.pdf
16. Rothstein R. The color of law: a forgotten history of how our government segregated America. New York, NY: Liveright Publishing Corporation; 2017.
17. Spikes T, Murden R, McKinnon II, Bromfield SG, Van Dyke ME, Moore RH, et al. Association of net worth and ambulatory blood pressure in early middle-aged African American women. JAMA Netw Open. 2022;5(2):1–13. https://doi.org/10.1001/jamanetworkopen.2022.0331.

18. Kershaw KN, Roux A, Burgard S, Lisabeth L, Mujahid M, Schulz A. Metropolitan-level racial segregation and black-white disparities in hypertension. Am J Epidemiol. 2011;174(5):537–45. https://doi.org/10.1093/aje/kwr116.

19. Chambers BD, Taylor B, Nelson T, Harrison J, Bell A, O'Leary A, et al. Clinicians' perspectives on racism and black women's maternal health. Womens Health Rep (New Rochelle). 2022;3(1):476–82. https://doi.org/10.1089/whr.2021.0148.

20. Hamer FL. Speeches of Fannie Lou Hamer, to tell it like it is. 1964. https://awpc.cattcenter.iastate.edu/2019/08/09/im-sick-and-tired-of-being-sick-and-tired-dec-20-1964/.

21. Albert M. Ignored in plain sight giving a voice to the weight of stress on cardiovascular disease risk in black women. Circ Cardiovasc Qual Outcomes. 2019;12(4):1–3.

22. Sternthal M, Slopen N, Williams DR. Racial disparities in health: how much does stress really matter? Du Bois Rev. 2011;8(1):95–113. https://doi.org/10.1017/S1742058X11000087.

23. Dhabhar FS. Enhancing versus suppressive effects of stress on immune function: implications for immunoprotection and immunopathology. Neuroimmunomodulation. 2009;16:300–17. https://doi.org/10.1159/000216188.

24. Ravi M, Miller AH, Michopoulos V. The immunology of stress and the impact of inflammation on the brain and behavior. BJPsych Adv. 2021;27(Suppl 3):158–65. https://doi.org/10.1192/bja.2020.82.

25. Osborne MT, Shin LM, Mehta NN, Pitman RK, Fayad ZA, Tawakol A. Distentagling the links between psychosocial stress and cardiovascular disease. Circulation. 2020;13(8):1–13. https://doi.org/10.1161/CIRCIMAGING.120.010931.

26. Chourpiliadis C, Aeddula NR. Physiology, glucocorticoids. In: StatPearls content is king. Treasure Island, FL: StatPearls Publishing; 2022.

27. Baumer Y, Pita MA, Baez AS, Ortiz-Whittingham LR, Cintron MA, Rose RR, et al. By what molecular mechanisms do social determinants impact cardiometabolic risk? Clin Sci. 2023;137:469–94. https://doi.org/10.1042/CS20220304.

28. Mozos I, Malainer C, Horbanczuk J, Gug C, Stoian D, Luca CT, Atanasov AG. Inflammatory markers for arterial stiffness in cardiovascular diseases. Front Immunol. 2017;8:1–16. https://doi.org/10.3389/fimmu.2017.01058.

29. Mitchell GF. Arterial stiffness and hypertension: chicken or egg? Hypertension. 2014;64(2):210–4. https://doi.org/10.1161/HYPERTENSIONAHA.114.03449.

30. Keith VM, Brown DR. African American women and mental Well-being: the triangulation of race, gender, and socioeconomic status from part II-the social context of mental health and illness. In: Scheid TL, Brown TN, editors. A handbook for the study of mental health. 2nd ed. Cambridge University Press; 2012. p. 291–305.

31. Geronimus A, Hicken MT, Pearson J, Seashols S, Brown K, Cruz T. Do US black women experience stress-related accelerated biological aging? Hum Nat. 2010;21(1):19–38. https://doi.org/10.1007/s12110-010-9078-0.

32. Simons RL, Lei MK, Beach SR, Philibert RA, Cutrona CE, Gibbons FX, Barr A. Economic hardship and biological weathering: the epigenetics of aging in a U.S. sample of black women. Soc Sci Med. 2016;150:192–200. https://doi.org/10.1016/j.socscimed.2015.12.001.

33. Vaughan AS, Quick H, Schieb LJ, Kramer MR, Taylor HA, Casper M. Changing rate orders of race-gender heart disease death rates: an exploration of county-level race-gender disparities. SSM-Popul Health. 2019;7:1–9. https://doi.org/10.1016/j.ssmph.2018.100334.

34. Tugade MM, Fredrickson BL, Barrett LF. Psychological resilience and positive emotional granularity: examining the benefits of positive emotions on coping and health. J Pers. 2004;72(6):1161–90. https://doi.org/10.1111/j.1467-6494.2004.00294.x.

35. Pearlin LI. The stress process revisited reflections on concepts and their interrelationships. In: Aneshensel CS, Phelan JC, editors. Handbook of the sociology mental health; 1999. p. 395–415.

36. Trudel-Fitzgerald C, Ouellet-Morin I. The cost of resilience: how allostatic load may jeopardize health through repeated demands for (successful) adaptation. Psychoneuroendocrinology. 2022;144:105874. https://doi.org/10.1016/j.psyneuen.2022.105874.

Telisa Spikes PhD, RN, is an Assistant Professor at the Nell Hodgson Woodruff School of Nursing at Emory University. Spikes' research interest focuses on the chronic stressors derived from the social environment and the impact of their embodiment related to accelerated biological aging and cardiovascular disease risk in early midlife adult African American women ages 30–44 years old, a group that has seen a dramatic increase in cardiovascular disease (CVD) morbidity and stagnating declines in CVD mortality. She has publications related to psychosocial stressors, hypertension medication adherence, and blood pressure reactivity in Black women and socioeconomic status and arterial stiffness in Black adults using both community-based and large epidemiological cohorts, with publications in high-impact clinical journals. Dr. Spikes has received funding from National Institute of Nursing Research (NINR), Sigma Theta Tau, National Heart, Lung, Blood, Institute, and is currently funded by

NINR. Dr. Spikes holds a Bachelor of Science in Nursing from Mercer University Georgia Baptist College of Nursing, Masters of Science in Nursing, and a PhD in Nursing Science from Emory University Nell Hodgson Woodruff School of Nursing. She completed a postdoctoral fellowship focused on research methodologies to eliminate cardiovascular health inequalities in vulnerable populations at the Rollins School of Public Health in the division of cardiovascular/social epidemiology at Emory University.

Disparities in Sociodemographic Factors of the Mother on Inequalities of Birth Outcomes in Low- and Middle-Income Countries

Hana Abera Hailemariam

Sociodemographic disparities have a profound impact on health outcomes worldwide. These disparities are particularly evident in low- and middle-income countries (LMICs) where resource limitations and social inequalities intersect [1]. Among the various health indicators, birth outcome stands as a critical measure of infant health and development. However, in LMICs, sociodemographic factors contribute significantly to disparities in birth outcomes, resulting in a disproportionate burden on disadvantaged populations [2]. LMICs encompass a diverse range of countries with varying levels of economic development, healthcare infrastructure, and sociocultural contexts. Within these settings, sociodemographic factors such as maternal education, income, maternal age occupation, and access to healthcare services exert substantial influence on birth outcomes [3–5]. Disparities in birth outcome can manifest in varies forms: The infant's adverse outcomes include preterm birth, low birth weight (LBW), death, congenital infections/anomalies, still birth and macrosomia [6–8].

H. A. Hailemariam (✉)
College of Health Science, Addis Ababa University, Addis Ababa, Ethiopia

Saint Pauls Millenium Hospital Medical College, Addis Ababa, Ethiopia
e-mail: hanna.abera@sphmmc.edu.et

1 Sociodemographic Factors that Influence Birth Outcomes

Maternal Education and Birth Outcomes. Maternal education, specifically, has been recognized as the key factor influencing birth outcomes that operates through a number of channels, including information accessibility, healthcare utilization, nutrition, and health-related behaviors. A study conducted in different developing countries showed that lower odds of poor birth outcome, such as LBW, are also seen among mothers with higher education levels outcomes compared to women with only a primary or secondary education [9–12]. A separate study conducted in Ethiopia revealed that infants born to mothers who had attended primary, secondary, and higher education experienced a 57%, 70%, and 55% reduction in the odds of small birth weight, when compared to infants born to mothers with lower levels of education [13].

Income and Birth Outcomes: Research conducted in developing countries highlights that infants born to lower-income mothers and ethnic minority groups often face disparities in birth outcomes. In countries like India, mothers from lower socioeconomic backgrounds frequently encounter poor birth outcomes. These disparities among women in LMICs are primarily attributed to restricted access to healthcare services due to inadequate sanitation, limited medical facilities, and a lack of modern amenities [3]. A study conducted in Pakistan revealed that mothers who were not compensated in cash for their work had a 1.41-fold higher likelihood of giving birth to LBW infants compared to those who received cash payments [11]. Studies from India corroborated the evidence that the economic status of mothers' families plays a role in birth outcomes. Specifically, mothers from the poorest wealth index had 1.11 times higher odds of giving birth to VLBW infants when compared to mothers from the wealthier wealth quintiles [14]. Furthermore, women belonging to the richest wealth quintiles had a 23% lower likelihood of experiencing birth weight inequalities when compared to those in the poorest category [15]. An Ethiopian study further reinforced the notion that mothers experiencing income inequalities often contend with inadequate sanitation, restricted access to medical facilities, and a lack of modern amenities. Notably, women with lower wealth, no access to toilet facilities, residing in rural areas, and using unprotected well water were significantly associated with a higher risk of perinatal death [16].

Maternal Age and Birth Outcomes: A mother's age significantly influences the likelihood of adverse outcomes during pregnancy, whether it's a very young or advanced age. When pregnancies are compared to those at the average childbearing age, we typically observe higher rates of low birth weight (LBW), preterm birth, and mortality. A study conducted in India and Korea further emphasized this connection, indicating that mothers aged 13–19 and those older than 35 had increased odds of VLBW compared to mothers at the average childbearing age [14, 17]. Ethiopian studies also provide compelling evidence, indicating that teenage pregnancies carry a 2.22-fold higher risk of low birth weight and a 2.87-fold higher risk of premature deliveries when compared to pregnancies in adults. Moreover, women aged over 35 years are independently associated with adverse perinatal outcomes, including newborn death and stillbirth [4, 18].

Maternal Occupation and Birth Outcomes: Maternal occupation encompasses a wide range of job roles and work environments, each with its unique challenges and potential impacts on pregnancy and childbirth. It is essential to consider various aspects, such as the physical demands of the job, workplace stressors, potential environmental exposures, access to prenatal care, and socioeconomic factors associated with occupational status. A systematic review conducted in sub-Saharan Africa showed maternal employment highly associated with preterm birth, LBW, and still birth [19]. Furthermore research from Ethiopia indicated that women whose partners were unemployed or engaged in agricultural occupations had a 1.54 times higher risk of giving birth to infants with low birth weight compared to those whose partners held formal jobs [13].

Access to Healthcare Services and Birth Outcomes: Access to healthcare services is a critical factor influencing birth outcomes, particularly in developing countries. Numerous studies have investigated the barriers that hinder healthcare access in these regions. A systematic review centered on sub-Saharan Africa revealed that women in this region face challenges stemming from both the demand and supply sides of healthcare access. On the demand side, obstacles include limited household resources, transportation limitations, indirect transportation expenses, and inadequate knowledge about healthcare services, social stigma, issues related to self-esteem, lack of birth preparedness, cultural beliefs, and a lack of awareness about essential obstetric healthcare services. Meanwhile, on the supply side, challenges encompass limited transportation choices, considerable distances to healthcare facilities, and financial constraints, all contributing to poor access to the healthcare services, which leads to adverse perinatal outcome [20]. Ethiopian studies have shown that insufficient access to services, such as the absence of dietary counseling, not utilizing family planning methods, having inter-pregnancy intervals of less than 24 months, and having hemoglobin levels below 11 g/dL had 11.24, 4.06, 5.21, and 4.86 times, respectively, higher risk of adverse birth outcomes [21]. Another Ethiopian study supported and revealed that inadequate ANC services significantly associated with the birth inequalities compared to mothers with adequate ANC [22].

The implications of sociodemographic disparities on birth outcomes in LMICs are significant. Adverse birth outcomes increase the risk of mortality, as well as short- and long-term health complications, such as stunted growth, developmental delays, and chronic diseases [23, 24]. These adverse birth outcomes not only impact individuals and families but also strain healthcare systems and perpetuate cycles of poverty and inequality.

In order to develop culturally relevant health inequities and sociodemographic disparities in birth weight outcomes within LMICs, it is essential to understand the multifaceted factors contributing to these disparities. Efforts to combat these disparities require tailored interventions that take into account the unique challenges and resources available within each LMIC. This includes improving access to quality prenatal care, enhancing maternal health education, and addressing the underlying social determinants of health. By focusing on these areas, we can work towards reducing sociodemographic disparities and improving birth outcomes for all mothers and children in LMICs [25].

Understanding the complex interplay between socioeconomic factors, healthcare systems, and cultural contexts is crucial for policymakers and healthcare providers in developing targeted interventions that promote equitable birth outcomes and improve maternal and child health in LMICs. By addressing sociodemographic disparities and working towards the achievement of sustainable development goals, we can ensure healthier futures for infants and their families in these countries.

2 Strategies to Address Sociodemographic Disparities in LMICs

Tackling the problem of sociodemographic disparities on birth outcomes in LMICs requires comprehensive strategies. This approach should encompass a strategy that includes enhancing healthcare access, advancing education, reducing socioeconomic inequalities, improving maternal support, enhancing access to high-quality prenatal care, bolstering maternal health education, and tackling the root causes of social determinants of health. The implementation of interventions targeting these factors is crucial for mitigating disparities and enhancing birth outcomes in LMICs. Addressing sociodemographic disparities in birth outcomes not only promotes health equity but also identifies vulnerable populations, guides public health interventions, supports prevention and early intervention efforts, and informs policy development. By proactively addressing these disparities, we can work towards achieving healthier birth outcomes and enhancing overall maternal and child health.

3 Community Resources to Reduce Disparities in Birth Outcomes

In LMICs where there are sociodemographic disparities in birth outcomes, several community resources may be available to address these disparities. The availability and accessibility of these resources can vary depending on the specific community and the local context. These resources include (1) primary healthcare facilities (prenatal care programs, maternal and child health services), (2) trained community health workers, (3) health education and counseling programs, (4) social welfare programs and nongovernmental organizations (NGOs), (5) maternal support groups and collaboration with traditional birth attendants (TBAs), (6) research institutions and data collection agencies, and (7) *government policies and programs.*

Primary healthcare facilities offer prenatal care programs and maternal and child health services to pregnant individuals. Prenatal care programs include regular check-ups, screenings, and interventions to monitor and address potential risks during pregnancy. The programs help to identify and manage health issues that may lead to adverse birth outcomes. Maternal and child health services provide vaccinations, nutritional support, postpartum care, and counseling on breastfeeding and infant care.

The programs offered through healthcare facilities address disparities by providing equitable access to healthcare services, regardless of residence, ethnicity, or social background. They offer culturally sensitive care and address the unique needs of different communities to reduce disparities and improve birth outcomes. The healthcare facilities also collaborate with community organizations and educational institutions to promote health education and literacy, providing information on reproductive health, prenatal care, and healthy behaviors during pregnancy. By improving health literacy and socioeconomic opportunities, they help individuals make informed decisions and access necessary healthcare resources, thus reducing birth outcome inequalities. Additionally, healthcare facilities recognize and respect cultural practices and beliefs, providing culturally competent care that incorporates evidence-based practices. By understanding and accommodating cultural practices, they foster trust and engagement within communities, leading to improved birth outcomes.

Trained community health workers (CHWs) are actively involved in delivering comprehensive maternal and child healthcare services. They provide a range of healthcare services including prenatal education, home visits, and assistance during deliveries, and postnatal support. CHWs also offer nutritional support programs, ensuring that pregnant women and new mothers have access to balanced diets, essential nutrients, and necessary supplements like iron and folic acid. They play a crucial role in educating and empowering pregnant individuals and families, promoting healthy behaviors, and improving birth outcomes. They are in the forefront of providing education, support, and advocacy, making a significant impact in maternal and child healthcare.

CHWs serve as a vital bridge between healthcare facilities and the community, providing outreach, education, and advocacy on various health topics including prenatal care and maternal and child health. Through home visits, community meetings, and workshops, they disseminate culturally appropriate information, address misconceptions, and promote healthy

behaviors, improving health literacy and empowering individuals to make informed decisions about their pregnancy and childbirth. CHWs also navigate complex healthcare systems, assisting with appointment scheduling, transportation, and insurance enrollment, while addressing barriers related to access and socioeconomic status to ensure individuals receive timely and appropriate prenatal care. Through collaborations with healthcare providers and community organizations, CHWs facilitate referrals and coordinate care, ensuring that pregnant individuals have access to necessary services, screenings, and interventions, ultimately reducing disparities in healthcare access, education, and socioeconomic status, and improving birth outcomes.

Health education and counseling programs in LMICs are powerful tools for reducing the disparities in birth outcomes. They empower women through the provision of knowledge, the promotion of healthier living, the consideration of cultural factors, and the enhancement of healthcare accessibility. These programs strive to heighten awareness, mitigate risk factors, advocate for timely prenatal care, enhance maternal well-being during pregnancy, and engage with local communities. By furnishing expectant mothers and their families with valuable insights into proper prenatal care and the importance of skilled birth assistance, these endeavors equip women to make informed choices and actively safeguard their own health and that of their infants.

Social welfare programs and nongovernmental organizations (NGOs) provide financial aid and health insurance to vulnerable populations, improving pregnant women's access to essential healthcare. NGOs actively engage in health education and counseling, promoting awareness about prenatal care, nutrition, and healthy pregnancy behaviors. Their strong community outreach, culturally sensitive approach, and respect for local customs ensure that healthcare disparities are minimized. These organizations invest in healthcare infrastructure development, including facilities, medications, and healthcare worker training. Additionally, NGOs advocate for policies prioritizing maternal and infant health, shaping effective healthcare policies and resource allocation to reduce sociodemographic disparities effectively.

Maternal support groups and collaboration with traditional birth attendants (TBAs) are among the resources aimed to improve outcomes and enhance care for pregnant women by providing emotional support, health education, and promoting positive health-seeking behaviors. Maternal support groups provide a platform for pregnant individuals and new mothers to come together, share experiences, and receive support from their peers. These groups often have a strong focus on education, providing information on prenatal care, nutrition, breastfeeding, and child development. By equipping women with knowledge and empowering them to make informed decisions, maternal support groups help bridge the gap in access to healthcare and education. Collaboration with TBAs, who are trusted and respected members of the community, is another valuable strategy. TBAs have deep cultural knowledge and experience in providing childbirth assistance. By partnering with TBAs, healthcare providers can work together to ensure safe and culturally appropriate care for pregnant individuals. TBAs can be trained to recognize danger signs during pregnancy and delivery, refer individuals to healthcare facilities, and support postnatal care.

Collectively, these collaborative efforts help address sociodemographic factors such as language barriers, cultural practices, and mistrust of the healthcare system. By integrating traditional practices with evidence-based care, maternal support groups and collaboration with TBAs improve access to healthcare services and promote positive birth outcomes. Additionally, these initiatives often focus on disadvantaged communities, providing resources and support to individuals with lower socioeconomic status and limited access to healthcare.

Research institutions and data collection agencies are responsible for the dissemination of information and knowledge. Researchers in these institutions publish research findings, reports, and guidelines that inform healthcare providers, policymakers, and communities about effective strategies to reduce birth outcome inequalities. This knowledge dissemination helps in raising awareness, shaping policies, and guiding interventions at various levels.

Research institutions conduct studies and gather data on factors like race, ethnicity, income, education, and healthcare access to understand the causes of birth outcome disparities. This information helps identify areas with higher rates of adverse outcomes and allows for targeted interventions. Data collection agencies monitor and evaluate the effectiveness of interventions and policies, using data on birth outcomes and related factors. This helps identify areas or communities in need of additional resources or interventions to improve birth outcomes. Collaborations with healthcare providers and policymakers are designed to develop evidence-based interventions and policies.

Government policies and programs ensure equitable access to healthcare services, promote health education, address sociodemographic determinants, and foster an environment conducive to fair birth outcomes. *Prenatal, maternal, and postnatal care* are made accessible and affordable through healthcare infrastructure expansion, cost subsidies, and insurance coverage for vulnerable groups. Implementing *educational programs* for disadvantaged populations empowers individuals with knowledge about proper prenatal care, nutrition, and healthy behaviors during pregnancy. Adequate *maternity leave and workplace accommodations* support expectant mothers' health and job security. *Policies* may also encompass nutrition assistance, data collection for identifying disparities, and community-based initiatives providing culturally sensitive health services. *Cultural sensitivity training* for healthcare providers, anti-discrimination measures, and collaborative efforts with various stakeholders further contribute to addressing sociodemographic disparities effectively.

4 Community Health Extension Program to Reduce Disparities in Birth Outcomes

The Health Extension Program (HEP) is a community-based healthcare delivery system that originated in Ethiopia and has been adopted and implemented in LMICs since 2002. The program aims to address health disparities and improve access to essential healthcare services, including maternal and child health, in rural and underserved communities. The program developed in response to the poor health outcomes and inadequate coverage of essential health care services, including low coverage of maternal and child health services. There was also a large disparity between rural and urban populations, and among demographic and socioeconomic groups. Moreover, there was a critical shortage of skilled health workers, and weak coordination of service delivery.

The Community Health Extension Program (CHEP) is one of the most innovative community-based health program launched by the Ethiopian Federal Ministry of Health to make health services accessible to rural communities by setting out women Health Extension Workers (HEWs) in rural Health Posts. Female HEWs who have completed tenth grade are recruited from the same community and trained in HEP modules for 1 year, after which they return home as salaried frontline healthcare staff.

HEWs are premised to provide basic, largely preventive, primary health services to rural villages, and the program gives special attention to children and mothers. Ethiopia's health service delivery is structured into a three-tier system: primary, secondary, and tertiary levels of care. The HEP is positioned, implemented, and managed under the umbrella of the primary healthcare unit (PHCU) [26, 27].

5 The Role of the Community Health Extension Program in the Community

The implementation of CHEP involved engaging key population with the communities, including Health Education Workers (HEWs), model households (MHHs), the Health Development Army (HAD), community members, and government representatives [28]. Community health extension workers (CHEWs) deployed in the community through the CHEP provide healthcare services at the community level. They are typically women selected from the local community, and they receive extensive training over a 12-month period on various health topics, including maternal and child health. In the community they delivered information in the form of health education and counseling for pregnant women focusing on antenatal care, healthy pregnancy practices, nutrition, family planning, and birth preparedness. These community workers also function to raise awareness about danger signs during pregnancy and childbirth, and encouraging women to seek timely care.

The HEWs conduct antenatal care visits in the community, offering essential services such as physical examinations, measuring vital signs, identifying high-risk pregnancies, and providing tetanus toxoid vaccinations. They also promote early initiation of antenatal care and encourage pregnant women to complete the recommended number of visits. HEWs promote skilled birth attendance and encourage pregnant women to give birth in health facilities or with the assistance of skilled birth attendants. They educate women about the benefits of safe delivery practices, including clean delivery techniques, infection prevention, and immediate newborn care.

Postnatal care is also a component of the services provided by HEW to both mothers and newborns. They provide postnatal visits, examine the mother and baby's well-being, provide breast-feeding support, diagnose and manage postpartum problems, and provide newborn care, immunizations, and family planning counseling. HEWs facilitate referrals and linkages between the community and formal healthcare facilities. They identify high-risk pregnancies, refer women for further evaluation or specialized care, and accompany them to health centers if needed. Then they in ensure continuity of care and seamless transitions between community and facility-based services. Along with the services they collect and report community health data by keeping records of antenatal care visits, deliveries, postnatal care, and other pertinent health information while providing services. This data is used to monitor health indicators, identify gaps, and support higher-level healthcare decision-making. The integration of all of these community-based activities given by community health workers has demonstrated encouraging results in improving maternal and child health outcomes in LMICs by minimizing the disparities.

CHEP addresses sociodemographic gaps and improves access to vital care for pregnant women by bringing healthcare services closer to communities, strengthening CHEWs, and promoting health education. As a result of comprehensive and context-specific interventions, supporting behavior changes and contributes to better health outcomes for pregnant women and their infants. For example, Ethiopia's maternal death rate fell from 728 to 357, with the combined effect of HEP and HDA accounting for 46% of the overall decrease [29]. The use of modern contraceptives among married women age 15–49 from 2005 to 2014 increased from 13.9% to 40.4%. Women who graduated as model families or worked towards graduation were 2.13 times more likely to use maternal health services. Increased program intensity scores increased the likelihood of receiving services, including ANC, birth preparedness, postnatal care, and breastfeeding. Visits by HEWs significantly correlated with ANC attendance and postnatal care attendance during the first 3 days.

6   Community Engagement with the Community Health Education Program

Community engagement is essential for inclusion in programs implemented to reduce the disparities in communities of LMICs. Community engagement through CHWs and local volunteers is crucial for community involvement. These individuals are trusted members of the community and play a vital role in delivering health services, providing education, and offering support to pregnant women and their families. CHWs act as a bridge between the program and the community, fostering trust and rapport. Training, supervision, and recognition of CHWs and volunteers helps to maintain their motivation and commitment to the program.

Health Education Program (HEP) is another community-based health service delivery program that employs the diffusion concept to gradually change community behaviors. In collaboration with Health Education Workers (HEWs), the goal of HEPs is to improve a health behavior by developing model families for others to follow. In the health system, HEWs are the first contact within the community. The HEWs' first tasks are to recruit Voluntary Community Health Workers (traditional birth attendants, health promoters, and reproductive health agents) to help HEWs in mobilizing the community to help implementing the program. These community volunteers are individuals who have had experience in community-based health services and are trusted to mobilize the community. Additionally, Model Households, Volunteer CHW, and Health Development Army (HDA) are used to involve the community in HEPs.

Model Households is an approach where families are recruited from the community to serve as examples of adopting healthy behaviors and practices related to maternal health. These model families are chosen based on their adherence to recommended health practices and receive training for 92 h and support from local health authorities and community health workers. Model families engage with the community through providing information, education, and support to other households, particularly marginalized or disadvantaged populations. They share their knowledge and experiences, addressing specific challenges faced by different sociodemographic groups. Promoting equitable access to healthcare services and acting as advocates addressing barriers and challenges faced by marginalized populations are the key roles of MHH. Through community outreach, health education, and counseling, model households work closely with local health authorities, community health workers, and health extension workers to develop and implement targeted interventions for different sociodemographic groups. Their involvement helps ensure that mothers from all backgrounds receive appropriate care and support.

Volunteer CHWs are community members trained by HEW to support the HEP. They play a vital role in health promotion, education, and disease prevention within their communities. Volunteer CHWs conduct home visits, provide screenings, and offer guidance on maternal and child health, family planning, and disease prevention. They also facilitate referrals to healthcare services, collect data, and report on community health. Their involvement strengthens the implementation of the HEP and improves health outcomes at the grassroots level.

The Health Development Army (HDA) is a collaborative movement promoting active learning and actions to improve health in the country since 2012 during the implementation of HEP. The government launched the HDA to strengthen HEP efforts, inspired by military structures and army discipline. The HDA involves women-centered community organizations and health development teams (30 households), the team further divided in to smaller group to form one-to-five networks. These groups work closely with health extension workers and local health authorities to promote health and deliver key messages within their communities. The HDA groups conduct door-to-door visits and community meetings and participate in events to disseminate health information and address specific

challenges faced by different sociodemographic groups. Their involvement ensures that interventions are tailored to the needs of marginalized populations and they act as advocates for adopting healthy behaviors. Overall, the HDA's involvement in the health extension program helps promote health education, awareness, and support targeted to marginalized populations.

Adopting a participatory approach involves active involvement of different community members in all stages of the project. This includes engaging them in the planning, implementation, monitoring, and evaluation processes. Community members can contribute their knowledge, experiences, and perspectives, ensuring that the program is relevant and tailored to their specific needs. Regular community meetings, focus group discussions, and participatory workshops are used to gather community input and ensure their active participation.

7   Reflection

Recognizing and addressing the sociodemographic factors affecting pregnant mothers are of paramount importance in enhancing birth outcomes. These factors exert a profound influence on a pregnant woman's health, overall well-being of newborn, and her access to healthcare services. Notably, disparities that exist among these sociodemographic factors have hindered mothers' healthcare access due to a lack of healthcare infrastructure, limited awareness, inadequate resources, and geographical barriers. Furthermore, limited-income households not only struggle to afford essential healthcare and nutritious food during pregnancy but also face compounded challenges due to inadequate access to maternity leave and workplace accommodations.

The CHEP serves as a vital bridge addressing the disparities and enhancing birth outcomes among vulnerable populations in LMICs, particularly in remote and underserved areas. This program has made significant progress in reducing adverse birth outcomes by improving healthcare accessibility and affordability, providing education and support, and addressing the complex challenges faced by pregnant women and their families. It empowers the population through increased awareness and decision-making abilities to encourage them to actively participate in healthcare-related decisions, including when to seek medical attention and how to access available healthcare services.

However, the implementation of programs in the region is not without its significant challenges and barriers. A primary obstacle is financial constraints, which limit the program's capacity to provide essential services, procure necessary medical equipment and supplies, and offer competitive salaries to healthcare workers. Inadequate healthcare infrastructure, encompassing a lack of healthcare facilities, essential medications, and medical equipment, can further hinder the comprehensive delivery of healthcare services through HEP. Secondly, geographical barriers, particularly in rural and remote areas, can exacerbate these challenges due to insufficient road networks and transportation options, making it challenging for healthcare providers to reach pregnant women and their families promptly. Additionally, ensuring the long-term sustainability of these programs beyond their initial implementation presents a formidable challenge. Disparities in levels of education related to health education within the population may hinder the comprehension of the importance of prenatal care and healthcare-seeking behaviors, impacting individuals' ability to understand and adhere to medical advice and recommendations. Cultural beliefs, traditions, and practices may discourage pregnant women from seeking timely and appropriate medical care, presenting challenges to HEWs through misconceptions and resistance.

To overcome program challenges and enhance its effectiveness, strengthening programs and addressing uncovered barriers is imperative, both requiring a collaborative and multifaceted approach. Strengthening programs involves increasing funding from both governments and international organizations and improving healthcare infrastructure. Additionally, there's a need for training and recruiting more healthcare work-

ers, particularly community health workers, as well as utilizing telemedicine and mobile clinics to reach underserved areas. Training healthcare workers should also include training for healthcare workers related to cultural, active community engagement, government commitment to healthcare as a fundamental right, international collaboration, and robust monitoring and evaluation systems. Together, these solutions help overcome workforce shortages, cultural barriers, resource limitations, and geographical challenges, ultimately enhancing healthcare access and outcomes in LMICs.

References

1. World Health Organization. Health inequities and their causes. 2018. https://www.who.int/news-room/facts-in-pictures/detail/health-inequities-and-their-causes. Accessed 27 July 2023
2. Khan A, et al. Environmental pollution is associated with increased risk of psychiatric disorders in the US and Denmark. PLoS Biol. 2019;17(8):e3000353.
3. Dongarwar D, Salihu HM. Place of residence and inequities in adverse pregnancy and birth outcomes in India. Int J MCH AIDS. 2020;9(1):53–63.
4. Kassa GM, Arowojolu AO, Odukogbe AA, Yalew AW. Adverse neonatal outcomes of adolescent pregnancy in Northwest Ethiopia. PLoS One. 2019;14(6):e0218259.
5. Muhe LM, et al. Articles major causes of death in preterm infants in selected hospitals in Ethiopia (SIP): a prospective, cross-sectional, observational study. Lancet Glob Health. 2019;7(8):e1130–8. https://doi.org/10.1016/S2214-109X(19)30220-7.
6. Asiki G, et al. Adverse pregnancy outcomes in rural Uganda (1996–2013): trends and associated factors from serial cross sectional surveys. BMC Pregnancy Childbirth. 2015;15(1):279. https://doi.org/10.1186/s12884-015-0708-8.
7. Gladstone M, Oliver C, Van Den Broek N. Survival, morbidity, growth and developmental delay for babies born preterm in low and middle income countries—a systematic review of outcomes measured E0120566. PLoS One. 2015;10(3):1–20.
8. Padhi BK, et al. Risk of adverse pregnancy outcomes among women practicing poor sanitation in rural India: a population-based prospective cohort study. PLoS Med. 2015;12(7):1–18.
9. Cantarutti A, et al. Mother's education and the risk of several neonatal outcomes: an evidence from an Italian population-based study. BMC Pregnancy Childbirth. 2017;17(1):1–10.

10. Hidalgo-Lopezosa P, et al. Sociodemographic factors associated with preterm birth and low birth weight: a cross-sectional study. Women Birth. 2019;32(6):e538–43. https://doi.org/10.1016/j.wombi.2019.03.014.

11. Jafree SR, Zakar R, Zakar MZ. Factors associated with low birth weight of children among employed mothers in Pakistan. Matern Child Health J. 2015;19(9):1993–2002. https://doi.org/10.1007/s10995-015-1708-z.

12. Parvin N, et al. Socioeconomic inequalities in the continuum of care across Women's reproductive life cycle in Bangladesh. Sci Rep. 2022;12(1):15618.

13. Kebede A, Kebede A, Belina S, Biratu Y. Trends and determinants of small birth weight in Ethiopia: further analysis of Ethiopian demographic and health surveys. Ethiop J Health Sci. 2021;31(2):299–310.

14. Jeemon P, et al. Determinants of very low birth weight in India: the national family health survey—4. Wellcome Open Res. 2022;7:20.

15. Zaveri A, et al. Maternal determinants of low birth weight among Indian children: evidence from the national family health survey-4, 2015-16. PLoS One. 2020;15:1–15. https://doi.org/10.1371/journal.pone.0244562.

16. Woldeamanuel BT, Gelebo KK. Statistical analysis of socioeconomic and demographic correlates of perinatal mortality in Tigray Region, Ethiopia: a cross sectional study. BMC Public Health. 2019;19(1):1301.

17. Kim Y-N, et al. Maternal age and risk of early neonatal mortality: a national cohort study. Sci Rep. 2021;11(1):814.

18. Abebe AM, et al. Teenage pregnancy and its adverse obstetric and perinatal outcomes at Lemlem Karl Hospital, Tigray, Ethiopia, 2018. Biomed Res Int. 2020;2020:3124847.

19. Ngandu CB, et al. The association between household socio-economic status, maternal socio-demographic characteristics and adverse birth and infant growth outcomes in Sub-Saharan Africa: a systematic review. J Dev Orig Health Dis. 2019;11(4):317–34.

20. Kyei-nimakoh M, Carolan-olah M, Mccann TV. Access barriers to obstetric care at health facilities in Sub-Saharan Africa—a systematic review. Syst Rev. 2017:1–16.

21. Hailemichael HT, et al. Determinants of adverse birth outcome in Tigrai Region, North Ethiopia: hospital-based case-control study. BMC Pediatr. 2020;20(1):10.

22. Degno S, et al. Adverse birth outcomes and associated factors among mothers who delivered in bale zone

hospitals, Oromia Region, Southeast Ethiopia. J Int Med Res. 2021;49(5):030006052110132.

23. Black RE, et al. Maternal and child nutrition 1 maternal and child undernutrition and overweight in low-income and middle-income countries. 2011.

24. UNICEF, WHO, and WBO. UN Inter-agency Group for Child Mortality Estimation (UN-Igme) Levels and Trends in Child Mortality Report 2020. 2020. https://www.unicef.org/media/79371/file/UN-IGME-child-mortality-report-2020.pdf.pdf.

25. Gezahegn T, Getachew D, Gessese T. Adherence to iron supplement intake during pregnancy and associated factors in Ethiopia: further analysis of a national based study. Food Sci Nutrit. 2023;11(9):5460–71.

26. Assefa Y, et al. Community health extension program of Ethiopia, 2003–2018: successes and challenges toward universal coverage for primary healthcare services. Global Health. 2019;15(1):24.

27. Negussie A, Girma G. Is the role of health extension workers in the delivery of maternal and child health care services a significant attribute? The case of Dale District, Southern Ethiopia. BMC Health Serv Res. 2017;117(1):641.

28. Wang H, Tesfaye R, Ramana GNV, Chekagn CT. 2016 Ethiopia health extension program: an institutionalized community approach for universal health coverage. World bank studies. Washington, DC. ISBN: 978-1-4648-0815-9; 97814644648081.

29. Rieger M, et al. Social science and medicine the impact of the Ethiopian health extension program and health development army on maternal mortality: a synthetic control approach. Soc Sci Med. 2019;232:374–81. https://doi.org/10.1016/j.socscimed.2019.05.037.

Hana Abera Hailemariam is a dedicated professional with a rich and diverse background in healthcare and education. With a career spanning from September 2004 to June 2017, she served as a clinical nurse at Addis Ababa University, Tikur Anbessa Specialized Hospital. Transitioning into the realm of education, Hana became a lecturer in June 2017 at St. Paul Hospital Millennium Medical College Nursing School, later advancing to the position of Assistant Professor by January 2023. Her academic contributions were multifaceted, involving classroom lectures, bedside mentorship for students, and advisory roles during research projects. Actively participating in clinical activities and demonstrated a commitment to bridging theory and practice.

Social Determinants of Maternal and Newborn Health: Engaging Communities in Botswana for Better Outcomes

Mabel Magowe and Onalenna Tsima

1 Social Determnants of Maternal and Newborn Health in Botswana: Engaging Communities for Improving Health Outcomes

This chapter entails an analysis of the contextual social determinants of maternal and newborn health in Botswana. Social determinants of health are nonmedical factors that influence health outcomes, including, the circumstances in which people are born, live, grow, and work. They include socioeconomic status, cultural factors and social norms, social policies and education systems, development agendas, political systems, neighborhood and physical environment, employment, and social support networks, as well as access to health care [1]. Because of their profound effect on people's lives, it is critical to understand social determinants of health in order to influence change that can reduce their negative effects on people.

Maternal health refers to the health of women during pregnancy, childbirth, and postpartum period [2]. According to the World Health Organization [3], in 2020, 800 women died due to preventable causes related to pregnancy and childbirth, with 2000 maternal deaths occurring every 2 min and a maternal mortality ratio (MMR) of 34 per 100,000 globally. The overwhelming majority 95% of these deaths occurred in low-income countries. Countries affected by conflict are the most attended [4]. Among nine countries facing the worst humanitarian crises, maternal mortality rates doubled up above the world average of 551 maternal deaths per 100,000 live births, compared to 223 globally [5, 6]. Disparities in health care access occur more in low- and middle-income countries, with detrimental impact on the health of the mother and neonate [5, 6]. In 2020, about 70% of all maternal deaths occurred in sub-Saharan Africa [1].

Newborn health refers to the health of a newly born baby or neonate, occurring during a neonatal period [7], which begins at birth and ends at 28 days post- delivery. This transitional period is a critical time for adaptation to life outside the uterus, with the most dramatic physiologic changes involving the respiratory and cardiovascular systems immediately at birth. These changes can be challenging and can lead to neonatal loss if not supported adequately. A UNICEF Report [8] indicated that in 2021, 2.3 million children died globally, and approximately 6400 of those were neonatal deaths that occurred every day. West, Central, Eastern, and Southern African regions were reported to have a combined neonatal mortality rate of 27 deaths per 1000 live births. Progress in neonatal mortality reductions has

M. Magowe (✉) · O. Tsima
School of Nursing, University of Botswana, Gaborone, Botswana
e-mail: magowem@ub.ac.bw; tsimao@ub.ac.bw

J. B. Hamilton, C. E. Moore (eds.), *Transforming Social Determinants to Promote Global Health*,
https://doi.org/10.1007/978-3-031-61160-5_9

been slow (2.4% decline from 1990 to 2021) compared to mortality among children 1–59 months with 3.3% decline. We explore some of the social determinants of maternal and neonatal health outcomes in Botswana and espouse the related cultural practices and the potential for community engagement in reducing the alarming and unnecessary loss of mothers and newborn babies.

2   Background

Botswana is a semi-arid landlocked country in the southern African plateau bordered by four countries; South Africa in the south-east, Zimbabwe on the east, Zambia on the north, and Namibia on the west. The country has a population of 2,346,179 [9], occupies a landmass of 581,730 km^2 (224,607 sq. mi), and is the 22nd biggest country in Africa and 47th worldwide next to France and Madagascar. With an occupancy of 4.4 inhabitants per km^2 it is one of the most sparsely populated countries on earth with (72%) of the population in urban and peri-urban areas [3, 8, 10–13]. The country enjoys political stability as a social democracy, with fairly good socioeconomic indicators (GDP 5.8% annually, 2022), and universal education and health care for all. The Government of Botswana through the Ministry of Health has made tremendous achievement in improving the health of women and newborn babies through improved access to health services and care.

Botswana's national health care structure is based on the Primary Health Care framework that advocates for community engagement. Communities have, over time, engaged in cultural health practices that have benefited them positively, before the advent of modern conventional medical practice. These cultural health care practices, if analyzed, understood, and documented, can be maintained or modified as necessary to reap their full potential for positive health outcomes. The country is inherently a communal society where family social support is part of the culture. Batswana (the people of Botswana) have a history of voluntary work that supports health care programs, especially during epidemics like HIV and AIDS where many people volunteered to participate in home-based care.

Communities inherently provided social and material support to affected families with resources like drinking water, firewood, and food. Some also volunteered as members of village health and village development committees that provided guidance for implementation of health care programs. Others participated individually in the provision of direct care to the sick such as bathing and feeding, with the guidance of health care professionals. Communities are still encouraged to provide such support to mothers and newborns where needed. We therefore present a scoping review of literature to explore determinants of maternal and newborn health from the perspective of culture, social norms, and policies, and how best communities can be engaged to improve maternal and newborn health outcomes.

Maternal and newborn health outcomes in Botswana are lagging behind, despite positive national developments. Botswana [14] reported a maternal mortality ratio (MMR) of 163 deaths per 100,000 live births in 2019. The Statistics Botswana brief (2020) also indicated that 76 maternal deaths were reported in 2020 from 58,244 live births yielding a Maternal Mortality Ratio (MMR) of 131 maternal deaths per 100,000 live births, showing a slight decline from 2019. The brief also indicated that maternal mortality has been fluctuating between 2014 and 2020 (151.6 in 2014, 127 in 2015, 154.6 in 2016, 143.2 in 2017, 133.7 in 2018, 166.3 in 2019, and 130.5 in 2020). Neonatal mortality rate fell gradually from 33.3 in 1971 to 21.9 in 2020 per 1000 live births [14]. The reports address deaths that mostly occur in health facilities. But there could be deaths that occur in homes that are not reported.

Given the persistently high maternal and newborn mortalities, it is imperative that national interventions commit to the Sustainable Development agenda of the United Nations General Assembly [15] that "no woman dies as a result of child birth," and by extension no newborn should die at the start of their lives. Botswana has signed the Ouagadougou

Declaration on Primary Health Care Renewal for the African Region, adopted in 2008. Declaration number 5.8 urges governments to build the capacity of communities to change behaviors, adopt healthier lifestyles, take ownership of their health, and be more involved in health-related activities. The country is also challenged to create an environment to empower communities in the governance of health care services in accordance with the Primary Health Care approach. Similarly, Declaration number 6 also commits states to encourage communities, including civil society, to seek recognition of their role in governance of health services, particularly in what relates to community-based, public health, and other health-related interventions. If implemented, sizable health care will take place within communities and families, with the potential to reduce overcrowding in health care facilities. This has seen the development of early discharge of women and their newborn babies within 24 h after a normal delivery and within 5 days after a Caesarian section, which shifted postpartum care to communities and families. However, there is evidence of inadequate follow up and supervision of delivered women at home to ensure positive recovery and early childhood adjustment to life.

Delivered woman means all women who have delivered, either at home or at a health facility, who have been identified and recorded as delivered. Almost all women (99%) deliver in health facilities, which include, maternity clinics, primary hospitals, district hospitals, national referral hospitals, and private hospitals. clinics. The 1% are those who deliver at home accidentally because of either precipitate labor, or delayed decision to reach health facilities, or very remote in the farming areas where there may not be midwives available on that day. Teams of nurses and midwives conduct mobile clinics three times a day in remote areas, especially in farming areas, and they may not receive every woman at the satellite stop on time. Botswana has not introduced domiciliary deliveries like other countries, and even domiciliary postpartum follow-up is very low at 9%. This is due to workforce shortages, transport, and other logistical problems, and it

should be one of the national priorities to reduce morbidities and mortalities in these population groups.

Improvements in clinical care have not reduced disparities in health outcomes and persist particularly with regard to social determinants of health [16]. In Botswana, clinical care interventions such as pre-service training of midwives and in-service training in emergency obstetric care (EMOC), which was revised to emergency obstetric and neonatal care (EMONC), have been the focus of attention. These, however, have not demonstrated commensurate benefit in addressing maternal and newborn health, as indicators remain high. While health determinants for clinical care have been adequately addressed, social determinants are not fully explored or documented, in Botswana. Nkhwalume and Mashalla [17] identified that there was inadequate community involvement in maternal newborn care, and minimal or no health education to communities, women, and their partners on sexual and reproductive health matters. The cultural perspectives and norms, community engagements, social support networks, and other socioeconomic contributions to the health of women and newborns have not been scoped and published. It is therefore critical to examine these social determinants of health in Botswana to provide policy and practice guidance for improvement.

3 Chapter Aims

3.1 Main Aim

This chapter presents an analysis of the contextual social determinants related to cultural practices of maternal and newborn health in Botswana. Specifically, the focus of the chapter is on culture and norms, social network support systems, and social and health policy.

Specific objectives
1. To identify cultural practices and norms related to maternal and newborn care, and their impact on maternal newborn health.

2. To explore social support systems and community engagement practices related to maternal newborn care.
3. To examine social and health policies that contribute to maternal and newborn health.
4. To draw implications and recommendations for improving maternal newborn health outcomes in terms of policy, practice, and research interventions.

4 Approach

We initially conducted a scoping review of literature on social determinants of health for maternal and newborn populations to contextualize them to Botswana and how the local communities are and can be engaged to improve health outcomes for the populations of interest. This entailed a preliminary assessment of the problem in past and current scientific research and gray literature and from unpublished reports and other documents that were available in the country. The aim of the review was to identify knowledge gaps, set research agendas, and identify implications and evidence for policy and practice decision-making relating to how communities are engaged to address social determinants of maternal and newborn health in Botswana. Our assumption was that a lot is happening that has not been explored, analyzed, and documented adequately, and the review would assist in putting things in perspective. In this chapter, we incorporated the findings from our review along with our experiences with working with this population. We draw conclusions based on our expertise and our review of the literature and make suggestions on how to strengthen community engagement to improve maternal newborn health outcomes.

5 Results

The focus of our discussion was on cultural and social norms and practices, community and social support networks, social and health policies to leverage on and improve community participation, and engagement in maternal and newborn health

care to achieve the Sustainable Development Goal for maternal and on newborn health. In the sections to follow, we describe key determinants of maternal and newborn health in Africa and Botswana. We conclude this section with by presenting implications for policy, practice, and research.

6 Key Determinants of Maternal and Newborn Health in Africa and Botswana

The greater focus of published literature regarding determinants of maternal and newborn health is largely on health-related issues. Therefore, fewer published studies that were retrieved focused on social determinants, especially cultural issues. A study by Adgoy [18] identified geographical location, transport, security, and access to health. Other social determinants included *age at marriage, gender inequity, maternal education and health literacy, material and human resources, lack of male involvement in health matters, health care worker attitude, and reliance on community and social networks*. We provide an analysis of these determinants from the Botswana perspective.

6.1 Geographic Location, Transportation, Cost, and Access to Health

The geographic spread of the country poses challenges in transportation for women to reach required health services. Most private buses and taxis operate during the day till 8 pm, and few taxis are available to be called at night. Anecdotal reports indicate that emergency medical services provided by the government are grossly inadequate to reach all who need them.

The health care system in Botswana is universal and free for all, provided by the Ministry of Health, within at least 2 km for most communities [12]. This includes pregnant and delivered women, and children. Cost is not a major issue for access to maternal and child health care because services are free. The national health care system provides mobile services two to three times a week to increase access in remote villages and farms. This, however, still leaves a small number of women without regular health care. Private clinics and hospitals also add to the availability of health services in peri-urban villages and cities, mostly accessed by people who subscribe to private health insurance. Mining companies also provide free services for mine workers and their families, and also provide coverage for surrounding villages.

Access to antenatal and delivery services is quite good. Approximately 98% of women attend antenatal care and 99.8% deliver in health facilities, under the supervision and care mainly by qualified nurse-midwives [14]. However, immediate postpartum follow-up within the first critical 10 days remains low at 9% coverage [19], which means 89% of mothers and their newborn babies do not have access to supervised health care during this period.

Many women attend antenatal care in the peri-urban villages and cities but still conform to the cultural practice of relocating to home villages immediately after delivery to be cared for by female family members. Some of the villages are rural in hard-to-reach areas in farms, and women are often seen by health care providers at 4 weeks when they bring their newborns for the first child welfare visit, or at 6 weeks when they come for the first postpartum check-up. The risk of unrecorded and unreported maternal and newborn morbidities and mortalities during this period cannot be ruled out under such circumstances. Additionally, some women may need to travel longer distances to access health services and this can contribute to lower utilization of the needed postpartum services.

6.2 Age at Marriage

Under the Botswana Marriage Act 2001, the minimum age of marriage is 21 years. A minor (a person under 21 years) may marry at the age of 18 years with parental or guardian consent. However, according to UNICEF [8], child marriage is any marriage or informal union under the

age of 18 years and is not acceptable. Statistics Botswana Report (2020) indicated that out of 6518 solemnized marriages that year, 0.3% were among brides below 21 years, indicating that the partners were older.

Child marriage is often entrenched in the economic status of women that disproportionately affects girls more than boys. Although early marriage is quite minimal in the country, such unions still take place despite being a violation of the law. Early marriages are a contributor to early sexual debut, early pregnancy, early parenting, and repeated pregnancies within shorter periods, contrary to the WHO-recommended minimum of 2-year interval, which have potential health risks for the mother.

Fan and Koski [20] purport that child marriage is a marker of gender inequality. This can be attributable to women's dependency on the older economically advantaged partner, and the control and potential abuses that can result. Such women are less likely to use contraceptives to prevent early pregnancy. This study also concluded that child marriage had the higher odds of longer time in pregnancies, giving before during their teen years, and having multiple births at an early age before they reached emotional and physical maturity. There is also an increased chance of having mis-timed and unwanted pregnancy with a threat of physical and emotional consequences, potential for abortions, miscarriages, and stillbirths. The use of maternal health services among these younger women may be inconsistent or lower, and they may be subjected to risks of untreated complications of pregnancy and childbirth. They are also likely to have poor nutritional intake, lifestyle-related health concerns, emotional turmoil and depression, obstetric complications like fistula due to difficult labor, and other postpartum complications like hemorrhage.

6.3 Gender Inequity

In a patriarchal society like Botswana, most family decisions are made by the older man in the family, who could be the father, elder brother, uncle, spouse, or partner. The decisions include matters of sexuality such as the number of children desired and their gender. Distribution of family wealth often favors the male child and thereby contributes to increased poverty among women. Additionally, preferential treatment for education also favors the boy child, because it is believed that the girl would get married to a different family and gain wealth from there or give her new family an advantage if she is gainfully employed. Women therefore remain poor and dependant on the male counterpart for livelihood, resulting in male partner potential dominance. All of these factors contribute to culturally perpetuated inequities in decision-making among couples.

Gender-based violence has increased because of the pressure on men to provide, and the cultural dominance over women reaching levels that are worrisome. The Gender Based Violence Indicators Study conducted by Machisa and van Dorp [21] indicated that 70% of women interviewed had experienced gender-based violence, 24 times higher than cases reported to the police in the previous year. The fear of violence restricts movement of women from accessing services at night often needed for delivery. This could contribute to noninstitutional births of 2%, and 3.7% of children born before arrival of a midwife, recorded in the Statistics Botswana Brief [14].

6.4 Maternal Education and Health Illiteracy

According to the literature reviewed, the lack of knowledge among those advising and caring for mothers was in most instances due to the lack of understanding of changes to the body brought by pregnancy, labor, and delivery, hence some of the grave errors that can lead to complications. Since the advent of modern health care, committee education has been undertaken robustly, leading to changes in attitude, behaviors, and practices that are aligned to modern health care, but gaps still exist in some communities here some cultural practices remain as part of the norms.

6.5 Human and Material Resources for Health

Shortage of health care workforce remains a concern for the Botswana health care system [22] with a ratio of 3.4 doctors and 28.4 nurses per 10,000 people. The health care workforce is dominated by nurses and nurse-midwives, who also extend outreach services to the most remote areas through mobile clinics. Nurse-midwives are essentially able to provide normal maternal and child health services, determine the need for collaborative care, and referral to an obstetrician in the urban and peri-urban health facilities. However, there is a critical shortage of nurse-midwives and scarcity of doctors, pharmacists, and other health workers. Most laboratory services in particular are centralized in cities and peri-urban villages. This necessitates movement of people who need these services, amidst transportation challenges. The development of the Faculty of Health Sciences at the University of Botswana in 2006 subsequently lead to the development of Faculty of Medicine in 2008 to improve supply of medical doctors, but is yet to meet the required numbers.

During the early years of primary health care in the late 1970s, the Family Welfare Educator cadre was developed and trained to provide family support through education, clean environments, and motivation of families to use health services. They visited newly delivered mothers and reminded them of required health visits. They also identified health concerns for delivered mothers and referred them to health services for further care. The cadre has been transformed to Health Education officers and the focus is more on communicable and noncommunicable diseases. This cadre can be strengthened to pay attention to maternal and newborn health concerns and to visit newly delivered mothers within the first 10 days, which are the most critical to achieve positive health outcomes.

Anecdotal reports and observations as we follow up with students during clinical teaching and on personal visits as patients are that there also is a critical shortage of basic equipment, drugs and supplies. For example, there is limited availability of blood pressure machines, thermometers, and weighing scales which are needed at the first level of assessment of a patient. Furthermore, available equipment is often inadequate or broken. Stock outs are frequent for long periods of months or even years. Basic drugs for maternity care are not available at peripheral clinics and this adds the need for referral to higher facilities along the continuum of primary health care. The majority of women are in the remote locations, and the infrastructure itself has not grown and kept up to meet the needs of women. Hence referrals are inevitable, necessitating unnecessary movement of patients, and the consequent loss of family support they need in order to continue to enjoy a safe and healthy pregnancy and postpartum recovery. The World Health Organization has an audit tool for maternity services that can provide detailed information about the status quo at all levels of the maternal and newborn health care system, and should be regularly utilized to identify areas that require attention.

6.6 Lack of Male Involvement in Health Matters

Davis et al. [23] reported that key informants who were policymakers admitted to the lack of male involvement in reproductive health matters due to cultural barriers. These matters were viewed as "women's business" in the Pacific region. Informants, however, underscored the importance of male involvement in reproductive health, as decision-makers in the family, to improve maternal and newborn health outcomes. Along a similar vein, in the Botswana context, Letshwenyo-Maruatona [24] reported that older married men were more comfortable communicating with their partners about reproductive health matters, child-care, family planning, pregnancy, and prevention of mother-to-child transmission services, but felt uncomfortable talking about sex, child-birth, and infertility, treating that as women's business. Communication is key in behavior change and therefore should be strengthened to benefit men's involvement for positive childbirth-related health-seeking behaviors.

6.7 Reliance on Community and Social Support Networks Related to Maternal Newborn Health

Botswana has a unique maternal health care practice not only reliant on the national health care system, but deeply rooted and entrenched in the culture, yet it is barely documented. Botswana's national Primary Health Care framework-based health system subscribes to community engagement. Communities have over time engaged in cultural health practices that have benefited them in terms of positive health outcomes before the advent of modern conventional medical practice. Some of these practices continue to prevail in some communities due to myriad factors such as low health literacy, inadequate health care resources, or simply because they still work better for them. These cultural health care practices, if analyzed, understood, and documented, can be maintained or modified as necessary to reap their full potential for positive health outcomes. It is hoped that the scoping review of literature and a reflection about some practices known to the authors will help in addressing these sociocultural determinants of maternal and newborn health from the perspective of culture, social norms, and policies, and how communities are and can be engaged to improve maternal and newborn health outcomes.

In maternal and child health, mothers were guided by older female relatives regarding the do's and don'ts that protect the life and health of the mother and the unborn child. Most of these entailed taboos that were deemed dangerous for fetal growth and development and labor outcomes. For example, women may be cautioned not to overeat to avoid overgrowth of the fetus, which presumably would contribute to a difficult delivery. The eating of eggs for example was prohibited for the same reason. There are many such myths and misconceptions that are given as helpful advice to mothers during pregnancy, labor, and delivery. Communities require the support of qualified health care providers to equip them with correct information, bearing in mind the common shared goal of positive safe pregnancy and childbirth.

Botswana has long embraced the Primary Healthcare Principles since 1978 and therefore all communities are encouraged to participate in activities that promote their health. Community participation or community engagement is a process in which the community voluntarily takes part in activities geared towards promoting their own health and that of another [13]. It also entails empowering families to provide care to sick family members at home under the guidance and support of health care workers. The implementation of effective social, behavioral, and community engagement (SBCE) interventions is critical for positive maternal and child health outcomes [25]. Training of health care providers, and other service providers, in skills and techniques related to communication, health education, and community engagement is also very important in promoting maternal and child health [25]. From a cultural perspective, communities have always been engaged in providing care to mothers during pregnancy, labor and delivery, postpartum period, and for childcare.

6.8   Care During Pregnancy Related to Social Networks

During pregnancy, the pregnant woman typically receives special care from an elderly woman in the family. A married woman would be taken care of by her in-laws, but towards the delivery, the mother-in-law asks the woman's parents to take over for care during and postpartum period. This was traditionally done because delivery was viewed as a sensitive period that required care by those women closest to the woman without being seen as abandoning her to her parents and shifting responsibility on the part of the in-laws. Hence the official consultation to hand her over to her parents. However, the in-laws would continue to provide material support like food and maternity clothing and anything that was required to meet her needs. Because of urbanization and individual preferences, many women leave with the spouses/partners, and attend modern health services at antenatal clinics. But some still relocate either towards the end of pregnancy or delivery to receive this home care in conjunction with modern health care.

The new mother receives total body massages as the pregnancy advances, to keep her healthy. A woman who was suspected of having an abnormal fetal lie or presentation (based on observation of the abdominal girth), receives abdominal massages from experienced traditional midwives to align the fetus for normal delivery (similar external cephalic version is done by obstetricians in modern health care system). People believed in this and deemed it to be working well for the health of the mother and her fetus. To this end, some people still continue to follow this tradition, especially if modern maternity can make a suggestion that the baby is in an abnormal presentation. Although it seemed to be successful for most women, the caretakers were not formally educated to identify such abnormalities, nor for appropriate interventions in case of any complications that might arise. Hence the risk of early rapture of membranes, placental separation, uterine rapture, tortion, and tightening of an umbilical cord around the fetal neck, which might occur with excessive manipulation, cannot be ruled out. Because of the lack of knowledge, there is also a greater likelihood of such events going unreported. The woman had to follow rules and regulations enforced by the caretaker that could affect her delivery. For example, she is typically expected to be seated during a meal, because eating while standing up was presumed to be responsible for any eventual poor progress during labor. The cultural practice of eating while standing refers to some of the culturally imposed rules for pregnant women, instructed by the older care takers who believe that if a woman eats in standing position, the labor will stand/stall or slow down, leading to delayed delivery with possible consequences on the mother and newborn, possibly maternal death or stillbirth (though this is never explained to that extent). They just say the labor will be slow. So the woman is expected to always eat in sitting position.

There were also choices as to what to eat and what not to eat. For example, eggs and offal meats were prohibited during pregnancy because they would make the fetus overgrow and cause difficult labor. Pregnant women are also prohibited from wearing tight maternity clothes because of the belief that this might suffocate the fetus. If packaged properly to emphasize the role of nutrition in maternal and newborn health, women and the fetuses/newborn babies would benefit from nutritional regulation of fetal growth and development, and maternal health during pregnancy and in the immediate postpartum period. The availability of health services countrywide has improved antenatal attendance in clinics to at least six times in line with health policies and practices, and the families have taken it on quite well. Attendance has risen to almost 100% for antenatal care and deliveries since availability of clinics countrywide.

6.9 Labor and Delivery Care Related to Social Networks

Once labor began, the mother would be placed in a secluded place in the home, usually a special hut at the back of the yard. She was advised not to make any noise or scream because it was shameful to be heard by neighbors or other people within the family compound. The women were given herbs that would speed up progress of labor and delivery, and many were instructed to bear down quite early. This unfortunately could bring the risk of maternal and fetal exhaustion or distress for a few women, who would end up being taken to modern health services to receive care for complications that might arise.

If membranes did not rapture during labor, they were raptured when the baby was delivered using a fingernail (of the grandmother conducting the delivery), which was risky for the spread of infection. The umbilical cord was also cut after delivery using a razor blade prepared while the woman was pregnant. The razor blade was not necessarily sterilized, leading again to the risk of infection. Families are not equipped with any modern equipment for maternal and newborn care, and therefore they use anything within their reach. Maternity call outs have also been drastically affected by shortage of nurse-midwives, basic supplies, and transport. The family practices cited, however, are no longer a common practice as many women deliver in modern health facilities under the supervision of qualified midwives. However, the risk cannot be ruled out for those who may need to deliver at home for several reasons such as precipitated labor or distance from a health facility.

In the cultural system of delivery, the umbilical cord is cut after delivery of the baby and the placenta. The newborn is just wiped clean with whatever cloth is available, and this may not necessarily be sterile. The baby is then wrapped up in warm clothes. The mother is laid to rest on some blankets or clothes that are not sterilized but cleaned prior to labor during the preparatory period. The umbilical cord is dried up using burned and cooled wood ash from a local hard wood tree called "*Motswere*" collected before the ash hits the ground to avoid contamination. This practice of using wood ash has been shown to have antiseptic and antibacterial properties and drying effects that promotes quick healing of the stump. Research is still needed to determine the components of the ash and its healing properties. But literature offers contradictory evidence regarding the role of ash in healing wounds.

6.10 Postpartum Care for the Mother–Baby Dyad Through Social Networks

The Botswana culture has always emphasized breastfeeding as the only way to support early childhood development. Newborns were initiated on breastfeeding immediately after delivery to benefit from the good hydration and rich nutrient support from breast milk. The family caretaker, who was usually the grandmother, great aunt, mother, or aunt, would ensure that the nursing mother remained well-hydrated and nourished to promote good flow of breast milk. The mother would receive total person-centered care in a secluded hut, where the caretaker ensured that she ate regularly, rested well between feeds while the baby was taken care of by the support person, who slept in the same hut, and she would usually determine who goes inside the room where the nursing mother and the newborn baby are resting. This practice promoted the newborn baby's health by minimizing the risk of infection. It also allowed the nursing mother to rest and concentrate on the baby so as to facilitate her recuperation.

The downside of it is that the husband or partner was not allowed to see the mother and her newborn baby until the baby was 3 months old, which causes separation anxiety for the couple. Traditionally men also used to believe that a newborn baby is solely the purview of the mother. This defeated the very essence of the positive impact on maternal and newborn health and early bonding for parents and the newborn baby from the early stages of child development and sharing of childcare responsibilities by both parents. But with an improved level of education, modern couples live together in the same household, especially with modern housing construction, and family support still being provided by someone older, mostly a mature woman coming in to support the couple. Men are now increasingly involved in the care of their children from pregnancy, through labor, delivery, and postpartum period and demand to be with their partners during the lying-in (postpartum) period. But there are some families which still hold on traditional cultural practices.

The newborn is cared for by the grandmother except during feeding times. This allowed the mother to rest. The newborn is bathed, massaged gently, and given passive exercises at frequent intervals to keep them healthy. This was believed to promote rapid growth and development. The growth and development of the child is a responsibility for all members of the family, and the child becomes a center of attraction to all, provided with all safety and security measures by all. The child is well fed, bathed, and assisted through all milestones such as sitting, crawling, walking, talking, and other similar developmental milestones. Recently, there are disruptions in these practices due to modernization and urbanization where young families are detached from the assistance of older and wiser family members, especially grandmothers. Hence some possible experiences of child neglect and malnutrition,

especially among disadvantaged unmarried women who bear sole responsibility for the care of their babies. However, some women still visit their families regularly, and send their children to visit grandparents during holidays to be in touch with their families, thereby keeping family networks in place to continue providing the support needed.

7 Implications for Policy, Practice, and Research

7.1 Practice Implications

An analysis of the literature and some anecdotal community reports have demonstrated a need for continuing education for families, including the mother and her support systems on the dangers of some of the cultural practices. Access to health services has dramatically improved service utilization and resultant positive health indicators for mothers and newborns. However, health education for mothers and families, including the role of fathers, needs to be strengthened to achieve improved universal coverage, improve health outcomes for mothers and newborns, and reduce maternal and newborn morbidity and mortality. Grandmothers and traditional birth attendants who may assist women during the childbearing cycle need to be reached with messages of caution when providing care. Some of the positive practices need to be acknowledged and supported. Therefore, midwives need to embrace outreach for maternal-newborn postpartum care and engage with family caregivers during pregnancy, labor, and delivery. The continued interaction through media discussions (radio, television, etc.) can be used to spread safety messages in case of emergency maternal and childcare.

7.2 Research Implications

Research is required to explore, understand, and document some of the cultural practices, and draw attention to those that are positive and need to be strengthened. Traditional birthing practices also need to be researched in order to preserve beneficial indigenous knowledge to determine strengths and weaknesses that need remedial action. Research on family support systems is also needed in order to strengthen systems where possible. The important role that family members play during pregnancy and postpartum period needs to be recognized and embraced.

7.3   Educational Implications

Health workforce shortages remain a concern, especially midwives and obstetricians to support childbearing women. Training of these cadres needs to be strengthened to increase the numbers that can reach out to women in all settings, especially community-based postpartum care. Strengthening of the importance of postpartum follow-up is necessary.

7.4   Policy Implications

Policies surrounding community-based maternal and child health services need to be strengthened to increase access to care in the most remote areas. Policy should introduce community and home-based antenatal care, postpartum care, and child welfare, which require minimal interventions, while deliveries can continue in the health facilities. Models have been demonstrated in other countries like the UK where midwives are assigned to conduct community antenatal, intrapartum, and postpartum services.

8   Reflection

Maternal and newborn health is still an area of concern in low- and middle-income countries because health care systems are not well-resourced to fully address challenges that lead to poor health outcomes for the mother and newborn. Interventions targeting social, behavioral, and community and family participation in the

health care of women need more research and when beneficial, used to promote maximal benefit for mothers and newborn babies. Male involvement in particular is very critical to support and bond with the new family.

Our personal observations working within clinical practice is that many of the determinants described above are real. Long queues at service points, shortage of essential but basic equipment, shortage of health care workforce, and self-reported gender-based violence are a reality that many women have to contend with on a daily basis. Many women have to walk far to access services. We started a domiciliary postpartum follow-up in one of the health care facilities working with students in the community. We experienced such a tremendous need and demand for providing deliveries because of perceptions in the community that this was what we were offering. This necessitated us to carry delivery packs while providing postpartum services. It was overwhelming to find that many women had to call on us for deliveries, which we had no choice but to conduct to save lives. Transportation was the biggest issue for women who lived in villages and needed to access services in peri-urban and urban centers. This was a true indication that home care is not just about postpartum follow-up or home-based palliative care for cancer and other chronic illness, but urgently needs to be expanded to all maternal and newborn health services in communities. It was also interesting to discover the profound commitment of mothers to saving their own lives and that of their babies, which seemed to supersede all the negative experiences, explaining the high attendance to available services. There is an urgent need to also study the attitude of health care providers and how things can be improved to promote respectful person-centered maternity care that meets women's and newborns' needs. This can hopefully improve service delivery and ensure availability of basic infrastructure and material as well as human health resource capital.

References

1. Dagher RK, Linares DE. A critical review on the complex interplay between social determinants of health and maternal and infant mortality. Children. 2022;9:394. https://doi.org/10.3390/children9030394.
2. WHO Report on Materna Health. World health statistics 2017. 2017. https://iris.who.int/bitstream/handle/10665/255336/9789241565486-eng.pdf.
3. World Health Organization (2023). Improving maternal and newborn health and survival and reducing stillbirth progress report 2023. https://www.who.int/news-room/events/d/improving-maternal-and-newborn-health-andsurvival-and-reducing-stillbirth. Accessed Jan 2024.
4. Roos N, von Xylander SR. Why do maternal and newborn deaths continue to occur? Best Pract Res Clin Obstet Gynaecol. 2016;36:30–44. https://doi.org/10.1016/j.bpobgyn.2016.06.002. Epub 2016 Jun 24. PMID: 27506412
5. WHO Report. A woman dies every two minutes due to pregnancy or childbirth: UN agencies. 2023a. https://www.who.int/news/item/23-02-2023-a-woman-dies-every-two-minutes-due-to-pregnancy-or-childbirth%2D%2Dun-agencies.
6. WHO Report. Trends in maternal mortality. 2023b. https://data.worldbank.org/indicator/SH.STA.MMRT?locations=BW
7. Doherty TM, Hu A, Salik I. Physiology, neonatal. In: StatPearls [Internet]. Treasure Island, FL: StatPearls Publishing; 2023. PMID: 30969662.
8. UNICEF Report. Levels and trends in child mortality. 2023. https://data.unicef.org/resources/levels-and-trends-in-child-mortality/
9. Statistics Botswana. Vital statistics. 2022. https://www.statsbots.org.bw/vital-statistics
10. WHO Africa Regional Office. Ouagadougou Declaration on Primary Health Care and Health Systems in Africa. 2008. https://www.afro.who.int/publications/ouagadougou-declaration-primary-health-care-and-health-systems-africa
11. Doherty M, Neilson S, O'Sullivan J, Carravallah L, Johnson M, Cullen W, Shaw SCK. Barriers to healthcare and self-reported adverse outcomes for autistic adults: a cross-sectional study. BMJ Open. 2022;12(2):e056904. https://doi.org/10.1136/bmjopen-2021-056904.
12. Ministry of Health. Botswana Primary health Care Guidelines 2016. Gaborone, Botswana: Government Printers; 2016.
13. WHO PHC Report (2021). Social determinants of Health. https://www.who.int/health-topics/social-determinants-ofhealth. Accessed 16 Feb 2024.
14. Statistics Botswana Brief (2020). Death Stats Brief. Statsbots.org.bw. https://www.statsbots.org.bw/sites/default/files/Deaths%20Stats%20Brief%2020.pdf. Accessed 19 Feb 2024.
15. United Nations General Assembly 2015. Health in the post – 2015 UN development agenda. https://www.un.org/millenniumgoals. Accessed 16 Feb 2024.
16. Whitman A, De Lew N, Chappel A, Aysola V, Zuckerman R, Sommers BD. Addressing social determinants of health: examples of successful evidence-based strategies and current federal efforts. 2022. https://aspe.hhs.gov/reports/sdoh-evidence-review.
17. Nkhwalume L, Mashalla Y. Health care workers experiences in emergency obstetric care following implementation of an in-service training program: case of 2 referral hospitals in Botswana. Afr Health Sci. 2021;21(Suppl):51–8. https://doi.org/10.4314/ahs.v21i1.9S. PMID: 34447424; PMCID: PMC8367308
18. Adgoy ET. Key social determinants of maternal health among African countries: a documentary review. 2018. https://doi.org/10.15406/mojph.2018.07.00219
19. Statistics Botswana Report (2017). Vital Statistics Report 2017. Statsbots.org.bw. https://www.statsbots.org.bw/sites/default/files/Deaths%20Stats%20Brief%2020.pdf. Accessed 19 Feb 2024.
20. Fan S, Koski L. The health consequences of child marriage: a systematic review of the evidence. BMC Public Health. 2022;22:309. https://doi.org/10.1186/s12889-022-x.
21. Machisa M, van Dorp R. The gender based violence indicators study. Ministry of Labour and Home Affairs, Women's Affairs Dept. Botswana. 2012. www.gov.bw.
22. Nkomazana O, Peersman W, Willcox M, Marsh R, Phaladze N. Human resources for health in Botswana: the results of in-country database and reports analysis. Afr J Prm Health Care Fam Med. 2014;6(1):716. https://doi.org/10.4102/phcfm.v6i1.716.
23. Davis J, Vyankandondera J, Luchters S, et al. Male involvement in reproductive, maternal and child health: a qualitative study of policymaker and practitioner perspectives in the Pacific. Reprod Health. 2016;13:81. https://doi.org/10.1186/s12978-016-0184-2.
24. Letshwenyo-Maruatona S. Who do batswana men prefer: male or female health providers? Am J Mens Health. 2017;11(6):1642–52. https://doi.org/10.1177/1557988315621727.
25. Chan HY, Kwok AO, Yuen KK, et al. Association between training experience and readiness for advance care planning among healthcare professionals: a cross-sectional study. BMC Med Educ. 2020;20:451. https://doi.org/10.1186/s12909-020-02347-3.

Mabel Magowe PhD, RN, is an Associate Professor and manages research activities for quantitative and qualitative studies, oversees operations for externally funded research grants, supports and leads internal and external grant applications, supervises graduate students' research, and serves as an examiner for graduate students' research in other regional universities. She also serves as a peer reviewer for several national, regional, and international scientific journals. As the Deputy Dean in the Faculty of Health Sciences, she oversees research development and stimulates and supports formation of departmental research committees that provide oversight for monitoring research proposals that meet standards for ethical approval and funding. Dr. Magowe is a reviewer for research proposals and grant applications for institutional review committees nationally, including the Ministry of Health Research and Development Committee. She has served as a reviewer for the University of Botswana Ethical and Scientific Review committee, as well as the Funding Review committee. She served in a panel of judges for grant proposals for the West African University at the African Association of Universities in Accra, Ghana (2019) for universities improvement projects sponsored by the World Bank.

Onalenna Tsima is a registered nurse, midwife, community health nurse specialist, and a PhD candidate (title: *Developing a programme for cancer service delivery in primary care settings: Botswana*). As a community health nurse, her focus is on health promotion across the lifespan and disease prevention. She engages communities and different stakeholders to develop different health promotion programs to support the needs of various groups in the community.

Using Strategic Communications to Inspire a Shared Vision for Black Women's Health

Kamila A. Alexander and Schenita D. Randolph

1   Introduction

Innovations in research and practice approaches are required to mitigate the disruptive effects of intimate partner violence (IPV) and HIV epidemics among Black women and their families. These epidemics often co-occur and can exacerbate one another because they are deeply rooted in adverse social determinants of health [1–4]. In the presence of IPV, many women find their ability to make safe sexual decisions with an abusive partner disrupted, thereby increasing their risk for HIV transmission or exacerbation of an already acquired infection [5]. Additionally, insufficient resources and support services can perpetuate IPV and HIV among Black women [6]. We use the term "Black" rather than African American in this chapter to refer to people of African descent living in the U.S. Thus, we aim to honor the diversity of cultures and ethnicities that make up the fabric of Black life disproportionately impacted by racial designations and the subsequent influential consequences to optimal health in our nation.

K. A. Alexander (✉)
School of Nursing, Johns Hopkins University, Baltimore, MD, USA
e-mail: Kalexen3@jhu.edu

S. D. Randolph
School of Nursing, Duke University, Durham, NC, USA
e-mail: Schenita.Randolph@duke.edu

Structural racism has created lasting, intergenerational negative consequences for Black individuals and communities with some of the highest burdens falling on Black women. For example, 24.6% of Black women in the U.S. live in poverty compared to 10.8% of White women [7]. Due to the disproportionately high poverty rates that Black women in the U.S. experience, they might access social services frequently and therefore are subject to experiences of stigma and discrimination [7]. Complicated applications and eligibility determination processes, lack of transportation, inconvenient appointment scheduling, and lack of information about how to enroll in programs all serve as barriers to access to social services [7]. Along with financial strain, unemployment, and disruption to daily routines, the COVID-19 pandemic decreased women's interactions with supportive services that could help them in situations of IPV [8]. Thus, many Black women have limited access to the resources that they need to be safe, healthy, and successful.

There is also ample research demonstrating that Black women across the spectrum of socioeconomic status experience HIV and IPV inequities disproportionate to other groups [9–11]. For example, healthcare provider bias influences clinical discussions about often stigmatized topics such as IPV, HIV, and sexual health, resulting in limited information-sharing, as well as opportunities for testing and screening, or access to pre-exposure prophylaxis (PrEP) among women with middle class means [12–14]. In fact, bias during clinical and community-based encounters with Black women can directly impact levels of trust and willingness to accept recommendations for PrEP [15, 16]. Findings from previous studies confirm that the complexity of interactions from both healthcare providers and their Black women clients can be influenced by beliefs and attitudes as well as expectations and judgments.

Ending the HIV epidemic and addressing IPV among Black women will require strategic interventions, programs, policies, and clinical and research engagement that prioritizes Black women's cultural and social life experiences. Communicating with partners and collaborators is critical to bringing awareness and execution of actions to transform health and advance equity for Black women. Thus, using strategic communications to facilitate this is urgent and necessary.

Strategic communications include approaches that describe the "purposeful use of communication by an entity to engage in conversations of strategic significance to its goals [17]. Researchers and practitioners use a variety of strategic communication methods to address important public health issues in communities. For example, public health entities use campaigns to provide education about infectious disease prevention such as HIV/AIDS and COVID-19 or to promote recognition of child sexual abuse and support the ways experts communicate about these sensitive and stigmatized topics [18–20]. Researchers can also use strategic communication approaches to disseminate study findings, cocreate messaging with community partners, engage in media stories, and to elicit input regarding next steps in a program of research designed to impact Black women.

We, the authors of this chapter, use strategic communications approaches in our programs of research to align with an ethos of health equity and community-engaged scholarship. As nurse scientists and leaders, our voices as nurses are often left out of the media on health topics and issues. In fact, in 1997 the Woodhull Study on Nurses and Media: Health Care's Invisible Partner, found that nurses were cited as sources in only 4% of health news stories in leading print media of the day [21]. Twenty years later, researchers conducted a replication of this study and found that nurses were cited as sources in only 2% of health news stories [22]. As nurse leaders, we recognize that strategic communications approaches are important not only for our programs of research but also for the discipline of nursing that is consistently recognized as the most trusted profession in the U.S. We aim to cultivate trust in the research process among community members, promote sustainability of health interventions, and support transparent cocreation of methodological approaches and interpretations of findings that can be translated into new or existing programs.

In this chapter, we discuss community-engaged approaches using strategic communications in two research studies focused on promoting safety and health among Black women. First, we describe each of these public health epidemics, IPV and HIV, in the context of Black women's health. Second, we describe how we came to our respective works, their overlap, and our strategic communications approaches to community-engaged work. Third, we each describe our programs of research and how we apply strategic communications to enhance engagement with our respective communities. Fourth, we provide researchers and practitioners with suggested steps for developing a strategic communication plan that is aligned within the community engagement continuum. We end the chapter with reflections on the meanings of our community-engaged work for moving an ambitious agenda that centers the needs of Black women forward with implications for policy, research, and practice.

2 Intimate Partner Violence and HIV: Global Syndemic Threats to Black Women's Health

Black cisgender women (hereafter, referred to as Black women for the purposes of this chapter) in the United States disproportionately experience intimate partner violence (IPV) and adverse sexual health outcomes, including HIV compared to cisgender women of other races and ethnicities. These syndemics (overlapping health epidemics) are leading causes of loss of quality-adjusted life years and occur within situational contexts influenced by environmental circumstances [23]. The intersection of these preventable syndemics among Black women is cause for grave concern among public health professionals because they are linked to long histories of social injustices that result in contemporary assaults on Black women's bodies.

2.1 Intimate Partner Violence and Black Women

Black women experience high rates of IPV victimization and subsequent consequences [24, 25]. Approximately 1 in 2 Black women report lifetime experiences of IPV compared to 1 in 3 White women [26]. Most women report experiencing IPV before the age of 25 [27, 28]. Black women experiencing IPV are more likely to experience repeated abuse, reproductive coercion, and other negative health outcomes including risks for HIV transmission and mental health consequences [10]. In fact, compared to White women, Black women report higher rates of severe IPV [26], greater IPV frequency [29], and are more likely to be murdered by an abusive partner in the U.S. [30].

2.2 HIV Prevention and Black Women

Despite prevention efforts and an overall decrease in HIV incidence, Black women remain dispro-

portionally impacted by HIV. Among all cisgender women, Black women account for 54% of new HIV diagnoses while only comprising 13% of reproductive-aged women. Black women in the United States South are even more disparately affected, accounting for 67% of new HIV diagnoses among women in the region.

Pre-exposure prophylaxis (PrEP) has been approved for the prevention of HIV since 2012. Although 99% effective in preventing HIV transmission when taken appropriately, only 10% of eligible women are prescribed PrEP, and Black women are four times less likely to start PrEP than White women [31, 32]. Several key factors create barriers to PrEP uptake for Black women. Socio-structural factors such as racism, housing instability, and poverty reduce access to prevention and care services and are associated with an increase in condomless sex, multiple sexual partners, and trading sex for money. Additional barriers to PrEP uptake—specifically for Black women—are a lack of awareness and knowledge about PrEP, medical mistrust, few marketing campaigns directed at Black women, misperception of individual risk, poor patient–provider communication, and stigma associated with PrEP and HIV [33–35]. Despite these barriers, Black women are interested in taking PrEP if they are aware of it and have access to it. Yet, PrEP uptake and adherence remain low among Black women. Increasingly, researchers are calling for community-based interventions that include local organizations that consider Black women's social networks. These social networks may serve as catalysts for positive changes in community social norms and behavior [13, 14, 36]. Culturally relevant interventions leveraging trusted venues, such as beauty salons, can overcome these barriers and are urgently needed to advance the national priority of ending the HIV epidemic by 2030.

2.3 Strengths and Resilience Among Black Women

Black women build on existing sources of strength and use safety behaviors to overcome the effects of IPV and prevent HIV [37–40]. Black women experiencing IPV draw on internal and external sources of strength and employ safety strategies to overcome IPV and HIV-related stigma and preserve or improve their health [39, 41, 42]. For example, women experiencing IPV have reported accessing sources of strength to gain motivation to change their situation, leave their abuser, or take care of their health. Internal sources of strength often include spirituality/religion or belief in God [43, 44], and self-reliance or belief in oneself [38, 39]. External sources sometimes include accessing informal and formal resources for support. Examples of informal support resources include friends or family who care about the women [45]. Formal support resources for Black women experiencing IPV included police or court systems, IPV organizations, and clinical providers within larger healthcare systems. Feelings of empowerment and resiliency derived from a shared identity, unique strategies for coping, and awareness of social and political meaning can preserve Black women's well-being in the face of adversity [46, 47]. To build on the existing numerous strengths of Black women, community engagement in research and practice can include a facile, culturally relevant communications strategy to facilitate trust and transparency along with inclusion, belonging, and ownership of processes to examine sensitive topics such as IPV and HIV prevention.

3   Authors' Positionality: What Brought Us to This Work

We are both Black women nursing scientists and members of the inaugural 2020 cohort of the Betty Irene Moore Fellowship for Nurse Leaders and Innovators (health.ucdavis.edu/nursing/NurseLeaderFellows). We are situated within two top nursing schools in the U.S., and both have more than 10 years of experience conducting community-engaged work with Black women.

3.1   Kamila A. Alexander

Dr. Alexander specializes in the effects of IPV and trauma on health among marginalized people most affected by the HIV epidemic. She is an advanced practice public health registered nurse; her research includes over a decade of community-engaged mixed methods and qualitative research studies examining the lives of Black women. Dr. Alexander uses health equity and social justice lenses to examine the complex roles that intimate partner violence, HIV resilience, societal gender expectations, and economic opportunity play in the experience of intimate human relationships.

3.2   Schenita Davis Randolph

Dr. Schenita Davis Randolph is an interdisciplinary trained (nursing and public health) health equity scholar with expertise in community-engaged research and extensive experience leading and collaborating on research teams addressing health inequities and social determinants of health (SDoH) in the Black community. She has addressed the health disparities of underserved populations and racial and ethnic minority communities in the United States (U.S.) through direct clinical practice, public health efforts, and research as a registered nurse for over 25 years. More specifically, she is currently conducting research that informs the development and implementation of culturally and socially relevant interventions that will reduce the incidence and prevalence rates of sexually transmitted diseases and HIV among minorities in the Southeastern region of the United States.

3.3   Descriptions of the Research

3.3.1   W.I.N.G.S. (Women Integrating, Networking, and Growing in Spaces)

While the scientific literature addressing the epidemic of IPV among young women has grown exponentially in the past 15 years and interventions have demonstrated favorable prevention effects at the individual level, there continue to be gaps in our knowledge that will hamper the development of culturally relevant interventions for Black young women. In the W.I.N.G.S. research study, we examined one of the most marginalized populations experiencing high rates of IPV and HIV in the U.S.—Black queer young women ages 16–24 living in Maryland. This population experiences multiple marginalizations due to race, sexuality, age, and gender expression. In fact, this group of young women often encounter multiple stressors including stigma, discrimination, economic instability, and depression that may change the course of their daily activities, the spaces in which they engage in those activities, and the social networks they encounter. Our study aims were to: (1) describe the daily routines and activity space characteristics among Black young women experiencing recent IPV, and (2) examine the associations between safety strategies employed by Black women and their activity space characteristics.

3.3.2 UPDOs Protective Styles (Using PrEP, Doing It for Ourselves Protective Styles)

There are few evidence-based interventions that have been developed to address the heavy toll HIV takes on Black women, especially when there is a safe, effective way to reduce HIV transmission. Pre-exposure prophylaxis (PrEP) is a pill that prevents HIV infection when taken as prescribed. Men who have sex with men have been a focus for PrEP for years, but cisgender women have not been prioritized, especially Black cisgender women. To fill this gap, researchers and clinicians have partnered with Black cisgender women and beauty salons to codevelop UPDOs Protective Styles. While the primary focus of UPDOs is HIV prevention, it takes a comprehensive approach to addressing women's overall health. UPDOs Protective Styles is a salon-based intervention and partnership with researchers and local community members. UPDOs has three components: Stylist Training, a mini-series called The Wright Place, and PrEP

Navigation. The project aims to promote awareness, knowledge, and uptake of PrEP among Black women in the Southern United States. UPDOs takes a comprehensive approach, addressing the overall well-being of Black women.

4 Research Purpose and Methodological Approaches

4.1 W.I.N.G.S.

We used a trauma-informed human-centered design approach to examine the social networks and activity spaces among Black queer young women experiencing IPV to understand how those spaces might confer sexual risks or protections. Activity spaces include social and place-based networks, informal or formal ties, relationships, and interactions with individuals or spaces within a consistent time. In this research, we assumed that social influences are embedded within the structures of place, underpinning Black young women's socio-spatial place in society. These critical social interactions occur at specific locations within the daily routine, influencing perceptions of a place and the ties connecting people and behaviors at those locations [48].

Human-Centered Design (HCD) is a problem-solving, participatory design process that we used to uncover the factors and context relative to IPV and sexual experiences among Black queer adolescent and young adult women [49]. As part of this process, we used strategic communications to focus on collaboration and on codesigning the methodological approaches with young women affected by IPV. Thus, we created a youth advisory board (YAB) to center Black queer young women survivors' experiences throughout the research process. This research was accomplished in three steps. First, we used mixed methods to elicit qualitative stories about the ways Black queer women survivors engage in the spaces they inhabit in their daily lives. Second, we developed a social network and activity space inventory to quantitatively capture the most common experiences described in the qualitative narratives. Third, we conducted virtual interviews and measured short-term changes in the characteristics of activity spaces and social networks.

4.1.1 UP-Dos Protective Styles

This multicomponent, mixed-methods study used a community-engagement approach to develop and pilot test a salon-based intervention, UPDOs. Study procedures have been reported elsewhere [50]. Eligibility criteria included for this study included the following: (a) age 18 years or older, (b) frequency of visiting the salon at least every 2 weeks, (c) self-identification as Black or African American, (d) self-identification as a woman, and (e) ability to speak and read English.

UPDOs consist of three components: (a) stylist training, (b) women-focused edutainment videos and modules, and (c) engagement of PrEP Navigator. First, virtual or face-to-face stylist trainings were provided to beauty salon stylists in the community who saw primarily Black women as their clientele. A pretest-posttest design was used to examine the knowledge and awareness improvement of PrEP among stylists. Upon full completion of training, stylists received a certificate of completion and "Ask Me about PrEP" signage for their beauty salons to facilitate conversations with women. Second, together with the community, an edutainment series (The Wright Place) was codeveloped with Black women and an established community advisory council [50]. The series uses culturally and socially relevant stories to highlight key messages about (a) HIV, (b) PrEP, and (c) Black women's social contributors to health. UPDOs Protective Styles considers the complex interplay between individual, relationship, and community factors that can influence decision-making for women to start PrEP. Quantitative measures were used in a pretest-posttest design to examine PrEP knowledge, awareness, risk, stigma, trust, and intentions.

5 Creating a Shared Vision Using Strategic Communications

Black women are often omitted from partnerships or their representation is minimized within research, which makes eliminating health inequities and improving health outcomes difficult [51, 52]. Well-documented historical abuses to Black Americans and communities by researchers and clinicians have prevented trust in the research process as well as in the healthcare system [53]. Additionally, ongoing societal racism and socioeconomic inequities act as barriers to research participation, including limited knowledge about research opportunities, transportation, or childcare if the women wanted to participate [13, 14, 54, 55]. Thus, partnering with Black women for these projects is a crucial step to promote a strong communications plan and can paint a big picture of what we as researchers aspire to accomplish by describing a compelling image of what the future could be like. As researchers, we developed strategic communications plans to convey our visions of a larger purpose by adopting strategies that conveyed our beliefs through shared planning and goal-setting aligned with the values that engaged our communities and other supporters. Effective communication was bidirectional during our research processes.

6 Community Engagement Using Strategic Communications

6.1 W.I.N.G.S.

6.1.1 Establish Trust with Communities: Developing a Youth Advisory Board

To focus on collaboration and designing with Black queer women affected by IPV and not for them, we created a youth advisory board (YAB) to center their experiences throughout the research. Thus, between June 2021–June 2023, we engaged with nine YAB members to inform the conduct of the research. We created an information page and Instagram posts that linked to a brief application. Questions on the application elicited interests and experience working in a team and discerned how much time the applicant had available to participate in quarterly meetings about the research. Two example questions on the brief application included:

1. Why are you interested in joining the YAB
2. What do you think are three important issues facing Black women's health in your community today?

Responses to questions about why they were interested in joining the YAB included desires to make connections with peers and help support women who share similar experiences. They also wanted to gain a deeper understanding of themselves, to increase their self-esteem, confidence, and strengthen their communication skills. We also asked about pressing issues that young Black women face. Many discussed important issues related to increasing Black women's self-esteem and overall mental health. They also noted a need to address poor medical and mental health services, sexually transmitted diseases, and high rates of sexual assault within the community.

We expected applicants to reflect the community context and lived experiences of Black queer young women; thus, the YAB consisted of Black queer young women with self-disclosed IPV histories. While our goals for the YAB included activities to inform our recruitment strategy, interpret results, and support dissemination of research findings to a wider audience, the success of these activities hinged on building community and facilitating relationships. Therefore, we aligned activities with their stated interests for joining the YAB by regularly using strategic communication with the members to reassess their aims for serving on the board, provide study updates, and offer professional development opportunities. We planned face-to-face meetings on a quarterly basis.

6.1.2 Strategic Communications Strategies with YAB

To maintain connection in-between face-to-face meetings, we created a bimonthly newsletter that included educational information, study updates, polls to elicit input about research processes, and other interactive engagement strategies. The YAB also received training and education about sexual health, relationship abuse, and advocacy. They used these skills during attendance at a statewide conference held by the Maryland Coalition Against Sexual Assault's Women of Color Network and to create educational social media posts on our team accounts.

6.1.3 Promoting Sustainability of Research: Using Strategic Communications to Contribute to the Research Process

We considered the YAB members as coinvestigators throughout the research to open avenues for communication about this valuable role in communities. Thus, YAB members supported our data collector training by serving as mock interviewees, helped us refine our questions and aims, and improved the data collection processes based on the outcomes of mock interviews, practice surveys, and providing systematic evaluation. Table 1 describes important methodological contributions and collaborative analyses activities identified as a conduit for trust-building among our group of researchers, new learnings about the research process, and communications skill-building that laid foundations for sustainability.

Table 1 YAB methodological contributions and collaborative analysis activities

	Methodological contributions	Collaborative analysis
Qualitative Interviews	Piloted survey Piloted in-depth interviews	Identified themes and insights through affinity mapping
Quantitative Social Network and Activity Space Inventory	Piloted demographic survey Piloted network inventory	Collective and individual ideation about future services for Black young women experiencing IPV

6.2   Qualitative Interviews

6.2.1   Methodological Contributions

In August 2021, the team held mock in-depth interviews with YAB members. This process involved practicing the interview and following a structured cognitive-interview guide to elicit feedback at each section. This served as a training opportunity for research assistants to conduct in-depth interviews, refine our demographic and interview questions, and improve overall data collection processes. For example, the YAB recommended we remove repetition in some parts, add labels to facilitate discussion during the mapping portion of the interview, and create an additional survey choice of "did not happen" to lessen the likelihood respondents "skip" answering a particular question.

6.2.2   Data Analysis

In January 2022, YAB members met with the study team to discuss and analyze preliminary data from the qualitative interviews. Using a word cloud built from the people and places participants reported during five in-depth initial interviews, the YAB discussed, categorized, and described the ways they make meaning related to each of the people and places. Over the course of multiple iterative discussions, we developed and revised the network inventory questions designed to capture the most common people and places where Black young women experience safety as well as the most common sites of violence experiences [2, 3].

7   Social Network and Activity Space Inventory

7.1   Methodological Contributions

The Social Network and Activity Space Inventory, hereafter called Network Inventory (NI), was designed to assess the characteristics of people and places in participant networks. We designed this data collection tool to be delivered by a research assistant and it was developed through an iterative revision process informed both by

qualitative interview data and YAB feedback. In June 2022, we worked together as a team to improve the demographic survey flow and refine the language. For example, one YAB member highlighted that language around our efforts to maintain confidentiality needed clarification. Furthermore, practicing the administration of the NI assisted the study team to improve the NI instrument and streamline our overall data collection protocols. This activity also maintained YAB members' connection to the larger goals of the research project and their role in moving it forward—a key strategic communications strategy.

7.2   YAB Personal and Professional Development

Professional development offerings were another feature of engagement as a team. The team solicited feedback from the YAB regarding types of professional development they might want. They expressed interest in networking, résumé development, and online professional courses. They also wished to locate health professionals from whom Black young women could confidently seek services and resources for LTBTQ+ health support. Some YAB members also expressed a need for community resources related to financial assistance, housing, mental health, and medical care. Thus, we expanded and refined our research team's resource guide to address a broad scope of needs as suggested by the YAB members. The tailored resource guide is part of an overall communications strategy for all study participants and community members and is featured on our website (threadsresearchlab.org).

7.3   Dissemination of Research Findings Back to Communities: Data Synthesis Through Community Conversations & Creative Workshops

We held two community conversations in collaboration with our community partner, Ballet

After Dark (balletafterdark.com), that provides somatic therapies to Black women survivors of violence. In response to the team's data, the workshops focused on community members identifying modalities for survivorship and healing spaces in Baltimore. We used arts-based strategic communications approaches designed to share some of our research findings and to elicit conversations about ways Black women can cocreate support within their social and activity-space networks. In each session, participants engaged in creative outlets such as movement and journaling in order to give input on future programming. We provided a meal as well as compensation for the time community members spent with us. All participants were identified as Black women survivors between the ages of 16 and 24 years old. In the first workshop, participants created affinity maps using text data collected from qualitative interviews. Each participant received a group of quotations and were asked to find patterns, group them, and identify a name that characterized each group. These quotes were placed as Post-its on a board that we referred to as Affinity Maps. We then asked them to select a quote that stood out for them and to create a collage to visually represent the Affinity Maps.

In-between workshop sessions, participants completed a photo-journal exercise responding to the following prompts (see Fig. 1):

1. Take a picture of somewhere that feels like a safe space.
   What makes it feel safe to you and why?
2. Take a picture that relates to one of the quotes or themes found in the research. How does it relate?

Participant photos described a range of spaces where they found safety including personal and private spaces such as their bedrooms and public spaces such as a nature trail (see Fig. 5). Rooms in private spaces are not shown due to privacy concerns.

In the second workshop, participants focused on ideation and developing prototypes to reflect on the previous activities (i.e., quotes, affinity maps, photo-journals, and collages). They were asked to determine what resources they would create to support queer Black women survivors of IPV and develop a visual representation of their ideas (see Fig. 2).

When asked to describe their prototypes, they described prototypes that ranged from a space that provided resources to women under one roof where respite, educational opportunities, and

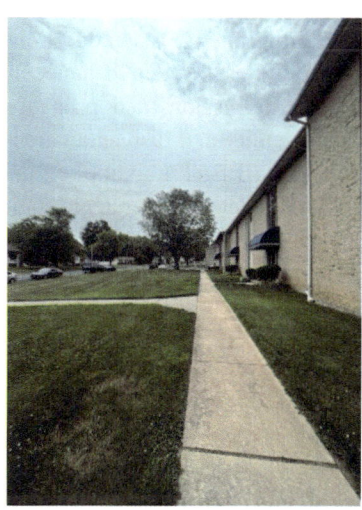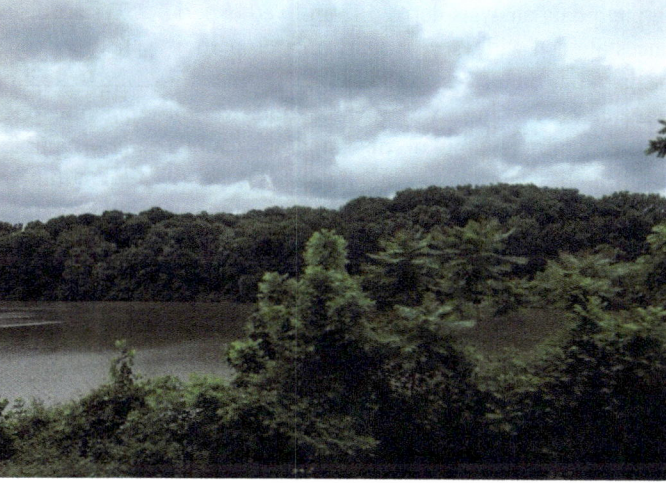

Fig. 1 Photos of Safe Spaces
Photo courtesy of Kamila Alexander

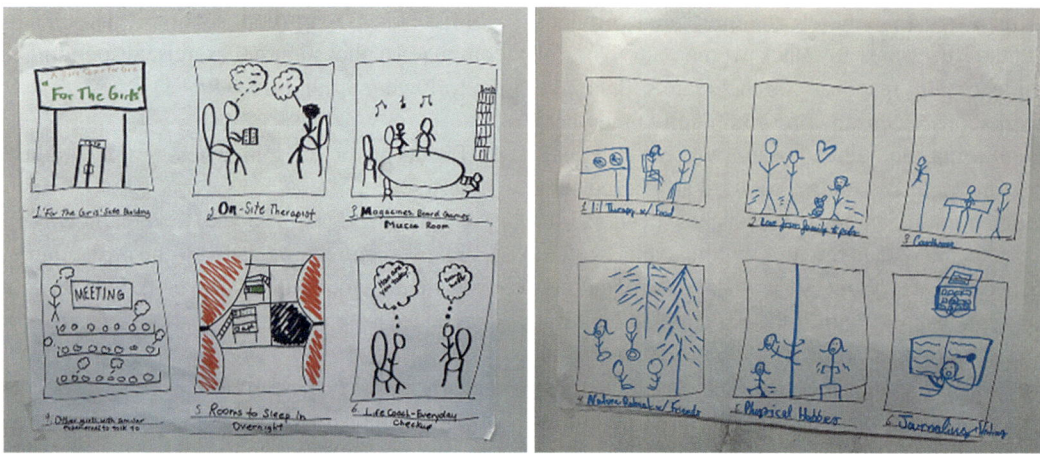

Fig. 2 Storyboard prototypes depicting visions of a safe future for black women and girls
Photo courtesy of Kamila Alexander

community with other women experiencing relationship challenges were priorities. Additional aspirations for their ideal spaces included self-care experts and a place to express hobbies through distraction such as with music or games. Some women wanted to transform existing spaces, such as the courthouse where they were expected to face the person who used violence against them, into a safer place to be heard.

In this study, W.I.N.G.S., strategic communications techniques were employed *within* the research process over time as a source of engagement for community and YAB members. The YAB purposefully communicated meaning through data analysis derived from lived experiences aligned with those of our research participants. They helped us validate and refine our research goals using a variety of methods to gain greater understanding of an important public health issue facing our communities. We cocreated messaging for materials, built community for the participants, and derived support for future interventions and programming that can make meaningful change for their peers. Use of strategic communications among our team of researchers enhanced our ability to create sustainable models for violence prevention that are culturally and experientially derived. In the next section, we discuss an exemplar that demonstrates the *external* application of strategic communications with partners.

7.4 UPDOs Protective Styles

The addressing Health disparities through Engagement, Equity, Advocacy, and Trust (HEEAT) Research Lab has prioritized effective strategic communications throughout the research process from development to dissemination. Using the 5Ws framework (see Fig. 7), we provided a retrospective analysis of the HEEAT Lab's experience using strategic communications in nurse-business partnerships (i.e., a community advisory council of salons and barbershops) in sexual health and HIV research with Black women living in the Southern United States. The 5Ws are categories representing lists of questions that function as a tool for assessment that encourage reflection, open discussion, and proactive planning to advance equity and dismantle structural racism [56]. The HEEAT Lab applied the use of this framework to develop a strategic communications plan that outlined strategies for communicating research throughout the research process from conception to dissemination of findings.

Table 2 outlines the 5Ws framework questions to consider ensuring an equity lens in community-partnered research and questions to consider in the development of a strategic communications plan. "Who" thoroughly examines inclusion and exclusion of "all parties involved in research from conception to dissemination." "What" inter-

Table 2 The 5Ws framework applied to strategic communications

	Framework questions	Framework applied to strategic communications
Who?	Who benefits? Who is harmed? Who is excluded? Who makes decisions? Who do systems prioritize? Who is made comfortable? Who is cited? Who is called an expert? Who can lead research?	Who needs to receive communications about research project/program?
Why?	Why is this project relevant? Why use this approach? Why should someone want to be involved? Why this research topic? Why this group of interest? Why you? Why not you?	Why is this communication relevant? Why is this strategic communication approach needed?
What?	What resources? What is the access? What values are prioritized? What languages are excluded? What are the accommodations? What variable are used or excluded?	What is important to communicate? What is important to communicate using specific communication strategies (videos, print, audio, etc.)?
When?	When did it become a priority? When do research activities occur? When is waiting acceptable, and for whom?	When is the best time to communicate with stakeholders?
Where?	Where does power sit? Where do you have to go? Where are resources shared? Where are findings shared? Where is this research going? Where does the money go?	Where do we want to communicate to ensure all stakeholders receive communication messages? Where are research findings shared?

rogates "the circumstances and extent of research activities" including the prioritization of resources that "reflect the research's equitable values" and leading to questions of "whether or not resources are deemed relevant, affordable, or valuable." "When" speaks to time and waiting or "whose time is prioritized" as time equity and autonomy are "often trivialized and overlooked" and are intimately connected to cost or money, acknowledgement, determination of scientific contribution, workload, and expectations. "Where" questions the nature of and decision-making around locations as sources of equitable access and participation, especially considering the "history of discrimination and disinvestment in Black and Brown communities" and how that context influences desire to and possibility of participation. As a result, "Where" probes beyond the surface to questions of the practical (logistics and convenience) and symbolic (authenticity and centering expertise). Finally, "Why" investigates intentionality through questions of status quo methodological design, implementation, and data analysis that focus on process combined with assumptions about race in process. The intersection of questions and responses across category are expected (see Fig. 3) [56].

Who needs to receive communication? The HEEAT Lab identified key stakeholders as being significant in needing to receive communication. These included the 10-member community advisory council (CAC), Black women who were eligible to participate in the research, beauty salons, and the broader community, which consists of lay members, policy makers, funders, and advocates. To effectively communicate with all stakeholders listed above, a website was developed: theheeatlab.org. This site was created with the community as a priority. Thus, we wanted to make sure that the graphics and layout of the site were culturally and socially acceptable and engaging. A short clip video was developed with input from the CAC. The video highlighted the UPDOs project purpose and significance. This video not only served as information-sharing but was useful for recruitment and dissemination at conferences and other community presentations. Throughout the research process we also prioritized informing the broader community of our engagement with community members as researchers. To do this, we shared our work in a community facing magazine, HUAMI (pronounced who am I). HUAMI magazine has a focus on highlighting individuals and businesses and connecting them with Black communities. The magazine is distributed in print to businesses throughout the community including barbershops and beauty salons where patrons can read while awaiting services. There is

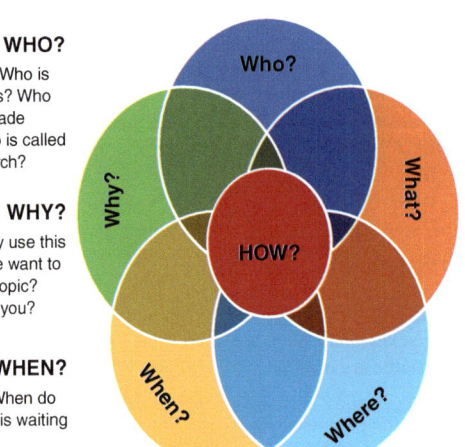

Fig. 3 5Ws of Racial Equity in Research Framework [56]

also an online version with a reach in multiple states in the southern region of the United States (North and South Carolina, Georgia, Texas, Florida) and California. See two articles here: https://issuu.com/terrywatson7/docs/issuu_may_2022/6?fr=sYjcyZjUwMTcyNjI

https://issuu.com/terrywatson7/docs/louisville2/s/24930527.

Why? When looking at the *why* applied to strategic communications, it is important to communicate to stakeholders the relevancy of the research and why the research topic is important. The *why* helps to communicate the vision and mission behind the work. To highlight the *why*, the HEEAT Lab's strategy for communication was the use of print media and audio such as a podcast. Communicating to the broader community about Black women and HIV inequities raised awareness to the community, advocates, policy makers, and funders about the significance of the problem. In the lab's communication plan, research was highlighted with journalists through news articles and podcasts. These communication strategies have a large impact due to the number of people who are reached and who would not read about the research in academic journals or attend conferences where research is often shared. Exemplars of news stories can be found on the heeatlab.org website under UPDOs Publications.

What? Linking *what* based on the 5Ws, it is important to not only know what to communicate, but also to consider what resources are available for a communications plan to be executed. Having the resources to engage a communication strategist or specialists, a website developer, and graphic designer adds great value to a research team. Through multiple funding mechanisms, the HEEAT Lab Principal Investigator and Founding Director was able to hire a communication strategist as an ad hoc member of the research team. The expertise of a communications specialist helps to translate research language into layperson's terms that will be understood by the community and create messages that are culturally and socially acceptable. It is a core value of the lab to disseminate research findings not only in peer-reviewed journals and conferences but also for every journal article submitted, wherein a communication is developed that can be disseminated back to the community. Using a QR code, the team placed the information in beauty salons that partnered in this work to allow community members to know the results of the study. This dissemination was also made available in the HUAMI magazine story. Finally, branding the HEEAT Lab with a logo (see Fig. 4) allows the community and other stakeholders to recognize research translation to address the community's most pressing challenges.

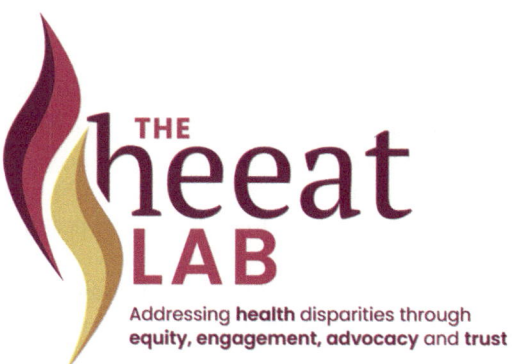

Fig. 4 The HEEAT lab logo

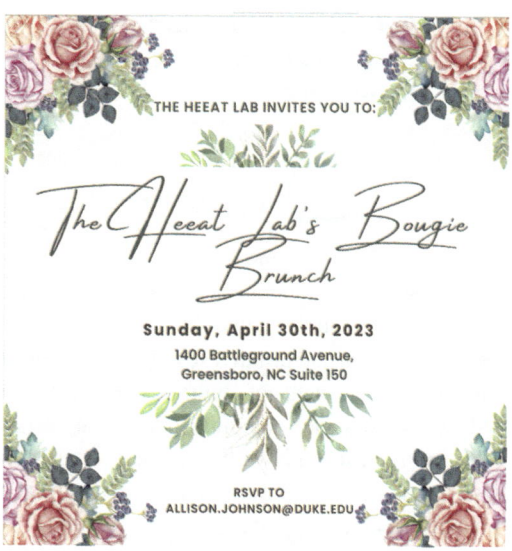

Fig. 5 Invitation for dissemination brunch

When? Aligning with the equity framework applied to strategic communications, knowing *when* to communicate with stakeholders is crucial to building and maintaining trust, sustaining programs and interventions, and measuring impact. One strategy in the lab's plan was to release communication messages during specific recognized months; for example, National Women and Girls HIV/AIDS Awareness Day. These messages could include a new story, invited guest on a podcast, or social media post. Communicating often and concisely keeps the community aware and engaged in the work. One of the main barriers for communities of color in research is that many researchers do not communicate with them after the data collection process; therefore, they often have no idea what happened with the work. This creates barriers for future research engagement and trustworthiness of the research process.

Where? Communicating to Black women and their communities of influence must be prioritized in order to have meaningful impact in addressing HIV and IPV among Black women. Researchers in academia cannot disseminate research findings solely in peer-reviewed journals and at academic conferences. The lack of dissemination back to communities perpetuates the structural and systemic racism, which is the foundation of many Black communities' reluctance to engage in research. Dissemination of research should include conferences and forums with and in communities. Intentional planning to reengage research participants after data collection and analysis promotes trustworthiness. An example of this is the HEEAT Lab's catered brunch that was organized with beauty salons and stylists' consultants. Women who participated in the UPDOs pilot testing were invited to attend the brunch and given the opportunity to invite one guest (see invitation, Fig. 5). At the brunch, the research team gave an overview of Black Women's health, HIV, and PrEP. Stylists' consultants shared their roles in the research and highlighted beauty salons as trusted partners in health promotion activities. Finally, results of the study and the next steps of the research were shared with attendees. There were 22 attendees, including four CAC members. We developed magnets with culturally appropriate photos to be displayed at stylist stations in the beauty salon or on mirrors in the bathrooms. This gave women the opportunity to learn about PrEP by scanning the QR code that gave an overview of PrEP, its use among Black women, and where to access PrEP if interested.

8   Reflections on Using Strategic Communications In Research

According to the Centers for Disease Control's principles of community engagement, there is a continuum of participation that describes increasing levels of involvement, impact, trust, and communication flow among community members. The overall goal of community engagement is to improve health promotion and health research. We described our common core value of community engagement and ways strategic communication approaches could be used to amplify the impact of research designed to support positive outcomes for Black women's health, safety, and overall well-being.

Communication flows at each step of the continuum are important markers of engagement (see Fig. 6). During the first step of the continuum—Outreach—communication flows from one to the other and is geared towards informing communities. The second step— Consulting— describes more community involvement and communication flows to the community and then back with a goal of seeking answers to pressing issues. In the third and fourth steps—Involve and Collaborate, respectively—communication flows both ways and is participatory across all parties

with increased intensity and touchpoints. The fifth and final step—Shared Leadership—features a communications flow that includes final decision-making at the community level. These different levels of communication provide opportunities for outcomes that have an increasing impact on connection, trust, and overall health.

In this chapter, we described diverse ways to develop and use strategic communications strategies to amplify messages with internal and external partners of two specific research projects. Common goals across these two research studies included meaningful strategies to engage with communities of Black women who are the most important partners in improving their health and in making decisions for themselves and their families. Strategic communications can include strategies internal to the research process and requires a plan for external dissemination to reach the broadest possible audience.

For example, during the time of the W.I.N.G.S. project, the Threads Research Lab became a reality through creation of a website (threadsresearchlab. org) for the research team to describe the team's activities, students, and staff, and, most importantly, convey our research mission and values. The YAB members became part of this process and are featured on the website. Our website and newslet-

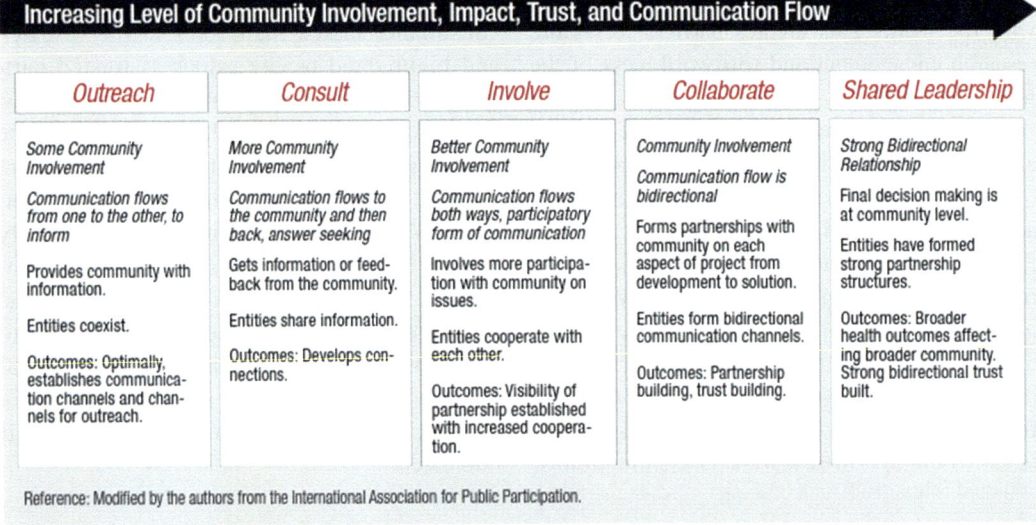

Fig. 6 Community engagement continuum

ter became part of a larger strategic communications strategy to convey a program of research focused on promoting the health and safety of Black women and girls. Our engagement in community activities is a shining feature of our work, cultivating sustainable trusting relationships.

The future for strategic communications as a community-engagement strategy is full of promise as a transformational approach to influencing research, practice, and policy. Integrating concepts such as anti-racism and cultural humility into community-engaged research are challenging yet compulsory activities that contribute to a broader social contract between the scientific endeavors we pursue as nurse scientists and our commitment to addressing the disproportionate health inequities experiences among Black women.

Using strategic communications approaches in our community-engaged research provides opportunities for broad impact by influencing policy, changing public opinion or informing debate, improving systems, designs, or processes that directly impact Black women and their communities. Our research demonstrates that trust and relationship-building are at the forefront of any strategic communications plan, and it should be directed towards internal and external stakeholders to cultivate urgency in meeting the goal of eliminating the injustices and health inequities that overwhelmingly affect Black women. Our communications plans are diverse in scope to maximize impact in many different realms. Internally, strategic communications approaches are a feature of cocreating a research plan that is equitable and sustainable for researchers and community partners. We generate interest in our research across mediums such as social media, traditional media outlets, and community-based conference presentations.

Using strategic communications strategies to promote health and safety for Black women requires a comprehensive approach that addresses broader and social health contexts. Thoughtful and culturally relevant strategic communication should be integrated into a holistic approach that aims to reduce health inequities and minimize structural harms.

Implications for Policy-Makers

- Advocate for policies that increase transparency of information sharing among Black women and service providers charged with serving them.
- Advocate for policies that support initiatives that incentivize using strategic communications strategies to package health programs and broaden their reach.
- Increase policy efforts that use strategic communications to reduce health inequities by making bold changes to mitigate the adverse social determinants of health that limit the potential for optimal health among Black women.

Implications for Researchers

- Engage community members, leaders, and organizations to enhance the effectiveness of health communication strategies and ensure they are culturally relevant.
- Invest in data collection and analyses processes that use specified techniques for engagement among Black women. Improved data can inform targeted health campaigns and improve experiences of research participation.
- Establish rigorous methods to monitor and evaluate the impact of strategic communications efforts to ensure that the approaches are working as they were intended.

Implications for Practitioners

- Promote health literacy and education among Black women to ignite existing knowledge and tools to make informed decisions about their personal health.
- Strategic communications can be powerful tools to influence changes from destigmatizing language about sensitive topics such as sexual health and relationship conflicts often associated with intimate partner violence.
- Encourage the media to depict accurate and positive images of Black women taking care of their health. This can influence perceptions of self-efficacy related to health.

Box 1 Developing a Strategic Communications Plan to Amplify Your Research

We offer the following five tips for developing an effective community-engaged communications strategy that is engaging and is aligned with principles of health equity:

1. Make sure all information about your research is communicated in a transparent way.

   The more you share and the easier you make information to understand, it is more likely that community partners will want to engage to understand your intentions, what their role is, and how it may affect them.

2. Communicate with your partners in a way that works for them. Recognize that each person or community is different and select the most suitable communication channel to reach them. Offer a variety of options to communicate and ensure they can access it to provide their input.

3. Do not judge what your community partners value. Instead, seek to understand why. Keep an open and curious attitude to help your team understand the history and concerns of the people you serve. This approach creates opportunities to be creative in finding solutions to overcome adversity using aligned values and interests throughout the process.

4. Provide feedback to community partners about how their interests and issues are addressed and resolved. Track commitments made and build in activities to ensure accountability.

5. Maintain a careful record of all aspects of your communication with community partners that occur over time. This action avoids miscommunication and is especially pertinent during multiyear projects where team members can change time.

References

1. Alexander KA. Social determinants of HIV/AIDS and intimate partner violence: interrogating the role of race, ethnicity and skin color. Rev Lat Am Enfermagem. 2020;28:e3280. https://doi.org/10.1590/1518-8345.0000.3280.
2. Alexander KA, Britton C, Warnke ES, McCree DS, Tobin KE. 44. Perceptions of safety: characterizing activity spaces among black adolescent young adult sexual minority women with intimate partner violence histories in Baltimore, MD. J Adolesc Health. 2023a;72(3):S29. https://doi.org/10.1016/j.jadohealth.2022.11.065.
3. Alexander KA, Mpundu G, Duroseau B, Osian N, Chambers S, McCree DJ, et al. Intervention approaches to address intimate partner violence and HIV: a scoping review of recent research. Curr HIV/AIDS Rep. 2023b;20(5):296–311. https://doi.org/10.1007/S11904-023-00668-8/TABLES/2.
4. Seth P, Wingood GM, Robinson LSS, Raiford JL, DiClemente RJ. Abuse impedes prevention: the intersection of intimate partner violence and HIV/STI risk among young African American women. AIDS Behav. 2015;19(8):1438–45. https://doi.org/10.1007/S10461-014-0940-7/FIGURES/1.
5. Phillips DY, Walsh B, Bullion JW, Reid PV, Bacon K, Okoro N. The intersection of intimate partner violence and HIV in U.S. Women: a review. J Assoc Nurses AIDS Care. 2014;25(Suppl. 1) https://doi.org/10.1016/j.jana.2012.12.006.
6. Leddy AM, Zakaras JM, Shieh J, Conroy AA, Ofotokun I, Tien PC, Weiser SD. Intersections of food insecurity, violence, poor mental health and substance use among US women living with and at risk for HIV: evidence of a syndemic in need of attention. PLoS ONE. 2021;16(5):e0252338. https://doi.org/10.1371/JOURNAL.PONE.0252338.
7. DuMonthier A, Childers C, Milli J. The status of black women in the United States; 2020. Retrieved from https://iwpr.org/wp-content/uploads/2020/08/The-Status-of-Black-Women-6.26.17.pdf.
8. Gosangi B, Park H, Thomas R, Gujrathi R, Bay CP, Raja AS, et al. Exacerbation of physical intimate partner violence during COVID-19 lockdown. Radiology. 2020:202866. https://doi.org/10.1148/radiol.2020202866.
9. Feinstein BA, Turner BC, Beach LB, Korpak AK, Phillips G. Racial/ethnic differences in mental health, substance use, and bullying victimization among self-identified bisexual high school-aged youth. LGBT Health. 2019;6(4):174–83. https://doi.org/10.1089/LGBT.2018.0229.
10. Holliday CN, Mccauley HL, Silverman JG, Ricci E, Decker MR, Tancredi DJ, et al. Racial/ethnic differences in women's experiences of reproductive coercion, intimate partner violence, and unintended pregnancy. J Women's Health. 2017;26(8) https://doi.org/10.1089/jwh.2016.5996.

11. Tekeste M, Hull S, Dovidio JF, Safon CB, Blackstock O, Taggart T, et al. Differences in medical mistrust between black and white women: implications for patient–provider communication about PrEP. AIDS Behav. 2019;23(7):1737–48. https://doi.org/10.1007/S10461-018-2283-2/FIGURES/1.

12. Fray NA, Caldwell KL. Communication between middle SES black women and healthcare providers about HIV Testing. J Natl Med Assoc. 2017;109(2):115. https://doi.org/10.1016/J.JNMA.2016.11.005.

13. Randolph SD, Golin C, Welgus H, Lightfoot AF, Harding CJ, Riggins LF. How perceived structural racism and discrimination and medical mistrust in the health system influences participation in HIV health services for black women living in the United States South: a qualitative, descriptive study. J Assoc Nurses AIDS Care. 2020a;31(5):598–605. https://doi.org/10.1097/JNC.0000000000000189.

14. Randolph SD, Johnson R, Meyers D, Washington D, Saint-Hillaire L. Leveraging social networks of Black women in beauty salons to improve uptake of pre-exposure prophylaxis. Health Educ J. 2020b;80(1):95–105. https://doi.org/10.1177/0017896920959383.

15. Jackson GY, Darlington CK, Van Tieu H, Brawner BM, Flores DD, Bannon JA, et al. Women's views on communication with health care providers about pre-exposure prophylaxis (PrEP) for HIV prevention. Culture Health Sexual. 2022;24(5):642–56. https://doi.org/10.1080/13691058.2021.1877824.

16. Sharpless L, Kershaw T, Hatcher A, Alexander KA, Katague M, Phillips K, Willie TC. IPV, PrEP, and medical mistrust. J Acquir Immune Defici Syndr. 2022;90(3):283–90. https://doi.org/10.1097/QAI.0000000000002956.

17. Macnamara J. A review of new evaluation models for strategic communication: progress and gaps. Int J Strategic Commun. 2018;12(2):180–95. https://doi.org/10.1080/1553118X.2018.1428978.

18. Fix RL, Busso DS, Mendelson T, Letourneau EJ. Changing the paradigm: Using strategic communications to promote recognition of child sexual abuse as a preventable public health problem. Child Abuse Neglect. 2021;117:105061. https://doi.org/10.1016/J.CHIABU.2021.105061.

19. Kreps GL. The role of strategic communication to respond effectively to pandemics. J Multicult Discours. 2021;16(1):12–9. https://doi.org/10.1080/17447143.2021.1885417.

20. Maibach EW, Kreps GL, Bonaguro EW. Developing strategic communication campaigns for HIV/AIDS prevention. In: Ratzan SC, editor. AIDS: effective health communication for the 90s. 1st ed. Routledge; 2014. p. 15–35. https://doi.org/10.4324/9781315061429-3.

21. Sigma Theta Tau International. The Woodhull study on nursing and the media: health care's invisible partner. Indianapolis: Center Nursing Press; 1997.

22. Mason DJ, Nixon L, Glickstein B, Han S, Westphaln K, Carter L. The Woodhull study revisited: nurses' representation in health news media 20 years later. Wiley Online Library. 2018;50(6):695–704. https://doi.org/10.1111/jnu.12429.

23. Sharps PW, Njie-Carr VPS, Alexander K. The syndemic interaction of intimate partner violence, sexually transmitted infections, and HIV infection among african american women: best practices and strategies. J Aggress Maltreat Trauma. 2019; https://doi.org/10.1080/10926771.2019.1667464.

24. Alexander KA, Volpe EM, Abboud S, Campbell JC. Reproductive coercion, sexual risk behaviours and mental health symptoms among young low-income behaviourally bisexual women: implications for nursing practice. J Clin Nurs. 2016;25(23–24):3533–44. https://doi.org/10.1111/jocn.13238.

25. Alexander KA, Willie TC, McDonald-Mosley R, Campbell JC, Miller E, Decker MR. Associations between reproductive coercion, partner violence, and mental health symptoms among young black women in Baltimore, Maryland. J Interpers Violence. 2019:886260519860900. https://doi.org/10.1177/0886260519860900.

26. Smith SG, Chen J, Basile KC, Gilbert LK, Merrick MT, Patel N, Waling J, Jain A. The national intimate partner and sexual violence survey: 2010–2012 state report. Centers for Disease Control and Prevention; 2017. Retrieved from https://www.cdc.gov/violenceprevention/pdf/NISVS-StateReportBook.pdf

27. Black MC, Basile KC, Breiding MJ, Ryan GW. Prevalence of sexual violence against women in 23 states and two U.S. Territories, BRFSS 2005. Violence Against Women. 2014;20(5):485–99. https://doi.org/10.1177/1077801214528856.

28. Breiding MJ, Smith SG, Basile KC, Walters ML, Chen J, Merrick MT. Prevalence and characteristics of sexual violence, stalking, and intimate partner violence victimization—national intimate partner and sexual violence survey, United States, 2011. Morbid Mortal Weekly Rep: Surv Summaries. 2014;63(SS08):1–18. Retrieved from https://www.cdc.gov/mmwr/preview/mmwrhtml/ss6308a1.htm?s_cid=ss6308a1_e#Table6

29. Mcdonnell KA, Gielen AC, O'campo P. Does HIV status make a difference in the experience of lifetime abuse? Descriptions of lifetime abuse and its context among low-income urban women. J Urban Health. 2003;80(3):494–509. https://doi.org/10.1093/jurban/jtg047.

30. Violence Policy Center. When men murder women: an analysis of 2015 homicide data; 2017. Washington, DC. Retrieved from http://www.vpc.org/publications.

31. Knight D, Saleem HT, Stockman JK, Willie TC. Experiences of black women in the United States along the PrEP care continuum: a scoping review. AIDS Behav. 2023;27(7):2298–316. https://doi.org/10.1007/S10461-022-03960-7/FIGURES/1.

32. CDC. Racism and Health. 2021. Retrieved September 6, 2022, from https://www.cdc.gov/healthequity/racism-disparities/index.html

33. Auerbach JD, Kinsky S, Brown G, Charles V. Knowledge, attitudes, and likelihood of pre-

exposure prophylaxis (PrEP) use among US women at risk of acquiring HIV. AIDS Patient Care STDs. 2015;29(2):102–10.

34. Nydegger LA, Dickson-Gomez J, Ko TK. Structural and syndemic barriers to PrEP adoption among black women at high risk for HIV: a qualitative exploration. Culture Health Sexual. 2021;23(5):659–73. https://doi.org/10.1080/13691058.2020.1720297.

35. Willie TC, Monger M, Nunn A, Kershaw T, Stockman JK, Mayer KH, et al. "PrEP's just to secure you like insurance": a qualitative study on HIV pre-exposure prophylaxis (PrEP) adherence and retention among black cisgender women in Mississippi. BMC Infect Dis. 2021;21(1):1–12. https://doi.org/10.1186/S12879-021-06786-1/TABLES/1.

36. Johnson R, Myers D, McKellar M, Saint-Hillaire L, Randolph SD. Perspectives of Black women in the United States on salon-based intervention to promote the uptake of pre-exposure prophylaxis (PrEP) for HIV. J Clin Nurs. 2021;30(21–22):3281–9. https://doi.org/10.1111/JOCN.15838.

37. Koch A, Ritchwood TD, Bailey DE, Caiola CE, Adimora AA, Ramirez C, et al. Exploring resilience among black women living with HIV in the Southern United States: findings from a qualitative study. J Assoc Nurses AIDS Care. 2022;33(2):224. https://doi.org/10.1097/JNC.0000000000000311.

38. Sabri B, Holliday CN, Alexander KA, Huerta J, Cimino A, Callwood GB, Campbell JC. Cumulative violence exposures: black women's responses and sources of strength. Social Work Public Health. 2016;31(3) https://doi.org/10.1080/19371918.2015.1087917.

39. St Vil NM, Sabri B, Nwokolo V, Alexander KA, Campbell JC. A qualitative study of survival strategies used by low-income black women who experience intimate partner violence. Soc Work (United States). 2017;62(1) https://doi.org/10.1093/sw/sww080.

40. West CM. Violence in the lives of black women: battered, black, and blue. Taylor and Francis; 2013.

41. Dailey AF, Johnson AS, Wu B. HIV care outcomes among blacks with diagnosed HIV—United States, 2014; 2017. Retrieved from https://www.cdc.gov/mmwr/cme/conted_info.html#weekly.

42. Lilly MM, Graham-Bermann SA. Ethnicity and risk for symptoms of posttraumatic stress following intimate partner violence prevalence and predictors in European American and African American Women. J Interpers Violence. 2009;24(1):3–19. https://doi.org/10.1177/0886260508314335.

43. Buseh AG, Stevens PE. Constrained but not determined by stigma: resistance by African American women living with HIV. Women Health. 2006;44(3):1–18. Retrieved from http://www.scopus.com/inward/record.url?eid=2-s2.0-33846625200&partnerID=40&md5=f6b0bf984b30644071289130aab92f02

44. Logie C, James L, Tharao W, Loutfy M. Associations between HIV-related stigma, racial discrimina-

tion, gender discrimination, and depression among HIV-positive African, Caribbean, and Black women in Ontario, Canada. AIDS Patient Care STDs. 2013;27(2):114–22. https://doi.org/10.1089/apc.2012.0296.

45. Geter A, Sutton MY, Mccree DH. AIDS care psychological and socio-medical aspects of AIDS/HIV Social and structural determinants of HIV treatment and care among black women living with HIV infection: a systematic review: 2005–2016. AIDS Care. 2018;30(4):409–16. https://doi.org/10.1080/09540121.2018.1426827.

46. El-Khoury MY, Dutton MA, Goodman LA, Engel L, Belamaric RJ, Murphy M. Ethnic differences in battered women's formal help-seeking strategies: a focus on health, mental health, and spirituality. Cult Divers Ethnic Minor Psychol. 2004;10(4):383–93. https://doi.org/10.1037/1099-9809.10.4.383.

47. Morrison KE, Luchok KJ, Richter DL, Parra-Medina D. Factors influencing help-seeking from informal networks among African American victims of intimate partner violence. J Interpers Violence. 2006;21(11):1493–511. https://doi.org/10.1177/0886260506293484.

48. Mennis J, Mason MJ. People, places, and adolescent substance use: integrating activity space and social network data for analyzing health behavior. Ann Assoc Am Geogr. 2011;101(2):272–91. https://doi.org/10.1080/00045608.2010.534712.

49. Chen E, Leos C, Kowitt SD, Moracco KE. Enhancing community-based participatory research through human-centered design strategies. Health Promot Pract. 2019;21(1):37–48. https://doi.org/10.1177/1524839919850557.

50. Randolph SD, Johnson R, Johnson A, Keusch L. Using PrEP and doing it for ourselves (UPDOs Protective Styles), a web-based salon intervention to improve uptake of pre-exposure prophylaxis among black women: protocol for a pilot feasibility study. JMIR Res Protoc. 2022;11(8):e34556. https://doi.org/10.2196/34556.

51. Chen MS, Lara PN, Dang JHT, Paterniti DA, Kelly K. Twenty years post-NIH Revitalization Act: enhancing minority participation in clinical trials (EMPaCT): laying the groundwork for improving minority clinical trial accrual. Cancer. 2014;120:1091–6. https://doi.org/10.1002/CNCR.28575.

52. Konkel L. Racial and ethnic disparities in research studies: the challenge of creating more diverse cohorts. Environ Health Perspect. 2015;123(12):A297–302. https://doi.org/10.1289/EHP.123-A297.

53. Washington HA. Medical apartheid: the dark history of medical experimentation on Black Americans from colonial times to the present. Doubleday Books; 2006. p. 501.

54. Bowleg L, Malekzadeh AN, Mbaba M, Boone CA. Ending the HIV epidemic for all, not just some: structural racism as a fundamental but overlooked social-structural determinant of the US HIV epidemic.

Curr Opin HIV AIDS. 2022;17(2):40–5. https://doi.org/10.1097/COH.0000000000000724.

55. Luebbert R, Perez A. Barriers to clinical research participation among African Americans. J Transcult Nurs. 2016;27(5):456–63. https://doi.org/10.1177/1043659615575578.

56. Bentley-Edwards KL, Jordan Fleming P, Doherty IA, Whicker DR, Mervin-Blake S, Barrett NJ. The 5Ws of racial equity in research: a framework for applying a racial equity lens throughout the research process. Health Equity. 2022;6(1):917–21. https://doi.org/10.1089/HEQ.2022.0042.

Kamila A. Alexander PhD, MPH, RN, is an Associate Professor, inaugural holder of the Natalie and Wes Bush Rising Professorship, and Director of the PhD and Postdoctoral programs at the Johns Hopkins School of Nursing. Her research examines the socio-structural determinants of trauma and violence on sexual, mental, and reproductive health outcomes among marginalized young people. She is the Director and Principal Investigator of the Threads Research Lab. Dr. Alexander is recognized for her scientific and community-engaged leadership as a member of the inaugural cohort of Betty Irene Moore Fellowships for Nurse Leaders and Innovators. Dr. Alexander earned a BS in Exercise Science from Howard University, a BSN and MSN/MPH from Johns Hopkins School of Nursing, and a PhD in Nursing Science from the University of Pennsylvania. Her goals are not only to promote health and prevent morbidities but to lead and create investigations that affect practice and policy on a global scale.

Schenita D. Randolph PhD, MPH, RN, FAAN, is an Associate Professor at Duke University School of Nursing, Inaugural Fellow of the Betty Irene Moore Fellowship for Nurse Leaders and Innovators, and Founding Director and Principal Investigator of The HEEAT Research Lab.

Part II

Cultural Pillar

Those customary beliefs, social norms, attitudes, values, and practices shared by a group of people (community or society) in a place and time with regards to health and healthcare.

Faith-Based Storytelling as SDOH to Promote Health: A Partnership with Marginalized Communities and Faith-Based Institutions

Jill B. Hamilton, Autherine Abiri, Charlyne Anne Nicolas, and Valarie Worthy

1 Storytelling in Interventions with African American Cancer Survivors

The purpose of this chapter is to describe the work of community-engaged research that eventually led to an NIH-funded study (R03 MD013509-01A1) *Faith-Based African American Cancer Survivorship Storytelling: A Culturally Relevant Intervention to Alleviate Psychological Distress*. The coauthors of this chapter, a Professor of Nursing at the Nell Hodgson Woodruff School of Nursing and a past president of Sisters Network Triangle, detail the ways in which their 16-year collaboration on qualitative research studies resulted in the pilot of an intervention study. The results of their study are published—*You need a song to bring you through: The use of religious songs to manage stressful life events. The Gerontologist; Reading the Bible for guidance, comfort, and strength during stressful life events. Nursing Research;*

and, *The use of prayer during life-threatening illness: A connectedness to God, inner-self, and others. Journal of Religion and Health.* Our intent of this chapter is to describe in detail the collaborations, the strategies to promote those collaborations, and the true partnership of identifying the issues with community members; designing, implementing, and disseminating community-engaged research.

2 Storytelling Through the Lens of an Academic Professor

The use of storytelling in interventions is emerging as a beneficial method for improving health outcomes among racialized minorities [1–4] and low literate populations [5]. In research among African American adult populations, storytelling interventions have resulted in increased health promoting behaviors such as adherence to follow-up care and quality of life among breast cancer patients [6], increasing self-care among diabetic patients and improvements to blood pressure [1, 2]. Interventions that incorporate culture, specifically dimensions of spirituality, in group discussions may not have lasting effects [7] while health educational interventions delivered in faith-based institutions exclude those individuals not religiously affiliated [8]. On the other hand, storytelling that incorporates the nar-

J. B. Hamilton (✉) · A. Abiri · C. A. Nicolas
Nell Hodgson Woodruff School of Nursing,
Emory University, Atlanta, GA, USA
e-mail: jbhamil@emory.edu;
Autherine.abiri@emoryhealthcare.org;
Charlyne.nicolas@emory.edu

V. Worthy
Duke Cancer Center, Duke University,
Durham, NC, USA
e-mail: Valarie.worthy@duke.edu

rative of religious songs to overcome psychological distress in life-threatening situations is interwoven into the culture of African Americans [9–11]. Additionally, in the U. S., African Americans are the most religiously affiliated population and likely to conceptualize their spirituality as a certainty that a Higher Power (God) exists [12] and that this sacred being has the ability to protect, heal, and deliver them from the sufferings of their worldly existence [13]. The outward expression of this spirituality has primarily been through African American storytelling and religious song, which continues to be an important aspect of their religious culture [13, 14]. During life-threatening situations, the narratives of these religious songs are used to encourage a positive sense of self through an identity as a child of God, to express a belief and faith in the promise of a life free of pain and suffering [13, 14] , and to promote social relationships among naturally occurring family networks [15]. Despite this strong cultural heritage of storytelling through religious song narrative, healthcare providers and researchers have yet to fully embrace and incorporate this coping strategy into supportive cancer care interventions.

3   An Exploration of Religious Songs Among African Americans in Response to Stressful Life Events

It was in 2008 that I attended the Homegoing Service for the mother of a long-time friend and colleague. This Homegoing Service was held in a small church and in a rural town in Eastern North Carolina. I had some trouble finding the church, so I was late when I arrived and had to take a seat near the rear of the church. The service was moving along smoothly with the usual words from the ministers, then a prayer, followed by a song from the choir. And then, came the time on the program for family and friends to share words of comfort with members of the family. An older man sitting behind me proceeded to walk to the front of the church. He walked over and whispered something to the family member sitting on the front pew. He then walked over to the mic just in front of the pulpit and started to sing. He was singing without any musical instruments and with his shaky and solid voice sang his song to the family. The lyrics of this song was his "gift"; his offering of support to comfort the family. There I sat, in the back of the church watching in amazement. Thinking, how beautiful the song, the singer, and this gift were of comfort to this grieving family. I also remember leaving church that day wanting to somehow capture that piece of African American culture and that piece of African American religious tradition that might be lost to future generations.

At this Homegoing Service, I also witnessed an older man singing a religious song about God's love to comfort a grieving family. I was later told by the family that this man was a long-time family friend, and singing this song was his way of comforting them during the loss of their mother. Although the name of the song is lost to memory, I recall realizing that this song was what this elder had *to give* and one that the family graciously received. Had I been able to interview the older man who sat in the back of the church, I likely would have found out the name of the song, its meaning, and why it was important to support the family in this way. I only knew that this was an amazing act, one that I wanted to explore more.

4   Getting Started: An Exploration of Religious Songs as Storytelling

Jill B. Hamilton

Armed with a research question, my initial steps were to seek out the help of collaborators. My plan was to solicit collaborators within the School of Nursing, but I also sought the advice of research mentors. Looking back on those days, I now laugh when I remember how everyone I approached in the academy to work with me said 'no.' One after the other, "No, No, No, and No again." But I believed the work important, and I was persistent. In spite of the negative responses,

I proceeded with initial steps to conduct this research with obtaining IRB approval to explore the use of religious songs among African Americans during stressful life events. The plan was to identify participants based on the criteria of self-identification as African American, age 50 or older, and having experienced a life-threatening situation. My focus on these sampling criteria was based on information from the Pew Forum that African Americans were religiously affiliated compared to other U.S. populations [12], more likely to experience high levels of psychological distress, less likely than other U. S. populations to seek mental health services [16] or to participate in hospital-based support groups [17]. I included interview questions related to Bible verses and prayers to be sensitive to religiously affiliated African Americans where religious song might not be emphasized in their worship services. With IRB approval in hand, I was ready to recruit appropriate individuals who could provide information that was data rich.

Recruiting Participants. Given my assumption that African Americans who were religiously affiliated would likely use a religious song during a stressful life situation, I initially contacted ministers in the community, hoping they could assist me with access to such individuals in their congregations, Bible study, or senior groups. My first contact was the late Rev. Dr. Marcus Ingram, my former professor, from NCCU School of Business and Pastor of the New Hope Baptist Church. I attended Dr. Ingram's church one Sunday morning and he introduced me to his congregation and invited me to talk about my study in front of the congregation. To my surprise, congregants began passing me notes with their names and phone numbers during the service (convenient sample). After the service, an older gentleman, a Deacon, and Senior Choir member, walked up and started singing a song to me.

During my recruiting efforts, I also reached out to religiously affiliated participants known to me who also had experienced a life-threatening illness. These individuals subsequently introduced me to their friends who also agreed to participate in the study (snowball sample). However, my greatest supporter (stakeholder) assisted in

introducing me into remote communities in Western North Carolina, was my Uncle, Deacon Marvin Hamilton and his childhood friend Presiding Elder, Rev. Herbert Grant. Through their introductions into the community, I was able to establish trust of participants and capture stories that would have otherwise not been possible. During the first phase, I captured the stories of over 60 older African Americans. I can remember being so happy that after all the no's from my colleagues in the academy, the community was saying, *yes, we are here, what you are doing is important to us, and we are going to help you.*

Although my initial plan was to gather a typology of religious songs, the participants in these interviews helped to refine and expand the interview. By the end of the fourth interview, I arrived at a framework to guide interviews, (1) identify their stressful life event, (2) identify the song used during that time, (3) derive the meaning from that song(s), and/or (4) note how the song made them feel. My research structure was consistent with the components of a story; the beginning, middle, and end along with the components consistent with the *Stress and Coping Theoretical Framework* that I had used in my previous research; a stressful life event, a coping strategy and an outcome [18].

Another source for the recruitment of African Americans came from my relationship with an African American breast cancer support group. In 2007, I served in a faculty position at my alma mater in Chapel Hill and knew that I wanted to connect with African American cancer survivors in the Triangle (Raleigh, Durham, and Chapel Hill). During my first year back in North Carolina, a childhood friend, distant cousin, and breast cancer survivor, Katherine Whittington Dubose, told me about Sister's Network and invited me to one of their monthly meetings. My initial goal for attending these meetings was to learn more about the survivorship experiences of these African Americans but to also learn how I could give back to the Black community, given my education and skills as a researcher. I was extremely fortunate to be welcomed into this group of sisters and to connect with other cancer survivors: Valarie Worthy, Priscilla Lewis, and Wadeeah

Beyah. These sisters have been my close colleagues for nearly 16 years and have shared their experiences as cancer survivors and helped to formulate my research questions, research design, assisted with recruitment, and more importantly, to ensure that my interpretations of any data collected accurately represents their stories when disseminated in peer-reviewed manuscripts or podium presentations. In the next paragraphs, my research partner for 16 years will share her story of how she began her journey in the community as a cancer survivor advocate and her involvement in this faith-based storytelling project.

5 Storytelling Through the Lens of a Breast Cancer Survivor, Patient Navigator, Community Leader

Valarie Worthy

I am a 20-plus-year survivor of breast cancer. In this chapter, I share my passion for storytelling to educate other African American women in my cancer prevention outreach work but also as a way to support other African American breast cancer survivors.

I can remember when I first realized that I was indeed a storyteller. I had been asked to speak at different venues, to emphasize different parts of my journey to different audiences. I didn't realize the power of telling stories for many years and only after I began speaking to groups. At one, a lady said, "Val, you know, I think I've heard you speak many of times, but I've never heard you tell the story that way." And for me, that was like God was saying, "You know, your conversations and what you say to people have to be tailor-made. You cannot use a cookie cutter approach sharing this kind of information." You have to look at your audience, pay attention to at who's out there, understand who can and cannot hold these deposits of information. You learn over time what worked well for different groups of people and, if you are patient and listen to the verbal and nonverbal cues, you can build the relationship with

the audience so they're listening to every word that you say because you are transparent and authentic. You must be mindful that the stories are informative and not frightening, a skill that develops over time Initially, people want to tell every single thing about their story but that can be frightening to people. In some situations, the survivor has to ask the question, "I'm doing this (telling this story) to inform people, to encourage people to get their care, or am I telling the story to get things off my chest?" There is a time for storytelling to get support and a time for storytelling to give support.

Over the years, I have found that sharing my story is a wonderful venue to help people help me. For example, when I was diagnosed, people would say to me, "Oh, I had an aunt that had *that* and she died." Finally, I got fed up with it. I said:

> Now, I know that person's intent is not to hurt me, it's because they have no manual about how to support a cancer survivor. I didn't get a manual on how to be a cancer survivor. We both need to learn. So, I need to teach this person how to help me and others. I would say to that person, "I know that you didn't mean any harm by that when you said your aunt died. But when you say things like that to a cancer survivor, it doesn't make us feel good. Because we think about that all the time, all you hear about is death, death, death, cancer, cancer, cancer. But if you say to us, 'you know what? I don't know much about cancer, and I've heard some things that's not true and some things that could be true, but I'm going to be praying for you, because I know God is a healer." I said, "that will mean all the world to us; don't tell me about your aunt that got sick and threw up, or died, or got the wrong chemo, or any of that, because everybody is different. Just tell us about the positive things, that's what we need to hear."

That's how I began educating people over a platform with storytelling. You're not doing it in a negative way; you're doing it in a positive way. We've learned that even when we set up our tables, and we had the breast models, some were turning away, because in the African American communities, such openness related to our bodies were prohibited, like a woman touching her breast. So, some women are not even looking at their body. This was my experience when I was diagnosed. I remember when my doctor was examining my breast saying to me, "How long have you had that dimple in your breast?" And I said, "I don't know. I don't do self-breast exams." Isn't that something? Me, a nurse. I said, "I don't know. I don't do self-breast exams." It never crossed my mind that at 40 years old, I would be diagnosed with breast cancer. Even if I had not touched my breast, just looked at it, I would've seen the dimple.

We haven't lived in a culture that encouraged stories around breast cancer. So, bringing breast models to our health fairs and literally having women touch the model so they know what a potential lump feels like, it blew people's minds sometimes. "Oh, is this how it feels? I was wondering how it felt." These were not conversations that we had in our communities. Sharing stories about breast cancer brings about self-awareness, not only for people who were not diagnosed, but for those of us that were diagnosed, who learned a lot of things because we certainly weren't talking about it at the kitchen table or even with our girlfriends. We didn't talk about breast health.

6   The Power of Healing Through Storytelling Through the Lens of a Breast Cancer Survivor, Patient Navigator, Community Leader

Valarie Worthy

I think the power of storytelling is evident when we are able to tell our stories about survivorship where the public could see their mother, sister, grandmother, girlfriend, in a way that was not negative. Sharing our stories of survivorship brought hope and not despair. People didn't pity us because we laughed, just like everybody else. Some women wore scarves, some wore wigs, some showed their hair, while others showed their bald head. Even though you had all black women, there was a lot of diversity in thoughts, their expressions, and different ways the women responded to the cancer experience. Our experiences spoke to different people's needs, we had

different people, different ages, and different perspectives. Some women were single and some were married. It was just a collection of stories, of God's gift to the community. I used to say that God handpicked us because He knew He could trust us, use us for His purpose. So that took us out of that victim position, we never saw that. We were always upbeat. That's what we showed to the non-cancer folk. I think they were drawn to that energy.

As African American breast cancer survivors, we have come through cancer diagnoses, surgery, losing our hair, and radiation. The cancer diagnosis, for many of us, became our litmus test. "If we survived this, hey, is there anything we cannot do?" I saw people get stronger. I saw women join our group for the first time and have difficulty saying they had a cancer diagnosis without crying, sometimes bawling. Each month I would see them get stronger and stronger, and they'd go through their treatment and get stronger and stronger. Then after a while, those very same women, who were crying at their first meeting, or maybe even the second one as well, take that box of tissues they once used and hand it to a new member and hug them. I would say it at our meetings sometimes, I would say, "girl, look at you. I remember when you were just boohoo…you couldn't even get the words out. And now you're providing comfort to other people."

That's what I liked about having a support group outside of an organized community, such as an academic center or cancer center. We were free to say God's name as many times as we wanted to; and for the African American experience, that's what we do. If they stifled us, we couldn't give God the glory for where we were at that particular time, like putting tape over our mouth, where we couldn't talk. The freedom of being outside of those constraints helped us in ways that I can't even begin to impart.

I've always believed that the church has not lived up to their responsibility in terms of helping people that have a diagnosis that is a taboo – such as a cancer diagnosis. People are still embarrassed to share that they have cancer. There has to be a way to normalize this in the church community and encourage those stricken to tell their stories in a way to express their fears and apprehension without being stigmatized or made to feel less than due to their cancer diagnosis. We know there is a better way to share our stories about breast cancer. One story is through the power of the hymn, or the power of talking about how a scripture, or how that that song carried them through the tough times.

7   The Development of a Faith-Based Storytelling Intervention

The development of a faith-based storytelling intervention was derived in three phases. *Phase 1* (Narrative Collection) and *Phase 2* (Narrative Review). In Phase 1, the Narrative Collection Phase, I drew from stories from 41 African American male and female cancer patients and their close family members from the qualitative research conducted for the purpose of exploring the use of religious songs in response to stressful life events. The findings from this study facilitated my understanding of African American experiences when diagnosed with cancer, the faith-based strategies used, and mental health outcomes. Participants in this study agreed to share their video recorded narratives in future intervention studies and for educational purposes. Patients and family members in this qualitative study were an average age of 65 (range 45-93), female ($n = 31$) and male ($n = 10$), married ($n = 24$) and unmarried ($n = 17$). The employment status was either retired ($n = 19$), employed ($n = 17$), or quit because of health reasons ($n = 5$). Religious affiliation was Baptist ($n = 27$), Methodist ($n = 5$), Pentecostal ($n = 2$), Catholic ($n = 3$), or nondenominational ($n = 4$) and geographical location was rural ($n = 22$) or urban ($n = 19$).

In this study, participants were asked to discuss the stress associated with a cancer diagnosis, the religious song or religious text they used, and their outcomes. Interview questions were "What was stressful for you? Was there a song, Bible verse or prayer that helped you through? How did you feel after using that song, Bible verse, or prayer?" Interviews were conducted in the privacy of participant homes or community churches and lasted from 15 to 45 min. *In Phase 2, Narrative Review*, members of the research team coded the transcribed narratives and derived five themes of survivorship stories. The categories from this coding process were validated with members of the target population. The five categories of stories from these 41 interviews are in Table 1.

In Phase 3, Professional Video Narrative Editing consisted of video editing with our multimedia expert. The video narratives that captured the diagnosis of cancer as a stressful life event, a coping strategy using a religious song, and an outcome were edited to capture components of the recordings most likely to be persuasive, rele-

Table 1 Themes from African American survivorship stories with religious songs and religious text

Theme	Faith-based meanings attached to stories
Stories of thanksgiving	Stories reflect expressions of thanksgiving to God for His past acts of goodness, mercy, grace. Stories are reminders to have faith in God's ability to strengthen and bring one through adversity
Stories of encouragement and guidance	Stories and lyrics of religious songs and religious text express what one should do when presently troubled; when sick; when feeling down. Stories offer encouragement to persevere hardships; a reminder that God has the ability to resolve health issues
Stories of the strength and endurance of forefathers	Stories, religious songs, and religious text connect individuals to a past time that was safe or to a person of strength
Stories of the power of prayer	Stories and lyrics of religious songs and religious text are expressions to God for some unmet need; desires for protection; need for healing; strength; help when in trouble; relief from pain and suffering
Stories of life continuing	Life is full of struggles that may not be overcome in this life. A religious consciousness of continued life in a better world that comes after death

vant, and emotionally engaging, for the target population. Our previous coding conducted by content experts and member of the target population has suggested the placement of these narratives (stories) according to five themes: (a) *Stories of Thanksgiving*, (b) *Stories of Encouragement and Guidance*, (c) *Stories of the Strength and Endurance of Forefathers*, (d) *Stories of the Power of Prayer*, and (e) *Stories of Life Continuing* (see Table 1).

During the video editing process, narratives (stories) were condensed into smaller segments, isolating those sections that highlight categories that were relevant and that had a greater likelihood of clarity and emotional engagement to participants. Those segments that captured the essence of the story as a whole (stressful beginning event, coping strategy used in response to stressful event, and benefit from strategy used) were given priority for inclusion into the intervention. Our final selection of video-recorded narratives considered representation of variations of age, gender, and types of cancer. Our professional multimedia expert oversaw the edits, so that all finished material was coherent and consistent with the mission of this study. The final selection of video recordings were uploaded into a social media site for patient and family caregiver access and viewing.

In a future Phase 4, Pilot testing will consist of a combined quantitative and qualitative methodology to examine usability and evaluation of transportation of the video-recorded narratives. Quantitative analysis of usability will include descriptive analysis (means and frequencies) from rating scales (higher scores = higher level of influence) to examine participant scaled responses on the following: clarity, persuasiveness, and ease of use. For evaluation of transportation and identity, we will examine means and frequencies to responses for: similarity to and identification; narrative engagement; and, the emotional engagement. We will use percentiles to rank the video recorded narratives. Narratives with higher levels of rankings (top 50%) will be retained for future feasibility testing.

Qualitative data collection and analysis will consist of open-ended interview questions will be explored according to usability and evaluation of transportation identity, engagement, and emotional response will be transcribed verbatim and uploaded into Atlas.ti for analysis. Guided by principles of conventional content analysis will consist of each participants' responses to the open-ended interviews and organized according to categories that emerge from the data [19]. Specifically, we will analyze interview data for *usability*: participant responses to perceived navigation (ease of use), content (video length, topics covered, presentation), persuasiveness (mood, encouragement), and value (time spent, future use, potential recommendations to others. We will also explore interviews for transportation and identity: similarity to and identification; narrative engagement; and, the emotional engagement of participants to selected recordings. We will use interrater reliability to validate themes emerging from the data.

The development of this faith-based African American cancer survivorship storytelling intervention assumes that African Americans will be receptive to an intervention that incorporates religious practices of using religious song and religious text to alleviate psychological distress. We have pretested the recordings with a small number of members of the target population and my community research partner, an African American breast cancer survivor. Although the video recordings included in this intervention are those that have previously been positively received, there is the possibility that one or more of the recordings will evoke a negative emotional response. This information will be helpful in our consideration of video recorded narratives selected for a future feasibility test of this intervention. We will notify patients' health care providers of those patients with high distress scores from our psychological distress measure Hospital Anxiety and Depression Scale (HADS) and National Comprehensive Cancer Network Distress Scale (NCCN). We will also refer overly distressed patients to their health care providers.

8 Reflections

The persistent narrative about cancer in the African American community is that this illness equates to an experience of emaciation, loss of hair, treatments that disfigure, and ultimately ending in a painful death. Historically, religious songs have been used to communicate a faith and hope of survival in the most dire circumstances; however, the lack of stories and positive images of African American cancer survivors has created heightened fears and psychological distress has been difficult to overcome. The Faith-Based Storytelling Intervention seeks to reverse that narrative through stories from survivors that show there is life after a cancer diagnosis.

The findings from this study have implications for advancing the science of intervention studies designed to improve psychological distress, leading to enhancements in supportive family relationships and ultimately quality of life during the diagnosis of and treatment for cancer.

References

1. Houston TK, Allison JJ, Sussman M, Horn W, Holt CL, Trobaugh J, et al. Culturally appropriate storytelling to improve blood pressure: a randomized trial. Ann Intern Med. 2011a;154(2):77–84. https://doi.org/10.7326/0003-4819-154-2-201101180-00004.
2. Houston TK, Cherrington A, Coley HL, Robinson KM, Trobaugh JA, Williams JH, et al. The art and science of patient storytelling-harnessing narrative communication for behavioral interventions: the ACCE project. J Health Commun. 2011b;16(7):686–97. https://doi.org/10.1080/10810730.2011.551997.
3. Kreuter MW, Holmes K, Alcaraz K, Kalesan B, Rath S, Richert M, et al. Comparing narrative and informational videos to increase mammography in low-income African American women. Patient Educ Couns. 2010;81(Suppl):S6–14. https://doi.org/10.1016/j.pec.2010.09.008.
4. Larkey LK, Lopez AM, Minnal A, Gonzalez J. Storytelling for promoting colorectal cancer screening among underserved Latina women: a randomized pilot study. Cancer Control. 2009;16(1):79–87. https://doi.org/10.1177/107327480901600112.
5. Larkey LK, Gonzalez J. Storytelling for promoting colorectal cancer prevention and early detection among Latinos. Patient Educ Couns. 2007;67(3):272–8. https://doi.org/10.1016/j.pec.2007.04.003.
6. Davis C, Darby K, Moore M, Cadet T, Brown G. Breast care screening for underserved African American women: community-based participatory approach. J Psychosoc Oncol. 2017;35(1):90–105. https://doi.org/10.1080/07347332.2016.1217965.
7. Kruizinga R, Hartog ID, Jacobs M, Daams JG, Scherer-Rath M, Schilderman JB, et al. The effect of spiritual interventions addressing existential themes using a narrative approach on quality of life of cancer patients: a systematic review and meta-analysis. Psychooncology. 2016;25(3):253–65. https://doi.org/10.1002/pon.3910.
8. Holt CL, Litaker MS, Scarinci IC, Debnam KJ, McDavid C, McNeal SF, et al. Spiritually based intervention to increase colorectal cancer screening among African Americans: screening and theory-based outcomes from a randomized trial. Health Educ Behav. 2013;40(4):458–68. https://doi.org/10.1177/1090198112459651.
9. Jones AC. Wade in the water. The wisdom of the spirituals. Maryknoll, N.Y.: Orbis Books; 1993.
10. Raboteau AJ. Slave religion. The "Invisible Institution". In: in the Antebellum South. New York: Oxford University Press; 1978.
11. Walker WT. Somebody's calling my name. Black sacred music and social change. Valley Forge, PA: Judson Press; 1979.
12. PewForum. A religious portrait of African-Americans. Pew Forum on Religion & Public Life; 2007. Retrieved from http://www.pewforum.org/religious-landscape-study/
13. Cone JH. Black theology & black power. Mayoll, NY: Orbis Books; 2006.
14. Raboteau AJ. Canaan land. New York: Oxford University Press; 2001.
15. Hamilton JB, Sandelowski M, Moore AD, Agarwal M, Koenig HG. "You need a song to bring you through": the use of religious songs to manage stressful life events. Gerontologist. 2013;53(1):26–38. https://doi.org/10.1093/geront/gns064.
16. Traeger L, Cannon S, Keating NL, Pirl WF, Lathan C, Martin MY, et al. Race by sex differences in depression symptoms and psychosocial service use among non-Hispanic black and white patients with lung cancer. J Clin Oncol. 2014;32(2):107–13. https://doi.org/10.1200/jco.2012.46.6466.
17. Somayaji D, Cloyes KG. Cancer fear and fatalism: how African American participants construct the role of research subject in relation to clinical cancer research. Cancer Nurs. 2015;38(2):133–44. https://doi.org/10.1097/ncc.0000000000000144.
18. Lazarus RS, Folkman S. Stress, appraisal, and coping. New York: Springer Publishing Company; 1984.
19. Hsieh HF, Shannon SE. Three approaches to qualitative content analysis. Qual Health Res. 2005;15(9):1277–88. https://doi.org/10.1177/1049732305276687.

Jill B. Hamilton PhD, MRPL, RN, FAAN, is Professor (tenured) and Senior Faculty Fellow of SDOH and Health Disparities at the Nell Hodgson Woodruff School of Nursing and Affiliate Professor at Candler School of Theology at Emory University in Atlanta, Georgia. Dr. Hamilton earned her BSN, MSN, and PhD in nursing from the University of North Carolina at Chapel Hill, a BS in Accounting from North Carolina Central University, postdoctoral training in the nursing care of older adults at the Oregon Health and Science University, and a Master's in Religion and Public Life at the Candler School of Theology. She previously held faculty positions at Johns Hopkins University and the University of North Carolina at Chapel Hill where she was a tenured Associate Professor. Dr. Hamilton's research interests include social determinants of health, health disparities, and the mental health promoting strategies used among older African American their families in response to life-threatening illness. Dr. Hamilton is Leading Editor of a text with Springer Nature titled *Integrating a Social Determinants of Health Framework into Nursing Education* published in 2023. She has done original research on the effects of storytelling that incorporates Black Sacred Music and scripture on psychological distress among older and younger African Americans. She was a Georgia Cancer Coalition Distinguished Cancer Scholar from 2003 to 2007 and a member of the 2014 Class of the UNC Thorp Faculty Engaged Scholars. Dr. Hamilton is currently a Fellow in the American Academy of Nursing and a Faculty Scholar of the Center for Spirituality, Theology and Health at Duke University. She was the recipient of the 2019 Distinguished Alumni Award from the School of Nursing at the University of North Carolina, the 2011 Oncology Nursing Society (ONS) Publishing's Division Award for Excellence in Writing Qualitative Research and the ONS 2023 Award for Excellence in Cancer Education. Dr. Hamilton was born and raised in the Southern Appalachian region of North Carolina.

Autherine Abiri DNP, RN, is an Assistant Professor at Nell Hodgson Woodruff School of Nursing. She is a certified family and emergency nurse practitioner. In 2009, Dr. Abiri obtained her Bachelor of Science in Nursing from the University of Wisconsin–Madison. She obtained her Master of Science in Nursing as a family nurse practitioner from Graceland University in 2015. Dr. Abiri graduated with her Doctor of Nursing Practice from Emory University in 2020 where she was recognized with the Nell Hodgson Woodruff School of Nursing Social Responsibility Award for breaking down barriers and creating an environment for diversity, equity, and inclusion. Additionally, Dr. Abiri has served as a national committee member of the American Academy of Emergency Nurse Practitioner's Diversity Equity and Inclusion Committee. With a focus on nursing education, she has served on educational work groups dedicated to integrating social determinants of health within nursing curricula. Dr. Abiri takes a special interest in research that centers on the impact of social determinants of health on patient outcomes and health disparities. She is passionate about providing patient-centered care and implementing processes that promote health equity.

Charlyne Anne Nicolas DNP, RN, is a recent Doctor of Nursing Practice and family nurse practitioner graduate of the Nell Hodgson Woodruff School of Nursing at Emory University in Atlanta, Georgia. She earned her Master of Nursing degree, also at Emory University, and was inducted into the Alpha Epsilon chapter of Sigma Theta Tau. She completed her undergraduate studies at the University of California, Los Angeles, in 2018, earning her Bachelor of Science in psychobiology and minor in global health. She is a published researcher in peer-reviewed, interdisciplinary journals, and her research interests include the impact of social determinants of health on patient outcomes and health disparities in marginalized and underserved populations.

Valarie Worthy MSN, RN, is Patient Navigator Manager at Duke University Health System and Co-Founder of TOUCH, the Black Breast Cancer Alliance, to bolster Black women's breast cancer clinical trial participation by 2025—with the goal of reaching 350,000 Black women and motivating 25,000 into trial portals. Valarie is a two-decade-plus breast cancer survivor, has been a nurse for more than 41 years, and worked at Duke for the past 20 years. Her hometown is Ahoskie, in northeastern North Carolina.

Engaged Scholarship on the Family's Role as a Proximal Health Resource for LGBTQ+ Adolescents

Dalmacio Dennis Flores, Anita Shubert, Tom McMahon, Alyssa Lagua, Connor Brandon, Abby Cabalbag, Caroline Dougherty, Christopher Krauze-Choi, Arielle Lewis, Aruna Rao, and Kim and John Otto

Adolescence is a period of transition between childhood and adulthood where individuals experience rapid physical, cognitive, and psychosocial growth. This transition is a period of both discovery and disorientation which can often lead to anxiety. This anxiety is usually exacerbated among lesbian, gay, bisexual, transgender, and queer (LGBTQ+) youth whose sense of identity and development may be asynchronous with their cisgender, heterosexual counterparts. For instance, some LGBTQ+ youth have an earlier sexual debut [1–3] and greater development of risky health behaviors. This pattern may be explained by a lack of adult guidance or age-appropriate LGBTQ+ media representation [4–6]. On the contrary, other LGBTQ+ youth have delayed adolescent milestones which may be explained by the fear and trauma related to chronic anti-LGBTQ+ stigma. These individuals often experience a second transitional phase in adulthood or "second queer adolescence" after fully developing and accepting an LGBTQ+ identity. Families play an integral role in adolescent development through rearing, instilling of values, and support of the LGBTQ+ youth [7].

According to the Gallup report, 7.2% of U.S. adults identify as LGBTQ+ in 2022 [8]. This is more than double the percentage when Gallup first started measuring LGBTQ+ identities a decade prior with 3.5% in 2012. Additionally, an increasing percentage of individuals identify as LGBTQ+ in younger generations with 19.7% of Generation Z compared to 11.2% of Millennials and 3.3% of Generation X [8]. However, despite these earlier self-disclosure trends, which portend to increase acceptance among parents and the larger society, blanket acceptance is still elusive for most LGBTQ+ youth, especially youth of color [9]. This precarious acceptance from proximal social determinants of health (e.g., fam-

D. D. Flores (✉) · A. Shubert · T. McMahon
A. Lagua · C. Brandon · A. Cabalbag · C. Dougherty
C. Krauze-Choi · A. Lewis
The University of Pennsylvania School of Nursing,
Claire M. Fagin Hall, Philadelphia, PA, USA
e-mail: dalmacio@nursing.upenn.edu;
Ashubert@umich.edu; Alyssrie@nursing.upenn.edu;
Cgb2001@nursing.upenn.edu;
Abigail.cabalbag@pennmedicine.upenn.edu;
Cardough@nursing.upenn.edu;
Ckc10@nursing.upenn.edu;
lewisari@nursing.upenn.edu

A. Rao
Desi Rainbow Parents & Allies Inc.,
Metuchen, NJ, USA
e-mail: aruna@desirainbow.org

K. a. John Otto
PFLAG Philadelphia, Philadelphia, PA, USA

ilies, schools, peers) has been closely linked with negative health outcomes for this population [10].

LGBTQ+ individuals have historically had poorer physical and mental health outcomes compared to their cisgender, heterosexual counterparts due to a multitude of factors including stigma; minority stress; and other behavioral, environmental, and structural risk factors [10]. Examples of these factors include historical medical maltreatment of this community (e.g., homosexuality deemed as a mental illness until the 1970s, delayed lifting of blood donation bans against MSM), targeted negative legislation (i.e., "Don't Say Gay" bills, prosecution of healthcare providers who provide transgender affirming care), improper government response to this community's needs (e.g., the U.S. federal government's slow recognition of AIDS in the 1980s), and persistent stigmatization in the public sphere.

1 The Inadequacy of Sexual Health Resources for LGBTQ+ Youth

The parent–child relationship is critical for the outcomes of a child's physical health. Studies have shown that the communication approach a parent takes with their child correlates with either positive or negative outcomes, including sexual and mental health. Children oftentimes feel uncomfortable discussing sexual health with their parents, which may prevent them from having these necessary educational conversations altogether [7]. Further, parents oftentimes have improper tools or information to educate their LGBTQ+ child on sexual health. Another issue is that some parents do not believe that sexual education is their responsibility; rather, they believe that the discussions of condom use, HIV, and STIs will be covered in the school setting [7]. However, the school system often fails LGBTQ+ youth in sexual education. When LGBTQ+ youth do not receive the proper sexual health education at home or in school systems, this leaves this population with the task of finding information

on their own. Not only does lack of parental and school guidance place LGBTQ+ youth at risk when it comes to HIV/STI infection, the silence around their health concerns may also lead to internalized stigma and negative mental health.

A Community Health Nurse's First-Person Perspective

Through my experience as a sexual health nurse out in the community, I have seen many teenagers and young adults come into my clinic scared and nervous beyond belief. For many this is their first time getting a full STI panel done, despite the fact that they have been sexually active for many years. The fear of STIs, HIV and what the testing itself entails, keeps young adults from knowing their status. These kids often have no knowledge of sexual health and if they do it was presented to them in a fear-based approach at their school. It's understandable that with a background like this, parents or mentors can be a crucial presence that changes adolescent mindset to become more health-seeking. Open and honest conversations with adolescents can make activities such as getting tested for STIs less scary, but a part of someone's health routine just as much as a yearly physical or dentist appointment. There is a taboo surrounding sex and sexual health that starts with messages communicated (or implied) from parents and trickles down to LGBTQ+ youth. It's time that sexual health become a normalized concern that anyone can talk about. Through inclusive family discussions, I believe we can create future generations that decrease the number of STIs and formulate a healthy outlook on sexual conversations and ultimately, sexual health.—Thomas McMahon, Sexual Health RN

To counter , parents are in an opportune position to provide much-needed resources. An open and nonjudgmental parent–child conversation about LGBTQ+ sexual health can facilitate positive health outcomes among adolescents. According to studies with heterosexual participants, effective parent–child sex communication can lead to an increase in condom usage, HIV/STI prevention strategies, and engagement with reproductive and sexual health services [11–13].

Expanding these initiatives to LGBTQ+ youth could positively impact the child's sexual health outcomes; for example, parents may educate their child about pre-exposure prophylaxis to take the initial steps to HIV prevention [14–16].

2 Development of Animated Videos and Website with Community

In this chapter, we describe the development of an original series of animated videos and a website cocreated with community members called Parents Advancing Supportive and Sexuality-Inclusive Sex Talks (ASSIST). Parents ASSIST focuses on inclusive sex communication education and skills for parents of gay, bisexual, and queer (GBQ) adolescent males. This work is premised on the idea that parents are potential HIV/STI prevention agents who can learn by observation and model their own behavior accordingly [17]. Through the Parents ASSIST videos and website, parents' self-efficacy is addressed to overcome perceived barriers (e.g., anticipated awkwardness of talks, sons' resistance to discussing sexuality issues) to sex communication. Furthermore, skill building strategies are modeled so parents can use the techniques with their sons. In this chapter, we present how we codeveloped Parents ASSIST and detail the lessons learned from this iterative intervention development process.

Focus on LGBTQ+ Health Disparities Outcomes: Cancer
The American Cancer Society (ACS) publishes annual reports on the reported and estimated cancer incidence, prevalence, survival, and mortality. Historically, there has been limited data regarding these statistics within the LGBTQ+ community. In fact, sexual orientation and gender identity data are not currently included in these reports and LGBTQ+ statistics have been extrapolated from general census data and cancer in the general population. This omission fails to capture the risks and incidence for certain cancers that the community faces.

Additionally, quantifying cancer risks and statistics in the LGBTQ+ community is challenging due to the perceived heterogeneity within the community. Existing data do suggest some known increased risks including anal cancer in gay and bisexual men, breast cancer in lesbian and bisexual women, and gonadal cancers with intersex individuals [10]. These elevated risks are likely due to socio-ecological factors including environment and access to competent care, individual factors including tobacco and alcohol use and increased rate of STI, and decreased screening due to a poor relationship with the healthcare system.

Issues with cancer screening include lack of awareness and avoidance of the healthcare system as well as inadequate screening tools for certain cancers. In "Out: The National Cancer Survey," 29% of LGBTQ+ respondents with cancer did not complete recommended age and organ-based cancer screening prior to their cancer diagnosis. Forty percent of those respondents were unaware of the screening and 35% noted that it was not brought up by their healthcare provider. Others were diagnosed before the recommended age of screening or did not have healthcare [18]. Cancer screening becomes more nuanced in the transgender community. Although there is insufficient evidence to state that there is an increased or decreased risk related to gender-affirming hormone therapy, transgender individuals should be screened for any particular body part or organ they possess that otherwise meets criteria for screening regardless of hormone use [19]. The University of California San Francisco (UCSF) has recommendations for cancer screening in transgender individuals in their "Guidelines for the Primary and Gender-Affirming Care of Transgender and Gender Nonbinary People." Discussions of individualized cancer risks, screening, and management approaches are contingent on a good relationship between the LGBTQ+ individual and their healthcare provider for shared decision-making.

In addition to the reduction of HIV/STI infection and internalized stigma, comprehensive parental sexual health education can play a role in reduction in certain cancers. The human papillomavirus (HPV) is the most common STI in the United States and spreads through skin-to-skin contact of affected areas. Certain high-risk strains of HPV (16 and 18) are known to cause certain cancers including cervical, anal, oropharyngeal, and penile cancers which disproportionately affect the LGBTQ+ community. The Papanicolaou (Pap) test is used to screen for HPV and precancerous/cancerous changes. It is widely used for cervical cancer screening; however, there are no reliable, recommended screening tools for other HPV-driven cancers. Anal pap may be done to high-risk populations including men who have sex with men living with HIV, however, it is not widely offered. HPV vaccination has been effective in the reduction of HPV-driven cancers and is most effective prior to sexual debut. It is recommended around age 12 but may be administered as early as age 9 and up to age 26. Through education regarding safe sex practices and HPV vaccinations, parents can play an integral role in reducing the incidence, morbidity, and mortality of HPV-driven cancers. Parents can also play a role in educating their children on the importance of HPV-driven cancer screenings and act as advocates in the healthcare setting for their LGBTQ+ youth.

3 Engaged Scholarship During Creation of Parents ASSIST

For the development of Parents ASSIST, we first convened and sought the input of our Parent Advisory Board and Clinician Expert Panel. Members of the Parent Advisory Board included local chapter leaders from PFLAG (formerly Parents and Families of Lesbians and Gays) and Desi Rainbow Parents, a national support group composed mainly of SouthAsian members. During consultations, we explained the study aims and presented the potential Parents ASSIST topics based on formative work with GBQ youth [20–23]. The advisory group shared their thoughts on existing resources, determined their intervention priorities, and identified any logistical concerns around the intervention work for the target population. The advisory group also shared ideas on how best to adapt *Cuidalos*, an evidence-based sexual education intervention for Hispanic families with heterosexual adolescents [24], for families with GBQ males. Parent Advisory Board members decided that a video-based intervention would appeal to other parents as a convenient way of learning about sexual health topics and communication strategies. Ultimately, the advisory groups guided screenplay development for the videos, provided content expertise, and helped ensure that topics recommended by GBQ adolescents were included throughout the development of the intervention [25]. Our trained research staff that included four gay, male research assistants from diverse racial/ethnic backgrounds facilitated the advisory group meetings throughout the video development process.

To maximize interactions with the advisory boards, we created and presented summaries of preliminary video contents into storyboards (e.g., *Rule-Setting and The Adolescent Male's Developing Brain during Puberty; Do's and Don'ts When Talking with Sons After They Come Out*). During subsequent meetings that were structured as focus groups, research staff asked advisory group members to react to the developed content using both written (e.g., whiteboard, easels) and verbal (e.g., group discussion) feedback (Image 1). Working with an in-house team of mHealth experts focused on LGBTQ+ health intervention work, we created the Parents ASSIST videos and website. Study staff created 12 animated videos produced on Vyond, a software program used to create professional, animated videos with an entertainment-education style. The central video for this intervention ("*Answering Questions*") runs for 12 min, and the remaining 11 videos range from 4 to 6 min in length. The cast of animated characters represent people from different cultural backgrounds through dress, gender, ethnicity, and age to reflect common and shared parenting concerns across diverse populations [26]. Previous research has found that culturally tailored eHealth videos could be used to increase awareness of HIV/STI prevention methods since the viewers may identify with the characters and lessen their resistance to the health message [26]. In addition, Bandura recommended that characteristics of the models should be similar to the viewers to increase the impact of educational modeling [27]. During subsequent meetings, advisory group members provided their suggestions on the characters' voices and on the conversations between central characters, and on the overall appeal of the videos. This cyclical engagement between advisory group members and program staff enabled the iterative codevelopment and refinement of a theoretically driven video series and website that is cognizant of the unique parenting challenges that our target audience face [28].

Sex communication topics and communication skills were determined from our previous studies with GBQ adolescents [20, 25] and preliminary work with parents. The communication approaches were refined with experts in family sex discussions, and the study design and protocol were codeveloped and approved by our parent advisory board and clinician panel [25]. Additionally, based on persuasion and attitudinal change literature that suggests communication features that include source, recipient, message, and context determines its effectiveness [29], the Parents ASSIST videos purposively features diverse racial/ethnic animated characters, at least

48 sexual health topics, six videos with fathers as central characters, and a multitude of family contexts to ensure its appeal to our target participants.

Description of Adapted Intervention. For this submission, Parents ASSIST's main aim is the initiation and maintenance of inclusive parent–child sex communication between parents and GBQ dyads. By inclusive, we focus on an often-studied domain in parent–child sex communication science: communication quality. Pertaining to the level of comfort, openness, and respect between dyad members, we add to our definition of communication quality an explicit acknowledgment of cisgender sons' sexual orientation (gay, bisexual, or queer). Penile-vaginal sex is not the de facto type of coitus throughout the Parents ASSIST modules and non-heteronormativity is normalized. Further, the intervention components explains and models sexuality-inclusive communication strategies pertinent to GBQ sons' attractions (e.g., recognizing attraction for another boy), behaviors (e.g., negotiating safe sex expectations with potential same-sex partners), and identities (e.g., asserting GBQ selfhood in heteronormative spaces).

In its adapted form, Parents ASSIST addresses the key barriers identified by GBQ youth and parents we interviewed. Communication challenges that parent–child dyads typically face (e.g. children's unenthusiastic reception to sex talks or corralling avoidant teenagers who are beginning to assert autonomy) are included to reflect common, sex talk roadblocks. Each parent will have access to over 10 h of intervention content (e.g., videos, activities) across 12 modules. Six modules center on communication-based content that makes a case for why parent–child sex communication is crucial to ensuring GBQ adolescent's health and how to initiate and sustain these talks. Six additional modules focus on topic-centered content to address the knowledge gap parents have reported regarding general LGBTQ+ concerns and specific GBQ adolescent issues and builds on the communication skills learned in the first set of videos. Table 1 details the contents of these modules.

Table 1 Parents ASSIST Modules and corresponding video content

Modules, theoretical domains, and descriptions

Welcome & overview—Introduction to Parents ASSIST and lists benefits of inclusive sex communication based on literature and pilot work

Communication-focused modules

1. Answering questions

Communication focus: *Hearing, Listening & Responding*—active listening and ways sons' questions can be answered in affirming ways

Interactive component: *Virtual troubleshooting*—typical family situations are presented, and parents identify whether practices have a positive or negative impact on GBQ youth

2. Gay, bisexual & queer adolescents 101—introduction to contemporary masculinities and different coming out narratives

Communication focus: *In Praise of My Teen*—listening, suspending judgment and supporting parents to verbalize approval of positive teen behavior ("That was a thoughtful thing you did…")

Interactive component: *Homework* about positive appraisals

3. Communication barriers and overcoming them—Clarifying misconceptions and troubleshooting communication roadblocks

Communication focus: *For the Record*—having parents clarify family values, safety messages, hopes and dreams for sons' future, and develop a timeline for when to share these thoughts with teen

Interactive component: *Case Scenario*—participants read about a parent paralyzed by communication barriers and they choose likely solutions

4. Myths & facts: why parents don't talk to their children

Communication focus: *Opening discussions*—ways to broach conversations (teachable moments, physical and social milestones, etc.) and address homophobic attitudes from extended family, school, and others

Interactive component: *Quiz*—parents identify from a series of scenarios myths and facts about home-based discussions

5. How do you think gay, bisexual or queer teenagers feel about themselves

Communication focus: *Two-Way Talks and Constructing I-Centered Sentences*—parents' feelings are made explicit to minimize negativity or blame away from teen ("I feel like we can talk things through…", "I feel confused when…")

Interactive component: *Report Back* three I-centered statements made in the last week

6. Now that you're talking: effective communication tips

Communication focus: *Tell me more, tell me more*—arming parents with reassuring skills to invite more teen participation (nonverbal open cues, nodding, restatement of teen words, open-ended questions, minimizing interruptions)

Interactive component: *Follow after me*—parents read aloud conversation enhancers and rank them based on ones they are most to least likely to say in real life, along with their self-edited versions that are more realistic for them

Information-focused modules

7. Before having sex

Communication focus: *Step by Step*—Parents help assess teen readiness to have sex by looking at options, making a choice (not making a choice is a choice, consulting a parent about choice)

Interactive component: *Choose Your Own Adventure*—parents contemplate steps they would take regarding two case studies and rehearse ways to communicate their decisions with teen

8. Consent: beyond abuse & victimization

Communication focus: *Safety Charades*—Parents examine tricky sexual possibility situations (when teen is pressured to have sex, when consent is not sought, when boundaries are crossed) and safe exit strategies are considered (letting a trusted person know plans, having them call at a specific time) *Interactive component*: *Case Scenario*—participant reads safety and security exemplars and have to choose likely solutions they can offer to teen

9. Demystifying HIV/STI testing as savvy healthcare consumers

Communication focus: *Normalizing Testing*—Parents explain why it's important to seek LGBTQ-competent care regularly, routinizing HIV/STI testing, and setting up medical appointments

Interactive component: *Parent Report* on how their dyad looked up LGBTQ-friendly testing centers; for dyads with older teens, successful accessing site

(continued)

Table 1 (continued)

Modules, theoretical domains, and descriptions

10. PrEP, HPV vaccines, & newfangled biomedical prevention
Communication Focus—A step-by-step explanation to parents of HIV/STI biomedical prevention modalities and FAQs; gives parents age-appropriate talking points on how to introduce and discuss with teens
Interactive Component: Current Events Quiz—Parents are quizzed on LGBTQ+ sexual health trends; scores are shown relative to other study participants' scores to encourage friendly competition and normalization

11. Safety, hooking up, & technology-based issues
Communication Focus: Provides language and discussion points around social media literacy (sexting, hook-up apps, online dating)
Interactive Component: *Report Back* two scenarios discussed in the last week

12. Details, not generalities
Communication Focus: *Rehearsing for Life*—showing parents how teach-backs ensure learning (having teens repeat back to parents what they talked about regarding condom use, practicing how to insist on condom use, extracting self from a condom-less sexual situation)
Interactive Component: *Homework* about how their actual conversation with sons about condoms went and troubleshooting tips

The end of the rainbow—Recap of Parents ASSIST
Final Message—Straight Talk About LGBTQ+ Health—a team of LGBTQ+ providers deputize straight parents to be the best sexual health educators for their teens, with examples from high profile supportive parents such as Magic Johnson, Dwayne Wade, Brandi Carlisle, and others

4 Seeking Expertise from Stakeholders of Color

While the participation and engagement from members of the Parents Advisory Group was impressive and sustained, our team was cognizant that the Board did not include any parents from communities of color. Despite our best efforts to recruit non-White parents, we were aware that extended participation in such a volunteer capacity was challenging for parents who might be juggling the demands of multiple jobs, hectic schedules, and general life stressors. To this end, we decided to instead seek out proxies for parents of color. Instead of demanding experts to show up at our laboratory, members of the team purposely sought out sexual health educators of color. With initial versions of the videos on hand, we shared these preliminary videos with stakeholders who had regular interactions with Black and Brown families in a process we have come to regard as *intervention road testing*. For the road-testing sites, we chose the annual Philadelphia Fight's HIV Prevention and Education Summit and the Center for Sex Education's national Sex Education Conference.

Event 1: HIV Prevention and Education Summit (Philadelphia, PA). The HIV Prevention

and Education Summit is an annual event organized by the nonprofit group Philadelphia Fight to provide ongoing training and updates to HIV prevention specialists. This event invites abstract submissions from community members that include staff from AIDS-service organizations, academic partners and other stakeholders. Our team submitted a workshop abstract that detailed our work in progress with language that invited HIV/STI prevention educators for a chance to view the prototype and provide feedback. Box 1 contains the accepted abstract with language about seeking additional feedback.

Box 1 Accepted Abstract
Parents Advancing Supportive and Sexuality Inclusive Sex Talks: Addressing the Questions of Gay, Bisexual, and Queer Youth for HIV/STI Prevention
Background:
In this workshop, we will share our preliminary study called Parents ASSIST (Advancing Supportive and Sexuality-Inclusive Sex Talks), which is an online animated video series that teaches parents how to talk about sexuality and health with their gay, bisexual, and queer (GBQ) ado-

lescent sons. GBQ adolescent males report a sense of obligation to their parents to stay healthy, but they often do not talk about sexual health with their parents. Research with heterosexual adolescents has shown that effective parent–child sex communication enhances youth's self-efficacy with using condoms, resisting pressure to have sex, initiating conversations about HIV/STIs prior to having sex, and accessing reproductive and sexual health services. Yet, little work has been done to incorporate parents in the sexual health education of their queer children. This workshop will describe the preliminary work we have conducted with local parents and health experts to assist parents be better sexual health educators for GBQ adolescent sons.

Objectives:

1. Describe the significance of parent-facilitated sexual health discussions in the home.
   (a) Through an interactive discussion, workshop participants will be able to verbalize 1–2 tangible outcomes of parent-facilitated conversations about sexuality and health with adolescent children.
2. Discuss the need for inclusive and targeted parent–child sex communication involving LGBTQ+ youth.
   (a) Through a small group activity, workshop participants will be able to identify 1–2 reasons why LGBTQ+ youth do not receive specific sexual health information that are pertinent to their emerging attractions, behaviors, and identities
   (b) Through reporting group discussion findings, workshop participants will identify the sexual health issues that they determine are crucial for parents to address at home.

3. Present six animated Parents ASSIST videos that inform and teach communication skills for parents to facilitate having inclusive parent–child sex communication.
   (a) Through group discussion, participants will critique each video presented and identify portions that are applicable/relevant and those that are non-applicable/irrelevant for families in Philadelphia
   (b) Through anonymous surveys, workshop participants will rank the videos' effectiveness and grade each video's appeal, approach, and relatability

Implications for Programs, Policy, and/or Research:

Health professionals need feedback from community members on new sex education programs like Parents ASSIST. Their feedback can inform HIV/STI prevention strategies for adolescents. It will also inform educational material for parents of GBQ adolescent males. This workshop at the 2019 Prevention Summit provides empirical basis for an intervention that engages parents in preventing HIV/STIs.

After receiving notification of abstract acceptance and prior to the summit, our team identified breakout sessions that were related to our topics based on the published titles and abstracts. This was done to learn about local emerging science, nonprofit workflows, and to identify potential intervention testers. During the actual conference, we attended the six related sessions where we also approached participants before and after each of those six breakout sessions to describe and invite them to our own session. Given that ours was scheduled during the final breakout session, we were able to generate interest and encourage experts' attendance in our session where we subsequently gathered their feedback.

During the first portion of our session, we provided the goals for Parents ASSIST, the sources of the preliminary data and the status of the video-creation process. We shared the website that was under construction at that time along with the 11 draft videos. A walk-through was conducted where audience members had a chance to see the project mock-up that was projected onto the conference screen along with each website tab being developed and a resource page for additional information. A portion of the main instructional video was played for the audience to provide a feel for the product under development.

As we ended the main presentation, we informed the audience about the lack of non-White members of the Parent Advisory Committee and our intention to collect inclusive feedback prior to pilot testing. As researchers of color, we explained our awareness of this shortcoming and invited them to stay behind after the formal presentation for two mini-focus groups. Audience members who opted to stay for the second portion were divided into two groups where a series of questions were asked. In these two smaller breakout groups, study staff played three videos each, solicited the group members' reactions to the videos (e.g., reaction to content, language, visual appeal) and probed about their opinions on how parents or members of the LGBTQ+ community would respond to the videos. Predetermined 1–2 min clips of the original videos were played. The two groups were asked questions similar to those of the Parent Advisory Board, but in a condensed format that reflected their expert background. The two study staff members who facilitated the mini focus groups were the P.I. and a doctoral trainee well-versed in human subject protection. No consent forms were required of the attendees and no incentives were offered as well. Both the two mini-focus groups lasted for about 45 min and were audio recorded after verbal consent was secured from participants.

Event 2: National Sex Education Conference (Newark, NJ). The National Sex Education Conference is a biannual gathering of sex educators in the US where they share research and best practices in the field of sexuality education and health promotion. Given that this was a larger event with attendees from all across the country compared to the HIV Prevention and Education Summit, we decided to forego the format above and decided to seek individual feedback from sex educators of color. Over 3 days, we approached conference participants in the lobby and other public spaces where they congregated, introduced the project aims, and asked if they would like to view some of the videos and provide feedback. To facilitate the viewing of videos, interested conference goers were provided an iPad and a paper survey to record their ratings and thoughts.

For this event, 8 of the 15 videos were shared. Five of those 8 videos were not shared with the Philadelphia testers and 3 were added as we felt they needed more feedback from a more diverse set of individuals. These 3 videos were deemed to contain more sensitive topics (e.g., Abuse and Victimization, Demystifying HIV Testing, and Overcoming Communication Barriers) and thus required as much expert feedback as possible.

5 Findings

Feedback from Sexual Health Educators of Color. The combined feedback from the two events yielded robust recommendations from the key stakeholders whose background differed from members of our Parent Advisory Board. Leveraging their personal backgrounds and professional training, we were able to accrue crucial insights for Parents ASSIST. Box 2 details key comments that were incorporated into the final intervention.

Box 2 Sample Suggestions from Sexual Health Educators of Color

1. Changing video titles to be more descriptive
2. Revision of video descriptions to be less academic and more brief
3. Changing icon images for each video to highlight diverse animated cast
4. Editing language and scripts to feature more accessible vernacular
5. Choosing more dynamic sound effects and audio instead of canned, stilted music
6. Increasing the number of characters from diverse backgrounds
7. Highlighting more realistic family scenarios (e.g., parent–child dyads having disagreements, discussions during family road trips)
8. Addition of more fathers in the vignettes
9. Providing feedback on the planned recruitment flyers to feature diverse dyads and not rely on staid academic recruitment language
10. Increasing planned study incentives to indicate value placed on future participants' time and effort

Feasibility and Acceptability of Parents ASSIST Videos. The Parents ASSIST video series consists of 15 total videos ranging from 4 to 6 min in length each, with the central video of the set titled "Answering Questions" running for 12 min. The videos feature parents of different cultural backgrounds tackling topics such as sex talks, coming out, and answering their child's questions related to sex, sexual orientation, and gender identity.

Once the videos and website were developed, we recruited an online sample of English-speaking parents whose GBQ adolescent sons were between the ages of 12–24 years to participate in online surveys. Participants were recruited nationally through advertisements on Facebook and Instagram and through word-of-mouth from community organizations local to Philadelphia. We initially aimed to recruit 30 parents in 6 weeks for the pilot study but ended up enrolling 54 parents in that time span, with 17 (31%) of parents from diverse racial/ethnic backgrounds. We recruited the majority of the sample online (83%), including mothers (55.6%) and fathers (44.4%) with about half having sons currently in high school (55.6%). The mean parental age was 44.5 years (SD 5.56) while sons' mean age was 16.98 years (SD 2.57).

Through the pilot study, it was shown that parents actively engaged with the video set from beginning to end. On average, it took parents 41 min to get through all of the required videos and answer pop-up questions along the way. Fifty-two out of 54 of the parents surveyed also completed the video series in one sitting. Feedback from the parents to the Parents ASSIST videos were overwhelmingly positive with the majority of parents rating each of the videos highly across four acceptability domains (e.g., relatability, likeability, utility, recommendability). Regarding relatability, 27.8% related to "most or all the characters" and 44.4% related to many of the characters. In addition, 20.4% found the videos "extremely interesting" and 61.1% found the videos "very interesting." In relation to likeability, 75.9% answered "definitely yes" when asked how much they liked what the main characters were saying, and 51.9% rated "very much" when asked how much participants liked the video series. In measuring knowledge utility, 87% answered "definitely yes" when asked if participants thought that watching the videos would help increase parent's knowledge about their son's health and sexuality. Majority of parents also reported that they would recommend these videos to parents of GBQ (gay, bisexual, and queer) adolescent males. 90.7% indicated that they would recommend the videos to other parents of GBQ adolescent males, and when asked if they would share the videos with their friends, 79.6% reported "definitely yes." When asked about the realistic quality of the videos, 64.8% parents reported "definitely yes" when asked if the videos seem realistic, and 75.9% answered "definitely yes" when asked if they would describe their situations as realistic. The pilot also asked about perceived potential impact on communication. 70.4% of participants answered "definitely yes" when asked if the videos would prompt parents to initiate inclusive conversations about health and sexuality with their sons, and 79.6% indicated "definitely yes" when asked if they thought that the videos could help parents learn how to handle conversations about health and sexuality with adolescent sons and broach issues/questions centers on same-sex attraction or behaviors.

Parents also provided qualitative feedback on each video. Many appreciated how the videos were relatable, easy to understand, and made it easy to initiate and discuss uncomfortable topics for them. The pilot study also included overall parental impressions. Many of the impressions were positive, some including simplicity of the step-by step instructions, short video duration for self-paced viewing and schedule flexibility, normalizing parental struggles with a nonjudgmental approach, character diversity and spectrum of family experiences and challenges, easy navigability, collection of parenting tips for improved communication, and acknowledgment that GBQ sons may sometimes know more than parents [30]. Some other positive feedback that the parents acknowledged included that the pilot addressed misconceptions about GBQ sexuality and barriers to talking about sex, showed a good range of typical family setting, covered the importance of nonverbal communication such as facial expressions, pauses, and head nods, provided reminders to fact check what sons claim to know about certain issues, and that the information provided came from an interdisciplinary team of health experts [30].

These preliminary findings from the pilot study demonstrate that GBQ parents had a positive experience utilizing the videos. Additionally in this pilot, 44% of parents recruited were fathers, which demonstrates high interest in this topic in not only mothers but with fathers as well [30]. At the end of the study, parents have also expressed interest in similar studies in the future and have indicated interest in participating in future Parents ASSIST research [30].

This pilot study shows that it is feasible for many other parents to complete this video set. If parents can carve out not even an hour of their day, they can watch the videos and gain the knowledge they wish to garner. Along with this, it shows that parents are open to receiving this type of information. The majority of the parents reported that their child had come out as gay, bisexual, or queer over 2 years ago. However, they were still seeking this information, proving that there is a lack of resources available to this group. A limitation to the feasibility of these videos is access to technology, as not every parent of a GBQ child has access to a phone or laptop computer that they can use to access the internet and complete the videos. Along with this, another limitation is that not every parent of a GBQ child is open to receiving this type of information. The parents who participated in the pilot study participated voluntarily, and not every parent is as open and accepting as those who participated. However, the findings of the study show that when parents are open to receiving such information, animated videos are a feasible method of delivering it. The overall positive reception from parents indicates that animated videos covering topics, including sexuality, health, and communication skills, is a feasible way to provide resources for GBQ parents to learn and also become a sexual health resource for their children.

6 Discussion

While the Parents ASSIST program provides a great resource for GBQ parents, there are state laws that prohibit discussion of same sex relationships particularly in the school curricula. Consequently, these laws and pending legislation can deter students and children, especially those figuring out their sexuality, from learning about safe sex practices [31]. While there are states that prohibit sexual orientation and gender identity discrimination, some states, such as Missouri and South Dakota, prohibit the inclusion of sexual orientation or gender identity in their school's anti-bullying and nondiscrimination policies (NASEM 2020). There are also states that have conflicting state laws in regard to curriculum and activity restrictions. States, including Alabama, Louisiana, Mississippi, Oklahoma, and Texas, prohibit discussion of same-sex relationships in sex education [10].

Since this research was conducted in a US-based context, future research should examine parent–child sex communication internationally. It would be especially important to examine places where LGBTQ+ youth do not have the same rights as those in the US. For instance, several countries, such as Sudan, Morocco, Zimbabwe, and Iran, criminalize sexual activity between males and/or the LGBTQ+ identity [32]. Criminalizing the LGBTQ+ identity creates an unsafe environment for GBQ adolescents. If LGBTQ+ youth cannot come out, they must navigate sexual education and communication much more cautiously. It is imperative to examine how and with whom LGBTQ+ youth communicate and learn about sexual health topics in these areas where they are not accepted. As such, a goal of future research could be to develop safe and accessible strategies for LGBTQ+ youth to gain sexual health knowledge across the globe in varying contexts.

Most of the research in this field focuses on cisgender male school age adolescents. Future research should expand to transgender, nonbinary and/or gender expansive (TNG) sexual health communication. The sexual communication and experiences of the TNG population likely differ from that of the cisgender male population. It is important to examine how parents can appropriately address the needs of TNG children, and create instructional videos that cater to them. Furthermore, examining this distinction combats the presumed heterogeneity of the LGBTQ+ community. In addition, expanding this research to older participants that are still developing and navigating GBQ sex could be very insightful. Different age groups may have different preferences and methods of sexual health communication. Some sexual health topics (e.g. hook up culture, polyamory, fetishes) may not be deemed age-appropriate until later in adolescence [30], which is important to explore.

References

1. Calzo JP, Antonucci TC, Mays VM, Cochran SD. Retrospective recall of sexual orientation identity development among gay, lesbian, and bisexual adults. Dev Psychol. 2011;47(6):1658.
2. Friedman MS, Marshal MP, Stall R, Cheong J, Wright ER. Gay-related development, early abuse and adult health outcomes among gay males. AIDS Behav. 2008;12(6):891–902.
3. Grov C, Bimbi DS, Nanín JE, Parsons JT. Race, ethnicity, gender, and generational factors associated with the coming-out process among gay, lesbian, and bisexual individuals. J Sex Res. 2006;43(2):115–21.
4. Avert. Young people, HIV and AIDS; 2018. www.avert.org/professionals/hiv-social-issues/key-affected-populations/young-people.
5. Bouris A, Guilamo-Ramos V, Pickard A, Chengshi S, Loosier P, Dittus P, Gloppen K, Waldmiller J. A systematic review of parental influences on the health and well-being of lesbian, gay, and bisexual youth: time for a new public health research and practice agenda. J Primary Prev. 2010;31(5–6):273–309.
6. Córdova D, Heinze JE, Hsieh H, Mistry R, Salas-Wright C, Cook S, Zimmerman M. Are trajectories of a syndemic index in adolescence linked to HIV vulnerability in emerging and young adulthood? AIDS. 2018;32(4):495–503.
7. Flores DD, Barroso J. 21st century parent–child sex communication in the United States: a process review. J Sex Res. 2017;54(4–5):532–48.
8. Jones JM. U.S. LGBT identification steady at 7.2%. Gallup.com; 2023. https://news.gallup.com/poll/470708/lgbt-identification-steady.aspx.
9. van Bergen DD, Wilson BD, Russell ST, Gordon AG, Rothblum ED. Parental responses to coming out by lesbian, gay, bisexual, queer, pansexual, or two-spirited people across three age cohorts. J Marriage Family. 2021;83(4):1116–33.
10. National Academies of Sciences, Engineering, and Medicine (NASEM). 2020. Understanding the Well-Being of LGBTQI+ Populations. Washington, DC: The National Academies Press. https://doi.org/10.17226/25877.
11. Crosby RA, Hanson A, Rager K. The protective value of parental sex education: a clinic-based exploratory study of adolescent females. J Pediatr Adolesc Gynecol. 2009;22(3):189–92.
12. Hall KS, Moreau C, Trussell J. Associations between sexual and reproductive health communication and health service use among US adolescent women. Perspect Sex Reprod Health. 2012;44(1):6–12.
13. Widman L, Evans R, Javidi H, Choukas-Bradley S. Assessment of parent-based interventions for adolescent sexual health: a systematic review and meta-analysis. JAMA Pediatr. 2019;173(9):866–77.
14. Adrian, H. (2020). Evaluating the association of parental insurance coverage on critical steps to HIV

pre-exposure prophylaxis uptake in young men who have sex with men.

15. Huebner DM, Barnett AP, Baucom BR, Guilamo-Ramos V. Effects of a parent-focused HIV prevention intervention for young men who have sex with men: a pilot randomized clinical trial. AIDS Behav. 2023;27(5):1502–13.

16. Thoma BC, Huebner DM. Parental monitoring, parent–adolescent communication about sex, and sexual risk among young men who have sex with men. AIDS Behav. 2014;18:1604–14.

17. Glanz K, Rimer BK, Viswanath K. Health behavior and health education: theory, research, and practice. John Wiley & Sons; 2008.

18. National LGBT Cancer Network. OUT: The National Cancer Survey; 2021. https://cancer-network.org/out-the-national-cancer-survey/.

19. Deutsch MB. General approach to cancer screening in transgender people. UCSF Transgender Care & Treatment Guidelines; 2016, June 17. https://transcare.ucsf.edu/guidelines/cancer-screening.

20. Flores DD, Docherty S, Relf M, McKinney R, Barroso J. "It's almost like gay sex doesn't exist": parent-child sex communication according to gay, bisexual, and queer male adolescents. J Adolesc Res. 2019a;34(5):528–62. https://doi.org/10.1177/0743558418757464.

21. Flores DD, Abboud S, Barroso J. Hegemonic masculinity during parent-child sex communication with sexual minority male adolescents. Am J Sexual Educ. 2019b;14(4):417–39. https://doi.org/10.1080/1554612 8.2019.1626312.

22. Flores DD, Meanley S, Bond K, Agenor M, Relf M, Barroso J. Topic recollections and recommendations for inclusive parent-child sex communication by gay, bisexual, and queer adolescent males. Behav Med. 2020a;47(3):175–84. https://doi.org/10.1080/089642 89.2019.1700481.

23. Flores DD, Blake BJ, Sowell R. "Get them while they're young:" Reflections of young gay men recently diagnosed with HIV. J Assoc Nurses AIDS Care. 2011;22(5):376–87. https://doi.org/10.1016/j.jana.2011.01.001.

24. Villarruel AM, Loveland-Cherry CJ, Ronis DL. Testing the efficacy of a computer-based parent-adolescent sexual communication intervention for Latino parents. Family Rel. 2010;59(5):533–43.

25. Flores DD, Rosario A, Bond K, Villarruel A, Bauermeister J. Parents ASSIST (Advancing Supportive and Sexuality-Inclusive Sex Talks): iterative development of a sex communication video series for parents of gay, bisexual, and queer male adolescents. J Family Nurs. 2020b;26(2):90–101. https://doi.org/10.1177/1074840719897905.

26. Bond KT, Ramos SR. Utilization of an animated electronic health video to increase knowledge of post- and pre-exposure prophylaxis for HIV among African American women: nationwide cross-sectional survey. JMIR Format Res. 2019;3(2):e9995.

27. Bandura A. Social cognitive theory and exercise of control over HIV infection. Preventing AIDS. Springer; 1994. p. 25–59.

28. Kreuter MW, Wray RJ. Tailored and targeted health communication: Strategies for enhancing information relevance. Am J Health Behav. 2003;27(1):S227–32.

29. Rogers AA. Parent–adolescent sexual communication and adolescents' sexual behaviors: a conceptual model and systematic review. Adolesc Res Rev. 2017;2(4):293–313.

30. Flores DD, Kornides M, Meanley S. Inclusive and age-appropriate timing of sexual health discussions at home according to gay, bisexual, and queer adolescent males. J Adolesc Health. 2023;72(5):754–62. https://doi.org/10.1016/j.jadohealth.2022.12.015.

31. American Civil Liberties Union. Mapping attacks on LGBTQ rights in U.S. state legislatures; 2023. https://www.aclu.org/legislative-attacks-on-lgbtq-rights.

32. Human Dignity Trust. Map of countries that criminalise LGBT people; n.d.. https://www.humandignity-trust.org/lgbt-the-law/map-of-criminalisation/.

Dalmacio Dennis Flores PhD, RN, FAAN, has a program of research focused on articulating the family's role as a proximal sexuality and mental health resource for adolescents who identify as LGBTQ+. This youth population has disproportionately been affected by HIV/STI infections, suicidality, depression, and a host of other negative health outcomes. His team's work at Penn Nursing is rooted in the commitment that, to eliminate these longstanding health issues, parents and the institutions they routinely interface with (e.g., schools, healthcare, local government) can effectively provide inclusive health education tailored to youths' emerging attractions, behaviors, and/or sexual and gender identities.

Anita Shubert is a senior pursuing a degree in both Psychology and Women's and Gender Studies at the University of Michigan. Her research interests include LGBTQ health with a focus on stigma and discrimination, sexual health, and mental health outcomes. After graduation, they plan to pursue a master's in public health, doctoral degree, and eventually a career in research.

Tom McMahon is a community-based sexual health nurse in Pennsylvania. He is passionate about public health and the ways nurses can mitigate negative outcomes for LGBTQ+ individuals.

Alyssa Lagua is an undergraduate student at the University of Pennsylvania School of Nursing in her senior year of the BSN program. She anticipates working in care settings dedicated to addressing access to care issues within communities of color.

Connor Brandon is a new nurse who graduated from the University of Pennsylvania School of Nursing. He is currently in Los Angeles working at Children's Hospital Los Angeles in the Cardiothoracic ICU.

Abby Cabalbag is pursuing her Masters in the Family Nurse Practitioner Program at the University of Pennsylvania School of Nursing. She is part of a graduate team contributing to Parents ASSIST (Advancing Supportive and Sexuality Inclusive Sex Talks) to create educational materials for parents of LGBTQ youth on selected health topics. She is a staff nurse at Penn Medicine in the liquid oncology floor. After graduation, she plans to work in an outpatient setting as a nurse practitioner.

Caroline Dougherty is a new nurse graduate from the University of Pennsylvania School of Nursing. She is eager to start a career in nursing with a focus on addressing issues that affect underserved populations.

Christopher Krauze-Choi is currently a staff nurse working in hematology/oncology and will be completing his family nurse practitioner with a minor in adult oncology from the University of Pennsylvania School of Nursing. His interests for future practice include the intersection between LGBTQ+ health, comprehensive sexual health including pelvic floor dysfunction, and oncology care.

Arielle Lewis is a new graduate of the School of Nursing at the University of Pennsylvania.

Aruna Rao founded Desi Rainbow Parents and Allies after a 20-year career in mental health advocacy and activism with a focus on the needs of immigrant families. She is the proud parent of a transgender young adult. She is also a member of the PFLAG National Board of Directors. She is the proud parent of a queer and transgender young adult and the founder and Executive Director of Desi Rainbow, which provides support, education, and advocacy for diasporic LGBTQIA+ South Asian Americans and their families. She has served on the PFLAG National Board and has over two decades of experience as a mental health advocate and nonprofit executive.

Kim and John Otto are previous Presidents of the Philadelphia chapter of PFLAG (formerly Parent and Families of Lesbians and Gays). They are involved in several LGBTQ+ initiatives in New Jersey and are members of the Parents Advisory Board of Parents ASSIST (Advancing Supportive and Sexuality Inclusive Sex Talks) at the University of Pennsylvania School of Nursing.

Structural Factors Affecting Mother–Baby Pairs to Access HIV Services in Malawi: A Case of Balaka District

Chifundo Colleta Zimba
and Alinane Linda Nyondo-Mipando

Human Immunodeficiency Virus (HIV) testing in adult population has progressed well in Malawi [1]. However, gaps remain in testing HIV-exposed children in Malawi and most of the sub-Saharan African countries to identify those living with HIV [2]. In Malawi, only a few HIV-exposed children received early infant diagnosis (EID) services prior to 2015 [3–5], secondary to a lack of health professionals and material resources [6–8]. The inadequate staffing levels in Malawi impeded a successful delivery of EID services, contrary to the desire of many health workers. As a result, these health care workers experienced high workload that led to stress and burnout [9].

In this chapter we present our efforts to address inequities in HIV testing through the Malawi MoH and Tingathe program (a partner to MoH). In this project, we worked with the Malawi MoH and Tingathe program to recruit Health Surveillance Assistants (HSAs), HIV Diagnostic Assistants (HDAs), and their supervisors, to explore the structural factors at community, facility, and policy levels. These levels of SDoH affected the mother–baby pairs' access to the HIV services in 14 health facilities of Balaka district—one of the pilot districts—in the southern part of Malawi. The HSAs were a lay cadre that were created by the Malawi MoH to be responsible for disease surveillance at the community level, and were also trained on HIV testing services, before creation of the HDA-cadre in Malawi. Our review of the literature revealed that although Malawi has excelled in its mother-to-child transmission of HIV program [1], there were challenges in identification of HIV-exposed infants [10], mainly due to inadequate human resource [9]. This led the Malawi MoH to create the HDA cadre to be responsible for HIV testing services at clinic level [11].

Our initial steps were to conduct a qualitative descriptive study in all 14 health facilities of Balaka district in Malawi. Balaka district is in the south-eastern part of the country with a catchment population of 524,113. The HDA program was supported by the Tingathe program [12] that worked under Baylor College of Medicine, a nongovernmental organization registered in Malawi that provides HIV services to children in the central and part of the southern region of the country, including the study sites. Prior to this qualitative descriptive study, the first author of this chapter interacted with managers responsible for the management of health services in Balaka and those from Tingathe program at Baylor College of Medicine in HIV studies, national thematic working groups, and

C. C. Zimba (✉)
University of North Carolina Project, and UNC-CH School of Nursing, Chapel Hill, NC, USA

A. L. Nyondo-Mipando
Kamuzu University of Health Sciences and University of Liverpool, Blantyre, Malawi
e-mail: lmipando@kuhes.ac.mw

© The Author(s), under exclusive license to Springer Nature Switzerland AG 2024
J. B. Hamilton, C. E. Moore (eds.), *Transforming Social Determinants to Promote Global Health*,
https://doi.org/10.1007/978-3-031-61160-5_13

conferences. This helped us to easily gain access to all the 14 health facilities in Balaka district. Of the 14 study sites, 13 were health centers and 1 was a district hospital. The 13 health centers included 8 government and 5 Christian Health Association of Malawi (CHAM) facilities. Malawi categorizes its health care delivery sys-tem into three levels: (1) primary or basic care is provided at health centers and community hos-pitals, (2) secondary or enhanced care is done at district and other CHAM hospitals that have capacity equivalent to a district hospital, and (3) tertiary or specialized care that is done at central hospitals [13].

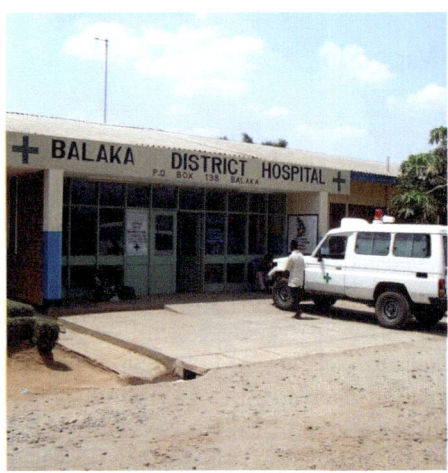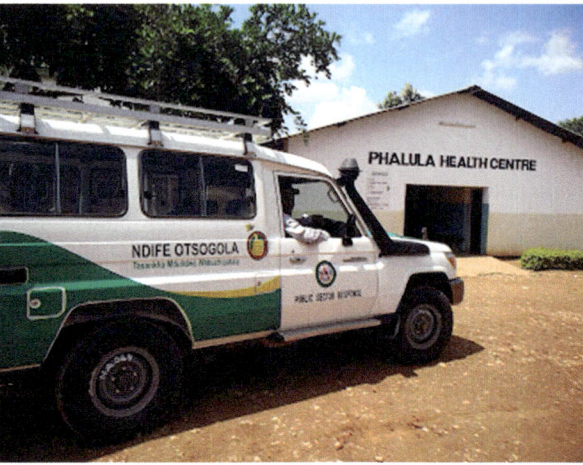

Fig. 1 Pictures of Balaka District Hospital and Phalula Health Centre
Balaka District hospital and Phalula Health Centre were part of the 14 study sites
Source: Downloaded from: https://web.facebook.com/people/Ministry-of-Health-Balaka-District-Hospital/100064557465305/?_rdc=1&_rdr

https://www.google.com/search?sca_esv=558765920&sxsrf=AB5stBhmHao6gt5dl2nxQlm138cbrVagAw:1692627702654&q=Phalula+Health+Centre&tbm=isch&source=lnms&sa=X&ved=2ahUKEwj6mtDH-e2AAxUNxAIHHVCkDNQQ0pQJegQIChAB&biw=1280&bih=603&dpr=1.5

1   Description of the HDA Program in Malawi

The HDAs are a lay cadre; trained outside of school, and similar to other lay cadres, such as the HIV counselors that most African countries use in implementing their HIV testing policies [11, 14–16]. The HDAs have a secondary school education and receive 3 weeks of classroom training and 1 week of practice focusing on HTS, ethical issues related to HIV, and documentation [11]. HDAs' responsibilities were limited to pre- and post-HIV test counseling, initial and confirmatory HIV testing, viral load testing, and Deoxyribonucleic acid-*Polymerase chain reaction* (DNA-PCR), and sample collection for infants for EID [11]. All facilities that offered HIV services were expected to have at least a minimum of two HDAs [11].

In coordination with the Malawi MoH and Tingathe district leadership, we identified the HDAs, HDA supervisors, and Health Surveillance Assistants (HSAs), to share their experiences working in the HDA program through in-depth interviews (N = 14 IDIs with supervisors and N = 10 FGDs—5 with HDAs and 5 with HSAs). Through working with already established structures within the health system and community, i.e., the Tingathe program and the MoH, we were able to establish trust with the participants (i.e. the HDAs, HSAs and all the 14 health facilities). This collaboration also enhanced our ability to access this setting and recruit participants, using their understanding of the social environment and the health systems in those environments. In total, 80 participants contributed to our findings; of these, 34 were HDAs, 32 HSAs, and 14 supervisors to HDAs. The overwhelming majority (66%) of participants in this qualitative study identified themselves as men; mean age of 37 years (range: 22–58 years), 72% were married,

and over 90% had at least some secondary school education.

1.1   Structural Factors Affecting Mother–Baby Pairs to Access HIV Services in Malawi: A Case of Balaka District

In the following sections, we describe the community, facility, and policy levels' structural factors affecting mother–baby pairs' access to HIV services in Balaka district of Malawi.

1.1.1   Community-Level Factors that Facilitated Access to HIV Services Include the Following

(1) Community health workers and HSAs that provide community health education and survey communities to identify onset of diseases and link them to heath facilities. If a mother and/or baby is HIV positive, community health workers follow up with them to remind them about their next scheduled visits;

(2) Outreach clinics that are organized by the facility staff in collaboration with the HSAs to provide community-based health services including HIV testing targeting both women and babies and linking HIV positive patients into care at the health facility;

(3) Supporting structures that include chiefs, community-based organizations, health and development village-based committees, and area development committees work hand-in-hand with the HSAs to inform these communities about the HIV services available at the outreach clinic or at a health facility; and,

(4) Health facilities used community radio programs as a platform to inform and sensitize people about the HIV services they offer.

1.1.2 Community-Level Factors that Were Barriers to Women and Their Babies to Effectively Accessing HIV Services Include These Services

(1) Geographical and financial challenges are a double-burden that impedes mother–baby pairs that live a far distance to health facilities. This burden of traveling is compounded by poverty resulting in lack of funds for transportation.

(2) Community norms that include lack of male engagement in HIV services, religious and cultural beliefs, and fragile families due to lack of mobility (most families are in the fish business). Culturally, men are decision makers in Malawi; women cannot make decisions regarding their own and their children's health. One of the prominent cultural underpinnings in Balaka are initiation ceremonies for both girls and boys. During these initiation ceremonies, taking about a month each year, women prioritize the associated events and fail to prioritize their health, rarely accessing services at health facilities. Some religious groupings within Balaka prohibit their congregants from accessing health services from facilities because they do not subscribe to western medicine. Lastly, self-stigmatization for some women and their babies contributes to their not accessing HIV services; to avoid shame, they hide their HIV status from the public.

1.1.3 Facility-Level Factors that Facilitated Utilization of HIV Services by Mother–Infant Pairs Include the Following

(1) Adequate human resources such as HDAs provide needed HIV services within the health facilities. Each facility has at least two HDAs to serve people seeking HIV services;

(2) Re-organization of HDA workflow to provide HIV services 6 days a week from 7:30 am to 5:00 pm. This gave women and their babies more options to choose a time that was conducive for them to access the services.

(3) HDAs' positive attitude towards clients created a more welcoming environment to those accessing their services without shame or fear.

(4) Availability of material resources in Balaka health area; there were no shortages of stock of the HIV materials such as testing kits and drugs. The availability of HIV testing kits and drugs made it possible for many women and their babies to access the HTS. If they tested positive, they were started treatment on time. Addition, every facility in Balaka had a dedicated room for the HIV services, where mother–baby pairs received integrated care.

(5) Institutionalization of the services among facilities in Balaka implemented several innovative strategies that eased the accessibility of HIV services such as the following:

- Synchronized appointment dates for mothers and babies through the implementation of the "Mother-Infant-pair (MIP) program." In this program, mothers and babies were matched with scheduled dates for services of the mother (e.g., refills of ARV drugs and contraceptives) baby (e.g., early infant diagnosis services, immunizations, growth and monitoring and refill of ARV drugs). This program enabled mother–baby pairs to reduce trips for services at a health facility.

- Implementation of Index case HIV testing is a strategy to test the children of any woman who tests positive for HIV. This strategy resulted in many children being tested and has facilitated access to HIV care services.

- Health education provided by HDAs through health education sessions ensures that HIV information is accessible to all people seeking health services.

1.1.4 The Facility-Level Challenges Include the Following

(1) Lack of support from senior healthcare workers.
(2) Lack of training to provide HIV services among health care professionals such as nurses and clinicians. This lack of training is especially evident among more advanced nurses and clinicians who otherwise would be available to perform in the role of an HDA.
(3) Inadequate workspace for HIV testing services affected patient confidentiality, as all HDAs at the facility delivered these services in one room.
(4) Competing interests that existed among religious institutions and health care facilities. For instance, Catholic hospitals that are main stakeholders of the MoH in Malawi do not offer condoms as one of the HIV prevention measures, leading to women deciding not to access all other HIV services from these facilities. Condoms are a critical component of the HIV services provided to this population.

1.2 Policy-Level Factors that Were Beneficial

Existing financing system policies were the main policy-level factor that facilitated utilization of HIV services by mother–infant pairs in Balaka health area. Balaka health facilities use collaborative health financing policies from both the Malawi MoH and its partner organizations to effectively deliver HIV services to women and their babies. All health care services, including HIV treatment in government hospitals, are free of charge, while those accessed at CHAM facilities have user fees. Therefore, the government of Malawi has a policy named "Service Level Agreement" with all CHAM health facilities to provide free HIV maternal and childcare services and direct their charges to the government that covers the cost.

Balaka health area also receives support from other partner organizations such as Tingathe, which pays the salaries of HDAs and that of the community health workers. Riders for Health (another organization) provides staff and motorcycles to transport EID samples from health centers to the laboratories, which are located at the district hospital or at Dream Centre, another partner organization within the district. *"Results Based Financing"* works with both health workers and community members by developing bylaws to meet targets in a given period of time. For example, health workers need to meet a certain percentage of people accessing HIV services at the facility, then they are given funds to buy the most needed item at their health facility to aid their work. For the community members, *Results Based Financing* signed bylaws with community leaders, giving them power so that all pregnant women could deliver at a health facility where they accessed HIV services. For women, *Results Based Financing* provides an award of the most needed mother–baby items to those women who do not miss their scheduled visits at the facility, and to all those delivering at a health facility. These policies helped women and their babies to effectively access HIV services from their nearest health facilities.

1.3 Policy-Level Factors that Were Challenges

A complicated EID sample management system that resulted in a lack of laboratories within health centers in Malawi. The EID sample is collected from babies in health centers, then is transported to either the district hospital laboratory or Dream Centre, whichever is closest to the district hospital, to be processed. If the result needs more analysis, the sample is then transported to the central laboratory in Lilongwe, more than 200 km away. This complex pathway—from sample collection to the delivery of results—significantly contributes to long turnaround times, which can lead to poor outcomes for some babies if HIV treatment is delayed.

2 Conclusion

Our work has shown that the newly created HDA cadre of healthcare providers positively contributed to improvement of HIV services targeting mother/baby pairs in Balaka district of Malawi. However, there are structural factors affecting mother/baby pairs to easily access HIV services in Balaka health area in Malawi. These factors arose from the community, facility, and policy levels. Finding ways to address the barriers and sustain the HDA cadre can help to improve the HIV services thereby contributing to the goal of eliminating HIV infections in infants in Malawi and globally.

Acknowledgment This work was supported by the National Institutes of Health, via the Fogarty International Center, National Institute of Nursing Research, and National Institute of Allergy and Infectious Diseases (D43 TW010060, D43 TW009340, K24 AI120796, P30 AI050410). The content is solely the responsibility of the authors and does not necessarily represent the official views of the National Institutes of Health.

We also acknowledge our mentors Professor Benjamin Chi and Dr. Nora Rosenberg for their support. A word of gratitude goes to the Research Assistants: Mercy Tsidya and Cecelia Masa for helping with data collection and transcription.

References

1. Ministry of Health Malawi. Malawi population-based HIV impact assessment (MPHIA) 2020–2021: summary sheet; 2022. Retrieved from Lilongwe: https://phia.icap.columbia.edu/malawi-summary-sheet-2/.
2. Teasdale CA, Zimba R, Abrams EJ, Sachathep K, Ndagije F, Nuwagaba-Biribonwoha H, et al. Estimates of the prevalence of undiagnosed HIV among children living with HIV in Eswatini, Lesotho, Malawi, Namibia, Tanzania, Zambia, and Zimbabwe from 2015 to 2017: an analysis of data from the cross-sectional population-based HIV impact assessment surveys. Lancet HIV. 2022;9(2):e91–e101. https://doi.org/10.1016/s2352-3018(21)00291-5.
3. Manzi M, Zachariah R, Teck R, Buhendwa L, Kazima J, Bakali E, et al. High acceptability of voluntary counselling and HIV-testing but unacceptable loss to follow up in a prevention of mother-to-child HIV transmission programme in rural Malawi: scaling-up requires a different way of acting. Trop Med Int Health. 2005;10(12):1242–50. https://doi.org/10.1111/j.1365-3156.2005.01526.x.
4. Moses A, Zimba C, Kamanga E, Nkhoma J, Maida A, Martinson F, et al. Prevention of mother-to-child transmission: program changes and the effect on uptake of the HIVNET 012 regimen in Malawi. AIDS. 2008;22(1):83–7. https://doi.org/10.1097/QAD.0b013e3282f163b5.
5. van Lettow M, Bedell R, Landes M, Gawa L, Gatto S, Mayuni I, et al. Uptake and outcomes of a prevention-of mother-to-child transmission (PMTCT) program in Zomba district, Malawi. BMC Public Health. 2011;11:426. https://doi.org/10.1186/1471-2458-11-426.
6. Cromwell EA, Dow AE, Low D, Chirambo C, Heyderman RS, Dube Q, Van Rie A. Barriers to successful early infant diagnosis of HIV infection at primary care level in Malawi. Pediatr Infect Dis J. 2015;34(3):273–5. https://doi.org/10.1097/inf.0000000000000625.
7. Donahue MC, Dube Q, Dow A, Umar E, Van Rie A. "They have already thrown away their chicken": barriers affecting participation by HIV-infected women in care and treatment programs for their infants in Blantyre, Malawi. AIDS Care. 2012;24(10):1233–9. https://doi.org/10.1080/09540121.2012.656570.
8. Nkhonjera J, Suwedi-Kapesa LC, Kumwenda B, Nyondo-Mipando AL. Factors influencing loss to follow-up among human immunodeficiency virus exposed infants in the early infant diagnosis program in Phalombe, Malawi. Glob Pediatr Health. 2021;8:2333794x211004166. https://doi.org/10.1177/2333794x211004166.
9. Schuster RC, McMahon DE, Young SL. A comprehensive review of the barriers and promoters health workers experience in delivering prevention of vertical transmission of HIV services in sub-Saharan Africa. AIDS Care. 2016;28(6):778–94. https://doi.org/10.1080/09540121.2016.1139041.
10. Herce ME, Mtande T, Chimbwandira F, Mofolo I, Chingondole CK, Rosenberg NE, et al. Supporting Option B+ scale up and strengthening the prevention of mother-to-child transmission cascade in central Malawi: results from a serial cross-sectional study. BMC Infect Dis. 2015;15:328. https://doi.org/10.1186/s12879-015-1065-y.
11. Flick RJ, Simon KR, Nyirenda R, Namachapa K, Hosseinipour MC, Schooley A, et al. The HIV diagnostic assistant: early findings from a novel HIV testing cadre in Malawi. AIDS. 2019;33(7):1215–24. https://doi.org/10.1097/qad.0000000000002159.
12. Kim MH, Ahmed S, Buck WC, Preidis GA, Hosseinipour MC, Bhalakia A, et al. The Tingathe programme: a pilot intervention using community health workers to create a continuum of care in the prevention of mother to child transmission of HIV (PMTCT) cascade of services in Malawi. J Int AIDS Soc. 2012;15(Suppl. 2):17389. https://doi.org/10.7448/ias.15.4.17389.
13. Makwero MT. Delivery of primary health care in Malawi. Afr J Prim Health Care Fam Med.

2018;10(1):e1–3. https://doi.org/10.4102/phcfm. v10i1.1799.

14. Bemelmans M, Baert S, Negussie E, Bygrave H, Biot M, Jamet C, et al. Sustaining the future of HIV counselling to reach 90-90-90: a regional country analysis. J Int AIDS Soc. 2016;19(1):20751. https://doi.org/10.7448/ias.19.1.20751.

15. Bemelmans M, van den Akker T, Ford N, Philips M, Zachariah R, Harries A, et al. Providing universal access to antiretroviral therapy in Thyolo, Malawi through task shifting and decentralization of HIV/AIDS care. Trop Med Int Health. 2010;15(12):1413–20. https://doi.org/10.1111/j.1365-3156.2010.02649.x.

16. Hu J, Geldsetzer P, Steele SJ, Matthews P, Ortblad K, Solomon T, et al. The impact of lay counselors on HIV testing rates: quasi-experimental evidence from lay counselor redeployment in KwaZulu-Natal, South Africa. AIDS. 2018;32(14):2067–73. https://doi.org/10.1097/qad.0000000000001924.

Chifundo Colleta Zimba PhD, GCGH, BCHN, RN, RM, is a Malawian Nurse/Midwife, Researcher, Systems Analyst and an Educator with PhD in Nursing-Health Care Systems, a Graduate Certificate in Global Health, Bachelor of Science in Community Health Nursing, and a University Certificate in Midwifery. Dr. Zimba is currently an Adjunct Associate Professor at the University of North Carolina at Chapel Hill (UNC), School of Nursing, NC, USA, a Faculty Affiliate at Center for Global Innovation Development within the School of Social work at UNC-Chapel Hill, NC, USA, and a project supervisor for the Innovations for Choice Autonomy (ICAN) project that is exploring means of empowering women to choose a contraceptive choice and build capacity of women to self-inject if they choose an injection method at Malawi University of Science and Technology (MUST), Malawi. Dr. Zimba received her PhD in Nursing-Health Care Systems from the University of North Carolina at Chapel Hill, School of Nursing, North Carolina, USA in 2016.

Alinane Linda Nyondo-Mipando PhD, MN-CH, BN-AP, RN, RM, is a Registered Nurse Midwife and an Associate Professor of Health Systems and Policy at Kamuzu University of Health Sciences in Malawi. She is a tenure track fellow at the University of Liverpool in the Department of Women's and Children's Health and based in Malawi at the Malawi Liverpool Programme. Her research interests are in Health Systems and Implementation Science Research with a focus on health service delivery including quality management. She is keen on redesigning health services with end-users, health care workers, and policy makers to ensure optimal delivery of health services. Her areas of interest are HIV and AIDS across different populations, Malaria, and Maternal and Newborn Health. Linda has vast experience in health systems strengthening, including improving delivery of health services and application of quality management techniques.

Developing Culturally Salient Assessment Tools and Interventions for Underserved and High-Risk Populations in the United States and Africa

Jacob K. Kariuki, Michael Ntim, and Moses Gitonga

This chapter broadens our work on noncommunicable diseases (NCDs) to draw attention to the rising prevalence of cognitive impairment and its connections to CVD risk factors in Sub-Saharan Africa (SSA). Through a pilot study in Kenya, we explore the feasibility of administering cognitive assessments in the region, highlighting challenges arising from cultural nuances and language disparities. We emphasize the need for contextually tailored cardiovascular and cognitive screening tools. Collaborative initiatives with local institutions, health authorities, and communities in SSA are pivotal to the success of our projects. We discuss our partnerships with health volunteers and existing healthcare platforms in Kenya and Ghana. Finally, we outline strategies to engage community leaders and leverage local resources to ensure successful recruitment, retention, and implementation of interventions. In conclusion, this chapter underscores the significance of culturally salient assessment tools and interventions, providing valuable insights into the development of strategies to mitigate health disparities.

1 My Story

I was born and raised in Kenya, where I did my BSN and worked in one of the referral hospitals for a year. Soon after, I got recruited to be a tutor in a hospital-based nursing program where I taught Human Anatomy, Cardiovascular Disease (CVD), and Research. Compared to classes focused on communicable diseases, my classes on CVD were considered to be more abstract because they focused on diseases that were thought to be rare in the local population. It was not uncommon to hear the classes being referred to as the time to learn about the diseases of the rich! Due to paucity of local data on CVD prevalence, incidence, and mortality, the teaching content was largely based on data derived from countries like the United States thus reinforcing the perception that CVD was mostly a problem associated with high-income countries.

J. K. Kariuki (✉)
Nell Hodgson Woodruff School of Nursing, Lillian Carter Center for Global Health and Social Responsibility, Emory University, Atlanta, GA, USA
e-mail: Jacob.kariuki@emory.edu

M. Ntim
Department of Physiology, School of Medicine and Dentistry, Kwame Nkrumah University of Science and Technology, Kumasi, Ghana
e-mail: ntim.michael@knust.edu.gh

M. Gitonga
School of Nursing, Dedan Kimathi University of Technology in Kenya, Nyeri, Kenya
e-mail: moses.gitonga@dkut.ac.ke

© The Author(s), under exclusive license to Springer Nature Switzerland AG 2024
J. B. Hamilton, C. E. Moore (eds.), *Transforming Social Determinants to Promote Global Health*,
https://doi.org/10.1007/978-3-031-61160-5_14

The healthcare systems were also underfunded, and the limited resources heavily invested in managing communicable diseases such as Malaria, HIV, and pneumonia. For example, between 2000 and 2010, most countries in sub-Saharan Africa (SSA) allocated <10% of their Gross Domestic Product (GDP) on healthcare, with only 20% of the limited budgets earmarked for managing all NCDs [1]. The World Health Organization (WHO) followed the same trend allocating only 12% of its budget for all NCDs [2]. These budgetary allocations influenced the clinical and research priorities in the region and perpetuated the perception that CVD was not a major concern in SSA. This skewed allocation of resources continues to date, and the healthcare systems remain fragile and overburdened by a double burden of communicable diseases and NCDs.

In Kenya, most people do not have a primary care provider and annual physicals exams are rarely done. The visits to the clinic or hospital are normally done when one is sick and the clinicians typically treat the presenting symptoms, without routine screening for NCDs. As a result, CVD risk factors such as high blood pressure remain undetected for extended periods of time, leading to missed opportunities for primary prevention. The diagnosis is usually made at the onset of major CVD events (e.g., stroke) when the disease has progressed to a stage where resource intensive interventions are needed to prevent death and manage the associated disabilities. Unfortunately, the healthcare systems in Kenya and most of the SSA region are not well equipped to manage advanced cases of CVD, leading to increased disability and premature deaths [3]. Due to cultural norms which encourage accepting death as the "will of God" and lack of optimal vital registration records, the cause of death is not always known in the region. This makes it difficult for clinicians, researchers, and policy makers to appreciate the scope of emerging health problems and risk factors that are associated with the rapid globalization and sociodemographic transition occurring in SSA.

In Kenya, all nursing students are required to take a community health class that culminates in a community diagnosis project. When we took the students for community assessment, most of the focus was on the home environment, sanitation, cleanliness, and nutrition. Almost everything we were doing was oriented on preventing communicable diseases, and the class projects focused on topics such as typhoid fever, malaria, and childhood conditions. Although we had the equipment to measure some CVD risk factors such as blood pressure, we did not consider CVD risk screening necessary especially in rural communities where we expected very low prevalence of the "diseases of the rich." This was the prevailing paradigm across the healthcare system.

Then, a team from the United States came to our college and requested to partner with us in conducting community based participatory research. As the research instructor, I was asked to be part of the team that worked with the Americans to identify research priorities and approach. They shared with us a growing body of evidence suggesting that NCDs are increasing in SSA, and CVD was projected to be the leading cause of death in the region by 2030. They suggested that we partner with the local clinics to sensitize them on screening and treatment of CVD risk factors. Our local team appreciated the informative data they had shared with us, but we reminded them that our college was in a rural area and our local communities could not possibly have a high burden of CVD risk factors. We contended that their data applied to affluent urban communities in SSA, and if they wanted to do anything focusing on diabetes or heart disease, they needed to implement the project in a big city where people are sedentary and probably rich.

The PhD trained nurse who led the American team suggested that we work together and do some initial screenings in the local community and use the data to inform research priorities. Of the 200 people we screened, about 14% of them had elevated blood glucose levels suggestive of diabetes and over 40% had high blood pressure. These data surprised all of us. Our local team was even more troubled because a good number of people we knew had blood pressures that were dangerously high and required urgent management to reduce the risk of stroke or heart attack. When we asked these individuals about their treatment history, many had never been diagnosed with high blood pressure. Others acknowledged having a history of hypertension but admitted to stopping taking their medications because of lack of obvious symptoms and financial constraints. They reported occasional headaches and dizziness which they self-treated with pain killers or occasional dose of their blood pressure medications. These data helped us realize that hypertension was such a big problem in our community, and we started doing health education sessions in churches and other community-based forums. As we taught local communities about CVD and how the risk factors can go undetected for a long time, people started recalling cases of family members or friends who appeared healthy until they had a sudden death or disability.

The community anecdotes were very powerful, but the existing literature had a premise that SSA was spared from the CVD epidemic sweeping across low- and middle-income countries [4]. This perspective was informed by very limited data because there were no vital statistic records for about 95% of deaths in SSA. The CVD estimates were based on statistical modeling and verbal autopsy which is affected by recall bias and literacy. Therefore, when the statistics were used without appreciating their limitations, conclusions were made that CVD was not a problem in SSA. These conclusions affected the allocation of resources and clinical priorities, leading to suboptimal screening and management of CVD risk. Our team contributed to addressing these challenges by working with the local clinicians to introduce CVD risk screening and management infrastructure. The initial screening focused on traditional risk factors such as blood pressure, weight, waist circumference, and blood sugars. Those diagnosed with the risk factors or CVD were initiated on the available treatments or referred to tertiary hospitals for further management.

My experience working with nurse scientists in my local community inspired me to pursue graduate education. While in graduate school, I worked with the Roxbury Heart and Sole team where we provided regular screening for CVD risk factors, health education, and physical activity training in one of the underserved neighborhoods in Boston. In this community, hypertension and obesity were prevalent and our initiatives were well received. We educated those who attended our sessions, but we also learned from them. One of the crucial lessons I learned was the importance of active listening and tailored solutions that address barriers that are important to the target population. While clinical visits are typically short, taking a few minutes to listen to the patient and their story makes it easier for the clinician to offer practical and acceptable solutions. Through active listening and questioning, we realized that some of the participants were using ultra-processed foods that were also high in sodium, thus increasing their risk of heart disease and diabetes. Others were embarrassed to do their physical activity in public spaces because of the stigma associated with obesity. We worked with each of these individuals to develop tailored plans that addressed their specific barriers, and the outcomes were very positive.

I worked with underserved communities in Boston in the Fall and Spring, but in the Summer, I worked with my mentor and other American volunteers in Kenya where we continued partnering with the local schools of nursing and clinicians in screening and CVD prevention initiatives. Most of those who volunteered to help in Kenya also committed to volunteer in the Roxbury Heart and Sole initiative for a year. It helped all who volunteered, including students, appreciate local and global problems, and innovate solutions that were practical in resource-constrained settings both in the United States and Africa. Many volunteers reflected on how one does not need a million dollars to make a difference in the community, and the need to leverage local resources such as churches and community organizations help people live healthier lives.

2   Making Cardiovascular Screening Practical in Underserved Communities

One of the biggest challenges we had in both United States and Kenya was access to convenient point of care CVD risk assessment tools that were validated in diverse populations. The CVD management guidelines recommended absolute risk assessment as the best evidence-based strategy for CVD prevention and risk surveillance [5]. The absolute CVD risk, also known as total or global risk, describes the probability that an individual will develop CVD within a given time frame, depending on the combination and severity of the risk factors present [6, 7]. This approach is preferred to the traditional approach where clinicians screened for and treated individual risk factors with arbitrary thresholds.

For many years, the available absolute CVD risk assessment algorithms were based on laboratory measures that are not readily available in resource-constrained settings or for individuals with limited access to care [8–10]. The development of non-laboratory-based algorithms, which could be used within one clinic visit presented opportunities for deploying them as first line of screening tools at the point of care. However, since the most robust algorithm, non-lab-based Framingham, was derived in a population that was 99.8% White [11], we determined that external validation of the screening tool in a diverse cohort was necessary to demonstrate its suitability for a diverse sample that included Black Americans.

We used the diverse Atherosclerosis Risk in Communities (ARIC) dataset to demonstrate the value of using the non-lab-based Framingham screening tool in a diverse sample of adults with no previous history of heart disease or stroke. In our analysis, there were no racial differences in performance of the screening tool and its risk stratification was comparable to that of the more resource-intensive lab-based screening tool [12]. We also evaluated the benefits a CVD prevention program guided by the lab- vs. non-lab-based Framingham screening tool in a sub-sample of Black Americans enrolled in the ARIC study. The main objective was to examine the associated economic and performance trade-offs. Are the savings realized from using BMI as a substitute for lab tests negated by a less effective screening process leading to more CVD events? This analysis was critical to appeal to policy makers and clinicians in resource-constrained settings. We reported that the non-lab-based screening approach was beneficial in both savings and accuracy because its costs were 11% lower and identified 6.5% for true positive cases compared with the lab-based approach [12].

Demonstrating the validity and benefits of the non-lab-based Framingham algorithm availed an important screening tool that could be deployed at any point of service in real time, without the need for follow-up visits to draw laboratory specimens or to review results. The convenience and time utility are critical for underserved and high-risk populations because every clinic visit provides an opportunity for timely risk mitigation.

2.1   Clinical Case Study on the Utility of Practical Screening Tools

Mr. Jones, a 64-year-old gentleman with no history of hypertension or diabetes, is visiting with his primary care provider for a routine physical exam. He denies ever smoking but admits to an unhealthy diet and a sedentary lifestyle. His key assessments include blood pressure of 138/78 mmHg and body mass index of 24 kg/m^2. Using the validated non-lab-based Framingham screening tool, these data are adequate to estimate the probability of Mr. Jones experiencing a cardiovascular event within a 10-year timeframe. If the lab-based Framingham screening tool were to be used with this patient, a blood draw is required to measure lipids. The laboratory measures for Mr. Jones included: high-density lipoprotein cholesterol of 1.11 mmol/L (43 mg/dL) and total cholesterol of 4.86 mmol/L (188 mg/dL).

The non-lab- vs. lab-based Framingham estimates were 21.3% vs. 20.1% suggesting that these additional measures did not make a big difference in the estimated risk profile of Mr. Jones. Therefore, the non-lab-based screening tool can be used as the first line of screening at the point of care, without significant tradeoffs in accuracy [12]. Both screening tools identify Mr. Jones to be at high risk of CVD and evidence-based guidelines would recommend intensive lifestyle modification and treatment of blood pressure to mitigate CVD risk [13, 14]. If the absolute CVD risk score was not computed using the evidence-based screening tools, only blood pressure meets a clinically meaningful cut point, but other major CVD risk factors do not meet their respective thresholds. Without the information provided by the absolute CVD risk screening tools, Mr. Jones may not be considered for intensive risk mitigation interventions.

As demonstrated in Mr. Jones' case study, moderate elevations in individual CVD risk factors can have cumulative detrimental effects that could be missed by focusing on individual risk factors. Although individual risk factors independently increase the likelihood of CVD events, the clustering of multiple risk factors is known to compound the risk [15]. Therefore, the validated absolute CVD risk assessment tools support clinical decision-making and facilitate the allocation of scarce resources toward those in greatest need of treatment while avoiding the expense of unnecessary treatment and associated adverse effects to those at low risk [16]. Individuals identified to be at high risk of CVD need evidence-based preventive interventions. In the US, numerous studies have reported the need for culturally salient interventions tailored for minoritized populations [17, 18]. In developing countries, especially SSA, few intervention-based studies have been conducted, and little is known about the utility of extant risk reduction strategies.

3 A Culturally Salient Cardiovascular Risk Mitigation Project in the United States

Black Americans report very low levels of physical activity (PA) and have the highest burden of CVD in the US [19, 20]. Our team recognized a critical need for culturally salient interventions that could be scaled to address barriers to PA that are more problematic for the black community, especially those with obesity. We appreciated the role of socio-environmental factors such as unsafe neighborhoods and limited access to fitness facilities in perpetuating the low levels of PA observed in Black Americans [21–23]. To mitigate these socio-environmental barriers, we endeavored to develop a culturally salient PA intervention that addressed socio-environmental barriers to PA.

Employing a focus group approach, the US team engaged our target populations to help us identify their preferred content to overcome the barriers. The participants were interested in a program that was convenient, fun to engage in, and featuring diverse individuals with varying body sizes, fitness levels, and age engaging in PA [24]. The cultural preferences varied by age and gender, with older women preferring religious-themed PA routines, while younger women and men did not want to mix religion with their PA regimen. Older women and men preferred slower-paced workouts with calm music, while younger women and men preferred fast-paced workouts with pop music in the background. The intervention development process was guided by the social cognitive theory's premise that observing similar others succeed can motivate action and help demonstrate a plan for success [25]. A subsequent study using the newly developed intervention demonstrated that the intervention was feasible and acceptable and helped a diverse sample of adults with overweight/obesity increase their PA.

4 Cardiovascular and Cognitive Risk Mitigation Projects in Sub-Saharan Africa

The US team reached out to colleagues in SSA and agreed to collaborate on projects focusing on addressing NCDs in the region. The team, including cardiovascular and brain health experts, reviewed data that described how the global increase in life expectancy and sedentary lifestyle is associated with increasing prevalence of CVD and age-related cognitive impairment [4, 19]. The data suggested that 80% of the global burden of CVD and 66% of the global burden of age-related cognitive impairment is in developing countries [4, 26] with fragile healthcare systems. The NIH Fogarty International Center also described cognitive impairment in SSA as an "impending crisis" and called for studies that characterized region specific risk factors and interventions designed to address them [27]. Based on these data, our team decided to prioritize a research program that addressed brain and heart health in the SSA region.

In SSA where the elderly population (≥60 years) is increasing at the fastest rates in the world [28, 29], few population-based studies focusing on cognition and/or cardiovascular health have been conducted [26, 30]. Moreover, the stigma associated with age-related cognitive decline, low public awareness, and failure to use state-of-the-art screening tools limits the accuracy of the available prevalence data [26, 30]. Notwithstanding these limitations, it is estimated that up to 25% of older adults in SSA are affected by cognitive impairment; while CVD is projected to be the leading cause of mortality in the region by 2030 [31, 32]. Considering that the prevalence of cognitive impairment and CVD is high and both chronic conditions tend to occur at an earlier age in SSA [28, 33], it was critical to examine the associated demographic and lifestyle risk factors.

Population-based studies, predominantly from the US suggest that midlife presence of major CVD risk factors, such as smoking and hypertension, predict age-dependent decline in cognition [34, 35]. Yet, there might be a differential impact of CVD risk factors across racial/ethnic groups. For instance, Gottesman et al. identified diabetes and hypertension as predictors of dementia in Black Americans [34]. In the age range of 55–64, Black Americans are four times more likely to experience cognitive decline compared to their age-matched White counterparts [36]. The increased risk of age-related cognitive decline has been attributed to higher prevalence of CVD risk factors, including diabetes, hypertension, and obesity [37]. There is also evidence suggesting that the prevalence of CVD and associated risk factors is rapidly increasing in SSA [38–40] but whether this increase is linked to increased rates of age-related cognitive decline remains unknown.

Our investigative team has initiated a pilot study in Kenya, to explore the connection between CVD and cognitive impairment and translational intervention strategies focusing on SSA. Our initial efforts have focused on developing a solid infrastructure and protocols for conducting population-based studies. We have worked with our local partners to establish effective communication strategies, collaborated in developing study protocols, coordinated regulatory requirements locally and in the US, and established a hybrid training program to ensure rigorous implementation of study protocols. The current project will provide a description of how lifestyle factors correlate with cognitive function, and the usability of CVD risk assessment tools and neuropsychological instruments in SSA.

The non-lab-based Framingham algorithm described earlier was used to estimate CVD risk, while a comprehensive neuropsychological battery was employed to measure cognitive health. The batteries included the cognitive portion of the NIH toolbox [41], Verbal fluency (VF), Wechsler Test of Adult Reading (WTAR), Repeatable Battery for the Assessment of Neuropsychological Status (RBANS), Trail Making Test (TMT), and Boston Naming Test (BNT). These cognitive batteries were selected due to their sensitivity to age-related cognitive changes and formative studies suggesting that they are sensitive to effects of PA. They are also routinely used in US-based studies with standardized procedures for monitoring the administration of tasks as well as cut-points for clinical threshold. Employing the same battery of tests in Kenya would allow us to make direct comparisons between performance on these tests in SSA and the US and tease out the influence of culture and literacy levels in the screening tools performance. In our subsequent studies, we will explore whether any low scores on cognitive function tests in SSA reflects true deficits or cultural differences in test taking or understanding of the tests. We plan to contribute to the ongoing efforts to develop screening tools and interventions that are culturally important and pragmatic in SSA.

The data we have collected so far suggest a high prevalence of CVD risk factors in a sufficiently active sample, with women more likely to have obesity and central adiposity compared to men. These preliminary findings have prompted us to start collecting additional data on lifestyle and atypical CVD risk factors, such as household air pollution which could be contributing to increased CVD risk among women due to the prevalent use of solid fuels for cooking in the region. Our team is also exploring cultural attitudes related to cognitive impairment and the perceived utility of interventions that prevent or delay the progression of cognitive decline. Based on the limited available data, we anticipate that the population in SSA may have less judgmental attitudes on obesity, and any intervention will need to be adapted to align with their preferences. The data from our ongoing project will provide important insights on the relevance and utility of the available screening tools and potential clinical cut points that may apply to the local populations. The overarching goal of the pilot study is to inform the development of culturally salient intervention, that will be beneficial in promoting heart and brain health.

4.1 The Community Resources Utilized in the Kenya Project

Nyeri County in Kenya, where our current projects are based, has a population of 759,164 and an area of 2361 km^2 [42]. It is one of the three counties in Kenya where the burden of NCDs has been reported to surpass the burden due to communicable diseases, maternal, neonatal, and nutritional causes [43]. The region's main economic activity is agriculture, but increasing land fragmentation has led to the conversion of agricultural land to settlements, which has promoted an urban lifestyle increasing the risks of NCDs. Utilizing the Kenyan community health strategy, the County government has enlisted community health volunteers (CHVs) whose primary mandate is to link health services to households. The CHVs play key roles including health promotion focusing on healthy lifestyles and environmental determinants of health such as sanitation and hygiene. They also address social-behavioral barriers to health by addressing health literacy and promoting health-seeking behaviors to facilitate timely detection of unmet health needs. The CHVs work closely with community leaders including chiefs, clergy, and county and national government. Our local partner, Dedan Kimathi University of Technology, tapped into the CHVs resource to gain community trust and buy-in, leading to successful recruitment and retention of all study participants. We will continue to nurture this collaboration in our future work.

4.2 The Community Resources to Be Utilized in the Ghana Project

After successfully completing our first SSA study in Kenya (East Africa), we plan to replicate the same model in Ghana (West Africa) so that we can have more balanced data and detailed insights on intraregional similarities and differences. In

Ghana, the Community-based Health Planning and Services (CHPS) program was introduced in 1999 as a national strategy to bring critical health services close to communities [44]. A CHPS zone is assigned for each community with a health facility known as the CHPS compound led by a nurse referred to as a Community Health Officer (CHO).

These nurses provide door-to-door services for the catchment area of their CHPS zone, as well as basic services at the community-based CHPS compounds [44, 45]. The use of CHPS as a platform for healthcare delivery in every community in Ghana has facilitated the implementation of many interventional studies. In our future project, we will leverage existing community resources, including the CHPS, to establish trust and community buy-in.

The community entry will start by engaging with the chiefs and community elders to secure their buy-ins. We will then request the chief to organize a community durbar where all members of the community were invited to attend. Because chieftaincy is revered and held in high esteem in Ghana, this approach will demonstrate our respect for the local customs, and the approval of the project by the community leadership will make it easy for the community to participate. Those interested in participating in the program will be invited at their local CHPS compound where the screening and assessments will occur.

5 Reflections

Though the CVD risk assessment tools used in the Kenya study were relatively easy to administer, the cognitive assessments posed various challenges. They required about 3 h per participant to complete, and several questions included in the screening tools lacked local context, making it difficult for the participants to understand the questions. For instance, in the MoCA questionnaire the word "Daisy" refers to a flower. Although all our participants were fluent in English, they thought "Daisy" could only be a woman's first name because that is how it is used in the Kenyan context. Other cognitive batteries

had pictures or references to weather conditions like snow which are not relatable to the local populations. We were able to address the long duration required to administer the cognitive batteries by providing breaks and refreshments. However, aligning cognitive batteries to the local context may require adaptation and validation studies. When publishing our study results, we will discuss how low scores in some cognitive batteries may be reflective of cultural differences in conceptualization of assessment questions rather than indicators of cognitive impairment.

Despite these challenges, our efforts to avail culturally salient risk assessment tools and interventions for underserved and high-risk populations in both the US and SSA have yielded notable successes. The CVD screening tool we validated has been used in many low- and middle-income countries including Kenya, Rwanda, Brazil, Iran, Qatar, and the Philippines. The tool is especially impactful in underserved communities and resource-constrained settings, as it is convenient and facilitates the implementation of evidence-based guidelines using resources that are readily available. When integrated as a regular screening tool into routine clinic visits, the tool can facilitate early risk detection and timely mitigation of risk.

Our work clearly demonstrates that successful implementation of robust research projects in SSA requires collaborative efforts, engaging local communities, leaders, and healthcare systems. Our emphasis on partnerships, such as leveraging community health volunteers and existing healthcare platforms, showcases the pivotal role of interdisciplinary collaboration and community engagement in promoting successful research programs which will lead to equitable health outcomes.

6 Future Plans

To address the challenges posed by cognitive assessments, we plan to apply for training grants that will allow us to adapt and validate current cognitive screening tools, ensuring that assessment questions and diagnostic thresholds resonate with the cultural backgrounds of participants. This approach will enhance the accuracy and relevance of the data we will collect in our future studies. Collaborative efforts with partners will continue to be a cornerstone, fostering contextual understanding and efficient protocol implementation. We will also continue with our efforts to enhance the local research capacity, culminating in locally initiated and led studies to address CVD and other NCDs in SSA.

In conclusion, this chapter sheds light on the complex interplay between CVD risk factors and cognitive health in underserved populations in the US and SSA. It underscores the significance of culturally salient assessment tools and interventions, providing valuable insights into the development of strategies to mitigate health disparities. By emphasizing collaborative partnerships, contextually tailored interventions, and the adaptation of assessment tools, we set the stage for addressing critical health challenges in underserved and high-risk populations.

References

1. World Bank. The growing danger of noncommunicable diseases: acting now to reverse course. The World Bank Human Development Network; 2011. p. 1–13. http://siteresources.worldbank.org/HEALTHNUTRITIONANDPOPULATION/Resources/Peer-Reviewed-Publications/WBDeepeningCrisis.pdf
2. Stuckler D, King L, Robinson H, McKee M. WHO's budgetary allocations and burden of disease: a comparative analysis. Lancet. 2008;372(9649):1563–9. https://doi.org/10.1016/S0140-6736(08)61656-6.
3. Kariuki JK, Stuart-Shor EM, Leveille SG, Hayman LL. Methodological challenges in estimating trends and burden of cardiovascular disease in sub-Saharan Africa. Cardiol Res Pract. 2015;2015:921021. https://doi.org/10.1155/2015/921021.
4. Alzheimer's Disease International. World Alzheimer Report 2018—The state of the art of dementia research: New frontiers. 2018.
5. Eckel RH, Jakicic JM, Miller NH, De Jesus JM, Sacks FM, Lee I, Smith SC, Lichtenstein AH, Svetkey LP, Loria CM, Wadden TW, Millen BE, Morgan LC. 2013 AHA/ACC guideline on lifestyle management to reduce cardiovascular risk a report of the American College of Cardiology/American Heart Association task force on practice guidelines. Circulation.

2013;129:S76–99. https://doi.org/10.1161/01.cir.0000437740.48606.d1.
6. Cooney MT, Dudina AL, Graham IM. Value and limitations of existing scores for the assessment of cardiovascular risk: a review for clinicians. J Am Coll Cardiol. 2009;54(14):1209–27. https://doi.org/10.1016/j.jacc.2009.07.020.
7. Hayman LL, Helden L, Chyun DA, Braun LT. A life course approach to cardiovascular disease prevention. J Cardiovasc Nurs. 2011;26(4 Suppl):S22–34. https://doi.org/10.1097/JCN.0b013e318213ef7f.
8. Beswick AD, Brindle P, Fahey T, Ebrahim S. A systematic review of risk scoring methods and clinical decision aids used in the primary prevention of coronary heart disease. London: Royal College of General Practitioners; 2008. http://www.ncbi.nlm.nih.gov/books/NBK55818/pdf/TOC.pdf
9. Gaziano TA, Young CR, Fitzmaurice G, Atwood S, Gaziano JM. Laboratory-based versus non-laboratory-based method for assessment of cardiovascular disease risk: the NHANES I follow-up study cohort. Lancet. 2008;371(9616):923–31. https://doi.org/10.1016/S0140-6736(08)60418-3.
10. Kariuki JKJKJK, Stuart-Shor EMEMEM, Leveille SGSGGS, Hayman LLLLL. Evaluation of the performance of existing non-laboratory based cardiovascular risk assessment algorithms. BMC Cardiovasc Disord. 2013a;13(1):123. https://doi.org/10.1186/1471-2261-13-123.
11. Framingham Heart Study. Cardiovascular disease risk. In: D'Agostino RB, Vasan RS, Pencina MJ, Wolf PA, Cobain M, Massaro JM, Kannel WB, editors. A general cardiovascular risk profile for use in primary care: the Framingham Heart Study; 2008. https://www.framinghamheartstudy.org/risk-functions/cardiovascular-disease/10-year-risk.php.
12. Kariuki J, Stuart-Shor EM, Leveille SG, Gona P, Cromwell J, Hayman LL. Validation of the nonlaboratory-based Framingham cardiovascular disease risk assessment algorithm in the atherosclerosis risk in communities dataset. J Cardiovasc Med. 2017;18(12):936–45. https://doi.org/10.2459/JCM.0000000000000583.
13. Arnett DK, Blumenthal RS, Albert MA, Buroker AB, Goldberger ZD, Hahn EJ, Himmelfarb CD, Khera A, Lloyd-Jones D, McEvoy JW, Michos ED, Miedema MD, Muñoz D, Smith SC, Virani SS, Williams KA, Yeboah J, Ziaeian B. 2019 ACC/AHA Guideline on the primary prevention of cardiovascular disease: a report of the American College of Cardiology/American Heart Association task force on clinical practice guidelines. Circulation. 2019;140(11):e596–646. https://doi.org/10.1161/CIR.0000000000000678.
14. Piepoli MF, Hoes AW, Agewall S, Albus C, Brotons C, Catapano AL, Cooney M-T, Corrà U, Cosyns B, Deaton C, Graham I, Hall MS, Hobbs FDR, Løchen M-L, Löllgen H, Marques-Vidal P, Perk J, Prescott E, Redon J, Verschuren WMMM. 2016 European guidelines on cardiovascular disease prevention in clinical

practice. Atherosclerosis. 2016;252:207–74. https:// doi.org/10.1016/j.atherosclerosis.2016.05.037.

15. Kariuki JKJK, Stuart-Shor EMEM, Hayman LLLL. The concept of risk as applied to cardiovascular disease. J Cardiovasc Nurs. 2013b;28(3):201–3. https://doi.org/10.1097/JCN.0b013e31828c3158.

16. Kariuki JK, Imes CC, Engberg SJ, Scott PW, Klem ML, Cortes YI. Impact of lifestyle-based interventions on absolute cardiovascular disease risk: a systematic review and meta-analysis. JBI Evid Synth. 2023;22:4–65. https://doi.org/10.11124/JBIES-22-00356.

17. Mendoza-Vasconez AS, Linke S, Munoz M, Pekmezi D, Ainsworth C, Cano M, Williams V, Marcus BH, Larsen BA. Promoting physical activity among underserved populations. Curr Sports Med Rep. 2016;15(4):290–7. https://doi.org/10.1249/JSR.0000000000000276.

18. Stuart-Shor EM, Berra KA, Kamau MW, Kumanyika SK, Stuart-Shor EM, Berra KA. Behavioral strategies for cardiovascular risk reduction in diverse and underserved racial/ethnic groups. Circulation. 2012;125(1):171–84. https://doi.org/10.1161/CIRCULATIONAHA.110.968495.

19. Benjamin EJ, Blaha MJ, Chiuve SE, Cushman M, Das SR, Deo R, de Ferranti SD, Floyd J, Fornage M, Gillespie C, Isasi CR, Jiménez MC, Jordan LC, Judd SE, Lackland D, Lichtman JH, Lisabeth L, Liu S, Longenecker CT, Muntner P. Heart disease and stroke statistics—2017 update: a report from the American Heart Association. Circulation. 2017;135:e146.

20. CDC. Facts about physical activity | physical activity | CDC. Centers for Disease Control and Prevention. 2014. https://www.cdc.gov/physicalactivity/data/facts.htm.

21. Henderson KA. Physical activity among African American women: change and ways of knowing. Quest. 2011;63:73–84.

22. Pekmezi D, Marcus B, Meneses K, Baskin ML, Ard JD, Martin MY, Adams N, Robinson C, Demark-Wahnefried W. Developing an intervention to address physical activity barriers for African-American women in the deep south (USA). Womens Health (Lond Engl). 2013;9(3):301–12. https://doi.org/10.2217/whe.13.20.

23. Siddiqi Z, Tiro JA, Shuval K. Understanding impediments and enablers to physical activity among African American adults: a systematic review of qualitative studies. Health Educ Res. 2011;26(6):1010–24. https://doi.org/10.1093/her/cyr068.

24. Kariuki JK, Gibbs BB, Davis KK, Mecca LP, Hayman LL, Burke LE. Recommendations for a culturally salient web-based physical activity program for African Americans. Transl J Am Coll Sports Med. 2019;4(2):8.

25. Bandura A. Self-efficacy: toward a unifying theory of behavioral change. Psychol Rev. 1977;84(2):191–215. https://doi.org/10.1037/0033-295X.84.2.191.

26. Roth GA, Johnson C, Abajobir A, Abd-Allah F, Ferede Abera S, Abyu G, Ahmed M, Aksut B, Alam T, Alam K, Alla F, Alvis-Guzman N, Amrock S, Ansari H, Ärnlöv J, Asayesh H, Mehari Atey T, Avila-Burgos L, Awasthi A, Murray C. Global, regional, and National Burden of Cardiovascular Diseases for 10 causes, 1990–2015. J Am Coll Cardiol. 2017;70:1–25. https://doi.org/10.1016/j.jacc.2017.04.052.

27. NIH Fogarty International Center. As dementia rises in Africa, urgent need for research—Fogarty International Center @ NIH. Global Health Matters Newsletter. 2018. https://www.fic.nih.gov/News/GlobalHealthMatters/september-october-2018/Pages/dementia-research-africa.aspx.

28. Guerchet M, Mayston R, Lloyd-Sherlock P, Prince M, Aboderin I, Akinyemi R, Paddick S-M, Wimo A, Amoakoh-Coleman M, Uwakwe R, Ezeah P, Prina AM. Dementia in sub-Saharan Africa: challenges and opportunities. ADI; 2018.

29. Hambleton IR, Caixeta R, Jeyaseelan SM, Luciani S, Hennis AJM. The rising burden of non-communicable diseases in the Americas and the impact of population aging: a secondary analysis of available data. Lancet Reg Health Am. 2023;21:100483. https://doi.org/10.1016/j.lana.2023.100483.

30. George-Carey R, Adeloye D, Chan KY, Paul A, Kolčić I, Campbell H, Rudan I. An estimate of the prevalence of dementia in Africa: a systematic analysis. J Glob Health. 2012;2(2):020401. https://doi.org/10.7189/jogh.02.020401.

31. Abbafati C, Abbas KM, Abbasi-Kangevari M, Abd-Allah F, Abdelalim A, Abdollahi M, Abdollahpour I, Abegaz KH, Abolhassani H, Aboyans V, Abreu LG, Abrigo MRM, Abualhasan A, Abu-Raddad LJ, Abushouk AI, Adabi M, Adekanmbi V, Adeoye AM, Adetokunboh OO, Amini S. Global burden of 369 diseases and injuries in 204 countries and territories, 1990–2019: a systematic analysis for the Global Burden of Disease Study 2019. Lancet. 2020;396(10258):1204–22. https://doi.org/10.1016/S0140-6736(20)30925-9.

32. Mavrodaris A, Powell J, Thorogood M. Prevalences of dementia and cognitive impairment among older people in sub-Saharan Africa: a systematic review. Bull World Health Organ. 2013;91:773–83. https://doi.org/10.2471/BLT.13.118422.

33. Keates AK, Mocumbi AO, Ntsekhe M, Sliwa K, Stewart S. Cardiovascular disease in Africa: epidemiological profile and challenges. Nat Rev Cardiol. 2017;14(5):273–93. https://doi.org/10.1038/nrcardio.2017.19.

34. Gottesman RF, Albert MS, Alonso A, Coker LH, Coresh J, Davis SM, Deal JA, McKhann GM, Mosley TH, Sharrett AR, Schneider ALC, Windham BG, Wruck LM, Knopman DS. Associations between midlife vascular risk factors and 25-year incident dementia in the atherosclerosis risk in communities (ARIC) cohort. JAMA Neurol. 2017;74(10):1246. https://doi.org/10.1001/jamaneurol.2017.1658.

35. Vu TT, Zhao L, Liu L, Schiman C, Lloyd-Jones DM, Daviglus ML, Liu K, Garside DB, Stamler J, Fries JF, Shih YT, Allen NB. Favorable cardiovas-

cular health at young and middle ages and dementia in older age—the CHA study. J Am Heart Assoc. 2019;8(1):e009730. https://doi.org/10.1161/JAHA.118.009730.

36. Potter GG, Plassman BL, Burke JR, Kabeto MU, Langa KM, Llewellyn DJ, Rogers MAM, Steffens DC. Cognitive performance and informant reports in the diagnosis of cognitive impairment and dementia in African Americans and whites. Alzheimers Dement. 2009;5(6):445–53. https://doi.org/10.1016/j.jalz.2009.04.1234.

37. Barnes LL, Bennett DA. Alzheimer's disease in African Americans: risk factors and challenges for the future. Health Aff (Project Hope). 2014;33(4):580. https://doi.org/10.1377/HLTHAFF.2013.1353.

38. Lozano R, Naghavi M, Foreman K, Lim S, Shibuya K, Aboyans V, Abraham J, Adair T, Aggarwal R, Ahn SY, AlMazroa MA, Alvarado M, Anderson HR, Anderson LM, Andrews KG, Atkinson C, Baddour LM, Barker-Collo S, Bartels DH, Murray CJL. Global and regional mortality from 235 causes of death for 20 age groups in 1990 and 2010: a systematic analysis for the Global Burden of Disease Study 2010. Lancet. 2013;380(9859):2095–128. https://doi.org/10.1016/S0140-6736(12)61728-0.

39. Mathenge W, Foster A, Kuper H. Urbanization, ethnicity and cardiovascular risk in a population in transition in Nakuru, Kenya: a population-based survey. BMC Public Health. 2010;10:569. https://doi.org/10.1186/1471-2458-10-569.

40. Seedat Y, Ali A, Ferdinand KC. Hypertension and cardiovascular disease in the sub-Saharan African context. Ann Transl Med. 2018;6(15):297. https://doi.org/10.21037/atm.2018.06.45.

41. Weintraub S, Dikmen SS, Heaton RK, Tulsky DS, Zelazo PD, Bauer PJ, Carlozzi NE, Slotkin J, Blitz D, Wallner-Allen K, Fox NA, Beaumont JL, Mungas D, Nowinski CJ, Richler J, Deocampo JA, Anderson JE, Manly JJ, Borosh B, Gershon RC. Cognition assessment using the NIH toolbox. Neurology. 2013;80(11 Suppl 3):S54–64. https://doi.org/10.1212/WNL.0b013e3182872ded.

42. Kenya National Bureau of Statistics. 2019 Kenya Population and Housing Census Results—Kenya National Bureau of Statistics. 2019. https://www.knbs.or.ke/2019-kenya-population-and-housing-census-results/.

43. Achoki T, Miller-Petrie MK, Glenn SD, Kalra N, Lesego A, Gathecha GK, Alam U, Kiarie HW, Maina IW, Adetifa IMO, Barsosio HC, Degfie TT, Keiyoro PN, Kiirithio DN, Kinfu Y, Kinyoki DK, Kisia JM, Krish VS, Lagat AK, Naghavi M. Health disparities across the counties of Kenya and implications for policy makers, 1990–2016: a systematic analysis for the Global Burden of Disease Study 2016. Lancet Glob Health. 2019;7(1):e81–95. https://doi.org/10.1016/S2214-109X(18)30472-8.

44. Nyonator FK, Awoonor-Williams JK, Phillips JF, Jones TC, Miller RA. The Ghana community-based health planning and services initiative for scaling up service delivery innovation. Health Policy Plan. 2005;20(1):25–34. https://doi.org/10.1093/HEAPOL/CZI003.

45. Awoonor-Williams JK, Tindana P, Dalinjong PA, Nartey H, Akazili J. Does the operations of the National Health Insurance Scheme (NHIS) in Ghana align with the goals of Primary Health Care? Perspectives of key stakeholders in northern Ghana. BMC Int Health Hum Rights. 2016;16(1):21. https://doi.org/10.1186/S12914-016-0096-9.

Jacob K. Kariuki PhD, RN, is a native of Kenya who graduated with a PhD in population health and health policy from UMass Boston in 2016. He was an Assistant Professor at the University of Pittsburgh School of Nursing for 6 years before joining Emory in November 2022. His program of research is focused on prevention of cardiometabolic diseases in high risk and underserved populations, and resource constrained settings.

Michael Ntim PhD, is a university lecturer at Kwame Nkrumah' University of Science and Technology in Kumasi, Ghana.

Moses Gitonga PhD, is a Kenyan epidemiologist and educator, boasting over 13 years of experience as a Lecturer at Dedan Kimathi University of Technology School of Nursing. Additionally, he served as a program officer and trainer at the Academic Model Providing Access to Healthcare (AMPATH) center in Eldoret, Kenya, for 6 years. Dr. Gitonga's educational background includes a Doctor of Philosophy in Epidemiology from Jomo Kenyatta University of Agriculture and Technology. Dr. Gitonga's primary research area centers on noncommunicable diseases, where his work significantly contributes to understanding the factors influencing their prevalence and impact within the Kenyan population.

Developing Resources for Caregivers of Persons Living with Dementia in English-Speaking Caribbean Countries

Glenna S. Brewster, Jodi Sutherland, Sylvia Gould, and Ishtar Govia

The Caribbean region is currently experiencing a significant demographic shift characterized by rapid population aging. In the year 2000, individuals aged 60 and older constituted only 10% of the population, but this figure is projected to increase to 25% by the year 2050 [1]. Moreover, the prevalence of dementia across the Americas is expected to nearly double every two decades, with estimates reaching 14.8 million cases by 2030 and a staggering 27.1 million by 2050. Notably, the rates of increase in Latin America and the Caribbean are anticipated to outpace the rates observed in North America. By 2030, the number of individuals living with dementia in Latin America and the Caribbean is predicted to surpass that in North America, and by 2050, this region is projected to have about 16.0 million persons living with dementia, compared to 11.0 million in North America [1].

By 2050, the Caribbean region is poised to witness a substantial increase in the number of people living with dementia, more than doubling from approximately half a million to 1.14 million [2]. Presently, dementia prevalence within the Caribbean spans from 9 to 23%, with most of these individuals residing in the community [3–5]. Between 2010 and 2050, the number of individuals living with dementia in the non-Latin Caribbean, including countries like St. Vincent and the Grenadines and Jamaica, is projected to surge by an astounding 237% [6]. In St. Vincent and the Grenadines, there is an expected 100% increase in the number of persons living with dementia, while Jamaica faces a projected 242% increase [6]. It is worth noting that estimates for St. Vincent and the Grenadines and Jamaica are around 9%, but these figures may be conservative due to factors such as limited access to healthcare providers for diagnosis, insufficient awareness regarding the signs and symptoms of dementia, and the stigma associated with a dementia diagnosis, which may deter individuals from seeking care when they exhibit signs of the disease [6]. While the prevalence of dementia is projected to increase significantly in the coming years, the available funding and resources in the Caribbean islands for identifying and managing this disease remain lim-

G. S. Brewster (✉)
Nell Hodgson Woodruff School of Nursing, Emory University, Atlanta, GA, USA
e-mail: glenna.brewster@emory.edu

J. Sutherland
Kingston, RI, USA

S. Gould
St. Vincent and the Grenadines School of Continuing Education, Kingstown, St. Vincent and the Grenadines

I. Govia
Amagi Health Ltd, London, United Kingdom

ited. For example, the estimated total costs of dementia in the Americas amount to US$236 billion. However, only a mere 11% of these costs, equivalent to $23 billion, are allocated to Latin America and the Caribbean, despite 44% of people living with dementia residing in this region [6].

The absence of residential long-term and assisted living facilities, the lack of long-term care insurance, and the inadequacy of primary care and caregiving programs for individuals living with dementia contribute to a heavy reliance on informal and unpaid family caregivers [7]. Typically, these caregivers are predominantly female relatives who bear the primary responsibility for caring for those living with Alzheimer's disease and related dementias. Often, these caregivers are simultaneously tending to other family members, juggling paid work commitments, and managing their own coexisting health issues as well as those of the individuals living with dementia [8]. Furthermore, on both islands, there is a dearth of resources that caregivers can access, with none specifically tailored to the unique needs of caregivers for persons living with dementia. Many Caribbean countries face a shortage of knowledge and awareness regarding dementia, coupled with a deficiency in financial, technical, and psychoeducational resources necessary for caregivers to provide adequate care [7]. Consequently, there is a growing urgency to develop, evaluate, and disseminate resources and interventions aimed at supporting this crucial yet vulnerable population of caregivers for individuals living with Alzheimer's disease and related dementias in the Caribbean.

1   My Experience with My Grandmother Living with Dementia

As a native of St. Vincent and the Grenadines, I grew up hearing about older adults "calling lists," and individuals showing symptoms of dementia being labeled as "senile." Consequently, when someone exhibited signs of dementia, they were often kept hidden away from the public eye, isolated from social interactions and the broader community. This not only allowed room for misconceptions and assumptions to grow but also subjected family members to the stigmatization associated with what, at that time, should have been recognized as dementia.

I had heard the whispers, but I never truly understood the emotional impact on family members until my grandmother experienced a stroke and was diagnosed with vascular dementia. My mother became her primary caregiver, and I supported her from a distance as a secondary caregiver (see Fig. 1). My grandmother was a devoutly religious person who attended church regularly, immersed herself in reading her Bible, and devoted herself to prayer. As a religious person, she believed in the Golden Rule and extended her care to many of our neighbors. Because of my research in the field of dementia and understanding of the importance of social interaction among older adults and persons living with dementia, we never isolated her from the community. Consequently, we felt that our family did not experience significant negative stigma commonly associated with a dementia diagnosis.

As the primary caregiver, my mother diligently cared for my grandmother, but the available resources for her as a caregiver were limited. For her, there was no caregiver-specific information about the disease nor guidance on how to care for my grandmother, who was living with dementia, nor information about how to take care of herself as the primary caregiver. While my

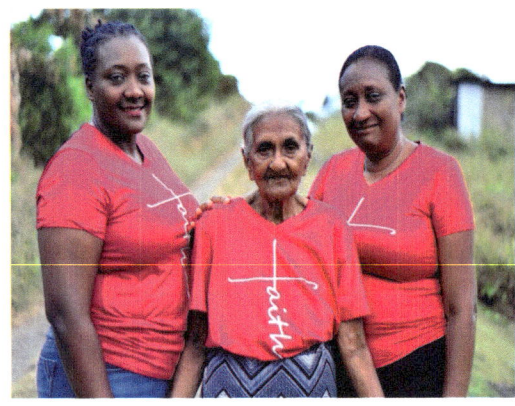

Fig. 1 Glenna Brewster with her mother and grandmother

grandmother did receive some assistance from a care worker who visited our home a few days a week to help with her daily activities, this caregiver had not received specialized training related to caring for someone living with dementia. Drawing upon my experiences as a researcher in the USA, where I have been consistently working with caregivers and individuals living with dementia, I was aware of the resources specifically developed for caregivers and used my knowledge and resources to guide my mother during this caregiving journey. I became determined to ensure that all caregivers in St. Vincent and the Grenadines and throughout the Caribbean, could access these invaluable resources.

2   Resources for Caregivers of Persons Living with Dementia

Jamaica: Established in 2012, the Jamaica Mental Health Advocacy Network (JAMHAN) provides community-based mental health services, conducting research consultancy, advocating for mental health issues, and organizing mental health promotion forums. This non-governmental organization (NGO) collaborates with both public and private sector entities in Jamaica and throughout the Caribbean. Within the broader context of a national policy shift from hospital-based models of care to community-based care, JAMHAN is a strategic partner for the Ministry of Health and Wellness. The organization actively contributes to destigmatizing mental and neurological disorders through its initiatives.

JAMHAN has also fostered partnerships with academic institutions in the Caribbean and beyond. Together, they have codeveloped and implemented funded grants while working to educate the public and healthcare professionals about dementia. The organization provides specific support and resources tailored to the unique needs of individuals dealing with dementia. These efforts encompass activities such as hosting support groups for caregivers of persons living with dementia and organizing educational webinars.

St. Vincent and the Grenadines: The Ministry of National Mobilization, Social Development, Family, Gender Affairs, Youth, Housing, and Informal Human Settlement arranges training programs for homecare workers called Roving Caregivers. These caregivers are subsequently assigned to assist older adults in their homes upon the request of family members. While these caregivers are trained to provide general care for older adults, they do not receive specific training regarding care for individuals living with dementia. Their primary responsibilities revolve around assisting with daily activities such as cleaning, cooking, and supporting the activities of daily living. Community Health Aides share similarities with Roving Caregivers in terms of their training. However, they are affiliated with district health centers and are tasked with visiting individuals who are ill or homebound. Their duties encompass conducting initial health assessments, administering basic healthcare procedures, and referring complex issues to District Nurses. Similarly, Community Health Aides receive education about care of the older adult with little specifics regarding care and assessment of persons living with dementia. The nursing programs offered by the Division of Nursing Education at the Community College include geriatrics/gerontology courses. However, even within these courses, there is limited emphasis on caring for individuals with dementia.

Private institutions also offer continuing education courses that teach participants how to care for older adults. Graduates from these programs are employed either in private settings, assisting families directly, or in nursing homes. These courses typically do not emphasize the care of individuals living with dementia, and graduates may not be adequately prepared to provide extensive care for people living with dementia. Overall, while there are some training programs and educational opportunities for formal caregivers and healthcare professionals in SVG, there appears to be a gap in specialized training and education specifically tailored for both formal and informal caregivers to the unique needs of individuals living with dementia.

The overarching goals of our research initiative were to tailor and/or develop resources explicitly designed to support caregivers of individuals living with dementia. In the following sections, we will provide illustrative examples from Jamaica and St. Vincent and the Grenadines to shed light on our efforts in this regard.

3 Demographics of Jamaica and St. Vincent and the Grenadines

As of 2023, Jamaica has an estimated population of 2,749,000 people, with roughly 55.7% residing in urban areas and 44.3% in rural areas [9]. Approximately 10% of the population are 65 years and older. Most of the Jamaica's population is of African descent, accounting for 92.1%, while individuals of mixed African and European heritage make up 6.1%. East Indian heritage represents 0.8% of the population, and the remaining 1.1% comprises various other ethnic backgrounds. Kingston, the capital city, stands as Jamaica's largest urban center. Most of the population is Protestant [9]. The official language is English but Jamaican Creole is widely spoken. In 2009, Alzheimer's disease was the eighth leading cause of death moving up to the seventh in 2019. Diabetes, stroke, and ischemic heart disease are the first, second, and fourth leading causes of death and disability in Jamaica and are all risk factors for vascular dementia [10].

St. Vincent and the Grenadines consist of a chain of islands, with the primary island being St. Vincent and 32 smaller islands collectively known as the Grenadines, situated in the southern Caribbean (see Fig. 2). The 2023 estimated population of St. Vincent and the Grenadines is 101,000 [11]. The island of St. Vincent has a diverse heritage resulting from its history of colonization by the English and French, who brought enslaved individuals to the island. The native Black Caribs also played a significant role in the island's history, engaging in conflicts with the British. After the abolition of slavery, Portuguese and Indian indentured servants arrived to work on plantations. Consequently, the population of St.

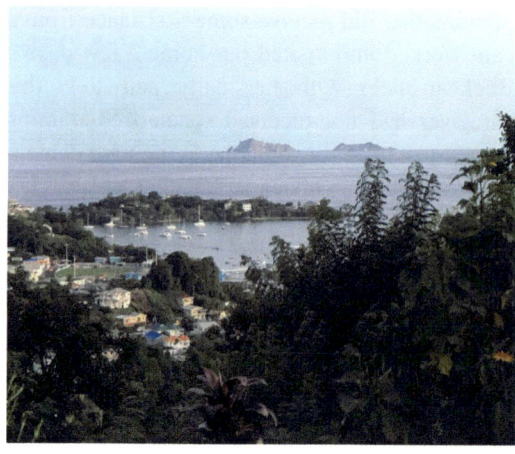

Fig. 2 Picture of a bay in St. Vincent with two Grenadine islands in the background

Vincent and the Grenadines reflects a mixture of these ethnicities, with around 71.2% of African descent, 23% mixed heritage, 1.1% East Indian, 1.5% European (primarily Portuguese), 3% Black Caribs or Kalinagos, and 3% from other ethnic backgrounds [11]. Additionally, there is a growing Syrian and Chinese population. English is the primary language, although most Vincentians also speak a creole or dialect. Most (75%) of the population identifies as Christian [11]. In 2019, dementia was the ninth leading cause of death in St. Vincent and the Grenadines, up from the 11th leading cause in 2009. Other leading causes of death and mortality in St. Vincent and the Grenadines include diabetes, heart disease, stroke, and hypertension, all of which are risk factors associated with vascular dementia [12].

4 Caregiver Interventions for Persons Living with Dementia

A wide array of interventions has been developed to support caregivers of individuals living with dementia. Psychoeducational interventions have shown significant positive effects on caregivers, including improved knowledge, reduced stress, anxiety, and depression, as well as an enhanced sense of self-efficacy [13–16]. Some studies have even indicated potential benefits of these interventions on the individuals living with dementia, such as improvements in their quality of life and reduction in neuropsychiatric symptoms [17].

Web-based interventions offer several advantages over face-to-face interventions due to their flexibility and accessibility [18–20]. Certain interventions, like the Savvy Caregiver program, have been adapted for virtual delivery [18], or tailored for African American communities [21], or rural populations [22]. Formative research has also been conducted to adapt the Savvy Caregiver program for use in India [23]. The Savvy Caregiver Program (SCP) is a structured program spanning 12 h, conducted by trained facilitators over a period of 6 weeks, with participants meeting for 2-h group sessions, each session focusing on specific content and goals [24]. The SCP curriculum recognizes the caregiving role as a clinical one, requiring specialized skills and knowledge [24]. Topics covered within the program encompass stages of dementia, cognitive decline, and corresponding caregiving strategies, the availability of community resources for caregivers, tailoring activities to align with tasks and activities, the roles of family members in caregiving, and self-care exercises [24]. It is important to note that none of these programs are currently available for caregivers of individuals living with dementia in Jamaica or St. Vincent and the Grenadines, and by extension, the wider Caribbean region.

5 SAVVYJA, An Intervention for Caregivers of Persons Living with Dementia

The initial project in Jamaica, known as SAVVYJA, focused on tailoring Savvy Caregiver, through a collaboration between Emory faculty and researchers at the University of the West Indies in Jamaica, in partnership with the Jamaica Mental Health Advocacy Network. The primary objective of this collaboration was to generate evidence to inform the adaptation of the SCP for the Jamaican target audience, with a focus on virtual delivery. The research incorporated a mixed-methods approach to assess the program's effectiveness, including the collection of data related to caregivers' levels of depression, perceived stress, and caregiver burden. Qualitative data obtained from focus groups and memos provided valuable insights from both caregivers and trainers, shedding light on the necessary modifications to both content and delivery methods to ensure the program's utility within the Jamaican cultural context.

Participants for the SCP were informal (unpaid) caregivers, typically family members or friends, caring for community-dwelling persons living with Alzheimer's disease or related dementias. These caregivers did not necessarily reside with the persons living with Alzheimer's disease or related dementias. After completing the SCP, the Jamaican team conducted four online focus groups via Zoom with caregivers, with each group consisting of four to six participants. The objective was to gather feedback about the program's content, how modules were packaged, and the mode of delivery. The project also trained researchers and volunteer caregivers as facilitators for the SCP, with the trainees providing valuable feedback on various aspects of the program. Approximately eight individuals completed a fully online SCP trainer program that included a standardized trainer's manual and audiovisual materials. These trained individuals played a crucial role in evaluating the cultural appropriateness of educational objectives, the agenda with time-linked sessions, and the content, talks, and exercises conducted in each session of the program.

This SAVVYJA feasibility study is built upon prior research involving informal dementia caregivers, which recognized the importance of adapting data collection tools and procedures. This earlier work was conducted as part of the Strengthening Responses to Dementia in Developing Countries—Jamaica (STRIDE JA) research project spanning from 2018 to 2022 [3]. Furthermore, it drew upon findings from the STRiDE Jamaica research, which highlighted significant challenges faced by caregivers of individuals living with dementia during the COVID-19 pandemic. These challenges included financial strain, inadequate coping strategies, and compromised emotional well-being [25]. In the STRIDE JA project, more than 50 stakeholders convened in Jamaica at the outset of 2018 to establish the project's impact objectives and the strategies to achieve them [26]. Additionally, prior to this initiative, the Jamaica team collaborated with colleagues at Manchester University and organized meetings with faith-based stakeholders and other influential community leaders. These meetings aimed to clarify needs and identify culturally appropriate approaches for enhancing the well-being of individuals living with dementia in Jamaica, while also ensuring that caregivers were not unduly burdened by costs.

The process of developing dementia care resources in Jamaica has involved knowledge exchange with individuals living with dementia and their support networks, as well as with healthcare professionals and policymakers. Initially, this effort relied on personal funding to support public education, awareness campaigns, and support programs. Advocacy and policy work, led by coauthor IG, stemmed from her personal experience seeking assistance for a family member. This work was built upon longstanding partnerships and collaborations formed over a decade with leaders of religious institutions, policymakers, and civil society organizations.

Subsequent stages were fueled by grant funding from academic institutions in the UK, allowing for deeper engagement with individuals living with dementia and their caregiving partners through the STRIDE JA research project, which ran from 2018 to 2022. These engagement strategies were employed in this project, along with valuable lessons learned regarding the active inclusion of individuals living with dementia [27].

6 Developing a Prototype for Vincentian Caregivers of Persons Living with Dementia

In St. Vincent and the Grenadines, the development of a prototype course for caregivers will employ a psychoeducation approach, rooted in Social Cognitive Theory [28] and the Sociocultural Stress and Coping Model [29]. To determine the content to be included in this psychoeducational intervention, we will actively engage caregivers through group and individual design-thinking exercises. Design thinking, a problem-solving approach centered on human needs, prioritizes observation, idea visualization, collaboration, and concept prototyping [30, 31]. This multistep iterative process of finalizing the caregiver intervention will involve five stages across multiple sessions:

- *Empathy*: This stage will begin with two focus groups with caregivers. Additionally, five healthcare providers will be individually interviewed to gather insights into the education they provide to caregivers. All focus groups and interviews will be audio-recorded, transcribed verbatim, and supplemented with field notes. Rigorous qualitative description techniques will be maintained, including cues for further participant input, clarifying probes, and member checks to validate interpretations [32].
- *Define*: A design-thinking team, comprising the Principal Investigator, collaborators, design-thinking and local consultants, and caregivers, will convene to identify common themes emerging from the collected data. These themes will be synthesized, combined, or narrowed down to reach a consensus on the specific issue(s) that the prototype should address.
- *Ideate*: The design-thinking team will engage in a creative brainstorming process to generate as many innovative solutions as possible for the identified issue(s).
- *Prototype*: The team will proceed to develop a prototype, specifying the content, form, delivery methods, and estimated duration of the program based on the ideas generated in the previous ideation phase. This is an iterative process, and feedback will be sought from caregivers and healthcare providers who were initially interviewed to make informed decisions about the final prototype's structure, flow, strategies, format, and content.

- *Test*: Through this comprehensive approach, we aim to create a caregiver intervention prototype that is both culturally sensitive and effective in addressing the unique needs and challenges faced by caregivers of individuals living with dementia in St. Vincent and the Grenadines.

7 Challenges and Opportunities in Dementia Caregiving

Stigma remains a persistent challenge in the context of dementia, primarily stemming from negative perceptions associated with the condition. An evident opportunity for intervention lies in the realm of education about the disease, offering a means to transform how individuals living with dementia are perceived and thus enhancing the available support for their caregivers. However, decision-makers with the authority to allocate funding for dementia-related projects may not consistently prioritize these initiatives, often facing competing demands and priorities. Consequently, dementia-related programs may not always secure the necessary resources to be disseminated. Despite these challenges, a significant number of caregivers have demonstrated a willingness to actively participate in research aimed at developing interventions that can provide support not only for themselves but also for future caregivers. International and regional collaborations present a valuable but nuanced opportunity. While there are cultural similarities across countries, subtle differences may necessitate careful consideration. As such, tailoring interventions to suit the specific needs and nuances of each country becomes imperative when fostering cross-border collaborations.

8 Conclusion

In many Caribbean countries, the landscape of dementia care is marked by a critical scarcity of knowledge, awareness, and resources. Caregivers, who play an essential role in supporting individu-

als living with Alzheimer's disease and related dementias, face numerous challenges due to these gaps in understanding and support [7]. This situation underscores the growing urgency to develop, test, and disseminate resources and interventions that can provide meaningful assistance to this increasing population of caregivers in the Caribbean.

The primary objectives of our research are to tailor and develop resources specifically designed to support caregivers of individuals living with dementia in the Caribbean, with particular focus on Jamaica and St. Vincent and the Grenadines. These endeavors have been marked by collaboration, innovation, and a commitment to improving the lives of caregivers and those they care for. In Jamaica, we leveraged existing networks and resources through the ongoing dementia care improvement project, STRiDE JA. This allowed us to gather critical insights to guide the adaptation of the SCP for Jamaican caregivers to be delivered virtually. Training researchers as facilitators for the SCP and seeking feedback from the program's end-users were pivotal elements of our formative research. In St. Vincent and the Grenadines, our approach involves the development of a prototype course. To ensure the content of the psychoeducational intervention resonates with end-users, we will engage them in both group and individual design thinking exercises.

We aim to bridge the knowledge gap and provide much-needed resources to caregivers in the Caribbean. Through empathy, collaboration, and the innovative development of tailored interventions, we strive to make a meaningful impact on the lives of those living with dementia and caring for persons living with dementia, ensuring that caregivers receive the support they need to provide compassionate care in a society that increasingly understands and values their vital role.

References

1. Quashie N, Jones F, Gény L, Abdulkadri A. Population ageing and sustainable development in the Caribbean: where are we 15 years post MIPAA? Int J Ageing Dev Ctries. 2018;2(2):128–48.

2. Guerchet M, Prince M, Prina M. Numbers of people with dementia worldwide: an update to the estimates in the World Alzheimer Report 2015. ADI; 2020.

3. Farina N, Ibnidris A, Alladi S, Comas-Herrera A, Albanese E, Docrat S, Ferri CP, Freeman E, Govia I, Jacobs R, Astudillo-Garcia CI, Musyimi C, Sani TP, Schneider M, Theresia I, Turana Y, Knapp M, Banerjee S. A systematic review and meta-analysis of dementia prevalence in seven developing countries: a STRiDE project. Glob Public Health. 2020;15(12):1878–93. https://doi.org/10.1080/17441692.2020.1792527.

4. Ribeiro F, Teixeira-Santos AC, Caramelli P, Leist AK. Prevalence of dementia in Latin America and Caribbean countries: systematic review and meta-analyses exploring age, sex, rurality, and education as possible determinants. Ageing Res Rev. 2022;81:101703. https://doi.org/10.1016/j.arr.2022.101703.

5. Davis G, Baboolal N, Mc Rae A, Stewart R. Dementia prevalence in a population at high vascular risk: the Trinidad national survey of ageing and cognition. BMJ Open. 2018;8(2):e018288. https://doi.org/10.1136/bmjopen-2017-018288.

6. Alzheimer's Disease International. Dementia in the Americas: current and future cost and prevalence of Alzheimer's disease and other dementias. 2013. https://www.alzint.org/resource/dementia-in-the-americas/.

7. Govia I, Robinson JN, Amour R, Stubbs M, Lorenz-Dant K, Comas-Herrera A, Knapp M. Mapping long-term care in Jamaica: addressing an ageing population. Sustain For. 2021;13(14):8101. https://www.mdpi.com/2071-1050/13/14/8101

8. Alzheimer's Disease International. Life after diagnosis: navigating treatment, care and support (World Alzheimer Report 2022, Issue). 2022. https://www.alzint.org/resource/world-alzheimer-report-2022/.

9. Central Intelligence Agency. The world Factbook: Jamaica. 2023a. https://www.cia.gov/the-world-factbook/countries/jamaica/.

10. Institute for Health Metrics and Evaluation. Jamaica. 2023a. https://www.healthdata.org/research-analysis/health-by-location/profiles/jamaica.

11. Central Intelligence Agency. The world Factbook: St. Vincent and the Grenadines. 2023b. https://www.cia.gov/the-world-factbook/countries/saint-vincent-and-the-grenadines.

12. Institute for Health Metrics and Evaluation. Saint Vincent and the Grenadines. 2023b. https://www.healthdata.org/research-analysis/health-by-location/profiles/saint-vincent-and-grenadines.

13. Han A. Effects of mindfulness-based interventions on depressive symptoms, anxiety, stress, and quality of life in family caregivers of persons living with dementia: a systematic review and meta-analysis. Res Aging. 2022;44(7–8):494–509. https://doi.org/10.1177/01640275211043486.

14. James T, Mukadam N, Sommerlad A, Guerra Ceballos S, Livingston G. Culturally tailored therapeutic interventions for people affected by dementia: a systematic

15. Kishita N, Hammond L, Dietrich CM, Mioshi E. Which interventions work for dementia family carers? An updated systematic review of randomized controlled trials of carer interventions. Int Psychogeriatr. 2018;30(11):1679–96. https://doi.org/10.1017/s1041610218000947.

16. Prince MJ, Acosta D, Castro-Costa E, Jackson J, Shaji KS. Packages of care for dementia in low- and middle-income countries. PLoS Med. 2009;6(11):e1000176. https://doi.org/10.1371/journal.pmed.1000176.

17. Meng X, Su J, Li H, Ma D, Zhao Y, Li Y, Zhang X, Li Z, Sun J. Effectiveness of caregiver non-pharmacological interventions for behavioural and psychological symptoms of dementia: an updated meta-analysis. Ageing Res Rev. 2021;71:101448. https://doi.org/10.1016/j.arr.2021.101448.

18. Hepburn K, Nocera J, Higgins M, Epps F, Brewster GS, Lindauer A, Morhardt D, Shah R, Nash R, Griffiths PC. Results of a randomized trial testing the efficacy of tele-savvy, an online synchronous/asynchronous psychoeducation program for family caregivers of persons living with dementia. Gerontologist. 2021;62:616. https://doi.org/10.1093/geront/gnab029.

19. Hopwood J, Walker N, McDonagh L, Rait G, Walters K, Iliffe S, Ross J, Davies N. Internet-based interventions aimed at supporting family caregivers of people with dementia: systematic review. J Med Internet Res. 2018;20(6):e216. https://doi.org/10.2196/jmir.9548.

20. Leng M, Zhao Y, Xiao H, Li C, Wang Z. Internet-based supportive interventions for family caregivers of people with dementia: systematic review and meta-analysis. J Med Internet Res. 2020;22(9):e19468. https://doi.org/10.2196/19468.

21. Brewster GS, Epps F, Dye CE, Hepburn K, Higgins MK, Parker ML. The effect of the "Great Village" on psychological outcomes, burden, and mastery in African American caregivers of persons living with dementia. J Appl Gerontol. 2019;07334648 19874574:1059. https://doi.org/10.1177/073346481 9874574.

22. Kally Z, Cote SD, Gonzalez J, Villarruel M, Cherry DL, Howland S, Higgins M, Connolly L, Hepburn K. The Savvy Caregiver Program: impact of an evidence-based intervention on the well-being of ethnically diverse caregivers. J Gerontol Soc Work. 2014;57(6–7):681–93. https://doi.org/10.1080/01634372.2013.850584.

23. Narayan SM, Varghese M, Hepburn K, Lewis M, Paul I, Bhimani R. Caregiving experiences of family members of persons with dementia in South India. Am J Alzheimers Dis Other Dement. 2015;30(5):508–16. https://doi.org/10.1177/1533317514567125.

24. Hepburn K, Lewis M, Tornatore J, Sherman CW, Bremer KL. The savvy caregiver program: the demonstrated effectiveness of a transportable dementia caregiver psychoeducation program.

J Gerontol Nurs. 2007;33(3):30–6. https://doi.org/10.3928/00989134-20070301-06.

25. Stubbs M, Govia I, Robinson JN, Amour R, Freeman E. The experiences of caregivers of persons living with dementia in Jamaica during COVID-19. Gerontol Geriatr Med. 2021;7:23337214211043384. https://doi.org/10.1177/23337214211043384.

26. Breuer E, Comas-Herrera A, Freeman E, Albanese E, Alladi S, Amour R, Evans-Lacko S, Ferri CP, Govia I, Iveth Astudillo García C, Knapp M, Lefevre M, López-Ortega M, Lund C, Musyimi C, Ndetei D, Oliveira D, Palmer T, Pattabiraman M, Sani TP, Taylor D, Taylor E, Theresia I, Thomas PT, Turana Y, Weidner W, Schneider M. Beyond the project: building a strategic theory of change to address dementia care, treatment and support gaps across seven middle-income countries. Dementia (London). 2022a;21(1):114–35. https://doi.org/10.1177/14713012211029105.

27. Breuer E, Freeman E, Alladi S, Breedt M, Govia I, López-Ortega M, Musyimi C, Oliveira D, Pattabiraman M, Sani TP, Schneider M, Swaffer K, Taylor D, Taylor E, Comas-Herrera A. Active inclusion of people living with dementia in planning for dementia care and services in low- and middle-income countries. Dementia (London). 2022b;21(2):380–95. https://doi.org/10.1177/14713012211041426.

28. Stajkovic A, Stajkovic K. Social cognitive theory; 2019. https://doi.org/10.1093/obo/9780199846740-0169.

29. Knight BG, Sayegh P. Cultural values and caregiving: the updated sociocultural stress and coping model. J Gerontol B Psychol Sci Soc Sci. 2010;65b(1):5–13. https://doi.org/10.1093/geronb/gbp096.

30. Meinel C, Leifer L, Plattner H. Design thinking: understand-improve-apply. Berlin: Springer; 2011. https://doi.org/10.1007/978-3-642-13757-0.

31. Micheli P, Wilner SJS, Bhatti SH, Mura M, Beverland MB. Doing design thinking: conceptual review, synthesis, and research agenda. J Prod Innov Manag. 2019;36(2):124–48. https://doi.org/10.1111/jpim.12466.

32. Milne J, Oberle K. Enhancing rigor in qualitative description: a case study. J Wound Ostomy Cont Nurs. 2005;32(6):413–20.

Glenna S. Brewster PhD, RN, FNP-BC, is a native of St. Vincent and the Grenadines who is an Assistant Professor at the Nell Hodgson Woodruff School of Nursing at Emory University. She is the founder of the St. Vincent and the Grenadines Alzheimer's Disease and Dementia Association. Her primary research focus has been the development of behavioral sleep interventions for persons in the preclinical/early stages of dementia and their caregivers. She has expanded her program of research to also tailor psychoeducational interventions specifically designed for caregivers in the Caribbean. Dr. Brewster holds an Associate of Science in Nursing degree from Broward College. She graduated from the University of South Florida with a Bachelor and Master of Science in Nursing, a Master of Arts in Gerontology, and a PhD in Nursing Science. She completed a post-doctoral fellowship with the Center for Sleep and Circadian Neurobiology at the University of Pennsylvania, School of Medicine.

Jodi Sutherland is a graduate student in the Behavioral Science program at the University of Rhode Island.

Sylvia Gould is a retired registered nurse. She is the founder of the St. Vincent and the Grenadines School of Continuing Education and teaches basic and advance courses in caring for the older adult.

Ishtar Govia PhD, is an award-winning social scientist, founder, and recognized leader focused on addressing the treatment gap in brain health and dementia, with a special focus on underserved and underrepresented communities worldwide. Dr. Govia is a nominated member of the World Dementia Council and a Senior Consultant with the WHO's Brain Health Unit. She held posts with the Caribbean Institute for Health Research at University of the West Indies, University College London, London School of Economics and Political Science, and the University of Michigan. Dr. Govia is the Vice President of the Caribbean Alliance of National Psychological Associations and a member of the Clinical Management Committee of Bellevue Hospital in Jamaica.

Expanding Primary Care Access in Multilingual Populations Using Flipped Visits and Telehealth

Quyen Phan and Caroline V. Coburn

The phone rang for Quyen Phan, a doctorally prepared family nurse practitioner. Mai (fictional name to protect individual's identity) was on the other end, panicky, desperate, unsure, and scared. "What should we do, *chi*?" (Chi means sister, an endearing but respectful way Vietnamese address other women.) Mai, the clinic office manager, explains that a clinic patient, Ms. N., has nowhere else to go because the clinic is closed indefinitely due to the newly discovered coronavirus. This phone call resulted in a chain of events that incorporated telehealth, student experiences, and creative ways of conducting patient visits.

1   The BPSOS Community

Dr. Phan, faculty in the Emory University School of Nursing, is also the co-founder and a family nurse practitioner volunteer at a free clinic in a large metropolitan area. The clinic serves uninsured, low-income families in the northeastern part of Atlanta, Georgia, in an area with a high concentration of refugees and immigrants who have diverse cultural and linguistic backgrounds.

This clinic is affiliated with a larger organization that addresses a specific need in the community. For many years, a group of Vietnamese healthcare professionals has been working with the nonprofit organization, Boat People SOS (BPSOS), to provide health screenings and health education to a growing community of Vietnamese former refugees and recent immigrants. Although BPSOS is a community-based service organization originally dedicated to providing healthcare and social services to former refugees from Vietnam, it has grown to include patients from various cultures and languages. Three major languages spoken at the clinic now are Spanish, Vietnamese, and Indonesian.

The Board for BPSOS is made up of business and faith leaders who oversee all the BPSOS initiatives: financial, social, as well as health. The financial and social initiatives of the parent BPSOS organization primarily are administered by the BPSOS Board, although social referrals are a frequent function of the clinic personnel. The health initiatives include providing annual physicals, chronic disease management, breast cancer prevention and screening, and treatment for urgent health matters. This health care for the community is conducted by the BPSOS clinic providers, all of whom are volunteers. The clinic administrative effort is donated by BPSOS administrative staff. Although the Board is not directly involved in the operations of the BPSOS clinic, the Board members provide input as needed.

Because this clinic has been in place for 11 years and is part of a service organization that

Q. Phan (✉) · C. V. Coburn
Nell Hodgson Woodruff School of Nursing,
Emory University, Atlanta, GA, USA
e-mail: qphan@emory.edu; ccoburn@emory.edu

has been around for 20 plus years, the community has come to trust the providers and staff. It is a measure of this trust, as well as the clinic's response to the need in the community, that the clinic has grown to serve a community much larger than the original focus of Vietnamese refugees. Ms. N's call to Mai was only one of the many examples of patients who rely on the BPSOS clinic for both ongoing and urgent health needs.

2   The Immediate Challenges of COVID-19

Mai's call came in April 2020, barely a month after the coronavirus pandemic spread to North America, shutting down schools, travels, offices, and clinics, including this clinic, and cutting off the only source of primary care for the diverse community we had been serving.

There also was another challenge to deal with: finding an alternative for our nursing students to have hands-on experience in primary care as part of a HRSA (Health Resources and Services Administration)-funded project. There were no clear guidelines at that early phase of the pandemic regarding safe clinic opening, so it was unclear how to provide treatment to our patients. Even patients with insurance, language skills, transportation means, and health literacy had trouble accessing primary care services during this unprecedented time, let alone uninsured, low-income patients with language challenges.

In Dr. Phan's conversation with Mai, it became clear that this was an opportunity to serve the community while also providing valuable experience for students in the HRSA grant. The use of telehealth was exploding as an option for patients in need of care when there were few to no clinics offering in-person visits. In responding to this need, students would gain valuable competencies in telehealth and have the opportunity to apply those competencies in the context of what has been described as a flipped or co-visit.

3   Flipped or Co-visits

As we studied various models of primary care nursing, the model of flipped or co-visits stood out as an opportunity for nurses to practice at the full scope of their licensure. However, we had not had the chance to put flipped or co-visit into practice. The flipped/co-visit is a team approach using RNs at the full extent of their education. Under this approach, there is evidence that patient outcomes are improved, both patients and providers report higher satisfaction, and providers are available to see more patients [1, 2].

Specifically, in the flipped/co-visit model, the RN takes the patient history and, as appropriate, makes a physical assessment (see Fig. 16.1). The

Fig. 16.1 Flipped/co-visit model utilizing RN to the full scope while releasing medical provider's time to see more complex patients. *MA* medical assistant, *pt.* patient, *VS* vital signs, *CC* chief concern, *HPI* history of present illness, *Subj* subjective assessment, *ROS* review of system, *cont. med* reconciliation, continued medication reconciliation

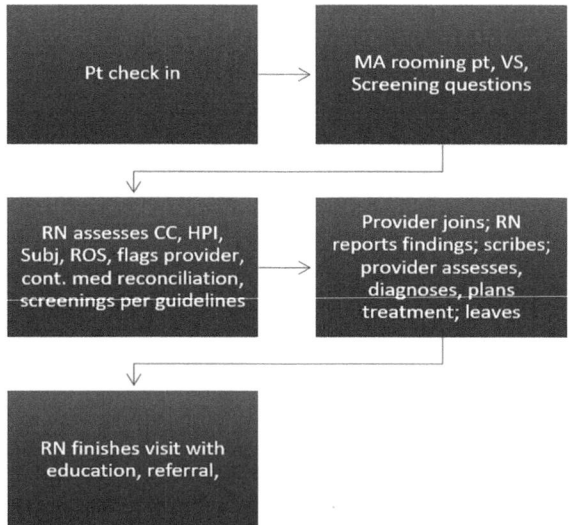

RN then reports to the provider and the provider continues the visit. After the provider finishes, the patient is turned back over to the RN for any follow-up or educational needs.

The flipped/co-visit model fits very well with the BPSOS clinic setting of a nurse practitioner (NP) provider in collaboration with pre-licensure nursing students and their faculty member. These nursing students, under the supervision of the faculty, could begin with the patient intake tasks (vital signs, reviewing chief complaint, conducting subjective assessment, and performing medication reconciliation). They then would report the findings to the NP provider, using a Situation, Background, Assessment, Recommendation (SBAR) format. The NP provider would conduct the objective assessment, make diagnoses, and prescribe treatment. Finally, the students, with faculty oversight, would finish with patient education and reinforcement of the care plan. This plan, for students in the primary care cohort of the HRSA grant, was to be implemented for in-person visits at BPSOS.

However, there was a major wrinkle in our flipped/co-visit plan. It was the dilemma described by Mai in the beginning of this chapter: the shutting down of in-person clinic visits that occurred in spring of 2020. As a result, we were faced with the challenge of providing a valuable clinical experience for our students without their actually laying hands on our patients. In response to COVID-19 restrictions, we quickly had to turn to a virtual or telehealth platform for care delivery, which required creative approaches to patient access and assessment.

4 Telehealth

In this discussion, the word "telehealth" will be used to describe health care that is delivered remotely. To provide context, the words "telehealth" and "telemedicine" are most widely used to describe any form of virtual healthcare, so "telehealth" is employed here in deference to common usage. However, we believe that the words "virtual healthcare" are a more accurate representation of modes that include audio, video, and even robotic types of methods to collect information and deliver care.

Telehealth as a platform for care delivery has both positive and negative aspects. Clearly, it allows providers to reach patients who have challenges to healthcare access. However, in one review of articles written prior to COVID-19, researchers noted that although there were documented benefits to what they described as digital health intervention (DHI), significant barriers also existed both in the delivery and in the patients' ability to access DHIs [3]. In other words, providers were limited in their visions of what might be possible, and patients were limited by technological issues such as bandwidth.

The onset of COVID-19 made the situation described above even worse. It brought what has been called the digital divide into sharp focus, increasing everyone's awareness of a significant area of health disparity [4]. The expression "digital divide" describes the discrepancy between specific populations and parts of the USA where groups of people have difficulty with Internet access and areas or populations where it is easily available. Suddenly, in clinics such as BPSOS, patients who had little to no resources for health care were left with almost no options. Fortunately, this was a wake-up call for the USA to address a problem that had previously been overlooked or underestimated. Unfortunately, because this *had* been overlooked, BPSOS and other clinics were scrambling for ways to provide care without increasing the dangers and risks of COVID-19.

While most patients had some type of Internet access, generally through their mobile phones, the infrastructure required to conduct effective visits that complied with privacy requirements was not in place. However, we quickly obtained the necessary software to meet HIPAA requirements. The next hurdle was determining how to involve the students. We had to address meeting the clinical requirements for pre-licensure BSN students while also giving them a crash course on how to conduct a patient visit online.

5   Virtual Clinic Visits

We had several goals for this clinical setting. The most urgent one was to open services for the clinic's existing 350 patients, who otherwise would not have received primary care. The secondary goal was to create a meaningful clinical experience for students whose educational world had been turned upside down. Finally, it was important to develop a process that would work as smoothly as possible while minimizing the stress and workload on the clinic support staff.

The immediate issue was technical: we had to implement a HIPAA-compliant platform that allowed both voice and video format, with a conference capacity of ten visitors at once to allow access for patient, students, provider, faculty, and in some cases, interpreter. Under this system, the patient would call into a secure, password-protected platform that would give them access to a virtual waiting room, where they would sign a telehealth consent form while waiting for admission into a virtual exam room with the provider. With patient permission, the provider would allow room access to students, faculty, and interpreter.

The rooms had video capability, and most patients were able to see and be seen, although some had cellphone issues that limited them to audio calls. Dr. Phan was the NP provider for the clinic, and Dr. Coburn was the faculty resource for the students. The clinic manager completed the consent (for those who did not speak English and could not complete the online consent while in the virtual waiting room) and set up mock virtual visits for first-time users. Students were provided with just-in-time training on virtual engagement, content on flipped/co-visits, and participated in a telehealth simulation prior to engaging with real patients on designated clinic days.

Two virtual rooms would run simultaneously, and students would stay in their assigned room. Dr. Phan and Dr. Coburn would change rooms as needed. Student experiences included conducting patient intake, observing Dr. Phan in patient care, providing patient education as needed, and col-

lecting population information such as clinic reports on hypertension. If needed, Dr. Phan or a clinic interpreter was available to the students when they conducted their intake or patient education. Table 16.1 provides an overview of the clinical schedule.

Table 16.1 Overview of clinical schedule

Time	Student group 1	Student group 2
1:00	Vietnamese-speaking pt. #1. QP as interpreter, working with students to do intake information and conduct visit	Students work with CC: clinic data related to population management, guidelines review, mammogram follow-up review, reports on HTN, DM
1:30	Students and QP finish with pt. #1—education needs, any clarification about orders	Pt #2—English-speaking. Students do visit intake: chief concern, HPI, PMHx, meds review with CC oversight
2:00	Group 1 break	QP goes to pt. #2. Performs pt. visit. students do post-visit education, clarification, etc.
2:30	Vietnamese-speaking pt. #3. QP as interpreter. Students do intake information and observe clinical visit	Group 2 break
3:00	QP as interpreter. Students finish visit with pt. #3 and provide education and care plan clarification	English-speaking pt. #4; students do Visit intake: chief concern, HPI, PMHx, meds review with CC oversight
3:30	Students work with CC: clinic data related to population management, guidelines review, mammogram follow-up review, reports on HTN, DM	QP goes to pt. #4 and performs exam; students provide education and order clarification
4:00	Post-conference, debriefing	

A "group" of students was no more than two and occasionally only one
HTN hypertension, DM diabetes mellitus, HPI history of present illness, PMHx past medical history, QP Quyen Phan, CC Caroline Coburn

6 Challenges in Implementation

The challenges that we encountered in this setting were twofold: related to the telehealth format of the visit and related to the social determinants of health (SDOH) specific to the population. As noted above, telehealth provides significant benefits but also relies on an assumption of technical resources. Some patients had significant difficulty with the video properties of their mobile phones, and there were times when clear connection was an issue as well. While we were not able to solve elements of the digital divide such as mobile phone or bandwidth limitations, we were creative in our responses to those issues. For instance, occasionally a patient was unable to connect to the platform. In this situation, the patient called the provider on a secure phone, who placed them on speaker phone to allow the students in the virtual platform to hear and participate in the visit.

As with in-person visits, a patient population with limited resources may have challenges simply getting to a visit, even a virtual one. In one instance, the patient had to work during the time of her appointment, but she did not want to reschedule and offered a solution. As a result, we were in the undesirable position of conducting the visit while she was alone in the break room of her place of employment, hoping that no one would walk in.

Language barriers sometimes added a further layer of complication. Due to trained interpreter shortages, family members sometimes assisted with both translation and troubleshooting of technology glitches such as poor video or audio quality. However, Dr. Phan is fluent in Vietnamese, and we usually had a clinic interpreter for Indonesian- or Spanish-speaking patients. For one patient we even involved a Russian-speaking student who acted as an interpreter when that student, witnessing the services the clinic provided, referred someone from her community who was struggling to find healthcare services.

As another example of working through challenges, in one situation a non-English-speaking patient with cellphone problems couldn't hear the interpreter or other people in the virtual room. So, the patient called the interpreter, who used a laptop to access the virtual room and placed her phone on speaker near the laptop so those in the virtual room could hear. The result was a technologically complicated three-way conversation between the patient, interpreter, and provider/students.

7 Results

In the immediate implementation of telehealth care after the clinic was closed due to COVID-19, the results were, naturally, 100% improvement in patient access. We were not able to determine how many patients may have chosen not to participate in care because of the telehealth limitation; however, approximately 40 patients were seen by student nurses during the initial semester of this flipped/co-visit program, fall of 2020. Prior to the fall semester, in the summer of 2020, the clinic visit platform was initiated, and students also saw about 40 patients as part of a clinical rotation focusing on mental health.

Since the fall of 2020, the clinic has continued to have student involvement during the school semesters and to support the patients with telehealth visits. In fact, the current clinic policy is that only new patients or those with urgent issues are seen in person. In concordance with supporting evidence, patients with chronic conditions are effectively managed through telehealth visits only, which may be conducted by an MD, NP, or RN. The number of volunteer providers seeing patients virtually also has increased to include an MD and another NP.

8 Impact on Students and Patients

The impact of this experience on the students has been documented by both their informal comments and their formal end of semester evaluations. In this setting, students had a powerful exposure to the challenges faced by patients who have multiple health problems that are even more complicated by language and access issues. They learned that providing affordable medications and affordable diagnostic testing may require creativity and persistence on the part of the provider and nurse. They found that a provider can obtain quite a lot of information without placing a hand on the patient, such as having the patient use a cellphone camera to show how far they can push a finger into the pitting edema on their ankle. Most important, they learned that, arguably, the most valuable tools a nurse can possess are active listening and empathetic responses.

9 Next Steps

In conjunction with other grants, Dr. Phan will be expanding care access for the BPSOS population to where they live, work, and play via mobile teams. This will incorporate telemedicine and involve developing partnerships with various community organizations such as those who work with refugees, persons with substance misuse, or unhoused individuals.

These ideas will require strategies to develop trust and collaboration, which have been and will continue to be encouraged. These strategies include:

- The long-term community involvement of Dr. Phan which opened the door for future engagement by other faculty and programs
- Pairing community partners with student/faculty support for various programs with mutual benefits such as health fairs, immunization campaigns, and breast cancer screening activities
- Providing letters of support for various grants initiated by the community organization and, in return, receiving letters of support for additional grants
- Supporting clinical agreements for student and faculty clinical rotations

10 Conclusion

While COVID-19-related restrictions placed significant obstacles in the delivery of patient care, in this primary care clinic, the faculty, students, providers, staff, and patients worked together to successfully provide help to an underserved population whose primary safety net had been pulled away. This success was the result of creative approaches to unexpected problems and a commitment to quality and, possibly equally important, flexibility.

Because the faculty also had a commitment to student learning, the telehealth format was implemented in the context of flipped/co-visits, a combination that encouraged learning on many levels. Students saw challenges of communication, inequity in resources, and the invaluable importance of active listening as they began to understand how RNs can collaborate to use their full spectrum of clinical understanding and critical thinking for a lasting positive impact on patient care.

In a recent *Tet* celebration (Vietnamese New Year) at the BPSOS office, Mai proudly presented evidence of the impact of the clinic on the underserved populations to a crowd of volunteer providers, pharmacists, board members, community representatives, and a new group of nursing and nurse practitioner students. At the end, she made a heart sign with her fingers, directed at the audience. Unlike in the initial phone call to Dr. Phan, she was no longer panicky, desperate, unsure, and scared. This time, Mai was confident, calm, reassured, and optimistic.

References

1. Bodenheimer T, Mason D. Registered Nurses: Partners in transforming primary care. In: Proceedings of a conference sponsored by the Josiah Macy Jr. Foundation in June 2016; New York: Josiah Macy Jr. Foundation. 2017.

2. Funk KA, Davis M. Enhancing the role of the nurse in primary care: the RN "co-visit" model. J Gen Intern Med. 2015;30(12):1871–3. https://doi.org/10.1007/s11606-015-3456-6.

3. Willis VC, Thomas Craig KJ, Jabbarpour Y, Scheufele EL, Arriaga YE, Ajinkya M, Rhee KB, Bazemore A. Digital health interventions to enhance prevention in primary care: scoping review. JMIR Med Inform. 2022;10(1):e33518. https://doi.org/10.2196/33518.

4. Etz RS, Solid CA, Gonzalez MM, Britton E, Stange KC, Reves SR. Telemedicine in primary care: lessons learned about implementing health care innovations during the COVID-19 pandemic. Ann Fam Med. 2023;21(4):297–304. https://doi.org/10.1370/afm.2979.

Quyen Phan DNP, APRN, FNP-BC, is a former Vietnamese refugee and an associate clinical professor specializing in nursing education, public health nursing, primary care, care of disfranchised populations, and community partnership building.

Caroline V. Coburn DNP, MS, RN, ANP-BC is an Associate Clinical Professor and adult nurse practitioner specializing in ambulatory care and chronic disease management, both in the USA and under-resourced islands in the Bahamas.

Using Human-Centered Design to Co-Create and Test an Integrated Group Postpartum and Well-Child Care Model in Malawi

Ashley Gresh, Esnath Kapito, Janet Mambulasa,
Nellie Ngutwa, Ellen Chirwa, and Crystal L. Patil

1 Maternal Mortality and Child Health Outcomes

Maternal mortality rates remain alarmingly high globally, and for every woman that dies due to pregnancy-related causes, many more experience life-threatening complication [1]. These high rates of maternal morbidity and mortality lead to poor maternal and child health outcomes and long-term health consequences [1, 2]. Malawi has some of the worst perinatal health outcomes globally; more than 439 women per 100,000 live births and 42 infants per 1000 live births die each year [3]. Women who experience severe maternal morbidity have been shown to have lower quality of life postpartum, increased risk of mortality, and increased risk of complications including from uncontrolled hypertension, cardiomyopa-

thy, or congestive heart failure [4, 5]. Other morbidities such as postpartum depression, urinary incontinence, obstetric fistula, and sexual dysfunction, although perceived as less severe, can be greatly distressing to women [6–8].

Women may additionally face intimate partner violence (IPV) and sexual and economic coercion in the extended postpartum period, which leads to increased socioemotional problems for both women and infants [9, 10]. In Malawi 17.8% of reproductive-aged women (15–49 years) are HIV positive [3]. After childbirth, women often disengage from care and, if HIV positive, drop off HIV treatment which leads to disease progression and sexual transmission [11]. The postpartum period, defined here for this study as the period from the delivery of the infant up to 12 months after delivery allowing for the variation in women's physical and psychological changes [12], is an important window for prevention and response across the maternal and child health continuum setting the stage for long-term health but is often neglected at the health systems level and by women [13].

Despite the recognition of the importance of the first year following childbirth, there are no standardized postpartum care packages for providers to follow beyond the first 6 weeks postpartum; thus no standard guidance exists to address ongoing maternal and infant morbidities and sup-

A. Gresh (✉)
Johns Hopkins University School of Nursing,
Baltimore, MD, USA
e-mail: ashley.gresh@jhu.edu

E. Kapito · J. Mambulasa · N. Ngutwa · E. Chirwa
Kamuzu University of Health Sciences,
Blantyre, Malawi
e-mail: ekapito@kuhes.ac.mw;
jmambulasa@kuhes.ac.mw; embweza@kuhes.ac.mw

C. L. Patil
School of Nursing, University of Michigan,
Ann Arbor, MI, USA
e-mail: clpatil@med.umich.edu

port the transition of the dyad from postpartum to primary care.

These high rates of maternal and infant mortality and morbidities are largely preventable through high-quality healthcare that leads to early identification and treatment of health issues and addressing social determinants of health. The goal of our work in Malawi was to fill this gap by identifying and co-creating solutions in collaboration with communities to design strategies to address social determinants of health and poor maternal and infant health outcomes.

2 Human-Centered Design

We used a human-centered design (HCD) approach to identify an intervention that has the promise to improve maternal and child health outcomes and then to subsequently co-design an intervention to address maternal and infant health with a holistic lens. Human-centered design (HCD) offers an approach to co-design and adapt evidence-based interventions safely, efficiently, and effectively to new contexts. HCD emphasizes the strengths, agency, and priorities of women and healthcare workers to build a model of care that is resilient and responsive to individual, dyad, and system needs. This approach reframes a research question from "what matters" to "what matters most" allowing for solutions that are human centered and context specific and fosters trust in each step of the process [14, 15]. Previous healthcare research supports the use of this approach, as participating in the co-design process increases self-efficacy for both patients and healthcare workers and leads to sustainable solutions to problems within the healthcare system [16, 17]. We used the Human-Centered, Evidence-Driven Adaptive Design (AHEAD) framework [14] that provided us with a practice research-based guide (see Fig. 17.1). We followed the five steps of the

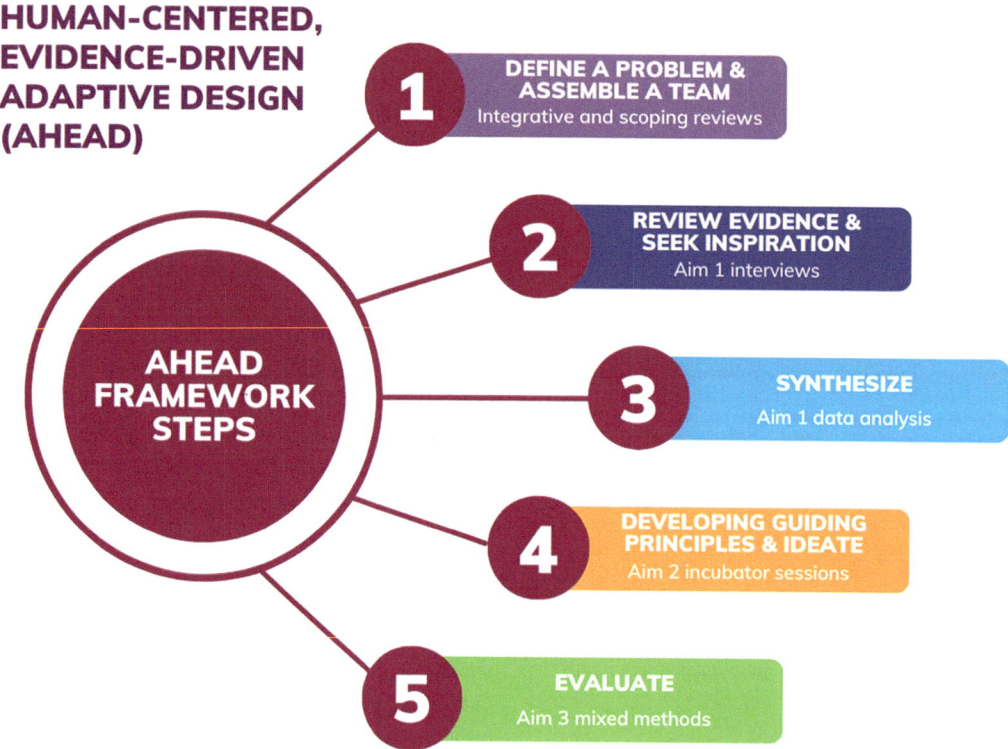

Fig. 17.1 Adapted AHEAD framework

AHEAD framework which we will describe which are as follows: (1) define the problem and assemble a team; (2) review evidence and seek inspiration; (3) synthesize; (4) develop guiding principles and ideate; (5) evaluate [14].

2.1 Step 1 Define the Problem and Assemble a Team

To define the problem, in-depth exploration of people's needs to identify a problem needing a solution is necessary [14]. Our initial step was to conduct an integrative review [18] to describe and evaluate current postpartum care content and service delivery models used throughout the African continent. Guided by the WHO's Maternal Morbidity Working Group's conceptual framework for healthcare interventions to address maternal morbidity, we also identified multiple gaps in care. We showed that noncommunicable diseases (NCDs), intimate partner violence (IPV) screening, mental health, and a rights-based approach to care are rarely included [18]. We

found that Malawi experiences high rates of maternal mortality and morbidities and poor quality or no postnatal care [19, 20]. Group care and integrated maternal and child health services models were identified as ways to improve maternal and child health outcomes.

2.1.1 Group Care

Group care, with its growing evidence base yielding positive results, is an innovative alternative to individual care that can address postpartum and well-child care gaps [21]. Prenatally, group care is an innovative service delivery model with a large body of rigorous evidence supporting effectiveness and feasibility for scale-up [22]. CenteringParenting, a model of group postpartum and well-child care, has three core components: healthcare in a group space, interactive learning, and community building (see Fig. 17.2 for the structure of a group session) [23]. These core components provide a structure to build capacity and enable nurses and midwives to provide efficient and effective care in the postpartum period. This model of care brings the same group

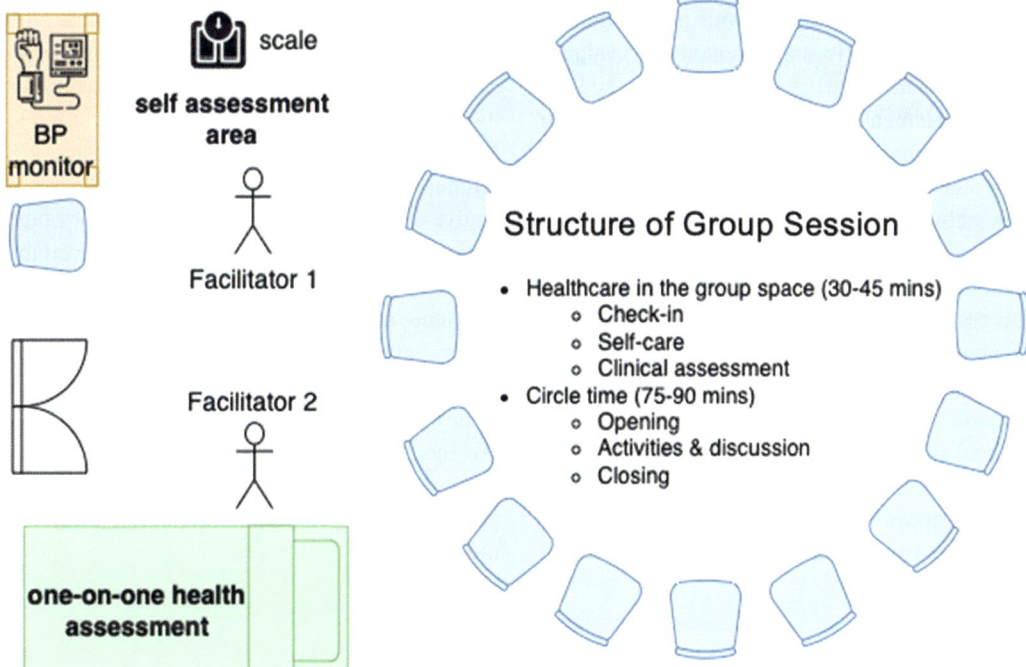

Fig. 17.2 Structure of a group session

of six to eight women and their infants, who are born within 1 month of one another, together for 1–2 years of healthcare. Each session is 120 min with the first 30–45 min consisting of self-care (measuring own infant's weight and length and taking their own vital signs) and standard health assessments of the infant and mother by a clinician in a separate section of the room. Mother and/or infant referrals are made if needed. This is followed by 75–90 min of interactive health promotion, skills building, and support activities. Group care has longer sessions than individual care and provides time and resources to support and address maternal and infant health needs, such as breastfeeding, family planning, depression, nutrition, child development, and infection prevention, and thus improves quality of care and has the potential to reduce maternal and infant morbidity and mortality [21]. Preliminary research shows that group care leads to increased well-child visit attendance, initiation and duration of breastfeeding, patient satisfaction, immunization rates, and parenting and clinician self-efficacy and has a positive impact on maternal psychological well-being [21].

Although the group postpartum and well-child model of care exists with promising outcomes, it has not been widely implemented nor evaluated in low-resource settings like Malawi. In addition when implemented, the model most often prioritizes the infant. Group antenatal care (ANC) has been adapted with success in low-resource countries including Malawi, Kenya, Nigeria, Tanzania, and Rwanda [24–26]. Based on existing ANC and postpartum and well-child group care model success, adapting and designing an integrated group postpartum and well-child care model that expands the continuum of care holds promise to improve maternal and child health outcomes in Malawi and other low-resource countries.

We concluded that an integrated group postpartum and well-child care model adapted for the Malawian context had promise to improve out-

comes. But to do that, we needed to continue to engage in the steps of HCD to co-design the adapted group care model for the Malawian context.

As a nurse-midwife and doctoral student at the time, I leveraged existing partnerships with my mentors and colleagues to continue the HCD process. Specifically I reached out to Sharon Rising, the nurse-midwife who founded Centering Healthcare, and currently leads Group Care Global, and she connected me with a team engaged in research related to group antenatal care in Blantyre District, Malawi. When I approached the team with the idea of exploring extending group care into the postpartum period, they were enthusiastic and ready to support and be a part of the work. Together we were able to leverage their existing research infrastructure, expertise, and momentum from their ongoing clinical trial "Group Antenatal Care: Effectiveness for Maternal/Infant and HIV Prevention Outcomes and Contextual Factors Linked to Implementation Success in Malawi" (ANC Trial, UIC IRB #00403255) that had been implementing and sustaining group antenatal care [27]. With a strong research and academic-community partnership already in place, this helped to facilitate exploring extending group care into the postpartum period. The location of the ongoing study was in Blantyre District, Malawi. Our work was conducted in three government-run clinics participating in the parent study; these were selected because they ranged in patient volume and number of staff available. These clinics allowed us to assess whether government-run clinics can implement group care under everyday conditions without major resource shifts [27]. See Fig. 17.3 for a map of Malawi and location of the clinics.

We then assembled an interdisciplinary team to guide the adaptation and development of an integrated group postpartum and well-child care model.

Fig. 17.3 Map of
Malawi with location of
clinics

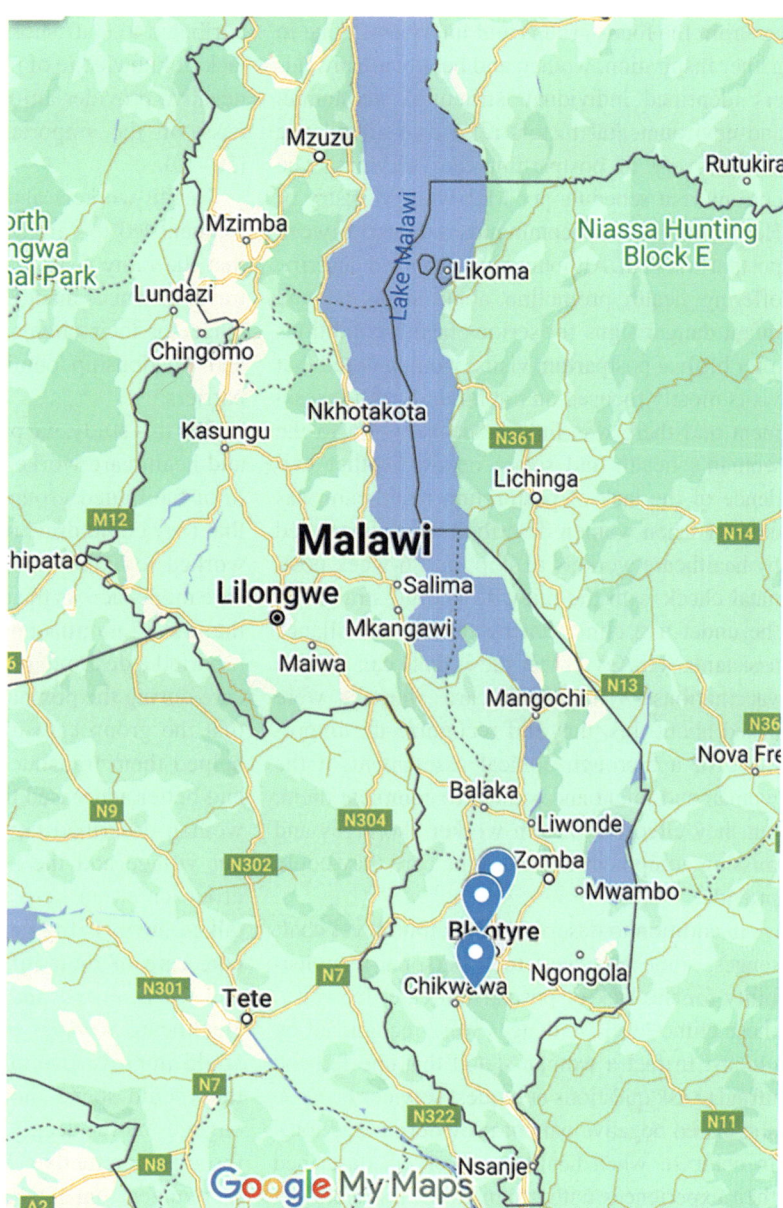

2.2   Step 2 Review Evidence and Seek Inspiration

In step 2, we conducted in-depth interviews with women and healthcare workers to explore their expectations for culturally appropriate postpartum and well-child clinic care. We identified five themes through interviews with women and healthcare workers: (1) maternal health assess-ments are not consistently completed; (2) challenges exist to postpartum and well-child care attendance and delivery of care; (3) postpartum and well-child health promotion topics are not standardized; (4) maternal and child health concerns included physical and psychological issues; and (5) there is buy-in for the group healthcare model from both women and healthcare workers.

From the focus groups and interviews done to gather inspiration, women and healthcare providers identified individual, structural, economic, and environmental factors related to attendance and delivery of postpartum care services. The current visit schedule per Malawian Ministry of Health guidelines recommends a 1- and 6-week postpartum visit. Although midwives did describe offering health promotion about maternal and infant danger signs for serious health conditions after birth at postpartum visits, women noted that visits mostly focused on the infant health assessment and there was little to no attention to the woman's health and social needs. Further evidence of the lack of postpartum healthcare was evident when women described being instructed by healthcare workers to skip their 6-week postnatal check with the midwife and go straight to the under-five clinic run by health surveillance assistants (HSAs) so that the infants can receive vaccinations. When healthcare workers were asked about this, they did recognize the importance of a thorough clinical assessment of the woman and infant and wanted to complete them, but they cited that health worker shortages and missing equipment impacted the care they could provide.

In addition to describing the clinic-level challenges, some midwives took personal responsibility for the lack of postpartum care. However, these clinic-level challenges were recognized by clients. In fact a woman stated that she felt too afraid to ask questions or request services because she feared negative patient-provider interactions. In contrast, when healthcare workers described their experiences with group ANC, they felt that they were able to spend more time with women and could complete thorough assessments; they recognized the higher quality of care they could provide. The results from engaging with women and healthcare workers reinforced findings from other studies that there are gaps in the availability and provision of postpartum care to women in Malawi [28]. These gaps in care provision are attributed to staff shortages, healthcare workers' lack of knowledge of postpartum care guidelines, negative provider attitudes, and a lack of awareness of the importance of postpartum care [28–30].

Health workers also described how the environment led to care access barriers. They noted that the rainy season, difficult terrain, and long travel distances made getting to the clinic a challenge for their clients. Others included poverty and relationship conflicts as additional access barriers.

For this study, we purposely included women and healthcare workers who either participated in or facilitated group antenatal care (ANC) so that they could draw on their experiences as we worked to extend the existing group antenatal care model across the care continuum to include the first 12 months postpartum. All participants reported a desire to participate in or offer group care during the postpartum period. Mothers felt that the group care model was supportive and helped them translate knowledge into practice and better addressed their health concerns. One woman described how emergencies happen in her village and the knowledge she learned in group care can help save lives. Other women talked about being eager to learn more how to take care of their infants when illnesses arise and themselves and their own well-being. Healthcare workers expressed that group care could improve overall quality of care because they could spend more time with women and engage more deeply with health promotion through interactive learning activities. They recognized that integrating maternal and child health services would be more efficient and ensure complete clinical assessments for both the mother and infant. They perceived that offering group care to the communities that they serve would ultimately translate into increased health service utilization for both women and infants and thereby improve maternal and child health outcomes.

2.3   Step 3 Synthesize and Step 4 Develop Guiding Principles and Ideate

We synthesized the findings from step 2 and presented these back to women and healthcare workers. We did so through a series of incubator sessions, which are similar to focus groups but focus more on brainstorming and co-creation ensuring the adapted model is tailored to the Malawian context. Using qualitative methods a range of physical, psychological, social, and behavioral issues were identified through free listing, grouped through pile sorting, and ranked to produce a set of priority health promotion topics (see Fig. 17.4 for a photo of the pile sorting and ranking). Topics included hygiene, exclusive breastfeeding, family planning (combined with return to sexual activity), nutrition (for both mother and infant), depression screening/mental health, growth monitoring and developmental

milestones, sexual health (including STIs and HIV), immunizations, danger signs of serious health conditions for mother and baby, IPV and relationship issues, mother's physical health (including anemia, hypertension, and cervical cancer screening), disease prevention and management (including COVID-19 and common maternal and child health concerns), and male involvement. An important outcome of this process was that there was a mismatch in the topics desired and prioritized to those promoted in current practice. Two major topics prioritized and desired were mental health and sexual health.

Across all three clinics, there was consensus about how the integrated postpartum and well-child care model be structured. They felt that a six-visit model would be ideal. They recommended that that recruitment occur at the 1-week postpartum visit and that the first group visit should be at 6 weeks postpartum. They also felt that the schedule should align with the child vac-

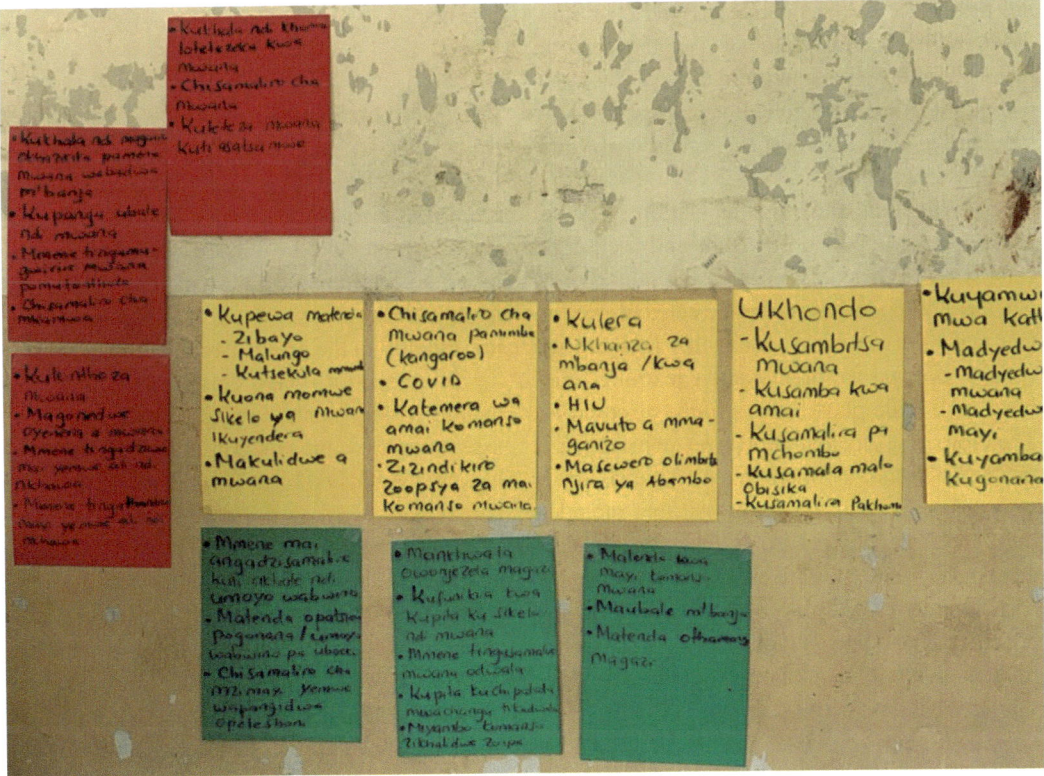

Fig. 17.4 Incubator sessions

cination schedule (6, 10, and 14 weeks and 6, 9, and 12 months) and that each 1–2-h group visit should be co-facilitated by a midwife and a health surveillance assistant (HSA). Participants noted that this schedule would likely increase vaccine uptake since vaccines would be administered at the end of each visit. Although a group size of no more than 12 is recommended for best practices for managing groups, responses varied for the ideal group size ranging from 8 to 15 mother/infant dyads.

Participants outlined a set of resources and materials needed to successfully provide high-quality care in a group format that included training of providers and equipment and supplies, such as an adult and baby weight scale, blood pressure equipment, thermometer, tape measure, an examination bed, mattress protectors, a mat to sit on, privacy screen for the room, physical assessment guidelines, hand sanitizer, laminated pictures of danger signs to show women, flip charts, toys for babies, and a storage basket. Further, many healthcare workers stated they did not have access to guidelines to perform standardized physical assessments. So, they recommended inclusion of written clinical maternal and infant assessment guidelines for each visit to standardize and improve the quality of these health assessments.

A curriculum and implementation structure prototype for group postpartum and well-child care was produced. In discussion about how women would like to receive the curriculum content and how providers would like to share the content, both preferred interactive learning activities with role-plays and group discussions. Therefore, the created prototype consists of a facilitator's guide outlining each of the six visits with a detailed plan for each visit that included the associated clinical guidelines for physical assessments and objectives and directions for each interactive learning activity reflecting the prioritized health promotion topics, as well as an implementation plan. For example, for the 6-week visit, interactive learning activities focus on danger signs of serious health conditions for mom and infant, physical and emotional adjustments after having a child, breastfeeding, and

family planning/resuming sexual activity. Each visit outlines all activities necessary to maintain fidelity to Centering-based group care's core components, such as healthcare in a group space, interactive learning, and community building.

Using a human-centered design (HCD) approach allowed for a collaborative process to create a group care prototype that is woman-centered and context specific. What we found during the co-design process was there were noticeable differences in health promotion topics desired and prioritized compared to current practice, particularly related to mental and sexual health, which highlight the need to transform the content and delivery of postpartum and well-child care to meet the needs of women and families. We were then able to create a prototype that included health promotion content that women and healthcare workers in Malawi perceived to be the most important to improve the health of women and infants in the postpartum period as well as suggested clinical guidelines to offer a tool for healthcare workers to standardize practice.

2.4 Step 5 Evaluate

Each of the six sessions was tested once at each clinic for a total of 18 pilot sessions. Overall, both women and healthcare workers reported group postpartum and well-child care was highly acceptable, appropriate, and feasible across clinics. Fidelity to the group care model was high.

Group sessions were designed to begin with health assessments which included self-assessments (women measured their own infant's weight, length, and head circumference and were taught how to take each other's blood pressure and weigh themselves) and clinical health assessments completed by a midwife for both the woman and infant. After health assessments were complete, facilitated discussion by the midwife and HSA with interactive learning activities occurred following the facilitator's guide with prioritized health promotion content for each session. Sessions were then to end with any services that were needed such as vaccinations or family planning and any follow-up that was needed for women and/or infants.

During the self-assessments, midwives were able to identify and treat health concerns, with the most common issue arising being hypertension. Other health issues identified during clinical assessments by the midwife included perineal pain, difficulty breastfeeding, and finger pain. Health issues identified among infants during clinical assessments included skin rash, cough or flu-like symptoms, abscess, inadequate weight gain, inguinal and abdominal hernias, and a skin mass. The most common health issue among infants was cough and flu-like symptoms. Follow-up and/or referrals were scheduled as needed.

Women reported gaining knowledge from facilitated group health promotion discussions and activities. They reported learning about mental health and how to deal with stress, danger signs of serious health conditions and when to go to the clinic to seek care, breastfeeding, hypertension, vaccinations, and the diseases they protect against, nutrition for both mother and infant, HIV and prevention of mother-to-child transmission (PMTCT), child health and development, family planning, hygiene and sanitation, growth monitoring, relationship conflict management, and cervical and breast cancer.

At the end of the group session, services that were received within the group space for women included family planning, mosquito nets (for the prevention of malaria), or medications (e.g., anti-hypertensives). The most common service received by women within the group space was family planning (the majority receiving Depo-Provera). Services that were received within the group space for infants included vaccinations, medications (e.g., antibiotics), and enrollment in a nutrition program for a malnourished child. The most common service received among infants was vaccinations. In total 51 people (including both women and infants) over the course of the 18 group sessions had a health issue that was identified and treated during health assessments or received a healthcare service or were referred to other providers for care at the end of the group session.

These are some reactions from a midwife facilitating and mother attending a group care visit.

"Women are happy because postnatal groups are a one stop shop, they can get their vaccines, family planning, medications, be assessed, get health education all in one place instead of us telling them to go here, go there on this day and then there on that day, so they are very happy."—Midwife, Clinic B

"I am happy to have learned about high blood pressure, now I know about hypertension and would like to continue with groups so that I can keep learning."—Mother, Clinic C

Health issues identified for women that participated in group sessions highlight unmet health needs in the 12 months postpartum. Noncommunicable diseases (NCDs) are a significant contributor to maternal morbidity and mortality, and the current state of maternal healthcare does not adequately identify or treat them as a part of routine care [31]. Hypertension was the most common health issue identified among women. Hypertension disorders in pregnancy are one of the leading causes of maternal morbidity and mortality, and this health issue can carry forward in the women's life course increasing their risk of chronic disease [1, 32]. Studies show a high prevalence of hypertension among women in the postpartum period in some African countries and missed opportunities to identify and treat it in the current state of postpartum care [33–35]. Studies in Malawi specifically reveal high prevalence of and risk for hypertension and the need for innovative interventions to prevent, treat, and control hypertension [36]. In addition to hypertension, opportunities exist within group care to increase screening for other NCDs such as diabetes, anemia, and mental health. Prevalence of postpartum depression among women in Malawi is estimated to be 19.8% [37], highlighting the need for targeted screening and preventive measures to support women experiencing it.

Health issues identified for infants also highlighted unmet health needs for infants. Factors leading to high rates of infant mortality and morbidities in Malawi include health service utilization, short birth intervals, malnutrition, pneumonia, preterm birth complications, diarrhea, and malaria [3, 38]. Current guidelines for well-child care in Malawi focus on vaccinations and growth monitoring and managing sick children. Group care creates an opportunity to do thorough assessments of infants, provide consistent follow-up to monitor their growth and development, maintain vaccination schedules, triage health concerns as they arise, and provide health education to parents through interactive learning activities.

3 Reflection

The COVID-19 pandemic caused us to reduce the group sizes that we piloted (we limited it to five dyads per session), however the ideal size for groups is six to eight dyads, and healthcare workers and women informed us that increasing the size would be acceptable and feasible to them. We relied mainly on measures of self-report which may introduce response biases. Our findings inform the implementation of group postpartum and well-child care at peri-urban and rural clinics in Malawi but may not be generalizable to other clinic populations. We evaluated implementation outcomes only and cannot comment on the effectiveness of the group postpartum and well-child care model compared to usual care. And finally, because we did not measure the model's effectiveness, we were unable to associate fidelity with outcomes.

With persisting high rates of maternal and infant mortality in Malawi, there is a call for integrating health services to improve both maternal and child health outcomes [39]. Group care provides an opportunity to fill a gap in the care continuum, identify and treat NCDs and other health issues, and assist in the transition from maternity care to primary healthcare services [31]. These promising results set the stage for rigorous research to examine the effectiveness of this model on maternal and child health outcomes in Malawi and other low-resource settings including the USA.

References

1. Geller SE, Koch AR, Garland CE, MacDonald EJ, Storey F, Lawton B. A global view of severe maternal morbidity: moving beyond maternal mortality. Reprod Health. 2018;15(Suppl 1):31–43. https://doi.org/10.1186/s12978-018-0527-2.

2. Firoz T, McCaw-Binns A, Filippi V, Magee LA, Costa ML, Cecatti JG, Barreix M, Adanu R, Chou D, Say L, Members of the WHO Maternal Morbidity Working Group (MMWG). A framework for healthcare interventions to address maternal morbidity. Int J Gynecol Obstet. 2018;141:61–8. https://doi.org/10.1002/ijgo.12469.

3. National Statistical Office. Malawi demographic and health survey 2015–2016. In: National Statistics Office The DHS Program. 2015. http://dhsprogram.com/pubs/pdf/FR319/FR319.pdf.

4. Ferreira EC, Costa ML, Pacagnella RC, Silveira C, Andreucci CB, Zanardi DM, Santos JP, Angelini CR, Souza RT, Parpinelli MA, Sousa MH, Cecatti JG. General and reproductive health among women after an episode of severe maternal morbidity: results from the COMMAG study. Int J Gynecol Obstet. 2020;150(1):83–91. https://doi.org/10.1002/ijgo.13161.

5. Soma-Pillay P, Makin JD, Pattinson RC. Quality of life 1 year after a maternal near-miss event. Int J Gynecol Obstet. 2018;141(1):133–8. https://doi.org/10.1002/ijgo.12432.

6. Andreucci CB, Bussadori JC, Pacagnella RC, Chou D, Filippi V, Say L, Cecatti JG, Parpinelli MA, Costa ML, Silveira C, Angelini CR, Ferreira EC, Zanardi DM, Santos JP, Souza RT, Cecchini GN, Firoz T, von Dadelszen P, Magee LA, Sullivan E. Sexual life and dysfunction after maternal morbidity: a systematic review. BMC Pregnancy Childbirth. 2015;15(1):307. https://doi.org/10.1186/s12884-015-0742-6.

7. Gon G, Leite A, Calvert C, Woodd S, Graham WJ, Filippi V. The frequency of maternal morbidity: a systematic review of systematic reviews. Int J Gynecol Obstet. 2018;141:20–38. https://doi.org/10.1002/ijgo.12468.

8. MacHiyama K, Hirose A, Cresswell JA, Barreix M, Chou D, Kostanjsek N, Say L, Filippi V. Consequences of maternal morbidity on health-related functioning: a systematic scoping review. BMJ Open. 2017;7(6):e013903. https://doi.org/10.1136/bmjopen-2016-013903.

9. Ahlfs-Dunn SM, Huth-Bocks AC. Intimate partner violence and infant socioemotional development: the moderating effects of maternal trauma symptoms. Infant Ment Health J. 2014;35(4):322–35. https://doi.org/10.1002/imhj.21453.

10. Mahenge B, Stockl H, Abubakari A, Mbwambo J, Jahn A. Physical, sexual, emotional and economic intimate

partner violence and controlling behaviors during pregnancy and postpartum among women in Dar es Salaam, Tanzania. PLoS One. 2016;11(10):e0164376. https://doi.org/10.1371/journal.pone.0164376.

11. Knettel BA, Cichowitz C, Ngocho JS, Knippler ET, Chumba LN, Mmbaga BT, Watt MH. Retention in HIV care during pregnancy and the postpartum period in the option B+ era: systematic review and meta-analysis of studies in Africa. J Acquir Immune Defic Syndr. 2018;77(5):427–38. https://doi.org/10.1097/QAI.0000000000001616.

12. Petersen E, Davis N, Goodman D, Cox S, Mayes N, Johnson E, Syverson C, Seed K, Shapiro-Mendoza C, Callaghan W, Barfield W. Vital signs: pregnancy-related deaths, United States, 2011–2015, and strategies for prevention, 13 states, 2013–2017. MMWR Morb Mortal Wkly Rep. 2019;68:423–9. https://doi.org/10.15585/mmwr.mm6818e1.

13. Fahey JO, Shenassa E. Understanding and meeting the needs of women in the postpartum period: the perinatal maternal health promotion model. J Midwifery Womens Health. 2013;58(6):613–21. https://doi.org/10.1111/jmwh.12139.

14. Fischer M, Safaeinili N, Haverfield MC, Brown-Johnson CG, Zionts D, Zulman DM. Approach to human-centered, evidence-driven adaptive design (AHEAD) for health care interventions: a proposed framework. J Gen Intern Med. 2021;36(4):1041–8. https://doi.org/10.1007/s11606-020-06451-4.

15. Mummah SA, Robinson TN, King AC, Gardner CD, Sutton S. IDEAS (integrate, design, assess, and share): a framework and toolkit of strategies for the development of more effective digital interventions to change health behavior. J Med Internet Res. 2016;18(12):c317. https://doi.org/10.2196/jmir.5927.

16. Aifah A, Okeke NL, Rentrope CR, Schexnayder J, Bloomfield GS, Bosworth H, Grover K, Hileman CO, Muiruri C, Oakes M, Webel AR, Longenecker CT, Vedanthan R. Use of a human-centered design approach to adapt a nurse-led cardiovascular disease prevention intervention in HIV clinics. In: Progress in cardiovascular diseases, vol. 63. W.B. Saunders; 2020. p. 92–100. https://doi.org/10.1016/j.pcad.2020.02.013.

17. Ippoliti N, Sekamana M, Baringer L, Hope R, Findings K. Using human-centered design to develop, launch, and evaluate a national digital health platform to improve reproductive health for Rwandan Youth. Glob Health Sci Pract. 2016;9(Suppl 2):S244–60.

18. Gresh A, Cohen M, Anderson J, Glass N. Postpartum care content and delivery throughout the African continent: an integrative review. In: Midwifery, vol. 97. Churchill Livingstone; 2021. https://doi.org/10.1016/j.midw.2021.102976.

19. Chimtembo L, Maluwa A, Chimwaza A, Chirwa E, Pindani M. Assessment of quality of postnatal care services offered to mothers in Dedza district, Malawi. Open J Nurs. 2013;03:343–50. https://doi.org/10.4236/ojn.2013.34046.

20. Pindani M, Phiri C, Chikazinga W, Chilinda I, Botha J, Chorwe-Sungani G. Assessing the quality of postnatal care offered to mothers and babies by midwives in Lilongwe District. S Afr Fam Pract. 2020;62(1):e1. https://doi.org/10.4102/safp.

21. Gaskin E, Yorga KW, Berman R, Allison M, Sheeder J. Pediatric group care: a systematic review. Matern Child Health J. 2021;25(10):1526–53. https://doi.org/10.1007/s10995-021-03170-y.

22. Grenier L, Lori JR, Darney BG, Noguchi LM, Maru S, Klima C, Lundeen T, Walker D, Patil CL, Suhowatsky S, Musange S. Building a global evidence base to guide policy and implementation for group antenatal care in low- and middle-income countries: key principles and research framework recommendations from the global group antenatal care collaborative. J Midwifery Womens Health. 2020;65(5):694–9. https://doi.org/10.1111/jmwh.13143.

23. Rising S, Quimby C. The CenteringPregnancy model: the power of group health care. Springer Publishing Company; 2016.

24. Grenier L, Suhowatsky S, Kabue MM, Noguchi LM, Mohan D, Karnad SR, Onguti B, Omanga E, Gichangi A, Wambua J, Waka C, Oyetunji J, Smith JM. Impact of group antenatal care (G-ANC) versus individual antenatal care (ANC) on quality of care, ANC attendance and facility-based delivery: a pragmatic cluster-randomized controlled trial in Kenya and Nigeria. PLoS One. 2019;14(10):e0222177. https://doi.org/10.1371/journal.pone.0222177.

25. Patil C, Klima C, Leshabari S, Steffen A, Pauls H, McGown M, Norr K. Randomized controlled pilot of a group antenatal care model and the sociodemographic factors associated with pregnancy-related empowerment in sub-Saharan Africa. BMC Pregnancy Childbirth. 2017;17:336. https://doi.org/10.1186/s12884-017-1493-3.

26. Sayinzoga F, Lundeen T, Gakwerere M, Manzi E, Nsaba YDU, Umuziga MP, Kalisa IR, Musange SF, Walker D. Use of a facilitated group process to design and implement a group antenatal and postnatal care program in Rwanda. J Midwifery Womens Health. 2018;63(5):593–601. https://doi.org/10.1111/jmwh.12871.

27. Chirwa E, Kapito E, Jere DL, Kafulafula U, Chodzaza E, Chorwe-Sungani G, Gresh A, Liu L, Abrams ET, Klima CS, McCreary LL, Norr KF, Patil CL. An effectiveness-implementation hybrid type 1 trial assessing the impact of group versus individual antenatal care on maternal and infant outcomes in Malawi. BMC Public Health. 2020;20(1):1–13. https://doi.org/10.1186/s12889-020-8276-x.

28. Duysburgh E, Kerstens B, Kouanda S, Kaboré PC, Belemsaga Yugbare D, Gichangi P, Masache G, Crahay B, Gondola Sitefane G, Bique Osman N, Foia S, Barros H, Castro Lopes S, Mann S, Nambiar B, Colbourn T, Temmerman M. Opportunities to improve postpartum care for mothers and infants: design of context-specific packages of postpartum interventions

in rural districts in four sub-Saharan African countries. BMC Pregnancy Childbirth. 2015;15(1):131. https://doi.org/10.1186/s12884-015-0562-8.

29. Sakala B, Chirwa E. An evidence-based policy brief: improving the quality of postnatal care in mothers 48 hours after childbirth. Malawi Med J. 2019;31(2):164–8. https://doi.org/10.4314/mmj. v31i2.12.

30. Sakala B, Kazembe A. Factors influencing the utilisation of postnatal care at one week and six weeks among mothers at Zomba central Hospital in Malawi. Evid Based Midwifery. 2011;9(4):113–36.

31. Firoz T, Pineles B, Navrange N, Grimshaw A, Oladapo O, Chou D. Non-communicable diseases and maternal health: a scoping review. BMC Pregnancy Childbirth. 2022;22(1):787. https://doi.org/10.1186/s12884-022-05047-6.

32. World Health Organization. Trends in maternal mortality 2000–2017: estimates by WHO, UNICEF, UNFPA, World Bank Group and the United Nations Population Division. World Health Organization; 2019. https://www.who.int/reproductivehealth/publications/maternal-mortality-2000-2017/en/.

33. Ishaku SM, Jamilu T, Innocent AP, Gbenga KA, Lamaran D, Lawal O, Warren CE, Olorunfemi OO, Abubakar HD, Karima T, Patience OO, Musa A, Azubuike OK, Baffah AM, Franx A, Grobbee DE, Browne JL. Persistent hypertension up to one year postpartum among women with hypertensive disorders in pregnancy in a low-resource setting: a prospective cohort study. Glob Heart. 2021;16(1):62. https://doi.org/10.5334/GH.854.

34. Larson E, Rabkin M, Mbaruku GM, Mbatia R, Kruk ME. Missed opportunities to improve the health of postpartum women: high rates of untreated hypertension in rural Tanzania. Matern Child Health J. 2017;21(3):407–13. https://doi.org/10.1007/s10995-016-2229-0.

35. Oyeneyin L, Ishaku S, Azubuike O, Agbo I, Dattijo L, Baffah A, Kayode G, Owa O, Odusolu P, Tunau K, Tukur J, Warren C, Abubakar H, Abdulkarim M, Franx A, Grobbee D, Browne J. Adherence to guidelines in postpartum management of hypertensive disorders in pregnancy in tertiary health facilities in Nigeria: a multi-centre study. Health Syst Reform. 2021;7(1):e1932229. https://doi.org/10.1080/23288604.2021.1932229.

36. Amberbir A, Lin SH, Berman J, Muula A, Jacoby D, Wroe E, Maliwichi-Nyirenda C, Mwapasa V, Crampin A, Makwero M, Singogo E, Phiri S, Gordon S, Tobe SW, Masiye J, Newsome B, Hosseinipour M, Nyirenda MJ, van Oosterhout JJ. Systematic review of hypertension and diabetes burden, risk factors, and interventions for prevention and control in Malawi the NCD BRITE consortium. Glob Heart. 2019;14(2):109–18. https://doi.org/10.1016/j.gheart.2019.

37. Chorwe-Sungani G, Wella K, Mapulanga P, Nyirongo D, Pindani M. Systematic review on the prevalence of perinatal depression in Malawi. S Afr J Psychiatry. 2022;28:1859. https://doi.org/10.4102/sajpsychiatry.v28i0.1859.

38. Ntenda PAM, Chuang KY, Tiruneh FN, Chuang YC. Factors associated with infant mortality in Malawi. J Exp Clin Med (Taiwan). 2014;6(4):125–31. https://doi.org/10.1016/j.jecm.2014.06.005.

39. Sakala JJ, Chimatiro CS, Salima R, Kapachika A, Kalepa J, Stones W. The integration of vertical and horizontal programmes for health systems strengthening in Malawi: a case study. Malawi Med J. 2022;34(3):206–12. https://doi.org/10.4314/mmj.v34i3.11.

Ashley Gresh PhD, MSN, MA, RN, CNM, is an assistant professor at Johns Hopkins University School of Nursing. She is both a certified nurse-midwife and a public health nurse, whose research focuses on addressing inequities in maternal and child health outcomes. Her current work examines the effects of perinatal group-based care on maternal and child health in the postpartum period and examines ways for adapting, implementing, and sustaining group care in Baltimore and globally. She is committed to co-creating solutions to issues in health care with the communities she serves by using a human-centered design approach; one that shifts power dynamics and centers the rights and well-being of childbearing people, their families, and communities. Dr. Gresh has a range of global and international health experience including being in the inaugural cohort of the Global Women's Health Fellowship, a joint venture between the Johns Hopkins School of Nursing, the Johns Hopkins School of Medicine, and Jhpiego. A foundational career goal for Ashley is to reimagine and redefine postpartum care to transform systems and delivery of care.

Esnath Kapito PhD, MScRH, BSc NsgEd, RNM, is a midwifery expert and nurse educator trained as a Registered Nurse Midwife. As a nurse leader, Dr. Esnath Kapito has growing interest in research implementation projects in maternal and neonatal care. Currently, she is the coordinator of Group Antenatal Care in Malawi under the Kamuzu University of Health Sciences in collaboration with the University of Illinois, Chicago. She chairs the Mulanje Mission College of Nursing and Midwifery Board of Directors and is the former publicity secretary of the Association of Malawian Midwives (AMAMI). Her passion is to promote the midwifery profession and the well-being of families especially mothers and babies including preterm infants.

Janet Mambulasa MSc RH, BSc, CHN, Dip NM, is both a certified nurse-midwife and a Reproductive Health Nurse Specialist whose focus is on improving the quality of maternal and neonatal care in the Public Health Service. Her current work involves testing possible solutions to address the quality-of-care gap in maternity and well-child care in Malawi. Her involvement in both Group Antenatal Care and Group Postnatal and Well-Child Care provides a wider spectrum of possible solutions to address the quality gap. Janet Mambulasa is committed to co-producing evidence-based solutions to issues in the health care system. She has experience in maternal and neonatal care, quality improvement processes, community health, and also implementation research. Her goal is to see healthcare providers embracing quality as a culture in service provision.

Nellie Ngutwa MscCH, BscNM, is a holder of a master's degree in child health. She has worked as a nurse educator in the Child Health Department. Her research work is qualitative in the child health field. Recently, she joined the research team working on adapting and implementing group postpartum and well-child health care.

Ellen Chirwa PhD, is a Malawian Registered Nurse Midwife and graduate of the University of Illinois at Chicago, where she earned her PhD in Nursing in 2007. She joined Kamuzu University of Health Sciences (formally Kamuzu College of Nursing) in 1990 and has mainly been teaching midwifery and reproductive in undergraduate and postgraduate programs. Professor Chirwa has a strong track record of leading international teams of research projects, including the National Institutes of Health funded project: Group Antenatal: Effectiveness for Maternal/Infant and HIV Prevention Outcomes and Contextual Factors Linked to Implementation Success in Malawi. Her research interests lie in quality improvement in maternal and neonatal health.

Crystal L. Patil PhD, is a Professor and Associate Dean for Research at the University of Michigan School of Nursing. She is an anthropologist and implementation scientist with qualitative and mixed methods expertise. She works to improve the health of women, families, and communities by using collaborative approaches to adapt evidence-based interventions for use in diverse community and clinic settings. Dr. Patil has adapted and implemented group healthcare models for prenatal and postnatal care, HIV prevention, the transition from pediatric to adult clinic for those with sickle cell disease, and for the uptake of PrEP among sex workers. Recently, she has joined teams working with EHR data to develop interventions and use AI to improve cardiovascular health. Dr. Patil is committed to collaborating with and mentoring colleagues, fellows, and students. In recognition of her approach to mentoring, she was awarded the 2022 UIC College of Nursing Distinguished Mentor of Faculty Award.

Implementing Culture as Treatment to Reduce Stress and Promote Well-Being in Reservation-Based Native American Head Start Teachers

Deborah H. Wilson, Adriann Ricker,
Hilary Gourneau, and Teresa N. Brockie

1   Introduction

Native Americans have a strong cultural identity, connection to traditions, and centuries of viewing health and well-being as a balance of physical, emotional, mental, and spiritual health [1–3]. Through strong ties to family, community, language, a deep spiritual connection to land and place, and traditional ceremonies and practices, Native Americans were able to be self-sustaining, healthy, and prosperous [4, 5]. However, the oppression of Native Americans through colonization which aimed to systematically wipe them out using federal programs such as forced reloca-

tion to reservations from sacred homelands, removal of children from their families placing them into boarding schools, outlawing Native languages and ceremonies, and forced acculturation through missionaries disrupted the natural balance that helped keep their communities healthy and prosperous [4, 5]. Instead, these federal policies and programs have resulted in extreme poverty, lack of access to quality education and health care, high rates of morbidity and mortality, and disproportionately high rates of preventable diseases such as diabetes and tuberculosis [4]. Native Americans also experience severe psychological distress at rates 2.5 times higher than the general US population [6].

These traumas affecting Native Americans have been passed down epigenetically through generations [7]. Research shows that the high rates of distress, substance and alcohol misuse, social dysfunction, and suicide among Native peoples can be connected to the intergenerational traumatic impact of the settler colonial policies outlined above [7, 8].

Further, the current woeful underfunding of the Indian Health Service by the Federal Government, contemporary discrimination and structural racism experienced by Natives when trying to access the health system, and inadequate access to culturally appropriate care continue to negatively affect Native American health and

Dr. Teresa N. Brockie is an enrolled member of the Aaniniiin Nation; Adriann Ricker is an enrolled member of Fort Peck Assiniboine and Sioux Tribes; Hilary Gourneau is an enrolled member of Fort Peck Assiniboine and Sioux Tribes.

D. H. Wilson (✉)
Auckland University of Technology,
Auckland, New Zealand
e-mail: debbie.wilson@aut.ac.nz

A. Ricker · T. N. Brockie
Johns Hopkins University, School of Nursing,
Baltimore, MD, USA
e-mail: aricker4@jhu.edu; tbrocki1@jhu.edu

H. Gourneau
Fort Peck Tribes Head Start, Poplar, MT, USA
e-mail: hgourneau@fortpecktribes.net

© The Author(s), under exclusive license to Springer Nature Switzerland AG 2024
J. B. Hamilton, C. E. Moore (eds.), *Transforming Social Determinants to Promote Global Health*,
https://doi.org/10.1007/978-3-031-61160-5_18

well-being [9, 10]. For many Native Americans, their experience of the Western health system is fraught with little or no recognition by staff which leads many Native Americans to feeling disrespected, unheard, ignored, or mistreated resulting in a disengagement with existing health services [9, 10]. There is urgent need for our medical system to view culture as a social determinant of health (SDOH) to help promote health equity.

2 Culture as a Social Determinant of Health

The importance of culture as a SDOH has contributed to a rise in research that demonstrates how reconnection with culture, cultural identity, and traditional practices can help return individuals and communities to balance, with a focus on optimizing individual and community health and well-being [5, 11]. Culture as treatment, which is defined as replacing mainstream models of health and policy interventions in research with the inclusion of cultural healing practices, traditional values, and messaging, may be useful for improving health outcomes among Native American communities [12]. Examples that have demonstrated positive findings include SACRED connections, a randomized control trial that found a statistically significant protective relationship between Native reliance and baseline and lifetime use of alcohol and marijuana [13] and a community-based mental health intervention implementing cultural sessions to improve the mental health of Native American youth which resulted in increased cultural identity, self-esteem, and demonstrations of positive coping strategies [14].

Another important component of culture as a SDOH is cultural safety. A term developed by indigenous Māori nurse, Irihapeti Ramsden, in Aotearoa (New Zealand), cultural safety highlights power imbalances between Indigenous patients and providers and how these imbalances can affect their well-being and identity [15]. The goal of cultural safety is to minimize disenfranchisement for members of minority cultures. This requires medical practitioners such as nurses to embrace continued learning and awareness of clients' cultures and how culture mediates determinants of health, to reflect on their own practice, to be aware of colonial structural inequities, and to be committed to advocacy in the face of these imbalances [15, 16].

Cultural safety, humility, and awareness are also imperative when conducting research with Indigenous populations. Many Native communities have been subjected to unethical research practices that have left them wary, mistrustful, and reluctant to engage with academics whom they view as researching "on them" rather than with or for them [17]. Community-based participatory research (CBPR) has proven to be a successful methodology when implemented by an academic-tribal partnership conducting research with urban or reservation-based Native American communities. It is key to centering Native American sovereignty and self-determination [18, 19]. It ensures that the research problem is identified by the community and works to ensure positive health outcomes or a decrease in health disparities for individual and community members. This framework also focuses on lessening the power imbalances inherent in academic-community partnerships, choosing to promote trust, partnership, and sustainability [17].

This chapter describes how CBPR was crucial to the implementation of traditional cultural practices as a treatment for reducing stress and promoting well-being in reservation-based Native American Head Start early childhood education (ECE) teachers working for the United States-based Head Start program.

3 Native American Head Start Teacher Stress and Well-Being

Early childhood education (ECE) has developed in industrialized countries in part due to research demonstrating that it helps strengthen childhood emotional social well-being and improve school achievement particularly for children from disadvantaged families [20, 21].

The largest federally funded public early ECE program in the United States is called Head Start. It aims to help break the cycle of poverty, by providing preschool children ages 3–5 from underserved, marginalized communities and families with a comprehensive program that meets their emotional, social, health, nutritional, and psychological needs [22]. Head Start consists of 12 regions. Regions I–X are geographically based and the other two are defined by the populations they serve. Region XI programs are administered by federally recognized Native American/Alaska Native[1] tribes, and Region XII serves migrant and seasonal workers and their families [22].

According to national data, consistent with teachers nationally, Head Start teachers report high levels of daily stress which affects their health, well-being, and performance resulting in burnout and high turnover affecting the socio-emotional outcomes of the children that they teach [23–26]. The American Indian and Alaska Native Head Start Family and Child Experiences Survey (AIAN FACES) provides nationally representative information on Region XI Head Start children and their families, teachers, and programs. According to this data, 65% of Region XI children's lead teachers experience some degree of depressive symptomatology [27]. To date research emphasis has focused on how stress or depression affects Head Start staff turnover or the academic and socio-emotional outcomes of the

children they teach, rather than valuing the teachers as individuals who themselves need psychological support and resources [25, 28–31].

Existing interventions such as mindfulness programs [32] that address Head Start teacher mental health and stress have not centered nor prioritized Native American culture nor valued their unique strengths when adapting and implementing health and wellness programs with reservation-based Head Start programs [31, 33, 34].

Based on community input, our academic-tribal partnership decided to adapt an existing intervention that used traditional cultural practices and implement it to promote well-being and resilience and reduce stress and depression in Fort Peck Reservation Head Start teachers.

3.1 Setting and Community Resources

In rural northeastern Montana, the Fort Peck Reservation spans 3200 square miles and is home to approximately 12,000 members of the Sioux and Assiniboine tribes [35]. Fort Peck has 6 Head Start programs with 21 teachers and teacher assistants funded to serve over 200 children ages 3–5. In a 2016 community health assessment in Fort Peck, multiple health disparities reflective of negative SDOH were found, e.g., 13% of youth had attempted suicide compared to 9% of youth in the rest of Montana, and 36% of households with children under 18 years live in poverty compared to 20% for the rest of the state. The median reservation household income is $34,345 compared to median household income of $46,766 in the rest of Montana [36]. The average mental health days reported in Fort Peck were 4.4 compared to 3.4 among other Montanans. This finding is concerning given the ratio of mental health providers to patients of 1 to 1030 on the reservation compared to 1 to 399 across the rest of the state. The reservation-based primary healthcare ratio is 1 provider to 5563 patients compared to 1 to 1312 patients in the rest of Montana [36]. See Photos 1 and 2 of Fort Peck.

---

[1]The term American Indian/Alaska Native is used by the Federal Government and US Census Bureau. For this chapter, however, the term Native American will be used throughout unless referring to a particular study that uses a different term.

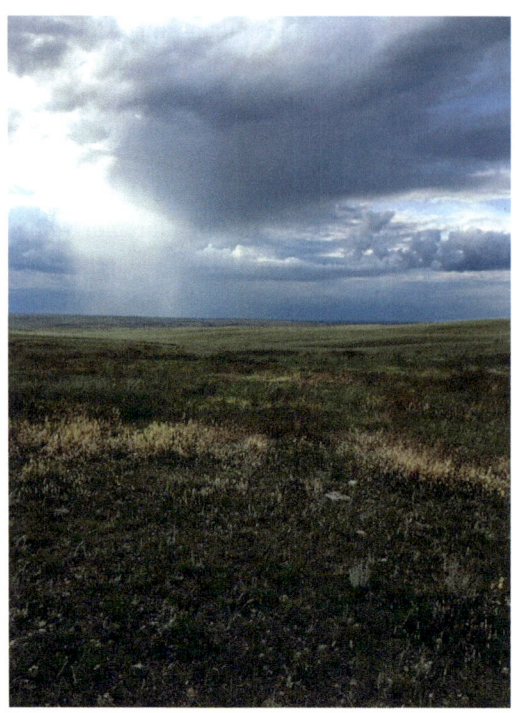

Photo 1 Fort Peck Reservation by Deborah H. Wilson

This lack of healthcare providers, a chronically underfunded Indian Health Service, and issues with access to health insurance, poverty, and stigma are all factors that necessitate the development and adaption of sustainable health and behavioral interventions that are community based and culturally informed. Existing cultural and community resources include the Fort Peck Community College; the Fort Peck Institutional Research Board (IRB); and the Fort Peck Buffalo Program that has successfully introduced buffalo back into the reservation [37].

3.2   Fort Peck Head Start Program

Fort Peck's Tribal Head Start administration anecdotally reports that most of the children enrolled in the program live in single-parent homes and 80% live in a household with incomes below the federal poverty level. They described to us how teachers report that many children exhibit signs of depression and behavior prob-

Photo 2 Fort Peck buffalo by Deborah H. Wilson

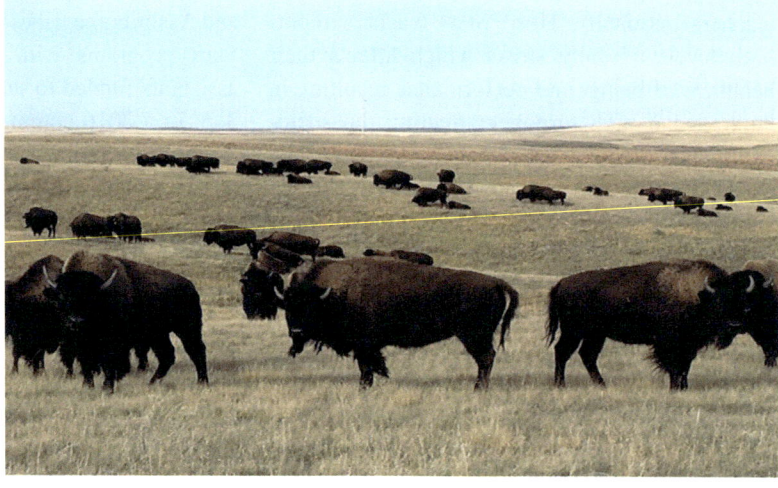

lems and that they feel a responsibility to address these issues so that the children may grow into healthy adults, despite little support from specialist services. The administration explained that the reasons for the lack of specialists to support the teachers and children include the remote location of the reservation, long waiting lists for services, and children being bumped from services because of others in crisis such as suicides. Furthermore, children often do not qualify for services if the issue is behavioral rather than special needs,[2] such as a learning disability.

Currently, the Head Start organizational support for teachers on the reservation is limited largely to trainings on trauma-informed care and working with autistic children. However, the program administration recognizes that the support has focused on how the teachers can better care for the children with no attention in training or services that address the health needs of the teachers. Thus, Fort Peck Head Start administration acknowledge that their teachers work in a stressful, remote, and under-resourced environment, with limited access to culturally informed interventions that promote teacher health and well-being. Therfore, they were interested to collaborate as we worked to implement a culturally informed intervention to reduce stress and promote the well-being of their teachers.

3.3   Community Collaboration and the Development of Trust

Crucial to the success of this research project was relationship building and collaboration. As the

lead researcher was not Indigenous, initial connection with the tribes was initiated by a cultural broker, a Native American academic researcher with ties to the reservation. By providing knowledge of the community needs and cultural differences and assisting the team in obtaining a formal agreement from the community for the research through a signed Tribal Resolution, we learned how cultural brokerage is imperative to consider when embarking on research with Indigenous communities. In addition, as non-natives with novice knowledge of the community, we completed graduate courses in Indigenous health and participated in a specially designed workshop led by tribal Elders and Native American faculty on how to best work with Native American communities. Ideally research in Native communities is led by a Native researcher, but when this is not possible, taking the time to learn the tribes and reservation history and relying on cultural brokerage are key to establishing a foundation of trust [33].

Respecting tribal sovereignty (the right of tribes to govern themselves and establish law) by formally obtaining the Tribal Resolution (#30-348-2020-03) and submitting our research plan to the Tribal IRB for approval established the rights of the tribes to the data, allowing them veto power of any materials produced because of the research. We also established a tribal advisory board (TAB) to help to continue to build trust and show respect for the self-determination of the tribe.

Our TAB consisted of community members, teachers, and cultural leaders. They were involved throughout the research process reviewing interview guides and discussing research findings and conclusions from the qualitative data, participated in all sessions as we worked on adapting the intervention to be a fit for Head Start teachers, and pilot tested the quantitative survey, providing feedback on order of the measures and how to introduce the survey. They were also available and able to answer questions from community members about the presence and purpose of the research team which helped increase the transparency of our work. We also meet regularly with the Fort Peck Head Start administration to update

---

[2]To be eligible for special education and related services, under the Individual with Disabilities Education Act (IDEA), a child must meet the criteria in two areas outlined in federal law: (1) the child must be identified as a child with a disability in one or more of the 13 categories defined below; and (2) the child's disability must adversely affect his or her educational performance. (Autism, deaf-blindness, deafness, emotional disturbance, hearing impairment, intellectual disabilities, multiple disabilities, orthopedic impairment, other health impairment, specific learning disability, speech language impairment, traumatic brain injury, visual impairment) (IDEA; P.L. 108–446)

them on experiences, findings, and complications. When the feasibility study was completed, we formally presented study results to the Fort Peck Tribal Executive Board which consists of Assiniboine and Sioux leaders. Prioritizing and adhering to tribal governance and protocols, while taking more time, helps to ameliorate the mistrust that has developed because of unethical practices in the past [33].

Hiring and training local staff was essential because we were implementing traditional cultural practices as an intervention. As one of the tribal Elders pointed out during a community discussion, "Natives are sick of white people telling them about their culture." While employing local staff can increase the credibility of the work and help to bridge the divide between the academic researchers and the community, it does place extra burden on community members. Research delays occurred because of traumatizing events that happened during the implementation period which placed strain on community members' capacity and resources. We had built into our National Institute of Nursing Research grant application the need for time to build relationships, to establish trust, and the potential need to account for strains on the local infrastructure. This meant we were able to accommodate delays in implementation when the community or local employees were dealing with competing demands.

4 Preparing the Research Study

To avoid pathologizing Native experience, we chose a conceptual model developed by Indigenous researchers—the Indigenist Stress-Coping Model [38]—and the Native American Framework of Health and Well-being [39]. Indigenous perspectives of well-being connect the individual, family, work life, community, spiritual, and cultural practices as integral parts of health and well-being that enable coping to allow a holistic return of balance in a person's life [40]. This model strategically enabled the exploration of well-being and resilience in the face of cultural-specific stressors such as historical loss and its impact on psychological health. It focused on the potential buffering effects of cultural activities and identity with the teachers [41]. This in turn could positively impact the teacher's stress and mental health and increase communal mastery, tribal identity, and resilience, thus improving a teacher's capacity to support and mentor students and collaborate with the parents, with the potential to promote a safer community and reduce the longer-term effects of trauma [7, 42].

We also used measurement tools that have previously been validated in Native American or Indigenous communities and employed mixed methods to collect and analyze data so that we could ensure that the quantitative findings were informed by participant experience. Too often Western evidence-based models of care are used in Indigenous communities when they have only been validated in larger general populations [33].

4.1 The Adapted Intervention

The development and implementation of our feasibility study occurred in three main phases. First, we conducted interviews and focus groups with Head Start administrative staff ($n = 3$), teachers ($n = 11$), parents with children enrolled in Health Start ($n = 8$), and ancillary staff ($n = 4$). The focus group and interview guides focused on identifying workplace stressors, support available to teachers through the program, teacher coping mechanisms, and interest in a culturally informed intervention.

Qualitative data findings were used to help guide us as we moved to the second phase which involved working with our TAB to adapt the four cultural lessons from an existing intervention called Wakȟáŋyeža (*Little Holy One*). *Little Holy One* is a randomized controlled trial of a 12-session intergenerational intervention designed to reduce stress and trauma-related symptoms among parent-child dyads of Head Start children ages 3–5 [41]. *Little Holy One* includes four cultural lessons designed to support the psychological health and well-being of parent-child dyads by (a) promoting tribal identity; (b) promoting communal mastery (group efficacy); (c) addressing contemporary and historical trauma; and (d) promoting smudging. We decided to adapt these four cultural lessons into a stress reduction intervention for the Fort Peck Head Start teachers. During the adaptation process, described in detail in a separate publication [43], a fifth lesson from the *Little Holy One* curriculum was added to the planned intervention. The fifth lesson, called Managing Your Emotions, is from the Common Elements Treatment Approach (CETA) and focuses on recognizing and dealing with depression, anger, and stress. CETA is an evidenced-based program designed to reduce mental health problems in low- and middle-income countries and can be delivered by community-based paraprofessionals [44]. The final result of the adaptation process was a five-session intervention ready for testing in a feasibility acceptability trial with Fort Peck Head Start teachers.

5   Traditional Activities to Decrease Stress and Improve Well-Being

Each of the four cultural sessions that we adapted (promoting tribal identity, smudging to reduce stress, healing historical trauma, and strengthening family and community) works to implement culture in ways to promote the health and well-being of the participants:

5.1   Promoting Tribal Identity

Promoting tribal identity involved activities that discussed connecting one to the Creator, worked on practicing greetings in Nakoda and Dakota languages, and discussed traditional naming ceremonies. As with many Indigenous languages, the Nakoda and Dakota languages of Fort Peck have been at risk of dying out [45]. The importance of reconnecting and preserving language is more than just being able to speak and understand the words. Many belief systems and con-

cepts that are inherent to the identity of one's tribe are communicated in language with ceremonial activities, prayers, and dances often being conducted in the traditional language [46]. There is growing evidence that those who can communicate in their Indigenous language are more likely to score higher in well-being indexes and less likely to consume alcohol or illicit substances at levels that negatively affect health and well-being [47]. Furthermore, lower levels of suicide in youth and decreased prevalence of diabetes have been found in those who are more connected to their traditional languages [38, 47]. Knowledge of and participation in cultural activities such as receiving a traditional name can enhance cultural identity and self-esteem and improve mental health [48].

5.2   Smudging to Reduce Stress

The Smudging module discusses how this therapeutic healing practice can help resolve unsettling feelings and thoughts. This was important to the team as we knew that we would be discussing difficult topics and needed a therapeutic practice to center everyone. Moreover, we were aware that making people cognizant of their disconnection to culture and language, the degree of assimilation that has occurred due to colonizing practices could potentially trigger feelings of sadness, loss, and shame [49].

5.3   Healing Historical Trauma

The module Healing Historical Trauma worked to identify the effects of historical traumas and discusses ways to cope. It includes an activity called the forgiveness exercise which allowed participants to process traumatic events that have affected them and discuss ways to heal and move on. The negative impact of historical trauma across generations is well documented [7, 8, 50, 51]. The prevalence of negative mental and physical health such as depression, substance misuse, and suicide has been correlated to the effects of historical trauma [8, 51, 52]. Through education and awareness and opportunities to process the effects of historical traumas, different healthy choices can be made as participants become aware of the internalized oppression that has been inflicted on themselves and their people through forced assimilation and racist policies such as boarding schools [53, 54].

5.4   Strengthening Family and Community

The fourth cultural lesson was strengthening family and community. This explored the therapeutic value of connecting to relatives and community and included an activity of filling out one's family tree and discussing it with the group. This module draws on evidence that has shown that for Indigenous communities healing happens through connections with family, community, and spirit [53].

Overall, these four lessons based on the cultural and traditional values and customs of the Assiniboine and Sioux tribes created a program designed to focus on the strength, resilience, and healing of reconnecting participants to their culture while supporting them through the process so that participant health and well-being could be improved at the individual, family, and eventually societal level.

6   Implementing the Feasibility Acceptability Study

In the spring of 2022, we implemented the 5-session adapted intervention with a sample of ($n = 18$) Head Start teachers and teachers' assistants over a period of 7 weeks on the Fort Peck Reservation, thus completing the final phase of the research study. Briefly we visited each Head Start center every week and provided a meal, and the Native American interventionist implemented the session with a researcher present to observe and take notes of fidelity to intervention content, participant attendance, participant reaction to

content, and any issues with lesson delivery. Each session lasted about an hour. To assess the effectiveness of the intervention, we administered a baseline and post-intervention survey to all participants measuring stress, depression, well-being, resilience, communal mastery, adverse childhood experiences, and historical trauma. The primary study outcomes were perceived stress and depression. Secondary outcomes were communal mastery, tribal identity, resilience, and satisfaction with life (well-being). Post-intervention focus groups were conducted with participants to provide depth and understanding of the quantitative findings, and to understand participant experience with the intervention, and explore benefits and suggestions for future use of the intervention.

The baseline and post-intervention surveys were analyzed using t-tests and Hedges' g to measure effect size. Although not powered to determine significance, the effect sizes for primary and secondary outcomes were determined to provide information for future planning of a larger trial of the intervention. The intervention effect demonstrated a decrease in the primary outcome of depression but not in perceived stress. The intervention effect on perceived stress was a small positive effect, indicating that teachers reported an increase in perceived stress post-intervention. For secondary outcomes of tribal identity, communal mastery, and resilience, the intervention had a small but positive effect, indicating that the intervention strengthened tribal identity, communal mastery, and resilience. There was no discernable shift in satisfaction with life. We go into detail about the findings in Wilson et al. [43] mixing the quantitative findings from the survey, the observational data, and results from the post-intervention focus groups. We also disseminated our findings to study participants 3 months after completion of the study, and their comments provided more insight into why the self-perceived stress measure showed an increase as well as expressed appreciation to the research team and the Fort Peck Head Start administration for the time and focus on their health and well-being.

Sharing manuscripts and data interpretation prior to publication with Tribal Head Start as well as the Tribal IRB ensured Indigenous perspectives on the data, helping us to prioritize resiliency and a strengths-based focus as it can be too easy to frame Indigenous experience within a Westernized deficit-based thinking approach. It also meant that we got feedback when our interpretation did not necessarily represent the community interpretation of the issue.

7   Reflection

By utilizing culture as treatment, we contribute to important emerging data on the effectiveness of culture as a SDOH that works to promote health and well-being of communities that have significant health disparities because of discrimination and colonization policies and programs. Our study findings indicate the promise of a group-based culturally informed workplace intervention delivered by a trained community-based interventionist in improving health and well-being of Tribal Head Start teachers. These promising findings justify plans for a larger rigorous pragmatic trial with other reservation-based Head Start schools.

Cultural brokerage from a Native American researcher, establishing partnerships with tribal members, and data ownership agreements as directed by the tribe were essential to ensure culturally safe research that centered the community and focused on capacity building. Furthermore, working closely with the community, we hope that we demonstrated respect for tribal self-determination and sovereignty further helping to promote health and a return to balance not only for study participants but the community. In conclusion this study was founded on the recognition that the SDOH includes the broader concepts of the importance of cultural connection and the harms that colonization has done to such cultural connections for Indigenous communities. See Photo 3 for Fort Peck community.

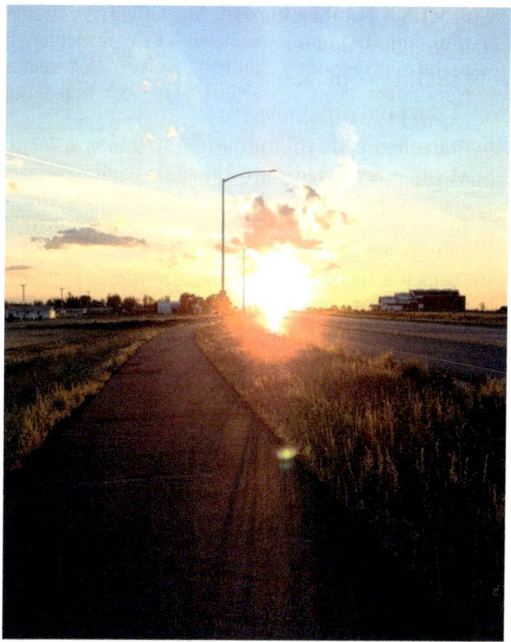

Photo 3 Wolf Point, Fort Peck Reservation at sunrise by Hilary Gourneau

References

1. Gone JP, Tuomi A, Fox N. The urban American Indian traditional spirituality program: promoting indigenous spiritual practices for health equity. Am J Community Psychol. 2020;66(3–4):279–89. https://doi.org/10.1002/ajcp.12436.
2. Moss MP. American Indian health and nursing. 1st ed. New York: Springer Publishing Company; 2015.
3. O'Keefe VM, Cwik MF, Haroz EE, Barlow A. Increasing culturally responsive care and mental health equity with indigenous community mental health workers. Psychol Serv. 2021;18(1):84–92. https://doi.org/10.1037/ser0000358.
4. Tuchman A. Diabetes and race in the USA over the past century. Lancet. 2022;399(10326):712–3. https://doi.org/10.1016/S0140-6736(22)00274-4.
5. Yamane CYEW, Helm S. Indigenous culture-as-health: a systematized literature review. J Prev. 2022;43(2):167–90. https://doi.org/10.1007/s10935-022-00666-3.
6. SAMHSA. Results from the 2019 National Survey on drug use and health: mental health detailed tables. Rockville; 2020. https://www.samhsa.gov/data/report/2019-nsduh-detailed-tables.

7. Brockie TN, Heinzelmann M, Gill J. A framework to examine the role of epigenetics in health disparities among native Americans. Nurs Res Pract. 2013;2013:410395. https://doi.org/10.1155/2013/410395.

8. Brave Heart MYH. The historical trauma response among natives and its relationship with substance abuse: a Lakota illustration. J Psychoactive Drugs. 2003;35(1):7–13. https://doi.org/10.1080/02791072.2003.10399988.

9. Fortney J, Kaufman C, Pollio D, Beals J, Edlund C, Novins D. Geographical access and the substitution of traditional healing for biomedical services in 2 American Indian tribes. Med Care. 2012;50(10):877–84. https://doi.org/10.1097/MLR.0b013e318268ab99.

10. Venner KL, Greenfield BL, Vicuña B, Muñoz R, Bhatt S, O'Keefe V. "I'm not one of them": barriers to help-seeking among American Indians with alcohol dependence. Cultur Divers Ethnic Minor Psychol. 2012;18(4):352–62. https://doi.org/10.1037/a0029757.

11. Institute of Medicine and Practice. Board on population health and public health, disparities, roundtable on the promotion of health equity and the elimination of health. In: Olson S, Anderson KM, editors. Leveraging culture to address health inequalities. National Academies Press; 2013. https://doi.org/10.17226/18496.

12. Green BL. Culture is treatment: considering pedagogy in the care of aboriginal people. J Psychosoc Nurs Ment Health Serv. 2010;48(7):27–34. https://doi.org/10.3928/02793695-20100504-04.

13. Morris SL, Hospital MM, Wagner EF, Lowe J, Thompson MG, Clarke R, Riggs C. SACRED connections: a university-tribal clinical research partnership for school-based screening and brief intervention for substance use problems among native American youth. J Ethn Cult Divers Soc Work. 2021;30(1–2):149–62. https://doi.org/10.1080/15313204.2020.1770654.

14. Goodkind J, LaNoue M, Lee C, Freeland L, Freund R. Feasibility, acceptability, and initial findings from a community-based cultural mental health intervention for American Indian youth and their families. J Community Psychol. 2012;40(4):381–405. https://doi.org/10.1002/jcop.20517.

15. Ramsden I. Cultural safety in nursing education in Aotearoa (New Zealand). Nursing Praxis in New Zealand Inc. 1993;8(3):4–10. https://doi.org/10.36951/NgPxNZ.1993.009.

16. Knibb-Lamouche J. Appendix A: culture as a social determinant of health. Leveraging culture to address health inequalities. National Academies Press; 2013. pp. 59–76.

17. Brockie TN, Dana-Sacco G, López MM, Wetsit L. Essentials of research engagement with native American tribes: data collection reflections of a tribal research team. Prog Community Health Partnersh. 2017;11(3):301–7. https://doi.org/10.1353/cpr.2017.0035.

18. Anastario M, FourStar K, Ricker A, Dick R, Skewes MC, Rink E. A preliminary needs assessment of American Indians who inject drugs in northeastern Montana. Harm Reduct J. 2017;14(1):22. https://doi.org/10.1186/s12954-017-0146-1.

19. Haroz EE, Ingalls A, Kee C, Goklish N, Neault N, Begay M, Barlow A. Informing precision home visiting: identifying meaningful subgroups of families who benefit most from family spirit. Prev Sci. 2019;20(8):1244–54. https://doi.org/10.1007/s11121-019-01039-9.

20. Friedman-Krauss AH, Raver CC, Neuspiel JM, Kinsel J. Child behavior problems, teacher executive functions, and teacher stress in head start classrooms. Early Educ Dev. 2014;25(5):681–702. https://doi.org/10.1080/10409289.2013.825190.

21. Kamerman SB, Gatenio-Gabel S. Early childhood education and care in the United States: an overview of the current policy picture. Int J Child Care Educ Policy. 2007;1(1):23–34. https://doi.org/10.1007/2288-6729-1-1-23.

22. Administration for Children and Families, [ACF]. Early childhood development. 2019. https://www.acf.hhs.gov/ecd. Accessed 19 Oct 2019.

23. Grant AA, Jeon L, Buettner CK. Relating early childhood teachers' working conditions and well-being to their turnover intentions. Educ Psychol. 2019;39(3):294–312. https://doi.org/10.1080/01443410.2018.1543856.

24. Harding JF, Connors MC, Krauss AF, Aikens N, Malone L, Tarullo L. Head start teachers' professional development, well-being, attitudes, and practices: understanding changes over time and predictive associations. Am J Community Psychol. 2019;63(3–4):324–37. https://doi.org/10.1002/ajcp.12327.

25. Jeon L, Buettner CK, Grant AA. Early childhood teachers' psychological well-being: exploring potential predictors of depression, stress, and emotional exhaustion. Early Educ Dev. 2018;29(1):53–69. https://doi.org/10.1080/10409289.2017.1341806.

26. Lever N, Mathis E, Mayworm A. School mental health is not just for students: why teacher and school staff wellness matters. Report on emotional & behavioral disorders in youth. 2017;17(1), 6–12. https://www.ncbi.nlm.nih.gov/pubmed/30705611, https://www.ncbi.nlm.nih.gov/pubmed/30705611.

27. American Indian and Alaska Native Head Start Family and Child Experiences Survey. Case Medical Research. 2019. https://doi.org/10.31525/ct1-nct04046965.

28. Kwon K, Ford TG, Jeon L, Malek-Lasater A, Ellis N, Randall K, Kile M, Salvatore AL. Testing a holistic conceptual framework for early childhood teacher well-being. J Sch Psychol. 2021;86:178–97. https://doi.org/10.1016/j.jsp.2021.03.006.

29. Li Grining C, Raver CC, Champion K, Sardin L, Metzger M, Jones SM. Understanding and improving classroom emotional climate and behavior management in the "real world": the role

of head start teachers' psychosocial stressors. Early Educ Dev. 2010;21(1):65–94. https://doi.org/10.1080/10409280902783509.

30. Roberts A, Kim H. To promote success in schools, focus on teacher well-being. Education + Development [BLOG]. 2019. https://search.proquest.com/docview/2220436981.

31. Wilson D, Plesko C, Brockie TN, Glass N. The well-being of Head Start teachers: a scoping literature review. J Early Child Teach Educ. 2022;44:747. https://doi.org/10.1080/10901027.2022.2147880.

32. Gold E, Smith A, Hopper I, Herne D, Tansey G, Hulland C. Mindfulness-based stress reduction (MBSR) for primary school teachers. J Child Fam Stud. 2010;19(2):184–9. https://doi.org/10.1007/s10826-009-9344-0.

33. Brockie TN, Hill K, Davidson PM, Decker E, Krienke LK, Nelson KE, Nicholson N, Werk AM, Wilson D, Around Him D. Strategies for culturally safe research with native American communities: an integrative review. Contemp Nurse. 2022;58(1):8–32. https://doi.org/10.1080/10376178.2021.2015414.

34. Wexler L. The importance of identity, history, and culture in the well-being of indigenous youth. J Hist Childhood Youth. 2009;2(2):267–76. https://doi.org/10.1353/hcy.0.0055.

35. Fort Peck Assiniboine and Sioux Tribes. Fort Peck Tribes. 2022. http://www.fortpecktribes.org. Accessed 1 Mar 2020.

36. Fort Peck Tribal Health Department. Fort Peck Community Health Assessment. Fort Peck: Fort Peck Tribes. 2016. https://mthcf.org/wp-content/uploads/Fort-Peck-CHA.pdf.

37. Fort Peck Pte Group, Fort Peck Buffalo Program. n.d.. http://www.fortpeckbuffalo.com/. Accessed 20 Apr 2023.

38. Evans-Campbell T, Walters KL, Simoni JM. Substance use among American Indians and Alaska natives: incorporating culture in an "indigenist" stress-coping paradigm. Public Health Rep. 2002;117(3):S104.

39. Cross TL. Understanding the relational worldview in Indian families. Pathways Practice Digest. 1997. http://www.nicwa.org/Relational_Worldview/.

40. Rountree J, Smith A. Strength-based well-being indicators for Indigenous children and families: a literature review of Indigenous communities' identified well-being indicators. Am Indian Alaska Native Ment Health Res. 2016;23(3):206–20. https://doi.org/10.5820/aian.2303.2016.206.

41. Brockie T, Haroz EE, Nelson KE, Cwik M, Decker E, Ricker A, Littlepage S, Mayhew J, Wilson D, Wetsit L, Barlow A. Wakȟáŋyeža (Little Holy One)—an intergenerational intervention for native American parents and children: a protocol for a randomized controlled trial with embedded single-case experimental design. BMC Public Health. 2021;21(1):2298. https://doi.org/10.1186/s12889-021-12272-9.

42. Baum N, Stokar Y, Ginat-Frolich R, Ziv Y, Abu-Jafar I, Cardozo B, Horenczyk R, Brom D. Building Resilience Intervention (BRI) with teachers in Bedouin communities: from evidence informed to evidence based. Child Youth Serv Rev. 2018;87:186. https://search.proquest.com/docview/2077077983.

43. Wilson DH, Nelson KE, Gresh A, Ricker A, Littlepage S, Krienke LK, Brockie TN. The pre-implementation process of adapting a culturally informed stress reduction intervention for native American Head Start teachers. Glob Implement Res Appl. 2023;3:16–30. https://doi.org/10.1007/s43477-022-00070-3.

44. Murray LK, Dorsey S, Haroz E, Lee C, Alsiary MM, Haydary A, Weiss WM, Bolton P. A common elements treatment approach for adult mental health problems in low- and middle-income countries. Cogn Behav Pract. 2014;21(2):111–23. https://doi.org/10.1016/j.cbpra.2013.06.005.

45. UNESCO. UNESCO atlas of the world's languages in danger. UNESCO; 2017.

46. Gonzalez MB, Aronson BD, Kellar S, Walls ML, Greenfield BL. Language as a facilitator of cultural connection. Ab-Original. 2018;1(2):176–94. https://www.jstor.org/stable/10.5325/aboriginal.1.2.0176.

47. Schanche Hodge F, Nandy K. Predictors of wellness and American Indians. J Health Care Poor Underserved. 2011;22(3):791–803. https://doi.org/10.1353/hpu.2011.0093.

48. Kading ML, Hautala DS, Palombi LC, Aronson BD, Smith RC, Walls ML. Flourishing. Society and Mental Health. 2015;5(3), 203–217. https://doi.org/10.1177/2156869315570480.

49. Biddle N, Swee H. The relationship between well-being and indigenous land, language and culture in Australia. Aust Geogr. 2012;43(3):215–32. https://doi.org/10.1080/00049182.2012.706201.

50. Gone JP, Alcántara C. Identifying effective mental health interventions for American Indians and Alaska natives. Cultur Divers Ethnic Minor Psychol. 2007;13(4).356–63. https://doi.org/10.1037/1099-9809.13.4.356.

51. Les Whitbeck B., Xiaojin Chen, Hoyt, D. R., & Adams, G. W. (2004). Discrimination, historical loss, and enculturation: culturally specific risk and resiliency factors for alcohol abuse among American Indians. Journal of Studies on Alcohol, 65(4), 409–418. 10.15288/jsa.2004.65.409.

52. Wendt DC, Hartmann WE, Allen J, Burack JA, Charles B, D'Amico EJ, Dell CA, Dickerson DL, Donovan DM, Gone JP, O'Connor RM, Radin SM, Rasmus SM, Venner KL, Walls ML. Substance use research with indigenous communities: exploring and extending foundational principles of community psychology. Am J Community Psychol. 2019;64(1–2):146–58. https://doi.org/10.1002/ajcp.12363.

53. Burrage RL, Momper SL, Gone JP. Beyond trauma: decolonizing understandings of loss and healing in the Indian residential school system of Canada. J Soc Issues. 2022;78(1):27–52. https://doi.org/10.1111/josi.12455.

54. Grayshield L, Rutherford JJ, Salazar SB, Mihecoby AL, Luna LL. Understanding and healing historical trauma: the perspectives of native American elders. J Ment Health Couns. 2015;37(4):295–307. https://doi.org/10.17744/mehc.37.4.02.

Deborah H. Wilson, PhD, MPH, RN CNE, is a senior lecturer at Auckland University of Technology in Aotearoa, New Zealand, and has been working as a registered nurse internationally for the last 25 years. Her specialties are emergency medicine and neuroscience, with a focus on trauma. Since 2004, Wilson has worked with Medicine Sans Frontiers (Doctors Without Borders) during global health emergencies such as Ebola, malnutrition, and cholera crises. She completed her PhD in 2023 at Johns Hopkins University School of Nursing in Baltimore, Maryland, USA. Dr. Wilson's focus of interest is the effect that reconnection to culture can have on the health and well-being of Indigenous peoples. She also works to incorporate Indigenous Ways of Knowing and cultural safety into nursing curriculums.

Adriann Ricker MPH, is a member of the Fort Peck Assiniboine and Sioux Tribes of Montana. She joined the Center for Indigenous Health as a Research Associate. She serves as the on-site coordinator for the Little Holy One Research Project. Prior to joining the center, Adriann worked in research in various capacities on her reservation for the past twelve years. In addition to her research experience, she has also worked as an adjunct faculty at the Fort Peck Community College and as a healthcare administrator for a local tribal program. Adriann holds a BS in Health Promotion from Montana State University Billings, an MPH from A.T. Still University, and is currently pursuing a PhD in Indigenous Health from the University of North Dakota.

Hilary Gourneau (Dakota, Annishnabae) Fort Peck Assiniboine and Sioux Tribes. Ms. Gourneau serves as the Head Start Director and is a member of the Fort Peck Assiniboine and Sioux Tribes, and she is a proud graduate of Poplar High School. She pursued a career in education at Montana State University-Billings, where in 2012, she received her Bachelor of Science degree in Elementary Education with a minor in Native American Studies. In June 2020, Ms. Gourneau graduated from Portland State University in Portland, Oregon, with a Master's in Counselor Education, with a focus on School Counseling and a certificate in Trauma-Informed Services. In August 2020, she accepted a position with the Fort Peck Tribes as the Head Start Director, where her love for learning initially began as a Head Start Graduate. Ms. Gourneau currently serves on the Board of Trustees at Poplar Public Schools, holds a position as an Ex-Officio Member of the Montana Advisory Council on Indian Education (MACIE), representing Tribal Head Starts, and serves on the National Indian Head Start Directors Association board as the Zone 8 Alternate. She has recently graduated from her local tribal community college, Fort Peck, with an Associates of Arts degree in Early Childhood Education.

Teresa N. Brockie research focuses on achieving health equity through community-based prevention and intervention of suicide, trauma, and adverse childhood experiences among vulnerable populations. A member of the White Clay (A'aninin) Nation from Fort Belknap, Montana, Dr. Brockie earned her PhD from the Johns Hopkins School of Nursing and completed a postdoctoral fellowship with the National Institutes of Health Clinical Center. In 2011, she led an all-Native American team to collect data to study suicidal behavior among reservation-based Native American youth.

Socio-cultural Barriers to Contraceptive Uptake and Its Consequences to Unintended Pregnancy in Ethiopia

Ayalnesh Zemene Yalew

1 Contraceptive Uptake and Unintended Pregnancies

Contraceptive uptake is a crucial social determinant of maternal, child, and society health. Recent evidence underscores its importance in improving various aspects of health and well-being. Contraceptive use plays a significant role in reducing maternal mortality and morbidity. Women who have access to and use contraceptives can better plan their pregnancies, leading to healthier intervals between births and reduced health risks associated with closely spaced pregnancies. Contraceptive uptake is closely linked to improved child health outcomes. Spacing pregnancies allows mothers to better care for their children, resulting in reduced child mortality and improved nutrition and development for each child [1–3].

Contraceptive use allows families to plan their children's numbers and timing, promoting economic stability. Smaller family sizes enable more investment in education, healthcare, and well-being. Access to contraceptive uptake slows population growth, enabling better resource management and sustainable development goals [4, 5]. Despite its various health importance, lack of access to and use of contraceptive methods is a serious public health problem particularly in resource-limited countries like that of Ethiopia. It exposes numerous women for unintended pregnancy and unsafe abortion.

1.1 Consequences of Unintended Pregnancy

Unintended pregnancies may lead to delayed or inadequate prenatal care, increasing the risk of maternal and child health complications. By reducing unintended pregnancies, maternal and child health outcomes can significantly improve. In regions with restricted access to safe abortion services, unintended pregnancies can result in unsafe abortion practices, leading to maternal morbidity and mortality. Access to comprehensive family planning services can help to prevent unintended pregnancies and reduce the need for unsafe abortions [6, 7].

Higher number of unintended pregnancies resulted in a strain to healthcare systems, particularly in low-resource settings, and perpetuated the cycle of poverty and poor health outcomes for future generations. Women with unintended pregnancies may experience delayed or inadequate care, increasing maternal and child health complications. Reducing unintended pregnancies can allocate resources more effectively, mitigate intergenerational impact, and improve maternal and child health outcomes. Empowering individ-

A. Z. Yalew (✉)
St. Paul's Hospital Millennium Medical College,
School of Nursing, Addis Ababa, Ethiopia

J. B. Hamilton, C. E. Moore (eds.), *Transforming Social Determinants to Promote Global Health*,
https://doi.org/10.1007/978-3-031-61160-5_19

uals and couples to plan their families can also help mitigate these issues [8–10].

2 Relevance of Addressing Socio-cultural Barriers to Contraceptive Use and Unintended Pregnancies

Unintended pregnancies have significant implications for individuals, families, and communities. High rates of unintended pregnancies can lead to adverse maternal and child health outcomes and overburdened healthcare systems and perpetuate the cycle of poverty. Addressing the socio-cultural barriers to contraceptive uptake is essential to reducing unintended pregnancies and improving public health. Unintended pregnancies are a global health concern affecting millions of people worldwide, especially in low- and middle-income countries. By understanding and addressing the socio-cultural barriers that influence contraceptive use, researchers and policymakers can contribute to global efforts to improve reproductive health and reduce maternal and child mortality. Sociocultural barriers can disproportionately affect marginalized and vulnerable populations, exacerbating health disparities. Working on this topic is a step towards promoting health equity and social justice by ensuring that all individuals have equal access to contraceptive options and family planning services. By studying socio-cultural barriers, interventions can be designed to empower individuals and communities to make informed decisions about their reproductive health. This includes promoting gender equality, fostering community engagement, and challenging stigmas surrounding family planning. In addition research conducted on socio-cultural barriers can inform the development of evidence-based policies and programs aimed at increasing contraceptive uptake and reducing unintended pregnancies. This can lead to more effective and targeted interventions that align with the needs and values of the affected communities. Moreover, addressing the socio-cultural barriers to contraceptive uptake

and unintended pregnancies has the potential to create a positive, long-term impact on population health contributing to bringing healthier and more prosperous societies.

Overall, the decision to work on socio-cultural barriers to contraceptive uptake and unintended pregnancy is driven by a commitment to improving public health, promoting health equity, and empowering individuals to make informed choices about their reproductive health. Researchers and policymakers recognize the importance of understanding and addressing these barriers to create positive and sustainable change for global health and well-being.

2.1 Socio-cultural Barriers and Unintended Pregnancies in Ethiopia

In Ethiopia, there are several socio-cultural barriers that hinder the uptake of contraceptives, leading to unintended pregnancies and their associated consequences. These barriers are deeply rooted in traditional beliefs, gender roles, religious norms, and social norms. A discussion of key socio-cultural barriers and their implication for Ethiopian populations is described in the following sections.

The decision to focus my scholarship and community work on socio-cultural barriers to contraceptive uptake and its consequences to unintended pregnancy comes from my exposure to this topic during my PhD work. The motivation behind focusing on socio-cultural barriers to contraceptive uptake and its consequences to unintended pregnancy during my PhD work was attributed to various factors. Firstly, my personal connection to the issue, witnessing its impact in my community or among friends and family, sparked concern and empathy, prompting me to delve into the topic. Secondly, I identified a research gap during my academic journey, which piqued my interest in addressing the understudied issue of socio-cultural barriers and unintended pregnancy. Additionally, my strong desire to make a positive social impact and recognize the implications of unintended pregnancies drove me to find solutions and promote access to effective contraception.

Moreover, understanding the intersectionality involved in contraceptive uptake and unintended pregnancies, particularly socio-cultural factors like gender, stigma and discrimination, social norms, religion, and culture, I inspired to explore this complex issue and advocate for evidence-based policies to improve access to and use of contraceptives. While I was working on my PhD project "Exploring reasons for unintended pregnancies," I came to understand that socio-cultural barriers are very common problems that affect the use of contraceptives leading to unintended pregnancies among women and school girls. These unintended pregnancies are the result of the underuse and lack of access to contraceptive methods.

2.2   Socio-cultural Barriers to Contraceptives

A significant socio-cultural barrier to contraceptive use in Addis Ababa is deeply rooted in traditional beliefs and cultural practices. Many communities in the city hold conservative views regarding family planning, associating large families with prosperity and social status. Women may be expected to bear as many children as possible, leading to a resistance towards contraceptive methods.

Second, gender roles and norms play a crucial role in the use of contraceptives. In some areas of Addis Ababa, decision-making power regarding family planning often lies with men. Women may face opposition from their partners or extended family if they wish to use contraceptives, making it challenging for them to access and use these methods.

Third, there is a prevailing stigma around discussions of contraception and reproductive health in some communities. Misconceptions and misinformation about contraceptive methods are widespread, leading to fear and reluctance to use them. Some individuals may believe that contraceptives have adverse health effects or that their use is morally wrong.

Finally, the underuse of contraceptives in Ethiopia is influenced by a diverse religious landscape. For example, faith-based communities may have reservations about contraceptive use due to religious doctrines or ethical concerns. For instance, majority of my study participants confirmed that conservative religious teachings may discourage or even prohibit the use of modern contraceptives, leading to lower contraceptive uptake among women from religious communities. In some cases, religious leaders may promote traditional family values and discourage any form of birth control, leading women to rely solely on natural methods or no contraception at all. This can result in a higher incidence of unintended pregnancies among women who adhere strictly to religious teachings regarding family planning. Moreover, religious norms and stigmas surrounding premarital sex or contraception may deter young unmarried women from seeking contraceptive services, making them more vulnerable to unintended pregnancies.

A lack of access to contraceptives is an additional socio-cultural barrier in Ethiopia. For example, adequate access to contraceptive services is limited in certain areas of Addis Ababa, particularly in slum settlements and marginalized communities. Health facilities may be far from people's homes, and transportation to these facilities can be a challenge. Additionally, awareness campaigns about the benefits and availability of contraceptives may not reach all segments of the population.

2.3   Setting/Community Where the Barriers Existed

Addis Ababa, the capital city of Ethiopia, is a diverse and bustling metropolis with a population of over four million people. It serves as the country's political, cultural, and economic center. The city has made significant strides in various areas, but like many developing regions, it faces challenges concerning reproductive health and family planning.

Addis Ababa is a melting pot of cultures, languages, and traditions. It attracts people from all over the country seeking better economic opportunities, education, and healthcare. The city's population includes individuals from various ethnic groups, such as Oromo, Amhara, Tigray, Gurage, Sidama, and others. This diversity contributes to a rich cultural tapestry but can also lead to different perspectives on family planning and contraception.

Although Addis Ababa generally has better access to healthcare facilities and services compared to rural areas, there can still be variations in accessibility within the city. Certain neighborhoods or districts might have limited access to family planning clinics and contraceptive resources. Traditional beliefs and cultural practices, along with conservative views regarding family planning and the association of large families with prosperity and status, act as significant barriers to contraceptive use in Addis Ababa. Gender norms and power dynamics also play a crucial role, with decision-making power often lying with men, making it challenging for women to access and use contraceptives. Stigma and misinformation about contraception are widespread, leading to fear and reluctance to use these methods due to concerns about health effects or moral considerations. Additionally, limited access to contraceptive services, particularly in marginalized communities, and diverse religious and ethical beliefs in Ethiopia further influence people's decisions regarding family planning.

2.4 Vulnerable Populations and Communities Affected by Contraceptives and Unintended Pregnancies

In the section to follow, I describe individuals and communities at risk for unintended pregnancies. These include school girls, women, married couples, marginalized communities, and religious and conservative communities.

School Girls: School girls are indeed a vulnerable population when it comes to socio-cultural disparities and the risks of unwanted pregnancies and abortions. Several factors contribute to their vulnerability: Limited access to comprehensive sex education can increase the likelihood of unintended pregnancies and risky behaviors in school girls. Socio-cultural stigma, gender inequality, and barriers to accessing contraceptive options can further hinder girls' decision-making power. Limited support systems, social isolation, and fear of judgment can further exacerbate vulnerability and increase the likelihood of unsafe abortion practices. Legal restrictions may also pose a risk to girls' health and lives, as they may resort to clandestine methods without proper medical care and supervision.

Women: Women and adolescent girls are most affected by socio-cultural barriers to contraceptives. They often bear the responsibility of managing family planning and face resistance from partners or family members when seeking to use contraceptives.

Married Couples: Couples seeking to control their family size and improve their economic prospects are impacted by the lack of access to contraceptives and prevailing cultural norms.

Marginalized Communities: Residents of slum areas and marginalized communities face additional challenges due to limited access to health services and lack of awareness about contraceptive options.

Religious and Conservative Communities: People living in communities with strong religious or conservative beliefs may find it more challenging to access and accept contraceptive services.

3 Programs Developed to Address Sociocultural Barriers and Promote Use of and Access to Contraceptives

In response to the socio-cultural barriers that hinder contraceptive uptake and access, various programs and initiatives have been developed with the aim of promoting family planning and reproductive health. This section explores some of the key programs that have been implemented to address these challenges and increase the utilization of contraceptives. From community-based awareness campaigns to culturally sensitive counseling services, these efforts highlight the significance of tailoring interventions to specific cultural contexts and empowering individuals to make informed choices about their reproductive health. By delving into these programs, we can gain valuable insights into the strategies employed to overcome social and cultural barriers, ultimately fostering better access to and utilization of contraceptive methods.

Family Guidance Association of Ethiopia (FGAE) (Addis Ababa Branch): FGAE is a well-established local organization that has been working on family planning and reproductive health services in Ethiopia since 1966. The Addis Ababa branch specifically focuses on providing contraceptive counseling, education, and access to contraceptive methods.

Addis Ababa Health Bureau: The Addis Ababa Health Bureau is a government agency responsible for the administration of health services in the city. They work on various health initiatives, including family planning and reproductive health. The bureau collaborates with local clinics and healthcare facilities to ensure access to contraceptive services and conducts awareness campaigns to address socio-cultural barriers.

Women's Health Project (WHP) (Addis Ababa University): The Women's Health Project at Addis Ababa University focuses on research and interventions related to women's health, including family planning. They conduct studies to better understand socio-cultural barriers to contraceptive use and develop targeted strategies to overcome them. Additionally, they collaborate with local health centers to implement evidence-based interventions.

Pathfinder International Ethiopia: Pathfinder International has been working in Ethiopia to promote family planning and reproductive health, including in Addis Ababa. They implement programs that involve community engagement and sensitization to address socio-cultural norms that might hinder contraceptive access and usage.

The Challenge Initiative (TCI): The Challenge Initiative, supported by the Bill & Melinda Gates Institute for Population and Reproductive Health, was active in Addis Ababa, among other cities in Ethiopia. TCI works with local governments and partners to design and implement evidence-based solutions for family planning challenges, including addressing socio-cultural barriers.

Population Council Ethiopia: The Population Council is an international organization that conducts research on reproductive health and family planning. Their Ethiopia office collaborates with local partners to generate evidence and develop interventions that can address socio-cultural barriers to contraceptive use in Addis Ababa and beyond.

3.1   Community Engagements in Implementation of Programs Existed to Prevent Unintended Pregnancy

Community involvement is essential for local programs aimed at reducing socio-cultural barriers to contraceptive use. By actively engaging the community, programs can ensure cultural relevance, build trust, overcome stigma, and identify sustainable solutions, leading to more effective and impactful family planning interventions.

To reduce socio-cultural barriers to contraceptive use, the following strategies are essential: First conduct community outreach and engagement activities, such as workshops and interactive sessions, to raise awareness about family planning and dispel misconceptions. Second, deliver culturally sensitive and tailored messages respecting the community's norms and values to enhance receptiveness towards family planning practices. For example, engaging religious and community leaders is crucial as they can play a significant role in advocating for contraceptive use within their communities. Third, the implementation of peer education programs and support groups empowering women and girls to openly discuss reproductive health and receive guidance on contraceptive use.

Collaborating with educational institutions like Addis Ababa University can facilitate comprehensive sex education and awareness-raising among students. Deploying mobile health clinics to remote and underserved areas provides access to contraceptive services. Engaging policymakers and stakeholders through advocacy efforts is vital for resource allocation and creating an enabling environment for family planning programs. Involving men in family planning discussions and addressing gender inequality are essential for empowering women to make informed reproductive health decisions. Lastly, regular monitoring and evaluation of program progress ensures evidence-based and impactful interventions.

4   Reflection

The concept of socio-cultural barriers to contraceptive uptake and its consequences on unintended pregnancy in Ethiopia highlights the critical role of family planning and reproductive health in improving maternal, child, and societal well-being. Contraceptive use is essential for reducing maternal mortality, improving child health outcomes, and promoting economic stability. However, limited access to contraceptive methods in resource-limited countries like Ethiopia poses a significant public health challenge.

The consequences of unintended pregnancies can be severe, leading to inadequate prenatal care, unsafe abortions, strained healthcare systems, perpetuation of poverty, and poor health outcomes for future generations. Addressing socio-cultural barriers to contraceptive use is crucial for mitigating these consequences and improving public health. Socio-cultural factors such as traditional beliefs, gender roles, religious norms, stigma, and misinformation play a significant role in hindering contraceptive uptake.

Understanding and addressing these barriers is essential for promoting health equity and social justice, ensuring that all individuals have equal access to contraceptive options and family planning services. By empowering individuals and communities to make informed decisions about their reproductive health, interventions can be designed to better align with the needs and values of the affected communities. Additionally, evidence-based policies and programs can be developed to increase contraceptive uptake and reduce unintended pregnancies.

In Ethiopia, where socio-cultural barriers to contraceptive uptake are prevalent, various organizations and programs are actively working to overcome these challenges. Community engagement, peer education, involving religious and community leaders, and collaboration with policymakers are among the strategies employed to promote access and use of contraceptives. By targeting vulnerable populations, such as women, married couples, marginalized communities, and school girls, these initiatives aim to create positive and sustainable changes in population health and bring about healthier and more prosperous societies.

Overall, addressing socio-cultural barriers to contraceptive uptake and unintended pregnancy is a vital step towards improving public health, promoting gender equality, and empowering individuals to make informed choices about their reproductive health. By fostering collaboration among researchers, policymakers, healthcare providers, and communities, Ethiopia can make significant strides in improving family planning services, reducing unintended pregnancies, and ensuring better health outcomes for its population.

By pursuing the following future plans, I hope to contribute significantly to the reduction of unintended pregnancies and the improvement of reproductive health outcomes in Ethiopia. Ultimately, I aspire to make a positive and lasting impact on population health, fostering healthier and more prosperous communities.

Continued Research: My future endeavors are driven by a commitment to conduct further research on the socio-cultural barriers that hinder contraceptive use and contribute to unintended pregnancies in different regions of Ethiopia. This research will provide valuable insights into the unique challenges faced by various communities, enabling the development of tailored interventions and programs. By understanding the specific barriers and cultural contexts, we can implement targeted strategies that effectively promote family planning and reproductive health.

Policy Advocacy: Engaging with policymakers at both the local and national levels will be a central focus of my future work. By presenting research findings and collaborating with relevant stakeholders, I aim to advocate for evidence-based policies that support family planning and reproductive health. Influencing policy decisions is crucial in improving access to contraceptives and family planning services, leading to better reproductive health outcomes for the Ethiopian population.

Program Implementation: I am dedicated to actively participating in or collaborating with organizations and programs that address socio-cultural barriers to contraceptive uptake in Ethiopia. My goal is to contribute to the design and implementation of culturally sensitive interventions that directly impact the accessibility and utilization of contraceptives. Through these efforts, we can work towards overcoming barriers and fostering a positive change in reproductive health practices.

Community Outreach: Emphasizing community engagement is vital in my future work. By working closely with religious and community leaders, local healthcare providers, and peer educators, I aim to create awareness and promote family planning practices. This will involve organizing workshops, seminars, and support groups to empower individuals with knowledge and resources to make informed decisions about their reproductive health.

Collaboration and Partnerships: Seeking to build strong partnerships with local and international organizations, research institutions, and governmental bodies is crucial for enhancing the effectiveness and sustainability of our interventions. Collaboration facilitates the exchange of ideas, resources, and expertise, enabling us to collectively address the challenges of family planning and reproductive health.

Advocating for Health Equity: My future work will be dedicated to reducing health disparities by ensuring that vulnerable and marginalized populations have equal access to contraceptive options and family planning services. By working to lessen the impact of socio-cultural barriers on these populations, we can promote health equity and inclusivity in reproductive healthcare.

Awareness and Education: I will continue to advocate for comprehensive sex education in schools and communities, as open discussions about reproductive health and family planning can challenge stigmas, dispel myths, and empower individuals to make informed decisions about their reproductive health.

Monitoring and Evaluation: Regular monitoring and evaluation of programs and interventions will be an essential component of my future work. By collecting data and analyzing outcomes, we can ensure that our efforts are evidence-based and result-oriented, allowing us to continuously improve and refine our approaches to family planning and reproductive health promotion.

References

1. America, Latin, Northern America, and Western Africa. Contraception evidence brief. 2017.
2. Mekonnen AG, Odo DB, Nigatu D, Amare NS, Tizazu MA. Determinants of adolescents' contraceptive uptake in Ethiopia: a systematic review of literature. Contracept Reprod Med. 2022;7(1):16.
3. Souza PD, Bailey JV, Stephenson J, Oliver S, Souza PD, Bailey JV, Stephenson J, Oliver S. Factors influencing contraception choice and use globally: a synthesis of systematic reviews. Eur J Contracept Reprod Health Care. 2022;27(5):364–72.
4. Beatty A, National Academies. Recent fertility trends in sub-Saharan Africa. 2016.
5. WHO. High rates of unintended pregnancies linked to gaps in family planning services: new WHO study. 2019.
6. Dingeta T, Oljira L, Worku A, Berhane Y. Low contraceptive utilization among young married women is associated with perceived social norms and belief in contraceptive myths in rural Ethiopia. PLoS One. 2021;16(2):e0247484.
7. WHO. Family planning/contraception methods. 2020.
8. Eastman A, Olunuga O, Moges T. Socio-cultural barriers influencing unplanned pregnancy in Mugombwa Refugee Camp, Rwanda: female adolescents' perspectives. Adolescents. 2023;3(2):259–77.

9. UN. 'Staggering number' of unintended pregnancies reveals failure to uphold women's rights. 2022.

10. Yazdkhasti M, Pourreza A, Pirak A. Unintended pregnancy and its adverse social and economic consequences on health system: a narrative review article. Iran J Public Health. 2015;44(1):12–21.

Ayalnesh Zemene Yalew MSc, PhD, is an Assistant Professor of Reproductive and Maternal Health at St. Paul's Hospital Millennium Medical College, Ethiopia, and a doctoral student at the Pan African University, University of Ibadan, Nigeria.

Addressing Sexual and Gender Minorities Intersecting Structural Stigma: An Evidence-Based Holistic Care

David Agor and Kenneth Daici

Sexual and gender minority (SGM or LGBTQIA+) is an all-inclusive term used in academic and research settings to refer to individuals who self-identify as nonheterosexual or cisgender. According to the National Institute on Minority Health and Health Disparities (NIMHD), SGM populations include individuals who identify as lesbian, gay, bisexual, asexual, transgender, Two-Spirit, queer, and/or intersex, as well as any individuals with same-sex or same-gender attractions or behaviors and those with a difference in sex development. SGMs have the highest psychiatric comorbidity; multimorbidity (co-occurring medical and psychiatric disorders) suicide is two to three times high among SGM populations compared to their heterosexual counterparts [1, 2]. The burden of HIV is highest among SGM populations: According to the CDC, in 2021, male-to-male sexual contact accounted for 70% of HIV incidence in the United States and 86% of estimated infections among all men [3]. The burden of HIV is higher for SGM with intersecting minoritized identities such as Black men who have sex with men (MSM). The CDC estimates that one in two African American MSM will be HIV positive within their lifetime despite Black MSM having health behaviors similar to other racial and ethnic SGM [1, 4, 5]. The constellation of the many health inequities confronting the SGM populations leads the National Institute on Minority Health and Health Disparities (NIMHD) to designate the SGM populations as a health disparity group in 2016. The best evidence from researchers and scholars attributes SGM health inequities to minority stress and different levels of stigma chronically experienced by the SGM populations.

This chapter describes SGM intersecting structural stigma and nuanced interventions for addressing minority stress and structural stigma. Many SGM individuals have multiple intersecting minoritized identities that compound their allostatic stress load which results in multimorbidity (medical and mental comorbidity). There are two major drivers of health inequities among SGM populations: (a) minority stress and (b) stigma.

1 Minority Stress Theory

The theoretical framework guiding our work on addressing sexual and gender minorities intersecting structural stigma is minority stress theory. Minority stress theory postulates that individuals from socially minoritized communities experience chronic stress in addition to everyday stressors experienced by the general population. These unique stressors experienced among minority indi-

D. Agor (✉)
The University of Pennsylvania School of Nursing, Philadelphia, PA, USA
e-mail: dagor@nursing.upenn.edu

K. Daici
Health and Human Biology and Photojournalism, Brown University, Providence, RI, USA
e-mail: kenneth_daici@brown.edu

© The Author(s), under exclusive license to Springer Nature Switzerland AG 2024
J. B. Hamilton, C. E. Moore (eds.), *Transforming Social Determinants to Promote Global Health*,
https://doi.org/10.1007/978-3-031-61160-5_20

viduals include those chronic stressors related to the stigmatization, marginalization, and discrimination of their minority identities [6, 7]. However, given that individuals who identify as sexual and gendered minorities at the intersection of racial and ethnic minority (REM) experience additional chronic stressors, we have incorporated the seminal work of Ilan Meyer. Meyer was the first to apply the minority stress theory to explain SGM health disparity concepts related to endemic chronic stressors among the SGM populations [6]. This seminal work titled Prejudice, Social Stress, and Mental Health in Lesbian, Gay, and Bisexual Populations: Conceptual Issues and Research Evidence is useful for our work on interventions

for SGM intersecting structural stigma in that it postulates that SGM health inequities are not inherent due to their identity but associated with higher allostatic chronic stress load emanating from stigma, discrimination, and homonegativity.

Hence, individuals who identify as SGM experience increased allostatic stress which predisposes them to increased stress-related mental illness (acute stress disorder, PTSD), depression, anxiety, substance use disorder, etc. Because of this chronic stress, there is an elevation of inflammatory markers causing low-grade chronic inflammation, HPA axis dysregulation, and increased cortisol, hence leading to immune dysregulation and metabolic syndrome (see Fig. 1).

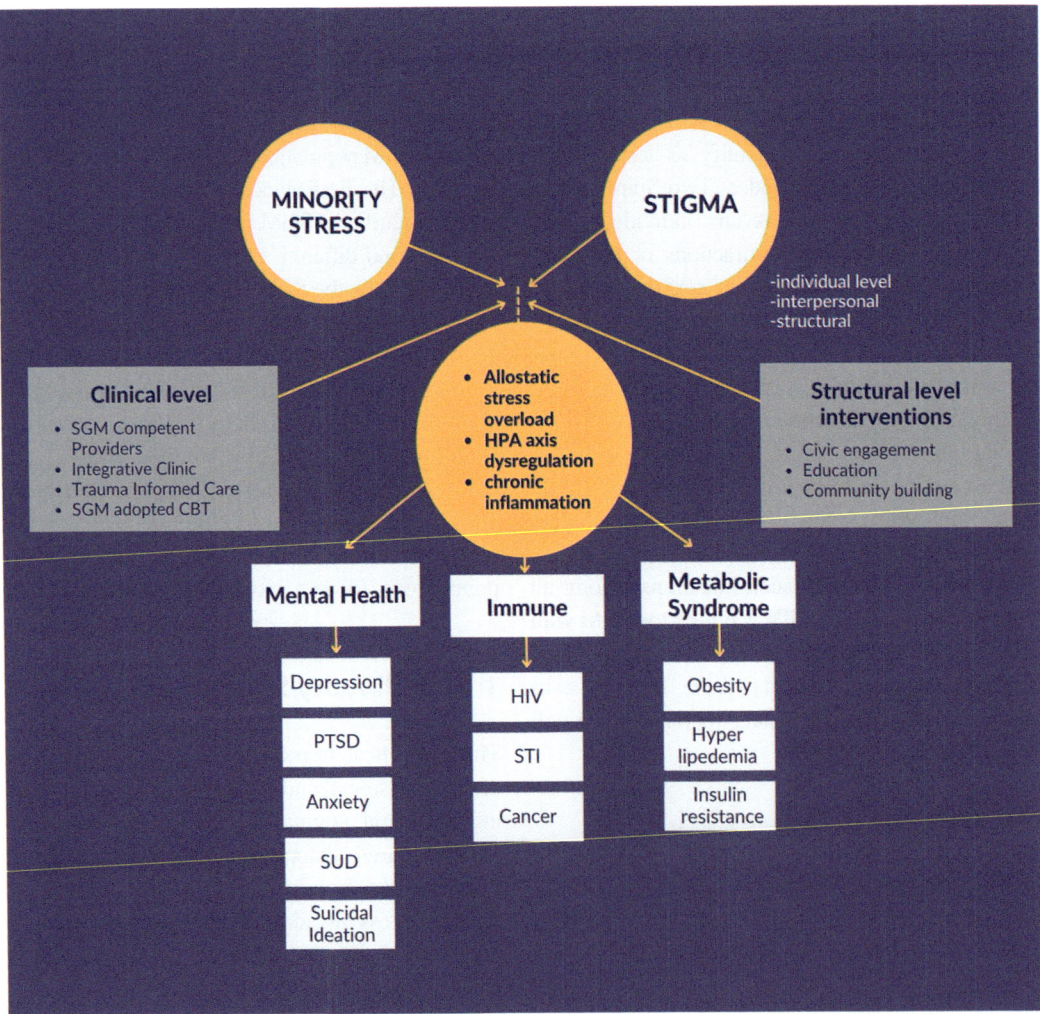

Fig. 1 Minority stress theoretical framework

Minority stress theory maintains that SGM populations experience unique stressors (e.g., stigma, homonegativity, microaggression, bullying, and discrimination) in combination with everyday stress experienced by the general populations [8]. These chronic stressors and compensating maladaptive coping mechanisms (substance use, survival sex work, condomless insertive sex without non-biomedical protection) contribute to the health disparities prevalent within the SGM community. The World Health Organization (WHO) in 2013 designated stress a social gradient in social determinants of health (SDOH). Collectively, minority stress theory—which is the theoretical underpinning for most SGM research and practice—is being used to guide our work to develop and test a culturally appropriate intervention to SGM intersecting structural stigma.

1.1 Sexual and Gender Minority Stigma

Stigma is a social construct within differing power dynamics; it devalues and dehumanizes individuals, groups, and communities based on perceived deviation from norms. It creates an ecosystem where health inequalities thrive because it leads to exclusion in many critical life domains vital for social determinants of health (SDOH), like housing, employment, education, interpersonal relationships, and healthcare [9, 10]. Agor [11] maintains that stigma is bidirectional: it drives health inequality, and health inequality drives stigma. Because of anticipated stigma and discrimination, the SGM populations may avoid healthcare systems; hence routine care and preventive care are delayed, which may worsen preventable health issues. For example, lesbian women and transgender men have the worst cancer outcomes because they are less likely to be offered routine gynecological cancer screening compared to their heterosexual counterparts [12].

For stigma to occur, a power differential must exist. It starts with labeling and distinguishing human differences → negative stereotyping of "others" → finally, a complete separation of "us" vs. "them" with an indelible social deviant mark ascribed. There are three levels of stigma: (a) individual, (b) interpersonal, and (c) structural stigma.

2 Individual Level/Self-stigma

These occur when a stigmatized person consciously or unconsciously accepts, internalizes, and manifests negative stereotypes—these can manifest through compensatory affective, emotional, and behavioral modifications such as concealment (being closeted) and self-isolation from communities. Self-stigma is affectively and cognitively harmful and can lead to psychopathology because it creates room for constant negative self-talk and impaired self-esteem. People can escape from the world around them, but they can't escape from themselves [13, 14].

3 Interpersonal Stigma

These are stigma individual-level homonegativity (negative emotions, feelings, attitudes, and behaviors towards SGM populations). Homophobia is not an evidence-based term because phobia is a psychopathology—which might excuse the behavior or perpetrator. This level of stigma includes overt, intentional, unintentional, and (micro)aggression actions and behavior from a privileged, non-stigmatized individual to a stigmatized individual. The privilege here refers to the power differential "normal" belonging to the majority heteronormative culture. This type of stigma happens between individuals: however, there needs to be an ecosystem that perpetuates its continuous existence [13, 14].

4 Structural Stigma

This is the highest level of stigma: these are policies, laws, regulations, and ordinances that legally and systemically exclude SGM individuals and negatively "other" them. These societal norms exclude SGM populations from participating and accessing essential elements necessary for social determinants of health (SDOH) [13, 14]. For example, as of June 2023, more than 530 anti-SGM bills have been proposed or passed around the US legislative bodies for the 2023 legislative calendar. Some of these laws aim to exclude gender minorities from accessing basic healthcare that affirms their personhood. Another good example is the FDA law that prohibited SGM populations from donating blood irrespective of risk behaviors. This FDA policy is not informed by evidence but rather by homonegativity that coined HIV as "gay-related immune deficiency" (GRID) or colloquially known as the "gay cancer/disease." It is difficult for the general populations to stop homonegative behaviors towards SGM populations when the government apparatus continues to reinforce homonegative attitudes and behaviors. This is because governmental policies have the power to normalize or denormalize any social phenomena. Other noteworthy examples of structural stigma with health implications include:

4.1 Healthcare Professional Education and Research

Healthcare professionals (nursing, medical doctors, pharmacist, and allied health) are undereducated or uneducated on SGM's unique healthcare needs. For example, most medical schools have SGM content as an elective [15]. A review study from Columbia School of Nursing exposed nursing perpetuation of SGM structural stigma by under-educating nursing undergraduate students on SGM competency [16]. Further, the National Institute of Nursing Research (NINR) has only funded 25 SGM-related studies since 1987–2018. Less than 1% of National Institutes of Health (NIH) funding focuses on SGM populations. These exclusions from policy, research, funding, and education of healthcare providers in and of itself are structural stigma. Further, licensed healthcare professionals with little or no experience with the unique needs of SGM populations can lead to re-trau-

matization for SGM populations within the healthcare system.

4.2 Elimination by Omission

Until 2021, the national census bureau did not collect any SGM status data; also, only 39 states collect SGM demographic data questions on the Behavioral Risk Factor Surveillance System (BRFSS): the largest continuous health survey in the world. BRFSS data are large data sets used by government officials to inform policy, and researchers also use those data for population-level studies. This trend is in concordance with national trends. According to the National Academies of Sciences, Engineering, and Medicine; Division of Behavioral and Social Sciences and Education; Committee on Population; Committee on Understanding the Well-Being of Sexual and Gender Diverse Populations [17], most national surveys do not collect SGM data. This governmental-level stigma (un)intentionally aiming to eradicate SGM populations by omission is an example of structural stigma. This paucity of national data also posed unique challenges, such as population-level research, and planning for SGM populations was almost impossible.

4.3 Social Determinants of Health

According to the World Health Organization (WHO), social determinants of health (SDOH) are the nonmedical factors that influence health outcomes. They are the conditions in which people are born, grow, work, live, and age, and the broader set of forces and systems shaping the conditions of daily life. These forces and systems include economic policies and systems, development agendas, social norms, social policies, and political systems (power and resource distributions).

The SDOH accounts for 80% of health outcomes—SDOH is the most important influencer of health inequities, the unfair and avoidable differences in health status seen within and between communities. Therefore, addressing SDOH is fundamental for improving health and reducing healthcare inequities prevalent among SGM communities. Interventions for SDOH must go beyond the walls of traditional healthcare—these need to happen where people are born, live, work, and play and must consider the resource and power distribution.

5   Components of a Culturally Appropriate Intervention for SGM Intersecting Structural Stigma

Our review of the literature and professional experience with SGM has led us to determine that necessary components for culturally congruent interventions to alleviate the unique chronic stress of SGM populations should include structural-level interventions and clinical interventions.

Structural-level interventions will target laws, policies, and regulations that significantly drive health inequalities among SGM populations. These upstream measures target SDOH that SGM populations are excluded from by structural stigma. Secondly, the clinical-level interventions are culturally congruent interventions by clinical workers at clinical or community setting to reduce barriers to accessing healthcare and improve clinical outcomes for the SGM populations.

6   Interventions for SGM Intersecting Structural Stigma

The interventions for SGM structural stigma capture SDOH because the major drivers of SGM health inequities occur within the context of built environment, laws, policies, and regulations that constrain SGM individuals from fully participating in essential elements of SDOH. In the following sections, we describe ways in which SDOH addresses structural stigma among SGM individuals.

6.1   Civic Engagement

Civic engagement is active participation in societal well-being and advancement. Civic engagement is altruistic—the collective betterment of all members of the society should be the guiding principle of civic engagement. Civic engagement includes helping people register to vote, voting, attending and engaging with town hall meetings, volunteering for local causes, advocating for social or political issues, participating in discussions and debates on matters of public concern, and holding elected officials accountable to campaign platforms. Civic engagement is vital for a healthy democracy. More importantly, civic engagement is quintessential for improving SDOH and structural stigma because it is created, enshrined, and maintained by policies and regulations made by people in positions of power and authority given to them by the people through civic engagement. Civic engagement is intertwined with politics because it affects political outcomes but is more holistic than politics.

Civic engagement plays a significant role in the distribution of resources and decision-making within a society which influences health outcomes—Harold D. Lasswell accentuated the impact of civic engagement in all facets of life with his classic definition of politics as who gets what, when, and how. Hence, public sentiment drives policy, and policy changes everything. This same sentiment has been echoed by research and healthcare professionals in the "voting is healthcare" movement [17, 18]. Data from Democracy Index shows that civically engaged communities have better health outcomes compared to less civically engaged communities.

The intricate connection between structural stigma and SDOH for SGM populations cannot be oversimplified: hence, intervention for structural stigma and SDOH must include modalities to positively influence policy outcomes for SGM populations. Healthcare professionals must go beyond advocacy by participating in the drivers of health inequality—laws, policies, regulations, ordinances, and distribution of resources that excludes some communities (SMG and racial and ethnic minorities [REM]) from elements of SDOH.

6.2   Education

Education is one of the most powerful tools for advancing health equity, addressing SGM structural stigma, and ameliorating the psychological effects of stigma among SGM individuals. Healthcare professionals can educate policymakers about the impact of the laws and regulations they enact. Policymakers will welcome our educated, unbiased opinion—especially when evidence is presented from a humanistic perspective. We can also educate our colleagues on evidence-based practice for SGM. Further, educating and advocating inclusive, atraumatic healthcare systems for SGM individuals at every healthcare entry point is crucial.

Finally, it is important to educate and engage with SGM communities on effective coping mechanisms for structural stigma. A good example is Dr. Bey's research at the University of North Carolina at Chapel Hill on the Inoculation Identity Vitality Pathology (IVP) [19]. She maintains that inoculation of identity is quintessential for moderating the effects of structural inequity-driven chronic stressors on health disparities. Healthcare professionals can educate SGM individuals to inoculate their identity by taking pride in their uniqueness and diverse identity to mitigate the pervasive nature of structural stigma.

6.3   Community Building and Allyship

The longest longitudinal study in the world on adult development is at Harvard: the study shows that quality relationship is the strongest predictor of well-being. Stigma alienates SGM individuals from their community and social bounds. Helping the SGM populations find and build community is critical for well-being. Therefore, interventions for structural stigma must include resources that help SGM individuals safely build and maintain affirming communities. For safety concerns and geographic restrictions, some of these communities might be virtual; see Table 1 for resources.

Table 1 SGM health resources for clinicians. These are clinical resources for referral, education, and point-of-care tools to enable clinicians to provide evidence-based care for SGM individuals

Resources (alphabetical)	Description
CDC SGM Health	SGM health services and clinics by state
Fenway Guide to Lesbian, Gay, Bisexual, and Transgender Health, 2nd ed	An encyclopedia for SGM healthcare
Gay Lesbian Medical Association (GLMA) Provider Directory	Searchable directory of SGM-competent providers
National LGBTQIA+ Health Education Center	Resources for the healthcare system and providers needing evidence-based training for SGM health equity
National Resource Center for LGBT Aging	A collection of guides and programs that aim to improve well-being, education, and healthcare access to SGM older adults and their caregivers/families

7   Clinical-Level Intervention for SGM Intersecting Structural Stigma

The pervasive nature of SGM health inequality demands a sense of urgency, with multifactorial and multisectoral intervention. The clinical-level intervention captures culturally congruent interventions by clinicians and community health workers within the clinical and community setting to advance health equity for SGM populations.

7.1   Referral to SGM-Competent Providers and Community Resources

Discrimination, microaggression, and interpersonal stigma contribute to SGM subpar clinical experience [20–22]. For example, Casey et al. [20] report that 18% of sexual minority and 22% of transgender adults have avoided healthcare because of anticipated stigma and discrimination, while 16% of SGM adults reported discrimination in healthcare encounters. This has led some SGM individuals to avoid or delay clinical care because of anticipation of discrimination and homonegativity [23]. Equally, the anticipation of discrimination and homonegativity triggered similar physiological and psychological effects as the actual event. Overwhelming evidence suggests that the SGM populations wants to be treated by SGM-competent providers. Cultural concordance between clinicians and patients significantly improve patient outcomes. SGM individuals are more likely to adhere to treatment recommendations if they trust the clinician and cultural concordance can enhance trust.

Therefore, referring SGM patients to SGM-competent providers is evidence-based practice. It is imperative for clinicians to know their local SGM resources to enable them to make good referrals. The CDC, Association of Gay and Lesbian Psychiatrists (AGLP), and Health Professionals Advancing LGBTQ+ Equality (GLMA) have a user-friendly clinical director for SGM-competent providers. See Table 1 for more resources. It might be challenging to find SGM competent in rural communities, and this will disproportionately impact health outcomes for REM SGM individuals. Equally, providers and health systems can leverage the educational materials from Fenway Health Institute to become SGM competent (see Table 1).

7.2   Integrative Clinic

Integrated clinics house various specialists under one roof (physically or virtually) like psychiatrists, cardiologists, psychologists, and oncologists. This improves streamlined referrals and efficient interoperability of electronic health records (EHR) between specialists. Integrative clinical models allow patient's different health needs to be addressed in one place.

Due to the high multimorbidity among SGM populations, most will need multiple specialists. However, SGM patients prefer integrative care models—it helps alleviate their anticipated discrimination and stigma. Also, it helps address

other SDOH elements like transportation. Clinicians committed to advancing health equity for the SGM populations should consider creating an integrative clinical model.

7.3   Trauma-Informed Care and Atraumatic SGM Welcoming Clinic

Trauma-informed care for all patients is best practice: especially for patients with significant trauma exposure like SGM individuals with intersecting minoritized identities (REM). Trauma-informed care is an evidence-based approach that recognizes the widespread impact of trauma on patients and aims to provide treatment and services in a way that avoids re-traumatization.

Further, all entry points of healthcare should be welcoming and atraumatic for SGM individuals. Including sexual orientation and gender identity in demographic data collection and employing SGM clinicians and auxiliary staff can communicate SGM belonging and inclusivity. This goes beyond putting a "Safe Zone" sign on the door to tangible and impactful action. Clinicians should leverage SGM individuals' lived experience, because lived experience in and of itself is expertise. Identity affirmation and shared experience are critical to enhancing sense of belonging and inclusivity: SGM individuals being represented among the staff improve affirmation and sense of belonging. Others include artworks, visuals, and pamphlets in the clinic that reflect SGM and REM inclusiveness.

7.4   SGM Culturally Congruent Cognitive Behavioral Therapy

Researchers and clinicians have highlighted the limitations of cognitive behavioral therapy (CBT) for SGM stress and stigma [2, 24, 25]. It does not address the actual chronic minority stress and stigma experienced by minoritized individuals [24]. Pachankis et al. [2] have developed SGM culturally competent CBT to target SGM minority stress and stigma. SGM culturally competent CBT effect was transdiagnostic as there were clinically significant improvements across different psychiatric comorbidities [2].

Hence, it will be quintessential for mental healthcare clinicians to educate themselves on the core tenets of SGM culturally competent CBT. SGM culturally competent CBT holds promise for advancing health equity for this population.

8 Defending Our Humanity

In a country where many towns and cities hold yearly Pride parades, gay marriage is legal, and many SGM films and shows are popular; it can be easy to assume that queer (SGM) people have achieved acceptance by society. But people's lived experiences combined with a great deal of empirical data prove that there is still substantial progress yet to be made for the US SGMs. A conversation between queer health researchers Dr. Agor and Mr. Daici demonstrates the need to continuously shed light on the struggles the SGM community faces, especially given how much things like heterosexism—the individual-, interpersonal-, and structural-level prejudice and discrimination against SGM people under the assumption that being straight is and should be the norm—manifest into poorer health outcomes.

8.1 The SGM Researchers and Their Aspirations

The two principal investigators for the work described in this chapter include Dr. Agor and Mr. Kenny Daici. Dr. Agor is a psychiatric mental health nurse practitioner (PMHNP) from the University of North Carolina (UNC) at Chapel Hill, where he implemented a psychometrics scale to assess multiple minority stress for SGM people of color in the clinical setting. He also researched structural issues that affect the mental health of SGMs and prevent them from accessing

healthcare. Now, as a Ph.D. student at the University of Pennsylvania, he examines policies affecting the clinical use of nutritional psychiatry for the SGM populations. Dr. Agor has been researching SGM health for approximately 5 years, and as he explains, "I want to help create the healthcare system I wish I had, as a Black gay man navigating the healthcare system." He wants to make things better not just for himself but for future generations as well. And as a Nigerian, he understands that SGM struggles and structural issues are often even worse outside of the United States, where SGMs, "especially in places like Africa, don't have the basic rights and access to freedom to be themselves." According to the Human Rights Watch, 33 of the 69 countries that criminalize same-sex relations are in Africa, usually due to laws that originated during colonial rule [26].

Mr. Daici, a premedical rising junior at Brown University from New Jersey, has been a researcher in SGM health for a year and half, and although he hasn't been in the field for as long as Agor, he has similar goals and levels of passion. He asserts that one of his main priorities is to "propel change that makes sexual and gender minorities safer," referring especially to youth, who make up the primary target community of his research. Daici is currently leading a systematic review on gender minority youth mental health disparities through the Columbia School of Nursing while also working with Dr. Agor on his review on mental health interventions for older sexual minorities living with HIV and with other researchers on studying LGBTQ+ cardiovascular health disparities. As a queer child of Romanian immigrants, Daici also understands the importance of advancing queer rights outside the United States, especially since places like Eastern Europe have substantial heterosexism and homonegativity—as polling data from the Pew Research Center suggest, the majority of the people in nearly all Eastern European countries oppose same-sex marriage [27]. Although they conduct research largely with US populations, Dr. Agor and Daici hope the impact of their work reaches all corners of the Earth.

8.2   A Multidisciplinary Approach to SGM Health

Many fields of health research involve relatively well-understood pathologies. For example, most people understand that smoking cigarettes increases the risk of cancer because tobacco products contain carcinogens that make DNA mutations more likely. However, what about the association between being an SGM and developing cardiovascular disease? As Daici explains, when "working with social data, it's not an immediately intuitive link." This is because having a stigmatized social identity often manifests as disease through a complex chain of events that begin at the societal level and eventually trickle down to the biological. Being an SGM increases the chance someone will experience life stressors like heterosexist prejudice, legal restrictions, and internalized stigma. This predisposes them to developing mental health conditions, health-harming behaviors such as drug use, and physiological changes like inflammation and decreased immune function, which can all collectively and independently eventually manifest into obesity, insulin resistance, and cancer (Fig. 1). The model includes the concept of allostatic load, which states that when someone is exposed to more stressors than they can cope with, the body's stress response becomes overactivated, leading to a shift in the body's physiological state (blood pressure, hormone levels, etc.) that is only exaggerated by other, more macro-level effects of stress, like low-quality sleep, poor diet, and drug use [28].

But of course, it's not having the identity itself that attracts poor health. "SGM is an identity, not a pathology," Dr. Agor explains. "It is what society is doing to the individual." The fact that SGM health is affected by such a diverse array of factors reflects its multidisciplinary nature and further illustrates that SGMs are often victims of the environment they are exposed to.

8.3   Challenges of Researching SGMs

Although conducting research with SGM populations is crucial to advancing their well-being, it is certainly not without setbacks. "I think everything makes it hard," says Dr. Agor. For one, there is a substantial gap in the availability of SGM data, primarily because many surveys and inventories do not ask questions pertaining to people's sexual and gender identities. Or, if they do ask these questions, they are very recent additions. This includes the US government's Census Bureau, which only started tracking SGM identities in 2021 with its Household Pulse Survey. Of course, it's a step in the right direction, but the data being very recent creates gaps in the data for anything prior to 2021 [29]. And there are still surveys like the American Community Survey (ACS) that still largely omit LGBTQ-related questions [30]. In the ACS, the only SGM data collected is whether a household is same-sex or different-sex based on cohabitation, which means that any sexual minority who doesn't live with a same-sex partner (youth, single SGMs, etc.) is ignored. "The fact that we do not ask these [SGM] questions, and that we do not have data in and of itself, is structural stigma, to erase an entire community by omission," Dr. Agor explains. This sentiment was also echoed by the seminal work from the National Academies of Sciences, Engineering, and Medicine *Understanding the Well-Being of LGBTQI+ Populations* (2020)—they maintained the need for population-level data, especially for subpopulation such as intersex, where almost no empirical data exist for them.

Even when a survey asks SGM-related questions, new problems arise. "It's a very new field of research," says Daici, which is exemplified by just how few SGM studies there are, and how narrow their focuses tend to be. In 2014, there were only 628 studies concerning SGM health funded by the National Institutes of Health (NIH), thus perpetuating SGM health inequities due to a lack of related research [31]. Of them 79.1% focused on HIV/AIDS; of course, studying HIV/AIDS is important, but the SGM populations experiences a vast array of health disparities that transcends stigmatizing STIs, such as in mental health, cardiovascular issues, metabolic syndrome, and cancer. SGM research is expanding in both depth and breadth, but there are still systemic barriers. The National Institute of Nursing Research (NINR), for example, has only funded 25 studies regarding SGM health from 1987 to 2018, a clear symptom of structural stigma [32].

8.3.1 Initial Steps to Develop Culturally Appropriate Measures to Evaluate SGM Culturally Congruent Interventions

How often is the data collected even reliable? According to a study conducted at Yale University, 83.0% of SGM individuals around the world conceal their sexual orientation from all or most people [33]. Societal stigma prevents many SGMs from answering truthfully about their sexual and gender identities even in confidential surveys, which "makes it a little bit challenging for what we know and what we can extrapolate about this [SGM] populations," says Dr. Agor. When SGM data only includes those who are confident and desensitized enough to disclose their personal identities, there are bound to be inaccuracies, particularly underestimation, in epidemiological information. For example, a survey seeking to quantify SGM mental health disparities may not depict the full picture since those who do not disclose their SGM identity may be more likely to be affected by stigma and heterosexism, and homonegativity, which predisposes them to health inequality prevalent among SGM populations.

SGM research is not easy on the researchers either since most of them are members of the SGM community themselves. "There can be burnout that comes with studying all these heavy topics that are about you," says Daici. "A lot of the time, I'll be reading about depression rates among SGMs, and it'll stress me out. And then I'll be thinking about any problems I have related to my queer identity, and it's a very easy hole to fall into." For queer researchers, it is very easy for the work they do to become very personal. It is often mentally taxing for them to read about the disparities, discrimination, and prejudice that they or their fellow friends in the SGM community struggle with.

Dr. Agor had a similar experience when examining psychometrics for suicidal ideation among SGMs at UNC at Chapel Hill. As one of the few people that did SGM work in the School of Nursing, it was easy for him to feel isolated without a solid community to use as an outlet for his stress. "Seeing myself in the data was really emotionally evoking," he explains. "So, I pulled myself back because I did not have the mental capacity and resources to continue to deal with this data on a daily basis."

But despite these personal struggles, it is crucial that members of the SGM community continue to make up the majority of SGM researchers. Daici expresses this sentiment, arguing that it would not be better for cisgender and heterosexual people to conduct this research, research that is not about them. "We understand the nuances of the experiences of being queer. It's not entirely our burden to do it, but if the research is going to be done properly, it will probably be done by a queer person," he says. It's a tough situation, one that often leads to SGM researchers being worked beyond their mental and emotional capacity, thus potentially decreasing productivity and retention in the field. But still, as Dr. Agor says, "nothing about us without us."

With all of these challenges that SGM researchers face, either on a systemic or personal level, it makes sense that SGM research is limited compared to other fields that don't deal with stigmatized identities. But this field isn't just grim and hopeless.

8.3.2 Rewards of Researching SGM

Aside from the many setbacks SGM researchers face, there are many benefits that come with working in this field. While the SGM research field may be small, this also creates a tight-knit and well-connected community of scholars who are all united with the common goal of improving the well-being of SGMs.

Both Dr. Agor and Mr. Daici are lucky to be involved with institutions with relatively large SGM research communities. Dr. Agor has just started his Ph.D. program at the University of Pennsylvania, where there is an entire floor dedicated to SGM work. "And we can support each other," Dr. Agor says, "whether it's [help with] research or emotional support, because those really count, especially when you need it most." This ecosystem of SGM researchers alleviates the burden that comes with working in a field that often brings personal stress since they can count on each other for support.

Even though Mr. Daici's research at Columbia University is virtual, he has experienced a similar level of support to Dr. Agor. "I've formed ties with people on the team," says Daici. "We talk about research, our lives, and it's a very nice community." Aside from the burden SGM researchers often experience, it can also be isolating being an SGM in general. Spaces such as SGM research centers thus serve as a comforting space for SGM researchers to relieve stress that comes not just from their emotionally taxing work but also from their emotionally taxing lives as SGMs in a society where SGMs are not always accepted. "You need a space where you don't have to debate your humanity. And I think people don't understand how exhausting it is to have to defend your humanity," says Dr. Agor, referring to the heterosexist prejudice that is too common in society. "I deserve to be my unique self."

The web of SGM researchers extends across institutions, something that only bolsters the SGM community and multiplies its stress-relieving benefits. After Mr. Daici mentions Dr. Billy Caceres, his research mentor at the Columbia School of Nursing, Dr. Agor can't help but grin. "I'm smiling because we actually met through Billy," he says. "Once you get plugged into that ecosystem, we support each other."

This network can be especially helpful for those who are not used to seeing fellow SGMs working successfully in prestigious academic or professional positions. When Dr. Daici first discovered Dr. Caceres' research in February 2022, he was amazed because of how many publications he had and how long he had been working in the field of SGM health. "He was such a decorated researcher," Daici says, amazed at the idea of an SGM like him surpassing all societal hurdles and succeeding in such a stigmatized field. "And he was so welcoming, so friendly," he says, smiling.

Ultimately, though, SGM researchers chose to study SGMs not just for themselves but also for all members of the community who truly need help, those who are the living humans behind the health disparity statistics. "I think of people that I know that have gone through similar experiences," says Daici, referring to the SGM challenges and health disparities he regularly reads about through his research. "The more exposure we get on these problems, the more interventions are going to be done to fix them." A rising tide lifts all boats, and improving SGM health will ultimately improve health outcomes for all. Dr. Agor shares the same sentiment. "It's worth it at the end of the day."

9 The Present and Future of SGM Health

Of course, SGM health has been and will continue to be a complex field that is shaped by a wide range of sociocultural factors and marked by many disparities that leave SGMs at a disadvantage. Even in 2023, there are still systemic issues that make acceptance of SGMs around the country more difficult. For example, the Don't Say Gay bill, passed in Florida in 2022, prohibits instruction on sexual and gender identity in schools before fourth grade and requires "age-appropriate" instruction of such topics for older ages.

But despite these setbacks, SGM health is making great progress in various areas. For example, according to Healthy People 2030, a list of national objectives to improve health and well-being over the next decade, there have been notable decreases in the bullying of sexual minority high school students, the number of new HIV cases, and the syphilis rate in men who have sex with men [34]. Although there is still substantial progress yet to be made in fields like mental health and illicit substance abuse, these changes should inspire hope for anyone who cares about SGM well-being. There have also been strides in the political and public opinion on SGM topics. In 2015, same-sex marriage was deemed a constitutional right through the Supreme Court case

Obergefell v. *Hodges*. And according to a Gallup poll, the American public has become increasingly supportive of most areas of SGM rights over time, especially marriage, with 71% of Americans believing that same-sex marriage should be legal in May 2023 compared to 59% in May 2013. A reflection of this increased acceptance is the expansion of SGM sensitivity courses and training for medical students and medical professionals, which allows for better treatment of SGM individuals in healthcare contexts [35]. Since a substantial cause of poor SGM health is the physiological manifestations of minority stress, changes like these that remove legal limitations, reduce stigma, and expand education inclusivity have been crucial to helping the realm of SGM health.

And with a growing nationwide network of SGMs and allied individuals that fight for SGM inclusion, equity, and well-being, SGM health will hopefully only improve over time. Aside from the aforementioned trends that show improvements across several health components for SGMs, there are many resources and interventions in place (listed in Tables 1 and 2) that will only accelerate progress. SGM individuals and clinicians alike are encouraged to utilize these resources so as to alleviate the stress and health effects that homonegative stigma has plagued the SGM community with. Only with increased inclusion and acceptance at all levels of society, from the government to the individual, can there be hope for SGM health disparities to disappear and for SGMs to finally stop needing to defend their humanity.

Table 2 Health resources for SGM individuals. These are clinical resources for SGM individuals to help effectively navigate healthcare and improve their health outcomes

Resources (alphabetical)	Description
BIENESTAR	A Los Angeles-based Latinx SGM health organization that increases access to medical care, HIV prevention and treatment, substance abuse management, sexual healthcare, and mental healthcare
Callen-Lorde	A New York City-based SGM community health center that provides primary care, sexual health services, and community outreach and prevention programs
Equality Federation	An advocacy organization that promotes SGM rights and healthcare access through policy work and social justice, on top of providing an up-to-date US SGM legislation tracker
Genders and Sexualities Alliances (GSAs)	School-based organizations that aim to build community among SGMs and allied youth and create a space where people feel safe and empowered to inspire social change
GLSEN	A network of educators that promotes SGM inclusion and well-being in K–12 schools
Human Rights Campaign (HRC)	An advocacy organization that promotes pro-SGM policies, empowers SGM to participate politically, and provides a host of programs that increase access to SGM education and health resources, two of which are highlighted below
HRC: HBCU Health Center Directory	Directory of sexual health services, particularly HIV testing, at historically Black colleges and universities
HRC: Long-Term Care Equality Index	An assessment tool for SGM inclusion in long-term care and elder housing communities that also provides resources for how to best provide culturally competent care to SGM older people
Lambda Legal	A law group dedicated to representing SGMs and people living with HIV in the court of law, dealing with issues in employment, healthcare, and family protection
LGBT HealthLink	A hub for health resources and community health centers that focus specifically on improving access to quality, inclusive care to SGMs
National Center for Transgender Equality	Provides resources for transgender people to access health
National Resource Center for LGBT Aging	A collection of guides and programs that aim to improve well-being, education, and healthcare access to SGM older adults and their caregivers/families

Table 2 (continued)

Resources (alphabetical)	Description
OutCare	Has a database of SGM healthcare providers, educates and trains people on SGM topics and issues, and provides healthcare materials to ensure SGMs receive quality care
PFLAG—Securing LGBTQ+ Health	A list of resources that help with SGM health issues, including anti-conversion therapy efforts and HIV/AIDS treatment and prevention
The Trevor Project	Youth-centric SGM resource hub: resources for mental health, suicide prevention, phone, and chat services
TRACE	An app created by and for trans people: to support and affirm them
You:Flourish	An app working to distribute wellness and affirming mental health resources to SGM people

References

1. He Y, Dangerfield Ii DT, Fields EL, Dawkins MR, Turpin RE, Johnson D, Browne DC, Hickson DA. Health care access, health care utilisation and sexual orientation disclosure among black sexual minority men in the deep south. Sex Health. 2020;17(5):421–8. https://doi.org/10.1071/SH20051.

2. Pachankis JE, McConocha EM, Reynolds JS, Winston R, Adeyinka O, Harkness A, Burton CL, Behari K, Sullivan TJ, Eldahan AI, Esserman DA, Hatzenbuehler ML, Safren SA. Project ESTEEM protocol: a randomized controlled trial of an LGBTQ-affirmative treatment for young adult sexual minority men's mental and sexual health. BMC Public Health. 2019;19(1):1086. https://doi.org/10.1186/s12889-019-7346-4.

3. HIV incidence | HIV in the US | HIV Statistics Center | HIV | CDC. n.d. https://www.cdc.gov/hiv/statistics/overview/in-us/incidence.html. Accessed 28 July 2023.

4. 2016 CROI Press release: lifetime HIV risk | CDC. n.d. https://www.cdc.gov/nchhstp/newsroom/2016/croi-press-release-risk.html. Accessed 15 Apr 2021.

5. English D, Smith JC, Scott-Walker L, Lopez FG, Morris M, Reid M, Lashay C, Bridges D, McNeish D. Feasibility, acceptability, and preliminary HIV care and psychological health effects of iTHRIVE 365 for black same gender loving men. J Acquir Immune Defic Syndr. 2023;93(1):55–63. https://doi.org/10.1097/QAI.0000000000003167.

6. Meyer IH. Prejudice, social stress, and mental health in lesbian, gay, and bisexual populations: conceptual issues and research evidence. Psychol Bull. 2003;129(5):674–97. https://doi.org/10.1037/0033-2909.129.5.674.

7. Sue DW, Capodilupo CM, Torino GC, Bucceri JM, Holder AMB, Nadal KL, Esquilin M. Racial microaggressions in everyday life: implications for clinical practice. Am Psychol. 2007;62(4):271–86. https://doi.org/10.1037/0003-066X.62.4.271.

8. Lawrence JA, Kawachi I, White K, Bassett MT, Priest N, Masunga JG, Cory HJ, Mita C, Williams DR. A systematic review and meta-analysis of the everyday discrimination scale and biomarker outcomes. Psychoneuroendocrinology. 2022;142:105772. https://doi.org/10.1016/j.psyneuen.2022.105772.

9. Hatzenbuehler ML. Structural stigma: research evidence and implications for psychological science. Am Psychol. 2016;71(8):742–51. https://doi.org/10.1037/amp0000068.

10. Link B, Hatzenbuehler ML. Stigma as an unrecognized determinant of population health: research and policy implications. J Health Polit Policy Law. 2016;41(4):653–73. https://doi.org/10.1215/03616878-3620869.

11. Agor DC. Nutritional psychiatry: transdiagnostic treatment model to provide a holistic care for gender and sexual minority youths. International society of psychiatric-mental health nursing 2022 annual conference. 2022.

12. Johnson MJ, Nemeth LS, Mueller M, Eliason MJ, Stuart GW. Qualitative study of cervical cancer screening among lesbian and bisexual women and transgender men. Cancer Nurs. 2016;39(6):455–63. https://doi.org/10.1097/NCC.0000000000000338.

13. Hatzenbuehler ML. Structural stigma and the health of lesbian, gay, and bisexual populations. Curr Dir Psychol Sci. 2014;23(2):127–32. https://doi.org/10.1177/0963721414523775.

14. Livingston JD, Milne T, Fang ML, Amari E. The effectiveness of interventions for reducing stigma related to substance use disorders: a systematic review. Addiction. 2012;107(1):39–50. https://doi.org/10.1111/j.1360-0443.2011.03601.x.

15. Manzer D, O'Sullivan LF, Doucet S. Myths, misunderstandings, and missing information: experiences of nurse practitioners providing primary care to lesbian, gay, bisexual, and transgender patients. Can J Hum Sex. 2018;27(2):157–70. https://doi.org/10.3138/cjhs.2018-0017.

16. Jackman KB, Bosse JD, Eliason MJ, Hughes TL. Sexual and gender minority health research in nursing. Nurs Outlook. 2019;67(1):21–38. https://doi.org/10.1016/j.outlook.2018.10.006.

17. National Academies of Sciences, Engineering, and Medicine; Division of Behavioral and Social Sciences and Education; Committee on Population; Committee on Understanding the Well-Being of Sexual and Gender Diverse Populations. In: White J, Sepúlveda MJ, Patterson CJ, editors. Understanding the well-

being of LGBTQI+ populations. National Academies Press (US); 2020. https://doi.org/10.17226/25877.

18. Brown CL, Raza D, Pinto AD. Voting, health and interventions in healthcare settings: a scoping review. Public Health Rev. 2020;41:16. https://doi.org/10.1186/s40985-020-00133-6.

19. Bey GS. The identity vitality-pathology model: a novel theoretical framework proposing "identity state" as a modulator of the pathways from structural to health inequity. Soc Sci Med. 2022;314:115495. https://doi.org/10.1016/j.socscimed.2022.115495.

20. Casey LS, Reisner SL, Findling MG, Blendon RJ, Benson JM, Sayde JM, Miller C. Discrimination in the United States: experiences of lesbian, gay, bisexual, transgender, and queer Americans. Health Serv Res. 2019;54 Suppl 2(Suppl 2):1454–66. https://doi.org/10.1111/1475-6773.13229.

21. Joudeh L, Harris OO, Johnstone E, Heavner-Sullivan S, Propst SK. "Little red flags": barriers to accessing health care as a sexual or gender minority individual in the rural southern United States—a qualitative intersectional approach. J Assoc Nurses AIDS Care. 2021;32(4):467–80. https://doi.org/10.1097/JNC.0000000000000271.

22. Quinn K, Dickson-Gomez J, Zarwell M, Pearson B, Lewis M. "A gay man and a doctor are just like, a recipe for destruction": how racism and homonegativity in healthcare settings influence PrEP uptake among young black MSM. AIDS Behav. 2019;23(7):1951–63. https://doi.org/10.1007/s10461-018-2375-z.

23. Casey EA, Lindhorst TP. Toward a multi-level, ecological approach to the primary prevention of sexual assault: prevention in peer and community contexts. Trauma Violence Abuse. 2009;10(2):91–114. https://doi.org/10.1177/1524838009334129.

24. Hays PA, Iwamasa GY, editors. Culturally responsive cognitive-behavioral therapy: assessment, practice, and supervision. American Psychological Association; 2006. https://doi.org/10.1037/11433-000.

25. Livingston NA, Berke D, Scholl J, Ruben M, Shipherd JC. Addressing diversity in PTSD treatment: clinical considerations and guidance for the treatment of PTSD in LGBTQ populations. Curr Treat Options Psychiatry. 2020;7:53. https://doi.org/10.1007/s40501-020-00204-0.

26. Reid G. Progress and setbacks on LGBT rights in Africa—an overview of the last year. Human Rights Watch. 2022. https://www.hrw.org/news/2022/06/22/progress-and-setbacks-lgbt-rights-africa-overview-last-year.

27. Poushter J, Kent N. The global divide on homosexuality persists. Pew Research Center's Global Attitudes Project. 2020. https://www.pewresearch.org/global/2020/06/25/global-divide-on-homosexuality-persists/.

28. Guidi J, Lucente M, Sonino N, Fava GA. Allostatic load and its impact on health: a systematic review. Psychother Psychosom. 2020;90(1):11–27. https://doi.org/10.1159/000510696.

29. File T, Lee JH. Phase 3.2 of Census Bureau survey questions now include Sogi, child tax credit, Covid vaccination of children. 2022. Census.gov. https://www.census.gov/library/stories/2021/08/household-pulse-survey-updates-sex-question-now-asks-sexual-orientation-and-gender-identity.html.

30. Deng B, Watson T. LGBTQ+ data availability. Brookings. 2023. https://www.brookings.edu/articles/lgbtq-data-availability-what-we-can-learn-from-four-major-surveys/.

31. Coulter RWS, Kenst KS, Bowen DJ, Scout. Research funded by the National Institutes of Health on the health of lesbian, gay, bisexual, and transgender populations. Am J Public Health. 2014;104(2):e105. https://doi.org/10.2105/ajph.2013.301501.

32. Bosse JD, Jackman KB, Hughes TL. NINR funding dedicated to sexual and gender minority health: 1987–2018. Nurs Outlook. 2020;68(3):293–300. https://doi.org/10.1016/j.outlook.2020.01.002.

33. Pachankis JE, Bränström R. How many sexual minorities are hidden? Projecting the size of the global closet with implications for policy and public health. PLoS One. 2019;14(6):e0218084. https://doi.org/10.1371/journal.pone.0218084.

34. Office of Disease Prevention and Health Promotion. LGBT—Healthy People 2030. LGBT. 2020. https://health.gov/healthypeople/objectives-and-data/browse-objectives/lgbt.

35. Dwilson SD. LGBTQ health care: a look at the present and future. Dignity Health. 2018. https://www.dignityhealth.org/articles/lgbtq-health-care-a-look-at-the-present-and-future.

Kenneth Daici As a queer person himself, a researcher focused on the health of sexual and gender minorities (SGM), and a junior at the Brown University, Kenny Daici understands the effects of societal and individual-level stigma all too well. Much of his research focuses on identifying and analyzing SGM health disparities, particularly in mental health and cardiovascular disease. Although, with substantial undergraduate coursework in the social determinants of health under his belt, he is interested in the way all types of social factors affect health, especially for disadvantaged populations. Kenny's parents are immigrants of Romania.

Part IIIa

Physical Environment

The part of the human environment that includes purely physical factors that contribute to health inequities and health disparities.

Community-Engaged Research with Agricultural Workers in Florida: Health and Climate Change

Roxana C. Chicas ⓘ, Jasmine Irish ⓘ,
Nezahualcoyotl Xiuhtecutli ⓘ,
and Abby D. Mutic ⓘ

1 Agricultural Workers in Florida: Health and Climate Change

An estimated two to three million agricultural workers in the United States (USA) [1] are exposed to an average summertime heat index of 94.7 °F [2]. An annual 702 deaths in the USA alone resulted from heat-related events between 2004 and 2018 [3]. Latino communities are disproportionally impacted by climate change because they not only live in states on the front lines of climate change but also work in outdoor industries that expose them to harsh environmental elements. Over two decades of data from the US Census of Fatal Occupational Injuries supports that Latino workers are at a significantly increased risk of heat-related death [4]. Agricultural workers, who are primarily Latino, have more than 35 times the risk of heat-related death than other occupational groups [5].

R. C. Chicas (✉) · J. Irish · A. D. Mutic
Nell Hodgson Woodruff School of Nursing,
Atlanta, GA, USA
e-mail: rchicas@emory.edu;
jasmine.irish@emory.edu; abby.mutic@emory.edu

N. Xiuhtecutli
Farmworker Association of Florida,
Apopka, FL, USA
e-mail: Neza@floridafarmworkers.org

Florida has the third highest Latino population in the USA and more than 100,000 agricultural workers, the majority of whom are Latino immigrants. Florida is also one of the top five states to experience increasingly destructive weather events fueled by climate change. Heat waves are projected to increase in frequency, intensity, and duration [6]. Specifically, the average heat index in Florida is projected to rise from 103.6 to 112.7 °F as a result of severe climate change [2].

In addition to environmental factors, agricultural communities face other social determinants of health that contribute to a disproportionate burden of heat-related illness (HRI) [7]. In general, agricultural workers face several social factors that make for precarious working conditions such as low wages, low levels of education and health literacy, and uncertain immigration status. Many agricultural workers labor in conditions where verbal, physical, or sexual abuse occurs. However, little reporting of such conditions occurs due to fear of retaliation, job loss, or deportation. This fear extends to US citizen agricultural workers who have likewise reported stress when speaking with immigration officials [8]. Accessing health care is a challenge for many workers due to a lack of health insurance, language barriers, and distrust in the US healthcare system. Underpinning these cultural, social, and environmental factors are policy determinants that continue to produce inequities and disadvantages. Agricultural workers are specifically excluded from protections to organize and form unions by the National Labor Relations Act (NRLA) of 1935. The Fair Labor Standards Act (FLSA) of 1938 denies agricultural workers the benefits of a minimum hourly wage, mandatory overtime pay, and child labor protections. Some states such as California, New York, and Washington have passed legislation allowing for agricultural workers to organize; however, no federal laws have been amended. Furthermore, federal heat protection standards are also lacking for outdoor workers. Immigration policies or immigration reform are essentially nonexistent for the largely undocumented agricultural workforce. The combination of these determinants of health highlights the extreme risk these workers face from the effects of climate change on health and well-being. The associated health implications call for urgent action on climate mitigation and adaptation, including raising awareness of climate-sensitive health risks and prioritizing agricultural workers through community-engaged research, community outreach, and advocacy.

2   Agricultural Worker Health and Climate Change

A meta-analysis of heat strain that included diverse populations, exposures, and occupations found a 15% incidence of acute kidney injury (AKI) or kidney diseases among those who work in high ambient temperatures for a minimum of 6 h per day, 5 days per week, for 2 months of the year [9]. Specific studies in the USA have shown an association between AKI and strenuous work in high ambient temperatures among agricultural workers [10–19]. A study of impaired renal function of US agricultural workers in California's Central Valley found that 11.8% had pre- to post-work shift increases in serum creatinine of at least 0.3 mg/dL or 1.5 times the pre-shift value (Kidney Disease: Improving Global Outcomes [KDIGO] criteria [20] for AKI [17]).

Our research in Florida determined that approximately 53% of 192 agricultural workers began their workday dehydrated (urine specific gravity ≥1.020) while 81% finished the workday dehydrated. On at least one of three workdays evaluated, 33% of workers developed AKI, and the odds of AKI increased 47% for each 5 °F increase in the heat index [15]. Piece-rate workers had higher workload intensity than hourly workers, spending nearly 2.5–4 h in moderate to vigorous activity per workday [21]. Our ongoing longitudinal Occupational Heat Exposure and Renal Dysfunction (OHEaRD) study estimates the prevalence of AKI in fernery workers with piece-rate compensation has increased from 10% in 2020 to 43% in 2022. In comparison, the rate of AKI in non-piece-rate workers remained unchanged at 10% from 2020 to 2022 indicating that piece-rate agricultural workers may be at higher risk for AKI due to their workload intensity.

AKI is a risk factor for chronic kidney disease and end-stage renal disease (ESRD). Two studies have reported "hot spots" of unexplained ESRD in agricultural areas in the USA [22, 23]. Chronic kidney disease in agricultural workers is a prevailing reason for weakening physical health, resulting in workplace absenteeism and reduced work output [24]. The $45 billion dollar US agricultural industry and its two to three million person labor force are in imminent danger of severe economic loss and poor health due to climate change and heat-related kidney dysfunction.

3   The Farmworker Community

The *Farmworker Association of Florida* (*FWAF*), founded in 1983 and incorporated in 1986, is a statewide, grassroots membership organization of more than 10,000 agricultural worker families in Florida from predominantly Mexican, Haitian, African American, Guatemalan, Honduran, and Salvadoran communities. FWAF's goal is to empower agricultural workers to respond to and gain control over social, political, economic, workplace, health, and environmental justice issues that affect their well-being. With five offices in the state, FWAF's work covers 15 counties. Since the early 1990s, FWAF has addressed pesticide exposure, field sanitation, and other health and safety issues by educating agricultural workers about their rights and securing the passage of Florida's Right-to-Know law to protect agricultural workers. FWAF helps its members file complaints for workplace safety violations, advocates for better enforcement of workplace safety, and participates as a research partner in farmworker health studies.

FWAF has collaborated with the Nell Hodgson Woodruff School of Nursing at Emory University since 2010 on community-engaged studies investigating the health effects of workplace exposures such as pesticides and heat. Initially, the collaboration started with survey research and has progressed to biomedical research to better understand, prevent, and treat health conditions experienced by agricultural workers. While the Hispanic population is widely underrepresented in biomedical research, FWAF has been instrumental in the establishment of a respectful and ongoing research program that is centered on agricultural health. The academic community partnership with FWAF codevelops research designs, crafts socially acceptable data collection methods to conduct the research in marginalized communities, and is critical for successful recruiting. This community-engaged research process has led to a strong long-term partnership between university researchers and community members that developed a comprehensive educational intervention for workers, supervisors, and healthcare providers on the hazards of heat exposure.

Our research program focuses on five communities that employ workers at various types of agricultural operations in Florida. Below, the communities are listed with their respective agricultural industries.

- Homestead (Miami-Dade County): mango and tomato harvests
- Fellsmere (Indian River County): melon, citrus, and watercress harvests
- Apopka (Orange County): nursery work, cucumber, and chili peppers
- Pierson (Volusia County): fernery work
- Immokalee (Collier County): tomato, squash, and zucchini harvests

Agricultural workers frequently move from one field to another depending on the agricultural abundance and growing season. Many work for multiple contractors or employers within an area to accumulate additional work hours and wages. Agricultural workers may have dangerous working conditions where they fear being fired by their employers as retaliation for participating in occupational research. These factors make it challenging to conduct research through partnerships with employers or in their workplace environment. However, over time, the FWAF has built a strong relationship with the community and their families by ensuring participant anonymity in research. Study visits are conducted outside of the workplace in a safe location. FWAF *promotoras* (community health workers) recruit agricultural workers in the five communities listed above. Participants are recruited through an FWAF-maintained roster of agricultural workers in their service area via telephone and home visits and during community outreach events.

4 Dissemination of Health Information to the Community

We believe it is imperative to provide research participants with the health information collected during the study. Therefore, we implement a research-to-practice (r2p) approach to disseminate findings to agricultural workers, healthcare providers, agricultural worker advocacy groups, and the agricultural industry. For each agricultural community studied, we develop graphics to translate aggregate findings and share them with community members during outreach events. These graphics are part of a corpus of training that is meant to raise awareness about the dangers of heat stress and ways to prevent illness for agricultural workers and their supervisors. Additionally, through a pedagogical approach that encourages storytelling, the training creates a setting where agricultural workers feel comfortable sharing their own stories of heat exposure with their coworkers. This storytelling and discussion setting allows workers to consciously process their lived experiences for the storage of positive memories. We have also created short videos tailored to general outdoor workers about the signs and symptoms of HRI and recommendations to prevent long-term health consequences. The short videos are disseminated via FWAF's social media channels, website, and organization newsletters and during community educational events and outreach.

We recognize the importance of including agricultural business owners and growers in the dissemination plan to increase their awareness of HRI and encourage their involvement in advocating for workplace safety and agricultural worker health. To that end, we are creating content specifically for agricultural employers and extension workers to promote renal health via our partnership with the Southeastern Coastal Center for Agricultural Health and Safety (SCCAHS) of the University of Florida.

Heat-related illness is the leading cause of climate-related death and is more prevalent due to the climate crisis. Healthcare education must be a key component in all primary care wellness visits. Healthcare providers are well equipped to identify individual risk factors and assess for heat-related sensitivities, and most importantly, they can provide individualized guidance to patients regarding their health and safety. We have created free web-based professional development modules to share our research findings on the Emory Nursing Experience learning platform for clinicians and community health workers to access at their convenience.

5 Community-Engaged Research on Heat and the Health of Agricultural Workers

We began to study how heat affects the health of agricultural workers after initial focus groups with agricultural workers identified heat exposure as a primary concern. Since that time, the community has continued to direct our research focus by asking questions and participating in the research (see Fig. 1). Each of the studies is

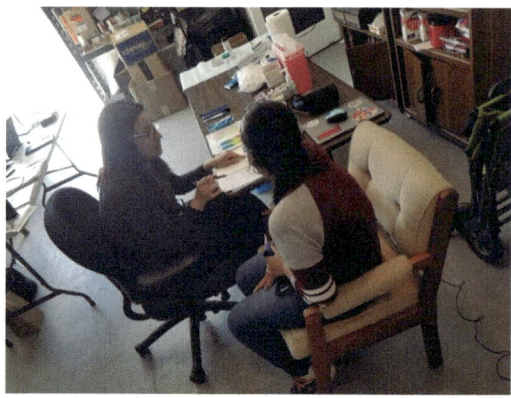

Fig. 1 A registered nurse provides results of point-of-care testing to an agricultural worker in Pierson, Florida

designed in collaboration with the FWAF to conduct research that is linguistically and culturally appropriate. We aim to minimize the research participant burden and collectively work to remove any barriers that may prevent workers from participating. More importantly, the continual feedback and improvements that FWAF provides ensure that our research is grounded in the realities of agricultural labor and centered on improving their health and well-being.

One example of incorporating FWAF feedback stemmed from a community member's request to include point-of-care testing that provides participants with a snapshot of their current health status. Therefore, a study nurse now provides each participant with his/her results that are immediately resulted, i.e., body mass index, blood pressure, urine specific gravity to assess hydration status, HbA1C, lipid panel, and measurements from the iSTAT® Blood Analyzer that include hemoglobin, sodium, potassium, blood urea nitrogen, glucose, and creatinine levels. Interpreting and communicating these results allows us the opportunity to engage participants in onsite health education at the conclusion of their individual study visits and refer them to additional health services as needed. This immediate wellness report serves to:

- Bring health equity to a marginalized, medically underserved population experiencing precarious working conditions

- Respond to the communities' requests to gain knowledge of their health status
- Improve the well-being of agricultural workers in the USA by encouraging agency and self-awareness
- Develop training that informs workers on how they can improve their health and better protect themselves against the dangers of heat stress
- Continue to build and strengthen the relationship between Emory University, FWAF, and its members
- Increase FWAF's outreach to more isolated communities, building the capacity and accessibility of FWAF's programming
- Increase FWAF's political efforts by motivating workers to bring greater attention to the dangers of heat stress

To date, we have provided individual results to over 500 agricultural workers participating in our Florida research program. FWAF has been an invaluable partner and advisor as we have gained the trust of agricultural communities and continue to advocate for safer workplace standards.

6   Reflections and Future Plans

The goal of our research program is to improve the working conditions of agricultural workers that perpetually tend to fields and nurseries in increasingly undesirable environments at the expense of their health. We actively use our research findings to inform legislation and have contributed to the newly proposed Occupational Health and Safety Administration (OSHA) heat stress standard (OSHA's Advance Notice of Proposed Rulemaking on Heat Injury and Illness Prevention in Outdoor and Indoor Work Settings; Docket No. OSHA-2021-0009). We will continue to work closely with FWAF and its membership to better understand the burden of HRI and kidney dysfunction among agricultural workers and explore innovative strategies to mitigate the burden. We are well-poised to build on our past findings through our existing partnerships and research infrastructure. We plan to devise

workplace interventions that protect the long-term health of agricultural workers and inform policy to advance environmental justice.

There has been an increasing national trend by the agricultural industry to hire more H-2A guest workers. Increasing the number of H-2A workers creates more workforce vulnerability because these workers rely largely on their employers to provide housing, transportation, and access to food. FWAF has more difficulty reaching H-2A workers given their limited autonomy and thus, the workers are deprived of FWAF resources. One solution to this challenge is for the Emory research team and FWAF to work more directly with employers to raise their awareness of heat stress and the need for standard worker protections. This arrangement in turn may present additional challenges if employers choose to downplay their role in implementing protections out of economic or efficiency concerns.

Political instability in places such as Venezuela has brought an influx of new immigrants to Florida entering the agricultural industry. The increased presence of Venezuelan immigrants has brought a more educated and diverse agricultural workforce to Florida, who have urban-related experience in the meat and produce packing industry and who confidently advocate for workers' rights. FWAF and Emory have been working on strategies to build solidarity between packing and field workers to support one another and reach out to transient H-2A workers.

To conclude, FWAF and Emory will continue conducting community-engaged research that informs policies to advance environmental justice for agricultural works and other outdoor workers exposed to rising temperatures due to climate change.

References

1. NIOSH. Agricultural safety. 2022. https://www.cdc.gov/niosh/topics/aginjury/default.html. Accessed 11 Sept 2022.
2. Tigchelaar M, Battisti DS, Spector JT. Work adaptations insufficient to address growing heat risk for U.S. agricultural workers. Environ Res Lett. 2020;15(9):094035.

3. Vaidyanathan A, Malilay J, Schramm P, Saha S. Heat-related deaths—United States, 2004–2018. MMWR Morb Mortal Wkly Rep. 2020;69(24):729–34.

4. Dong XS, West GH, Holloway-Beth A, Wang X, Sokas RK. Heat-related deaths among construction workers in the United States. Am J Ind Med. 2019;62(12):1047–57.

5. Gubernot DM, Anderson GB, Hunting KL. Characterizing occupational heat-related mortality in the United States, 2000–2010: an analysis using the Census of Fatal Occupational Injuries database. Am J Ind Med. 2015;58(2):203–11.

6. Dahl K, Spanger-Siegfried E, Licker R, Caldas A, Abatzoglou J, Mailloux N, Cleetus R, Udvardy S, Declet-Barreto J, Worth P. Killer heat in the United States: climate choices and the future of dangerously hot days. Union of Concerned Scientists; 2019. https://www.ucsusa.org/resources/killer-heat-united-states-0.

7. Mutic AD, Mix JM, Elon L, Mutic NJ, Economos J, Flocks J, Tovar-Aguilar AJ, McCauley LA. Classification of heat-related illness symptoms among Florida farmworkers. J Nurs Scholarsh. 2018;50(1):74–82.

8. Sabo S, Lee AE. The spillover of US immigration policy on citizens and permanent residents of Mexican descent: how internalizing "illegality" impacts public health in the borderlands. Front Public Health. 2015;3:155.

9. Flouris AD, Dinas PC, Ioannou LG, Nybo L, Havenith G, Kenny GP, Kjellstrom T. Workers' health and productivity under occupational heat strain: a systematic review and meta-analysis. Lancet Planet Health. 2018;2(12):e521–31.

10. Chicas R, Suarez J, Elon L, Xiuhtecutli N, Houser MC, Berra L, Sands JM, Hertzberg V, McCauley L. Hydration interventions among agricultural workers: a pilot study. J Occup Environ Med. 2022;64(5):e357–9.

11. Garcia-Trabanino R, Jarquin E, Wesseling C, Johnson RJ, Gonzalez-Quiroz M, Weiss I, Glaser J, Jose Vindell J, Stockfelt L, Roncal C, Harra T, Barregard L. Heat stress, dehydration, and kidney function in sugarcane cutters in El Salvador—a cross-shift study of workers at risk of Mesoamerican nephropathy. Environ Res. 2015;142:746–55.

12. Glaser J, Lemery J, Rajagopalan B, Diaz HF, Garcia-Trabanino R, Taduri G, Madero M, Amarasinghe M, Abraham G, Anutrakulchai S, Jha V, Stenvinkel P, Roncal-Jimenez C, Lanaspa MA, Correa-Rotter R, Sheikh-Hamad D, Burdmann EA, Andres-Hernando A, Milagres T, Weiss I, Kanbay M, Wesseling C, Sanchez-Lozada LG, Johnson RJ. Climate change and the emergent epidemic of CKD from heat stress in rural communities: the case for heat stress nephropathy. Clin J Am Soc Nephrol. 2016;11(8):1472–83.

13. Hansson E, Glaser J, Weiss I, Ekström U, Apelqvist J, Hogstedt C, Peraza S, Lucas R, Jakobsson K, Wesseling C, Wegman DH. Workload and cross-harvest kidney injury in a Nicaraguan sugarcane worker cohort. Occup Environ Med. 2019;76(11):818–26.

14. Laws RL, Brooks DR, Amador JJ, Weiner DE, Kaufman JS, Ramirez-Rubio O, Riefkohl A, Scammell MK, Lopez-Pilarte D, Sanchez JM, Parikh CR, McClean MD. Biomarkers of kidney injury among Nicaraguan sugarcane workers. Am J Kidney Dis. 2016;67(2):209–17.

15. Mix J, Elon L, Thein Mac VV, Flocks J, Economos E, Tovar-Aguilar AJ, Stover Hertzberg V, McCauley LA. Hydration status, kidney function, and kidney injury in Florida agricultural workers. J Occup Environ Med. 2018;60(5):e253–60.

16. Moyce S, Armitage T, Mitchell D, Schenker M. Acute kidney injury and workload in a sample of California agricultural workers. Am J Ind Med. 2020;63(3):258–68.

17. Moyce S, Joseph J, Tancredi D, Mitchell D, Schenker M. Cumulative incidence of acute kidney injury in California's agricultural workers. J Occup Environ Med. 2016;58(4):391–7.

18. Moyce S, Mitchell D, Armitage T, Tancredi D, Joseph J, Schenker M. Heat strain, volume depletion and kidney function in California agricultural workers. Occup Environ Med. 2017;74(6):402–9.

19. Wesseling C, Aragon A, Gonzalez M, Weiss I, Glaser J, Bobadilla NA, Roncal-Jimenez C, Correa-Rotter R, Johnson RJ, Barregard L. Kidney function in sugarcane cutters in Nicaragua—a longitudinal study of workers at risk of Mesoamerican nephropathy. Environ Res. 2016;147:125–32.

20. Khwaja A. KDIGO clinical practice guidelines for acute kidney injury. Nephron Clin Pract. 2012;120(4):c179–84.

21. Mix JM, Elon L, Thein Mac VV, Flocks J, Economos J, Tovar-Aguilar AJ, Hertzberg VS, McCauley LA. Physical activity and work activities in Florida agricultural workers. Am J Ind Med. 2019;62(12):1058–67.

22. Anand S, Staniec A, Montez-Rath M, Vlahos P. Using GIS mapping to track hot spots of kidney disease in California. N Engl J Med. 2020;382(23):2265–7.

23. Bragg-Gresham J, Morgenstern H, Shahinian V, Robinson B, Abbott K, Saran R. An analysis of hot spots of ESRD in the United States: potential presence of CKD of unknown origin in the USA? Clin Nephrol. 2020;93(1):113–9.

24. van Haalen H, Jackson J, Spinowitz B, Milligan G, Moon R. Impact of chronic kidney disease and anemia on health-related quality of life and work productivity: analysis of multinational real-world data. BMC Nephrol. 2020;21(1):88.

Roxana C. Chicas PhD, RN, FAAN, is an Assistant Professor at Emory University's Nell Hodgson Woodruff School of Nursing. Dr. Chicas's research is shaping the future of climate and occupational health science, two pressing fields of scientific inquiry. A sought-after scientist with features in Bloomberg

News, NPR, and The World, she conducted the first field-based intervention study of methods to reduce core body temperature using real-time biomonitoring equipment among farmworkers in the United States. As a bilingual bicultural nurse scientist, she is committed to conducting research that informs policy to advance environmental justice.

Jasmine Irish MPH, is a Project Manager/Special Assistant at the Nell Hodgson Woodruff School of Nursing. She holds an MPH in Global Health from Emory University and has experience in global health program management and qualitative research. She currently manages an HRSA-funded grant that focuses on the Social Determinants of Health in nursing training.

Nezahualcoyotl Xiuhtecutli PhD, is the General Coordinator/Executive Director of the Farmworker Association. He has actively engaged research partners and community members in the dissemination of research results through heat stress and pesticide training.

Abby D. Mutic DNP, FNP-BC, MPH, is an Assistant Tenure Track Professor at the Nell Hodgson Woodruff School of Nursing with a clinical and translational research background in perinatal and pediatric environmental exposures. She earned a BS in Biology and Psychology from Drury University, a BSN in Nursing from Saint Louis University, an MSN in Nurse Midwifery from Vanderbilt University, and a PhD in Nursing from Emory University

Mapping and Modeling the Social and Ecological Determinants of Vector-Borne Disease Risk: A Case Study of Human African Trypanosomiasis

Demetrice R. Jordan, Matthew H. Bonds, and Ashton M. Shortridge

Human African trypanosomiasis (HAT), colloquially called African sleeping sickness, is one of several neglected tropical diseases (NTDs) that affects the livelihood and subsistence of poor, rural inhabitants of 36 countries in sub-Saharan Africa. Both the vector (tsetse) and the parasitic organism (trypanosomes) have been a source of economic hardship, impacting multiple industries in sub-Saharan Africa and creating development barriers [1–3]. Tsetse and trypanosomiasis are a substantial threat to the subsistence of pastoralists dependent upon the African bush for herd grazing activities, thus exacerbating conditions for poverty among remote rural populations [4–6].

African trypanosomiasis is an inherently multiscale global health problem, with a spatially and environmentally constrained vector, a transnational disease distribution, two distinct disease strains (East and West Africa), and innumerable human and animal reservoirs, and deeply entrenched in social determinants [7]. Specifically, the effects of government policies that spur political instability in endemic regions leading to population displacements, economic inequality and the occurrence of famines, poor community infrastructure and healthcare system engagement, and the collapse of other sociocultural institutions worsened for inhabitants in remote rural settings [7]. A disease of those in mostly rural settings, the full extent of the health burden of African sleeping sickness remains poorly understood; despite more than 100 years of research [8, 9], the case fatality rate of African sleeping sickness is near 100% if left untreated. Yearly, 60 million Africans are at risk of infection [10, 11]. Currently no vaccine or test of cure exists [12]. Because the trypanosomes require an ectothermic insect vector as part of its life cycle, it is necessarily constrained by environmental factors, such as temperature and rainfall that determine habitat suitability for the vector. But social factors determine several key aspects of the disease burden, including exposure to the vector, proximity to other reservoir species, such as livestock that people rely on for subsistence, as well as rates of detection and treatment.

The endemicity of African trypanosomiasis is driven by ecological determinants. In humans, African trypanosomiasis has two distinct disease

D. R. Jordan (✉) · M. H. Bonds
Department of Global Health and Social Medicine, Harvard Medical School, Boston, MA, USA
e-mail: Demetrice_jordan@hms.harvard.edu;
Matthew_Bonds@hms.harvard.edu

A. M. Shortridge
Department of Geography, Environment and Spatial Science, Michigan State University, East Lansing, MI, USA
e-mail: Ashton@msu.edu

J. B. Hamilton, C. E. Moore (eds.), *Transforming Social Determinants to Promote Global Health*,
https://doi.org/10.1007/978-3-031-61160-5_22

systems, and the symptoms vary based on the causative agent of infection, which differs by geographic region, i.e., East Africa or West Africa [13]. West African trypanosomiasis, caused by infections from human-derived *Trypanosoma brucei gambiense* (*T.b. gambiense*) [14], is responsible for the chronic illness with symptoms including swollen lymph nodes (Winterbottom's sign), headache, fever, and joint pain. People infected with this variant have a life expectancy of 3 years post-exposure [15]. The *gambiense* human African trypanosomiasis (g-HAT) infections account for 98% of the reported human African trypanosomiasis cases [16, 17]. East African sleeping sickness, in contrast, is caused by infections from *Trypanosoma brucei rhodesiense* (*T.b. rhodesiense*). Rhodesian human African trypanosomiasis (r-HAT), the rarer of the two strains, is an animal-derived infection and is more virulent and lethal in humans [18, 19]. Human hosts of r-HAT usually die within 6 months of infection [20].

This chapter focuses on the outbreak of r-HAT infections in the East African country of Malawi starting in 2019. Since the early 1990s, the country of Malawi has reported an average of 30 cases

yearly (Fig. 1). In 2019, diagnosed r-HAT infections increased to a record 91 cases, higher than any period since 1992 (see Fig. 1). The transmission of HAT requires the presence and interaction between human or animal hosts and trypanosome-infected tsetse fly [21, 22]. Given that the primary reservoir of r-HAT infections is livestock, transmission typically follows an animal-tsetse-human pathway whereby the virulent trypanosomes are passed to the human via the saliva of the tsetse during a blood meal [23].

1   A Spatial Approach to Understanding Human African Trypanosomiasis Risk in Malawi

Human African trypanosomiasis must be microscopically detected through spinal fluid [24] requiring engagement with the healthcare system. Therefore, prevalence may be higher than current estimates due to unreported cases among persons unable to access the healthcare system. Nevertheless, the sudden elevation in laboratory-confirmed r-HAT signals that interactions among

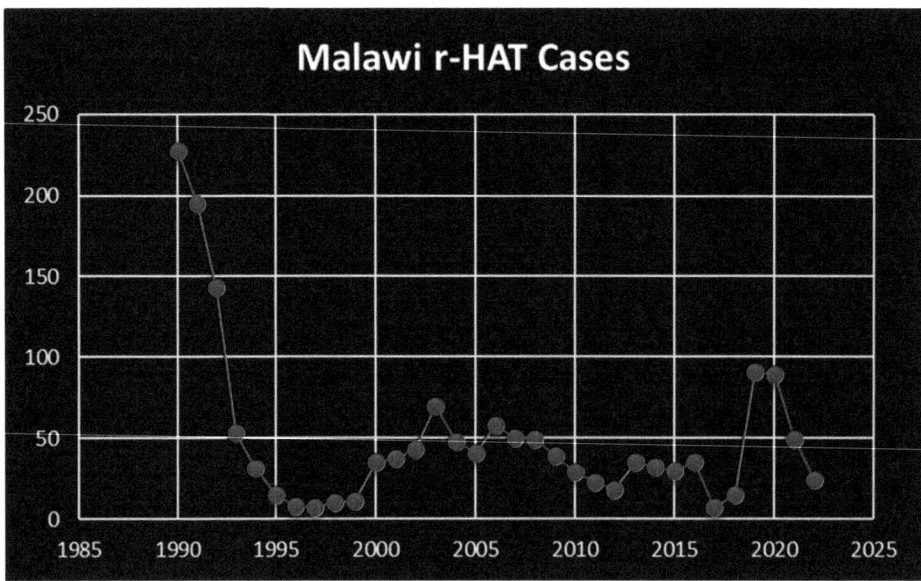

Fig. 1 Diagnosed cases of r-HAT in Malawi from 1990 to 2022. (Source WHO Global Health Observatory. https:// apps.who.int/gho/data/node.main.A1637?lang=en)

animals, tsetse, and humans have likely intensified, suggesting a change in social and ecological conditions across the rural landscapes of Malawi. Shifts in these dynamics could be attributed to expansions of tsetse habitat due to climate change reducing the distance between grazing lands, fly reservoirs, and villages, or fluctuations in residential settlement or movement patterns among human inhabitants due to conflicts and social unrest in neighboring countries leading to refugee migration. Understanding the nature of these changes in Malawi and their policy implications can be improved with detailed spatial models of core factors in tsetse and human ecology for the region.

The Simulated Models for Areas at Risk for Trypanosomiasis or SMART combine social factors such as the distribution of human and animal populations across a county's landscape with environmental and climate indicators such as temperature, soil moisture, and vegetation types suitable for the propagation of tsetse species across affected countries. Merged within a Geographic Information System (GIS) and leveraging the outcomes of the tsetse ecological distribution model for Google Earth Engine (GEE-TED) developed by Peter and Messina [25], these factors are used to produce a per-pixel map depicting the risk landscape in order to visualize areas of increased exposure risk for HAT infections at a 1-km spatial resolution every 16 days. Precision mapping such as the SMART approach could improve the accuracy of location targeting for tsetse control programs in low- and middle-income countries where funding may be limited. In those instances, modeling and mapping may substantially improve decision-making on where to locate tsetse control interventions. Spatial risk models thereby may reduce the likelihood of exposure and lessen the disease burden through development of control and public awareness campaigns. Reducing the presence of tsetse could preserve life and increase economic activity and development in remote areas of Malawi.

2   Authors' Interest in Human African Trypanosomiasis

The first author became aware of African sleeping sickness as a child, while reading a book on tropical medicine. Several decades later, tsetse and trypanosomiasis would become the topic of her doctoral dissertation. Through reviewing the literature and time spent in several countries where the disease is endemic including Malawi, she learned firsthand how severely under-resourced tsetse and trypanosomiasis control programs were and how they have been deprioritized since the early 1990s in most countries. The difficulties with control and eradication of tsetse are complex and require both the elimination of the fly and a reduction in the prevalence of the pathogen among human and animal reservoirs. Due to the sustained incidence rates of HAT, and the feasibility of disease control, the World Health Organization (WHO) sought to make the eradication of tsetse and the control of trypanosomiasis a global health priority. To spur research and support in this area, the WHO set a target priority of the elimination of sleeping sickness as a public health concern and the eradication of tsetse by 2030.

While this new focus elevated the status of HAT cases, much of the efforts have been focused on g-HAT, the chronic variant which affords more opportunities for breakthroughs in case detection and treatment. The acute nature of the r-HAT infection makes it less amenable to lengthy public health surveillance campaigns and interventions. However, the recent spike in prevalence of r-HAT increases the urgency with strategies needed to identify areas at risk of exposure—where human populations, animal reservoirs, and the insect vector converge—in order to prioritize control efforts. Exposure risk pathways are reliant upon and intensified by the interplay between the physical, ecological, and social determinants. Identification of at-risk areas can be done through the SMART riskscape maps, which support those whose daily activities regularly require engaging with tsetse habitats, at times when tsetse are active, such as cattle grazing, water procurement, and other household chores. Given that risk is not uniform, ubiquitous, nor homogenous through time or across landscapes, we need methods that help prioritize areas for control and intervention with specific granularity. This project contributes to WHO's 2030 control and elimination target priority by providing an approach for strategic site selection to maximize chance of treating patients and interrupting disease transmission within a time frame relevant to both decision-makers and the vulnerable populations.

3   A Brief Overview of Malawi

Malawi is a small republic in sub-Saharan Africa located in the southeastern region of the continent roughly located around 13.2° S, 34.3° E. The country is landlocked, surrounded by Tanzania to

the northeast, Mozambique to the southeast, Zimbabwe to the southwest, and Zambia and the Democratic Republic of the Congo (DRC) to the northwest (Fig. 2). Topographically, Malawi is relatively flat with a mix of plateaus and plains. The climate is semiarid with variable humidity (see Figs. 3 and 4).

Economically, Malawi is one of the poorest countries in the world with two thirds of the population living below the international poverty line. A primarily agrarian population, more than 90% of the population engages in subsistence farming including pastoralism (see Figs. 5, 6, 7, and 8).

There are approximately 21 million people in Malawi with an average life expectancy of 67 years for both men and women. The primary languages are English and Chichewa. As a severely under-resourced nation, Malawi relies on international aid and foreign assistance. Due to the limited resources, policies that focus on neglected tropical diseases such as human

Fig. 2 The country of Malawi and surrounding countries

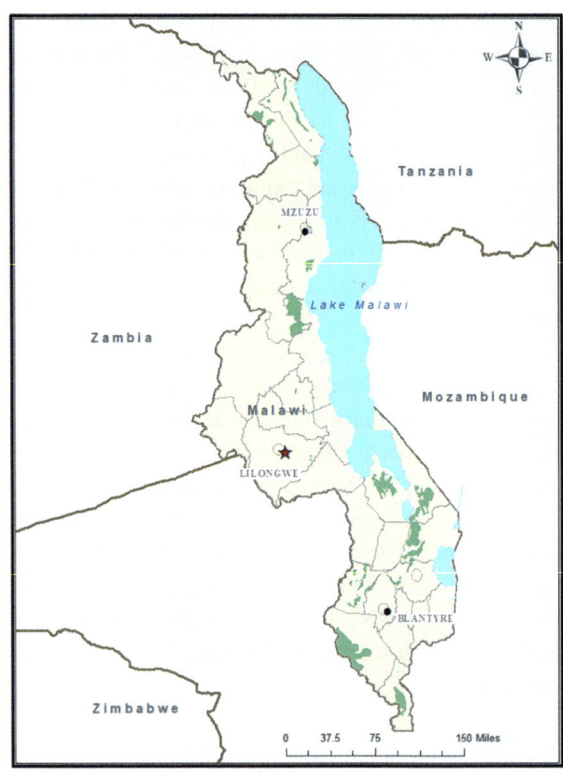

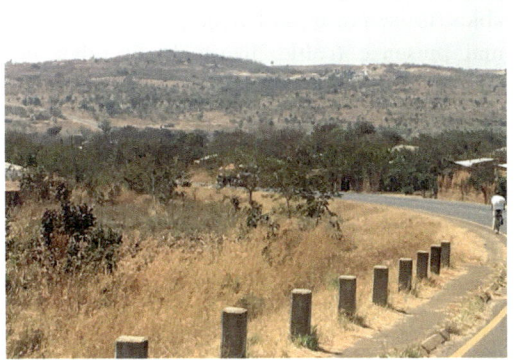

Fig. 3 Malawi's landscape has a mix of plateaus and plains. (Photo taken by Demetrice Jordan)

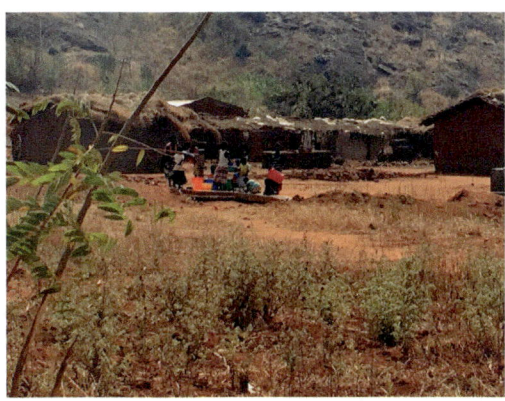

Fig. 6 Village in rural Malawi. (Photo taken by Demetrice Jordan)

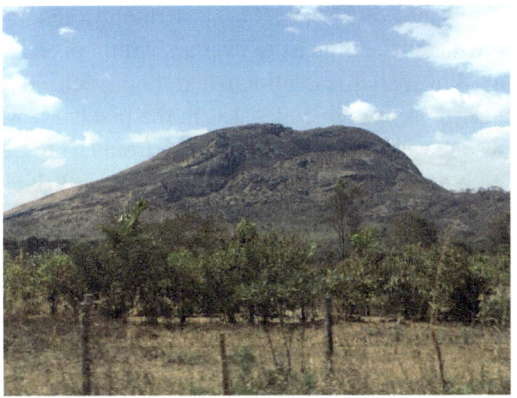

Fig. 4 Malawi topography includes hills peppered across the landscape. (Photo taken by Demetrice Jordan)

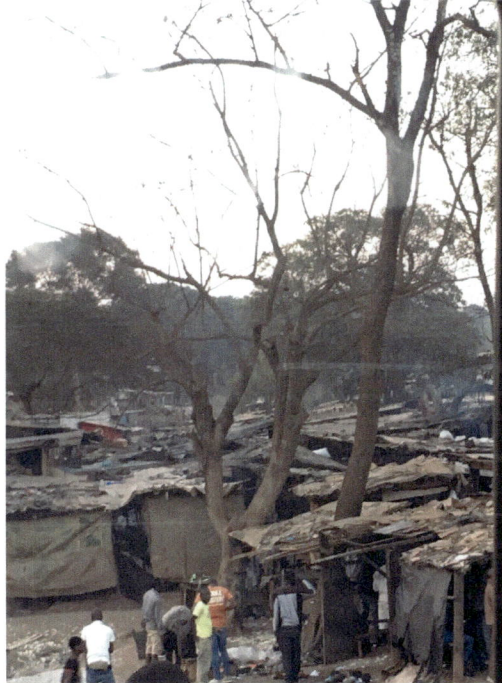

Fig. 7 Shanty town in Malawi. (Photo taken by Demetrice Jordan)

African trypanosomiasis are underfunded. WHO's call to action increased research on the disease. However, countries like Malawi with stable and sustained low levels of the infection receive less funding for control and eradication programs in favor of hot zones such as the DRC.

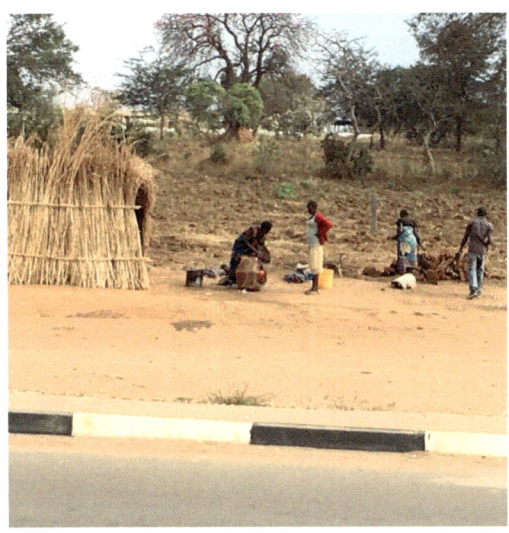

Fig. 5 Villagers conducting daily chores in rural Malawi. (Photo taken by Demetrice Jordan)

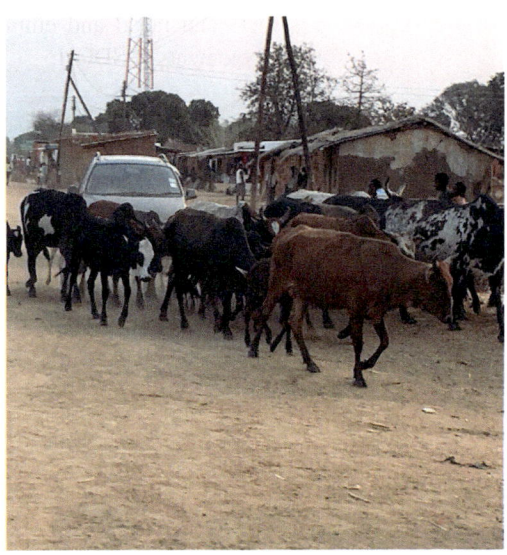

Fig. 8 Pastoralist moving cattle herds to graze in rural Malawi. (Photo taken by Demetrice Jordan)

4   The Simulated Models for Areas at Risk for Trypanosomiasis (SMART)

The Simulated Models for Areas at Risk for Trypanosomiasis (SMART) are interaction models that provide an exposure risk ranking over large regions (riskscape) to determine geographic areas with a confluence of factors that increase trypanosomiasis transmission risk. This spatially disaggregated approach aids countries like Malawi with limited resources for tsetse and trypanosomiasis control to prioritize the areas for interventions at a granular level, which is valuable when budgetary constraints do not allow for broad area-wide insect control operations. The SMART can allow practitioners to conduct a low-cost feasibility analysis to select and target sites where risk is the highest.

The SMART require three parameterized variables: tsetse presence, human presence, and animal presence (cattle, livestock, or other host animals) available at a per-pixel spatial unit across the region of interest. The models offer three variants depending on the subject of interest to the practitioner. The host model weighs the presence of animal and human hosts, the vector model weighs the presence of tsetse across a region, while the combined model weighs the presence of both host and vector equally. The models assign a risk magnitude level based on the presence or absence of the parameterized variables.

The combined model (see Fig. 9) weighs the abundance of tsetse and hosts across the geography and detects areas of overlap, within pixels at a 1-km spatial resolution where both vector and host presence are collocated in the pixels across the area. The outcomes will range from HH to LL with a risk magnitude range from Level 3 (high risk) to Level 0 (no risk).

The ability for analytical tools, such as the SMART, to be truly effective requires integration with the communities they are intended to serve. Accordingly, a series of interviews were conducted with local stakeholders to capture their perspectives on the development of a community-driven framework for tsetse and trypanosomiasis control. Historical top-down strategies to tsetse control included population displacements, land development, game culling, bush clearing, and other policies with largely negative consequences to local communities and the environment. Methods to include local voices, such as the Political, Economic, Socio-cultural, and Technological (PEST) analysis, support community participatory policy development using a decision matrix and create the opportunity for meaningful engagement with local stakeholders across different scales. The PEST analysis has been utilized for HAT control

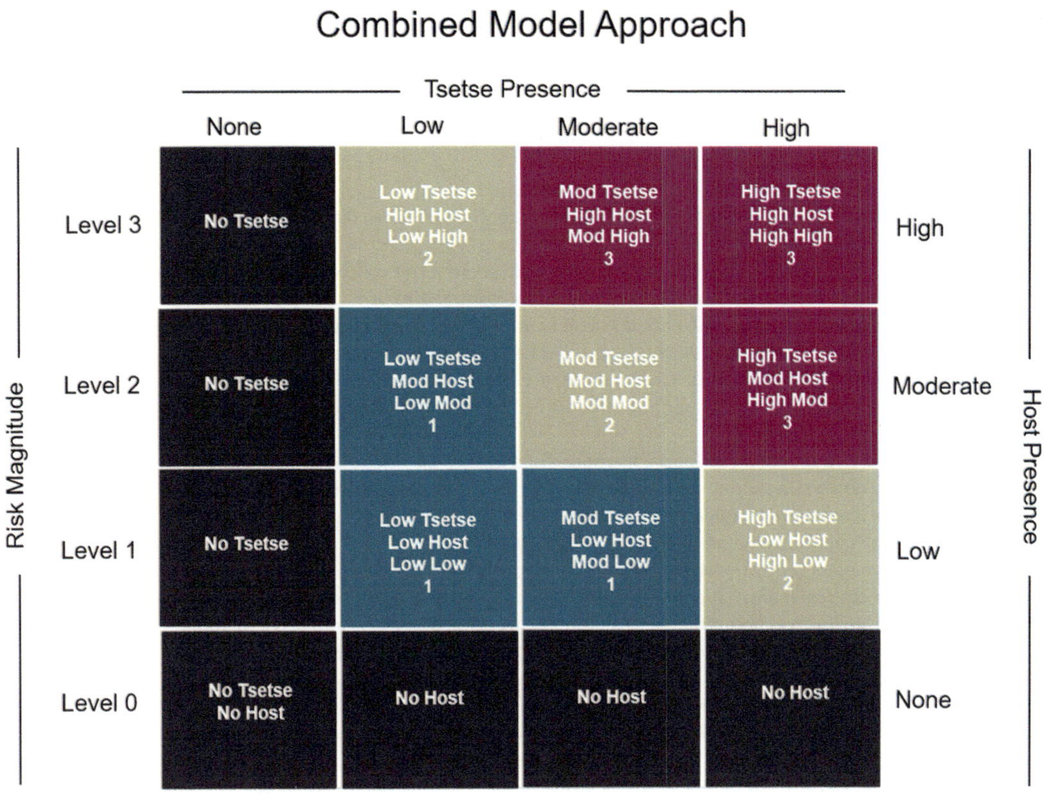

Combined Model Approach

Fig. 9 Conceptual diagram of the combined model equally weighing vector and host presence. (Adopted from Jordan [7])

interviews in Senegal and Tanzania—both tsetse-endemic countries. Therefore, its prospective use in Malawi is feasible.

5 Community Participation in Tsetse and Trypanosomiasis Control

Engaging the community to share their perspective on strategies to improve tsetse control in East and West Africa included the collection of information through participant interviews. The multidisciplinary and cross-sectoral interviewees included representatives from development, international aid agencies, regional and local elected officials, agricultural extension workers, animal and human health, and the academy. Survey participants were selected due to their history of involvement in tsetse and trypanosomiasis control; role in nongovernmental organizations; national government appointments; expertise in subject matter research at local, regional, or national levels; and leadership in the local community.

The structured interviews consisted of 16 questions to understand attitudes toward and perceptions of tsetse control programs and to docu-

Interview Questions

1) How long have you been working in tsetse control?
2) What type of tsetse control programs have you been involved with?
   a. Past
   b. Current/Active
3) What barriers have you faced implementing control strategies (i.e. political, resource and technological)?
4) Which agencies have/are supervising the past/present control programs you have been involved with? What different agencies are funding the control efforts?
5) How have policies helped or hurt tsetse control efforts in your district/regionally/nationally?
6) What type of resources do you feel would help with tsetse control?
7) Do you think coordinated PanAfrican supervision of tsetse control would work?
8) Which tsetse control strategy do you feel is the most optimal approach with the greatest chance of sustainable results?
9) What's your opinion on local governance of and local participation in control efforts?
10) How do you feel about the level of administrative support and assistance received from your local government, regional government etc for control efforts?
11) What's your opinion on current control programs?
12) Do you feel control information is shared widely and effectively between the districts/regionally/nationally (i.e. best practice, successes, failures)
13) How do you feel about the WHO's target elimination of trypanosomiasis as a public health concern by 2020 and the eradication of tsetse by 2030? Do you think the goal will be reached why/why not?
14) Have your programs achieved success in control? Explain.
15) In your opinion what components would a good policy for T&T control require to achieve long-term success?
16) What are the most significant or common tsetse control program errors you have seen/made?

Fig. 10 Stakeholder structured interview questions [7]

ment local stakeholder opinions on the components necessary to achieve long-term tsetse and trypanosomiasis control (Fig. 10). While pure consensus was not achieved in any one thematic area, most of the participants desired stronger tsetse control policies, an equitable distribution of resources for control programs, to move toward innovative and hi-tech control options, and a combined suppression and elimination strategy, not elimination alone. Another impediment discovered through the PEST analysis was the lack of local participation and feelings of being marginalized during the initial policy construction and development phases. Most stakeholders agreed the best way to alleviate these concerns is through participatory policy development.

5.1 Reflection

Addressing neglected tropical diseases such as human African trypanosomiasis is always challenging due to low status, political will, and the lack of influence of the poor, rural, populations that are most impacted. However, these challenges are surmountable. In global health priority setting such as the target elimination of tsetse and trypanosomiasis by 2030, the WHO sponsors help provide economic resources that spur innovation and research to control these often-fatal diseases. For instance, recent developments by Drugs for Neglected Diseases Initiative (DNDi) have improved HAT treatment, making them more accessible and less lethal. Where previous HAT medications caused fatalities in around 10%

of those being treated, these pharmaceutical advances reduce deaths from the disease and make it possible for infected people to take the pills at home. The existence of such technologies places even more importance on quickly identifying those who are at risk for treatment and prevention. Following successful implementation and validation in Senegal and Tanzania, Malawi is a natural next destination for the SMART given the recent uptick in cases, its heterogenous human and animal landscapes, and its low level of public health resources. As temperature and precipitation patterns shift due to global climate change, the geographic patterns of the tsetse riskscape are also changing.

Monitoring and forecasting will be critical to identifying the shifting riskscape of vector-borne parasitic diseases such as human African trypanosomiasis. As with other NTDs, the reliance on insect vectors and alternative reservoirs means that the dynamics of HAT are necessarily determined by environmental drivers including temperature and rainfall. Paradoxically, this makes the disease especially dependent on social determinants because the poor are vulnerable to external conditions. It is the subsistence livelihood strategies in poor rural areas that expose humans to the disease. The acute manifestations in r-HAT require that rapid detection and treatment are essential, especially challenging for these communities who also suffer the greatest social and geographic barriers to diagnosis and treatment. SMART can thus serve as a valuable tool for intervention planning in low-resource settings reducing the burden of HAT, one of the deadliest of neglected tropical diseases.

References

1. Alsan M. The effect of the tsetse fly on African development. Am Econ Rev. 2015;105(1):382–410. https://doi.org/10.1257/aer.20130604.
2. Grant C. The politics of knowledge: whose knowledge matters in trypanosomiasis making in Zambia. Brighton: STEPS Centre; 2014.
3. Grant C, Anderson N, Machila N. Stakeholder narratives on trypanosomiasis, their effect on policy and the scope for one health. PLoS Negl Trop Dis. 2015;9:e0004241. https://doi.org/10.1371/journal.pntd.0004241.
4. Ilemobade AA. Tsetse and trypanosomosis in Africa: the challenges, the opportunities. Onderstepoort J Vet Res. 2009;76:35–40.
5. Lachenal G. The Lomidine files: the untold story of a medical disaster in colonial Africa: EBSCOhost. JHU Press; 2017.
6. Namangala B, Odongo S. Animal African trypanosomosis in sub-Saharan Africa and beyond African borders. In: Magez S, Radwanska M, editors. Trypanosomes and trypanosomiasis. Vienna: Springer; 2013.
7. Jordan DR. A risk reduction approach to tsetse and trypanosomiasis control case study: the CANVAS method. Michigan State University; 2020.
8. Bouteille B, Oukem O, Bisser S, Dumas M. Treatment perspectives for human African trypanosomiasis. Fundam Clin Pharmacol. 2003;17(2):171–81. https://doi.org/10.1046/j.1472-8206.2003.00167.x.
9. Maudlin I, Eisler MC, Welburn SC. Neglected and endemic zoonoses. Philos Trans R Soc B Biol Sci. 2009;364(1530):2777–87. https://doi.org/10.1098/rstb.2009.0067.
10. Franco JR, Simarro PP, Diarra A, Ruiz-Postigo JA, Jannin JG. The journey towards elimination of Gambiense human African trypanosomiasis: not far, nor easy. Parasitology. 2014;141(6):748–60. https://doi.org/10.1017/S0031182013002102.
11. Simarro P, Diarra A, Ruiz-Postigo JA, Franco JR, Jannin JG. The human African trypanosomiasis control and surveillance programme of the World Health Organization 2000–2009: the way forward. PLoS Negl Trop Dis. 2011;5(2):e1007. https://doi.org/10.1371/journal.pntd.0001007.
12. CDC. CDC—African trypanosomiasis—treatment. CDC; 2023. https://www.cdc.gov/parasites/sleeping-sickness/treatment.html.
13. Mulenga P, Boelaert M, Lutumba P, Kelen CV, Coppieters Y, Chenge F, Lumbala C, et al. Integration of human African trypanosomiasis control activities into primary health services in The Democratic Republic of the Congo: a qualitative study of stakeholder perceptions. Am J Trop Med Hyg. 2019;100(4):899–906. https://doi.org/10.4269/ajtmh.18-0382.
14. Mulenga P, Chenge F, Boelaert M, Mukalay A, Lutumba P, Lumbala C, Luboya O, Coppieters Y. Integration of human African trypanosomiasis control activities into primary healthcare services: a scoping review. Am J Trop Med Hyg. 2019;101(5):1114–25. https://doi.org/10.4269/ajtmh.19-0232.
15. Kennedy PGE. The continuing problem of human African trypanosomiasis (sleeping sickness). Ann Neurol. 2008;64(2):116–26.
16. Headrick DR. Sleeping sickness epidemics and colonial responses in East and Central Africa, 1900–1940. PLoS Negl Trop Dis. 2014;8(4):e2772. https://doi.org/10.1371/journal.pntd.0002772.

17. Mulenga GM, Likwa RN, Namangala B. Assessing the capacity to diagnose human African trypanosomiasis among health care personnel from Chama and Mambwe districts of eastern Zambia. BMC Res Notes. 2015;8(1):433. https://doi.org/10.1186/s13104-015-1403-6.

18. Van Den Berghe L. The form of trypanosomiasis seen in fishermen at Lake Tumba, Belgian Congo. Ann Soc Belg Med Trop. 1956;36(2):185–9.

19. Edwards DP, Sloan S, Weng L, Dirks P, Sayer J, Laurance WF. Mining and the African environment. Conserv Lett. 2014;7(3):302–11. https://doi.org/10.1111/conl.12076.

20. Kennedy PGE. Clinical features, diagnosis, and treatment of human African trypanosomiasis (sleeping sickness). Lancet Neurol. 2013;12(2):186–94.

21. Aksoy S, Weiss BL, Attardo GM. Trypanosome transmission dynamics in tsetse. Curr Opin Insect Sci. 2014;3:43. https://doi.org/10.1016/j.cois.2014.07.003.

22. Courtin F, Camara M, Rayaisse JB, Kagbadouno M, Dama E, Camara O, Traoré IS, et al. Reducing human-tsetse contact significantly enhances the efficacy of sleeping sickness active screening campaigns: a promising result in the context of elimination. PLoS Negl Trop Dis. 2015;9(8):e0003727. https://doi.org/10.1371/journal.pntd.0003727.

23. Semayat O, Maireg H. Review on prevalence of bovine trypanosomosis in Ethiopia. Afr J Agric Res. 2018;13(1):1–6.

24. Smith Knox Byrd J. Sleeping sickness the Castellani-Bruce controversy. Notes Rec R Soc Lond. 1973;28:93–110.

25. Peter B, Messina J. GEE-TED: a tsetse ecological distribution model for Google Earth engine. Harvard Dataverse; 2022.

Demetrice R. Jordan PhD, is an Instructor in the Department of Global Health and Social Medicine. She holds a dual-PhD in Health Geography and Environmental Science and Policy from Michigan State University (MSU), a Master of Public Health in Global Health, and graduate certificate in Global Infectious Diseases from Harvard T.H. Chan School of Public Health. Her research focuses on the spatial-ecological determinants of disease risk for vector-borne parasitic diseases and Neglected Tropical Diseases of sub-Saharan Africa and the tropics.

Dee also examines issues related to health equity, health disparities, social and environmental justice. She is a council member of the American Geographical Society (AGS) and the creator of the Celebrating Black Geographers anthology, hosted online by AGS. She is a diversity, equity, and inclusion (DEI) consultant and offers strategic planning, educational, and leadership development programs, and DEI training. Dee is the founder of the Advancing Geography Through Diversity Program (AGTDP), a cohort-based recruitment and retention program which seeks to address the persistent underrepresentation of African Americans, Latinx Americans, and Native Americans in US geography doctoral programs and provides fully funded graduate education opportunities.

Matthew H. Bonds is an associate professor of global health and social medicine at Harvard Medical School, and co-founder of Pivot, a global health NGO that partners with the Madagascar government to establish a district level model health system. He holds a PhD in economics and a PhD in ecology from the University of Georgia. His research focuses on (1) the ecology of poverty and economic development; (2) infectious disease modeling, and (3) the science of implementing global health delivery systems. With novel data systems at all levels of care (community, primary and secondary care), Pivot has generated some of the most rigorously evaluated population level impacts of a local health initiative in Africa. His work has been supported by Pivot, the NIH, the NSF, the Gates Foundation, James S. McDonnell Foundation, and the Mulago Foundation, among others.

Ashton M. Shortridge PhD, is Professor and Chairperson of the Department of Geography, Environment, and Spatial Sciences at Michigan State University. He is a geographer with research and teaching focii in spatial statistics, geocomputation, and geographic information science, with applied science interests in coupled human and natural systems and health geography. His prior engagement with geographic information systems (GIS) in the government and private sectors has provided critical perspective throughout his academic career. His professional research strategy has been to seek out application domains that couple substantial challenges in spatial data science with the opportunity for significant scientific and societal impact.

Communities in Action: Creating a Path to Environmental Health Equity in Southeast Indian Country

Jada Lynn Brooks and Jefferson Currie II

Water—an integral facet of many Indigenous people's lives and cultural identities—is a key determinant of Indigenous health [1, 2]. As the source and sustenance of all life, many Indigenous belief systems consider water a living, spiritual element of sacred importance that extends beyond a material resource [3, 4]. Its significance is multifaceted, encompassing economic, political, sociocultural, and spiritual dimensions [5]. Centuries of colonial practices following European arrival to the Americas fundamentally altered every aspect of the natural environment, severing Indigenous people's life-sustaining relationships with water [4, 6]. With the chronic contamination of water sources across tribal lands, Indigenous people face insurmountable challenges in accessing clean water [4, 7, 8]. Such severe water insecurities both threaten Indigenous people's overall well-being and amplify the persistent health inequities they collectively experience [9–11]. This chapter highlights specific water conflicts confronting tribal communities in the southeastern region of the United States of America (USA), as well as solutions driven by these communities to combat such issues.

Water quality deterioration is a widespread issue affecting tribal communities throughout the USA. The Southeast, however, faces persistent challenges unique to the region. In 1513, the Southeast became a popular land attraction for European settlers. Over the next century, human and economic activities, such as agricultural production and extraction of natural resources, swept through the Southeast, permanently altering the region's landscape. Rapid ecological changes—widespread deforestation, biodiversity loss, and erosion of ecosystems—produced by Western industrial practices ultimately disrupted Indigenous Peoples' complex and expansive relationships with water. Despite these vast geographical changes, the Southeast remains one of the most biodiverse and resource-rich regions globally and, as such, one of the most vulnerable. Thus, the Indigenous people inhabiting this land are especially susceptible to the changes it has undergone—primarily because the wetlands they have long occupied serve as a crucial source of physical and spiritual sustenance. Despite enduring centuries of systemic harm from ecological degradation, Indigenous Peoples' resilience and adaptation to shifting environments have ensured their survival. To protect future generations and the ecosystems they will inherit, we must respect Indigenous perspectives, knowledge systems, and the life-preserving gifts they offer.

To this end, tribal communities are taking deliberate steps in applying such principles to

J. L. Brooks (✉)
School of Nursing, University of North Carolina at Chapel Hill, Chapel Hill, NC, USA
e-mail: jada@email.unc.edu

J. Currie II
Winyah Rivers Alliance, Laurinburg, NC, USA
e-mail: LumberRK@winyahrivers.org

recover and preserve waterways in the Southeast. As people deeply embedded in this context, we are acutely aware of the need to address the water issues impacting southeastern tribal territories, including the Lumber River.[1] Jefferson Currie II, the Lumber Riverkeeper, partners with local activists and leaders to protect the Lumbee River Watershed and improve water quality for the diverse communities living along its waterways. As a nurse scientist with more than 20 years of practical experience working with and within Indigenous communities, I, too, am committed to addressing health inequities and environmental issues affecting Southeast tribes. We are both enrolled members of the Lumbee Tribe of North Carolina. Jeff sought education in American Indian Studies, while I studied public health and nursing. Jeff and I met about 2 years ago on what was supposed to be my first canoe trip down the Lumber River. Our planned river excursion ended memorably with what locals would call an icy river baptism. From there, we formed a collaborative relationship, joining forces to combat community water challenges and concerns within Indian territory. We have teamed up in this chapter to present an illustrative example based in the southeastern region of North Carolina that applies community-based participatory research approaches and principles from the Equity, Access, Usability, and eXchange (EAUX) framework [12]. We hope that this example will model ways to protect and restore water sources in Southeast Indian Country and, in doing so, create a path to environmental health equity.

1 Illustrative Example: Mercury Contamination in the Coastal Plain Region's Rivers

1.1 Introduction to the Lumbee River

Of the many rivers flowing through the flat Coastal Plain of south-central North Carolina, the Lumbee River bears cultural and symbolic significance for Indigenous people who first and now inhabit the region. For some 6000–10,000 years, the Lumbee River has been vital in linking people, communities, and trade across the region. The river's headwaters lie in the wooded, hilly land of the Sandhills ecoregion, originating as a small stream flowing through gravelly sand known as Drowning Creek.[2] Its name, first assigned by European settlers, remains in use. The Lumbee River, named a black water river for its inky black hue, winds and meanders through expansive floodplains that stretch from the Hoke County–Scotland County border through the North Carolina–South Carolina state line (see Fig. 1). Its tea-stained waters derive from its steady flow through densely wooded terrain, where decaying leaves and flora accumulate in the watercourse, gradually releasing tannins that impart the signature deep coloration (see Fig. 2). The river's complex architecture reflects an intricate network of waterways and swamps that weave throughout the region, revealing large fields of row crops connected by ribbons of deep green. Functioning as a natural irrigation source, the river has allowed nearby occupants to benefit economically from regional agriculture and farming practices for centuries. Its enigmatic waterways also acted as maritime channels, facilitating the extraction and exchange of valuable resources, including timber. The dense wood of longleaf, loblolly, and other pines on drier land complement the bald cypress, swamp tupelo, and

---

[1] Before 1809, the Lumber River and its headwaters were known as Drowning Creek. In 1809, John Willis, a prominent community figure in Lumberton, persuaded government officials to change its name to Lumber River to better attract investors to timber and other businesses. This chapter uses the term Lumbee River as the reclaimed ancestral name of the Lumber River.

---

[2] Drowning Creek was once erroneously considered the Little Pee Dee River headwaters. Drowning Creek is the headwaters of the Lumbee River.

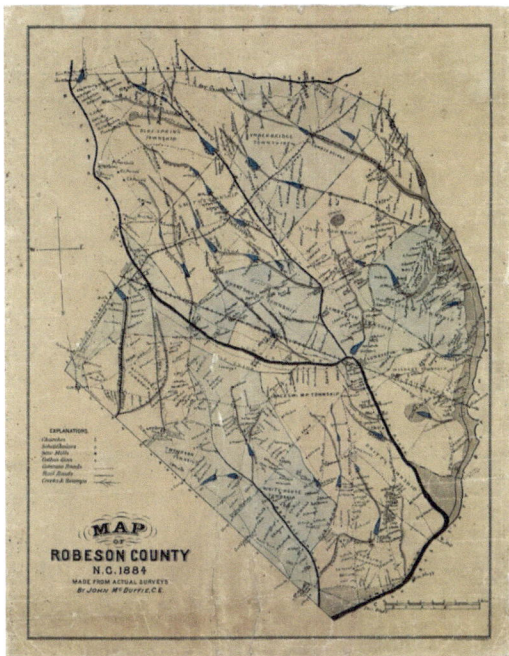

Fig. 1 1884 McDuffie Map of Robeson County, North Carolina. (Photo courtesy of State Archives of North Carolina)

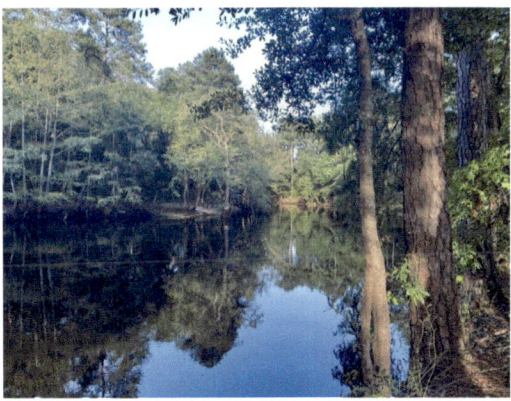

Fig. 2 Bottomland swamp forest draped in Spanish moss bordering the Lumbee River with bald cypress (*Taxodium distichum*) in the center. (Photo courtesy Jada L. Brooks, 2021)

features. They are known as the People of the Dark Water.

2 Lumbee: People of the Dark Water

During the first 300 years of colonial aggressions—ravaging epidemics, devastating wars, enslavement, and land seizure—Europeans used many legal and covert maneuvers to subdue, detribalize, assimilate, and enculturate Indigenous people. The goal of these reprehensible efforts was the targeted erasure of the population. Indigenous people across the Carolinas and Virginia who survived the destructive impacts of settler colonialism often relocated to seek refuge from European encroachment. Uniting with others dwelling along tributary rivers in the Carolina region, many Indigenous Peoples, speaking disparate languages, permanently settled along the swampy waterways of the Lumbee, Little Pee Dee, and Waccamaw Rivers, which flow south/southwest into the Great Pee Dee River. In a 1754 report about county militias in North Carolina, the growing Indigenous population was characterized as "50 families a mixt Crew, a lawless People, [who] possess the Lands without patent or paying quit rents; [and] shot a surveyor for coming to view vacant lands being inclosed (sic) in great swamps."[3] The sophisticated nature of the watershed's dense swamps and wet ecosystems protected and sheltered Indigenous settlements along the waterways. A form of natural seclusion, the swamps allowed Indigenous Peoples to maintain community and preserve aspects of their culture despite a growing colonial presence in the region. In 1773, Indigenous communities continued to operate independently, without permission from the king, governor, or

black gum guarding the river's edge. Low-hanging branches and fallen snags drape the river, serving as picturesque adornments while offering refuge to a rich tapestry of diverse plant and animal life. Long-standing Indian communities overlay the river's expansive swamplands, blending with its

[3]Before 1800, most maps did not include the Lumbee River or were mapped incorrectly (None 1754). Due to the large number of dense swamps around the main streamline of the river, it is believed that early colonists did not comprehend the size and extent of the river. As noted, in 1754, the Indigenous community on Drowning Creek shot at a surveyor coming to map out the area, so there were likely few existing depictions.

lord's proprietor, which settlers, including Archibald McKissack JP, considered unacceptable. Petitioning the House Assembly on October 13, 1773, he referred to the group as rogues, asserting that he had submitted "a list of the mob raitously (sic)[4] assembled together in Bladen County…living on the Kings' land."[5] Among the names from McKissack's petition were surnames common to Indigenous Peoples in the Carolinas and Virginia in the late eighteenth century. These surnames, some inherited by the Lumbee, suggest that many Indigenous people now living in the region descended from this organized group.

Lumbee diaspora has historically (in the last 250 years) included Indigenous people and communities connected through complex cultural, familial, and tribal relationships living around or near the North Carolina–South Carolina state line. Because of the growing need to establish tribal sovereignty, the Lumbee sought and received recognition by the state in 1885. With the 1956 Lumbee Act, the Congress formally recognized the Lumbee, which partially secured their tribal status. Because the government was terminating its relationships with Indian tribes during this era, the Lumbee were not afforded federal benefits. The Lumbee Nation remains the only tribe not to have had such benefits restored. Now, with more than 55,000 enrolled members, the Lumbee are the largest tribe in North Carolina and the largest east of the Mississippi River. Indian families with deep ties to the area reside primarily in Lumbee Territory, which includes Robeson and adjoining counties.

Intertwining with the inland swamps, freshwater rivers, and nearby coastal sounds and beaches, the Lumbee's relationship with the riv-

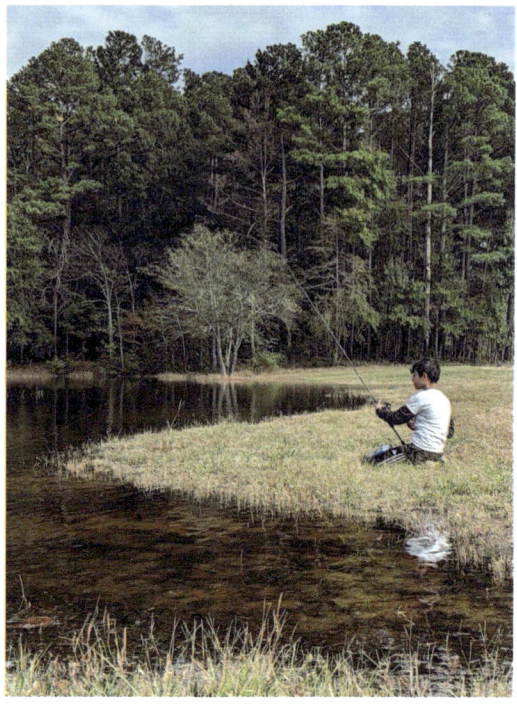

Fig. 3 A young Lumbee angler fishing on the riverbank in Robeson County, North Carolina. (Photo courtesy Jada L. Brooks, 2022)

ers of the Great Pee Dee River Basin is braided into their culture and history (see Fig. 3). The bounty of foods they gathered from the aquatic ecosystems and other diverse habitats provided sustenance that allowed the Lumbee to exist and thrive in their rapidly changing climate. Lumbee elders interviewed in the late 1960s and early 1970s through the University of Florida, Gainesville, attest to the diversity of cultural activities connected to the waterways in the region. Both Crossie Lowry and Herman Barton spoke keenly about fishing in the Lumbee River and how they would snag catfish, "redbreast, "robins," perch, and other fish.[6] Elisha Dial and Ellie Lowry Revels described how families would make trips to the coast to catch fish and salt them before making the journey back to Robeson County, which Mr. Dial said they did by way of mule and wagon.[7] Born primarily in the late nine-

---

[4] Jeff C. and others believe the word "raitously" is an alternate spelling for "riotously." Given his name, McKissack, and that southeastern North Carolina was heavily settled by Scottish colonist, the petitioner was likely of Scottish or Scots–Irish descent. The website Dictionaries of the Scots Language Online shows wide variation in the spelling of the word riotously before and after 1700. This supports that the spelling of raitously is in keeping with other colonial records, which also show variation in spelling for many words during, before, and after this time period (Dictionaries of the Scots Language Online, 2023).

[5] McKissAck (1773).

---

[6] Lowry (1973) and Barton (1973).

[7] Revels (1971) and Dial and Rogers (1971).

teenth century, these elders connect our community to precontact traditions. The preservation of sacred fishing traditions through centuries of colonialism that actively suppressed Indigenous cultural practices demonstrates cultural resistance to such stark obstacles. Such traditions extend beyond fishing. Lumbee elder Colon Brooks explained how the branches, swamps, and rivers in the Lumbee diaspora were tangible resources that bound the Lumbee to the watershed's ecosystems, telling an interviewer how his grandfather, Big Arch Locklear, "dug [his father's first boat] out of a cypress log."[8] From the sustenance and cultural renewal of seasonal freshwater fishing catches on the coast to the shelter and transportation provided by the dense hardwood bottomland cypress, Lumbee's ties with water have shaped their identity and persistence for centuries. Accumulating threats in recent decades from industrialization and poor land-use practices within its watershed have compromised the Lumbee's connection to and dependence on the river. Heightened sedimentation, stemming from erosion along poorly managed riverbanks or mismanaged forested and agricultural lands, poses a grave danger to the flora and fauna of the river [13]. Further, decades of polluted runoff laden with pesticides, fertilizers, and synthetic chemicals have contaminated the waters, imperiling the myriad organisms reliant on the river system.

3 Contamination of the Lumbee River

The relentless invasion of American industry in the Southeast accounts for much of the legacy pollution that lurks and persists in the Lumbee River. The insidious remnants of past industries hide among vacant buildings, slowly leaking contaminants into the region's soil, groundwater, and surface waters. Pollution remains an ongoing—not just historical—concern across the region. Government agencies' lack of interference (e.g., oversight and enforcement of environmental regulations) enables profit-driven industries to treat the river's watershed as a dumping ground for toxic chemicals. Systemic destruction of the river's ecosystems and pollution of precious habitats are perpetuated by the colonial mindset that humans and other species are separate from the natural world in which they live. By valuing capitalistic gain over the environment's health, companies continue to enact harm through ongoing contamination.

Mercury is one of the many harmful toxins contaminating the Lumbee River and its diverse fish species. Although the element mercury occurs naturally, the geological conditions usually creating such situations are absent in the Lumbee River Watershed. Thus, it is deposited into the ecosystem through anthropogenic sources. At room temperature, mercury is a heavy metal often used to fabricate products such as light bulbs, dental fillings, and batteries. When mercury in its metallic form is heated, it becomes a colorless and odorless gas. As a gas, it is emitted into the air and deposited on land and surface waters. Scientists agree that the major source for toxic levels of mercury in fish in the Lumbee River Watershed and throughout waterways in Eastern and Piedmont areas of North Carolina occurs from the release of mercury while burning fossil fuels, primarily coal, for energy production.[9] After being deposited in the waterways, mercury often changes into a form called methylmercury, which organisms absorb. When fish ingest these organisms, the mercury becomes stored in their tissues. As larger fish consume smaller fish, the mercury level bioaccumulates in the tissue of the larger fish, which can increase over time. Mercury levels can also vary based on the habits and diet of different fish species and their position on the food chain. Largemouth bass are popular game fish, although some folks consume them. As a large predator, largemouth bass eat other fish, such as medium-sized black crappie—also a predator—which is high in mercury. Thus, due to their diet, largemouth bass can have very high levels of mercury. Because mercury binds to a protein in fish muscles that is not weakened or destroyed through washing or cooking,

---

[8] Brooks and Brooks (1969).

[9] Mercury in Fish Q&A (2023).

anglers who overconsume these fish are at increased health risks. There are no signs in the Lumbee River Watershed to warn anglers of fish contamination, illustrating the long-standing neglect and disinvestment in Indigenous people's habitats, health, and livelihood at multiple levels.

4   The Disappearance of Fish Consumption Signs

When Jeff attended the University of North Carolina at Pembroke[10] during the 1990s, advisory signs were common at boat landings and "honey hole" fishing spots throughout the watershed. The signs cautioned anglers that rivers in the Great Pee Dee River Basin, including the Lumbee, Little Pee Dee, and Waccamaw, were under state and federal fish consumption advisories and that certain fish contained high levels of mercury. Consumption advisories varied based on a person's sex or age. For men, the advisory recommended limiting consumption of certain contaminated fish to a weekly or monthly basis. For women of childbearing age and children, the advisories were more restrictive, instructing minimal consumption of some fish and no consumption of certain species of contaminated fish. Over the last 25–30 years, the number of advisory markers has dwindled and become scarce. Questions about what happened to the signs are among the most frequent that locals ask. Most often, the questions come from Indian anglers

concerned about water quality and its impact on community health. Over the years, the fish consumption advisory signs weathered badly; some could not be read anymore, others likely fell from their location, and some were removed for unknown reasons. It is rare to find any signs still posted anywhere along the Lumbee River.

Concerned about people[11] who regularly consume fish high in mercury, Jeff decided to learn more about the current aspects of Lumbee fishing culture. Whether out sampling at the river or on a paddling trip, Jeff prioritized talking with anglers about their fishing habits. Gathering anecdotal information over the last few years, he learned that many anglers have favorite fishing spots while others explore the watershed to try out different swamp and river locations friends or family have recommended. Some folks release all the fish they catch, while others consume most. Many anglers devote one or more days a month to fishing, purposely taking time off work to relax and do something they enjoy. Jeff also gathered anglers' insights on the fish advisory signs in the Lumbee River Watershed. Some folks believed the lack of posted fish consumption advisory signs indicated that the mercury problem had been resolved or that the fish contamination levels were safe. Many assumed that even with fish contaminated with mercury, officials would not bother replacing the signs.

5   Community-Led Monitoring of the Lumbee River Watershed

At first glance, the disappearance of the fish consumption signs fails to call attention to the full scope of the problem—authorities' failure to monitor and report on water contamination. For Lumbee who frequent the waterways in the tribal homeland to fish for a meal as their ancestors did, there is little accessible and available information

---

[10]The University of North Carolina at Pembroke (UNCP) was founded in 1887 as a school for American Indians in Robeson County, North Carolina, known as the Croatan Normal School. Over the next century and with minimal input from the local Indian community, the North Carolina General Assembly changed the institution's name to Indian Normal School of Robeson County (1911), Cherokee Indian Normal School of Robeson County (1913), Pembroke State College for Indians (1941), Pembroke State College (1949), Pembroke State University (1969), and University of North Carolina at Pembroke (1996). From 1939 to 1953, the institution was the only state-supported 4-year college for Indians in the country (University of North Carolina at Pembroke, 2023).

[11]Although mercury fish contamination in the Lumbee River Basin affects many racial/ethnic groups, including Black, White, Latinx, and Tuscarora, this chapter focuses on the Lumbee people in the region who fish the river.

about levels of mercury contamination, the least and most dangerous fish to consume, the amount of fish consumption that is safe, and the people most vulnerable to excess consumption. To advocate for cleaner water and improved health protections, locals—including the Lumbee Riverkeeper—have taken actions to better understand, manage, and restore the Lumbee River Watershed. In his work, Jeff blends Indigenous and Western methods to assess the water quality and gather traditional knowledge from Indigenous folks. He often draws on his knowledge of collaborative ethnography, a research method emphasizing a conscious, engaging, and equitable ongoing dialogue and collaboration between a folklorist and an individual or community consultant(s). He also applies community-based participatory research (CBPR) principles, a model approach for working with Indigenous communities and growing effective partnerships [14]. CBPR is an inclusive and collaborative process where communities equally contribute to all aspects of a research project, including the design, interpretation, and dissemination of data [15]. From an Indigenous perspective, CBPR respects the following principles: (1) Indigenous knowledge is valid and valued; (2) culture is always part of research; thus, research cannot be culturally neutral; (3) responsible stewardship includes learning how to interpret and understand data and research; (4) tribes must exercise sovereignty when conducting research and managing data; (5) research must benefit Native people.[12]

Using principles related to CBPR, the Equity, Access, Usability, and eXchange (EAUX) framework offers a similar yet unique way of addressing contamination issues through a water-related lens [12]. The water-focused acronym EAUX encapsulates the significance of equitable and ethical approaches to collaborating with Indigenous communities, particularly when weaving together Indigenous and Western knowledge systems. In "EAUX," the "E" signifies "equity," emphasizing the significance of respecting diverse knowledge systems. This involves

maintaining humility, being receptive to various ways of understanding, and questioning colonial structures prioritizing Western knowledge. "A" stands for "access," indicating that collaborative projects should honor data sovereignty and cultural and intellectual property to ensure access for all. "U" represents "usability," signifying that the project aims to benefit Indigenous Peoples, with partners responding to community needs. Lastly, "X" underscores the significance of partnership "eXchanges." This emphasizes the need for continuous communication among project partners, prior and ongoing informed consent, and the building and nurturing of relationships.

Applying these principles, Jeff is partnering with the tribal community in response to a community-specific need related to mercury contamination, a serious water issue endangering the lives and livelihoods of the Lumbee. Because of their historical presence and complex connections with ancestral waterways in the region, approval and input from the tribal community in the planning and design were critical in shaping the water project. Prioritizing tribal input in these early stages guarantees the project's relevance, credibility, and benefit to the tribal community. It also ensures the *usability* of information in collective decision-making when investigating and addressing water-related issues in tribal areas. Grounded in reciprocity and shared responsibility, this collaborative approach forges an *equitable* partnership with Indigenous peoples that honors and preserves traditional knowledge and tribal sovereignty. It also encourages equal power among partners. Employed by a nonprofit, non-Native-led organization[13] based outside of a tribal community, Jeff has learned the importance of navigating power imbalances in his relationships with partners. In addition to anticipating and balancing power structures, Jeff has worked to build and cultivate meaningful and trusting relationships. He has found that establishing trust requires physical, mental, and emotional effort, which translates to being transparent, present, and willing to participate, share, learn, and inter-

---

[12]For, NCAI Policy Research Center and MSU Center (2012).

[13]A Lumbee Tribal Member serves on the Board of Directors.

act with the community. It demands time, patience, humility, and the willingness to let go of self (ego) and notions (likely flawed) of what must be and how things should proceed. Working as partners also requires the continuous *eXchange* of information throughout a project's entire process. Jeff relies on ongoing and open dialogue with tribal communities in co-developing sampling protocols and procedures and determining data ownership, management, and sharing agreements. Sharing power and project ownership demonstrates respect for Indigenous data sovereignty. It also ensures tribal *access* and community rights to relevant findings that are accurately interpreted, which helps protect tribal communities from the enduring harms of unethical research. This illustrative example draws on the overlapping principles of CBPR and EAUX, which, we firmly believe, lays the groundwork for ethical and equitable community-led water projects in Southeast Indian Country.

Water is vital to Indigenous People's health and well-being, yet this critical element is often disregarded in programmatic efforts to address avoidable health inequities. In response to the growing challenges tribal communities encounter in securing clean water, Indigenous scientists and activists are acting to tackle water-related issues within these communities. Here, we demonstrate the use of Indigenous-aligned principles (i.e., CBPR and EAUX) in a collaborative planning project to address mercury contamination of fish and fish consumption guidelines in the Lumbee River Watershed. In this example, collaborative and continuous engagement with the tribal community helped ensure the project reflected the historical, social, and cultural underpinnings of fishing and water-related activities in the area. It was crucial that its impact reach deep into the community of Indigenous anglers who fish the waterways from boats, banks, or bridges. This example illustrates one approach to applying such principles to support community-led programs that restore culturally significant waterways and improve the health and well-being of Indigenous people. Overall, this chapter is intended as a resource for scholars, academics, and community partners engaged in the co-production of projects that aim to protect water, restore ecosystems, and sustain cultural resources. We consider the outlined principles foundational in water-related projects. They are an essential first step in ethical and responsible work, ensuring respect for Indigenous Peoples' connections with water systems. Applying these principles is crucial in bringing together diverse partners with varying knowledge systems to yield a well-designed project focused on understanding the community's needs and priorities. Ending with Jeff's words, we can then "better respond to any water quality impacts on the health and well-being of Indigenous people and the places they value."

References

1. Christensen L, Damon S. Social determinants of health and response to disease associated with health outcomes of American Indian and Alaska Native patients. JAMA Netw Open. 2022;5(3):e224827. https://doi.org/10.1001/jamanetworkopen.2022.4827.
2. Institute of Medicine (US) Committee on Assuring the Health of the Public in the 21st Century. The future of the public's health in the 21st century. Washington, DC: National Academies Press (US); 2002. https://www.ncbi.nlm.nih.gov/books/NBK221239/.
3. Craft A, King L. Building the Treaty #3 Nibi declaration using an Anishinaabe methodology of ceremony, language and engagement. Water. 2021;13(4):1–15. https://doi.org/10.3390/w13040532.
4. Martin C, Simonds VW, Young SL, Doyle J, Lefthand M, Eggers MJ. Our relationship to water and experience of water insecurity among Apsáalooke (Crow Indian) People, Montana. Int J Environ Res Public Health. 2021;18(2):582. https://doi.org/10.3390/ijerph18020582.
5. Parsons M, Fisher K. Indigenous peoples and transformations in freshwater governance and management. Curr Opin Environ Sustain. 2020;44:124–39. https://doi.org/10.1016/j.cosust.2020.03.006.
6. Whyte K. Settler colonialism, ecology, and environmental injustice. Environ Soc. 2018;9:125–44. https://www.jstor.org/stable/26879582.

7. Credo J, Torkelson J, Rock T, Ingram JC. Quantification of elemental contaminants in unregulated water across western Navajo Nation. International Journal of Environmental Research and Public Health. 2019;16(15):2727. https://doi.org/10.3390/ijerph16152727.

8. Powers M, Yracheta J, Harvey D, O'Leary M, Best LG, Black Bear A, MacDonald L, Susan J, Hasan K, Thomas E, Morgan C, Olmedo P, Chen R, Rule A, Schwab K, Navas-Acien A, George CM. Arsenic in groundwater in private wells in rural North Dakota and South Dakota: Water quality assessment for an intervention trial. Environmental Research. 2019;168:41–47. https://doi.org/10.1016/j.envres.2018.09.016.

9. Billiot S, Mitchell FM. Conceptual interdisciplinary model of exposure to environmental changes to address indigenous health and well-being. Public Health. 2019;176:142–8. https://doi.org/10.1016/j.puhe.2018.08.011.

10. Meltzer GY, Watkins BX, Vieira D, Zelikoff JT, Boden-Albala B. A systematic review of environmental health outcomes in selected American Indian and Alaska Native populations. J Racial Ethn Health Disparities. 2020;7(4):698–739. https://doi.org/10.1007/s40615-020-00700-2.

11. Tanana H, Combs J, Hoss A. Water is life: law, systemic racism, and water security in Indian country. Health Secur. 2021;19(S1):S78–82. https://doi.org/10.1089/hs.2021.0034.

12. Mehltretter S, Longboat S, Luby B, Bradford. Indigenous and western knowledge: Bringing diverse understandings of water together in practice (Technical Report), Global Commission on the Economics of Water, Paris. 2023. Retrieved from https://www.waterjusticehub.org/wp-content/uploads/2023/03/Mehltretter.pdf.

13. Maxwell W. The Back Swamp drainage project, Robeson County, North Carolina: biopolitical intervention in the lives of Indian farmers. Water History. 2017;9:9–28. https://doi.org/10.1007/s12685-016-0176-8.

14. Saunkeah B, Beans JA, Peercy MT, Hiratsuka VY, Spicer P. Extending research protections to tribal communities. Am J Bioethics. 2021;21(10):5–12. https://doi.org/10.1080/15265161.2020.1865477.

15. Israel BA, Schulz AJ, Parker EA, Becker AB. Review of community-based research: assessing partnership approaches to improve public health. Annu Rev Public Health. 1998;19:173–202.

Jada Lynn Brooks, PhD, MPSH, RN, FAAN, is an Associate Professor at the University of North Carolina at Chapel Hill School of Nursing and the Carol Morde Ross Distinguished Term Scholar of Psychiatric-Mental Health Nursing. She holds a PhD and ABSN from Duke University, an MSPH from the University of North Carolina at Chapel Hill, and a BS in Biology and Chemistry with Biomedical Emphasis from the University of North Carolina at Pembroke. She completed postdoctoral training at the University of North Carolina at Chapel Hill. As an enrolled member of the Lumbee Tribe of North Carolina, Dr. Brooks conducts community-engaged research focusing on environmental conditions that shape health outcomes and inequalities among American Indians. Dr. Brooks is recognized for her scientific contributions and nursing leadership in advancing Indigenous health equity as a Fellow of the American Academy of Nursing and a member of Class VII (2018–2020) of the UNC Thorp Faculty Engaged Scholars program. She is also co-Director of UNC Rural, an Office of the Provost program founded in 2019 that connects rural community-campus partners across North Carolina.

Jefferson Currie II, an enrolled member of the Lumbee Tribe of North Carolina and a native North Carolinian, holds a BA in American Indian/Native American Studies from the University of North Carolina at Pembroke. He is pursuing an MA in Folklore Studies at the University of North Carolina at Chapel Hill. Jefferson worked for over 10 years at the North Carolina Museum of History in Raleigh as a curator, historian, and researcher for exhibits and educational programs. He has worked on projects about textile mills, civil rights, music, fishing traditions, plants and gardening, and labor communities, many of them with North Carolina's seven state-recognized tribes. Currently, Jefferson is the Lumber Riverkeeper working with local community partners to protect and improve water quality for the health of the Lumber River watershed, its imperiled ecosystems, and the diverse communities of people living along its waterways. Tackling an onslaught of polluting industries from CAFOs to biomass and biogas projects while working for clean and healthy groundwater and surface waters, Jefferson's work is grounded in the principles of inclusion, collaboration, equity, and justice. He is thankful that he can work in his tribal territory along the branches and swamps of the Lumber River, in diverse communities, with folks who teach him daily about important things such as passion, patience, and persistence.

Community-Based Environmental Protection: Grassroots Approaches to Advance Environmental Justice and Health Equity

Na'Taki Osborne Jelks

What if our society was sustainable and just—one in which access to basic amenities like clean air to breathe and clean water to drink, access to healthy foods, and healthy living and working environments were afforded to every member of our society regardless of race or class? No one, and particularly those in economically disadvantaged households, would have to make trade-offs with respect to paying for utilities, such as electricity and water, over providing food for their families. Broad-based, strategic, and solutions-focused action to address the root causes of climate change would be underway, and those who contribute the least to the problem would no longer suffer the most from it. In this society, one's zip code would not be the best determinant of health status, educational attainment, and wealth, and the informal community designation, "the other side of the tracks," would have no meaning except a literal one. Imagine our society with no disparities in access to quantity and quality of public services and amenities, and those most impacted by the implementation of policy and urban and rural practice are meaningfully and authentically engaged in decision-making. In our society, race would no longer be a valid predictor

in identifying the location of toxic and hazardous wastes, and everyone would have a fair and just opportunity to achieve their full health potential.

While efforts to advance health equity, address the climate crisis, fight environmental racism, and reduce the wealth gap are supported with an intensity and intentionality never seen before on the federal level, this just and sustainable society is still more possible in our imaginations than it is in reality. As a community leader, activist, and environmental justice researcher with Mississippi roots and lived experience in Louisiana's "Cancer Alley" corridor, I am keenly aware that place matters. This rings true in terms of the location of pollution-generating facilities; which communities have access to quality schools; the existence of amenities such as parks, green space, and open space; and investment in infrastructure in communities. Furthermore, as a 20-plus-year West Atlanta, Georgia, resident and self-proclaimed "Westside griot," I can attest to stories of place, space, and inequities that more than affirm this notion and a closely related concept—all places were not created equal. In urban spaces, the built environment—man-made settings that shape human activity (from infrastructure and buildings, parks, and planned green space to restaurants and grocery stores)—can have a significant impact on the health of communities. The way that communities are designed, their unique features and characteristics, and the opportunities that exist therein for physical activity, recreation,

N. O. Jelks (✉)
Department of Environmental and Health Sciences, Spelman College, Atlanta, GA, USA

West Atlanta Watershed Alliance, Atlanta, GA, USA
e-mail: noborne@spelman.edu

and healthy food consumption can impact individual choice and behaviors that, in turn, influence health outcomes.

1   The Peril of Place

Social and environmental determinants of health are place-based phenomena that can either promote or detract from health. A growing body of evidence points to the zip code as the single best predictor of one's future health, wealth, and well-being [1]. Data from across the United States has revealed huge differences in life expectancy in neighborhoods in the same geographic locales, particularly in urban settings—in many cases revealing the wicked problem of intersecting racial, spatial, and health disparities [2–4].

Dr. Camara Phyllis Jones, a physician, public health expert, and leading scholar on the study of racism and health, writes about the three levels of racism: institutionalized, personally mediated, and internalized racism. Of these three, institutionalized racism, because of its far-reaching and systemic nature, is the most pervasive. Jones [5] defined institutionalized racism as "…differential access to the goods, services, and opportunities of society, by race" (p. 1212). It is ubiquitous in American society in that it has been codified in our institutions of custom, practice, and law. Identifying a specific culprit is not necessary. Jones further describes institutionalized racism as inaction in the face of need. It manifests itself both in material conditions and in access to power such as differential access to quality education, healthy housing, steady employment that pays a livable wage, suitable medical facilities, and a clean environment. It is further operationalized as differential access to information (including one's own history), resources such as wealth and organizational infrastructure, and voice (including voting rights, representation in government, and control of the media). Institutionalized racism explains the association between social class and race—an association that originated with distinct historical events. It persists, however, because of present-day structural factors that perpetuate historical injustices (p. 1212).

1.1   The Indelible Imprint of Redlining

Redlining, a practice codified into law by the US government-sponsored Home Owners' Loan Corporation (HOLC), is a demonstration of institutionalized racism at play. It refers to the practice of denying access to credit based on the demographic composition of one's neighborhood [6]. In the wake of the Great Depression as a part of President Franklin Delano Roosevelt's New Deal, the US government created the HOLC as an emergency agency to implement measures to limit foreclosures and stabilize the housing market. The HOLC did this, in part, through loaning billions of dollars to thousands of American homeowners and transforming and standardizing the manner in which property was appraised. Most notably, the HOLC established a system to assess neighborhood creditworthiness that was tied to the creation of HOLC residential security maps for more than 200 US cities to identify and rank the riskiness of lending across neighborhoods therein [7]. As a result, neighborhoods were systematically ranked based on risk-based housing-related factors such as age of housing stock, quality, occupancy, and prices, along with access to transportation, and proximity to amenities like parks or environmentally unwanted land uses such as polluting industries. Furthermore, non-housing-related demographic factors were considered such as neighborhood racial and ethnic composition, immigration status, and socioeconomic status as well as the employment status of residents and the percentage of renters in the community [6–8]. In essence, the HOLC's system for assessing neighborhood creditworthiness and the value of the homes therein was largely influenced by the documentation of specific social factors such as race, ethnicity, and economic class. Neighborhoods were graded by an A to D designation with the lowest ranking areas in each city identified as "hazardous." These undesirable areas were colored in red on the maps, and they were largely correlated with the areas with the highest percentage of Black residents. Other neighborhoods were color-coded in green for the "best" locations, while blue was used to designate those areas that were, "still desirable," and the areas colored in yellow were characterized as "definitely declining" [7].

Although the HOLC was rendered defunct by 1954, and the Fair Housing Act was passed in 1968, the effects of redlining persist. The Fair Housing Act also eliminated racially restrictive covenants, language inserted into warranty deeds to prevent people of color from purchasing or even occupying certain properties; however much of the segregation in housing that these practices created continues to exist today across the country [9, 10]. These types of racially motivated policies and practices that were implemented decades ago, shape place, spatial, racial, economic, and health inequities—essentially serving as pre-existing conditions that render places, populated by people of color and low-income populations, toxic and degraded sacrifice zones [11].

1.2 Environmental Racism, Residential Segregation, and Health

According to Dr. Robert Bullard, widely acknowledged as the father of environmental justice, environmental racism "…refers to any environmental policy, practice or directive that differentially affects or disadvantages (whether intended or unintended) individuals, groups or communities based on race or color" [12]. While some scholars believe that there must be a consensus on definitions with respect to how environmental racism and injustices manifest themselves to adequately address these challenges, others argue that environmental racism and injustices are contextual and that they are understood and experienced differently across community types, geographies, and social, political, and institutional contexts. Furthermore, environmental racism spans beyond disproportionate exposure to environmental toxicants and environmentally unwanted land uses that Black and other people of color in the United States experience. It also refers to inadequate investment in community infrastructure and long-term divestment of public resources in urban neighborhoods and rural spaces heavily populated by people of color, lax code enforcement, and gentrification and displacement in the aftermath of community cleanup and revitalization [13].

Due to the influence of racism on both urban and rural planning in the United States, many US communities are segregated along racial and economic lines. Residential segregation has been associated with differential experiences of community stress, exposure to pollutants, and access to community resources [14]. Furthermore, there is evidence that demonstrates that racial residential segregation is a fundamental determinant of racial disparities in health [15]. Authors of the 2020 study, *Poisonous Homes: The Fight for Environmental Justice in Federally Assisted Housing*, indicated that an estimated 70,000 federal public housing residents are at risk from environmental health threats because of where they live. Of the more than five million families across the United States who live in federal public housing, the majority are Black, Latinx, children, people with disabilities, and other groups who are most vulnerable to exposure to environmental hazards. The study also reported that although the US Environmental Protection Agency (EPA) and the US Department of Housing and Urban Development (HUD) released data in 2017 that more than 70% of this country's Superfund sites were located within 1 mile of federal public housing [16], little has been done to protect the residents in these environmentally degraded communities.

Public health and social science studies have shown that living in close proximity to environmental hazards including hazardous waste sites, industrial sites, high traffic roadways, and gas stations and repair shops leads to an increased risk for adverse health outcomes [17–20]. Low-income and communities of color often live in the worst conditions that subsequently impact the intensity of poor health outcomes therein [21]. Poor environmental quality found in communities of color has the most significant impact on those whose health status is already at risk [22]. Exposure to unhealthy environmental conditions contributes greatly to producing and maintaining health disparities.

2   Community-Based Environmental Protection: A Primer

In response to the rampant inequality that dots both the United States and our global landscape, particularly with respect to environmental factors, countless communities have long taken these critical matters into their own hands. They have not waited on government to solve their problems. They have not accepted the status quo as their destiny and have challenged the current limitations of their realities with the understanding that the just, sustainable society they seek is only achieved when those who are most vulnerable to environmental racism and other societal ills can prosper. In the context of environmental injustice, this resistance to the toxic realities that many communities experience has been embodied, in part, as community-based environmental protection by community residents, leaders, grassroots organizations, activists, and advocates. In alignment with the fourth principle of environmental justice that "...affirms the fundamental right to political, economic, cultural and environmental self-determination of all peoples" [23], communities have built power and used diverse strategies, tactics, and approaches to advance self-determined environmental and community change outcomes.

According to the US Environmental Protection Agency (US EPA), community-based environmental protection (CBEP) is "...action that local individuals and groups take to address their own environmental concerns" [24]. Low-income and communities of color and other historically environmentally overburdened communities have often found that such actions are their only recourse in the wake of disproportionate exposure to environmental hazards, a long history of unequal protection despite the existence of environmental laws and policies [25], lack of authentic community engagement on the part of government actors, and exclusion from environmental decision-making processes [26]. In its resource book on CBEP, US EPA also asserts that strategies and plans using this approach consider local social, economic, and environmental conditions alongside community values—creating a sense of local ownership of issues and solutions, thereby encouraging accountability and long-term community support [24].

The cries of community-based organizations and individuals living in neighborhoods disproportionately affected by environmental hazards and the vestiges of racism in planning and public policy align with the concepts of CBEP and the premise that those most affected by environmental and racial injustices are at the forefront of developing the solutions. Yet, often, these same groups and individuals are denied access to decision-making tables and left completely out of implementing the change processes that will remedy what ails them. Those most impacted then have no other choice but to act on their own—building community power and leadership; diagnosing their challenges; advancing innovative approaches to shift the dusts of change in the places where they live, work, play, worship, and learn; and creating just sustainable and healthy futures. In this chapter, we will specifically discuss four approaches to community-based environmental protection pursued by local residents and community-based organizations working to secure self-determined community outcomes: (1) environmental justice advocacy, (2) environmental education, (3) environmental stewardship, and (4) community science and other participatory approaches to research.

3   Environmental Justice Advocacy

The US Environmental Protection Agency (US EPA) defines environmental justice as "...the fair treatment and meaningful involvement of all people regardless of race, color, national origin, or income, with respect to the development, implementation, and enforcement of environmental laws, regulations, and policies" [27]. The US EPA also asserts that environmental justice is realized when all people can achieve "the same degree of protection from environmental and health hazards, and equal access to the decision-making process to have a healthy environment in which to live, learn, and work" [28].

Commonly, grassroots justice organizations and environmentally overburdened consider a wholistic definition of the environment—noting both the natural and built environments and the manner in which the physical conditions of the spaces in which people live, work, play, worship, and learn can impact health and well-being. In this context, environmental justice advocacy is focused on the right that all people, regardless of race, ethnicity, income level, or geography, have to breathe clean air, drink clean water, consume healthy and affordable food grown in healthy soils, work in toxic-free workplaces, live in toxic-free communities, be protected from environmental harms in schools and places of worship, have an equitable share of health-promoting amenities in their communities, and have a place at the decision-making tables that create and inform policies that govern our everyday lives.

The environmental justice movement was catapulted into the national spotlight in 1982 with protests, mass acts of civil disobedience, and over 500 arrests in Warren County, North Carolina, as Black residents in this rural and predominantly Black community laid their bodies across a road to block the delivery of hazardous wastes into a landfill and the subsequent publication of *Toxic Waste and Race in the United States* [29], the landmark publication and first cross-sectional study to demonstrate the positive association between demographics and the location of uncontrolled hazardous waste facilities. The study revealed that race was the strongest predictor of where said environmentally unwanted land uses were located—topping out all other factors examined including income level [29, 30].

Environmental justice advocacy can also be traced back to the last mission of Dr. Martin Luther King, Jr prior to his death. When Dr. King was assassinated in Memphis, Tennessee, on April 4, 1968, he had been there in support of Black sanitation workers who were striking because of hazardous working conditions and low wages [30]. Lesser-known accounts of environmental justice advocacy abound in both popular culture and peer-reviewed literature that

amplify the leadership of grassroots environmental justice leaders and organizations fighting for the human right to safe drinking water and sanitation, the cleanup of hazardous waste sites located in close proximity to communities, elimination of toxic air emissions from polluting industries, denial of permits to site pollution-generating facilities in low-income and communities of color, and anti-gentrification and anti-displacement strategies when community greening projects threaten the well-being of long-time residents. Before the term community-based environmental protection was coined, communities disproportionately exposed to environmental stressors were enacting strategies to reduce or eliminate said harmful exposures as well as gain access to the decision-making tables whose actions help determine the fate of their communities.

4   Environmental Stewardship

Environmental education is commonly touted for its potential to instill a sense of stewardship toward the environment. Environmental stewardship, responsible use and protection of natural resources through conservation, active restoration activities, and other sustainable practices [31, 32], is often associated with the modern-day US conservation movement; however, its roots can be found in the ways that Indigenous people have previously lived in harmony with and cared for the land and waters of their traditional homelands [33]. Environmental stewardship practices can benefit both ecosystem and human health and can encompass a wide range of actions and activities such as, but not limited to, planting and replanting trees, restoring wildlife habitat, creating protected areas, establishing and maintaining community gardens, reducing harmful consumption behaviors that cause pollution and other activities that deplete natural resources faster than they can be regenerated, land and waterway cleanups, restoring environmentally degraded areas, and removing invasive plants. Furthermore, in the context of environmental stewardship, the concept of stewardship science refers to actions taken by individuals or groups to collect and report data obtained through monitoring environmental conditions to inform management of the applicable nature resource (i.e., water, air, or soil quality, etc.) [34].

In communities fighting environmental harm and degradation, environmental stewardship can take on a triple role of protection, conservation, and restoration of the natural resources in the context of specific geographic areas. It encompasses active management of land and waterways. Environmental stewardship in communities can look like creating community gardens for purposes of community greening, beautification, and meeting local food security needs. It is practiced through community-based monitoring of air and water resources as well as soil testing to identify potential contaminants. Planting and replanting trees is sometimes pursued to help cool communities by helping to reduce the urban heat island effect in cities, a phenomenon, that often disproportionately affects historically redlined and other communities with large populations of people of color [35].

5   Environmental Education

In addition to environmental justice advocacy and environmental stewardship, environmental education is also a tool that is critical to the enactment of community-based environmental protection. The US Environmental Protection Agency defines environmental education as "…a process that allows individuals to explore environmental issues, engage in problem-solving, and take action to improve the environment" [36]. There are five key components to environmental education: (1) awareness and sensitivity to the environment and environmental challenges, (2) knowledge and understanding of the environment and environmental challenges, (3) attitudes of concern for the environment and motivation to improve or maintain environmental quality, (4) skills to identify and help resolve environmental challenges, and (5) participation in activities that lead to the resolution of environmental challenges. Unlike environmental and environmental

justice advocacy, no particular viewpoint or course of action is advocated for in the delivery of environmental education; however individuals are taught to critically consider competing perspectives associated with an issue or challenge—a process that both enhances problem-solving and decision-making skills [36].

While environmental education is generally associated with K–12 audiences, particularly given efforts across the United States to integrate it into state-level and national education standards, the delivery and engagement of environmental education programs can span across age ranges. Dominant approaches to environmental education tend to place a disproportionate emphasis on environmental problem-solving from a perspective of individual behavior change and choice versus a more collective or community-relevant approach [37]. Historically, however, environmental education initially focused more broadly on themes such as, but not limited to, pollution, depletion of natural resources, and environmental degradation [38]. In the context of community-based environmental protection, the field's historical roots align with the potential for environmental education to play a key role in raising public awareness about pressing environmental concerns as well as fostering engagement in problem-solving and action for change to address said concerns from a community perspective and not solely from an individual perspective.

6   Community Science and Other Participatory Research Approaches to Research

When conditions are appropriate, communities can empower themselves to advance just, resilient, healthy, and sustainable futures through community-engaged processes such as community-owned and community-managed research, community-based participatory research, collaborative problem-solving, and partnerships between communities and healthcare providers [39]. Promising practices implemented by community-based organizations and a myriad of partners, from academic institutions to health practitioners, have yielded success in helping to secure basic amenities in underserved communities; address unequal climate change burdens; connect kids and families to nature as a tool for health promotion; and revitalize polluted spaces into healthy landscapes.

Federal agencies such as the National Institute of Environmental Health Sciences and the US Environmental Protection Agency have begun to acknowledge the role and potential of participatory approaches to research. The US EPA defines participatory science as an approach that "… engages the public in advancing scientific knowledge by formulating research questions, collecting data, and interpreting results" [40]. Of the benefits of participatory science approaches, those that are most salient in the context of community-based environmental protection include the potential to fill in important gaps in knowledge with respect to environmental challenges impacting communities, improving public understanding of environmental issues and the actions needed to address them, as well as creating stronger and more inclusive networks to advance environmental problem-solving.

Other terms such as community science have been used to define the leadership of communities impacted by environmental injustices and related public health challenges to engage in research endeavors that seek both to advance generalizable knowledge and to advance environmental, community, or systems change. Community science starts with challenges and research questions of importance to communities and elevates local community knowledge, traditional ecological knowledge, and the lived experiences of community members over that of academics and other experts [41].

Before recent terminology to describe these activities that both improve community capacity to engage in research and help to democratize the practice of science, communities have been on the ground advancing a diverse range of approaches to lessen the gap with respect to environmental health disparities.

7 Community-Based Environmental Protection: Leadership from the Grassroots in Atlanta, Georgia

In the United States and particularly in the Southeast, low-income and communities of color are disproportionately impacted by climate change hazards and risks in addition to a plethora of overlapping environmental injustices associated with cumulative exposures to environmental hazards, disproportionate exposure to extreme heat in historically redlined neighborhoods, pre-existing conditions in the form of aged wastewater systems and inadequate stormwater infrastructure, social vulnerability produced by centuries of institutionalized racism codified through urban planning and practice, and exclusion from meaningful access to decision-making tables where solutions are being developed to address long-standing wastewater and stormwater challenges, advance climate resilience, and improve health and quality of life. Atlanta, Georgia, and, in particular, West Atlanta communities are both a demonstration of these phenomena and also an important site of resistance, community-informed policymaking, and action to advance environmental, policy, and systems change.

Atlanta is known by many names, "Hotlanta," the Black Mecca, birthplace of the Civil Rights Movement, and the city too busy to hate, and the list continues. Despite these monikers, Atlanta has been a posterchild for income inequality—in fact, it is the worst in the nation [42], and this distinction has persisted for at least a decade [43]. Stemming from historic and systemic racial discrimination, the legacy of redlining and other discriminatory public policies has compounded this reality. West Atlanta communities have been ground zero for income inequality and many of its associated challenges such as disproportionate exposure to environmental hazards [44] and the lowest life expectancy in the Atlanta region [2]. In direct response to these realities, community-based organizations on Atlanta's

Westside have sought to address these long-standing atrocities [45].

The work of community-based organization, the West Atlanta Watershed Alliance (WAWA), is illustrative of a four-pronged approach to operationalizing community-based environmental protection, particularly through environmental justice advocacy, environmental education, environmental stewardship, and community science and other forms of participatory research. WAWA serves low-wealth and communities of color in the Proctor, Utoy, and Sandy Creek Watersheds of Northwest and Southwest Atlanta—those overburdened with environmental stressors but often least represented at environmental decision-making tables. Established in the aftermath of successful community efforts to change the course of discriminatory wastewater treatment practices in West Atlanta, WAWA has grown to become an impactful force in community-centered sustainable development. For over 25 years, WAWA has pioneered efforts to advance environmental education, community science efforts, community engagement in watershed and green space protection and stewardship, and climate and environmental justice in Northwest and Southwest Atlanta neighborhoods. WAWA helps to set conditions that enable residents to empower themselves and elevate their voices to be advocates for their communities and press for environmental, community, and systems change. While WAWA and much of its work are locally based, the organization sits at important regional, statewide, and even national tables where its impact is felt and acknowledged.

WAWA's mission is to improve the quality of life within the West Atlanta Watershed by protecting, preserving, and restoring the community's natural resources. The organization believes that a healthy environment is a key ingredient for a healthy community, and its grassroots approach to organizing, research, community science, and education elevates local community knowledge and lived experiences, enabling residents to diagnose and solve their environmental challenges. WAWA envisions (1) a community that protects their watersheds and recognizes and *appreciates* their important connections to these vital resources; (2) informed and engaged residents who fully participate in decision-making on issues that impact environmental quality, health, and community well-being; and (3) strong and equitable environmental protections. The organization also seeks to be a trusted thought leader and primary resource for West Atlanta communities seeking to advance environmental, community, and systems change.

WAWA gets results for and with West Atlanta communities through grassroots organizing and advocacy; creating and delivering placed-based, culturally relevant and responsive environmental education to Pre-K to gray community audiences; engaging in community science and other participatory research approaches; and facilitating community-led environmental protection strategies and hands-on land and watershed stewardship.

7.1 Advancing Environmental Justice on Atlanta's Westside

Since its start, WAWA's goals and objectives have been designed to elevate the voices, harness collective grassroots power, and increase the efficacy of West Atlanta residents to advance self-determined outcomes for environmental community challenges in the context of pollution and the hyperlocal impacts of climate change and poor infrastructure including increased precipitation, urban flooding, polluting wastewater systems, and inadequate stormwater management. WAWA was founded by and continues to be led primarily by Black community members from Northwest and Southwest Atlanta—communities that are highly impacted by income inequality, disproportionate exposure to environmental hazards, inadequate public education, and health disparities. Its origin story is tied to a history of racialized politics and policies that have shaped current-day inequities with respect to wastewater and stormwater infrastructure, economic development, public education investments, enforcement of environmental policies, utility burden (water and energy), food insecurity, and a host of other factors that render West Atlanta communities vulnerable in the face of new urban development schemes and climate change.

Upon its founding, WAWA engaged in environmental justice advocacy in the tradition of Southwest Atlanta residents in Atlanta's Utoy Creek Watershed who successfully advocated to avert both the siting of a mini wastewater treatment plant in a community park and the construction of an 8-mile sewage tunnel slated to convey wastes from the north side of town and a neighboring jurisdiction through Southwest Atlanta for treatment. Building on these major victories, WAWA later joined forces with West Atlanta residents and partners from across Atlanta neighborhoods to successfully advocate for the closure of one of the Proctor Creek Watershed's combined sewer overflow control facilities and the separation of the sewer system in a portion of the watershed such that Proctor Creek, a waterway in West Atlanta that flows through and near residential yards, school grounds, and public parks, would no longer receive overflows of raw, untreated sewage during heavy rain events in the affected area.

In the vein of helping to shape infrastructure improvements in West Atlanta communities, WAWA also collaborates with community members to advocate for and invest in the cultivation of public-private-community partnerships to influence how public and private dollars are spent on projects that impact environmental quality, health, and quality of life in target watersheds. In line with its historical leadership of community-based efforts to clean up, protect, and restore Atlanta's Proctor Creek Watershed for its residents and downstream neighbors, WAWA was instrumental in getting the Proctor Creek Watershed designated as a US Environmental Protection Agency (US EPA) Urban Waters Federal Partnership site in 2013. Persistent advocacy, education of grasstops, and partnership cultivation with the US EPA led to the nomination and ultimate selection of Proctor Creek for the urban waters federal designation. This partnership is meant to "…reconnect urban communities, particularly those that are overburdened or economically distressed, with their waterways by improving coordination among federal agencies and collaborating with community-led revitalization efforts to improve our Nation's water systems and promote their economic, environmental, and social benefits," [46]. Proctor Creek is one of the most impaired waterways in Metro Atlanta, and its watershed is plagued by numerous social, economic, and health disparities. From 2013 until 2020, the urban waters designation brought new resources from a diverse array of federal agencies to focus on restoration of the watershed. New and previously unlikely partnerships began as agencies and national-level nonprofit organizations collaborated with WAWA and watershed residents to leverage financial and staff resources to prioritize community-led initiatives that address the watershed's varied environmental, economic, and social challenges [47]. Furthermore, as community members advocate for the implementation of community greening initiatives and other efforts aimed at improving the environmental conditions in their neighborhoods, WAWA has been a voice for equitable development and policy measures to slow down gentrification and displacement of legacy residents who deserve to reap the benefits of community change, in place, without being forced out after experiencing years of neglect and disinvestment.

7.2 Community-Led Environmental Stewardship in West Atlanta Communities

WAWA was established on the heels of the aforementioned two community victories to halt sewer infrastructure projects deemed harmful by Southwest Atlanta residents. As a twin strategy to its environmental justice advocacy efforts, WAWA began its environmental stewardship efforts through hosting intergenerational stewardship events—core activities in WAWA's work and community engagement efforts. Specific projects and their associated events have included neighborhood and creek and neighborhood cleanups in West Atlanta communities to address illegal dumping and nonpoint source pollution on the land and in local streams; storm drain stenciling (with "Don't dump…drains to stream" messages painted on neighborhood storm drain surfaces), adopt-a-drain efforts (cleaning out clogged storm drains), water quality monitoring, and watershed-focused service-learning initiatives for youth.

WAWA also trains community members to serve as stewards of the natural resources in their neighborhoods. Activating "Watershed Warriors" who learn how to conduct chemical, biological, and bacterial monitoring of local creeks and streams has been a long-standing role for the organization—helping it to enact community-based protection not only through environmental stewardship but also through environmental education and community science. Community efforts to monitor water quality and other environmental conditions have been instrumental in helping to bring government-funded cleanup efforts to West Atlanta communities.

Although water infrastructure issues were central to WAWA's formation, its watershed approach to environmental stewardship includes land stewardship. In 2008, WAWA signed a Memorandum of Understanding with the City of Atlanta Bureau of Parks, Recreation, and Cultural Affairs to operate the Atlanta Outdoor Activity Center (OAC) and to manage and serve as stewards of the 22-acre urban forest and a nature center, located in the heart of a low-to-moderate income, somewhat environmentally degraded, and underserved community in Southwest Atlanta. Active maintenance was severely lacking, and community programming was on life support when WAWA entered into its agreement with the City of Atlanta to operate the OAC. With the help of community residents, youth and community groups, corporations, foundations, and government agencies, WAWA has turned the forecast for the OAC around. Engaging hundreds of volunteers annually in tens of thousands of volunteer hours to help manage the OAC grounds, WAWA operated primarily on a sweat equity model to provide stewardship for the 22-acre urban forest and its accompanying nature center before growing the financial capacity to hire staff. Even, now, engagement of volunteers in

monthly Service Saturday programs as well as corporate service days and mass engagement service activities such as the annual MLK Day of Service help to greatly extend the capacity of staff members who work on a day-to-day basis to manage the OAC building and grounds. Under the supervision of WAWA staff members, volunteers remove invasive plants, plant trees, maintain hiking trails, plant in and maintain wildlife and food gardens, and repair bridges and boardwalks among other tasks. As an enhancement of its land stewardship activities, WAWA and local college students established an UGRO (Urban Garden Resiliency Oasis) Initiative to bring urban agriculture to the neighborhoods surrounding the OAC. During the COVID-19 pandemic, WAWA increased its food production to distribute fresh produce to food-insecure households in Bush Mountain, Oakland City, and other nearby Southwest and South Atlanta communities. This work has continued, and WAWA collaborates with community partners who also contribute fresh produce to help support WAWA's mutual aid efforts in the local community.

7.3 From Pre-K to Gray: Connecting West Atlanta Kids and Families to Nature Through Environmental Education

While WAWA's environmental stewardship efforts preceded its robust engagement in environmental education, it's approach to engaging kids of all ages in place-based, culturally relevant education about the world around us, and our relationship to the planet that sustains us, undergirds its work across all spectrums—from environmental justice advocacy to environmental stewardship and participatory approaches to research. Using the urban environment as a teaching tool, WAWA helps youth and adults connect to nature in their own backyards and in parks and green spaces across the Atlanta landscape. WAWA's stewardship role at the OAC goes hand in hand with its efforts to grow the site into a leading urban ecology center. WAWA's steward-ship and environmental education efforts at the OAC and other nearby green spaces are inextrica-bly linked to one another.

Established in 1975 as the Bush Mountain Outdoor Activity Center, the initial purpose of the OAC was to involve children and adults in environmental issues through education about conservation, ecology, and the natural environ-ment. Located just a few miles from downtown, the center had, in past years, been integral to the Atlanta Public Schools System as a location for field trips. Historically, the facility has been an asset and amenity as urban forest land within the largely single-family communities of Bush Mountain and Oakland City. The OAC is owned by the City of Atlanta's Department of Parks, Recreation, and Cultural Affairs but has histori-cally been operated by a third-party steward. Before WAWA became stewards of the space, the facility had operated marginally for nearly a decade under previous third-party stewards, and in 2007, the City of Atlanta Parks Department approached WAWA to move into the OAC to operate the community and school-based envi-ronmental education and civic engagement pro-gramming that it had been successful at for over 12 years without a permanent physical site from which to operate.

Because of WAWA's track record of working with a variety of groups from within the Black community as well as groups from the outside community to achieve significant conservation, environmental education, and environmental pro-tection victories, WAWA was seen as the most appropriate organization to revitalize the OAC and to make it the quality community and envi-ronmental education resource that it was long ago envisioned to be. Suffering from years of being under resourced and in some cases neglected, when WAWA moved into the OAC, the building and an outdoor tree house classroom were in des-perate need of repair. Furthermore, overgrown trails and acres of invasive plants covered the for-est, and no environmental education or other pro-gramming accessible to the surrounding community could be found. WAWA has breathed

new life into the OAC through both its environ-mental stewardship and environmental education efforts.

Building on the site's legacy, WAWA has worked to re-establish the OAC both as a site for nonformal education, through annual community events and programs, and as a site at which local schools can extend teaching from the classroom and into the outdoors. WAWA routinely conducts guided hikes, hands-on, inquiry-based learning experiences for local schools and youth groups, nature-based festivals, a nature-based camp pro-gram for youth, cultural programs that illuminate Black and Indigenous environmental practices, and outdoor recreation programs such as an annual family-centered overnight camping expe-rience. WAWA has also replicated its environ-mental stewardship and education programs to neighboring green spaces. In 2012, WAWA launched the Atlanta Children's Forest Network (ACFN) in collaboration with the USDA Forest Service and the US EPA to increase visitation to and provide nonformal environmental education, hands-on land and water stewardship, and pro-grams that promote physical activity in the out-doors for underserved communities on over 355 acres of publicly owned green space in Southwest Atlanta. This network of sites includes the OAC, the 135-acre Cascade Springs Nature Preserve, and the 200-acre Hampton-Beecher Preserve. As an all-volunteer group, WAWA spearheaded efforts to save the 200-acre Hampton-Beecher Preserve from development and raised over $2.5 million to do so before becoming a 501c(3) organization.

WAWA worked for 14 years to provide public access to the Cascade Springs Nature Preserve, a vibrant, 135-acre, city-owned green space that was previously only open to the public on Monday through Friday from 8:00 am to 3:00 pm when most members of the surrounding commu-nity do not have the opportunity to visit. WAWA petitioned the City of Atlanta Parks Department to open the preserve on evenings and weekends so that the surrounding community could have access to it. When they said that their budget would not allow for additional personnel to open the gates on Saturdays and Sundays, WAWA board members appealed to city officials to allow them to do it. After significant negotiating, the City turned over the keys, and WAWA board members showed up at the gate every Saturday and Sunday at 7 am and 7 pm to open and close the gate—completely changing access to this green community asset that was previously only open when members of our community were at work or school. When it first opened, countless stories were heard from neighbors of the preserve who lived in the community for 20–30 years who had never had an opportunity to go inside because it was never open when they weren't working or when their kids or grandchildren were not in school. More recently the City installed an electronic fence so WAWA board members no longer have to show up on Saturdays and Sundays to provide the community and broader public with access. WAWA also now partners with the newly formed Cascade Springs Nature Conservancy to co-steward the site as WAWA continues to provide education and outdoor recreation programs for surrounding communities and people from across the Atlanta region.

7.4 Taking Science to the Streets: Community Science and Other Participatory Approaches to Research in West Atlanta Communities

As a key approach to its community research, WAWA engages West Atlanta residents in environmentally overburdened neighborhoods to bring their local community knowledge and lived experiences to bear along with monitoring local environmental conditions to generate actionable data for community change. In doing so, WAWA and West Atlanta residents seek to develop effective interventions that revitalize toxic, degraded spaces into healthy places. Government agencies have not always been responsive to community concerns about pollution and infrastructure challenges and the health impacts that they influence. Through engaging in community science and other participatory approaches to research, com-

munity members both lead and collaborate with WAWA staff and academic partners in efforts to collect water and air quality data as well as well map the locations of environmental hazards, areas that routinely flood, and areas where the stormwater infrastructure is inoperable or otherwise compromised [48]. For example, WAWA, in collaboration with Proctor Creek Watershed residents and Georgia State University students, developed a Proctor Creek Citizen Science App. This Global Positioning System (GPS)-enabled digital data collection tool is used to spatially and visually document meaningful yet "hidden" street-level, environmental hazards in the Proctor Creek Watershed. Through a participatory approach, joint community-university teams used the app to map important attributes of the built environment that often go unaddressed in communities yet negatively influence environmental quality, health, and quality of life [49]. These hazards were not captured in publicly available databases and therefore received no attention by city, state, or federal authorities. Spatial narratives created with community-generated data exposed "hidden hazards" and helped West Atlanta residents get problem areas addressed.

In a related participatory research effort, West Atlanta residents used the photovoice method to explore local community knowledge and community perceptions of environmental health risks, assets, and community strengths in the Proctor Creek Watershed. Visual data was captured through photographs taken by ten Proctor Creek Watershed residents (Proctor Creek Watershed Researchers), and this data has been used to influence the development of policy recommendations and strategies to mitigate environmental risks to help improve health and quality of life in the Proctor Creek Watershed. These and other participatory research efforts have demonstrated the benefits derived from using community-generated visual and spatial data to examine community concerns [48]. Such approaches can help democratize decision-making and can alter power relations by putting powerful data in the hands of community residents to help prioritize and leverage action when issues go unseen or are consistently unaddressed. WAWA has also introduced participatory research approaches to staff at federal agencies—transforming a community-located biological monitoring project in the Proctor Creek Watershed to one that ultimately engaged community residents and local college students [50].

8   Conclusion

In the context of systemic racism, neglect, and disinvestment in low-income and communities of color that are overburdened with environmental hazards and risks, community-based environmental protection is often a necessary practice to help advance on-the-ground change in service of environmental justice and health equity. By leveraging assets and resources both within and outside of communities, individuals and grassroots organizations can integrate tools such as advocacy for environmental justice, environmental stewardship, environmental education, and participatory research to both envision and achieve cleaner, greener, healthier, and more sustainable futures.

True to its roots, WAWA continues to invest in efforts to develop grassroots leaders to play significant roles in advancing environmental justice and health equity. The organization's pursuit of justice, health, and well-being for West Atlanta communities is undergirded by its intergenerational environmental education and environmental stewardship work. WAWA is an example of a small, community-based organization that has leveraged its expertise, community assets, and partnership with community residents, stakeholders, and other community partners to become an impactful force in community-led and community-driven sustainable development.

References

1. Graham G. Why your ZIP code matters more than your genetic code: promoting healthy outcomes from mother to child. Breastfeed Med. 2016;11(8):396–7.
2. Brasch B, Peebles J. By neighborhood: how long on average a person lives in metro Atlanta. Atlanta J Constit. 2019; https://www.ajc.com/news/local/neighborhood-how-long-average-person-lives-metro-atlanta/n3FI2Ki1UfysL38SqS4kXK/.
3. Lartey J. 'It's totally unfair': Chicago, where the rich live 30 years longer than the poor. The Guardian. 2019; https://www.theguardian.com/us-news/2019/jun/23/chicago-latest-news-life-expectancy-rich-poor-inequality.
4. NYU Langone Health. City health dashboard. 2019. https://www.cityhealthdashboard.com/.
5. Jones CP. Levels of racism: a theoretic framework and a gardener's tale. Am J Public Health. 2000;90(8):1212–5. https://doi.org/10.2105/ajph.90.8.1212.
6. Aaronson D, Hartley D, Mazumder B. The effects of the 1930s HOLC "redlining" maps. Federal Reserve Bank of Chicago; 2019.
7. Mitchell B, Franco J. HOLC "redlining" maps: the persistent structure of segregation and economic opportunity. National Community Reinvestment Council; 2018. https://ncrc.org/wp-content/uploads/dlm_uploads/2018/02/NCRC-Research-HOLC-10.pdf.
8. ATLMaps. Home Owners' Loan Corporation. n.d. https://atlmaps.org/layers/e9i49.
9. Nelson RK, Ayers EL, editors. Mapping inequality. In: American panorama. Washington, DC: Racial Justice. https://dsl.richmond.edu/panorama/redlining/. Accessed 14 Oct 2023.
10. Bakelmun A, Shoenfeld SJ. Open data and racial segregation: mapping the historic imprint of racial covenants and redlining on American cities. In: Hawken S, Han H, Pettit C, editors. Open cities | open data. Singapore. Retrieved from:: Palgrave Macmillan; 2020. https://doi.org/10.1007/978-981-13-6605-5_3.
11. Lerner S. Sacrifice zones: the front lines of toxic chemical exposure in the United States. MIT Press; 2010.
12. Bullard RD. Dismantling Environmental Racism in the USA. Local Environ. 1999;4(1):5–19. Retrieved from:. https://doi.org/10.1080/13549839908725577.
13. Kern L, Kovesi C. Environmental justice meets the right to stay put: mobilising against environmental racism, gentrification, and xenophobia in Chicago's Little Village. Local Environ. 2018;23(9):952–66.
14. Gee GC, Payne-Sturges DC. Environmental health disparities: a framework integrating psychosocial and environmental concepts. Environ Health Perspect. 2004;112(17):1645–53.
15. Williams DR, Collins C. Racial residential segregation: a fundamental cause of racial disparities in health. Public Health Rep. 2001;116(5):404–16.
16. Coffey E, Walz K, Chizewer D, Benfer EA, Templeton MN, Weinstock R (2020) Poisonous homes: the fight for environmental justice in federally assisted housing. https://www.povertylaw.org/wp-content/uploads/2020/06/environmental_justice_report_final-rev2.pdf.
17. Brender JD, Maantay JA, Chakraborty J. Residential proximity to environmental hazards and

adverse health outcomes. Am J Public Health. 2011;101:S37–52.

18. Barnett AG, Plonka K, Seow WK, Wilson L-A, Hansen C. Increased traffic exposure and negative birth outcomes: a prospective cohort in Australia. Environ Health. 2011;10:26. Retrieved from: http://www.ehjournal.net/content/10/1/26

19. Canadian Institute for Health Information (CIHI). Urban physical environments and health inequalities: Factors influencing health. Ottawa: Ontario; 2010. Retrieved from: http://www.healthequity.umd.edu/documents/cphi_urban_physical_environments_en.pdf

20. Evans GW, Katrowitz E. Socioeconomic status and health: the potential role of environmental risk exposure. Annu Rev Public Health. 2002;23(1):303–31.

21. Bell J, Rubin V. Why place matters: building a movement for healthy communities. PolicyLink; 2007. http://www.policylink.org/sites/default/files/WHYPLACEMATTERS_FINAL.PDF.

22. Centers for Disease Control and Prevention (CDC). (2010). Environmental health. Healthy people 2020. Retrieved from: http://www.healthypeople.gov/subtopics-sdoh/environmentalhealth.

23. United Church of Christ Commission for Racial Justice (UCCCRJ), Nelson RK, Winling LD, Marciano R, Connolly N, et al. The Proceedings of the First National People of Color Environmental Leadership Summit. United Church of Christ Commission for Racial Justice; 1991.

24. United States Environmental Protection Agency (U.S. EPA). (1997). Community-based environmental protection: a resource book for protecting ecosystems and communities, (EPA 230-B-96-003), Washington, DC.

25. Lavelle M, Coyle M. Unequal protection: the racial divide in environmental law, a special investigation. Natl Law J S2, col. 1. 21 Sept 1992.

26. Jelks NO. Sewage in our backyards: the politics of race, class, + water in Atlanta, Georgia. Projections MIT J Plann. 2008;8:173–88.

27. United States Environmental Protection Agency (U.S. EPA). Learn about environmental justice. 2020. https://www.epa.gov/environmentaljustice/learn-about-environmental-justice.

28. United States Environmental Protection Agency (U.S. EPA). Environmental justice. 2021. https://www.epa.gov/environmentaljustice.

29. United Church of Christ Commission for Racial Justice (UCCCRJ). Toxic waste and race in the United States: a national report on the racial and socio-economic characteristics of communities with hazardous waste sites; 1987.

30. Bullard RD. Environmental justice in the 21st century: race still matters. Phylon. 2001;49(3/4):151–71.

31. Bennett NJ, Whitty TS, Finkbeiner E, Pittman J, Bassett H, Gelcich S, Allison EH. Environmental stewardship: a conceptual review and analytical framework. Environ Manag. 2018;61:597–614.

32. Chapin FS, Carpenter SR, Kofinas GP, Folke C, Abel N, Clark WC, Olsson P, Smith DMS, Walker B, Young OR, Berkes F, Biggs R, Grove JM, Naylor RL, Pinkerton E, Steffen W, Swanson FJ. Ecosystem stewardship: sustainability strategies for a rapidly changing planet. Trends Ecol Evol. 2010;25(4):241–9. Retrieved from:. https://doi.org/10.1016/j.tree.2009.10.008.

33. Fletcher MS, Hamilton R, Dressler W, Palmer L. Indigenous knowledge and the shackles of wilderness. Proc Natl Acad Sci. 2021;118(40):e2022218118.

34. National Oceanic and Atmospheric Administration (NOAA). Stewardship definitions: educating people in environmental stewardship practices. 2022. https://www.noaa.gov/office-education/noaa-education-council/monitoring-resources/common-measure-definitions/stewardship-definitions.

35. Hoffman JS, Shandas V, Pendleton N. The effects of historical housing policies on resident exposure to intra-urban heat: a study of 108 US urban areas. Climate. 2020;8(1):12. MDPI AG. Retrieved from. https://doi.org/10.3390/cli8010012.

36. United States Environmental Protection Agency (U.S. EPA). (2024). What is Environmental Education? US EPA. Retrieved from: https://www.epa.gov/education/what-environmental-education.

37. Bellino ME, Adams JD. A critical urban environmental pedagogy: relevant urban environmental education for and by youth. J Environ Educ. 2017;48(4):270–84.

38. Gough A, Gough N. The denaturation of environmental education: exploring the role of ecotechnologies. Aust J Environ Educ. 2016;32(1):30–41. Retrieved from: https://www.jstor.org/stable/26422911

39. Wilson S, Campbell D, Dalemarre L, Fraser-Rahim H, Williams E. A critical review of an authentic and transformative environmental justice and health community—university partnership. Int J Environ Res Public Health. 2014;11:12817–34.

40. United States Environmental Protection Agency (U.S.EPA).(2022).Using participatory science at EPA: vision and principles, Washington, DC. Retrieved from: https://www.epa.gov/participatory-science/epa-vision-participatoryscience.

41. Heaney CD, Wilson SMM, Wilson OR. The West End Revitalization Association's community-owned and -managed research model: development, implementation, and action. Prog Community Health Partnersh. 2007;1(4):339–49. https://doi.org/10.1353/cpr.2007.0037.

42. Community Foundation of Greater Atlanta (CFGA). What is wealth inequality and who does it effect? 2023. https://cfgreateratlanta.org/2023/04/17/what-is-wealth-inequality/#:~:text=Atlanta%20has%20the%20worse%20income,%2C%20About%20Racial%20Wealth%20Gap.

43. Jackson D. Atlanta's income inequality is the highest in the nation. Atlanta J Constit. 2022; https://www.ajc.com/news/investigations/atlanta-has-the-highest-income-inequality-in-the-nation-census-data-shows/YJRZ6A4UGBFWTMYICTG2BCOUPU/. https://www.governing.com/community/atlantas-income-inequality-is-the-highest-in-the-nation.

44. GreenLaw. The patterns of pollution: a report on demographics and pollution in metro Atlanta. Atlanta, GA: GreenLaw; 2012.

45. Jelks NO. Environmental justice: how pollution is ruining our planet and our Health—and what we can do about it. AFT Health Care; 2022.

46. United States Environmental Protection Agency (US EPA) (2014). Urban waters federal partnership. https://www.epa.gov/urbanwaterspartners

47. US Environmental Protection Agency (US EPA). (2014). Urban waters and the proctor creek Watershed/Atlanta (Georgia)|US EPA. https://www.epa.gov/urbanwaterspartners/urban-waters-and-proctor-creek-watershedatlanta-georgia.

48. Jelks NO, Smith DO, Hawthorne T, Fuller CH, Dai D, Stauber CE. Participatory research in Northwest Atlanta's Proctor Creek Watershed: using photovoice as a tool to explore environmental health risks at the water's edge. Health Place. 2020;66:102444.

49. Jelks NO, Hawthorne T, Dai D, Fuller C, Stauber C. Mapping the hidden hazards: community-led spatial data collection of street-level environmental stressors in a degraded, urban watershed. Int J Environ Res Public Health. 2018;15(4):825. Retrieved from:. https://doi.org/10.3390/ijerph15040825.

50. Johnson T, Jelks NO. Implementing community-engaged ecological research in Proctor Creek, an urban Watershed in Atlanta, Georgia, USA. Ecol Appl. 2023;33(5):e2792. Retrieved from. https://doi.org/10.1002/eap.2792.

Na'Taki Osborne Jelks PhD, is an Assistant Professor of Environmental and Health Sciences at Spelman College in Atlanta, GA, and Co-founder of the West Atlanta Watershed Alliance (WAWA), a community-based organization dedicated to growing a cleaner, greener, healthier, and more sustainable West Atlanta.

Might be further defined as the surroundings (social settings and institutions) that are influenced by humans that contribute to health inequities and health disparities.

Culturally Relevant Community Engagement Strategies for Promoting Cervical Cancer Prevention Among Black Women

Kayoll Galbraith Gyan (ID),
Stephanie Devane-Johnson, Preeti Khanal,
Jane Kimani, Rosette Serwanga,
Emmanuel Owusu, Cherice Escobar Jones,
Deborah Effiong, and Karrington R. Johnson

1 Small Beginnings

For who hath despised the day of small things? for the LORD rejoices to see the work begin— Zechariah 4:10

In this chapter, I (Kayoll Gyan) describe how my career in academia began and my experience conducting cervical cancer research among Black women. This report is from my personal perspective and so the reader will note usage of 'my' and 'I' throughout to indicate the first author's voice. However, in the spirit of community-engaged participatory research, I am deeply aware that my work does not take place in isolation. As such, I include my community partners, research assistants and colleague who supported this work within the authorship section of this chapter. My research focusing on cervical cancer prevention among Black women was sparked from an undergraduate experience in the Ronald E. McNair Scholars program at the State University of New York at Binghamton. While completing my Bachelor of Science in Nursing, I conducted research with faculty members in Nursing and

K. G. Gyan (✉)
Phyllis F. Cantor Center for Research in Nursing and Patient Care Services, Dana-Farber Cancer Institute, Harvard Medical School, Boston, MA, USA
e-mail: Kayoll_gyan@dfci.harvard.edu

S. Devane-Johnson
Vanderbilt School of Nursing, Vanderbilt University, Nashville, TN, USA
e-mail: stephanie.devane-johnson@vanderbilt.edu

P. Khanal
Department of Social and Behavioral Sciences, Harvard T.H. Chan School of Public Health, Boston, MA, USA
e-mail: Preetikhanal@hsph.harvard.edu

J. Kimani
Uhai for Health, Inc., Worcester, MA, USA

R. Serwanga
Tyngsborough, MA, USA

E. Owusu
African Bridge Network, West Newton, MA, USA
e-mail: Emmanuel@africanbn.org

C. E. Jones
College of Social Sciences and Humanities, Northeastern University, Boston, MA, USA
e-mail: jones.ch@northeastern.edu

D. Effiong
Department of Pharmaceutical Sciences, Northeastern University, Boston, MA, USA
e-mail: Effiong.d@northeastern.edu

K. R. Johnson
Department of Biology, Spelman College, Atlanta, GA, USA
e-mail: karringtonjohnson@spelman.edu

J. B. Hamilton, C. E. Moore (eds.), *Transforming Social Determinants to Promote Global Health*, https://doi.org/10.1007/978-3-031-61160-5_25

Human Development. My professors had given me the liberty to explore any topic of interest to conduct research on during the summer. This was around 2006, when the human papillomavirus (HPV) vaccine was first approved for use in adolescent girls. I would often see the "One Less" Gardasil commercials on television but did not know what HPV was or its connection to cancers or sexually transmitted infections [1]. As a Jamaican immigrant, I wanted to conduct a project that could be of help to my community. This desire drove my summer project to focus on understanding Caribbean women's awareness and perceptions of HPV and the HPV vaccine. Although this was a small student project, it made me realize that not only were Caribbean women unaware of HPV and its connection to cervical cancer but that, culturally, there was much skepticism around the HPV vaccine's effectiveness. This experience was the impetus for my pursuit of a BSN to PhD in Nursing Research, in which my dissertation examined the role of culture among Black women's HPV vaccination acceptance. I didn't realize the value of that undergraduate research experience at the time, but it was the seed from which my career in cervical cancer prevention among Black women was birthed.

In building my program of research, the PEN-3 cultural model (Fig. 1) has been a useful conceptual framework to ground my research in culture [2]. The PEN-3 cultural model was developed by Dr. Collins O. Airhihenbuwa to bring attention to the role of the sociocultural context

in assessments of communities and in developing community health interventions [3]. Culture is defined by this model as shared values, norms, and codes that collectively shape a group's beliefs, attitudes, and behavior through their interaction in and with their environments [4]. The model identifies culture as a central factor facilitating or deterring an individual's engagement in preventive health behaviors and centers culture in developing, implementing, and evaluating interventions. The letters, P, E, and N, are acronyms referring to constructs within three interrelated and intersecting domains of the model (Relationships and Expectations, Cultural Empowerment, and Cultural Identity).

While there are three domains within the PEN-3, my work has predominantly incorporated two domains in particular: the Relationships and Expectations and Cultural Empowerment domains. These two domains are used during the assessment phase of a study to explore the factors that influence a population's health behavior change. Once my program of research transitions into the intervention development phase, I will incorporate the Cultural Identity domain to determine the best point of entry the intervention should take, either at the individual, extended family, or neighborhood level. The Relationships and Expectations domain [3] examines the Perceptions, Enablers, and Nurturers that influence health behavior. Perceptions include knowledge, attitudes, and beliefs that may prevent or promote performing a health behavior. Enablers are community or structural factors that prevent or promote performing a health behavior. Nurturers are family or members of kinship networks who prevent or promote performing a health behavior. The Cultural Empowerment domain examines whether the constructs of the Relationships and Expectations domain (Perceptions, Enablers, and Nurturers) are considered Positive, Exotic (or unique), or Negative. Beliefs or behaviors identified as positive promote a health behavior and should be viewed as an asset; beliefs or behaviors identified as exotic are not harmful and can be continued; and beliefs or behaviors identified as negative prevent performing a health behavior [3]. I have used aspects of this model in most of my studies on culture

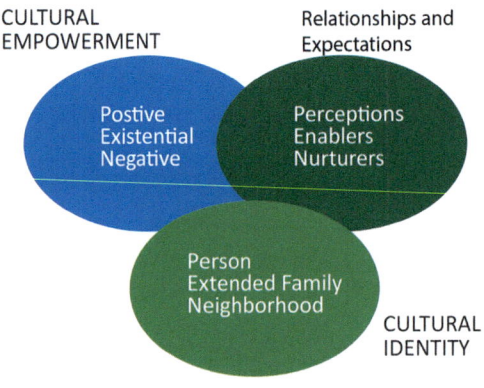

Fig. 1 The PEN-3 cultural model

because it has helped me to conceptualize the problem of cervical cancer disparities among Black women and provided a way forward in intervention development.

2 Integrating Qualitative Methodologies with a Culturally Oriented Framework

An understanding of a people's unique cultural experiences and their social context provides important insight into their health decisions and health behaviors. Combining the PEN-3 cultural model with qualitative methodological approaches within my research studies has allowed me the space and opportunity to ask relevant questions of my research participants and of my data during qualitative data analysis. Qualitative methods are a good fit when studying culture because it facilitates getting to the inner experiences of participants, to determine how meanings are formed through and in their culture, and to discover rather than test variables [5]. I am able to listen to participants tell me their stories about their history, how it shapes them as individuals, and how it informs their views on health conditions like cancer. The following paragraphs describe two qualitative studies in which the PEN-3 cultural model guided my line of inquiry: (1) my dissertation study that examined the role of culture among African American mothers and their daughters' HPV vaccination acceptance (AMDHA study) and (2) the Black immigrant women cervical cancer screening study (BICCS study). In this chapter, Black women is defined as native-born women of African descent whose ancestors were brought to the USA involuntarily as slaves (African Americans), and Black immigrants include recent immigrants from Africa and the Caribbean [6]. In the BICCS study, Caribbean women were recruited; however, this chapter will discuss findings relevant to African immigrant.

Case Study 1 In the AMDHA study, grounded theory techniques were used to explore cultural factors that influenced the acceptance of the HPV vaccine among African American mothers

($n = 28$) and their daughters ($n = 34$). The study's inclusion criteria were (1) African American/Black ethnicity by self-report, (2) parent or guardian of an adolescent daughter, and (3) having daughters between the ages of 12 and 17 years. Participants were recruited from two health departments serving low-income families in Guilford County, NC (Greensboro Department of Health and Highpoint Health Department), and from churches, hair salons, and public libraries in New York City. Recruitment was enhanced through partnerships with community stakeholders, such as nurses from Guilford County health department (HDs), pastors, and directors of community organizations that serve inner city youths, to identify and recruit eligible parents and daughters for this study. Recruitment strategies involved publishing advertisements within the health departments' newsletter, distributing flyers, receiving referrals from community stakeholders, and word of mouth

The interview guide was developed based on the constructs of the PEN-3 cultural model and included questions about factors that influenced HPV vaccine acceptance. During data analysis, descriptive summaries were written for each participant that included a summary of their experiences with cultural factors and included exemplar quotes. Theoretical sampling and constant comparative analysis were used to sample specific factors among mothers and daughters that influenced HPV vaccine acceptance.

Case Study 2 The BICCS study came from two influences. One was the gap in the literature on studies that examined subgroups of Black women's cervical cancer screening experiences. The second influence was to be of service to the African immigrant community I was immersed in after relocating to Boston for postdoctoral training. An emerging body of literature examining differences between African American women and African immigrant women documents varied factors that may contribute to differences in their cervical cancer risks. This literature identifies that over half of cervical cancer deaths in the USA occurred in foreign-born women and that African immigrant women may experience more structural barriers that impede their access to cervical cancer screening, such as lack of health insurance, less timely contact with the healthcare system, and other sociodemographic factors [7, 8]. However, much of the cervical cancer data available is aggregated. To address this gap in the cervical cancer literature and to be of service to the diverse African immigrant community in Boston, I conducted this study.

A qualitative descriptive approach was used to interview $N = 19$ African immigrant women to examine barriers and facilitators to cervical cancer screening. A semi-structured interview questionnaire guided by the PEN-3 cultural model was developed to examine the barriers and facilitators experienced in obtaining cervical cancer screening and examine their perceptions toward Pap testing (cytology-based testing) and emerging HPV DNA self-testing. Participants were recruited from four high-density immigrant communities in Massachusetts (MA) to target four of the top ten Black immigrant groups that migrate to the USA and have large enclaves in MA: (1) Worcester, MA (Ghanaian population); (2) Lowell (Kenyan population); (3) Waltham (Ugandan population); and (4) Boston (English- and French-speaking Caribbean/Haitians). The study's inclusion criteria were women who (a) self-identified as being Ghanaian, Kenyan, Ugandan, Caribbean-English speaking, or Haitian, (b) are English speakers, (c) are foreign-born, and (d) are between ages 25 and 65 years old. Exclusion criteria were women who (a) were already diagnosed with cervical cancer, (b) had a hysterectomy, and (c) do not communicate effectively in English language.

An academic-community partnership with two community organizations, the African Bridge Network (ABN) and Uhai for Health, Inc., and an African immigrant community health advocate, Rosette Serwanga, facilitated recruitment and engagement with community members. The ABN, located in Boston, MA, provides support to African immigrants across Massachusetts to navigate the challenges that accompany integrating into the US workforce [9], while Uhai for Health, Inc., is a nonprofit organization that was founded with the mission of empowering African immigrants, refugees, and other underserved communities to become healthy and self-sufficient [10]. Both organizations have relationships with other community organizations. We obtained letters of support from the president of both organizations and discussed a recruitment approach that was feasible and appropriate for each organization and their resources. Our recruitment entailed distributing study flyers and informational brochures through each organization's directory through email, WhatsApp, their social media platforms, and newsletters. Study staff attended community events where we discussed the study. We also used snowball sampling to refer network members to the study and word of mouth. Flyers were also posted at other community settings within the African community such as grocery stores, restaurants, churches, and hair salons.

The next sections will discuss the problem of cervical cancer disparities among Black women based on findings from the two studies described above and from the larger cervical cancer literature.

3   Discussion of the Problem According to the Nell Hodgson Woodruff School of Nursing Social Determinants of Health Framework

The American Cancer Society (ACS) estimates that about 13,960 new cases of invasive cervical cancer would be diagnosed in 2023 and be responsible for an estimated 4310 deaths [11]. Cervical cancer is unique in that it is the only cancer that is preventable through vaccination and one of only two cancers that can be prevented through screening [colorectal cancer being the other]. In the last century, major advancements have occurred in the fight against cervical cancer. First in 1943, with the publishing of the landmark book, *Diagnosis of Uterine Cancer by the Vaginal Smear*, the Papanicolaou (Pap) test (cytology-based testing) became the gold standard for screening for cervical cancer [12]. The development of the Pap test led to significant decreases in cervical cancer deaths in the USA by more than 70% between 1955 and 1992 alone [13, 14].

In 2006, the quadrivalent human papillomavirus (HPV4) vaccine was developed for use among females and later males as young as 9 up to 26 years old. The HPV vaccine (HPV-9) is a safe and effective prevention strategy against persistent infection with high-risk HPV strains and high-grade cervical lesions that lead to cancer [15]. The quadrivalent HPV vaccine prevented infection from high-risk strains 16 and 18, known to cause the majority of cervical cancers, in addition to low-risk strains 6 and 11, which caused over 90% of genital warts. In 2014, a 9-valent vaccine offering protection from additional high-risk strains (31, 33, 45, 52, and 58) was licensed, increasing cervical cancer protection from 70% to 90% [16, 17, 18].

In 2020, the ACS updated their cervical cancer screening guidelines to include the use of high-risk HPV DNA-based testing (no cytology) as a primary screening method for detecting high-grade cervical dysplasia in women at average risk age 25 up to 65 years old [19]. Currently, ACS recommends cervical cancer testing begins at age 25 and women aged 25–65 should have a primary HPV test every 5 years, or screen with a co-test that combines HPV testing with a Pap test every 5 years, or a pap test alone every 3 years [20]. Primary HPV testing has already been used widely outside the USA, in Europe, and in low- and middle-income countries as a cost-efficient and effective screening method [21]. Unlike cytology-based screening, HPV DNA testing relied on viral detection rather than morphologic interpretation by a trained individual, making the results less ambiguous being left up to human interpretation [22].

Through equitable delivery of HPV vaccination, organized screening programs, and timely quality treatment, cervical cancer is indeed a cancer that can not only be prevented but eliminated completely. Reviewing the comprehensive cervical cancer screening programs of countries like Sweden, Denmark, and Finland that are on track to eliminate cervical cancer by 2030, we see that this goal is indeed possible [23]. However, the full benefits of these cervical cancer prevention milestones, while significant, have not been equitably experienced by Black women.

In the next sections, I draw from two of the four pillars—social and cultural—of the Nell Hodgson Woodruff School of Nursing Social Determinants of Health Framework to briefly describe the conditions that contribute to the disparate cervical cancer burden experienced by Black women.

4 Social Conditions Contributing to Cervical Cancer Disparities

According to the Nell Hodgson Woodruff School of Nursing Social Determinants of Health Framework, social conditions are those factors that occur in society due to systemic (structural) racism and imbalances in power, environmental resources, education, and access to quality care that influence the overall wellness of an individual or lack thereof [24]. These conditions represent factors that place people of color at increased risk for poor health outcomes and overall well-being [24].

4.1 Racial and Ethnic Cervical Cancer Disparities

Race and ethnicity is a telling indicator for who gets cervical cancer and who dies from cervical cancer. Although Hispanics have the highest overall cervical cancer incidence rates, Black women have the second highest incidence rate, which is 30% higher than non-Hispanic white women [25]. Racial disparity in cervical cancer incidence has narrowed in the last several decades; this decrease has slowed among Black women [26]. Black women also experience the highest cervical cancer mortality rate (3.3 per 100,000 women) compared to non-Hispanic white women (2.0 per 100,000 women). In fact, non-Hispanic Black women are 80% more likely to die from cervical cancer than non-Hispanic white women [25]. A pivotal study by Beavis et al. that corrected for hysterectomy prevalence concluded that the mortality rate among Black women was underestimated with corrected mortality rate being significantly higher [27].

Black women also experience a higher incidence of distant stage disease when compared to non-Hispanic white women. Additionally, the 5-year relative survival rate is lower among Black women than white women, with 58% of Black women surviving cervical cancer after 5 years compared to 68% of white women [28].

4.2 Socioeconomic Factors

Cost is one of the largest obstacles to accessing high-quality cancer care. One's level of insurance coverage is linked to employment. Black people have an increased likelihood of receiving inadequate health insurance even with employment [6]. Studies show that people with health insurance have a usual source of care, utilize preventive services, and seek care when it is needed [29]. Individuals without health insurance are more likely to be diagnosed with advanced cancer and have a higher risk of cancer death compared to people who are privately insured [29]. This pattern holds true for cervical cancer as well, where women who are uninsured or do not have a regular healthcare provider experience increased risk for developing cervical cancer [30, 31]. Hence, lack of insurance impacts cervical cancer treatment options and further contributes to Black women's lower 5-year survival rate for cervical cancer.

Having insurance is not a certainty of receiving quality care or treatment for cervical cancer either. A study by Churilla et al. found that cervical cancer patients with Medicaid and those without any insurance had increased odds of having advanced-stage cervical cancer disease at diagnosis, receiving suboptimal therapy, and experiencing an increased risk of overall mortality, compared to those with private insurance. In this same study, Black women were more likely to have Medicaid or lack health insurance [30]. We know that cervical cancer is highly preventable through screening and treatment, yet Black women are more likely to be diagnosed with advanced-stage cervical cancer and are less likely to receive timely and adequate cervical cancer treatment [32]. Surgery is the standard of care for treating cervical cancer. However, a recent study by Markt et al. found that non-Hispanic Black women were more likely to receive radiation and less likely to receive surgery for early-stage disease [33]. Hence, Black, poor, and low socioeconomic status women experience significant socioeconomic barriers in obtaining high-quality and timely cervical cancer screening and follow-up care.

4.3 Low Knowledge About HPV and HPV Vaccination

Race/ethnicity and socioeconomic position are important indicators of HPV knowledge. A consistently reported barrier to HPV vaccination uptake is gaps in knowledge related to HPV infection and the HPV vaccine [34]. Gaps in HPV knowledge is often an underlying factor influencing HPV vaccination hesitancy and overall acceptance among non-Hispanic Black adults [35]. Studies show that non-Hispanic whites are more likely to have higher cervical cancer knowledge compared to non-Hispanic Blacks and Hispanics, and this was also found among Blacks from high socioeconomic position [36, 37]. Gaps in knowledge among African Americans have been found on the link between HPV causing cervical cancer and its causative role in other HPV-associated cancers such as oropharyngeal, anal, and penile cancers. Granted, awareness of HPV has increased since HPV vaccination licensure; however awareness has been associated with either being diagnosed with HPV, cervical dysplasia, or cervical cancer or having someone within their network diagnosed with HPV or cervical cancer [38, 39]. Younger age was also associated with awareness of HPV and willingness to vaccinate adolescent boys and girls [40]. Greater efforts to increase knowledge and awareness of HPV and its link to cancers prior to exposure are needed among Black women.

5   Cultural Conditions

Cultural conditions are those customary beliefs, social norms, attitudes, values, and practices shared by a group of people (community or society) in a place and time [24]. Religion and spirituality and medical mistrust are two salient cultural determinants that have been influential in Black women's cervical cancer prevention behaviors.

5.1   Religion and Spirituality

There are mixed findings on whether religious beliefs act as a barrier to HPV vaccination uptake. Many studies focused on African American parents' HPV vaccination decisions identified that when parents can separate their religious beliefs from their HPV vaccination decisions, they are more likely to accept HPV vaccination for their daughters [41]. Their HPV vaccination decisions are based on information they receive from their healthcare provider. However, for those unable to make that distinction, their religious beliefs on the doctrine of no premarital sex were a barrier to their HPV vaccination acceptance [35]. These findings are consistent with other studies in the HPV vaccination literature [42–44].

5.2   Medical Mistrust

The history of exploitation and abuse of the Black body, originating, perhaps most saliently, with slavery but persisting long after, may manifest today in feelings of mistrust in western institutions, including healthcare and research. During slavery, this exploitation was complete and inclusive of all domains of life. The following themes of mistreatment have been well documented and are posited here as *related* to present-day medical mistrust among Black people: (1) violence against those enslaved; (2) medical experimentation on Black people, which played a particularly insidious role in the lives of some enslaved people, and Black women, which impacted enslaved women and their infants [45, 46]. Mistrust has carried over in their use of vaccination for health promotion. The most prominent example of this is the case of Henrietta Lacks, an African American woman with cervical cancer in 1951, who was provided suboptimal care for her medical condition and had her medical records forged [47]. What we now recognize as informed consent to participants in medical research was absent leading up to the collection of Lacks' cells or in the years that followed as use of those cells continued and expanded. The Lack's family never received compensation for the use of her cells until 2023 [48] when her family filed a lawsuit against a biotech company and won an undisclosed amount of money. The Emancipation Proclamation (1865), enacted almost a century before Lacks sought care for cancer, did not shield Lacks from the exploitation that Black bodies experienced while entrenched in American culture. This case illustrates that the medical exploitation of Black women's bodies can diminish their control over their body and in so doing perhaps disrupt their sense of personhood. Today, many African Americans are reluctant to participate in research studies and clinical trials due to fears that the medical community may abuse their power by taking advantage of the poor, weak, and powerless [49].

6   Strategies for Engaging the Community and Allowing Community Members to Tell Their Story

Until the lion tells the story, the hunter will always be the hero.—African proverb

Throughout my work in cervical cancer prevention, my population of interest has always been Black women from diverse ethnic groups. I examine how differences in social and cultural backgrounds influence women's cervical cancer prevention behaviors and treatment decisions. I do this because I hold the perspective that peoples' social and cultural backgrounds greatly inform their identity and contribute to their health decisions and health behaviors. As such, my studies have included native-born African Americans from the Southern USA, Caribbean women, and African immigrant women. The participants in the AMDHA study were recruited from rural communities in North Carolina and from urban neighborhoods in Brooklyn, NY. In the BICCS study, which examined the cervical cancer screening barriers and facilitators experienced by African immigrant women, I collaborated with churches and community-based organizations in MA to recruit African and Caribbean immigrant women in the study. Principles of community-engaged research have been a consistent strategy implemented to ensure culturally responsive recruitment efforts in most of my studies. Below, I describe the community engagement strategies that have been successful in the scope of my research thus far.

7   Steps to Engage the Community

1. **Tap into your established relationships**. Tapping into existing community relationships has been an integral strategy for me to successfully conduct research among Black women and their daughters. For example, to recruit participants for AMDHA study, I relied heavily on existing relationships with community members and stakeholders that were first established during my teenage years growing up and working in the inner city of Brooklyn, NY. As a teenager, I was also involved with the Police Athletic League, as a Camp Counselor in the Brownsville section of Brooklyn. I fostered relationships with staff members and counselors and later returned as a college student to conduct community health outreach programs and volunteer within the same organization. So, when recruiting for the AMDHA study, the community stakeholders I reached out to trusted me and my intentions toward the work I envisioned within the community.

This trust was fundamental in obtaining their assistance to recruit African American mothers and their adolescent daughters into my study.

2. **Assess your new surroundings**. My career path has led me to travel and reside across the USA. Changing cities can be a real challenge when conducting community-driven research. It takes time to establish new relationships and build trust among community members as a new resident. When I moved to Boston, MA, I learned about the city and its history while meeting key stakeholders working in the field of cancer disparities and vaccine uptake. It was vital to be courageous and learn to put myself and my work on display for community members to get to know me and build trust. Joining a diverse church of African and Caribbean immigrants was an integral aspect that allowed me to build strong relationships with the diverse Black community within the city of Boston.

Black Americans tend to be more religious than the general American public. This is evident by their religious affiliations, engagement in religious practices, and the frequency in their belief in God or a Higher Power [50]. The Black church, for example, has had a long-standing and integral role within the Black community [51]. A recent study noted that religious participation served as an asset in sustaining a sense of hope and meaning and was associated with strengthened psychosocial resilience by fostering a sense of peace and positive outlook and promoting social connectedness [52]. When traveling to a new location, a long-standing advice passed down is to be sure to find a church. This was not only for the religious and spiritual fellowship that the church provides but also for the practical, social, and civic resources of the church for Black people [53]. With that in mind, when I moved from North Carolina to Massachusetts, that was the first thing that I did.

Joining a diverse church allowed me to build genuine relationships with pastors and other Black women in a new city. To engage potential participants from my church, I introduced my research study first to my Pastor during the grant writing stage where I obtained a letter of support for the grant submission. I also obtained permission to speak to church members upon activation of the study. Although not always possible, the earlier you can obtain buy-in and support from the pastor and clergy for your study, the better the recruitment process can be. I used this strategy for my dissertation study, as well as during my most recent study on understanding the cervical cancer screening barriers and facilitators among Black immigrant women.

3. **Build new relationships with researchers and members already integrated within your community of interest**. Another way in which I have been successful in recruiting diverse African American women into my research studies is by attending various community events and networking with members already integrated within my community of interest. For me, this meant (1) attending events held by organizations that served the African immigrant community in Massachusetts, like the African Bridge Network and Uhai for Health, Inc., (2) meeting one on one with the leaders of those organizations to introduce myself, and my work, and (3) discussing potential collaborative opportunities in which my expertise in cancer prevention could be of service to their organization's mission and programs. It was important for me to introduce myself and be known by these community leaders and members to build trust, establish a working relationship, and more importantly, obtain opportunities to understand the needs of their organization and the individuals they served. By attending events and co-hosting programs, I was able to organically become part of the community.

8 Challenges and Special Considerations When Engaging Black Women into HPV Vaccination and Cervical Cancer Prevention Research

8.1 Time Intensive

One consideration worth discussing is the time it takes to build relationships to conduct community-engaged research effectively. As a researcher and a woman with young children, being able to attend community events meant that my children often accompanied me. While juggling these two things can be challenging, I have found some benefits during this process. Involving my children in my outreach efforts allowed community members to view me not only as a researcher or an academic but also as a working mother and a "real" person interested in them living healthy lifestyles. This strengthened the personal connections that allowed me to be seen as a trusted member of the community, despite being new. Given the privilege and responsibility of being welcomed into the community, I stayed intentional in my efforts and leveraged my Research Assistants (RAs) to attend events in circumstances where I was unable to. When hiring RAs, take time to hire students who are genuinely interested in conducting community-engaged research. You can create a calendar of community events and pair students up to attend and disseminate information about a particular study. You can attend these events with your students or have them attend and report back during weekly meetings.

One strategy for hiring RAs is to hire students at various professional levels if possible (e.g., undergraduate, graduate, and postdoctoral). By hiring an RA from each level, you can delegate project management responsibilities to an experienced student while they oversee the work of a recent graduate or a student hoping to enter the research sector. This approach allows less experienced RAs to learn from those more experienced and provides you the opportunity to focus on other work demands, such as teaching, grant writing, and publishing. Finally, this approach allows you to build a collaborative and supportive team in which various experiences, knowledge, and interests amalgamate.

8.2 Balancing the Focus of Your Study with the Priority of Your Community of Interest

During my postdoctoral fellowship at Harvard T.H. Chan School of Public Health/Dana-Farber Cancer Institute, I was part of a study to understand the perspective of community leaders and program coordinators from community-based organizations on how to implement HPV evidence-based practice programs within medically underserved communities in MA [36, 37]. In that study, participants were asked whether HPV vaccination and cervical cancer were considered priority health concerns by the community-based organizations they worked in or within the communities of color they served. The study identified that community-based organizations' priorities were set based on funding allocation for community members which encompassed individuals with other types of cancers and chronic health conditions rather than on cervical cancer prevention and HPV vaccination among adolescents.

As my research transitioned from focusing on native-born African Americans from the Southern USA to focusing more on African immigrant women, the need for dissemination of awareness around cervical cancer prevention became more apparent. My study included Black immigrant women in MA from Ghana, Kenya, Uganda, and the Caribbean. These women were indeed aware of the importance of cervical cancer screening but underwent other social challenges in their daily life that delayed their engagement in the screening and vaccination uptake. I learned that the major barriers to cervical cancer screening among African immigrant women were related to the following issues: (1) navigating challenges of their immigration status for those who were

undocumented or were in the USA on a student visa; (2) navigating their new experiences as a Black immigrant and the perceived racism and discrimination this new identity brought; (3) navigating experiences of racism and discrimination they experienced themselves or experienced by others within their network; (4) navigating challenges to communicate due to their accent, language, and cultural differences; and (5) navigating how to use health insurance (manuscript in preparation). For example, one 28-year-old married Kenyan woman who had been in the USA for 4 years reported the following in my study:

I actually was just closed-mouthed to not be mocked because she was [a] white lady and I'm not really close to white people like that due to what I've heard about racism and discrimination by white people. I'm not really close to my doctor. I don't really relate to my doctors very well...Due to what I have heard about white nurses treating black people, I feel I don't really have to go there [to the hospital], because I don't want to be treated bad because of my skin color.

The study clarified the potential misalignment of research priorities with the target population given the constant concern of other social challenges many immigrants undergo in this country. It is vital to be aware and intentional while working with immigrant population to understand the challenges they face during the study that may not be related to the research topic. Creating a safe space for women to share their concerns and assisting them to alleviate their stress within the scope of research can make a difference when recruiting for long-term research studies despite the difference in priorities between the research topic and population of interest.

8.3 Challenges Discussing Sensitive or Taboo Health Topics

In the same study, we also found that HPV vaccination was a sensitive topic to discuss for community members due to the vaccine protecting against STIs and the cultural stigma surrounding topics of sexuality among adolescents. Though research studies showed that HPV vaccination does not increase harmful sexual behavior [54], community members held the misconception that HPV vaccination was an unspoken permission for adolescents to have sex [35]. Topics of sex and sexual risk are not a regular topic in many Black households, so engaging the parents requires a culturally sensitive approach.

Few strategies that have been effective in my line of study for overcoming Black women and adolescent girls feeling uncomfortable discussing HPV are listed below:

- Reframing the HPV vaccine as a cancer prevention
- Ensuring that conversations occur in the participant's choice of private and safe space
- Having female researchers conduct all interviews
- Establishing a sense of relatability and shared cultural experience by providing personal examples
- Being cognizant of the placement of sensitive questions within the interview guide (sometimes it takes some time before the participant feels comfortable enough to share)
- Recognizing the stigma around sexual health and empathizing with participants and reminding them of their choice to answer questions

As a Jamaican woman familiar with the stigmas surrounding HPV vaccination, I have found being honest and empathetic with my participants to be a repeating strategy in building a trusting relationship. However, it is vital to recognize that creating each community strategy requires an individualized and culturally responsive approach. Regardless of similar background, one size does not fit all, and you cannot always utilize the same textbook strategy in every research setting. Thus, I encourage you to view the recommendations in this chapter not as prescriptive, but as guidance as you determine the most appropriate and feasible strategy to engage with your population of interest. Your adaptation of the strategies discussed will look different from my own; and that is a good thing.

9   Intervention Components Important to African American Mothers and Daughters and African Immigrant Women

As I transition my program of research in cervical cancer into the intervention phase, the findings from my formative research will inform my intervention development. Below, I present a summary of the findings and suggestions for important intervention components to potential interventions targeting HPV vaccination acceptance among African American mothers and cervical cancer screening promotion among African immigrant women.

9.1   AMDHA Study Major Findings

In the AMDHA study, the major study findings were that positive attitudes toward vaccination stemmed from the belief that the HPV vaccine has cancer prevention benefits and from a general belief in the protection conferred by vaccines against infectious diseases. Negative attitudes, on the other hand, stemmed from beliefs that the HPV vaccine was too new and not effective and that daughters may be too young to get vaccinated against HPV. Negative attitudes toward vaccination also stemmed from the belief that vaccines are not "one size fits all interventions." While spirituality and religion are core aspects of African American culture and experience [55], and weighed on African Americans' HPV vaccine acceptance [56], the AMDHA study found that religious doctrine did not impede African American mothers and daughters' HPV vaccination decisions. Regardless of HPV vaccination status, both mothers and daughters felt they needed more information about HPV, and HPV vaccine safety, side effects, and effectiveness. This finding is again highlighted in mothers' dissatisfaction with the information shared by their healthcare providers about HPV and the vaccine. Lastly, this study found that social network members were a source for HPV vaccination information and played an important role in whether parents held positive or negative attitudes and beliefs about HPV vaccination.

An intervention with the aim of promoting HPV vaccination acceptance among African American mothers and daughters may include the following components:

- *Consider targeting the intervention to African American mothers.* While fathers are important pillars within the family, our study found that mothers were the primary decision-makers for health decisions for their children.
- *Address knowledge gap.* Many mothers and daughters reported not having adequate information about HPV or HPV vaccination. One consideration to address this is to develop culturally tailored materials to be mailed or delivered electronically to parents and adolescent girls. In addition to educational materials, I would include a consultation with a patient navigator or cervical cancer health educator in advance of the HPV vaccination appointment to answer any questions that parents and their daughters may have. By doing this, parents and daughters will have the opportunity to ask questions that arise from their review of the information and can address any concerns.
- *Address concerns related to sexual promiscuity.* A minority of mothers within this qualitative study reported that a barrier to HPV vaccination is due to their belief in no premarital sex and concerns the vaccination would lead to promiscuity. Studies show that HPV vaccination does not promote sexual activity among adolescents. Highlighting this point within the educational materials during consultation may be beneficial.
- *Conduct intervention within a healthcare setting.* Research provides evidence that including the HPV vaccination with other childhood recommended vaccinations promotes uptake of the HPV vaccine. By conducting an HPV vaccine intervention within a health clinic, nurses can provide the HPV vaccination immediately once parents decide they are ready to proceed.

9.2 Major Findings in the BICCS Screening Study

Our study found low awareness and knowledge about HPV vaccination and cervical cancer screening. Themes identified as barriers to cervical cancer screening included navigating a new identity as a Black immigrant and perceived racism and discrimination this new identity brings, concerns related to their accent and language barrier, navigating health insurance system, experiences of racism and discrimination by self or others, and cost of transportation. Facilitators of cervical cancer screening were having knowledgeable network members to support identifying a doctor, receiving a doctor recommendation, and having student health insurance. We also found that African immigrant women were interested in HPV self-testing but had concerns about whether they could collect the sample correctly and the quality of the self-test outside a hospital/clinic setting.

An intervention to promote cervical cancer screening among African immigrant women in the USA could include the following components.

- *Partnering with community partner to develop and tailor the intervention.* In developing an intervention, I would be sure to work with the same community-based organizations I worked with during my formative research. This consistency in collaboration is one way to build trust within the community of interest and allows community partners to be invested in the impact the intervention could potentially have.
- *Include a community nurse navigator within the intervention.* The community nurse navigator role is designed to support patients in finding their way through health and social care systems, help them overcome barriers to accessing services, and to help them promote early detection of diseases [57]. Including a community nurse navigator within an HPV self-testing intervention could help African

immigrant women overcome barriers of navigating health insurance, cost of treatment, and finding a trusted healthcare provider. Our study also found concerns about collecting an HPV self-sample incorrectly and concern about the quality of the self-sampling test if used outside of a hospital setting. To mitigate HPV self-testing barriers reported earlier, integrating a community nurse navigator within a community-based HPV self-testing intervention could bolster patients' self-efficacy in collecting a sample and could facilitate African immigrant women's engagement within the healthcare system to return for timely follow-up care for abnormal results.

- *Tailor educational materials for cultural norms and language.* Concerns about language differences and communicating effectively with healthcare providers were concerns identified in the Afro-immigrant study. Tailoring educational materials for specific subgroups of African immigrants, a part of the community you work in is an important component of a successful intervention. I would recommend working with community partners to recruit community members during the intervention development period to support the translation process.

- *Consider social norms and cultural stigmas.* Within the African American and African immigrant community, conversations around cancer, sex, and sexually transmitted infections are considered taboo. These topic areas are difficult to discuss and can be challenging to engage women into conversations around these personal and stigmatized topics. Because of this stigma, perceptions on risk for cancer or HPV can often be underestimated. In interventions focused on these topics, ensuring that participants are comfortable, in a safe and private space, and being interviewed by another female has been important in having these types of conversations with research participants. Attention to the setting in which interviews are conducted, who the interviewer is, and phrasing of the interview questions is highly encouraged.

10 Reflection

A growing body of literature indicates that attitudes and beliefs shaped by culture play a prominent role in HPV vaccine acceptance among African Americans. Factors such as mistrust of healthcare providers and the healthcare system, religion, and social norms related to appropriate sexual behaviors were identified as factors that play a role in HPV vaccination decisions among African Americans. Addressing these factors with culturally tailored interventions unique to the African American historical and lived experience mitigates the myths and mistrust about the HPV vaccine itself.

The predominant focus of HPV vaccination uptake has largely targeted women but recently, more studies inclusive of males are being conducted. Ensuring the inclusion of males within HPV prevention initiatives is important in reducing and eliminating cervical cancer in women as well as other HPV-associated cancers prevalent in men and women. Including males in HPV preventive initiative shifts the burden of HPV prevention from being solely on females to being one that males play an active role in preventing as well. Considering that oropharyngeal cancer related to HPV rose 2.8% in men from 2015 to 2019, shifting the way HPV vaccination is framed may increase the odds of eradicating HPV and decreasing cancers associated with HPV infection [58].

The launch of the Cervical Cancer Elimination Initiative by the World Health Organization in November 2020 underscored the importance of all countries coming together to eliminate cervical cancer. According to the initiative, countries must reach and maintain an incidence rate of 4 per 100,000 women if not less, and there are three key pillars in achieving this goal [59]. One of the main pillars targets vaccination rates across the globe where 90% of girls must be fully vaccinated with the HPV vaccine by the age of 15 [60]. Despite the accessibility of HPV vaccination in the USA relative to the rest of the world, this should be a target for all minority groups across the USA. Given how the recent COVID-19 pandemic has exacerbated the delay of many health programs, we should ensure HPV vaccination and cervical cancer screening are accessible and acceptable through culturally tailored community engagement strategies.

References

1. Grantham S, Ahern L, Connolly-Ahern C. Merck's one less campaign: using risk message frames to promote the use of Gardasil® in HPV prevention. Commun Res Rep. 2011;28(4):318–26. https://doi.org/10.1080/08824096.2011.616243.

2. Airhihenbuwa CO, Iwelunmor J, Munodawafa D, Ford CL, Oni T, Agyemang C, Mota C, Ikuomola OB, Simbayi L, Fallah MP, Qian Z, Makinwa B, Niang C, Okosun I. Culture matters in communicating the global response to COVID-19. Prev Chronic Dis. 2020;17:E60. https://doi.org/10.5888/pcd17.200245.

3. Iwelunmor J, Newsome V, Airhihenbuwa CO. Framing the impact of culture on health: a systematic review of the PEN-3 cultural model and its application in public health research and interventions. Ethn Health. 2014;19(1):20–46. https://doi.org/10.1080/13557858.2013.857768.

4. Airhihenbuwa CO. A conceptual model for culturally appropriate health education programs in developing countries. Int Q Community Health Educ. 1990;11(1):53–62. https://doi.org/10.2190/LPKH-PMPJ-DBW9-FP6X.

5. Corbin JM, Strauss A. Basics of qualitative research: techniques and procedures for developing grounded theory. SAGE Publications; 2008.

6. Giaquinto AN, Miller KD, Tossas KY, Winn RA, Jemal A, Siegel RL. Cancer statistics for African American/Black People 2022. CA Cancer J Clin. 2022;72(3):202–29. https://doi.org/10.3322/caac.21718.

7. Cudjoe J, Turkson-Ocran R-A, Ezeigwe AK, Commodore-Mensah Y, Nkimbeng M, Han H-R. Recruiting African immigrant women for community-based cancer prevention studies: lessons learned from the AfroPap Study. J Community Health. 2019;44(5):1019–26. https://doi.org/10.1007/s10900-019-00677-y.

8. Lim JNW, Ojo AA. Barriers to utilisation of cervical cancer screening in Sub Sahara Africa: a systematic review. Eur J Cancer Care. 2017;26(1):525. https://doi.org/10.1111/ecc.12444.

9. African Bridge Network. Mission and approach | Massachusetts. 2023. https://africanbn.org/mission-and-approach. Accessed 16 Aug 2023.

10. Uhai for Health Inc. About us. 2022. www.uhai.org. Accessed 1 Aug 2023.

11. American Cancer Society. Cervical cancer statistics | Key facts about cervical cancer. 2023. https://www.cancer.org/cancer/types/cervical-cancer/about/key-statistics.html. Accessed 15 Aug 2023.

12. Tan S, Tatsumura Y. George Papanicolaou (1883–1962): discoverer of the pap smear. Singapore Med J. 2015;56(10):586–7. https://doi.org/10.11622/smedj.2015155.

13. Arbyn M, Castellsagué X, de Sanjosé S, Bruni L, Saraiya M, Bray F, Ferlay J. Worldwide burden of cervical cancer in 2008. Ann Oncol. 2011;22(12):2675–86. https://doi.org/10.1093/annonc/mdr015.

14. McGraw SL, Ferrante JM. Update on prevention and screening of cervical cancer. World J Clin Oncol. 2014;5(4):744–52. https://doi.org/10.5306/wjco.v5.i4.744.

15. Pils S, Joura EA. From the monovalent to the nine-valent HPV vaccine. Clin Microbiol Infect. 2015;21(9):827–33. https://doi.org/10.1016/j.cmi.2015.05.001.

16. Petrosky E, Bocchini JA, Hariri S, Chesson H, Curtis CR, Saraiya M, Unger ER, Markowitz LE, Centers for Disease Control and Prevention (CDC). Use of 9-valent human papillomavirus (HPV) vaccine: updated HPV vaccination recommendations of the advisory committee on immunization practices. MMWR Morb Mortal Wkly Rep. 2015;64(11):300–4.

17. Joura EA, Giuliano AR, Iversen O-E, Bouchard C, Mao C, Mehlsen J, Moreira ED, Ngan Y, Petersen LK, Lazcano-Ponce E, Pitisuttithum P, Restrepo JA, Stuart G, Woelber L, Yang YC, Cuzick J, Garland SM, Huh W, Kjaer SK, et al. A 9-valent HPV vaccine against infection and intraepithelial neoplasia in women. N Engl J Med. 2015;372(8):711–23. https://doi.org/10.1056/NEJMoa1405044.

18. Serrano B, Alemany L, Tous S, Bruni L, Clifford GM, Weiss T, Bosch FX, de Sanjosé S. Potential impact of a nine-valent vaccine in human papillomavirus related cervical disease. Infect Agents Cancer. 2012;7(1):38. https://doi.org/10.1186/1750-9378-7-38.

19. Fontham ETH, Wolf AMD, Church TR, Etzioni R, Flowers CR, Herzig A, Guerra CE, Oeffinger KC, Shih Y-CT, Walter LC, Kim JJ, Andrews KS, DeSantis CE, Fedewa SA, Manassaram-Baptiste D, Saslow D, Wender RC, Smith RA. Cervical cancer screening for individuals at average risk: 2020 guideline update from the American Cancer Society. CA Cancer J Clin. 2020;70(5):321–46. https://doi.org/10.3322/caac.21628.

20. American Cancer Society. Guidelines for the prevention and early detection of cervical cancer. 2021. https://www.cancer.org/cancer/types/cervical-cancer/detection-diagnosis-staging/cervical-cancer-screening-guidelines.html. Accessed 15 Aug 2023.

21. Georgalis L, de Sanjosé S, Esnaola M, Bosch FX, Diaz M. Present and future of cervical cancer prevention in Spain: a cost-effectiveness analysis. Eur J Cancer Prev. 2016;25(5):430–9. https://doi.org/10.1097/CEJ.0000000000000202.

22. Chrysostomou AC, Kostrikis LG. Methodologies of primary HPV testing currently applied for cervical cancer screening. Life (Basel, Switzerland).

2020;10(11):290. https://doi.org/10.3390/life10110290.

23. Vaccarella S, Franceschi S, Engholm G, Lönnberg S, Khan S, Bray F. 50 years of screening in the Nordic countries: quantifying the effects on cervical cancer incidence. Br J Cancer. 2014;111(5):965–9. https://doi.org/10.1038/bjc.2014.362.

24. Hamilton JB, Swan BA, McCauley L, editors. Integrating a social determinants of health framework into nursing education. Springer International Publishing; 2023. https://doi.org/10.1007/978-3-031-21347-2.

25. American Cancer Society. Cancer facts & figures for African American/Black People. 2022. https://www.cancer.org/research/cancer-facts-statistics/cancer-facts-figures-for-african-americans.html. Accessed 15 Aug 2023.

26. DeSantis CE, Miller KD, Goding Sauer A, Jemal A, Siegel RL. Cancer statistics for African Americans, 2019. CA Cancer J Clin. 2019;69(3):211–33. https://doi.org/10.3322/caac.21555.

27. Beavis AL, Gravitt PE, Rositch AF. Hysterectomy-corrected cervical cancer mortality rates reveal a larger racial disparity in the United States. Cancer. 2017;123(6):1044–50. https://doi.org/10.1002/cncr.30507.

28. SEER*Explorer. An interactive website for SEER cancer statistics [Internet]. Surveillance Research Program, National Cancer Institute; 2023. https://seer.cancer.gov/statistics-network/explorer/. Data source(s): SEER Incidence Data, November 2022 Submission (1975–2020), SEER 22 registries (excluding Illinois and Massachusetts). Expected Survival Life Tables by Socio-Economic Standards. https://seer.cancer.gov/statistics-network/explorer/application.html?site=57&data_type=4&graph_type=6&compareBy=race&chk_race_1=1&chk_race_6=6&chk_race_5=5&chk_race_4=4&chk_race_9=9&chk_race_8=8&chk_race_3=3&chk_race_2=2&hdn_sex=3&age_range=1&stage=101&advopt_precision=1&advopt_show_ci=on&hdn_view=1&advopt_show_apc=on&advopt_display=2#resultsRegion1. Accessed 15 Aug 2023.

29. Tolbert J, Drake P. Key Facts about the Uninsured Population. KFF; 2022. https://www.kff.org/uninsured/issue-brief/key-facts-about-the-uninsured-population/.

30. Churilla T, Egleston B, Dong Y, Shaikh T, Murphy C, Mantia-Smaldone G, Chu C, Rubin S, Anderson P. Disparities in the management and outcome of cervical cancer in the United States according to health insurance status. Gynecol Oncol. 2016;141(3):516–23. https://doi.org/10.1016/j.ygyno.2016.03.025.

31. Cowburn S, Carlson MJ, Lapidus JA, DeVoe JE. The association between insurance status and cervical cancer screening in community health centers: exploring the potential of electronic health records for population-level surveillance, 2008–2010. Prev Chronic Dis. 2013;10:E173. https://doi.org/10.5888/pcd10.130034.

32. Holt HK, Peterson CE, MacLaughlan David S, Abdelaziz A, Sawaya GF, Guadamuz JS, Calip GS. Mediation of racial and ethnic inequities in the diagnosis of advanced-stage cervical cancer by insurance status. JAMA Netw Open. 2023;6(3):e232985. https://doi.org/10.1001/jamanetworkopen.2023.2985.

33. Markt SC, Tang T, Cronin AM, Katz IT, Howitt BE, Horowitz NS, Lee LJ, Wright AA. Insurance status and cancer treatment mediate the association between race/ethnicity and cervical cancer survival. PLoS One. 2018;13(2):e0193047. https://doi.org/10.1371/journal.pone.0193047.

34. Blake KD, Ottenbacher AJ, Rutten LJF, Grady MA, Kobrin SC, Jacobson RM, Hesse BW. Predictors of human papillomavirus awareness and knowledge in 2013. Am J Prev Med. 2015;48(4):402–10. https://doi.org/10.1016/j.amepre.2014.10.024.

35. Galbraith KV, Lechuga J, Jenerette CM, Moore LAD, Palmer MH, Hamilton JB. Parental acceptance and uptake of the HPV vaccine among African-Americans and Latinos in the United States: a literature review. Soc Sci Med (1982). 2016;159:116–26. https://doi.org/10.1016/j.socscimed.2016.04.028.

36. Galbraith-Gyan KV, Lee SJ, Ramanadhan S, Viswanath K. Disparities in HPV knowledge by race/ethnicity and socioeconomic position: trusted sources for the dissemination of HPV information. Cancer Causes Control. 2021a;32(9):923–33. https://doi.org/10.1007/s10552-021-01445-x.

37. Galbraith-Gyan KV, Ramanadhan S, Viswanath K. Community stakeholders' perspectives on introducing human papillomavirus vaccination and biobanking evidence-based programs within medically underserved communities: a community-engaged approach. Int Q Community Health Educ. 2021b;41(3):315–23. https://doi.org/10.1177/0272684X20942071.

38. Davlin SL, Berenson AB, Rahman M. Correlates of HPV knowledge among low-income minority mothers with a child 9–17 years of age. J Pediatr Adolesc Gynecol. 2015;28(1):19–23. https://doi.org/10.1016/j.jpag.2014.01.109.

39. Thompson EL, Wheldon CW, Rosen BL, Maness SB, Kasting ML, Massey PM. Awareness and knowledge of HPV and HPV vaccination among adults ages 27–45 years. Vaccine. 2020;38(15):3143–8. https://doi.org/10.1016/j.vaccine.2020.01.053.

40. Maness SB, Reitzel LR, Watkins KL, McNeill LH. HPV awareness, knowledge and vaccination attitudes among church-going African-American women. Am J Health Behav. 2016;40(6):771–8. https://doi.org/10.5993/AJHB.40.6.9.

41. Galbraith-Gyan KV, Lechuga J, Jenerette CM, Palmer MH, Moore AD, Hamilton JB. HPV vaccine acceptance among African-American mothers and their daughters: an inquiry grounded in culture. Ethn Health. 2019;24(3):323–40. https://doi.org/10.1080/13557858.2017.1332758.

42. Shelton RC, Snavely AC, De Jesus M, Othus MD,

Allen JD. HPV vaccine decision-making and acceptance: does religion play a role? J Relig Health. 2013;52(4):1120–30. https://doi.org/10.1007/s10943-011-9553-x.

43. Thomas TL, Strickland O, Diclemente R, Higgins M. An opportunity for cancer prevention during preadolescence and adolescence: stopping human papillomavirus (HPV)-related cancer through HPV vaccination. J Adolesc Health. 2013;52(5):S60–8. https://doi.org/10.1016/j.jadohealth.2012.08.011.

44. Thomas TL, Strickland OL, DiClemente R, Higgins M, Haber M. Rural African American parents' knowledge and decisions about human papillomavirus vaccination. J Nurs Scholarsh. 2012;44(4):358–67. https://doi.org/10.1111/j.1547-5069.2012.01479.x.

45. Devane-Johnson S, Williams R, Woods Giscombe C. Historical research: the history of African American breastfeeding in the United States. J Hum Lact. 2022;38(4):723–31.

46. Washington HA. Medical apartheid: the dark history of medical experimentation on Black Americans from colonial times to the present. Doubleday Books; 2006.

47. Skloot R. The immortal life of Henrietta Lacks. New York: Random House Audio; 2010.

48. Holpuch A. Family of Henrietta Lacks settles with biotech company that used her cells. The New York Times. 2023; www.nytimes.com/2023/08/01/science/henrietta-lacks-cells-lawsuit-settlement.html.

49. Gibson P, Abrams L. Racial difference in engaging, recruiting, and interviewing African American women in qualitative research. Qual Soc Work. 2003;2:457–76. https://doi.org/10.1177/1473325003024005.

50. Pew Research Center. A religious portrait of African-Americans. Pew Research Center's Religion & Public Life Project; 2009. https://www.pewresearch.org/religion/2009/01/30/a-religious-portrait-of-african-americans/.

51. Gates HL Jr. The Black Church: this is our story, this is our song: an American history. Penguin Random House; 2022.

52. Chen Y, Koh HK, Kawachi I, Botticelli M, VanderWeele TJ. Religious service attendance and deaths related to drugs, alcohol, and suicide among US health care professionals. JAMA Psychiatry. 2020;77(7):737–44. https://doi.org/10.1001/jamapsychiatry.2020.0175.

53. Mitchell T. 5. Churches and religion in Black American life. Pew Research Center's Religion & Public Life Project; 2021. https://www.pewresearch.org/religion/2021/02/16/churches-and-religion-in-black-american-life/.

54. Brouwer AF, Delinger RL, Eisenberg MC, Campredon LP, Walline HM, Carey TE, Meza R. HPV vaccination has not increased sexual activity or accelerated sexual debut in a college-aged cohort of men and women. BMC Public Health. 2019;19(1):821. https://doi.org/10.1186/s12889-019-7134-1.

55. Taylor RJ, Chatters LM. Importance of religion and spirituality in the lives of African Americans, Caribbean Blacks and non-Hispanic Whites. J Negro Educ. 2010;79(3):280–94.

56. Thomas T, Blumling A, Delaney A. The influence of religiosity and spirituality on rural parents' health decision making and human papillomavirus vaccine choices. ANS Adv Nurs Sci. 2015;38(4):E1–E12. https://doi.org/10.1097/ANS.0000000000000094.

57. Budde H, Williams GA, Scarpetti G, Kroezen M, Maier CB. What are patient navigators and how can they improve integration of care? European Observatory on Health Systems and Policies; 2022. http://www.ncbi.nlm.nih.gov/books/NBK577640/.

58. American Society for Clinical Oncology. Cancer.Net: Oral and oropharyngeal cancer statistics. American Society for Clinical Oncology; 2023.

59. World Health Organization. Cervical Cancer Elimination Initiative. 2023. https://www.who.int/initiatives/cervical-cancer-elimination-initiative. Accessed 15 Aug 2023.

60. eClinicalMedicine. Global strategy to eliminate cervical cancer as a public health problem: are we on track? EClinicalMedicine. 2023;55:101842. https://doi.org/10.1016/j.eclinm.2023.101842.

Kayoll Galbraith Gyan PhD, RN, is a Nurse Scientist in Medical Oncology and the Associate Director of the Phyllis F. Cantor Center for Research in Nursing and Patient Care Services at Dana-Farber Cancer Institute. She is also a Member of the Faculty of Medicine at Harvard Medical School. Her program of research focuses on cervical cancer prevention among Black women, with a specific focus on social cultural determinants of health, such as social support, and religion and spirituality. Her work also examines the cancer experience of young Black women diagnosed with breast and cervical cancer and the role of spirituality and religion as coping mechanisms among this population. She is a 2021 NIH Loan Repayment Award recipient and a 2018 NIMHD Research Scholar. She is also a member of the American Cancer Society's National Roundtable on Cervical Cancer's (ACS NRTCC) Patient/Consumer Education Workgroup.

Stephanie Devane-Johnson PhD, CNM, FACNM, is an Associate Professor in the Midwifery Department at Vanderbilt University School of Nursing. She received a PhD in Nursing from the University of North Carolina at Chapel Hill. Dr. Devane-Johnson has been a Certified Nurse-Midwife for 25+ years and has worked in private practice settings as well as academic institutions, providing care for women from all ethnic and socioeconomic backgrounds. In her 25 years, she has caught over 2500 babies. Dr. Devane-Johnson's research is focused on breastfeeding and health disparities among African Americans.

Preeti Khanal MPH, completed her Master of Public Health at Harvard T.H. Chan School of Public Health. Her research interest centers on access to health and education among women and children in marginalized communities of South Asia. Preeti strives to translate research into evidence-based solutions for public health issues, particularly in cancer prevention and vaccine uptake, while emphasizing health and gender equity.

Jane Kimani is the Founder and Executive Director of Uhai for Health Inc. Uhai is a nonprofit organization located in Worcester, MA, that works to promote the health of African refugees and immigrants in Massachusetts.

Rosette Serwanga is a community health advocate and patient navigator with over 20 years of experience serving and advocating for the Ugandan community in Massachusetts.

Emmanuel Owusu is Founder and Executive Director of the African Bridge Network (ABN). The ABN is a non-profit organization that works to support highly skilled, foreign-trained professionals build careers in Massachusetts.

Cherice Escobar Jones PhD, earned her doctorate in English at Northeastern University. Her research focuses on the rhetoric of race at the intersection of language, writing, and health.

Deborah Effiong is an undergraduate student at Northeastern University majoring in Pharmaceutical Sciences with a minor in Health Science Entrepreneurship.

Karrington R. Johnson is an undergraduate student at Spelman College majoring in Biology/Pre-Med.

Addressing SDOH in Communities: Perceptions from Faith-Based Institutions

Keith Lipsey, Herbert Grant, Lavonia C. Ray, Brent La Prince Edwards, and George K. Logan

1 New Bethel AME Zion Church and Surrounding Community

Keith Lipsey

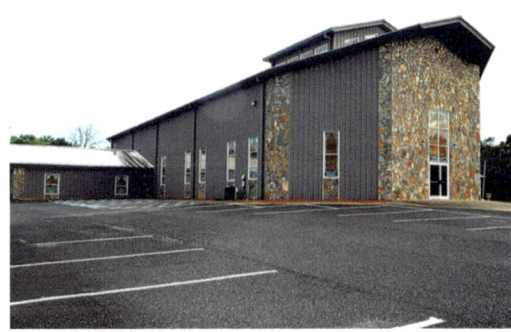

K. Lipsey (✉)
New Bethel AME Zion Church, Blue Ridge AME Zion Conference, Forest City, NC, USA

H. Grant
Goodes Temple AME Zion Church, Blue Ridge AME Zion Conference, Strawberry Plains, TN, USA

L. C. Ray
WNC Baptist Fellowship Church, Asheville, NC, USA
e-mail: contact@wncbf.org

B. L. P. Edwards
St James African Methodist Episcopal Church, Asheville, NC, USA

G. K. Logan
New Day Christian Church, Morganton, NC, USA
e-mail: pastorlogan@newdaycc.com

I am the pastor at a church located in Forest City, North Carolina. It's in the foothills, nestled between the Piedmont and the western portion of the mountains of North Carolina. I'm in an area which is better known as Grahamtown. It was a very affluent African American neighborhood some years ago. I remember coming up in this area after I got out of the military in 1989 and by that time, a lot of Black-owned businesses had gone away, and what was left was basically just the cotton and textile mills, and things of that nature. The area had changed tremendously. Now, it's basically just churches, and whatever it is that you do for work, the work is limited. A lot of jobs are gone now, and a lot of people are unemployed, and a lot of them turned to drugs and alcohol as a result of unemployment. However, there's a small remnant that still believes in the Lord.

Today, as you travel from church to church, you'll find that there aren't many people actually living in or attending church in their neighborhoods. One reason is that as they've grown older, they've moved away to attend college and educated themselves, and they've moved on. Those who remain here have a heart and love for the church and are churchgoers. I said all that to say this: there's not much going on in Rutherford County or in Forest City today.

In my time serving as pastor, I see that there are plenty of needs in my community. The former pastor who was here at New Bethel AME Zion Church, Reverend Leroy Staley, pastored the church for 26 years. As a matter of fact, the church has a rich history. My grandfather, Reverend George M. Lipsey, pastored there years ago in the late 1960s. There's a lot of history there about New Bethel AME Zion Church. It burned down twice, I think. After being rebuilt from the first fire, the old church burned down a second time. What stands there now is Thompson's Mortuary or Thompson's Funeral Home. Just below it, on Forest Street, is the newly built church, which is New Bethel. That's where Reverend Leroy Staley—who was a double amputee before he passed away 2 years ago—went out to the streets and knocked on doors. Back then, this community was infested with drugs and alcohol, but Pastor Staley went door-to-door. The next thing you know, he had a church full of over 300 members. A lot of them were former drug dealers, alcoholics, bootleggers, gamblers, and some of everything else. He was able to win them over for the Lord and get them in the church.

I arrived 5 years ago in 2018. I became the pastor knowing that I would have to become the community pastor, just as Reverend Staley was, but I don't mind. New Bethel is the largest African American church in Forest City. I have about 116 members, but I only see half of that. Some come this Sunday; some come another Sunday. With that being said, this is a community church that everybody uses at some point in time, whether it be for funerals, baby showers, or marriages.

1.1 New Bethel AME Zion and Community Engagement

Since I have been at New Bethel, I have been able to do some good things in the neighborhood. Within my first year, I connected with the Chase Cornerstone Ministries, which is located in the Chase area. We call it the Chase area, but the address is still Forest City. They have a food pantry, and we were able to unite with them and collaborate to be able to serve our community on several occasions. Even when it wasn't at our church, we were able to go to other churches because the food pantry moved around. That was one way of having some camaraderie among ourselves and in our community.

To make a long story short, the food pantry allowed us to feed people. We were also able to give away clothing for the children as well as adults in the community. There were people needing help to pay their light bills. So we collaborated with the United Way, a nonprofit organization, for funds that supported our ability to distribute essentials for babies like Pampers diapers, wipes, and things of that nature—on top of food, on top of the utility bills being paid to the community. That was one of the highlights of our community engagement since I have been at New Bethel.

1.2 Social and Health Problems in the Community

We are centrally located in the community and focus on the social and health problems we see as vital to the survival of our members and the communities in which they live. We also work in partnership with the local health department to address health issues in our community.

As pastor, I was able to join forces with the Rutherford County Health Department and Blue Ridge Health to set up outdoor COVID testing on several occasions. They thought the church would be a good location for COVID testing because you can drive all the way around the church, giving the people easy access. People could also drive up to the front of the church and park in the parking lot and someone would come out and test them in their cars. The nurses would come out and test them and then read off their test result a couple of days later.

That's how I first got connected with the United Way. Because I'm partnering with them, now they come down to New Bethel on a monthly basis. These monthly meetings have led to workshops where we are able to talk about health disparities in the community. We talked about the COVID outbreak and what we can do for our community. From there, we were able to work with Blue Ridge Health to develop strategies to alleviate some of these disparities related to COVID.

1.3 Partnerships Among New Bethel AME Zion Church and Healthcare Agencies

Our partnership with other organizations came as a result of the United Way reaching out to Blue Ridge Health and saying "Hey, we got this guy, this church, this pastor that we've connected up with, and he's got the facility for it, no problem." That's how it all started. We were able to get a partnership with the Rutherford County Health Department, and from there, others in the community heard that something was going on at New Bethel. We then allowed Blue Ridge Health to come onboard to also engage with our community.

As a result of these partnerships, we were able to do COVID tests and then administer the vaccines, both the first and second shots. The turnout in the community was great. It was just a marvelous sight to be there as the pastor in the community and seeing Blacks as well as whites coming out for these services. The majority that came though were Caucasians because, you know, we [African Americans] are skeptical about coming out, about getting vaccinations, and all the stereotypes that come along with it. But we were always sounding the trumpet and trying to get these services to our people because we're right there in the neighborhood; in an all-Black neighborhood.

Despite the turnout [*for COVID services*] being mostly white, we were still able to reach people in our community. People came because it was so hard to get the vaccine. There was a time when there were a lot of inconveniences to accessing the testing and vaccines; you had to wait in line, when you had to come back with another appointment, whereas here at New Bethel services were on the spot. You just go online, put your information in, and drive to the church. During those days, accessing these services through your regular doctor or healthcare provider was impossible. At New Bethel, we were trying to place these resources where people could come and easily access them. Everything that they needed was right there in our community. We were blessed to be able to do that.

Later on, we were able to receive funding by a grant because we were a location that provided the COVID vaccine and tests. They gave us a little $500 stipend for taking these services online. As we went online, we were able to give my name, location, and what we're doing. We were recipients of this funding twice during COVID. Through our collaboration with Blue Ridge Health, you just went online and put in your information, and that was it. Once you pulled up, you told them your name, and they gave you what you needed.

When the community came to us for COVID services, they were already fully staffed. Blue Ridge Health brought 10–15 people with them to do the work. They brought the computers and they set them up for the next time they were there. They took down the person's information and gave them another date when they could come back to get what they needed. That was key because if they don't have computers at home, they can't get on for the second time—or, who knows, perhaps not even for the first time. Computer access depended on somebody helping them, or they may have gone to Blue Ridge Health, and they may have been able to get on there [the computer] by having some other assistance.

Those were really some highlights of our community work that I'll never forget. I'll always cherish these successes even though funding ran out or ran slim for COVID as we looked at it as being over, post-pandemic. But now, we're seeing those numbers rise again. If they continue rising, we'll go back to wearing masks and other PPE, but the good news is that we'll be able to make ourselves available again to do that ministry.

1.4 Reflection: Moving Forward

As we talk about meeting the needs of our community, there was an African American school by the name of Dunbar, up the street from Thompson's Mortuary. Dunbar is located at the place known in the community as the playground on Hardin Road in Forest City. Many of the people in the community were educated there, such as in nearby places such as Black Mountain and in Asheville. However, most of the people who once lived here in this community have moved on. It would be great to see this former African American school returned to its former state. Dunbar is a historical landmark for the African American culture of Grahamtown, and many teachers and students still reminisce about their employment and education here at Dunbar.

Dunbar is a place where people from all over the USA continue to come to be reunited with their community of family and friends. To restore the school would provide educational, recreational, and social purposes to involve the children and youth who are missing a sense of oneness. Dunbar is a staple of the community other than the churches, and that's all that African Americans here in this town have to claim that belongs to the community. Even today, many activities are observed on the playground and basketball court, there is a Grahamtown Reunion every Labor Day weekend on Saturday, and it's all day. Others still operate that building and sometimes they'll have events in the winter and they're trying to start up a Black museum. These types of educational and cultural activities would greatly benefit our community.

Secondly, I think we still need to be looking at drug use in our community and to focus our ministry on addressing substance use and abuse. There's still a lot of substance abuse going on—meth, amphetamines, pills, things of that nature. At one point, every time you turned around, someone was dying of overdosing. These were social issues here and just recently, within the last 6 months; now we are seeing a lot of issues with fentanyl. A lot of people are playing around with fentanyl, and they are losing their lives due to drug overdose from this substance.

Third, there are other needs in our community such as clothing, affordable housing, and food. A lot of our churches don't have food pantries or food ministries, which is one we're somewhat undermanned in, and here at New Bethel, we haven't been able to provide these services either. Those who normally have the soup kitchens, like

Oak Grove Missionary Baptist Church around the corner, continue to provide hot meals for persons who are less fortunate in the Forest City, Grahamtown area. Other than that, there are not really a lot of resources located in our community, so people are forced to travel to distant cities like Asheville and places like that.

Fourth, there is the persistent issue of HIV/AIDS in our community. These individuals have to travel far just to receive the services they need. Many of those affected with HIV/AIDS don't have the means to travel, or the transportation, so a lot of them don't have the needed resources to deal with their situations on a day-to-day basis. Some of them don't even have affordable healthcare or even know how to sign up for it.

Finally, although there are a lot of ministries providing access to nutritious foods out there, it would be nice if the church I'm serving had a food pantry, for example, being able to say "the food pantry at New Bethel is going to be open on such and such day. Here's a bag of groceries." There is one other food ministry in the neighborhood, it's called the "G Team," and it deals with the Grahamtown area. They are doing great work and led by Wilfred McDowell who is a member of New Bethel. The G Team grows vegetables and distributes them out to the community. They also provide resources or can turn people toward resources. The G Team is funded and I meet with them when I can on Tuesdays. The mayor is there, police officers are there—they sit around the table discussing social and health issues that are affecting our community.

1.5   Future Goals

Prior to COVID, I started a ministry and haven't yet restarted it, but it was called "Am I my brother's keeper?" I had just begun to get an open forum going, bringing in police officers, the mayor, other dignitaries, and other members of churches with Black and white congregants. I also brought in those who were victims of physical violence from gunshots or those who had committed crimes. We had one discussion inside the church, and then we had another session outside in the community. However, when the COVID pandemic kicked in, that ministry was shut down. This ministry was important because I wanted to bring the community together because there was always a shooting. I was trying to grab the Black male and bring him in off the street. Get him acclimated to somebody's church; get the guys to put down the guns; stop the violence; let's think about this. I wanted to educate them as well.

There are so many things that we are doing, small things, that can really make a huge difference in our community.

2   Goodes Temple AME Zion and Straw Plains, Tennessee

Herbert Grant

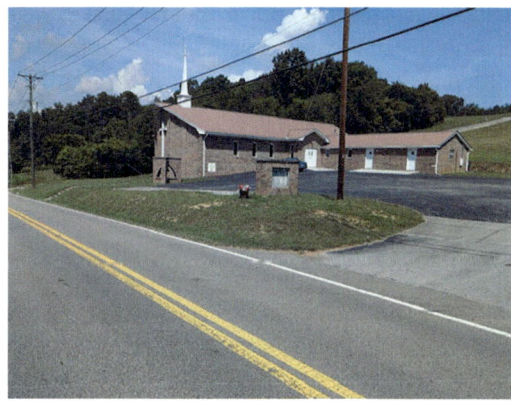

The first AME Zion church when you cross the North Carolina line going west into Tennessee is in Newport, which is Cocke County. It's a nice community. The next church is the Belmont Church, which is in Dandridge. It's in a rural area and much more of a family church. The Newport church is family, too. The people there—Black and white—are well connected to one another. The church in Dandridge has a minister who grew up in that church, so they get along really well. They have a lot of support.

The areas from Newport to Dandridge are well mixed, Black and white. You don't see too many issues there. The next one is Morristown,

Tennessee, and that church is family and mixed. Basically all the churches in Tennessee have a mixed congregation. The next one is in New Market, which is in Jefferson City. It's right there in the heart of Carson-Newman University. A lot of the students attend services at the New Market church. I know they used to, some may still, but not as prevalent as it used to be. It's a good congregation.

The church where I'm at is in Straw Plains, commonly called Strawberry Plains, Tennessee. It's about 7 miles this side of Knoxville. It is a family church, but it's like all the other churches, racially mixed. The people are kind; it's a nice community. I do have a relationship with a lot of the white churches in the area because we do Holy Week services together every year. Churches in Tennessee appear stronger than churches in North Carolina. I would say people in the churches of Tennessee are more appreciative of the ministry than North Carolina.

2.1   Minister Relationships with Congregation and Community

I was always taught by my mentors—men like the late Reverends J. F. Wills and Jesse Williams—they always said, "If you have an idea or something you want to do, a program you want to get across, something you want to put forth, then kick it around with your officers like your chairman or trustee board." They might see it from a different angle, and if they do, they might have a twist to it that they want to try. If they run with it, and if the people want it, the people will support it.

Most of the time, as pastors, we'll come up with a solution to a problem, and the people will say, "Well, Reverend, you know…" and when they start humming around, then you know it's something they don't want to do. But because they have respect for the preacher, then what they'll do is say, "Well, Reverend, that's good," but when it comes time for the program, the people don't show up. You're there by yourself, and you can't get mad at them because it's what *you* wanted—not them. It's important to get your membership on board with any initiative that you want to do. Remember, as the pastor, you may only be there for a short period of time; it's the members who will always be there.

2.2 Community Engagement in Goodes Temple AME Zion and Straw Plains, Tennessee

In the area of Tennessee where my church is, some people work in education, others in the local factory, and some at medical facilities, but the rest of them are pretty much retired.

The churches in Tennessee are strong in their congregant participation. In my experience, churches in Tennessee don't struggle with their (financial) obligation or responsibility to the conference like the churches on the North Carolina side. So, in that regard, the people are more intentional about their church and so their attendance and membership are better. In addition to being pastor at Goodes Temple AME Zion, I am also the Presiding Elder of the Asheville District of the Blue Ridge AME Zion Conference. Since I'm in two states, if I have a district meeting in Tennessee, then the next meeting has to be on the North Carolina side. When the meeting is in Tennessee, the churches are pretty well packed out. But when it comes to North Carolina, that's not necessarily the case.

2.3 The Church and Engaging with Today's Youth

I've always given my young people, say, 5 or 10 dollars as an incentive when they attend church on Sunday. Then it dawned on me—because I had children getting ready to graduate from high school and some already in college—that we needed to do something more, something so that when they finish high school, we'll be able to give them some financial support when they get ready to go to college.

I talked to my young people about making good grades and always asked, you know, "What kind of grades are you making in school?" Most of them are making As, and they may have a B or two. I told them, "Well now, if you keep your A's and B's up, if you don't fall below that, then at the end of the school year, the pastor's going to reward you." So, that's what I do. I don't draw from the Youth Investment Fund for these incentives because our goal is to have at least $10,000, or more, in that fund. So I use other resources for these incentives.

The other thing I do is allow them to do some activities that they want to do. They may have a yard sale or a car wash. Because they did well with their yard sale last year, they raised about $1800 for their Investment Fund. The youth are currently organizing for another fundraising event this year.

I always try to incorporate them into the Sunday morning worship service, too, and make them a part of it. I share with my older church congregants that children are not inclined to want to sing the traditional hymns because there's a different beat. And the hymns really have no meaning to them. But then, you know, when they listen to songs of artists like Donnie McClurkin, that's the kind of contemporary form that has meaning to them, because this is the present age we're serving and the lyrics of these songs reflect the things they find themselves going through.

One of my mentors had shared with me that he had some unruly kids in church when he was pastoring in Morganton, NC. He shared his wisdom with me, so when I went to Mount Zion in Marion, North Carolina, in the fall of 1983 or 1984, I had some young men that I knew how to handle. There were about 10 or 12 of them, but there was always one who seemed to be the ringleader. What he did, the others did. So, I corralled the leader of the group here, and I talked to him, and I said, "Now, listen…" I appointed him over the rest of the group, and I said, "Now, if you all come to Sunday School, and you're all supportive of the church, and vacation bible school, etcetera, this is what the pastor is going to do." So, I would give him a little more money as an incentive. The leader had higher earnings than the rest of them. Once I established that, you would be surprised what he did. He kept the rest of them in line.

But you always have to pick out the ring-leader, the one that kids mostly follow who seems to be the leader of the group. You have to observe and see who's who. Once you discover who the leader is, the one they're following, the one who has control, then the leader will cause the rest of them to fall in line. The late Reverend J. F. Wills taught me that, and that money would do the trick. Nowadays, you know, you have to pull out a 10, but I don't mind. I'm never empty. I always have more to give. And I tell them all the time: I wished I had 100 kids where I could give out $10 to every Sunday, to every child that comes to church.

My church office is filled with all kinds of piggy banks. Whenever a young person comes, whether they come just to visit or they're regular attendees, I'll tell one of the kids that brought their friend to church, "You take them in the office and you let them pick out a piggy bank." And then when I give them their funds, I'll tell them, "Now, the pig only eats greens. Pigs don't eat coins. The pig only eats greens." So, you feed the pig greens…your goal is to stuff the pig until you can't stuff it anymore. If you come every Sunday, you'll get something, but if you don't come on Sundays, you don't get it.

This money for the piggy bank comes out of my pocket, my own personal funds, but it ultimately comes from the Lord. I hate to say that, but I'm serious. Because I don't have it, but the Lord has it. Whenever I get to church, whatever I do, regardless of how many children I have, I'm always blessed in that I still have more than I started out with, even after I paid my tithes.

These strategies I put into place for our youth just came about by having them in the church and seeing that it won't be but a few years before they're going off to some university. I want us to be able to support them with their future educational and career goals. These strategies will also keep them rooted and grounded in the church because they'll be able to say, "This is what my church has done or what the church did for me." And hopefully, in return, they will come back when they graduate, and get jobs, and continue to be supportive of their home church.

2.4 What Most Influenced the Strategies to Engage Today's Youth in Church Activities?

I grew up in an area where people recognized in me what I did not recognize in myself. I was sought out in the ministry, and they gave me respect. They allowed me to preach at churches in my local community: Mills Chapel Baptist, New Salem Baptist, Macedonia AME Zion. They knew my mother and knew she raised seven children by herself. So, to see me in the ministry, and not having a criminal record, they gave me a lot of words of encouragement that have always kept me humble. I benefited tremendously from the fellowship that we had with one another. It's the people that pour into your life, people that pour into your ministry, that keep you in touch and keep you humble.

For the most part, I try to attend all the home-going services in my community if I'm not busy. There are some that I can't attend because I have regional or national meetings with the church that I have to be a part of. But for most of them, I always do. Like I said, this is home. We all grew up together. Most of the ones that have gone on, they were part of that fellowship with one another. After graduating high school, I left for the military, but I came back home to the Swannanoa Valley and started preaching in 1980. So, these are just things that you do. We learned to respect one another.

Sunday school gives us the foundation. Even when church is over, Sunday school is open, and kids are required to attend—that's what we had when I was growing up. Sunday school gave us a sense of who God is. It gave us a sense that there is a higher being. The sense that you learn to respect your elders and you learned to have respect for one another.

2.5 Establishing Respect and Trust in the Community

In this age that we find ourselves in now, that's one of the things that is missing: young people need to learn to have respect for themselves and for their neighbors. They need to learn how to have respect for others even though you may not know them. When you go into the mall or to restaurants, you practice good manners.

That's the one thing that Sunday school and church did for us. It taught us to be on our best behavior. So, even when you're not in church—and that's the one thing I try to get over to young people—your name and your character is all you have. You don't have anything else. And if you mess that up, then you pretty much write a whole lot of things off. But if you keep your name clean, if you keep your character intact, people will respect you.

None of us are perfect, you know. I have to share that with them. None of us are perfect, but if you try your best, you do your best. I always tell my youth that if they have any problems whatsoever—because, sometimes, children are not able to talk to their parents—my door is always open. I tell them, "Listen, your pastor is always available. You call me. Don't make no difference what time of day or whatever. You call me. If there's something going on in your life that you can't discuss with anybody else, I want you to know that my door is open. Whatever you share with me, we'll keep it in strict confidence, unless it's something that I know that we have to sit down and talk about and share with your parents."

One thing I've learned too is the value of being consistent. You can't be one thing today and something else tomorrow and then expect children to respect you. So, whatever you are today, you have to be that tomorrow, next week, this year, next year—because children are watching us. A lot of children, if we're not careful, will imitate us. So, you have to be careful how you walk, what you do, and what you say. The last thing you want is to offend one and cause them to fall from grace, as scripture teaches us, because that would be devastating.

The other thing is that young people have to have confidence in you. That's the key, that is, the youth need to know they can trust you and that they can put their confidence in you. And anytime—not just in children, but the adults as well—once that confidence is gone, you might as well just move to another area.

I always show an interest in young people and ask them if they have thought about what they want to do in the next 10 years. Have they given any thought to what they want to do or where they want to be in the next 10 years? My mentor, the late Reverend Wills, raised that question with me one day and I hadn't given it any thought. Since then, when he asked that question, I started thinking about that. I would love to see every young person that has crossed my path in ministry to go on and become leaders and excel. One of the things I share with the young people is that if they learn to save—and this is one of the problems that a lot of us have, even as adults—they start now, and if they give the Lord His 10%, and set 10% aside for themselves, they can do whatever they want with the remaining 80%. By the time they reach 25 or 30, they shouldn't have to work for anybody—if they make good investments.

Moving forward, that's one of the things that we'll be doing this year, bringing in some investors to share with the youth, to drop that seed in their spirit of saving. Even if we reach just one, then what we have done will not be in vain.

I remember growing up poor and not having anybody to teach us how to save. We worked though; they taught us how to work but not how to save or invest. That kind of experience does influence your thinking in terms of how it was for us and how it could be different if these kids were taught those skills much earlier in life.

2.6   Value of Working with Today's Youth

One of the joys is watching our young people grow and develop through our teaching and preaching. Because when you reach the youth, then you know you've done your job. The only thing we can do is try our best and at the end of the day, we let the Lord do the rest.

When we were kids, everybody in our community was part of our family no matter what.

Our neighbors helped raise us. Whether we understand it or not, we had a rich life back in those days. We didn't have to worry about any shootings. If you went to a dance, the only thing that may happen is a fist fight. Even after you had a fist fight, within 5 or 10 min, you were friends again.

Nowadays, that's not so. Nowadays, I teach these kids how to respond to police. I tell them the same thing I told my children. Anytime you are approached by an officer of the law, you stop, you listen, and you use good manners. Whatever question they ask you, you need to be on your best behavior. One of the keys is good manners. *Yes, ma'am. No ma'am. Yes sir. No sir.* It goes a long way. I always tell the story about my oldest son who was stopped by the police in Weaverville, and he had some underage people in the car, and they had alcohol. When the sheriff called me, he said, "Mr. Grant, you'll have to come and secure the car because I need to take him to Buncombe County." The officer said my son was just as nice as he could be, and that went a long way. When it came time for my son to go before the judge, the same officer shared with the judge that my son had good manners and that was the thing that got him off.

I try to teach these young people, "Think before you speak." Because once the milk is spilled, you can never reclaim that. "Look before you launch." I tell them, "Listening doesn't cost you one red cent." Whether you agree with it or not, it doesn't bother you to listen. Listening is very important in the life of every individual. If we learn to listen, it will cause big dividends for us in the end, because it will always come back. Once you hear it, it's in your memory bank. You may not know it or use it for a whole year, but then something will happen, and you'll say, "Oh, that's what they were talking about! I really appreciate that."

2.7 Reflection

We have to start teaching our youth now, while they're young, when we can shape them. Once they get past 16, there may not be much you can

do for them. If you start early, you can shape them and mold them into a pattern that will be beneficial for them years later down the road.

When we were young and growing up in the Swannanoa Valley, everybody was working, sometimes two jobs, just trying to make it. Community was very important because everybody had to chip in and help raise the kids, help discipline the children. Nowadays, no one wants to do that. That's why church is so important. It's not perfect, but it's all we as a people have. It's still the main institution in our community, and it's important.

3 The Black Community in Asheville, North Carolina

Brent La Prince Edwards

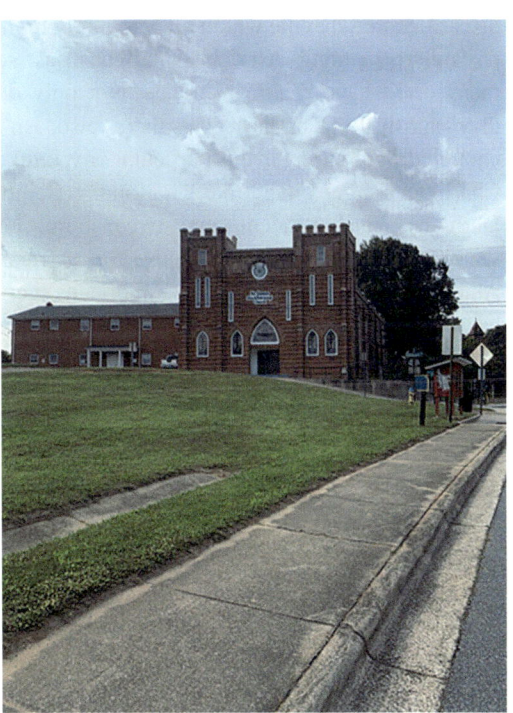

Asheville, North Carolina, is located in Buncombe County and is an unusual place. It's predominantly Caucasian, and our population is only about 11% African American and it's a very expensive place to live. People move here from all over the world because it's beautiful in the mountains. It's in Western North Carolina, and it's one of the fastest-growing cities—I call them big towns—in this part of North Carolina.

The problem about living here is that it's so expensive. The job market is terrible, unless you are in a type of profession like a doctor, or something like that. The job market is especially terrible for African Americans. With that being said, the economy here is horrible, and to live here is just very expensive, so we have a small percentage of African Americans here.

3.1 Lack of Health Insurance and Access to Healthcare Affecting African Americans in Asheville, North Carolina

One of the problems we've noticed is the health disparities in Asheville which are very, very high, particularly among African Americans, as so many don't have health insurance. Not only do they not have insurance, but there also isn't enough programming in this particular city, unlike Charlotte. Larger cities, like Charlotte, Raleigh, Durham, Winston-Salem, and Greensboro, all seem to have better programs for African Americans. Very few African Americans here have health insurance, and there's not enough health education toward our people in this city.

3.2 Programs Implemented in St. James AME Church to Address Social Issues and Health Disparities

What our church has done is that we have something called the Rosa Walker Advancement Initiative, Inc. It's not only an educational and mentoring program, but it also addresses health disparities. We educate the community on health disparities. We bring in healthcare professionals. We help people in the community who could not

get health insurance and things like that. We point them in a direction where they can get that by partnering with health organizations in the city. We partner with one of the major hospitals here and also with other groups in the city, and that has proven to be an effective approach to addressing health disparities in our community. This program is still growing, but it's proven to be effective because we're having discussions with African Americans. It's not limited to just African Americans, but that's one of our top priorities because we're the unreached group of people.

The Rosa Walker Advancement Initiative has helped to educate our people on how to stay on top of their health; how to get health insurance; how to do blood pressure checks, HIV testing, diabetes testing, and precancer screenings; and all those different types of things.

3.3 Health Disparities in Asheville, North Carolina

When I first came to Asheville in 2010, I didn't know all these problems were in Asheville because I had always heard that "Oh, Asheville is such a beautiful place." Everybody talks about the Biltmore House and all these other things, and I didn't know the disparities here were this bad. No one emphasizes the issues with affordable housing, employment, and access to healthcare among African Americans in our communities.

I'm actually part of the Asheville Buncombe County Land Trust Board. We also help with housing, to get people affordable housing. I've only been here 10 or 12 years now, and I have seen so many changes because it seems every time I turn around, something new is being built here. Since I've been here, there are almost hardly any African Americans downtown at all. They're all being pushed way out. What's happening is a lot of people are leaving Asheville. The older people are staying, but a lot of people are leaving because of what's going on here.

3.4 Social and Health Issues Informed by the Black Community

I was informed about social issues that exist in Asheville first by people in the community because when I initially came here, I wasn't aware of these issues since I didn't grow up here. So, I didn't know what was really happening in the underbelly of Asheville. I've really learned the status of Asheville through the community and then through my involvement with a lot of organizations in the city. In my role as pastor, I have worked closely with social action, a lot of political groups, and some social action groups. By being in these meetings, and then just from the church members themselves, that's how I was informed.

I also learned about health issues primarily through our affiliation with a large healthcare provider in Asheville. We've had health organizations come to us and ask if they could use our facility. I remember once Mission Hospital wanted to use our facility to host a citywide health meeting. I attended and I learned so much from that about health-related issues affecting the people of Asheville.

3.5 Experience with Healthcare Institutions to Address Access to Care

Our collaboration with Mission Hospital was a positive experience. The focal discussion with this healthcare provider was opioid usage because there is a lot of that, and meth and things. We had a lot of people here in Asheville, both Black and white, to die from this opioid usage. So, that was the main discussion during our meetings and I wanted to be nosey, to be honest. I wanted to learn of what our white counterparts were doing to address the opioid pandemic. I thought, well this is a good opportunity for me to see what they're thinking and what can I learn from them that will help my congregants.

So, it was a positive experience, even though Mission is now going through a big transition. They changed their administration, and a lot of people are complaining because Mission is making a lot of mistakes. They have lawsuits and things against them. We even had a member of our church pass away from a misdiagnosis.

What made my experience with Mission Hospital so positive is that there were a lot of Black organizations that were present in our community meetings with them that kind of balanced things out. For example, we partner with an organization called Asheville Buncombe Institute for Parity Association (ABIPA), and they have been very instrumental in addressing health disparities in Asheville. ABIPA has been one of the four leaders to work with our church and the community that really helped us navigate our way through all the health-related issues in Asheville. We don't have that type of relationship with Mission Hospital anymore since their new administration has taken over, but we do have a strong relationship with other organizations.

Prior to the new administration at Mission Hospital, we were asked to permit them to talk to my congregation about the opioid crisis in Asheville. During their presentation of the opioid situation, we were allowed to ask questions. I took what we learned from that, and I reshaped what I learned from that meeting for information that would be relevant to our community.

During those initial meetings, Mission presented information to us about the problem. They didn't come with solutions, only there to discuss the problem with us. I thought, okay, we know what the problem is. Now what…Give us our next steps. What should our response be to this problem? However, the solutions Mission Hospital did come up with were tailored to the white community. It's a known fact that white people have better health insurance. They have better access to healthcare. Of course, you have white people who don't have health insurance at all but not like our people.

Following our initial meetings with Mission Hospital which we called meeting "A," we did our own part "B" meeting. During our part B meeting, we did not include them. We adapted what we learned from them and came up with our own strategies to help our community. How can we help our community with this? And not only address the opioid issue but also the other health disparities that relate to issues like poor prenatal care with Black American females. So, we just took the information we learned from Mission and said, "Well, this is what we're going to do, and this is how we're going to shape this…."

3.6 Developing Our Own Strategies for Our Community

One of the things that we did was canvas the community. We're in the East End of Asheville, which is one of the very few remaining historically Black areas in Asheville, and that's being gentrified. So, our church is right at the top of Martin Luther King and College streets which is at the end of downtown.

Our church started canvassing the community through ABIPA, having conversations with the locals, particularly African Americans—starting the conversations, reaching out to them, getting them to talk about it, and then pointing them to resources: "If you're having this problem, this is what you can do." Or "If you're having this experience, this is what you can do." And "If you don't have resources, this organization over here can help you get the resources that you need."

That's one of the main things that we have done to pull people in, because it's almost like when it comes to the Black community, it's like "Okay, *we're [healthcare systems]* not even going to reach out to you all." You know, what our community suffers most with, particularly in Asheville, is the lack of information. They don't know how to get these resources or where to start.

Then we also had a group of nurses and RNs and others to teach people about healthcare—staying on top of your blood pressure, making sure that you're getting mammograms, making sure men get prostate exams, all different types of things. And we actually do blood pressure checks and prostate exams and things on a regular basis.

3.7 Addressing the Issue of Trust in the Black Community in Asheville, NC

Our efforts to address health disparities are still a work in progress because the trust is still not there. People say, "No matter what you're saying, we don't trust it." We've almost had to give them the educational tools to know how to go into the belly of the beast and how to work to get the resources they need. It's like we've been teaching them to understand what their rights are and what their rights may not be. So that when they go into these areas, even though they may not trust these institutions, they'll have the knowledge to know how to navigate them.

Unlike Charlotte and other places, I can only think of maybe two Black doctors here. There may be more, but in Charlotte, there are Black doctors everywhere. There are Black health clinics, and even at a white health clinic, there are African Americans throughout. Here in Asheville, you almost have no choice but to go to a lily-white health institution.

It's like that saying "If you can't be with the one you love, love the one you're with." It's kind of like that. We say, since we have to, since we're in a position in these mountains to love the one we're with, "This is what you do with this. Know what your rights are. Know what you're legally entitled to."

Most of the nurses that we work with are from our community. In our congregation, we have registered nurses but most of them came through ABIPA. Some are CPAs and other levels of nurses as well, but most are RNs. Then, of course, ABIPA has another level of resources for registered nurses. They did a dynamic job. They canvassed all the churches. Our church isn't the only church they canvas; they canvas all the churches and African American churches in Asheville. In doing that, they've taken leadership, and as an incentive, the church that has the most blood pressure checks or the most to participate in the program gets $1000. Our church has won several times because we need the money to pay off the AME conference claims. So, I tell them, "I know you got your blood pressure checked last week. Get it checked again."

One of my favorite organizations here in Asheville was started by Kenyon Lake. He's the son of one of the Harlem Globetrotters. His organization is called "My Daddy Taught Me That." He's a hero in this city. His program has lasted through the test of time. They kind of started when I came here around 2010 and he has all these young men that he mentors, makes sure they go to school, and teaches them life skills. He's like a father to the men in this city. He was a social worker here, and he actually quit his job in social work to pursue this organization. He's recognized by the city and they even made a "Kenyon Lake Day" to celebrate the work he is doing here in Asheville.

3.8   Reflection

One of main challenges is that the white world, in essence, doesn't do much for African Americans. It's almost like they do "enough" so they can check the box off to say that they have [helped] a certain number of minorities. You know, "Well, we did help *this* minority group." Everything here, as is across America, is more white-centered to benefit the white community. So, that's the first challenge.

The next challenge is getting our people to support something that's not their own. It's almost like we have the same problems, but there are these cliques. You know, "I'm going to stick with the Baptist side," or "I'm going to stick with the Presbyterian side." So, one of the main challenges we have is trying to get our people to see that it doesn't matter the name of the bricks; we need to work together.

Then, funding, funding, funding. We've been doing pretty good with funding, amazingly, and that's because we have some good grant writers. The former mayor of Asheville, who is African American, Terri Bellamy, is on our grant writing board. She doesn't attend our church, but she's on our board, so she knows where all the bodies are.

Finally, I wanted to add that I've written a children's book called *You Can't Bully Me Anymore*. When you think about health, bullying has an effect on it. We've had several children in

Asheville commit suicide because of bullying since I've been here. So, they're using this book in elementary schools here. It's written specifically for elementary school-age children, and it gives the next steps to bullying. Through the Rosa Walker Advancement Initiative, we were able to purchase around 4000 books and give them out for free to the schools.

You Can't Bully Me Anymore is a book written for the mind of a child because a lot of times it's difficult for children to articulate trauma. This book draws out that bullying is real so that children can begin to have the discussion with parents or guardians. We're doing a remake of the first book—called *You Can't Bully Me*—because in it, I didn't include LGBTQ children. And they're some of the most bullied. Whether people agree with the same lifestyle or not, every human being deserves respect.

4   A Historical Perspective: The Black Church and Community Engagement in Asheville, North Carolina

Lavonia C. Ray

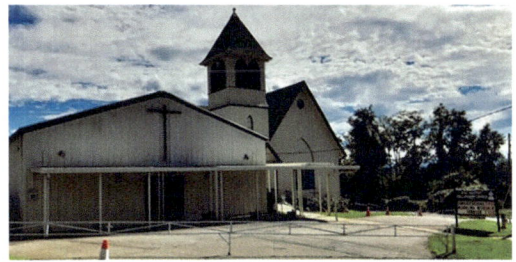

I am the oldest serving minister in the city and the county overall. I have been preaching here in Western North Carolina for about 56 years. Before we organized the WNC Baptist Fellowship Church here in downtown Asheville, I pastored in Fletcher for 38 years. I have served as President of the Baptist Ministers' Union and worked in many education and community projects here in Asheville. I have also been the director and board member of the YMI Cultural Center (Young Men's Institute), the one located on Eagle and Market Street, but I guess one of my more interesting roles in the Asheville community was when I was Director of Shaw University, one of their satellite Divinity Schools in the 1980s. I have also been a Board Member of the National Baptist Convention and attended meetings with other Baptist clergy and leaders throughout the Southeastern USA in places like North Carolina, New Orleans, and Texas. However, as I previously mentioned, I was Director of the Shaw Divinity Distance Program that was in operation for about 11 or 12 years before they dissolved the program.

Shaw University's Divinity Program in Western North Carolina and Asheville in particular was important because it was instrumental in the education of a ministerial workforce in Asheville for a cohort of Black Baptist Churches who could meet the religious and social needs of the Black community. Many pastors of the Black Baptist Churches in Asheville were graduates of Shaw's Divinity Program. Over the years, I have had the opportunity to work alongside ministers like Dr. Mosely of Nazareth, Dr. Avery of Hill Street, Dr. White at Mount Zion, and, prior to Dr. Mosely, Dr. Dunn. All of whom came out of Shaw University. Shaw University is located in Raleigh, North Carolina, and is among the oldest HBCUs in the USA and affiliated with the Baptist Church. Shaw's Divinity School is especially known for educating a number of individuals to enter into ministerial professions.

When I look back over the years that I have been pastoring in Asheville, I am fortunate to have worked alongside with colleagues many of whom came out of high school with me. These are colleagues that have known each other as children growing up and have had very close relationships with each other throughout our lives and in our careers as pastors of the Baptist Churches in Asheville. Some of them have died, like Dr. Charles Mosley, pastor of Nazareth Baptist Church. Pastor Mosely and I came out of high school together. He was a Shaw Divinity graduate and taught for me in the Shaw Divinity satellite program here in Asheville. And although

I went to Mars Hill College, I was very much involved in the Shaw Divinity Program here in Asheville. Black Churches like Nazareth and Mount Zion Baptist, St. James AME, Hopkins Chapel AME Zion, and Berry Temple United Methodist Church are all located in the East End neighborhood of Asheville. These churches were the center of the community, raising money and sponsoring programs and other special projects to support the Black community. These churches are still standing but gentrification of the East End community has led to a decrease in the membership of these communities. These churches like other traditional congregations are adapting to support their older members while attracting younger members.

4.1 The Value of the YMI Cultural Center to Asheville's Black Community

When I look back on another important role I have taken on in the community, it would have been back in the early 1980s when I was Director of the YMI Cultural Center, which is still there although you don't hear a lot about it today. But back in the early 1980s, the YMI Center was so important because it was a place that many of us (African Americans) could identify with. It was the Center for Black culture. Some wealthy whites in Biltmore Forest put the money into the YMI because they knew that it had a rich history. During those times, the YMI Cultural Center identified itself with George Vanderbilt, a wealthy philanthropist that lived in Biltmore Forest. Mr. Vanderbilt and other whites from the Asheville community contributed funds for the renovation of the YMI for the purpose of maintaining a cultural center in the Black community. It was right there in the heart of Eagle Street, so to speak. You know, I remember when I was growing up my mom would tell me, "Now don't you go down on Eagle Street" since at times there were some tough people hanging around that area. But there were also a lot of Black-owned businesses in the area with a rich history. A lot of rich history was there on Eagle Street. You know, I remember walking through the area to the high school I attended, Stephens-Lee. Back in those days we walked to school, and some 50 years ago, this was during the period of segregation and Jim Crow and is really where Blacks couldn't be anywhere else.

Thinking back on those days, I'm quite sure a lot of parents did think the YMI Cultural Center was the hope of people, who invested and were engaged in the YMI. The hope among the community was that by having a place to house the history of the culture of the people served as a reminder of the history of the people of Asheville—a reminder of the culture that people could identify with and something that was positive that would help shape and maybe reduce crime in the area. The YMI displayed positive images of Black people and provided information whereby parents could instruct their children. Parents could tell their children positive stories of the ancestors that paved the way for them.

4.2 Current Needs of the Black Community in Asheville, NC

We have a saying now that since we're in the twenty-first century or whatever, things are not like what they used to be. Pretty much everything is based on the same level now than it was back in the late 1970s and early 1980s. But what I see now is that we're missing so much from our culture and history that sustained us during those earlier years. Soon, I'll be with a group of preachers who have transitioned on, and my fear is that our grandchildren, my grandchildren, will not, I feel, be able to meet certain levels of understandings necessary to be successful because we really hadn't left some of the proper things for them to be able to handle the persistent racism that persists in our society. I don't know of any really important educational things we're leaving for the children, for future generations, especially for those that want to achieve the levels of success of my generation. I don't quite see it. Um, it could happen, and I pray that it does. But around here in Western North Carolina, I don't see a lot that

we're doing. I just don't see it. We could do more. We need to do more. It could happen, but I don't see it happening. Now, I guess, because of integration, we're saying that everybody is equal now, and that's not true. We're so far from that. Even as clergy, as a minister, I don't see where many of our young people are advancing.

One issue for the next generation is that they do not know their history. They do not know of influential Blacks who paved the way for them. It's a tough situation, and where some of us have been equally successful, that's not paying the toll. And then sometimes we are so happy that we made it up here that we forget all about it. It just doesn't come across our mind that we need to put strategies for everybody to be successful. So, I find that as a minister, as a clergyman, you know I can look back at the successes that I've had in my life and although there are many, we cannot depend on one person to lead and be a part of everything. If we continue with that attitude, we will continue to have problems. We'll never get where we need to be and the whites will always have a heads up above us because only a few of us will have achieved the levels of success as leaders in our communities. The progress of our community will take more than a few leaders; it will take the efforts of everybody. Everybody needs to be on the same page but I just don't see that happening.

A prevailing thought is that we're not dealing with racism and segregation now. With integration, the thought is that everybody's equal, but I don't think that's true. We're so far from that. And because the system has said, "Well, you can't do this anymore [discriminate against Blacks]," Blacks are still marginalized and oppressed. And many of our fine young men and women are at a point that it'd be hard for them to reach a certain level maybe where others are, because maybe people thought that once we became integrated, racism would no longer exist—that once segregation ended, we could go and sit at the table and there were no racial barriers, that since there were no Black-white water fountains, somehow racism wasn't there anymore. I think a lot of us thought that. That once segregation was done away with, everything would be okay. And I get it. I thought it, too—that once that's done away with, naturally, everybody would be equal, but that's not the case. We're so far from that. And we [individuals of my generation] can look back, and we can see it; however the younger group, like your son and others, my kids, and so forth, just don't quite catch it. They know it, but they don't quite catch it. And they'll say, "Oh Mom, oh Dad, that's old. That's old. It's a different day today." And that's true, it is a different day. But the racism is still there. They still feel, "We're better." But we are not.

5   Social Issues and New Day Christian Church in Morganton, NC

George K. Logan

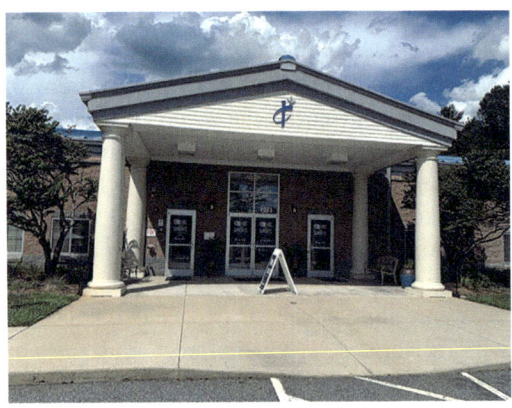

The breakdown of the family as a whole goes back farther than just what has happened recently in the Black community. A lot of times when you talk about social issues in our communities, you'll hear white people say "Well, you know, they need to get their families to help." And honestly, my pushback would be "Well, where did the breakdown of the family begin for us? It began out of slavery." So, if we're really going to talk about the breakdown of the family, we have to talk about where it began—the origin of it. I do think that we need to take responsibility, but not

be dismissive about the role that early slavery had on the destruction of many, many Black families. It's a wonder, to be quite honest, that Black families have remained as intact as they have.

One of the things we've done to somewhat address that issue here in our church over the past 15 years is we've said, "How can we do ministry in an environment where even church is not readily received as it once was back when we were growing up?" So during the summers, for 8 weeks, we started having church on Monday. We invite people and families to attend our church and to participate in our basketball league. There are more people sometimes here on Monday nights throughout the night than on Sundays. And it's young people, too. It's guys with their girlfriends and their parents and it's like one big get-together. I think it kind of reminds me of what community used to be like when I was growing up in Black Mountain, NC.

5.1   The Demographics of Morganton, North Carolina

The demographics here in Morganton, NC, historically, had a pretty good number of Black people. I would say, and I don't know the exact numbers, somewhere between 10% and 13% in the community. Over time, Blacks have left the communities because manufacturing went down and there was a loss of jobs. This is really a blue-collar town which has had a lot of factory jobs. During the time that I have been here, that has changed because manufacturing took a big hit, and even though some of it has come back, jobs aren't as plentiful as they once were. What has sustained the community is the state jobs like J. Iverson Riddle for disabilities, and we have a few prisons here, and of course there is Broughton Hospital which is a regional psychiatric hospital operated by the state of North Carolina.

The community as a whole, because of the manufacturing, and of course now the chicken business, has a lot of Hispanics that live here in Morganton as well. That's probably the community that has grown the most. So, I say overall for

Burke County and Morganton, the demographics are probably somewhere in the 60% for whites, and then other racialized minorities would be about 40% or so.

5.2 Advocating for Change and Racial Justice in Morganton

So Morganton is a predominantly white community, and I kind of put my neck out there when attempting to attract attention to the insensitivities that have occurred in our community. For example, they have a confederate monument and statue, and someone asked me if I would speak about it to the county commissioners. This opportunity came at a perfect time because I had just read a book by Jemar Tisby called *The Color of Compromise*. That book enlightened me on things that I did not know about the history of the church, racism, and prejudices and ways in which some churches are really complicit and silent regarding these issues. When I speak of the church, I speak of the whole church but specifically those of the lighter hues. They're complicit and silent about taking up their cause to make the house of God a place to address the racism and prejudice that occur in our society. I became more aware of these issues after reading that book and seeing factual and historical information of how the church treated Blacks during that time, and then the symbolism in the statues, and confederate monuments, and confederate flags. We have confederate flags at both ends of our county, literally. There is a major interstate running through our town, and there are two confederate flags on display, highly visible to travelers going east and west. So, that made me address the issue, not so much as a Black man, but as a Christian and as a believer who is saying to my brothers who are also Christians: "This is not right. Especially when you know the history. There is something that should be done. We should not have a symbol of hatred in our community." Not if we're saying that we are inviting *everyone* into our community.

5.3 Value for Engaging Youth in Religious Activities and Building Character

Basketball, to me, is just a tool. We use it and we get to have an opportunity to have some inroads into a lot of parents and kids. You'd be amazed at who comes out on Monday nights. It's almost like "Where are you guys at in the community? Where? Where are you?" But they come out, we treat them as royal as we can, we provide a good environment, and we share the gospel with them, of course. Our primary goal is sharing the gospel, but we also want to create some relationships.

I think, fundamentally, it's in relationships where change is made. I believe that there are some things that can systemically happen within society. Policies change, those types of things can help move the needle, but I think the biggest change happens within the context of relationships.

I read something recently about a young man who grew up with a Black father and a white mother, but he was estranged from his mother. So, in the community where he lived in Baltimore, Maryland, he distanced himself from that side of the family as they seemingly did to him. Then, as he grew up, he got to know his aunt who he thought abandoned him and realized that there were a lot of nuances that he wasn't aware of. But what changed the game for him is he learned about *contact theory*. Basically, the premise is that the closer we are to one another, the less there will be -isms.

Without knowing that was a theory, I think we kind of model that principle ourselves at the church. As how we can create inroads to grow closer to people, and the basketball league is just one of them. We have a crossover camp that happens as well. Then, just going on throughout our regular ministry is just trying to get to know one another. Today, we're reluctant for people "to get into my business." Because that's what it boils down to: I don't want you in my business. But if someone knows me and I know that person, and they know me well enough to speak into my life, that's where change happens. So much has happened in my life and if someone knows me well enough, then I respect them enough to tell the truth to me. Sometimes it's hard. It's kind of hard to receive truth about oneself, but it's needed. Because that's the only way we can really change, and that's important.

5.4 Moving Forward After the COVID Pandemic

We're engaged in strategic planning in our ministry right now. We're coming out of COVID, and we don't want to go back to normal. You know, what is normal now? We wanted to think deeply about where to go from here on out and we're addressing those things. One strategy is *reaching* people and another is *growing* people—reaching people, meaning, "how do we get to people who may have been estranged from the community?". How do we bring them back into the community? And once they're here, how do we grow together? How do we create an environment where people can grow?

I've always felt that if you can get young people on the grounds and integrate faith inside of something that they really want to do and really enjoy doing, then we've got a winning combination. With the camps that we do, although we stopped during COVID, we're back on it again. We teach them *leadership skills* and *devotionals*. We go through those two things all day every day for a week. That came from what vehicle we could use to teach faith, and ours was through activities in the gym. When building our church, we built the gym first; then we built the sanctuary. Some people would probably balk at that, but we wanted it to be functional from the gate. That's how it came about initially, and it has been extremely successful. As a matter of fact, when we didn't do the camps for a couple of years, we got all kinds of "When are you starting back? When can I get my kid in there?"

I believe the idea for the camps was something from God. He says, "Here's an opportunity; let's use it. What do you have in your hands? You have a gym; okay, then use it for the glory of God. What else do you have in your hands? Well, we

have a group of kids that do well in basketball. Use them." I think that's how it all came about.

We grew up in Black Mountain which at that time was a community where I think we may have taken a lot of things for granted. Like, we never thought that there's another world out there where they don't honor family, people, and elders. So, when we came into this community, we found—even more so than Black Mountain—this place is riddled with breakups of family.

This is my own hypothesis, these are my own thoughts, but I think it's because back in the mountains where we lived, there were no real cash crops. There were former slaves, but they're almost like family members. You know, they were domestics, and I think they were treated a little differently than former slaves who may have been out in the fields for work. I think that Morganton was kind of the beginning. I do know that Morganton has a history of being one of the beginnings of the agricultural cash crop.

So, we see here the longtime systemic breakdown of the traditional family structure. I have many people in the church who came from broken families. They didn't have a father in the home. We realized going into this situation that even as my mom and dad came down here, and my sister with her husband, we were modeling something. We were modeling family. We're modeling this thing that, if you really think about it, I didn't realize I was doing from the beginning. I thought we were just coming together to teach the word. But I think the bigger picture now that I look back was that we were modeling family. We were modeling relationships; we were modeling closeness; we were modeling love; we were modeling forgiveness. We were modeling all those things and I think people in our church picked up on it.

I think maybe at first people in this area thought we were an aversion to what they had known as family. They probably looked at us and thought "Man, these people are weird. They love one another; they like sticking around with one another. What's wrong with these folks?" But I think throughout time, you've seen that this is where it's at—this nuclear family, this loving, caring, and forgiving family. We modeled that.

My parents come down every Sunday and Wednesday and have for many years, just to support me. I didn't ask them to; I didn't tell them to leave their home church. But they're like "What else? What else would we do for our family?" You know, for 30 years congregants in this church have seen parents that really, truly, are faithful and are there for their child. Some may have even felt like we were too close, but I don't know if you could be too close. When you do have a breakdown and a communal breakdown, that's what breeds suspicion and distrust.

5.5 Community Collaborators

One of the things God has really favored us with while I've been here these 29 years is that a lot of people have sought to help us out. We provide food for the kids, so everything from supplying scholarships for kids, or local restaurants giving us food or a discount on food—there have been a lot of people who have been involved throughout the years, not just with our camps, but overall.

I mean, I'm sitting in a paid-for building right now. It's debt free completely. A lot of it was because not only our neighbors of the church but even other people outside of the church have sown generously. We have a playground; I don't know what it's worth, but probably a hundred thousand plus. It sits right in front of our building on a pad that we were responsible for, so we may be paid $20,000 for it. But an agency came looking for a place where kids can come and play and said, "Would you all like to be a part of that?" So, we got a big team going, and in one day, we built the playground. It's top notch, but it took a lot of community involvement to do that.

5.6 Successes in Strategies Implemented

I think what made us successful is that we've been consistent. We try to put out our very best. One of the things that we sought to do is make it different than regular basketball camps. We want to celebrate each child, and we do. There are children that come to camp over the past years who didn't know anything about basketball, and they're immersed with kids who have been playing basketball for a long time. But they all come out like "This is different." We had people that sent their kids to Carolina and said they preferred our camp because of the connectiveness. For us, it's not just about your child playing basketball. We really want them to develop, and cultivate, and we want to bring out gifts and talents in your child.

We have one part in our basketball camp that is like old school Vacation Bible School. They don't do crafts like they used to, but they're learning scriptures. They'll go on to learn and memorize scriptures and learn something from it. Then, they come to me, and I teach them how to stand in front of people and talk, project their voices, look people in the eyes, and introduce themselves.

We give them several different types of phrases to memorize. One of the things we do to build a good habit is we say, "Repetition easy, easy pleasure, pleasure often, often habit." They'll repeat that over, and then we'll start singing that. I had a kid who came back who has long since left the camp because of age and he says, "I still remember my repetition. I still remember how to change a bad habit into a good habit." One time I thought we might need to change it, but we haven't.

5.7 Challenges Encountered

I think the first challenge is just coming into a new area and starting a new church and not knowing anyone in the community. My wife is from here, so we have some family here, but that was not really the impetus for us to come here. It really was just—and I don't know why He said it—but God spoke to me and told me to start the ministry here.

In April 1994, we started our church with a mission to deliver the word of God in a simple but yet practical way and to positively impact all of Morganton, Burke County, and this nation through the message of Jesus Christ. However, I think we weren't readily embraced because of our newness, the novelty, and perhaps the fear that we were taking other churches' members— with other churches questioning our real purpose for being here. Even though those fears and suspicions still exist, I think it is important for us to stay true to our mission and continue to grow our ministry. So, from a standpoint of wanting to be embraced by everyone, it was a challenge. But that was to be expected.

Once it starts moving, there are challenges, just to be quite honest. I think the old issue of *racism* becomes an issue as well. I know for us getting a bank loan to build the church was difficult. I was in banking, so I kind of knew our numbers were good, I thought our ratios were good, but we got turned down one after the other, after the other, after the other. Nobody would give us a loan. And so, God spoke to me and said, "What are you putting your confidence in? Are you putting your confidence in them telling you, yes, based on your knowledge of numbers and what you got, or are you putting your confidence in me?" And he arrested me on that part, and I'm like "I think I've been trusting in what I know more than I trust You."

I would have told people I was trusting God, but I was really trusting what I saw on paper. Once I gave that up, literally, then I said, "Alright. I repent. I ask for forgiveness for trusting in man and our numbers." It didn't matter if they told me yes or no. I don't care if you tell me no a thousand times; I still trust God. So, it doesn't really matter now.

Believe it or not, I was in a restaurant at a little snack bar with a friend of mine who happened to be a pastor. He saw the president of the local bank that holds our money. For me, it was a lot of money; it was a lot of money for our church. But that was also the same bank that turned us down. He knew we had the money, and they turned us down. So, my friend, who happens to be a white man, a white pastor, said to the president of the bank, "That's my friend George. You need to consider him." Next thing you know, I'm getting a phone call from the same bank that denied us three times, saying, "Can you come back in? We want to see what we can do for you." So, the bank ended up giving us the loan to build the building. We paid it off before it was due. There was never

a risk. But I just kind of felt like that was probably God.

When God speaks to me, it's almost like when you go fishing and you put the little bobbers on and the fish takes the bobber and it'll go underwater. Then, it'll come back up. And it'll go back under. That's kind of how it is. The thought won't go. It won't leave. So, I'm like "Okay, God, You must be speaking to me on this." And that's kind of how that happened to me. Sometimes it's clearer than that. Sometimes it's like three, four, or five in the morning, and I'll get clarity. I'll know exactly what I'm supposed to do.

When God asks us to do something, it's much like when Moses said, "Well, how do you want me to do this?" And God said, "What do you have in your hand?" And he had a staph in his hand. That's all he had. So, I think about that myself. When God speaks to me, He's speaking to me because there's something that I have access to at the time. It may just be my voice; it may just be going and asking someone for something, or making a phone call, or whatever it is. There is always something. We can't make a first step unless we have feet, and if we have feet, then we can make a first step. He's only going to ask us to take a step because he knows we have something that we can move on.

I am reminded of something I was reading in a book written by someone who had attended a missions' conference. In this book, there was one lady walking around and the author asked the question "What do you want to do today?" and she said, "I'm going to save Africa. Yeah, I'm going to save Africa." And the author replied to her "Well, I don't know about all that." But then in the book the author asked the same question of someone else, and that person says, "All we're going to do is believe that God is calling us to fund businesses in Africa." The takeaway from this book is to follow God's direction and take baby steps. Their first step in starting this ministry was to send a letter to everybody that was on our wedding registrar to see if they would send a little bit of money to support our mission. Now, it's a multimillion-dollar ministry, and that's how it started.

Keith Lipsey is Pastor of New Bethel AME Zion Church in Forest City and Treasurer of the Hendersonville District of the Blue Ridge AME Zion Church Conference. He holds an Associate of Science degree in Social Work from Walters State Community College, Morristown TN, and a Bachelor of Social Work degree from Mars Hill University. Currently, Rev. Lipsey is attending Gardner Webb University School of Divinity, Boiling Springs, North Carolina, with a concentration in Pastoral Care and Counseling. Rev. Lipsey is the newly elected president of the Rutherford County NAACP Branch #5444. He was born and raised in Forest City, Rutherford County, North Carolina, where he continues to reside.

Herbert Grant is Presiding Elder of the Blue Ridge AME Zion Church Conference (Asheville District) and Pastor of Goodes Temple AME Zion Church in Strawberry Plains, Tennessee. Rev. Grant was born and raised in Swannanoa, North Carolina, where he still resides. He is a lifelong member of the AME Zion Church and a member of the Macedonia AME Zion church. Rev. Grant has been a minister for over 40 years.

Lavonia C. Ray is Senior Pastor at WNC Baptist Fellowship Church in Asheville, North Carolina, United States. Rev. Ray is one of the oldest surviving ministers from the Asheville, North Carolina region. He is a graduate of Mars Hill College and formerly taught in the Distance Program for Clergy with the Divinity School of Shaw University.

Brent La Prince Edwards is Pastor of Waters AME Church in Baltimore, Maryland, and former Pastor of St James AME Church in Asheville, North Carolina. Rev. Edwards is currently a graduate student in the School of Divinity at Duke University, Durham, North Carolina.

George K. Logan is a native of Black Mountain, North Carolina. He earned his bachelor's degree in industrial relations at the University of North Carolina at Chapel Hill in 1986. While at Chapel Hill, Logan participated in Army ROTC and was later commissioned into the US Army as a Chemical Corp Officer. After fulfilling his military training, Logan sensed God's call to ministry and decided to attend Ministry School in Los Angeles, CA. At Crenshaw Christian Center Ministry Training Institute, he graduated from the program in 1992. While in Los Angeles, Logan was actively involved in New Life for Old Prison Ministry, serving in jails, prisons, and youth camps. Pastor Logan now resides in Morganton, NC, where he founded New Day Christian Church in 1994. He is very involved with his community serving on a variety of boards as well as coaching, mentoring youth, and volunteering for NC Dept. of Corrections. He was awarded Dept. of Corrections volunteer of the year and the 2013 Morganton Rotary Club Man of the Year for his service in the community. He was also awarded a Doctorate of Letters from Montreat College in 2020.

Expansion of Family Networks and Social Interactions to Facilitate Successful Navigation of Health Care Systems for the Management of Cognitive Impairment

Kalisha Bonds Johnson, Megan Gilligan, Manka Nkimbeng, Shanae Rhodes, Dawnita Michelle' Brown, and Kimesha Grant

1 Navigation of the Health Care Systems for the Management of Cognitive Impairment

Navigating the health care system for the diagnosis, treatment, and management of a chronic disease can be challenging. Navigation can include scheduling and attending appointments within the health care system, engaging with many health care professionals (e.g., physicians, nurse practitioners, nurses, social workers, speech therapists, occupational therapists, and medical assistants), managing medications (e.g., having prescriptions filled, taking medication as prescribed, and monitoring for side effects), and reporting back to the health care team. To successfully participate in the tasks associated with navigating the health care system, individuals need to have a certain level of agency, health literacy, and knowledge about the health care system [1].

One chronic condition that further complicates the navigation of a health care system is the diagnosis of cognitive impairment, such as Alzheimer's disease and related dementias (ADRD). ADRD is a progressive brain disease that results in a person's inability to care for oneself [2]. Health care navigation is essential for the treatment [3], management [2, 3], and quality of life of persons living with ADRD [4–6]. As the

K. Bonds Johnson (✉)
Nell Hodgson Woodruff School of Nursing, Emory University, Atlanta, GA, USA
e-mail: kalisha.bonds@emory.edu

M. Gilligan
Human Development and Family Science, University of Missouri, Columbia, MO, USA
e-mail: mgilligan@missouri.edu

M. Nkimbeng
Division of Health Policy and Management, University of Minnesota School of Public Health, Minneapolis, MN, USA
e-mail: manka@umn.edu

S. Rhodes
The University of Texas Health Science Center at San Antonio School of Nursing, San Antonio, TX, USA
e-mail: rhodess@livemail.uthscsa.edu

D. M. Brown
Hey Caregiver!®, Baltimore, MD, USA

The Binti Circle, Baltimore, MD, USA
e-mail: dawnita@heycaregiver.com

K. Grant
Johns Hopkins University School of Nursing, Baltimore, MD, USA
e-mail: Klinton8@jh.edu

disease progresses, the person living with ADRD will be unable to provide an accurate medical history, describe their symptoms, or determine the best course of action regarding their treatment plan. For individuals living with moderate to severe stages of ADRD, there is often a need to have someone else (e.g., family member) involved in the navigation of the health care system on their behalf.

The characteristics of the family members can influence the ease of navigating the health care system on behalf of the person living with cognitive impairment. For example, spouses tend to have easier access to medical records, health care providers, and involvement in the creation of a treatment plan when compared to adult children. Families with multiple children may experience additional complications because there are more individuals trying to navigate the health care system together [7]. The racial and/or ethnic identity of the family members can also influence the ease of navigating the health care system for a person living with ADRD [8]. African American persons living with ADRD experience low rates of health care use [9, 10], health disparities in receiving quality health care [2, 4, 9], underdiagnosed [11, 12], and undertreatment of ADRD symptoms [4, 13], which result in greater morbidity [2, 4] and worse quality of life for African American persons living with Alzheimer's disease and related dementias [5, 6].

African American family members face a myriad of trials as family caregivers and are grossly underrepresented in the caregiving space [14]. African American family caregivers report experiencing racism during interactions with the health care system [15], miscommunication with health care providers [8], and misunderstanding of insurance coverage [8, 14]. While 75% of all caregivers are women [16], only a small percentage of programs are geared to meet the needs of female minority caregivers [17], which may result in these family caregivers experiencing poorer health outcomes due to

a lack of health care support and increased barriers to accessing culturally competent services. For example, African American family caregivers desire more family involvement when making health care decisions for African American persons living with cognitive impairment [18], which often does not align with how health care systems deliver care. Thus, African American caregivers tend to exhaust family resources before engaging with the health care system [19], considering the system as a threat (rather than support) [20]. While African American women bear a disproportionate share of the burden of caregiving [2, 19, 21], it is critical to address the underrepresentation of Black women in caregiver research.

For families who migrate to the United States (USA), navigation of the health care system reflects a complex interaction of social and cultural factors. Immigrant-related social factors include language barriers and immigration status. Cultural factors implicated in navigating the health care system and accessing resources for persons living with ADRD from immigrant communities are (1) cultural perceptions and meaning norms (e.g., meaning and translation of caregiver and dementia in different African languages) and (2) cultural norms and values (e.g. familism/filial piety) [22].

This chapter will focus on the experiences of one social scientist, two nurse scientists, and a community partner with community-engaged research that focuses on the expansion of family networks. These family networks include the following: (1) siblings caring for their parent(s) living with ADRD, (2) a specific focus on African American adult daughters caring for their parent with ADRD, and (3) the family networks of Black immigrant families in the USA. We will share firsthand accounts of the problem and goals, the community settings and partners, the programs being developed, and our reflections on how the strategies we provide are working, as well as future implications.

2 Firsthand Accounts of the Problems and Goals

2.1 Siblings and Their Parents

2.1.1 Social Scientist (MG)

In my project, *Siblings Caring for Parents with Dementia*, I seek to examine the role of sibling relations on adult children caregivers' physical health and psychological well-being by considering the network in which caregivers are embedded. Nearly all previous research on family caregivers of older adults with ADRD has taken the perspective of a single primary caregiver. However, studies have shown that caregiving is usually a "family affair" negotiated among siblings. Siblings can be a source of both support and stress to each other during parental caregiving. *Siblings Caring for Parents with Dementia* seeks to extend previous caregiving research by considering the perspectives of multiple adult children in the same family.

I relied primarily on previous literature when designing this first project. Previous caregiving research indicated that spouses were often the first sources of support for older adults living with ADRD, and adult children typically become primary caregivers when spouses were not available (e.g., widowhood). However, the voices of research participants further shaped this research during data collection. For example, when I started interviewing families, it became clear to me that these individuals were often providing care in much more complicated networks than indicated by the previous literature that focused on a single primary caregiver. In other words, spouses and adult children are sometimes providing support together to manage work schedules and other personal responsibilities.

To be intentional about including African American families in my recruitment, I relied on partnerships with experts working with African American caregivers of older adults living with ADRD. These partnerships have included the Community Advisory Board at the Wisconsin Alzheimer's Institute, Roslyn Thibodeaux Goodall, Founder of the Hopeful Alzheimer's and Caregivers Symposium, and Dr. Fayron Epps, Director of Community and Research Engagement at the Nell Hodgson Woodruff School of Nursing at Emory University. I formed these partnerships in year 3 of the project when I was actively recruiting participants. Through these partnerships, I have been encouraged to consider how caregiving networks are defined and how I might broaden the definition of caregivers to better reflect the lived experiences of diverse families. In the future, I intend to form these types of partnerships earlier in the project so that work can benefit from this input at the inception of the project.

Taken together, the work on this project thus far has taught me that we should be careful to consider those voices that have been included in as well as those voices excluded from research studies. The voices of those underrepresented are critical in the interpretation and design of programs that are culturally relevant for diverse populations.

2.2 African American Adult Daughters and Their Parents

2.2.1 Nurse Scientist (KBJ)

My passion for understanding issues related to caregiving of persons living with cognitive impairment was ignited during a literature review while in my PhD studies. A literature review is often one of the first projects assigned to a PhD student. With this assignment, the student reviews the literature to see what has been studied on their topic of interest as well as identifies gaps in the existing literature. My literature review project highlighted two gaps that I still focus on in my work today—the lack of rigorous and thoughtful work in African American caregiving research and the lack of inclusion of African American persons living with cognitive impairment in the research using dyadic analysis. Dyadic analysis is defined as research that involves two people. In my work, these two people are identified as the person living with cognitive impairment and their caregivers. In my current project, *Daughters and Their Parents*, the dyad is the African American adult daughter and their parent living with cognitive impairment including ADRD. Regardless of the severity of the impairment, the goal of my current project is to empower these African American parent-adult daughter dyads to make health care decisions that will contribute to improved quality of life.

To reach African American adult daughters across the USA for this project and ensure their voices are heard, I partnered with several community organizations (i.e., Daughterhood.org, Parenting UP!, Zeta Phi Beta Sorority, Inc., and the Binti Circle) and created a community advisory board affiliated with my lab. Ms. Dawnita Brown is the Founder and Executive Director of the Binti Circle. I was introduced to Ms. Brown by Dr. Fayron Epps, Director of Community & Research Engagement at the Nell Hodgson Woodruff School of Nursing at Emory University. Dr. Epps connected me to Ms. Brown because of our passion to improve caregiving experiences for African American daughters. The community advisory board affiliated with my lab consists of African American women who are health care professionals (i.e., physicians, nurses, respiratory therapist), current and past caregivers of a family member living with ADRD, and older adults. Refer to Sect. 3 for more information about these community partnerships.

2.3   African and Black Immigrants' Families

2.3.1   Social Scientist (MN)

I have a long history of community organizing and engagement. Having served in cultural community organizations starting in high school, I observed firsthand the challenges and barriers that members of the African and Black immigrant communities faced in accessing health care and services. As a result, I partner with community-based organizations to conduct all my research projects. Community members often want to be considered and involved in research projects, but researchers do not approach them or approach them in an inappropriate manner, which results in them feeling hurt and distrustful of researchers. After hearing these stories, I sought

to conduct research through a community-based participatory research (CBPR) lens and actively engage in educating the next generation of researchers to practice CBPR principles in research and programs with diverse communities. Community-based participatory research is often described as a continuum with the involvement of the community increasing as one progresses across the continuum. I conduct research across the entire continuum. For example, my dementia research, *African Immigrant Memory Loss Project*, incorporated community voices and partners through a three-armed leadership structure of community partners, academic research team, and community advisory board. See Sect. 3 for more information.

3   Community Involvement

In this section, the social scientist and nurse scientists will describe when they partnered with community organizations and how the timing of these partnerships influenced their projects. This section will end with a firsthand account from one of our community partners. Ms. Dawnita Brown, our community partner, will share her reason for starting the organization and the need for organizations that center the voices of the African American and Black women.

3.1   Scientists and Community Partnerships

As mentioned in the previous section, I, (MN), am working in partnership with a community partner, established a community advisory board and worked with them from project inception through implementation on two projects. Indeed, the community advisory board first identified the need for dementia education, which we subsequently collaborated on together. Our first project, *African Immigrant Memory Loss Project*, was a three-way collaboration with community partners, academic research, and the community advisory board. The community advisory board led all project activities, which meant community advisory board agreement on decisions was necessary prior to any project implementation. For example, the community advisory board helped to develop and approve interview guides for interviews conducted with participants recruited to the project, approved survey instruments that were used to collect quantitative data from participants, and conducted community conversations. Community conversations (i.e., community focus groups) were led by the advisory board members. In addition, the project findings were shared with the community advisory board and community partners prior to dissemination to the academic and scientific community. There was great enthusiasm from the community advisory board about their role in the research projects despite logistic challenges (e.g., parking and scheduling of meetings) related to attendance from all community advisory board members.

On the other hand, we (KBJ and MG) partnered with the community later in the project progression. I (KBJ) established a community advisory board associated with my lab *after* I wrote the grant proposal, received the notice of the award, and requested ethical approval by the institutional review board at Emory University. As a result of establishing the community advisory board after starting recruitment, there were challenges that may not have occurred if I had been working with a community advisory board from the inception of my project and thus working together through the entire process. The community advisory board members support the mission of my lab and voice the importance of the work. However, the marketing and branding of my lab, including the lab name and the flyers I used initially to recruit, were questioned by the community advisory board members. For example, my lab name is the D.E.C.I.D.E. Research Lab. D.E.C.I.D.E. is an acronym, which initially stood for **D**ementia **E**xperiences for **C**ulturally **I**nclusive **D**ecision-Making **E**ngagement. A few of the members did not like how the acronym flowed from the tongue. Another member was concerned the word "engagement" would lead the community to think my research was about marriage. After thoughtful discussion, the name has been changed to **D**ementia **E**xperiences:

*Culturally **I**nclusive **D**ecision-Making* for **E**ldercare. While "eldercare" is a favorable term in many African American communities, there has been concern in gerontology and geriatric spaces regarding the negative connotation associated with the term "elder." We discussed whether it was more important to appeal to the masses or to appeal to our community of interest. It was decided to lean toward our community of interest. This example is one of several conversations that I have had to negotiate. It can be time-consuming and delay deadlines because consensus must be reached. It is also uncomfortable at times to be vulnerable and allow others to critique what I've created. Although I know that to appeal to the needs of the community, I must have a diverse group of voices at the table. Their suggestions have only improved the projects coming from the D.E.C.I.D.E. Research Lab.

3.2 Firsthand Account of a Community Partner

3.2.1 Community Partner (DB)

The Binti Circle is a nationwide intergenerational supportive network comprised of over 90 unpaid former and current long-term African American and Black daughter caregivers. Binti means daughter in Swahili, and the circle symbolizes unity, commitment, love, and community. The Binti Circle members, affectionately known as "bosisi," which means "sisters" in siSwati, make up a diverse community of African American and Black daughter caregivers in various ages and life stages, each navigating their unique caregiving journeys. The ability to access vital resources, such as useful tools, methods, and knowledge, lightens the burden of their caregiving journey. The Binti Circle members are at various stages of life and caregiving. Many of the Binti Circle members are caring for or have previously cared for family members with ADRD. Since its inception in 2021, membership has increased by 846% and continues to grow.

The Binti Circle was born from my (DB) lived experience. On August 5, 2018, while serving as a Community Health Peace Corps volunteer in

Eswatini, Africa, I learned that my mother was on life support and needed to have a brain craniotomy immediately or she would die. After landing on USA soil, the next day I became a caregiver in every sense of the word. After navigating the caregiving journey primarily on my own, I noticed a lack of accessible and relevant resources for caregivers. This lack was particularly in the context of African American and Black communities, so I felt compelled to create a space where others in similar situations could find solace, understanding, and guidance. This transformative personal experience fueled my dedication to building a community that serves as a source of strength, knowledge, and connection for African American and Black daughter caregivers.

To address these gaps, the Binti Circle is shifting the narrative by offering culturally tailored resources, direct support, and respite. The Binti Circle curates culturally tailored direct support and respite through monthly "Feel Good" Friday meetings offered in a hybrid format (i.e., live and virtual) group chat, educational workshops with a focus on caregiver holistic wellness, an annual all-expense-paid restorative respite retreat, and respite scholarships that provide self-care opportunities for caregivers and home care for the person receiving care. Workshops led by subject matter experts cover an array of crucial topics, including mental health, estate planning, financial well-being, yoga, meditation, resilience, and ADRD care.

4   Programs and Projects Through Community and Academic Partnerships

In this section, we will describe in greater detail some of the projects and programs we are working on with our community partners. Our community partner will also share about programs and projects in which she is partnering with academic institutions. The projects and programs are in different phases—being developed, currently being implemented, or being evaluated—and are related to either the expansion of the family net-

work, social interactions among caregivers, or the navigation of the health care system.

The *Siblings Caring for Parents with Dementia* project is in the development phase. We are in the process of completing data collection on approximately 100 families (two adult children per family) in which an older parent is living with ADRD. I (MG) am currently working with colleagues to translate the emerging findings from this project to develop a caregiving program designed to improve the interpersonal relationships of ADRD caregiving network members. For the development of the caregiving program, my colleagues and I plan to work with the community advisory board at the Wisconsin Alzheimer's Institute at the earliest stages of the projects so that we can incorporate their input into the program design and evaluation from the start of the project.

The *African Immigrant Memory Loss Project* is in the evaluation phase. I (MN) worked with community partners and a community advisory board to develop and pilot test a culturally tailored dementia and caregiver education program. To do this, we begin by conducting key informant interviews with community leaders to explore cultural domains to consider. The key informant interviews were followed by conversations with community members. These interviews and conversations informed the cultural domains and aspects incorporated into the educational curriculum. During this iterative process, we worked with the advisory board and community partners to finalize the program content. We then worked with our community partners to identify other community-based organizations and community events where the education will be pilot-tested. We finished pilot testing the curriculum with over five community-based organizations in 1 year. Next, we will assess how the curriculum influenced the participants' knowledge.

The *Daughters and Their Parents* project led by the first author (KBJ) is in the development phase. The project aims to develop and create—with community advisory board members—a program to empower African American adult daughters to navigate the health care system for an African

American parent living with cognitive impairment. The project will take at least 5 years to complete and has two phases. The first phase is to collect quantitative and qualitative data from African American dementia dyads across the USA. The first phase will end when quantitative data has been collected from approximately 70 dyads and qualitative data from a nested sample has been collected from approximately 15 African American dyads. The second phase of the project is to use data from phase one to create and test the program. The creation of the program will be with the community advisory board and key informants. Key informants are defined as African American parent-adult daughter dyads from diverse backgrounds (e.g., geographic region, socioeconomic status, years of caregiving) who comfortably navigated the health decision-making for their parent with ADRD.

In addition to several daughters from the Binti Circle participating in the first author's (KBJ) *Daughters and Their Parents* project, I (DB) have partnered with academics to conduct three projects including:

- First, *The Binti Circle: Yoga and Journaling Workshop for Black Daughter Caregivers* is focused on examining the use of a culturally tailored yoga/journaling workshop to decrease the caregiving burden and stress of Black daughter caregivers. Through a community award from Morgan CARES (**C**ommunity **A**ligned **RE**search **S**olutions), the Community Engagement Core component of the Center for Urban Health Disparities Research and Innovation at Morgan State University (RCMI@Morgan), I and Morgan State University academic partner, Dr. Valerie Odero-Marah, curated a retreat for 19 Black daughter caregivers to evaluate the impact of respite on health through the practice of yoga and journaling. I led this project with the first

author (KBJ) assisting with quantitative design and analysis.

- The second project *Empowered Voices: Exploring the Impact of Storytelling on Black Daughter Caregivers* is a continuation project of the yoga and journaling workshop and aims to explore if storytelling can provide African American and Black daughter caregivers with a therapeutic holistic approach to self-care, emotional well-being, and reduction of caregiving intensity and stress. This project will begin in November 2023, and the first author (KBJ) will assist with quantitative and qualitative design and analysis.

- The third project *Co-Designing a Program to Improve the Quality of Life for Black Daughter Caregivers* is advancing my research interests. This project, led by Morgan State University academic partner Dr. Valerie Odero-Marah and co-led by me, will evaluate the present curriculum of the Binti Circle and identify the specific challenges, stressors, and resource gaps experienced by African American and Black daughter caregivers. The overall impact of this project will be to develop the core components of a culturally tailored curriculum that can address the health disparities faced by African American and Black daughter caregivers. The first author (KBJ) is again assisting with quantitative and qualitative design and analysis.

Collaborating with academic partners enables the Binti Circle to participate in grant-funded research initiatives and collect vital data. This data serves as the foundation for developing evidence-based interventions and strategies aimed at providing essential support to African American and Black daughter caregivers. These collaborative efforts unlock opportunities and insights that would otherwise be unavailable to us as African American and Black daughter caregivers.

5   Concluding Reflections

To assuage health disparities in the navigation of health care systems for individuals living with cognitive impairment, there is a need to partner with communities in whom the research will impact. Han et al. [23] found in their study that community partners echoed a need for dialogue between researchers and community partners to begin in the earlier stages of research [23]. While these partnerships are encouraged to be established sooner rather than later, we hope our chapter shows that there is an opportunity to make positive changes even if these partnerships are started later. For those who may be interested in engaging with community partners but are hesitant about where to begin, models for engaging communities in research have been identified. For example, the Network, Give, Assess, Give again and Evaluate (NGAGE) models stresses that engagement with the community begins through networking, then giving (e.g. volunteering with the organization), and followed by evaluating readiness for research, more giving, and evaluating the outcomes and process of collaboration [24]. This process and CBPR recommend engaging in activities and practices that can facilitate a trusting relationship between the academic institution, researcher, and community to engage in work that is mutually beneficial [25]. Expanding family networks and social interaction to improve the health and well-being of all involved and considering these networks in the navigation of the health care system for a person living with cognitive impairment is challenging, but with thoughtful community partnerships, academic institutions and researchers are working to make this process better.

References

1. Haggerty JL. Ordering the chaos for patients with multimorbidity. Br Med J. 2012;345:e5915. https://doi.org/10.1136/bmj.e5915.
2. Alzheimer's disease facts and figures. Alzheimers Dement. 2023;19(4):1598–695. https://doi.org/10.1002/alz.13016.
3. Dilworth-Anderson P, Hilliard TS, Williams S, Palmer MH. A contextual conceptualization on transitions of care for older persons: shaping the direction of care. Annu Rev Gerontol Geriatr. 2012;31:1–14.
4. Chin AL, Negash S, Hamilton R. Diversity and disparity in dementia: the impact of ethnoracial differences in Alzheimer disease. Alzheimer Dis Assoc Disord. 2011;25(3):187–95. https://doi.org/10.1097/WAD.0b013e318211c6c9.
5. Dubois B, Padovani A, Scheltens P, Rossi A, Dell'Agnello G. Timely diagnosis for Alzheimer's disease: a literature review on benefits and challenges. J Alzheimers Dis. 2016;49(3):617–31. https://doi.org/10.3233/jad-150692.
6. Hinton L, Franz C, Friend J. Pathways to dementia diagnosis: evidence for cross-ethnic differences. Alzheimer Dis Assoc Disord. 2004;18(3):134–44. https://doi.org/10.1097/01.wad.0000127444.23312.ff.
7. Yun S, Weber K, Ferszt G, Dieker J, Qualls S. Different experiences of adult child and spousal caregivers with family conflict. Innov Aging. 2021;5(Suppl 1):792. https://doi.org/10.1093/geroni/igab046.2921.
8. Alexander K, Oliver S, Bennett SG, Henry J, Hepburn K, Clevenger C, Epps F. "Falling between the cracks": experiences of Black dementia caregivers navigating U.S. health systems. J Am Geriatr Soc. 2022;70(2):592–600. https://doi.org/10.1111/jgs.17636.
9. Dilworth-Anderson P, Pierre G, Hilliard TS. Social justice, health disparities, and culture in the care of the elderly. J Law Med Ethics. 2012;40(1):26–32. https://doi.org/10.1111/j.1748-720X.2012.00642.x.
10. Dilworth-Anderson P, Williams IC, Gibson BE. Issues of race, ethnicity, and culture in caregiving research: a 20-year review (1980–2000). Gerontologist. 2002;42(2):237–72. https://doi.org/10.1093/geront/42.2.237.
11. Gianattasio KZ, Prather C, Glymour MM, Ciarleglio A, Power MC. Racial disparities and temporal trends in dementia misdiagnosis risk in the United States. Alzheimers Dement. 2019;5:891–8. https://doi.org/10.1016/j.trci.2019.11.008.
12. Lennon JC, Aita SL, Bene VAD, Rhoads T, Resch ZJ, Eloi JM, Walker KA. Black and white individuals differ in dementia prevalence, risk factors, and symptomatic presentation. Alzheimers Dement. 2022;18(8):1461–71. https://doi.org/10.1002/alz.12509.
13. Zuckerman IH, Ryder PT, Simoni-Wastila L, Shaffer T, Sato M, Zhao L, Stuart B. Racial and ethnic disparities in the treatment of dementia among Medicare beneficiaries. J Gerontol B Psychol Sci Soc Sci. 2008;63(5):S328–33. https://doi.org/10.1093/geronb/63.5.S328.
14. Cothran FA, Paun O, Strayhorn S, Barnes LL. 'Walk a mile in my shoes': African American caregiver perceptions of caregiving and self-care. Ethn Health. 2020; https://doi.org/10.1080/13557858.2020.1734777.

15. Cothran FA, Chang E, Beckett L, Bidwell JT, Price CA, Gallagher-Thompson D. A landscape of subjective and objective stress in African-American dementia family caregivers. West J Nurs Res. 2022;44(3):239–49. https://doi.org/10.1177/01939459211062956.

16. https://www.caregiver.org/resource/caregiver-statistics-demographics/#

17. Smits CH, de Lange J, Dröes RM, Meiland F, Vernooij-Dassen M, Pot AM. Effects of combined intervention programmes for people with dementia living at home and their caregivers: a systematic review. Int J Geriatr Psychiatry. 2007;22(12),1181–93. https://doi.org/10.1002/gps.1805.

18. Bonds K, Lyons KS. Formal service use by African American individuals with dementia and their caregivers: an integrative review. J Gerontol Nurs. 2018;44(6):33–9. https://doi.org/10.3928/00989134-20180509-06.

19. Potter EC, Roberto KA, Brossoie N, Blieszner R. Decisions, decisions. Res Aging. 2017;39(4):476–500. https://doi.org/10.1177/0164027516655581.

20. Pharr JR, Dodge Francis C, Terry C, Clark MC. Culture, caregiving, and health: exploring the influence of culture on family caregiver experiences. ISRN Public Health. 2014;2014:689826. https://doi.org/10.1155/2014/689826.

21. Dilworth-Anderson P, Williams SW, Cooper T. Family caregiving to elderly African Americans: caregiver types and structures. J Gerontol B Psychol Sci Soc Sci. 1999;54(4):S237–41. https://doi.org/10.1093/geronb/54b.4.s237.

22. Knight BG, Sayegh P. Cultural values and caregiving: the updated sociocultural stress and coping model. J Gerontol B. 2009;65B(1):5–13. https://doi.org/10.1093/geronb/gbp096.

23. Ilan II-R, Xu A, Mendez KJW, Okoye S, Cudjoe J, Bahouth M, Reese M, Bone L, Dennison-Himmelfarb C. Exploring community engaged research experiences and preferences: a multi-level qualitative investigation. Res Involve Engage. 2021;7(1):19. https://doi.org/10.1186/s40900-021-00261-6.

24. Denny A, Streitz M, Stock K, Balls-Berry JE, Barnes LL, Byrd GS, Croff R, Gao S, Glover CM, Hendrie HC, Hu WT, Manly JJ, Moulder KL, Stark S, Thomas SB, Whitmer R, Wong R, Morris JC, Lingler JH. Perspective on the "African American participation in Alzheimer disease research: effective strategies" workshop, 2018. Alzheimers Dement. 2020;16(12):1734–44. https://doi.org/10.1002/alz.12160.

25. Gilmore-Bykovskyi A, Croff R, Glover CM, Jackson JD, Resendez J, Perez A, Zuelsdorff M, Green-Harris G, Manly JJ. Traversing the aging research and health equity divide: toward intersectional frameworks of research justice and participation. Gerontologist. 2022;62(5):711–20. https://doi.org/10.1093/geront/gnab107.

Kalisha Bonds Johnson PhD, RN, is an assistant professor at Emory University's Nell Hodgson Woodruff School of Nursing in Atlanta, Georgia, and a psychiatric mental health nurse practitioner at Emory University's Integrated Memory Care, a primary care clinic tailored to the care of persons living with dementia and their families. She graduated from the University of Tennessee at Martin with a Bachelor of Science in Nursing, graduated with a Master of Science in Nursing from Vanderbilt University, and graduated with a PhD from Oregon Health and Science University. She completed her postdoctoral training (or training after completing a PhD) at Emory University. Dr. Bonds Johnson's research focusing on improving health care decision-making processes for African American persons living with dementia and their family care partners as well as improving the communication between primary care providers and these families through the development of culturally-tailored interventions.

Megan Gilligan PhD, is an associate professor in the Department of Human Development and Family Science at the University of Missouri. She received a Dual-Title PhD in sociology and gerontology from Purdue University in 2013. She is a Fellow of the Gerontological Society of America. Dr. Gilligan's research focuses on family relationships and well-being, with particular interest in parent-child and sibling relationships in the middle and later years. Much of her recent work has focused on family caregiving. She is the Principal Investigator on a K01 award from the National Institute on Aging on the health impact of sibling relations on caregivers for parents with dementia. Her work has been published in the *Journal of Gerontology: Social Sciences*, *The Gerontologist*, *Journal of Marriage and Family*, and *Journal of Family Theory and Review*.

Manka Nkimbeng PhD, MPH, BSN, is a nurse scientist and assistant professor at the University of Minnesota School of Public Health and an Affiliate Assistant Professor in the University of Minnesota School of Nursing. Prior to that, she was a Robert L. Kane Postdoctoral Fellow in the Division of Health Policy and Management at the University of Minnesota School of Public Health. She received her PhD in nursing from Johns Hopkins School of Nursing, her MPH from Boston University School of Public Health, and Bachelor of Science in nursing from the University of Massachusetts Amherst. She works with communities to develop and test culturally appropriate interventions that can be translated into health policies and clinical practice to improve health and eliminate health inequities for older adults.

Shanae Rhodes is a registered nurse specializing in adult care and a PhD candidate at the University of Texas Health Science Center at San Antonio School of Nursing. Ms. Rhodes is the founder of My Sister's Keeper, a virtual health-education platform dedicated to women of color.

Ms. Rhodes is committed to a career in community service and research that advocates for underserved and marginalized communities. Ms. Rhodes' current research is focused on gaining a more in-depth understanding of the experience of African American women who are dementia caregivers and their mental health and wellness.

Dawnita Michelle' Brown   is the founder and CEO of Hey Caregiver! Hey Caregiver! is a lifestyle brand that educates, equips, and encourages Black family caregivers to live a life of "selfullness" (i.e., the sweet spot between selfish and selfless) during their caregiving journey. Ms. Dawnita Brown is the founder of "The Binti Circle," a nationwide intergenerational supportive network of Black daughters who are caring or who have cared for their parents. Ms. Brown is also the host of The Selfull Caregiver Podcast. Ms. Brown is the sole caregiver to her totally dependent mother, Mama Joan. In 2021, Ms. Brown became a Certified Caregiving Consultant™, Educator™, and Facilitator™ to combine her caregiving experience with education to better serve her fellow caregiving community. Throughout her caregiver journey, she has learned the importance of caring for herself so she can better care for her mother. This philosophy, known as "selfullness," has become her divine mission. Ms. Brown envisions a community of holistically well caregivers… mind, body, and spirit.

Kimesha Grant   is a Doctor of Nursing Practice-Family Nurse Practitioner student at Johns Hopkins University School of Nursing. She has worked in settings spanning mental health, community primary care, public health surveillance, and health services research. She obtained a Bachelor of Science in Biology and Neuroscience from Florida Atlantic University. She obtained a Bachelor of Science in Nursing from Emory University. She also received a Master of Public Health in Global Health Epidemiology and Disease Control from George Washington University. She is committed to supporting integrated care models and improving mental health outcomes for racial and ethnic minority populations.

SDOH and School Nurse-Led Interventions: Improving Health and Education Outcomes Among School-Aged Children and Adolescents

Nakia C. Best and Cassidie S. Thomas

1 Becoming a Researcher and Advocate for School Nurses

Nakia C. Best

I never expected nor planned to become a researcher who focused on the impact school nurses have on child and adolescent health and education outcomes. My clinical background was in adult cardiothoracic critical care and my research interests included how we used electronic health records to communicate care. By chance, or some would say by divine intervention, my dissertation chair introduced me to the North Carolina (United States) state school nurse consultant supervisor, Ann Nichols, MSN, RN, NCSN, FNASN, that totally changed my trajectory. This introduction turned into my first opportunity to collaborate with a community partner. The school nurses in North Carolina had been conscientiously collecting data about school nursing and all the services they provided for students who attended public schools since the 1990s. Ann had been searching for a research partner to analyze the data, but as I said earlier, my experience was with providing nursing care for adults in the hospital. I knew *nothing* about

school nursing and had never worked with kids. But here I was considering this opportunity, I'm fortunate to have parents that encourage me to try new things. I've discovered throughout my life that I am less afraid to try something because I know I have their support. So, I went to meet the school nurse consultant supervisor to express my enthusiasm and to show her she could trust me with the school nurse story. After the meeting, I was convinced I had found my calling. I wanted to use this data to tell a story about how the healthcare services school nurses provide keep *all* children and adolescents in a safe learning environment and help them be healthy. I read everything I could about school nurses and school health, worked with my mentors and Ann to complete my research, and earned my PhD. Now, I use my knowledge, experience, and resources to work with school nurses in North Carolina and across California. I leverage data to inform how school nurse interventions mitigate the effects of social determinants of health (SDOH) and improve child and adolescent health and education outcomes.

In the next paragraph, you will meet one of my current community partners, Cassidie Thomas, DNP, APRN, FNP, PHN. Cassidie is an experienced school nurse in Los Angeles County, California. We met when Cassidie was accepted to the Doctorate in Nursing Practice (DNP) program at the Sue & Bill Gross School of Nursing, University of California, Irvine. It was a casual

N. C. Best (✉) · C. S. Thomas
Sue & Bill Gross School of Nursing, University of California, Irvine, Irvine, CA, USA
e-mail: nbest@hs.uci.edu; csthomas@hs.uci.edu

© The Author(s), under exclusive license to Springer Nature Switzerland AG 2024
J. B. Hamilton, C. E. Moore (eds.), *Transforming Social Determinants to Promote Global Health*,
https://doi.org/10.1007/978-3-031-61160-5_28

zoom meeting where I talked about my research to new DNP and PhD nursing students. It was there I discovered Cassidie was a school nurse, and she discovered my passion for school nurse and school health research. We immediately decided we were going to do great things together. Cassidie's voice and expertise as a practicing school nurse is extremely important to our partnership and research. Cassidie brings her knowledge and expertise of working as a nurse in the school setting and the health services school nurses provide. Her invaluable experience is key to understanding contextual nuances that are relevant and applicable to real-world circumstances, allows us to delve deeper into complex issues, and enhances the credibility and impact of our findings.

2 Becoming a School Nurse

Cassidie S. Thomas

I've been affiliated with the same pre-K-6 school in Los Angeles County for the past 7 years. However, since starting my doctoral program, I also occasionally work as a substitute school nurse at other schools in Los Angeles County. Seeing how school nursing functions differ in these schools and getting exposure to diverse student populations in Los Angeles County have helped develop my understanding of the variation in school nursing practice and school health policies. It has also helped me gain insight into the issues that impact the communities I care for to better inform my efforts to support school nurses.

My interest in becoming a school nurse started in high school when I began exploring health careers through the Regional Occupations Program (ROP), which allowed students to learn about different careers and volunteer in a professional setting in their area of interest before school each day. Growing up on a farm in a small, rural town, I had limited exposure to potential careers requiring university degrees and hadn't given much thought to my future until college applications began approaching. Through ROP, I began

to develop my interest in nursing, and I think that this was primarily shaped by the instructor of the program—the school nurse at my school. The school nurse was an absolute superhero. She taught the ROP course for several hours a day with such commitment to her students, juggled caring for students on campus as a school nurse, had a wonderful family, and maintained her bedside skills at the local community hospital. I was drawn to her positivity, balance, and professionalism, and I still consider her an inspiration today, as we've kept in touch over the years.

Although I didn't immediately start my nursing career in school health, it was always in the back of my mind, as it was the environment in which my love of nursing was fostered as a teen. I struggled with my nursing identity and wondered if I needed to work bedside to utilize my degree fully. However, I think how I grew up drives my approach to nursing, and I was always meant to work in a community setting. Having grown up in a small town, my goal has been to bring the same level of investment and awareness of the interconnectedness of individuals to my practice that exists in rural communities. Sometimes, that can be challenging in densely populated, urban areas, but this mindset guides my practice in school nursing. Caring for my school community and watching the students grow up over the years have been so rewarding and motivated me to continue the work to improve the health of my community.

3 What Do School Nurses Do?

School nurses (SNs) are healthcare providers in the school setting charged with advancing student well-being and academic achievement [1, 2]. Grounded in public health, SN responsibilities include supporting student emotional, behavioral, physical, and social health well-being [3]. This is accomplished through activities and services such as direct acute care, management of chronic health conditions, program and policy development, education programs for school staff, students, and families, health promotion and disease prevention, and care coordination between student, family, school, provider, and home [4, 5].

School nurses help students with health issues, such as asthma, diabetes, and severe food allergies. School nurses may care for multiple grade levels, such as children in pre-K, while simultaneously caring for elementary, middle, or high school students. In younger student populations, school nurses may care for students with newly diagnosed conditions that present in early childhood. Besides common chronic health conditions, school nurses may also encounter students with new conditions they have never seen before. That is where the school nurse community comes into play. Local and national school nurses stay in touch, share information, and help each other safely care for students with rare congenital conditions. School nurses collaborate to figure out the best evidence-based plan of care to ensure all students can safely attend school.

While caring for students with acute and chronic health conditions and navigating new student diagnoses continues through the adolescent student population, school nurses working with adolescents must also be prepared to address the social-emotional and developmental aspects that impact this age group. Thus, nurses in these settings develop an additional skillset related to managing concerns like substance use disorder, sexual and reproductive health, and the psychosocial complexities that impact this student population.

School nurses are also often on the frontlines of the identification and management of student mental and behavioral health conditions, such as: anxiety, depression, attention-deficit/hyperactivity disorder, and autism spectrum disorder. School nurses may sometimes see signs of mental or behavioral conditions in students at an early age, which can be challenging. This is because it can take a while for students to get assessed and properly diagnosed. When addressing student mental and behavioral health needs, school nurses can be the liaison between the parents, teachers [and outside resources], to ensure there is a good line of communication and that the student's needs are being addressed.

A school nurse may be the only healthcare professional in a school setting [6]. School nurses assess and interpret student health status and identify trends in symptoms and student responses [7]. School nurses can help increase the amount of time students are in the classroom and improve school attendance by assisting students to better manage their chronic health conditions and advocating for students and families to receive support and appropriate health resources [7, 8]. School nurses and the services school nurses have provided have been associated with decreased hospitalizations and healthcare costs [9], positive return on investment [10], and improved quality of life [4].

4   How Do Social Determinants of Health Impact Children and Adolescents?

SDOH have a major impact on the health, wellness, and quality of life of children, adolescents, and their families. SDOH include access to education and good schools, healthcare, and healthy foods, and safe housing and neighborhoods [11]. During the 2020–2021 school year, 10.1 million US students were chronically absent (missing 10% or more of school days), a considerable increase from the over eight million students who were chronically absent pre-covid in the 2018–2019 school year [12]. Unstable housing, unsafe living conditions, and acute illness are just a few of the factors that may lead to chronic absenteeism. Chronic absenteeism has been linked to health conditions, such as asthma, diabetes, obesity, and anxiety [8]. Regular attendance in school is critical to develop children and adolescents into successful, productive citizens [12]. The presence of a school nurse has been associated with reduced absenteeism [3, 13]. To successfully decrease chronic absenteeism, it is essential that students have access to school nurses and that school nurses are integral members of school attendance teams [3, 14].

Lack of access to healthcare, safe housing, and safe places to play are SDOH [11] that may increase the likelihood of risk factors such as obesity and type 2 diabetes in children and adolescents [15–17]. Prevalence of obesity among US children and adolescents (2–19 years) has risen in the last two decades from 13.9% to 19.7%. Type 2 diabetes has also become prevalent. Between 2002 and 2015, the rate of type 2 diabetes increased by 4.8% each year [18]. These widespread alarming trends of obesity and type 2 diabetes are compounded by racial/ethnic disparities [6, 19]. School nurses may be the only consistent healthcare provider students see [20], placing school nurses in a unique position to help mitigate the effects of SDOH, particularly among racial/ethnic minoritized populations.

School nurses practice in schools throughout the USA, providing evidence-based healthcare to students and families who are impacted by SDOH. Many studies have shown the remarkable and substantial beneficial effect of school nurses on child and adolescent health and well-being [7]. School nurses are public health specialists and are positioned to lead healthcare in schools to holistically address the needs of students, families, school staff, and the community. They bring a diverse skill set to student health and wellness, community health promotion, and disease prevention. They are uniquely qualified to manage the health and safety of the entire school community [21].

5   Why Is the School Setting the Ideal Place to Positively Change Children and Adolescents' Lives?

Although varied by country, educational level, and specific school policies, on average elementary school students may spend 25–30 h in school per week, while middle and high school students may spend 30–40 h per week [22]. Because children and adolescents spend such a significant amount of time in the school setting, schools have the opportunity to positively influence students' quality of life and connectedness to peers and school staff, playing a crucial role in fostering their health.

Schools provide an environment for students to:

- Access education, learning, and skills critical to their intellectual and lifelong personal growth, future careers, and adulthood.
- Socialize and interact with peers to develop social skills, empathy, teamwork, navigate challenges, and the ability to work and communicate effectively with others.
- Establish a daily routine that instills discipline and time management, organizes tasks, sets goals, and manages their time effectively later in life.
- Participate in extracurricular activities such as sports, arts, music, drama, and clubs.
- Be inspired, guided, and supported by school staff to help build self-confidence, character, and resilience.
- Learn about different cultures, histories, and perspectives.
- Access support services that can address various challenges they might face, including academic difficulties, personal issues, and emotional struggles. These support services can help children develop coping mechanisms and build emotional intelligence.
- Access health and nutrition that contribute to their well-being and receive health services to help them manage acute and chronic health conditions [23–25].

Schools aim to provide a safe and secure environment for students. Together, school nurses, school staff, and families can work together to build school environments that are safe and supportive for students [26].

6   The School Setting as a Social Determinant of Health

There is a strong connection between education and health and well-being. Evidence supports education as a significant factor influencing health, with a notable impact on life expectancy, health-related behaviors, and overall quality of life. Educational attainment not only affects health outcomes but also influences opportunities, employment, and income. Education is a pivotal tool for breaking the cycle of poverty, addressing socioeconomic disparities, and promoting equality in various spheres of life [27].

Schools play a crucial role in the holistic development of children and adolescents. They serve as environments fostering social and emotional growth, offering opportunities for physical activity, and ensuring safety. Additionally, schools act as a support system for those coming from challenging backgrounds, providing refuge for those from impoverished, violent, or abusive homes.

Essentially, healthier children are better students, and better education yields better health outcomes. This connection makes schools the perfect setting to address the impacts of SDOH on children and families and to help them connect to community resources.

Research indicates that children and adolescents attending subpar schools lacking adequate health resources, experiencing higher levels of violence, and having an unfavorable school atmosphere are prone to developing deteriorated physical and mental health. As marginalized racial and ethnic minoritized students are often enrolled in such schools, addressing schools as a SDOH becomes crucial in efforts to eliminate disparities in child and adolescent health [28].

7 Why Is Research About School Nursing Significant?

We hope that we have convinced you that school nurses are critical to ensuring the health and well-being of children and adolescents. Daily access to school nurses is key to providing a school environment that is safe and equitable [21]. Research on how school nurse interventions improve the health of students and school communities are important to further the science of school nursing and to keep students safe, healthy, and ready to learn. We cannot advocate for a school nurse in every school without providing evidence of the positive impact school nurses and the services they provide [29].

All nurses, regardless of their practice area, collect data. School nurses collect data to record (document) something that currently exists or that happened, to report on something, to count something, etc. The planned structure for purpose directed data is usually completely based on the most efficient way to obtain, record, report and store the desired information. School nurses collect all kinds of data including physical assessments (for students with acute illnesses, injuries, chronic health conditions), screenings (hearing, vision, dental), immunizations, medication administration, health conditions and care for students (services provided, diagnoses and outcomes, education, case management), and school nurse workforce (type of degree, certifications, number of students responsible for). These data are typically used at the local level (e.g., school level) to assist with developing school health programs and quality improvement. As you can see, student health and the services school nurses provide have a large scope and are extremely complex. And with this scope and complexity comes lots and lots of data (unpublished presentation by Ann Nichols and Nakia Best 2022).

So, what is the problem? To demonstrate how school nurse health services improve student health and education outcomes and advocate for all students to have daily access to a school nurse, data need to be shared beyond the local level. To do this successfully, we suggest practice/community and academic partnerships.

8 Mutual Collaboration Between Practice/Community and Academic Partners Is Vital!

Research in practice/community settings has traditionally progressed in one direction:

- Academic researchers conceptualize research projects with minimal (or perhaps without any) input from community stakeholders→
- Implement projects or programs, often without a plan for sustainment in the communities→

- Obtain data and information from community members→
- Disseminate the newly gained knowledge and information to peers and colleagues rather than to members of the community.

Following this process can lead to research failing to be translated from university-based to "real-world" settings and program implementation and community stakeholders experiencing a lack of investment in the research and left with needs different from those being addressed by the researchers. Thus, partnerships between academic researchers and practice/community are essential to improve the translation of research into practice.

Improved partnerships between practice/community and academic researchers are bidirectional:

- Everyone has meaningful strengths and expertise to improve collaboration.
- Practice/community stakeholders can provide relevant firsthand knowledge and insight that could help to identify critical concerns and to design and implement research projects.

To build thriving partnerships with school nurses in North Carolina (North Carolina Department of Health and Human Services) and California (School Nurses of California Foundation, Orange County School Nurses Organization), we had multiple discussions about what each of us wanted to accomplish. Doing this allowed us to develop a list of shared vision and goals. We utilized effective communication to examine expectations, so that all of us were on the same page. We developed clearly defined roles and functions for each partner. We also wrote grants together that included monetary compensation for the school nurse partners and incentives for the school nurse study participants. These activities facilitated our practice/community and academic researcher partnership and led to trust and respect between us, dissemination of work in journal articles and state/national presen-tations, and positive impact on school nurse prac-tice, resulting in mutual benefit for all partners.

Our work with the school nursing communi-ties in North Carolina and California has demon-strated the feasibility of strengthening partnerships between practice/community and academic researchers. By adopting partnerships like this, schools across the country can break the cycle of the traditional practice/community approach to research and encompass a mutually beneficial process for improving school health services.

9 Final Thoughts

School nurses work on the frontlines, bridging health and education. They serve as a vital link for students and their families to community resources. School nurse health services (e.g., acute care, case management for chronic health conditions, health education, screenings) can help mitigate SDOH (e.g., lack of access to healthcare, safe housing, and healthy foods) that impact students and families. All children and adolescents deserve to thrive and live their healthiest lives possible. We believe investing in schools and school nurses, where students may spend 25–40 h a week, is an opportunity to ensure a safe and equitable environment where students can learn.

Our work has been rewarding because we get to contribute to a body of knowledge that recog-nizes the importance of school nurses in the lives of children and adolescents.

Additionally, through practice/community partnerships, our work can have a lasting impact on students, families, and the larger communities they are a part of. In the future, we hope to use school nurse-reported data to develop innovative interventions to address the SDOH that impact youth across the country. School nurses are uniquely positioned to positively impact stu-dents' long-term health and success, and we look forward to continuing our work supporting school nurses as they carry out their transforma-tive role in community health.

References

1. American Academy of Pediatrics (AAP) Council on School Health. Role of the school nurse in providing school health services. Pediatrics. 2016;137(6):e20160852. https://doi.org/10.1542/peds.2008-0382.

2. National Association of School Nurses. School nursing: scope and standards of practice. 4th ed. NASN; 2022.

3. Best NC, Nichols AO, Oppewal S, Pierre-Louis B, Waller AE, Zomorodi M, Travers D. The impact of school nurse health services and school nurse-to-student ratios in North Carolina public schools, 2011–2016. J Sch Health. 2021;91(6):473–81. https://doi.org/10.1111/josh.13025.

4. Best NC, Oppewal S, Travers D. Exploring school nurse interventions and health and education outcomes: an integrative review. J Sch Nurs. 2018;34:14–27. https://doi.org/10.1177/10598404517745359.

5. National Association of School Nurses, Tanner A, Griffin R, Stanislo KJ, Hinkley T, Walsh CA, Clark E, Graf K, La Point R, D'Souza-Vazirani D. A contemporary framework update for today's school nursing landscape: introducing the School Nursing Practice Framework™. NASN School Nurse. 2024;39(3):140–7. https://doi.org/10.1177/1942602X241241092.

6. Centers for Disease Control and Prevention. CDC healthy schools. School nurses help keep students healthy. n.d.-a. https://www.cdc.gov/healthyschools/features/school_nurse.htm. Accessed 19 Aug 2024. Last reviewed 27 Apr 2023.

7. NASN Position Statement: student access to school nursing services. NASN Sch Nurse. 2022;37(4).223–4. https://doi.org/10.1177/1942602X221098463.

8. Jacobsen K, Meeder L, Voskuil VR. Chronic student absenteeism. NASN Sch Nurse. 2016;31(3):178–85. https://doi.org/10.1177/1942602X16638855.

9. Wang LY, Vernon-Smiley M, Gapinski MA, Desisto M, Maughan E, Sheetz A. Cost-benefit study of school nursing services. JAMA Pediatr. 2014;168(7):642–8. https://doi.org/10.1001/jamapediatrics.2013.5441.

10. Ohneck MC, Dake JA, Maughan ED, Telljohann SK, Glassman T. A cost-benefit analysis of school nursing in one large urban school district. J Sch Nurs. 2023; https://doi.org/10.1177/10598405231197836.

11. Hamilton JB. Integrating a social determinants of health framework into nursing education. In: Hamilton JB, Swan BA, McCauley L, editors. Integrating a social determinants of health framework into nursing education. Springer; 2023. p. 9–53.

12. Chang H, Balfanz R, Byrnes V. Pandemic causes alarming increase in chronic absence and reveals need for better data. Attendance Works; 2022. https://www.attendanceworks.org/pandemic-causes-alarming-increase-in-chronic-absence-and-reveals-need-for-better-data/.

13. Yoder C. School nurses and student academic outcomes: an integrative review. J Sch Nurs. 2020;36(1):49–60. https://doi.org/10.1177/1059840518824397.

14. Rankine J, Goldberg L, Miller E, Kelley L, Ray K. School nurse perspectives on addressing chronic absenteeism. J Sch Nurs. 2021;39:496. https://doi.org/10.1177/10598405211043872.

15. Chung ST, Onuzuruike AU, Magge SN. Cardiometabolic risk in obese children. Ann N Y Acad Sci. 2018;1411(1):166–83. https://doi.org/10.1111/nyas.13602.

16. Powell-Wiley TM, Baumer Y, Baah FO, Baez AS, Farmer N, Mahlobo CT, Pita MA, Potharaju KA, Tamura K, Wallen GR. Social determinants of cardiovascular disease. Circ Res. 2022;130(5):782–99. https://doi.org/10.1161/CIRCRESAHA.121.319811.

17. Robson SM, Lozano AJ, Papas M, Patterson F. Food insecurity and cardiometabolic risk factors in adolescents. Prev Chronic Dis. 2017;14:170222. https://doi.org/10.5888/pcd14.170222.

18. Stierman B, Afful J, Carroll MD, Chen T-C, Davy O, Fink S, Fryar CD, Gu Q, Hales CM, Hughes JP, Ostchega Y, Storandt RJ, Akinbami LJ, et al. National Health and Nutrition Examination Survey 2017–March 2020 prepandemic data files—development of files and prevalence estimates for selected health outcomes (158). CDC National Center for Health Statistics; 2021. https://stacks.cdc.gov/view/cdc/106273.

19. Centers for Disease Control and Prevention. Childhood obesity facts n.d.-c. https://www.cdc.gov/obesity/php/data-research/childhood-obesity-facts.html. Accessed 19 Aug 2023. Last reviewed 2 Apr 2024.

20. Johnson K. Healthy and ready to learn: school nurses improve equity and access. Online J Issues Nurs. 2017;22(3):1–10. https://doi.org/10.3912/OJIN.Vol22No03Man01.

21. NASN Position Statement: safe, supportive, equitable schools. NASN Sch Nurse. 2023;38(4):213–4, 10.1177/1942602X231168706.

22. National Center for Education Statistics. Minimum number of instructional days and hours in the school year, minimum number of hours per school day, and school start/finish dates, by state: 2020. National Center for Education Statistics; 2020. https://nces.ed.gov/programs/statereform/tab1_1-2020.asp. Accessed 17 Sept 2023.

23. McCabe E, Best NC. The significance of social development support in schools: the critical role of school nurses. NASN Sch Nurse. 2022;38(2):62–4. https://doi.org/10.1177/1942602X221128227.

24. National School Climate Center. What is school climate and why is it important? National School Climate Center; n.d. https://schoolclimate.org/school-climate/. Accessed 17 Sept 2023.

25. Centers for Disease Control and Prevention. CDC healthy schools. School nutrition. n.d.-b. https://www.cdc.gov/healthyschools/nutrition/schoolnutrition.htm. Accessed 19 Aug 2024. Last reviewed 3 Mar 2023.

26. McCabe EM, Davis C, Mandy L, Wong C. The role of school connectedness in supporting the health and well-being of youth: recommendations for school nurses. NASN Sch Nurse. 2022;37(1):42–7. https://doi.org/10.1177/1942602X211048481.

27. The Lancet Public Health. Education: a neglected social determinant of health. Lancet Public Health. 2020;5(7):e361. https://doi.org/10.1016/S2468-2667(20)30144-4.

28. Huang KY, Cheng S, Theise R. School contexts as social determinants of child health: current practices and implications for future public health practice. Public Health. 2013;128(Suppl 3):21–8. https://doi.org/10.1177/00333549131286S304.

29. Best NC, McCabe E. Learning from the past and moving forward: implementing school nursing research priorities. J Sch Nurs. 2023;39(1):3–5. https://doi.org/10.1177/10598405221143495.

Nakia C. Best PhD, RN, is an Assistant Professor in the Sue & Bill Gross School of Nursing at the University of California, Irvine. Dr. Best earned her BSN from Winston Salem State University, MSN in Nursing Education from the University of North Carolina at Greensboro, Post Master's in Applied Health Informatics from Johns Hopkins University, and PhD in Nursing from the University of North Carolina at Chapel Hill. Dr. Best advocates for all students to have daily access to a school nurse. She leverages data to provide valuable insights on how school nurses and the services they provide improve student health and education outcomes.

Cassidie S. Thomas DNP, APRN, FNP, PHN, is a clinical instructor in the Sue & Bill Gross School of Nursing at the University of California, Irvine and a school nurse in Los Angeles, California. Dr. Thomas earned her BSN and DNP-FNP from the University of California, Irvine. Dr. Thomas has dedicated her career to supporting school nurses through continuing education and professional support to facilitate best practices in school nursing that positively impact students' long-term emotional and physical health.

Assessing Global Community Oral Health Efforts to Promote Well-Being

Charles E. Moore and Rueben C. Warren

1 Oral and Systemic Health Among Global Communities

Oral and systemic health are synergistic and complimentary. Both are essential to promote well-being. Thus, oral health care should be available, accessible, and acceptable whenever comprehensive health care is provided. African American dentists have historically focused their attention on improving health by addressing relationships between oral and systemic diseases. In fact, Clifton O. Dummett, Sr., in his book entitled, "NDA II: The Story of America's Second National Dental Association," describes the evolution of African American physicians, dentists, and pharmacists bonding together under one organizational umbrella to enhance the health of African Americans and other underserved populations. The coming together of these health professionals was partially due to discrimination, prejudice, and racism and resulted in a multidisciplinary approach to health care delivery. Because they were forced to work together, many of their clinical, behavioral, economic, and public health decisions influenced both oral and systemic health outcomes. Many of the patients whom African American health care providers served, and continue to serve, did not have full geographic nor economic access to advances in health care. Thus, a multidisciplinary approach by African American health care providers was necessary to navigate through the maze of the health delivery system. Unfortunately, many of the same challenges still exist.

It is important to consider strategies to ensure that underserved populations, in every global setting, will be included, from the outset, in all public and private efforts to improve oral and systemic health. Some scientists and health care providers believe that the approach is new. However, historically, oral and systemic health care were developed simultaneously to promote and assure the well-being of individuals, groups, and communities. From years of clinical experiences, African American health professionals view this strategy as a "renewed paradigm," at best. Much of the published research continues to report racial and ethnic disparities in health, particularly for African Americans, which apply to both oral and systemic diseases and conditions. Current research suggests biologically plausible associations between oral and systemic diseases. However, clear cause-and-effect relationships have not been substantiated. Some researchers suggest providers have noted anecdotal associations between oral and systemic health, as well as compounding adverse effects of oral and sys-

C. E. Moore (✉)
Department of Otolaryngology, Emory School of Medicine, Emory University, Atlanta, GA, USA
e-mail: cemoore@emory.edu

R. C. Warren
National Center for Bioethics in Research and Health Care, Tuskegee University, Tuskegee, AL, USA

temic diseases and dysfunctions. A more comprehensive clinical, behavioral, economic, and public health decision-making process related to overall health and well-being in the health care setting should include, but not be limited to, maximizing prevention services during all health care visits, considering oral and systemic treatment plans, maximizing reimbursements, and assuring oral and systemic health care follow-ups.

Oral health is integral to overall health and well-being. You cannot be healthy without oral health. Oral health and systemic health operate synergistically and should not be interpreted as separate entities. Oral health is a critical component of overall health and well-being and must be included in the provision of heath care and the design of community programs [1, 2].

Oral health disparities among select groups of people in the United States include those groups with the poorest oral health status—generally ethnic and racial minority populations, particularly African Americans [1, 3–6]. Ethnic and racial disparities also exist in systemic health. In the 1985 federal publication, "Report of the Secretary's Task Force on Black and Minority Health," the former Secretary of the US Department of Health and Human Services, Margaret Heckler, writes:

> There is a continuing disparity in the burden of death and illness experienced by Black and other minority Americans as compared to our Nation as a whole. That disparity has existed ever since Federal record keeping began more than a generation ago and although our health charts do itemize steady gains in the health of minority Americans, the stubborn disparity remains...an affront to both our ideals and to the ongoing genius of American medicine. [7]

In response to, in December 2000, the National Dental Association Foundation, the National Dental Association, Inc. (NDA), the National Institute of Dental and Craniofacial Research, and the Colgate Palmolive Company cosponsored a symposium entitled, "Exploring the Relationship Between Oral Health and Systemic Health Within the African American Population." The symposium addressed oral and systemic health, oral and systemic diseases, dysfunctions

and premature deaths, and the relevant behavioral and socioeconomic factors that disproportionally affect the health of African Americans and other underserved populations [8].

2   Oral Health Disparities Among Global Communities

Oral health disparities are also prevalent globally. Many of the issues identified in the aforementioned symposium are evident in global communities. Even with the broad-based recommendations from the Task Force, the restructuring of many federal, state, and local public health agencies and more than a decade of financial support for creative research and intervention programs in both the public and private sectors, racial and ethnic health disparities remain [9]. In fact, since the 1985 Task Force Report, some of the racial and ethnic health disparities are the same or have worsened. While some of the health gap is a result of socioeconomic status, race and ethnic backgrounds remain essential in accounting for the disparities. Some of the disparities can be explained by inequalities in the health delivery system, such as differences in accessibility, use, quality of care, or benefit derived [10–13]. Unfortunately, most of these variables can be chronicled by race and ethnicity [14–17]. Regardless of the interventions to close race/ethnic health disparities, the problem remains. Health disparities, diseases, dysfunctions, and premature deaths continue to be recorded based on race and ethnicity, even when other factors are held constant. More aggressive efforts must be made if eliminating health disparities is expected [18].

Edwin Nichols, PhD, a psychologist in Washington, DC, has taught medical and dental students for many years [19]. He discussed cultural and social barriers that influence oral and systemic health among US populations consisting primarily of people from Europe, Africa, Asia, and Native Americans. Although US populations come from different parts of the world, common ethnic worldviews are shared. It is precisely this common ethnic worldview that has shaped cultural and social influences on oral and systemic health. Although Nichols did not fully develop the construct of worldview as culture, he described European culture as another example of a particular ethnic worldview. For example, the ethnic relationship in European culture is subject-object oriented. The highest value for Europeans lies in the object or its acquisition. For Africans, the highest valued group experience is in the relationship [20]. People of African descent see themselves to be of equal worth or value. If a person of African descent is treated less than equal or with disrespect, the relationship has been destroyed. Regardless of the external circumstances (employer/employee, teacher/student, etc.), the relationship must be mutually respectful, or it will be destroyed. In transmitting knowledge in the European context, one transmits the object or data. The data are the literature or what the research has reported. However, for other ethnic groups, the object may not be the most important element. A personal relationship must be established to effectively transmit knowledge, particularly about health. To effectively transmit the object or data, a trust relationship must first be established, i.e., a patient will likely comply with instructions/treatment if they trust the clinician.

2.1 Gaining Access to Diverse Communities and Patient Populations

The United States is becoming more and more diverse. Many health care providers must, therefore, consider serving a more diverse patient population. These new patient populations will bring their cultural norms with them. For example, Nichols' description indicates that in the Asian culture the highest value is in the cohesiveness of the group. The goal is consensus, not only among individuals, but consensus in "your heart and mind." He says that the word group, from the Asian (Chinese) perspective, has two meanings and includes two components—king and sheep.

To be a group, there must be a leader and followers. In this scenario, sheep are viewed as conformist animals or followers. Therefore, to respond to patients from this group, providers must seek and receive consensus or approval from local leaders and the local community residents themselves. It is a community decision within the hierarchy of the group. Providers will have to reach out to this group by understanding that a consensus or group discussion will determine the individual decisions concerning oral health care.

In European culture, according to Nichols, pedagogically the individual parts comprise the whole. Things are presented in a linear and sequential pattern—A is followed by B, B is followed by C, C is followed by D, etc. If a linear and sequential pattern is used, the parts will equal the whole. For some people, the individual parts do not make the whole. The data or correct information may be provided, but this linear sequential thinking may not be employed or relevant to diverse populations; thus, a different conclusion may be reached. Medicine is practiced in a linear and sequential form (i.e., taking pills in a specific time sequence). There is often noncompliance by diverse and underrepresented groups, because of different cultural or ethnic norms. For example, if the highest value is the relationship, symbolic imagery and rhythm are used. Rhythm means function. If the heart is out of rhythm, it is not functioning properly, thus taking medicine will not solve the problem.

Disease is viewed as a dysfunction or being out of rhythm. So, action or behavior is a sign used to determine disease state. In many non-European cultures, differing from European culture, one looks for rhythms or how an individual is acting. These varying cultural perspectives must be understood if health is to be improved and if health care is to be effectively delivered. Linear and sequential thinking requires a different set of learning and teaching tools than does holistic thinking. Not good or bad, just different. These different perspectives only become value-laden when they are misunderstood.

2.2   Social Determinants of Health, Oral, and Systemic Health

Social determinants of health such as social, behavioral, cultural, and economic factors provide the context for improving oral and systemic health. Matters of discrimination, prejudice, sexism, and racism based on differing worldviews, cultural backgrounds, and experiences will increase as the nation becomes more diverse. If obtaining and maintaining oral and systemic health in the United States are expected, a more holistic public health perspective must be strongly considered. More importantly, the commitment to addressing issues that challenge long-held beliefs, outdated traditions, and systems barriers must be addressed. Oral health and systemic health for all are both possible and expected if the United States intends to ensure, among all who live in the country and abroad, a healthy world for the next generation.

For many reasons, individuals, groups, communities, and health care providers and health care systems often overlook oral health. Factors that have contributed to this phenomenon include limited exposure to oral diseases, oral prevention, and treatment modalities in medical and nursing school curricula; virtually no continuing medical education for health care providers in identifying, treating, or referring oral diseases; and a lack of understanding of the association between oral and systemic diseases and/or conditions. The high costs of oral health care, the lack of public and private dental insurance for adults, and limited public insurance for children also lead to a low priority for oral health. All these factors combined with a lack of oral health literacy contribute to poor oral health.

Despite these factors that contribute to poor oral health, much can be done to improve the quality and appropriateness of oral health care as well to reduce the costs, particularly for those who have limited financial access to the care they so badly need. Oral health is important for overall health and well-being. Physically, eating and talking require anatomical and functional coordination of hard and soft tissues in and around the oral cavity. Psychologically, self-esteem and self-worth are negatively impacted by one's appearance. Social engagement is influenced by appearance and the mouth is the initial focal point to assess the value of that social interaction. A smile or frown is a revealing sign of approval or disapproval of social interactions. Acts of eating, speaking, smiling, or frowning have social components at school for children and youth, at work for adults, and in other settings for people of all ages. Untreated caries and periodontal (gum) disease also can lead to tooth loss and/or be associated with systemic diseases such as diabetes [7].

Poor oral health in low-resourced communities and communities of color is a tremendous challenge for children, youth, and adults. Although a global challenge exists in assuring oral health equity, this chapter features the city of Atlanta and the state of Georgia to highlight the challenges and what is being done to resolve them. For example, Atlanta is an urban area with low-resourced communities in Georgia with pockets of severe health and income disparities. The issues faced by Atlanta are prototypical to many US urban and global countries. A 2014 Georgia Department of Public Health report outlines the following dental health disparities in Georgia. These disparities contribute to poor dental health outcomes in the state of Georgia. The Georgia Department of Public Health has identified the following five dental outcomes in Georgia that need to improve:

- The presence of dental caries in young children aged 2–5 years and children in third grade
- Untreated dental decay
- Sealant on molars
- Early detection of oral and pharyngeal cancers
- Oropharyngeal cancer mortality

Frequently cited barriers to reducing oral health disparities and the above dental outcomes include a shortage of dentists in areas of the state, unwillingness of dentists to participate in the Medicaid Entitlement Program due to low reimbursement rates and perceived high no-show rates, limited adult Medicaid dental benefits, cost of care, and unresolved patient education issues. These barriers contribute to a lack of access to oral health care in low-income communities throughout the state. Beyond the public health consequences of poor oral health are outcomes that affect the financial, educational, and workforce aspects of families and communities. This can lead to a self-reinforcing cycle that prevents families from improving their socioeconomic status and overall quality of life.

Studies have found that toothaches are the number one reason for school absenteeism. Toothaches are given as a reason for school absence seven times more than asthma. Missed school days limit a student's access to education and education outcomes are essential to moving out of low-income status. Parents miss work when their child cannot attend school due to toothaches, which limits their ability to earn income on those days. Missed productivity of workers also affects the companies and businesses that employ them.

In addition to school absenteeism, poor oral health can lead to increased emergency room visits. "The proportion of non-Hispanic Black and Hispanic high school students who visit an emergency room (ER) or urgent care center for oral or dental problems (10.3% each) is twice the proportion of non-Hispanic white high school students, who visit an ER for the same problems (4.9%)." "Adults earning $50,000 or more per year are significantly more likely to visit a dentist than adults with income less than $15,000 a year (85% vs. 39%)"[21]. Finding ways to improve oral health in low-income communities is essential to overall health and helps individuals move from poverty to middle-class status. Improving oral health requires a collaborative effort of a diverse array of health care workers to ensure equitable outcomes that lead to overall health.

2.3 Programs to Address Oral Health Disparities

One initiative, Oral Health in Communities and Neighborhoods (OHICAN), addresses poor oral health in low-income communities. Poor oral health is a burdening problem that inflicts significant burdens on children, youth, and adults alike. The communities in which we work continue to have wide disparities in untreated tooth decay and restricted activity days for children. The lack of trained providers who can address these problems from both a definitive treatment approach and a preventive perspective is at the heart of the issue. The need for increased oral health literacy among people of all generations throughout the state adds to the disparity. To help close existing gaps in care, knowledge of oral health and diseases needs to be incorporated into the fabric of the health care system (i.e., health care professionals who are not in oral health care disciplines) across the lifespan.

OHICAN seeks to increase access to oral health services and improve community knowledge on the importance of preventive oral health care in low income and minority neighborhoods in Atlanta. Our intent is to work locally to demonstrate what can be done and deploy the successes and products nationally and internationally. The OHICAN program is composed of the following initiatives:

- Increasing community knowledge of preventive oral care
- Expanding existing oral health care capacity in local communities (includes training and education initiatives and incorporating oral health into care protocols for medical care providers)
- Creating new points of access
- Advocating on behalf of evidence-based strategies to expand care and lower costs
- Rolling out/disseminating results of the OHICAN project and transitioning it to an initiative for deployment nationally and internationally

The Oral Health in Communities and Neighborhoods (OHICAN) project is part of the Urban Health Initiative (UHI) at Emory University in Atlanta, Georgia. Leadership for the OHICAN project was provided by an interdisciplinary team from the Robert Wood Johnson Clinical Scholars program and supported by numerous community and academic partners. Our immediate goal was to increase access to oral health services in three target low income and minority neighborhoods in the Atlanta area. Our longer-term goal is to develop a blueprint of solutions including documented approaches/ways of work, tools, and resources that could be expanded into a program for addressing poor oral health in communities and neighborhoods outside the project area.

2.4 Development of Oral Health in Communities and Neighborhoods (OHICAN) Project

The impetus for the OHICAN project to address oral health disparities came from a 2013 community needs assessment (CNA) done by Dr. Moore and the Emory Rollins School of Public Health faculty, staff, and students in a marginalized community of West Atlanta composed of zip codes 30311, 30314, and 30318. This community has approximately 65% of families that live below the poverty line. Most families are single-parent/grandparent or caretaker homes. This region is also a known food desert. According to the West Atlanta Oral Health Community Needs Assessment, lack of equitable access to care was among the top reasons for poor oral health in underserved and other vulnerable populations. Our values guiding this work included (1) health equity; (2) cultural sensitivity and relevancy; (3) products developed that would be empowering, easy to use, informative, and self-gratifying; (4) work that would bridge education and training, clinical practice, research, and health policy and be provided at no cost to users; and (5) reflection of a desire to serve multiple elements of the health care system, such as providers and stu-

dents, patients and families, stakeholders, and partners.

Our initial step was to perform a community needs assessment in our three target zip codes. We engaged students from the Emory University Rollins School of Public Health to work with our team. Together, technology can be used to bridge clinical practice, education and training, research, and health policy. Integrating medical and oral health efforts will increase access to preventive care. Changes to improve access to oral health care can take place in a relatively short period of time when all who care about and are impacted by this continued unmet oral health need work together. The needs assessment was combined with information gleaned from interviewing patients, providers, and members of the community we planned to serve. The CNA was based on the OHIP-14 guidelines. The assessments were through in-person interviews using a digital platform. There were also focus groups led by experienced public health professionals that contributed to the knowledge obtained.

In addition to confirming results of the 2013 Community Needs Assessment, our assessments pointed out the need to involve and engage local community members and partner with other individuals and organizations with interests in oral health and whose work aligned with our goals. We formed a community advisory board (CAB) composed of people representing the diversity of the community from faith-based, private, and public including nonprofit organizations. Additionally, individuals with an interest in oral health that resided in the community were included in this CAB. The age span was from 16 to 74 with primarily female representation. Over time, we have expanded our team to include partners from nonprofits, public health organizations, business, professional associations, and universities.

Once we had information from community needs assessments, we partnered with the Georgia Center for Nonprofits to develop a strategic plan. This assessment informed us of whom we served, impacts on those we served, and indicators of success. We were also able to develop an overall strategic plan with key actions, funding strategies, and community engagement strategies and decide on our next steps. The strategic plan further served as the basis for a monitoring and evaluation plan, which we jointly developed with students from the Emory Rollins School of Public Health. The plan included our program goal, objectives, specific subactivities, process and output indicators, baseline data, target data, source of data collection and means of verification, frequency of data collection, and responsible team members. In year 2 of the project, we modified the monitoring and evaluation plan with the assistance of the Robert Wood Johnson Foundation Clinical Scholars Evaluation team.

We adopted essentially two strategies for program implementation. The first strategy was community engagement through personal contact. Examples of community engagement activities included building relationships, delivering hands-on trainings in oral health screening and preventive care, and working with the CAB and our partner organizations. On the academy side, we collaborated with professional organizations and universities, advocated for and supported evidence-based strategies to expand care and lower its cost, engaged medical care providers in our efforts, served on boards relevant to our goals, disseminated findings through lectures and presentations to appropriate audiences, and published manuscripts in peer-reviewed journals.

The second strategy expanded the reach of our personal contact work and incorporated technology solutions to broaden the scope of our innovative changes to make them transformative and sustainable. With this second strategy, we also explored various transformative health care models that included technology-based solutions and focused on creating innovative change at the system level but found none that embraced the values we espoused. Therefore, we decided to incorporate the values stated above in our development of technology-based interventions. We called our approach the 2 Transformative Technology Evaluation and Assessment Model or 2TEAM. We employed both strategies (personal contact and technology) in addressing five initiatives described in the following section.

2.4.1 Initiative 1: Increasing Community Knowledge of Preventive Oral Health Care

In this first initiative, strategies to enhance personal contact included (1) educating our CAB of the importance of oral health care; (2) developing and conducting a dental provider needs assessment; (3) engaging our CAB in discussions regarding best ways to increase community knowledge and seeking their input and feedback on plans, activities, and educational brochures; (4) working with local medical providers to increase their willingness and capability to incorporate basic dental preventive education into their patient encounters and learn the appropriateness of knowing when more extensive dental care was needed; and (5) developing a brochure called OHICAN in which we introduced ourselves and the OHICAN program, listed service locations, services available, and contact information, defined who was eligible to access the services, and provided facts and information about oral health care. We distributed 750 copies of the OHICAN brochure to schools and community organizations through community events in the target area. At these events, we measured the baseline level of knowledge of the respondents then had a brief educational intervention followed by a post survey. These educational interventions to raise community awareness were done in-person.

In addition to the distribution of educational brochures, we developed two technology-based solutions that contribute to increasing community knowledge of preventive oral care. One was a culturally sensitive website to improve communication and provide information on free resources and local opportunities for dental care. The brochure discussed above is featured on this website.

The second technology-based solution is a smartphone app (OH-I-CAN) available for download on the website. The phone app has two questionnaires, the OHIP (Oral Health Impact Profile) and the ECOHIS (Early Childhood Oral Health Impact Scale). The OHIP measures people's perceptions of the impact of oral health disorders on their well-being and includes questions regarding dysfunction, discomfort, disability, and handicap resulting from oral health conditions. The ECOHIS measures the quality of oral health-related quality-of-life of preschool children and their families.

2.4.2 Initiative 2: Expanding Existing Oral Health Care Capacity in Local Communities

This second initiative addresses the need for increased literacy about the importance of oral health as only part of a comprehensive solution. However, once people are aware, they need places to go to obtain dental care. Lack of adequate capacity to care for populations in low-income and minority areas is a major issue. During the work of personal contact, we expanded dental health care capacity to include (1) identifying, engaging, and training nontraditional dental care providers to perform oral exams and apply fluoride when indicated; (2) training providers to be aware of the requisite steps to address oral health issues and enhance preventive oral health measures in communities (approximately 1000 non-dental health care professionals were educated and trained in this area); (3) educating hygienists of recent changes in licensing laws that allow their profession to provide preventive care under general supervision; (4) educating stakeholders (primarily dentists) of the implications of the changes in dental hygienists' practice laws (approximately 325 dentists were educated in this area); (5) supporting implementation efforts for the expanded role for hygienists; and (6) integrating medical and dental efforts to increase access to preventive care.

In the expansion of our in-person intervention efforts, we used technology primarily through the development of the OHICAN website. The OHICAN website has educational tools for providers, training modules, provider protocols, videos, a toolkit, and other resources and connects to a metadata repository that gathers information from the quality-of-life questionnaires on the smartphone app. Using the website as a repository database for educational tools, providers can examine the oral health-related quality of life of individual patients at discrete points or review an individual patient's status over time. As the repository builds and appropriate safeguards are put in place, providers can compare results with others on national and international levels. The repository will enable providers and researchers to uncover information including hidden patterns, unknown correlations, and customer/patient preferences that can help providers make better-informed clinical decisions. The app, repository, and database will also allow for population-based studies revealing need(s) based on zip code, age, illness, and other parameters.

2.4.3 Initiative 3: Creating New Points of Access

The goal of this third initiative was to increase community capacity for providing dental care through new points of access. To this end, we (1) partnered with dental residency programs to expand the number of residents at existing sites and establish new ones; (2) worked to establish and support new dental clinics in marginalized neighborhoods; (3) supported the establishment of oral health programs at school-based health centers; and (4) supported efforts to attract dental practices and practitioners to areas with high unmet needs.

Establishing oral health practices can be quite expensive. To aid practitioners and stakeholders in determining financial requirements for establishing new points of access in underserved areas of Georgia, we engaged the Office of Business Practice Improvement, Emory University's Internal Consulting Group, to develop an oral health business plan. The model includes specific service and staffing costs, unreimbursed costs, time for client education, team meetings, referral coordination, training of staff, and supply and technology costs. Any new program or practice must be fiscally sound; therefore, our model allows the consideration of costs, identification of payment opportunities, and development of cost containment strategies. The business model allows for an individual or practice to accurately apply the conditions of their unique environment and elicit the costs of running a program within that environment. The financial model also includes cost projections based on volumes and projected revenue and can provide pro-forma financial statements to give an idea of how the actual statement would look if the underlying assumptions held true. The interactive business plan is available on the OHICAN website.

2.4.4 Initiative 4: Advocating on Behalf of Evidence-Based Strategies to Expand Care and Lower Costs

In this fourth initiative, and throughout our team's project, we personally engaged in advocacy efforts at the individual, regional, state, and national levels to build support for our program. One example was our work in supporting the Dental Hygiene General Supervision for Preventive Care Bill. It was passed into law on January 1, 2018, with the goal of increasing access to preventive oral health care for children and adults in under-resourced areas. In collaboration with the Georgia Dental Hygiene Association, Georgia Dental Association, and the Grady Health System Advance Education in General Dentistry Residency (AEGD) program, we created an implementation toolkit to assist providers in both public and private sectors implement the law. The OHICAN team continues the work of advocacy in roles such as chairing the general supervision implementation subcommittee and with team leaders serving as board members of the Georgia Oral Health Coalition.

On the OHICAN website, we included a tab specifically for advocacy in which we post relevant articles, white papers, and other items of interest to advocates. Additionally, the Toolkit for Incorporating General Supervision in Dental Private Practice and Safety Net Settings in Georgia is available on the website.

2.4.5 Initiative 5: Rolling Out/ Disseminating Results of the OHICAN Pilot Project and Transitioning It to an Initiative for Deployment Nationally and Internationally

In this fifth and final initiative, we employed both in-person and technological strategies in rolling out and disseminating the results of the OHICAN project. We designed and implemented a social media rollout (Facebook, Twitter, Instagram) to share information about OHICAN and its purpose and uses, results, and tools. A critical part of dissemination included educating medical providers (physicians, nurse practitioners, physician assistants, nurses) and oral health professionals about the website and its learning opportunities, specifically additional training and education modules, toolkits, videos, and further information on the OH-I-CAN app available on the website. Attendees were instructed through presentations, seminars, and skills workshops. Included in educational sessions was an introduction to the OHICAN website and the downloadable app and its purposes and uses. Additional dissemination efforts were accomplished through the publication of aspects of this work in peer-reviewed journals and via radio and other media appearances, and we plan additional publications for the immediate future. We also incorporated concepts of the OHICAN project in an interprofessional course titled Social Determinants of Health and Health Equity, developed in collaboration with Emory University.

2.5 Our Recommendations to Address the Inequitable Access to Oral Care

Oral health is an essential component of optimal health. Not only is the oral system the primary way we take nutrients into our bodies through the food we consume, but the health of that system is also critically associated with other health outcomes. Appropriate oral health care and taking preventative measures to protect against diseases of the oral cavity, craniofacial diseases, and cancer are critical elements of optimal health. However, poor oral health and lack of access to care among low-income, minority, and other vulnerable populations are significant contributors to health disparities for these populations. The personal contact and technology-based strategies implemented through the OHICAN project were especially designed to address the lack of equitable access to care.

A myriad of factors contributes to poor oral health and inequitable access to oral care. Lack of dental insurance and/or transportation to a dental facility both impact an individual's ability to obtain oral health care. Services provided by insurance and public programs must be expanded. For instance, in Georgia, adult Medicaid recipients have access only to emergency care and extractions. The disparity between the privately insured and uninsured populations is even larger for children and older adults. Unmet oral health care needs continue to be highest among individuals without insurance.

Secondly, training programs for health care professionals have neither exposure to identifying oral health issues, nor do they have educational opportunities for learners to develop the ability to identify and definitively treat oral health issues. The development of training videos in conjunction with specific algorithms for providers should provide health care workers, and non-dental health care workers, with tools to assist in the treatment of their patients with oral health issues. Likewise, providing in-person trainings for non-traditional oral health care providers in nursing schools, physician assistant schools, and other medical health care training programs should help equip future providers and also expand oral health care to underserved populations.

Third, an increased level of oral health literacy among the general public and across the lifespan is needed. In an ideal situation, oral health would be initiated at the stage of infancy. Training parents or caretakers on the expected oral health milestones and appropriate strategies to deliver optimal oral care, in a similar manner as is done with the stages of crawling to walking from infancy to toddler stage, to the teenage years, young adult, to senior years, would be an excellent start. Oral health messages and healthy practices can also be reinforced through the creation of new access points that will allow more people to receive care.

A fourth issue in increasing access to oral health in marginalized communities includes advocacy efforts to change legislation that in turn creates opportunities for providers to perform at the top of their licenses. Additionally, advocacy efforts are needed to create funding sources for seniors to receive required care such as the inclusion of dental benefits for Medicare recipients.

A fifth recommendation is for more research focused on costs associated with oral health to provide evidence-based strategies for expanding care and lowering costs for patients from marginalized communities. Additionally, the collection of quality-of-life data related to oral health would be useful and could also be used to expand the evidence on a more global platform. For example, more knowledge is needed on similarities and differences in patients' experiences which could be used to compare and contrast experiences across differing age groups, sex, geographic location, and other parameters. Expanding research to these sociodemographic, cultural, and environmental determinants on a more global platform should help provide the basis for evidence-based work to effectively address the burden of poor oral health in low-resourced communities.

Finally, the number of oral health care providers willing to work with underserved populations needs to be increased. The shortage of these providers is even more pronounced in rural communities. Minority dentists are more likely to practice in communities that have larger minority populations. Also, African American and Hispanic American dentists disproportionately serve African Americans and Hispanic Americans, respectively, in their private practices and patients are more likely to seek health care from professionals of a similar culture or background. However, racial and ethnic minorities are underrepresented in the dental profession. As the general population continues to have significant increases in ethnic and racial groups, there will be an ever-increasing need for a more diverse dental workforce.

2.6 Global Perspectives on Oral Health and Addressing Inequities in Oral Care

From an international perspective, several factors contribute to inequities in oral health and accessing oral care. Generally, these factors relate to the resources (human and fiscal) available to these populations. For example, when addressing a lack of resources, much of the work believed impossible in low-resourced countries is being done with efficacy and efficiency. These findings about what is working well in these countries suggest that inequities in oral health and oral care require an understanding of the strengths of underserved populations and creative approaches to meet the oral health care needs of these populations.

When the factors relate to human resources, internationally, nurses are advising and providing preventive services such as oral hygiene education, screening, and referral networks that are far more efficient than those of higher-resourced countries. However, while there have been many successes in lower-resourced, global countries, it is important to note that the provision of care is limited to the skills of the provider (both oral and non-oral care clinicians). For example, non-oral health clinicians will extract teeth to relieve pain because these clinicians do not have the necessary skill set to practice clinical dentistry. It is important to acknowledge that these general practice clinicians could possibly do more to alleviate disparities in oral care, particularly for preventative care, should their current license be expanded to oral screening and health education. Given the limitations in training and/or skill set related to the delivery of oral care, problems that could be detected and treated early when patients are seeking care for other health issues might be detected. If training for oral care available to nurses and other health care providers could be expanded to include oral screening and diagnosis of oral conditions, more serious health problems originating from oral health issues such as bleeding or inflamed gums might be detected earlier.

However, in some instances, fiscal issues tend to override the positive benefits from human resources. In Tanzania, for example, dental therapists have been doing much of the work that dentists are doing, which has tremendous positive oral health outcomes for this population. However, the costs of some treatments continue to be inaccessible to populations with limited fiscal resources. An example of advances in treatment not being available to populations with limited fiscal resources occurs with the use of amalgam fillings. In African countries, particularly in southern and eastern Africa, they are "phasing out" amalgams because of the systemic health problems. These countries are more advanced in this "phasing out" process than in the United States. In the United States, they are "phasing down," as opposed to phasing out the use of amalgams. The economic benefits of producing amalgam by the dental trade industry support the continued use of amalgam by the American Dental Association (ADA) and slowed the process of "phasing out" amalgam. Instead, a slower process of "phasing down" amalgam is recommended by the ADA and others. In the United States, this phasing down rather than phasing out approach to the use of amalgam for fillings is an additional social justice issue because African American and Hispanic American, Native American children, and low-income children of all races and ethnicities have more dental caries than their middle- and upper-class non-Hispanic counterparts. Thus, there is a greater likelihood that they will receive amalgam fillings. Thus, the disproportionate use of amalgam has both social injustice and ethics violations considerations.

Another example of inequities related to fiscal resources relates to the rewards or disincentives to provide oral health care to populations in under-resourced communities. Given the increased expense of oral health, a greater emphasis is placed on other needs, such as food, clothing, and shelter. Public oral health insurance usually focuses on pregnant women and children. Private oral health insurance for children, youth, and adults is very limited. Unless the clinical provider has a passion and commitment to work in under-resourced communities, the support systems to provide the same quality of care that more-resourced communities have at their disposal are disconcerting. All too often, individuals from under-resourced communities only seek oral health care, as a last resort. Oral health issues may be further aggravated in a situation where there are no resources. For example, when there are resources to support oral screenings in schools, dental caries, and early detection of oral disease, treatment options are more available and less costly. Moreover, when there is no disease, preventive care can be provided, oral health literacy can be taught, and health education about the synergy between oral health and systemic health can be implemented. Whatever oral education can be provided in school settings is an added value to complement the health care delivery system. Whereas, in many cases, private schools are the major educational institutions on the African continent, these educational institutions are equipped to synergize the health and formal educational systems, particularly with oral health education. As a result, the formal education system becomes the ideal place to educate students about health and provide health services. Building schools to include health in a broad sense like fresh running water and school health systems with expanding nursing services to include oral health will surely enhance the overall health of children, youth, and families. Similarly, the United States should consider expanding school-based health programs, particularly in low-resourced and rural communities to accomplish this goal.

2.7   Reflections

Expanding the duties of the nurse and possibly other clinical practitioners is an untapped resource in addressing disparities in oral health care. He/she is respected by the community and his/her colleagues. Specifically, expanding the duties of the school nurse to address oral health care under the indirect supervision of a dentist will provide more access points for oral health care.

Reframing oral health, which includes all health providers, is critical. Increasing the consciousness about the importance of the synergy between oral health and systemic is essential to improving overall health, well-being, and quality of life for children, youth, and adults. A paradigm shift from dental health to oral health will expand

the thinking of all clinicians and thereby expand the opportunity without overwhelming health care providers. A shared load in assuring oral health by all health care professionals will improve overall health. If thinking oral health, then evaluating the entire cavity as opposed to dental health where there is a greater focus on the teeth will benefit patients' overall well-being. This expanded thinking will result in an improved physical, social, and psychological well-being of the individual, group, and community. This new way of thinking will require additional training and advance the opportunities to address long-standing disparities in oral and systemic health in underserved and under-resourced communities.

Providers serving low-resourced communities see the impact of oral and systemic conditions far more than those that do not. There is an automatic crossover due to the exposure and lack of other resources to address those issues. Transdisciplinary continuing education should be across disciplines. Providing Continuing Medical Education (CME)/Continuing Education Units (CEU) on oral health for all primary care providers is essential. Likewise, CME/CEUs for oral health providers is also essential to learn more about systemic manifestations of oral diseases and dysfunctions.

References

1. National Institutes of Health. Oral health in America: a report of the surgeon general. US Department of Health and Human Services, National Institutes of Health, National Institute of Dental and Craniofacial Research; 2000.
2. National Institutes of Health. Oral health in America: advances and challenges. US Department of Health and Human Services, National Institutes of Health, National Institute of Dental and Craniofacial Research; 2021.
3. Centers for Disease Control and Prevention. Healthy people 2020: oral health objectives. n.d. https://www.cdc.gov/oralhealth/about/healthy-people-2020.html#:~:text=The%20overall%20goal%20of%20the,on%20social%20and%20economic%20conditions. Accessed 20 Sept 2023. Last reviewed 2 Dec 2020.

4. Centers for Disease Control and Prevention. National hospital ambulatory medical care survey: 2010 emergency department summary tables. 2010. https://www.cdc.gov/nchs/data/ahcd/namcs_summary/2010_namcs_web_tables.pdf. Accessed 20 Sept 2023.

5. Davis EE, Deinard AS, Maïga EWH. Doctor, my tooth hurts: the costs of incomplete dental care in the emergency room. J Public Health Dentistry. 2010;70(3):205–10. https://doi.org/10.1111/j.1752-7325.2010.00166.x.

6. Patel R, Miner JR, Miner SL. The need for dental care among adults presenting to an urban ED. Am J Emerg Med. 2012;30:18–25. https://doi.org/10.1016/j.ajem.2010.09.011.

7. Centers for Disease Control and Prevention. Oral health fast facts. 2016. https://www.cdc.gov/oral-health/fast-facts/index.html. Accessed 20 Sept 2023. Last reviewed 25 Jan 2021.

8. Georgia Department of Public Health. Georgia comprehensive cancer registry: policy and procedure manual. 2014. http://dph.georgia.gov/reporting-cancer. Accessed 20 Sept 2023.

9. National Association of Dental Plans/Delta Dental Plans Association. 2013 NADP/DDPA joint dental benefits report: enrollment. 2014. https://www.nadp.org/about-dental-plans-care/understanding-dental-benefits/.

10. Attendance Works & Healthy Schools Campaign. Mapping the early attendance gap: charting a course for student success. 2015. https://www.attendanceworks.org/mapping-the-early-attendance-gap/. Accessed 30 Sept 2023.

11. Dye BA, Li X, Thorton-Evans G. Oral health disparities as determined by selected healthy people 2020 oral health objectives for the United States, 2009–2010. NCHS Data Brief. 2012;104:1–8.

12. Georgia Health Equity Initiative. Health disparities report 2008: a county-level look at health outcomes for minorities in Georgia. Georgia: Georgia Department of Public Health; 2008.

13. National Association of Dental Plans/Delta Dental Plans Association. 2012 NADP/DDPA joint dental benefits report: enrollment. 2012. https://www.nadp.org/about-dental-plans-care/.

14. Finegold K. New census estimates show 3 million more Americans had health insurance coverage in 2012. Office of the Assistant Secretary for Planning and Evaluation; 2013. https://aspe.hhs.gov/reports/new-census-estimates-show-3-million-more-americans-had-health-insurance-coverage-2012-0. Accessed 20 Sept 2023.

15. Lee HH, Lewis CW, Saltzman B, Starks H. Visiting the emergency department for dental problems: trends in utilization, 2001 to 2008. Am J Public Health. 2012;102(11):e77–83. https://doi.org/10.2105/AJPH.2012.300965.

16. National Research Council. Improving access to oral health care for vulnerable and underserved populations. Washington, DC: The National Academies Press; 2011. https://doi.org/10.17226/13116.

17. Ramraj C, Sadeghi L, Lawrence HP, Dempster L, Quiñonez C. Is accessing dental care becoming more difficult? Evidence from Canada's middle-income population. PLoS One. 2013;8(2):e57377. https://doi.org/10.1371/journal.pone.0057377.

18. McCormick AP, Abubaker AO, Laskin DM, Gonzales MS, Garland S. Reducing the burden of dental patients on the busy hospital emergency department. J Oral Maxillofac Surg. 2013;71(3):475–8. https://doi.org/10.1016/j.joms.2012.08.023.

19. Nichols E. The cultural and social barriers and enablers influence oral and systemic health. In: Paper presented at: Exploring the Relationship Between Oral Health and Systemic Health Within the African American Population, Washington, DC; 2000.

20. Dixon WH. White conquest (the Black heritage library collection). New Hampshire: Ayer Company Publisher; 1976.

21. Okobi E, Okobi OE, David AB, Ofochukwu VC. Oral health considerations for adults aged 18 years or more seeking dental care in the past year: A CDC Oral Health Data Analysis. Cureus. 2024;16(1):e52200. https://doi.org/10.7759/cureus.52200. PMID: 38347992; PMCID: PMC10860365.

Charles E. Moore received a Bachelor of Science from Union College and his medical degree from Harvard Medical School. He subsequently completed residency training in Otolaryngology—Head and Neck Surgery and fellowship training in Craniomaxillofacial— Cranial Base, Facial Plastic, and Reconstructive Surgery at the University of Michigan. Dr. Moore is a Professor at Emory University and the Chief of Service in the Department of Otolaryngology—Head and Neck Surgery at Grady Health System. Dr. Moore has a longstanding and profound commitment to the training and development of learners from all backgrounds. His research focus has been in the investigation of factors involved in healthcare disparity with a particular focus on head and neck cancer incidence in medically underserved communities. He is the President and Founder of Health Education, Assessment and Leadership (HEAL), Inc. Through this organization, he strives to educate the community on health issues, assess its needs, and in the process, build leaders from within the community to address those issues. This traveling resource has grown into the Healing Community Center (HCC), one of Atlanta's newest Federally Qualified Healthcare Centers. This center is a free and affordable medical facility with four separate locations, which provide general adult medical care, pediatric medical care, specialty medical care, dental services, as well as mental health services for the uninsured and disadvantaged. The HCC is focused on those who fall in the gap between public funded health care and the privately insured. A primary emphasis is on preventative health, nutrition, and wellness. This center incorporates all of the major Atlanta academic institutions and community organizations in an integrated fashion to provide service-learning experiences while also providing the necessary care to those in need.

Rueben C. Warren DDS, MPH, DrPH, MDiv, is former Director of the National Center for Bioethics in Research and Health Care and former Professor of Bioethics at Tuskegee University in Tuskegee, Alabama. From 1988 to 1997, Dr. Warren served as Associate Director for Minority Health at the Centers for Disease Control and Prevention (CDC). Dr. Reuben C. Warren earned his undergraduate degree from San Francisco State University and his dental degree from Meharry Medical College. He also earned his MPH and PhD from the Harvard School of Public Health, as well as a Master of Divinity from the Interdenominational Theological Center.

Part IV

Policy

Guidelines, principles, legislation and political activities that affect the living conditions conducive to the welfare of individuals, communities, societies quality of life.

Using Policy to Combat SDOH: Establishing Coalitions in Low-Resource Communities

Ernest J. Grant

1   On Becoming a Nurse Scientist and Political Advocate

Usually, when people ask me what made me want to become a nurse, my response is, "I really didn't want to become a nurse. I think nursing found me." By that I mean, when I was in high school, my dream was to be an anesthesiologist and drive a lime green 1968 Mercury Cougar with a red interior. My high school guidance counselor knew that there probably weren't a lot of scholarships for a Black male to not only go to college but then especially to go on to medical school. He suggested that I consider going into nursing and becoming a nurse anesthetist. Then, if I still wanted to be an anesthesiologist, I could work my way through medical school as a nurse anesthetist and not have educational loans to repay. When I thought about it, it seemed like that was a good idea. He said, "Well, you may not like nursing either," so he suggested I go to the local technical institute at that time—(nowadays they're called community colleges)—and he said, "They have a 1-year nursing program, so you can try that and if you don't like it, that's fine, or if you do, you could easily transition into their

E. J. Grant (✉)
Diversity Equity and Inclusion, Duke University
School of Nursing, Duke University,
Durham, NC, USA
e-mail: Ernest.grant@duke.edu

second-year program and still graduate as an RN." So, I decided to go to the LPN program, and probably about 3 months in, I realized that nursing was my calling and that I wanted to be able to do more for my patients. The role of the LPN at that time was very limited. You were mostly considered to be a medication nurse. Yes, you did hands-on patient care, but it was not as effective as I was seeing the registered nurse colleagues were able to do.

I was working in the ICU at Memorial Mission Hospital in Asheville, North Carolina, and that is a major referral center for Western North Carolina. We would get a great mix of patients coming in, and you would begin to look at the type of community they came from, obviously a very underserved community, very rural, and very poor. Seeing some of the things that patients were encountering, you began to realize that had there been someone in their community that could give them ongoing healthcare, it could've prevented them from coming to the hospital at the last minute. Their healthcare could've been managed more effectively.

That was something that drove me to want to achieve my Baccalaureate degree, so that I could do more for the patients—not only from a hands-on perspective but also from a policy perspective as well. Advocating on their behalf, the possibility of clinics being opened in local communities or the fact that maybe we need more checks and balances on the patients' care and seeing how they're doing. I'd also have a better understanding of who they are from the different cultures because it isn't that you were just seeing people from the Black community. You were also seeing a little bit of the Hispanic community, the Native American community, and the White community as well. This is rural Appalachia, so you had a great mix of people from all different walks of life.

Upon graduating from the LPN program, I immediately started taking courses toward my Baccalaureate degree and subsequently moved to the Durham-Chapel Hill area to complete my BSN. During my years at North Carolina Central University, the feeling of wanting to be more of an advocate and to drive for policy change was reinforced by my professors in the nursing program there. On almost a daily basis, they drilled into our heads that if you are going to consider yourself a professional nurse, you need to do a couple of things. One is to join your professional nursing association as well as the American Nurses Association—and not only join but also be an **active** member. It's one thing to have your name on the roll: it's another to be an active member.

One of the things that reinforced that in my mind was that I'm sure every nurse out there has been given an assignment when you were a nursing student, to go to your regional or state nurses' association meeting and see what's going on. What are the hot topics in nursing or within health care that may be affecting the practice of nurses? We were given that assignment as well. The unique thing was that when I got there, I saw my professors, and they weren't just there checking the roll. They were going up to the microphones, asking challenging questions, or they were chairing committees. In other words, they were showing us how it should be done. It just seemed like a no-brainer that once you graduated, your next step—in addition to sitting the licensure exam—was to join your state nurses' association, which is what I promptly did. Even with getting the Baccalaureate degree, I still realized that in order to be taken more seriously when interacting with policymakers at local or state levels, even at the national level, the higher

degree you have, the more credibility. I realized that just having the BSN, sometimes people would listen to you, but there was that credibility factor that seemed to be lacking. Even though you could talk about the experiences you had and what you saw your patients going through, that still is not quite enough. I got the impression that those who were in control (legislators, policy makers, lobbyists, payers, etc.) ignored your concerns. So that drove me to want to get my master's degree as well, which I did probably within 3–5 years of getting my Baccalaureate degree. Acquiring a master's degree also made me realize that people with a doctorate degree were treated and accepted as more credible than those with a Baccalaureate or master's degree. Being the patient advocate that I was, this further drove me to eventually get my doctorate, too.

2   Patient Advocacy Through Legislative Coalitions

Some of my earlier experiences as a political advocate started with my role as a registered nurse in the Jaycee Burn Center at UNC Hospitals. It was during that time that I began to see a lot of ways in which policy could be used to help reduce burn injuries. A couple of ways I did that was to lobby the legislature to make it mandatory that all hot water heaters sold in the state be set at 120 °F and have information placed on those heaters that if you adjust the dial and turn it up, you risk a scald injury. Another piece was to restrict the sale of fireworks to individuals 16 years of age and older. Prior to that, when the state first passed fireworks legislation, there was no age limit, and we were encountering young kids as young as —6-, 7-, or 8-year-olds—who were having fireworks-related injuries. Either loss of their eyesight, their hands, or other burn injuries, so it just seemed like a no-brainer to restrict giving those kids fireworks—it's almost like giving them a loaded gun. I think another one of the most important pieces of legislation that was passed was the law that required smoke alarms in rental property. Smoke alarms are an early warning device that can alert you that there may be a fire and that you and your family need to leave. The passage of this piece of legislation alone saved many lives. Another important piece of safety legislation was getting the law passed for the sale of fire-safe cigarettes in the state of North Carolina. We know that a lot of the house fires that we encountered were the result of smoldering cigarettes. The fire-safe cigarette is one that extinguishes itself if it's not inhaled at certain points. Once that law was passed, we saw a dramatic reduction in the amount of not only house fires but also burns as a result of house fires that could've happened because of cigarettes.

So, again, having that credibility, not only going in and talking with the legislatures; having the facts and figures based on my experiences; but also having that credibility factor and expertise as someone with a master's degree who has published a lot of papers regarding fire and burn injuries—those are the things that help to drive policy change. The end result…the citizens of North Carolina are much safer because of these policy changes.

3   Patient Advocacy Through Local, State, and Federal Legislative Branches

Those are just a few examples of how we as nurses can use the knowledge that we have to draw attention to prevention or to things that will help keep our patients safe in so many different ways. The challenge is that when you go before legislators—either at the state or national level— you have to remember that you're going against individuals. You're going to be going against folks on the other side, lobbyists for industries that will have their interests at heart also.

Take the afore mentioned hot water heater legislation, for example. You would think that it would be a no-brainer that it's important to want to reduce the risk of a burn injury, particularly to older adults and young children. Many of their scald injuries happen in the bathtub or shower when they accidentally turn on the hot water valve and get instantly scalded because the heater temperature is set too high. Part of my argument

was that obviously these two groups are very vulnerable because of how thin their skin is, and they have difficulty escaping the bathtub or shower if that were to happen. There was likely to be a long hospitalization period as a result of their injuries…not to mention the additional expense associated with that hospitalization and rehabilitation. You compare that to the fact that by reducing the hot water heater temperature, you're reducing the possibility of this person sustaining a significant or life-changing, or even life-threatening injury. On the other side were lobbyists for the hot water heater industry and the electric industry, such as Duke Energy. Their rationale was that if you reduce the temperature setting, you extend the life of the hot water heater by maybe 1–3 years. That means that by doing that, their sales are going to go down. For the electric industry, it means saving on electricity, which will lower the person's electric bill. As a result, the electric company will have less money coming in, and perhaps less profit for their shareholders. So, that creates a conundrum.

I thought about going into the legislature, arguing the statistics, showing them horrible pictures of burned kids and older adults, the hospital costs, etcetera, that would reign supreme, but obviously, it was an uphill battle. We finally won by working out a compromise. Pointing out that one of the things the electric industry or hot water industry could do is come at this issue from the consumer perspective—we want you to be safe, you and your family to be safe, using positive messages. Yes, it may mean that it prolongs the life of the water heater, but by doing that, it also means that chances are when the person does need to replace the hot water heater, they'll go with the same brand they had before. Because they figure that, "Hey, it lasted, 10, 15 years, so it's a good brand." Taking that spin proved very positive, and subsequently, the law was passed.

If you look at the fireworks-related legislation, again, you would think it would be a no-brainer. We ran into lobbyists for the fireworks industry who had pretty deep pockets, so to speak, who were making contributions to the reelection campaign of various members of the legislature, both at the state and national level and on both sides of the isle. You know my pockets are dry! They would also proport that fireworks were safe and same. Again, showing them the results of what could happen and how children who are injured;, people who we anticipate being future productive members of society, are now unable to do that because they've lost a hand or lost their eyesight, so now they're dependent members of society. They're going to rely on disability and maybe require more assistance than someone else at such a young age. So, those are some of the ways to persuade our legislators to look at restricting the sales to those 16 years of age and older. You would think that someone at age 16 would have the conscience enough to realize or think about the consequences of their actions, as opposed to someone much younger who might just think about the enjoyment of watching that device explode. And they don't realize that "Hey, once I light this, I need to throw it away so that, I am not harmed." A lot of times, what happens is that these kids will hold it in their hands, not realizing that it stood the opportunity to explode or that it could possibly cause a house fire if it is thrown in a very dry area.

So, those are some good examples of how you have to consider the other side. If you're going to be an advocate, you have to think about what your opponent may be saying and how they may frame their arguments. You have to come back a little bit better than they are, or at the very least offer the potential of compromise or consensus. You give some; they give some. Nobody's really winning, but hopefully, it's the consumer who is going to be a lot better off as a result. You know, these are just an example of consumer issues.

4 Patient Advocacy to Promote Healthcare Access

If we were to talk about healthcare-related issues, some of the things to think about is the potential of putting a clinic in an undeserved area and giving attention to people that are likely to come to your healthcare facility and who may need to travel by bus, even a couple buses, or walk a great distance. Maybe there isn't a drugstore in their

area. We've heard of food deserts; they may also have a drugstore desert as well, so it's difficult for them to get the medications that they need in order to try to be as healthy as they can. It's important that we know and understand the communities where our patients come from so that we can advocate. So, if we find there is no drug store, there is no routine transportation, then we need to bring the health resources to them, into their community. We can also petition the local town council or county commissioners to offer incentives to get a drug store placed in the underserved community.

You know, we also should ask ourselves, "Why do we only have clinic from 8 in the morning 'til 4:30 or 5 in the afternoon? Why can't we have it all the way 'til maybe 8:30, 9, or 11 at night?" That gives people who work the opportunity to still go and work so that they can keep their jobs, put food on their tables, pay their bills, etcetera, but once they get off work, they can still come and seek the healthcare they need. It will probably enhance compliance to treatment from patients, knowing that they can still go to work and go to the doctor once they get off work. We can bring the clinics to them, to their communities, using local houses of worship, setting up clinics in their dining halls, or even in their sanctuaries or local community centers.

4.1 Gaining the Trust of the Community Is Extremely Important

One way to gain the trust of the community is to collaborate with using community advocates or community leaders to get the word out that clinics will be held in such-and-such place, at such-and-such time. This collaboration allows us to keep better tabs on what's going on with the individual, with their family, and, most importantly, within the community itself. There is also the need to have a discussion with the community leaders to find out what is needed in the community. No one knows the community or its needs better than those who reside there. Questions such as what are the community resources that may be lacking so that we can have a discussion with the city council, or the county commissioners, or even the local state representatives? Even our national representatives and, our US senators, because they can appropriate funding from the federal government to build a freestanding clinic within that community, or lobbying to get a drugstore or something like that within the area, to help serve the underserved community.

Patient advocacy is all about looking, doing an assessment, and seeing what is needed. Asking questions: What resources do we have? What do we need? And how do we champion those to be able to get where we want to be?, Getting members of the community involved, letting them know that they have a voice, that we want to hear their thoughts regarding what they need within their community. After all…it is their community, and they should have a say about the services that are needed.

5 Shared Experiences with Populations from Low-Resource Communities

My background from growing up in a small community in the Southern Appalachian Region of Western North Carolina has shaped the way in which I approach patient advocacy for individuals from low-resource communities. When I remember growing up in Swannanoa, North Carolina, I think there was probably a population of 5000 at the time. There were only two physicians there, Dr. Clapp and Dr. Folson, both of whom were White. I still remember the segregated waiting rooms that they had for a while. Both doctors made house calls, so they would come to your home, if you were too sick to come into their office. When they would come into the Black community, resources were obviously very different from what they may have seen in the White communities. In some places, there was still the use of outhouses. You grew your garden, and you shared what you grew with your neighbors. You picked fresh fruits that grew on the trees like cherries and apples. There was a lot of

canning (preserving of fruits and vegetables). Back then, the paint still had lead in it, but we didn't know at the time that it could pose a problem to the health of individuals. Of course, you couldn't always afford to pay the doctor in cash, so you paid him in fruits and vegetables, or when you killed a hog and gave him a ham or something like that to help pay off your bills and stuff.

Then, you also had women who were nurses in the community. I think of women like Aunt Thelma or Ms. Johnny Morehead, and I don't know if Annabelle Daniels was a nurse or not, but many of them worked at the local Sanatorium in Black Mountain. That was the hospital that treated patients with TB; many of these ladies were LPNs who worked there.

I also need to mention the role of the Black church in the community, how members of the church would visit the homebound and clean their homes, check their medications, make sure they were up to date, and things like that. It was a way to keep tabs on how well the person was doing from so many different perspectives. I frequently tell people that when we had the old nurse midwives, their primary responsibility was for the mother and the baby, but then they were also responsible for the family and everything else that was going on because that affected the mother's ability to care for the infants. And you wanted to make sure that the infant was growing up in a house that was safe—that didn't have roaches or big gaps where the wind would come through in the wintertime, or mold, or lead paint and stuff like that.

When women started having babies in hospitals, all of that went away. You just assumed or took it for granted that they were going back to a safe environment. However, it wasn't until the social workers came into the community that the attention was given to the environment and began to drive change. But the nurse-midwives were very quick to pick up on things that were going on in the community and would be the drivers of change much needed in our communities. They were very creative in trying to get and use the limited resources they had at their disposal. Even with segregation and stuff going on, they were able to look at whatever federal or state resources that were available and use those in the Black and Brown communities.

6 Role of Political Advocate as Past President of American Nurses Association

In 2018, I was elected President of the American Nurses Association. That was a historical moment because I became the first male and only the third African American to serve in that role. At that time, it was in the 124-year history of the American Nurses Association.

6.1 Diversifying the Profession

When I assumed the office of president, there were six goals that I had, and one of them was to increase diversity within the profession. I had long recognized that nursing needed to have more people of color and more men. We know that we have better patient outcomes when patients can look up and see someone who looks like them, who is from their same culture, who understands them, etcetera; knowing that that person can advocate on their behalf, educate other members of the healthcare team about how the patient's cultural views health or healthcare; getting the patient to open up more and to talk about their resources and things they have at home that they may be a little hesitant to share with individuals they view as strangers.

One of my other goals was to increase public awareness of who we are as nurses and what we do—not just thinking of nurses as being those individuals who work at the local health center but that nurses are everywhere. Yes, we work at the local hospital, but we are also in community health, we're in the schools, and we have our own businesses. We're entrepreneurs. We work in industry…and most importantly, we are a part of the community…meaning that whatever happens in the community affects us and our family as well!

6.2 Advocating for Protective Gear for Nurses

A little bit after taking office in 2019, obviously the thing that happened was the onset of COVID-19 and how that literally shut the whole globe down within a week's time. One of the things that I began to realize was that I needed to put on my advocacy hat, not only for the public being affected by this virus that at the time we knew very little about but also for members of the healthcare team as well and particularly for nurses. Nurses by far were more disproportionately affected by COVID than any other member of the healthcare team. That's because of who we are and what we do—that we're there 24/7 with the patients and their families. I'm sure everyone can recall the numerous stories of nurses being there to hold the hands of a dying patient because their family members couldn't be there or holding the phone for the family members so they could say their final goodbyes to their loved ones.

During the COVID-19 pandemic, one of the things that we began to realize was that there was a failure in the supply chain with the protective gear the nurses were relying on for their safety in the workplace. There were N-95 masks that had been in mass storage for such occasions as this, but they were not rotated properly, so many had dry rotted and were ineffective…meaning that they no longer met the NIOSH filtration protection standard. Another issue was related to healthcare facilities buying masks on the black market that did not meet the NIOSH standard, yet they were expecting members of the healthcare team to wear them.

As President of ANA and advocate for the profession, I had to go before a Senate subcommittee to talk about what I was hearing from nurses in the field. I also made it a point to speak with 60 nurses from around the country, on a regular basis during the pandemic, who worked at the grassroots level. These nurses worked in many different areas, either at the bedside or in nursing education or community health, just to get an idea of what's going on. What were they seeing? Because obviously, if it's happening in their community, it's going to bubble up to the national level as well, and this was a way for us to be prepared. By calling the senator's attention to several issues: (1) that counterfeit masks were being bought by healthcare facilities; (2) that the national supply and distribution chain was failing; (3) that people were failing to rotate the products the way that they were supposed to; (4)

that the nurses lives were at risk as a result of this; and, (5) without nurses, we wouldn't have anybody to take care of the patients as they continued to get sick. Our efforts resulted in more focus on the national supply chain, getting more up-to-date masks, gowns, and gloves. A lot of the gloves had dry rotted too, so it was important that they understood that as well. It was also important that they cracked down on the counterfeit masks that were coming in that did not meet the OSHA or NIOSH standards. The nurses couldn't get close to their patients and have masks that weren't doing what they were designed to do. That was extremely important that we brought this to their attention.

6.3   Educating the Public About Masks and Vaccines

The other big challenge obviously was educating the public about their need to wear masks as well. Subsequently, once the vaccines were available, educate the public about the efficacy of the vaccines and how important it was that they get the vaccines and follow-up boosters. Particularly, when you look at the marginalized communities, we realized the trust that nurses had with patients—we needed to use that [trust] to educate the marginalized communities that these vaccines are safe and effective and encourage the patients to get them. It was important to take the time out to answer their questions, and listen to their concerns.

I think one of the greatest advocacy moves that I could use was the fact that I participated in the clinical trial of one of the vaccines. So, I could tell them firsthand, "I took it before we knew if it was going to be effective." Once they learned that I was a guinea pig, so to speak, and that things worked for me, I could help alleviate the fears and concerns they had. I also could use that opportunity to encourage them that we needed to get more people of color in research, in these clinical trials so that when the next pandemic comes along—or even just other illnesses like cancer or rare diseases—we need to have that specific data on how it affected the Black and Brown communities in relation to that illness or disease that may be there. It was quite a challenge, and it was done through several different ways, either going on multiple TV or radio shows, doing commercials, using social media, and speaking at various conferences. I spoke at a few church conferences to get the word out again that the vaccines were safe and about other things people needed to do in order to help keep them and their family members safe from potentially contracting the virus as well.

7   Policy Issues for the Future

The pandemic has opened the door for nurses to be able to advance who we are as a profession. Prior to the pandemic, particularly for the advanced practice nurse, there was always some question of do we need to have a physician supervision for some things that we do,... the scope of practice? Then, when the pandemic came about, for 2-plus years, there was a declared emergency, which meant that states that restricted the full practice authority for advanced practice nurses had to lay that aside. We can look at that data and see that there was no harm done to the public like had been feared or preached by our physician colleagues. You couldn't ask for a better experience or experiment than that.

I think, moving forward, there are a couple of things that nursing needs to do. One, be more proactive as far as having our seats at the table and demanding our seats at the table. If a seat is not offered, then we need to bring our own seat to the table! When laws or regulations are being proposed that will affect nursing and our ability to practice to the full extent of our education, we need to be that voice at the table and say who we are and what we can or cannot do. No other profession, I think, is regulated more by people outside of the profession than nursing. We need to take ownership back of what we are capable of doing as nurses. We can't continue to let individuals who are far removed from nursing such as payers, CFO's, state, and federal agencies dictate how our profession should be governed. I'd like to stress to our physician colleagues that we don't want to be physicians. But we want to be treated as colleagues. Giving us the opportunity to have full practice authority is the best thing that you can, or you will be able to do. There's an old quote that I love to use when discussing nurse advocacy about the profession, "If you're not at the table, then you're on the menu"!

Embracing innovations and technology that will help to make the work that we do much easier and allow us to spend more time with the patient will help us as well. Right now, we spend so much time checking boxes because our employers have put it in our minds that if you didn't check the box, it wasn't done. And if it wasn't done, then you're going to be dinged about it or they (the employer) may not get reimbursed for it. They don't quite understand that maybe I didn't check that box because I needed to hold that patient's hand as they were just told that they were diagnosed with cancer, or that a family member died, or something like that. You shouldn't be punished for doing the work of nursing just because you didn't check a box so that the facility can get reimbursed for that procedure by the payers. We need to really look at what is more important. Is it the patient who we're supposed to be taking care of or is it checking the box so that the hospital can get their reimbursement?

I also think nurses should be able to find their voice and advocate that we should be able to charge for the care that we bring instead of being included in room and board. If our physician colleagues can charge for what they do—physical therapists, respiratory therapists, pharmacists, and occupational therapists—all of them charge for the services that they bring. Yet nursing, the most intensive area within a hospital, is thought of as a commodity, listed under room and board. You know, that is a slap in the face as to who we are as a profession. We have our own body of work. We do our research. We are held to higher standards. We have practice guidelines, etcetera, yet we don't have the ability to charge for the services that we provide. There's something wrong there. Obviously, we know what it is, that healthcare facilities feel like they're going to be missing out on money. In actuality, there have been a few places where through pilot studies of allowing nurses to charge, the facilities are still able to reap a profit. So, there's no reason why this could not be enacted.

Finally, I think nurses need to have their seat at the table in the boardrooms of healthcare facilities in addition to the chief nursing officer. There need to be other nurses that are there who can talk about what is happening right there at the bedside. Sometimes, administrators get far removed from the actual place where healthcare is taking place hands-on. Nurses need to be at the table to talk about the experiences that they are having, what the consumer wants, and what they bring to the table could mean a more efficiently run facility, as opposed to things being dictated to you from the top down.

It's important that nurses feel that their voices are being heard. Not only heard but that some of the suggestions and things they are proffering are being enacted—which could be a savings for everyone. I'm sure we would be able to see that there will be better patient outcomes also. Of course, we have a lot of evidence-based practice to prove that, so we need to continue to push the envelope of nurses being able to have their voices heard.

Nurses need to be well-versed in how to become political activists, if you will. Even though we have Nurses Night at the Legislature, and visits on Capitol Hill, etcetera, there are some other things that nurses can do. Volunteer to be a health consultant for a candidate. Usually we, as nurses, know somebody who knows somebody. So, if it's a subject we're not familiar with, we know somebody who probably might be an expert on it. When you stop and think that for a lot of politicians, their healthcare expert is someone who either works for a lobbying company or pharmaceutical company. The information they may have will either reflect the opinion of the company that would benefit from the legislation passage (or non-passage) or they have gotten their information from Wikipedia or somewhere else. They're not getting the full picture. I think by having nurses volunteering to serve as a healthcare consultant, they can provide a broader view of "If you enact this legislation, this is how it's going to affect people in your community that you represent." Give them the other side of that, so that they can understand.

I think it also is important that nurses themselves get involved. I mean, heck, run for office! Be the change that, you know, we'd like to see. In the North Carolina legislature, I think we have three nurses—two in the House and one in the Senate. Yet, we have eight physicians in the legislature. So anytime a health bill comes up, they're going to run to the physicians first. Yes, they will consult the nurses, but they run to the physicians first and get their opinions. It would be great if we had more nurses, there that can in essence sort of cancel out the votes of the physicians if needed, so that it means getting better care for the patients or the community.

When I look at our state, we're one of the last states to implement Medicaid or Obama Care for our citizens. Even though they passed it, they kept delaying implementing it. It's been tied to the budget, hoping the budget will get passed. Right now, they're saying the budget was supposed to be passed in June, then it went from June to July, and now it's gone from August to maybe late September or October. Already, we've gone 4 months since that piece of legislation was passed and the possibility of 600,000 North Carolinians getting Medicaid. They're missing out on that now. The federal government is dropping more and more people from Medicare roles as a result of COVID-related legislation ending. That means that people who were getting healthcare are now just left in limbo. These are the things that nurses need to be aware of and bring to the attention of the legislatures.

8 On Policy as Essential to Community Engagement

A politician is not going to be willing to change things unless they hear from enough people who could influence their opinion. It goes back to what I was talking about as an undergrad at Central, a

professor saying, "You've got to be an *active* member of your Association. Not just having your names on the roll." Because again, it's that activity that makes them sit up and think, "Okay, maybe there is enough opposition here or enough call here that we do need to enact this piece of legislation," or whatever it may be. Usually, unless they don't hear something against it, their thing is, "Well, this guy from the pharmaceutical company is going to grease my hand and…" Or whatever the industry may be. So, they need to be able to hear how the vote that they're about to make will affect the people that they are voting on behalf of, when they may be doing some harm. Because those guys, especially on the national level, our senators and our US representatives, they have some of the best healthcare for the rest of their lives. They only have to serve one day, and they get the best healthcare. They get additional perks as well just because of the office that they held. They forget that they are our employees, not the other way around. So, they need to hear from their employer every once in a while, when things are going awry.

The other thing is getting more nurses to understand the power that they have. There are roughly about 4.4 million registered nurses in the country. That's a significant number. I know when I was president and I went up on Capitol Hill, I would say, "I represent the nation's 4.3 million registered nurses." Well, the first words out of some of the elected official mouths … especially the Republicans were "And how many of them are in my state?" or "How many of them do you know will vote for me?" Because that's all they care about. The bottom line is voting. So, it's important that the nurses realize the power that we have and that if you gain the public's trust, all it takes is for nurses to be out in public saying, "This guy or this woman is wrong," "This is how this is going to affect your family," or "We need to get clean air and water and get lead paint removed." We have to be that activist as well as that healthcare provider. We must find and use our voice!

Ernest J. Grant PhD, RN, FAAN, is the Vice Dean for Diversity, Equity, Inclusion, and Belonging at the Duke University School of Nursing. He is also the immediate past president of the American Nurses Association (ANA), the nation's largest nurse's organization representing the interests of the nation's 4.3 million registered nurses. He is the first man to be elected to the office of president of the ANA in its 127 years of existence. A distinguished leader, Dr. Grant has more than 30 years of nursing experience and is an internationally recognized burn-care and fire-safety expert. He also serves as adjunct faculty for the UNC-Chapel Hill School of Nursing., For the past 4 years in a row, Dr. Grant has been recognized by Modern Healthcare Magazine as one of 50 Influential Clinical Executives in Healthcare and as one of 100 Most Influential People in Healthcare. He has been nationally recognized for his work addressing racism, equity, and inclusion within the nursing profession. In 2002, President George W. Bush presented Grant with a Nurse of the Year Award for his work treating burn victims from the World Trade Center site. He was inducted as a fellow into the American Academy of Nursing in 2011. Grant holds a BSN degree from North Carolina Central University and MSN and PhD degrees from the University of North Carolina at Greensboro.

How Community Should Inform Policy and Ultimately Policy Should Improve Community as It Relates to SDOH

Jasmine Clark

1 Community Informing Policy

1.1 Serving in the Legislature with a Science Background

In 2017, fresh off the heels of a presidential election that would have profound impacts on our country going forward, I sat in a room with other science-minded individuals, and we collectively decided that we should have a March for Science in Atlanta, GA. The March for Science was a call to action after the new administration had adopted some troubling policies on climate change science. While I was not a climate scientist, I was a concerned individual who felt that policy should be embracing science and addressing climate change concerns, not abandoning it and writing those concerns off. By the end of a series of meetings, it was decided that the March for Science would be held on Earth Day of that year and I was democratically chosen to lead the march. I had no idea what I was in for, as I had never done anything like this, but this moment would become a "sliding door" moment for me, that would change the trajectory of my life. Prior to these convenings, going into politics in any way was not a part of any of my long-term goals. Even in that moment, I did not know that a year from then I

would be on the campaign trail running for elected state office. But that's exactly what happened. The March for Science in Atlanta was a resounding success, with over 10,000 people marching for scientifically sound and evidence-based policymaking. After the march, I started doing social justice work with a local organization. And by the beginning of the next year, 2018, I was making phone calls and considering running for office. When I put my name on the ballot that year, I ran on bringing a science voice to the GA legislature. I would be the only PhD microbiologist to serve in the legislature. In November of 2018, when I won in a very tight race, my mindset now had to shift from running for office to being an effective legislator. How would I be able to effectively use my science background in this new role?

There were pros and cons to being a political newcomer. Because my background was in science and my career is teaching future nurses, I went into the role thinking that good policy was enough to make good things happen. I quickly learned the difference between policy and politics. Same prefix but the suffix can be worlds apart. Having a good policy is not enough. You must be able to get 256 individuals (or at least 50% +1 of them) to see *why* or *how* the policy is good. I also learned what drives a lot of the decisions that ultimately get made (or not made). One of the major driving factors of policy change is public input. While it is not the only factor, it is vital to the process.

J. Clark (✉)
Nell Hodgson Woodruff School of Nursing, Emory University, Atlanta, GA, USA
e-mail: jrainey@emory.edu

2   Who/What Is Community?

For the purposes of this chapter, I want to emphasize that when I refer to "community" I am referring to both individuals that live in the community,
as well as a group of people that share a common
interest or goal. For example, if a community in
rural south GA is concerned that the lack of
healthy food options is affecting their health, and
they would like to advocate for access to fresh
fruits and vegetables in their area, they could
reach out to someone at the state level to see what
programs or policy could be implemented to
address this critical need. In 2022, residents from
Juliette, GA came to the Capitol to express concerns that chemicals from coal ash in Georgia
Power's unlined coal ash pits were seeping into
the groundwater supply and leading to adverse
health outcomes in their community. These residents constituted a community, with a common
concern and a common objective—making sure
they had access to clean drinking water. They
came to the Capitol, dressed in matching shirts,
and spoke with legislators that represented their
town and they were able to get legislation passed
that would require that their water supply be
monitored for cancer-causing contaminants.

The community does not have to just be a
group of neighbors or a town. Often, we will have
groups of people come to the Capitol donning
white coats, and we know that they are there to
represent healthcare workers in some capacity.
Sometimes it is a group of medical students that
are expressing concerns about how certain legislation could impact their future careers.
Sometimes it is nurses coming to the Capitol to
advocate for policies that will make it easier for
them to serve their patient populations in a safe
manner. Sometimes there are communities within
a given community. For example, early in my
career, we would often hear from midwives in
GA—both certified nurse midwives and community midwives. While they were both advocating
for making the practice of midwifery in GA more
accessible to Georgians, as individual communities they also had unique perspectives and objectives that they sought.

3   Community-Informed Policymaking

There are no requirements to get elected to office
outside of the age requirements, a qualifying fee,
and the ability to get people to vote for you.
Consequently, many, and arguably most, lawmakers are not policy experts. While they may
have institutional knowledge in a limited field or
niche, they rely on information from others to
inform their decisions. Some sources of that
information include lobbying firms, subject matter experts, organizations, and community input.
Generally, lobbying firms are hired by a client,
usually a corporation, to speak on their behalf
and for their interests. Subject matter experts provide targeted, often data-driven information
about specific policies. Additionally, many organizations and associations may provide subject
matter expertise on policy or can also speak on
behalf of a community or population. Lastly,
community input is an integral part of public policymaking and democratic institutions rely on
input from the public when making informed
decisions on policy. This chapter will focus on
how the community has the ability to inform policy, particularly at the state level, to influence
social determinants of health, and improve health
outcomes for their community.

As a first-time legislator, mere weeks after the
election was certified in 2018, I was approached
by a parent in the district who wanted to speak to
me about the sex education curriculum being
taught in Gwinnett County. When we met, she
spoke with me about the work she had been doing
to advocate for more comprehensive sex education because of the experience her daughter had
using the current curriculum. Upon meeting her,
I learned that the curriculum being used by
Gwinnett County (and several other counties in
the State of GA) was an abstinence-only curriculum that emphasized virginity pledges. This
purity-centered curriculum may have seemed
innocuous to the untrained eye. If, like many legislators, you do not have school-aged children, it
may be difficult to grasp why it may be troubling
to approach sex education this way. When this

parent sat down and talked to me, she explained how the curriculum could have dire, even if unintended, consequences for children who were being abused. For example, a curriculum that teaches girls that their vagina was "ruined" and no one would want it if they were not a virgin might cause a child to be ashamed to tell others that they are being molested. Additionally, we also found parts of the code section that were using outdated language. As a person with a PhD in Microbiology with expertise in retrovirology, I found it disturbing that schools in GA were only required to teach about AIDS and not HIV. While most people may not understand that there is a difference between the two, or understand why the difference between the two should matter, I recognized that focusing on an end-stage disease (AIDS) versus the causative agent of the disease (HIV) left too much room to leave out important information. For example, a school could state "if you have sex, you can get AIDS, and die," and that would have been sufficient to cover the requirements in the State law. But that explanation completely leaves out the infectious process, prevention of transmission, testing and diagnosis, and treatment. In a state that unfortunately boasts some of the highest numbers of new HIV cases in the country, this information is necessary and transformative. So along with seeking to make sex education evidence-based, science-based, and medically accurate, this interaction with my constituent led us to also seek to update the language in the Georgia code to teach "HIV prevention."

This is just one of example about how someone's lived experience was transformed into a legislative bill that would be introduced in the Georgia General Assembly. In this instance, the policy was brought to a legislator so that a bill could be drafted from scratch. The individual reached out to their state representative, presented a policy idea, and then helped craft the language of a bill. The community can inform policy this way, and they can also inform policy by providing public comment on existing policy that is already being considered by the legislative body. If a person has concerns about a bill that has been introduced in the state legislature, they

have the ability to bring their concerns to the committee in which the bill is being heard, or they can bring their concerns to their individual elected officials prior to them voting on passage. Both methods of communication, however, strengthen the legislative process.

What are the consequences of the community *not* engaging in the policymaking process? When community voices are not available or heeded when making policy, often the consequences can lead to bad or worse outcomes for those within the community. There can be a disconnect between what the community's actual needs are and what policymakers the community needs. This disconnect can lead to laws being passed that make existing disparities more disparate or that are contrary to the will of the people most affected by the policy. Additionally, policies that could reduce disparities and improve health outcomes may never get introduced or passed by the respective legislative body.

4   Why Does the Community Not Engage in the Policymaking Process?

Given the benefits of community-informed policymaking, why don't more people get involved in the process? Many in the community do not know who to engage; do not know how to participate; do not think that have enough knowledge or expertise; face barriers to participation or lack the resources necessary to participate; or do not believe the process makes a difference.

When I was running for office for the first time, I would knock on doors to tell people about myself and ask them for my vote. One thing I found interesting was the number of people who were not familiar with the state legislature. They thought I was running for Congress, and when I explained that I was running for the state-level equivalent of Congress, they would look perplexed. Even if people had driven down the highway and seen the shining Gold Dome many times, they were completely unaware that laws were being made underneath it. If they do not know that the state legislature exists, or what the state legislature does, then they will not know to engage them on matters where the state legislature can impact their lives. In 2022, when the Supreme Court overturned *Roe v. Wade* and ruled that access to abortion care would be up to each individual state, more people became aware of the existence of, and importance of, the state legislature.

There are times when people have legitimate concerns and they would like to engage with elected officials to discuss solutions, but they are not sure which level of government is best to handle that situation. For example, when I was first elected one of the biggest complaints I received in my office was not about legislation I was proposing or about laws that were being considered at the Capitol. The biggest complaint I got was about trash collection. People would contact my office to tell me that their trash had not been picked up, or that their cans were strewn haphazardly in the street or the middle of driveways. I shared in their frustrations, as I was experiencing some of the same issues, however, it was not my office that was responsible for trash collection. Trash collection is handled by the local government (county commissioners or city council members). Additionally, when someone needs a passport, and they didn't give themselves enough time and the passport has not arrived in time for their flight, they are often told to contact their elected official, and they may end up calling my office instead of their congressperson.

While some individuals do not get involved in the policymaking process because of a lack of knowledge of how or with whom to engage, there are some within our communities who want to participate but do not feel they have enough expertise to have valuable input. This is a common misconception that is usually born from the illusion of grandiosity of the State Capitol. Once, when I was walking from my office in the Coverdell Legislative Office Building to the State Capitol across the street, I was stopped by an individual who asked me who was "allowed" to go into the building. This was before 2022, when a large, black fence was erected outside of the building, making it even more intimidating to those who might want to enter. Within the rooms

and chambers of the State Capitol, we refer to the place as "The People's House," yet the truth is many do not feel they are invited within.

Once inside, the committee hearing process can also feel uninviting. Many people do not realize that you do not have to be representing an organization, a subject matter expert, or a special invited guest to speak on a policy that is important to them. The committee hearing process is open to the public, and anyone can sign up to speak. While individuals are often concerned that they are not subject matter experts or that they may not have enough knowledge to speak to a legislative body, there is evidence to show that storytelling has the ability to change minds [1]. This is important in policymaking because the storyteller (a member of the community) is only expected to be an expert on their lived experience and the policymaker, who is often also not a subject matter expert, is presented with information that is easy to understand, and for some policymakers, relatable.

Committee hearings are the opportunity that the public has to give elected officials information about how certain policies can have an impact on their lives. Speakers are usually given a few minutes to speak to the members of the committee and make their case as to why a certain policy should or should not be implemented. They can also bring up specific issues or suggest specific changes to legislation being heard in that committee. This is just one way the community can get involved in the process.

Additionally, members of the community are able to request meetings with legislators to discuss policy in detail. They may suggest a policy be introduced (like the sex education bill proposed by my constituent), or they can speak to elected officials about how policies that have been introduced could have an effect on their lives. There are no college degrees or specific expertise required to take these steps.

Another issue that can lead to a lack of involvement by community members affected by public policy is the lack of resources. The State of Georgia stretches almost 300 miles north to south, and almost 250 miles west to east. If a person who lives in Valdosta or Savannah, GA, wants to come to the State Capitol to speak at a hearing or to meet with their legislator face-to-face during the legislative session, they would need to drive 3.5–4.5 h, respectively to do so. In addition to the distance, some legislative hearings are held first thing in the morning. This may require a person wanting to come to the State Capitol to also secure lodging. Both transportation and lodging come with a significant cost, and for some, could be cost prohibitive. This is where social determinants can have an impact on the ability to advocate for one's health or the health of their community.

Lastly, every now and then, I hear from a member of a community that states that the reason why they do not get involved is because they do not feel that participation will make a difference. For some, they believe, systemically, that all of the outcomes have already been decided and trying to impact the process is an exercise in futility. For others, they may feel like they cannot influence the process because the political party they align with is not the political party in power in the State Capitol, and therefore have a very hard time getting good or necessary policy passed, or are unable to stop bad or harmful policy from crossing the finish line. On this last point, ironically, it is usually community input that can help the minority caucus make the case for why policy should or should not be passed. They can come to the Capitol, tell their stories, and speak to lawmakers from a perspective that is based on real-life experiences. Hearing from your constituents can, in some cases, be *more* compelling than hearing from your colleagues who do not live in your community and can only speak about the impact of the policy tangentially.

5   Who Should the Public Engage?

Just as important as how a person engages with elected officials is with whom they engage. If an individual is interested in introducing legislation that has not been introduced already, it is best to engage with their elected representative or sena-

tor (or both). While this would be easiest if there were a uniform system for making these types of requests, in the State of GA, this does not exist. The easiest way to schedule a meeting with an elected official is to reach out to their administrative assistant who will facilitate the process. The administrative assistant's contact information is available on the legislator's profile page on the Georgia General Assembly website (legis.ga. gov). When preparing to meet with the elected official about a policy you would like to see implemented in the state of Georgia, it is best to start with your story of why it is important to you, and then go into why the elected official should care. This should include information about how the policy you would like to be implemented would affect their constituency, their own community, or an industry within their community. Also, consider the legislator's background when preparing. If you are going to speak to them about healthcare policy, and by all indications, they do not have any healthcare experience, then the way you approach it may be different than if they are a trained healthcare professional.

If a community member is concerned about a particular policy that has already been introduced and assigned to a standing committee in the State House or State Senate, they can reach out to the Chair of that standing committee as well as all the members of that committee. Just because a bill is introduced and assigned to a committee does not mean it will get a hearing. Which bills get heard in committee is up to the discretion of the Chair of that committee. During the 2023 legislative session, of the over 800 bills introduced in the GA State House, less than 20% were actually heard in their respective committee. Given this, it is possible that the bill one is concerned about may not get a hearing. This is also true for policies that you believe would be good for your community. If the bill of concern is not scheduled for a hearing, then it is best to reach out directly to the Chair of that committee to inquire as to whether or not the bill will be heard. If, however, the bill has been scheduled for a hearing, then reaching out to the Chair as well as *all* the members of the committee would be most effective. The hearing allows the opportunity for community members to engage with the committee, in-person, through public comment.

If an individual or organization is speaking on behalf of a community, then another way to engage in the policymaking process is to meet with the different caucuses within the Capitol. The two main causes are the democratic and republican caucuses of each chamber. Additionally, there are several other caucuses. The Georgia Legislative Black Caucus (GLBC), the largest state black caucus in the nation, could be engaged when speaking on issues that will have a disproportionate impact on Black Georgians. For example, groups have met with the GLBC to discuss maternal mortality, prostate cancer, triple-negative breast cancer, and other issues that have had an outsized impact on Black people or Black communities across the state. If there are policies that would impact women more so than men, there is a Women's Caucus in the Georgia General Assembly as well. There are many smaller caucuses that are identified by ethnic group, specific industries, or even age. If there is an issue that would be of importance to members of these groups, then reaching out to them for a meeting is a great way to engage many elected officials at once.

6   How to Get the Community More Involved in the Policymaking Process

Given the consequences of a lack of community input in the policymaking process, it is important that the community is involved. How, then, do we increase community engagement with elected officials? I think it is incumbent upon members of the community or organizations that advocate on behalf of community members to inform community members that they can participate in the legislative process, and, additionally *how* they can engage. Community involvement and input do not always have to be in the form of speaking into a microphone to a committee, although that is one way that individuals can engage elected officials during the policymaking process. For example, at the Georgia State Capitol, anyone

with a vested interest in a bill being heard in a standing committee can sign up to give public comment. Usually, the people who show up to speak are a part of an advocacy organization, speaking on behalf of a community. This opportunity, however, is not limited to organizations. Individuals who will be impacted by the policy being heard could sign up to speak as well, where they can tell their stories. If a person does not feel comfortable with public speaking, they can still engage their public officials through email, phone calls, and letter writing. Individuals can also engage their elected officials one-on-one instead of speaking to an entire committee. They can ask their elected official for a meeting, or they can call their elected official (at the Georgia State Capitol) out "to the ropes"—an area designated for the public just outside of the House and Senate chambers—to speak with them about a bill that may be being voted on that day, or to speak about an issue that is being considered during the session.

In addition to what members of the community can do to increase public engagement in the legislative process, I think it is important that legislative officials and others in positions of power make the State Capitol building and the processes that occur within it more accessible. In 2021, when the pandemic shifted the way we operated in the State Capitol for that legislative session, the Capitol was much more accessible to many people because legislators and the public could participate in the hearing by Zoom. The public had to sign up to speak in advance, but once signed up, they were given the Zoom link and able to submit public comments virtually. For those within Georgia who may not have had a vehicle to drive to the Capitol, or the money to pay for a hotel, the hearing process became much more accessible. Unfortunately, after the 2022 session, when pandemic fears lessened and pandemic protocols were relaxed, the leadership in the Capitol chose to abandon this access and return to the policy of requiring individuals to comment at hearings, in person. Those barriers to participation, that were removed out of necessity for safety during the pandemic, were subsequently reerected. But, while requiring in-person public comment can limit who is able to participate in committee hearings, the public can still use electronic means (or even snail mail) to communicate with elected officials. Many elected officials will meet with constituents via Zoom. Also, most elected officials have community town halls, which gives community members the opportunity to engage with their legislators within the community (as opposed to driving to the State Capitol).

Organizations that represent a community can also invite legislators to meet with them. Often, during and after the legislative session, community groups and organizations will schedule meetings with groups of legislators to outline their legislative priorities or express their concerns about specific legislation that is being considered or that has just passed. Since these organizations are representative of the communities they serve, this is a great way to get the community's message to the policymaker. In this way, a community that may be 200 or 300 miles away from the State Capitol can still have their voices heard in the State Capitol. These organizations can also help community members who want to engage themselves through advocacy education or help familiarize community members with the process.

7 Emphasizing Advocacy in Nursing Education

Nurses have a unique ability to advocate for their personal community as well as their patient population. Despite this, many nurses do not participate in public policy discussions. This presents an opportunity for nursing education programs to introduce advocacy into their nursing curriculum. I recently had the opportunity to teach a course for DNP students that emphasized health policy. As a part of the requirements for the course, students were asked to identify their elected officials, identify a policy issue important to them, and advocate for that policy to their elected officials. During our first meeting of the course, I realized that many of the students in the course had never looked up their elected officials

at each level of government. Additionally, I discovered that many students were not aware of which level of government was responsible for specific policies. For example, Medicare is a federal-level program, and advocacy involving Medicare would be directed toward congress people and U.S. senators, while Medicaid is a state-level program, where advocacy would be directed toward a state representative, state senator, or the governor. As a final project for the course, students were required to fully immerse themselves in the public policy advocacy space by advocating for a specific policy. Students were required to identify which elected official would be responsible for the policy they were advocating for; meet with the elected official and present a one-pager of information about the policy, and then reflect on their experience. At the end of the semester, many students expressed that this was their first time doing anything of this sort. Some students found the assignment difficult (as the process was so new to them), while other students worked with a local nursing organization to continue their work after the class had ended. Overall, as the instructor of the course, I saw tremendous value in students learning how to engage, and as an elected official, I saw why it was important for my colleagues who do not have nursing backgrounds to hear from these students.

Reference

1. Krakow MM, et al. Comparing mediational pathways for narrative- and argument-based messages: believability, counterarguing, and emotional reaction. Human Commun Res. 2018;44(3):299–321. https://doi.org/10.1093/hcr/hqy002.

Jasmine Clark PhD, was at the Nell Hodgson Woodruff School of Nursing at Emory University from 2014 to 2024 and is now currently working as an Assistant Teaching Professor at the Emory College of Arts and Science Biology Department. In addition to her work at Emory, she also serves as the GA State Representative for GA's House District 108, which is located in Gwinnett County, GA, and covers parts of Lilburn, Lawrenceville, and Stone Mountain. She was first elected in 2018 and is currently serving a third biennial term (2023–2024).

A Community-First Technology Model to Help Ameliorate Social Determinants of Health

Hope Haynes Bussenius and Rose Hayes

This chapter describes an integrated, community-first technology model that nurses can leverage in their practice, research, and policy work. The 2TEAM2GO® Model stands for the Transformative Technology Evaluation Assessment Model.[1] The 2TEAM2GO® Model can help to ameliorate social determinants of health (SDOH) by facilitating the development and implementation of community-centered, technology-enabled health solutions. To be "community- or communities-centered" means honoring the priorities of local stakeholder groups as guiding strategic priorities; it means continually engaging with stakeholder groups throughout the technology implementation lifecycle.

This paper contextualizes the 2TEAM2GO® Model by describing nurses' role in the evolving health technology landscape. Nurses are uniquely positioned to earn stakeholder trust and collaboratively implement health technology solutions [1–4]. We describe the features of the 2TEAM2GO® Model and its flexible and scalable approach to healthcare innovation. As part of this discussion, we highlight two use cases developed within the 2TEAM2GO® Model: the Pedia BP® (Pediatric Blood Pressure) and OH-I-CAN® (Oral Health in Communities and Neighborhoods) applications. These apps illustrate how 2TEAM2GO® can inform and enable the implementation of community-first health solutions. We share the story of the development, testing, and implementation of the apps, as well as their limitations and future possibilities. We conclude with a discussion on the responsible use of health technologies in community settings.

1 Background and Context

The healthcare landscape is evolving rapidly, with new technologies emerging globally, hour-by-hour, designed to increase the speed, ease, and accessibility of healthcare services [5]. Healthcare providers immersed in daily clinical realities often cannot keep pace with transformative technologies—and everyday people often cannot afford or access technology solutions either. Incredible health resources are becoming available to help reduce gaps in care, but many people and communities do not benefit from those resources due to social, financial, logistical, and other barriers to technology access [5, 6]. In this way, access to technology can both contribute to and function as a social determinant of health.

For instance, at a basic level, 22.3% of people living in rural areas and 27.7% of people living

---

[1] The "2GO" refers to the fact that it builds upon the previous 2TEAM model, with an expanded emphasis on "on-the-go" and app-based solutions for community health settings.

H. H. Bussenius (✉) · R. Hayes
Nell Hodgson Woodruff School of Nursing, Emory University, Atlanta, GA, USA
e-mail: hhaynes@emory.edu;
rose.kathleen.hayes@emory.edu

J. B. Hamilton, C. E. Moore (eds.), *Transforming Social Determinants to Promote Global Health*,
https://doi.org/10.1007/978-3-031-61160-5_32

on tribal lands do not have access to broadband Internet [7, 8]. Residents of rural areas are less likely than residents of urban areas to own a smartphone, tablet, or computer as well [9, 10]. These factors limit access to care coordination, on-demand nursing services, and virtual clinic visits [11, 12]. Technological limitations can interfere with the ability to search for health answers on Google or look up local health resources. Not having a cell phone/service can pose a barrier to calling emergency services (9-11) or the National Suicide Prevention Lifeline (9-88) when needed. Geographic isolation—combined with communication barriers—can keep people experiencing violence, abuse, or human trafficking from accessing information and help, to name some impacts of technological barriers to care [13, 14].

Even as access to technologies like broadband is limited in certain US communities, remarkable technologies are becoming available in others [9, 10, 15]. Pocket-sized EKG monitors can give people with certain cardiac syndromes peace of mind at home, instead of at the emergency room (ER) [16]. Smart inhalers can monitor lung health for people with asthma [17]. Smart contact lenses can track blood sugar levels and eye health for people with diabetes [18–20]. Pregnant people can perform pocket-sized ultrasounds on their own [21]. While app-based services are often low-cost or free (except for introductory app and product fees), their in-hospital equivalents can be invasive, time-consuming, and exponentially more expensive [22, 23].

The implementations of such technologies tend to take place through the lens of marketing science and mass distribution—advertising to people with enough income to purchase products. Meanwhile, models for implementing health system technologies tend to focus on changes at the institution or system level. Too often, the importance of translating and disseminating breakthroughs with/among stakeholders, such as clinicians, patients, and communities, goes overlooked [24, 25].

Even as clinicians who entered practice 3-5 years ago may be unfamiliar with or hesitate to adopt basic concepts in data science and technology. Certain advancements simply may not have existed when these professionals were completing their education. Studies indicate clinicians can be resistant to new technologies that are seen as adding to clinical burden, distracting from patient care, and/or lacking clinician buy-in [26]. Likewise, patients may be unfamiliar with health conditions, let alone the technologies emerging to help manage those conditions. When technology implementations fail to continuously involve stakeholders, therefore, the result is often that broad swaths of people never receive help or relief, even when it is readily available [5, 24–26].

Nurses are afforded unique levels of trust and access within communities; they are, therefore, well-positioned to help patients explore the power and potential of health technologies [27]. Given the holistic, person-centered approach of nursing care, nurses can work with people to create tailored solutions to technological challenges. Likewise, nurse leaders can advocate for technology and data-informed solutions in their roles on interdisciplinary care teams [28, 29]. The nursing process of "assessment, diagnosis, planning, implementation, and evaluation," aligns well with best practices in technological implementation [28, 30]. Like the nursing process, models for healthcare innovation (such as agile or design thinking) tend to emphasize continuous improvement [31, 32]. Such models often involve similar steps as the nursing process, even if they use different verbiage. The following section provides an overview of the 2TEAM2GO® Model and how it can assist nurses in their development of community-centered technology solutions.

2 The 2TEAM2GO® Model Addresses SDOH

The 2TEAM2GO® Model is an integrated, community-first approach to technology implementation. It is integrated in that it does not only consider the development of technology, but its translation, dissemination, and adoption by different stakeholders, at different levels of scale. It is also integrated in that it emphasizes the importance of creating educational assets to help facilitate technical adoption, such as web and video resources. Furthermore, it considers the strategic use of population health data, not only for clinical research purposes, but also for public health and policy reform efforts.

This model is different from other technology implementation models for important reasons. Not only is it nurse-led, but it positions each local community as the foundation, or "bridge," that informs, connects, and benefits from every phase of the technology lifecycle. Figure 1 offers an

illustration of the 2TEAM2GO® "bridge." As a result of this community-first approach, the same technology might exist differently (i.e., carry different cultural significance, clinical applications, policy implications, etc.) in each new location. Other technology models often include stakeholder engagement at the start of the technology lifecycle; however, many such models reapply the same stakeholder insights, over and over, in different locations as the project scales up. In contrast, 2TEAM2GO® involves working with local community members and leaders on a continual basis. Project teams take a fluid and flexible approach, assessing each new community's needs, and reconsidering their approach in each new location.

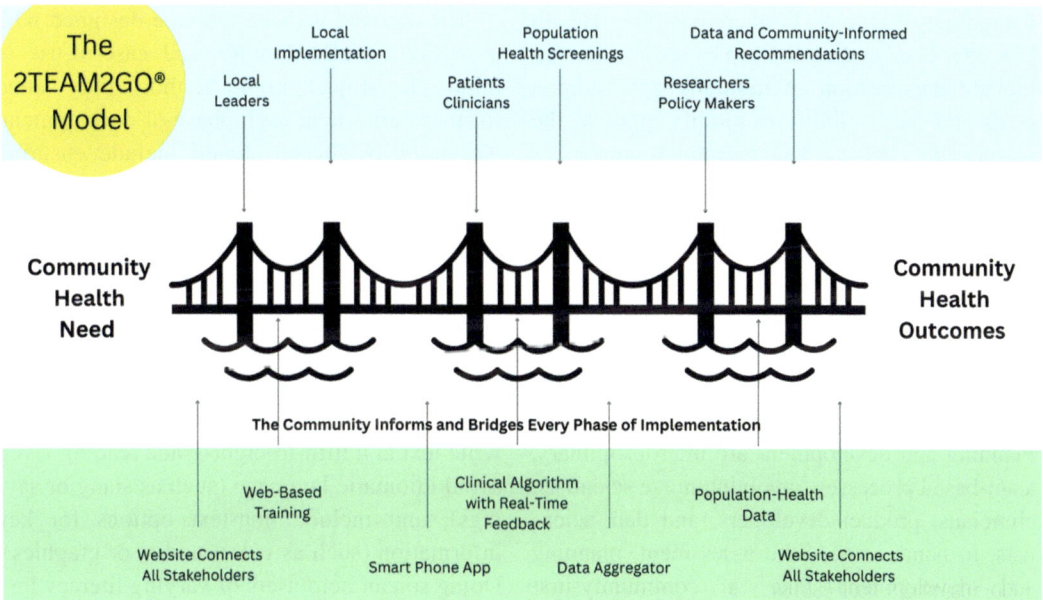

Fig. 1 Above is a depiction of the 2TEAM2GO® Model. The figure should be read from left to right. The process starts with a community health need. People and stakeholders (pictured above the bridge) are supported by different technology components (pictured below the bridge) in their efforts to improve community health. For instance, local leaders (which might include local clinician-leaders, depending on the project) complete web-based trainings to create local implementation plans; the smartphone app helps clinicians to screen patients; a clinical algorithm provides real-time feedback that streamlines and enables effective population-health screenings, etc. The community itself informs and "bridges" each phase of the implementation process. The process leads to improved community health outcomes when project teams and communities "get to the other side"

2.1   Assessment

The 2TEAM2GO® Model starts with assessment. The nurse leads an interdisciplinary project team in partnering with a community to understand its barriers to health surrounding a particular issue or condition. Typically, within the 2TEAM2GO® Model, the condition of focus is one that is often overlooked or incorrectly treated within the community. The reason for this approach is a recognition of technology's capacity to reduce care and knowledge gaps surrounding such conditions. The project team and local stakeholders work together to assess community needs and brainstorm technology-based solutions that might help to improve health outcomes. Discussions follow the Guiding Principles for Partnership, developed by the Community-Campus Partnerships for Health [33, 34]. The Guiding Principles for Partnership include the creation of mutually agreed-upon goals and the flexibility to modify goals as the partnership evolves. The principles emphasize resource sharing, mutual capacity building, and continuous feedback. The full list of guiding principles can be found at cpphealth.org.

2.2   Planning and Development

Next comes product planning and development. Planning and development are interdisciplinary, team-based processes, involving nurse scientists, clinicians, product developers, and data scientists, to name some. Like assessment, planning and development take a community-first approach, with local input and buy-in at every step [35]. Projects should ideally have a community advisory board with members who review and approve each iteration of the product or project. Products, such as health applications, should undergo formal testing by clinicians, community members, and people with lived experience, as well. Testing should include pilot testing (where users try the app in the real world and provide feedback) and focus group testing (where a group of users try the app in a controlled setting and then discuss their experience with group leaders).

Users should be offered opportunities for both open dialogue and anonymous feedback after each iteration [36, 37].

Typically, a 2TEAM2GO® project includes at least the following components: (1) a mobile application with an accompanying website for educational purposes and (2) a data aggregator to help download and organize app data for use in research and policy matters. (A data aggregator is a type of tool or mechanism that helps to automatically compile and organize data [38].) These elements are integrated with one another so that end-users can have a streamlined and comprehensive user experience, regardless of whether they begin their user journey via app, web, or data aggregator. Rationales for the use of mobile app and web-based tools are discussed under the Sect. 3.

The app and website must be designed with accessibility, affordability, and ease-of-use in mind. The project should be thoroughly vetted for these criteria at each phase of development. Accessibility checks should include ensuring that text size, font, images, and screen reader compatibility are in compliance with the Americans with Disabilities Act [39, 40]. The US Department of Justice and Civil Rights explains what these checks mean in practical terms and provides information on how to implement them at https://www.ada.gov/resources/web-guidance/. The team should write text at a fifth-to-eight-grade reading level, avoid idiomatic language (such as slang or sayings), and include non-text options for key information (such as video, audio, or graphics). Doing so can help users of varying literacy levels and people who speak English as a second language to access the technology. Microsoft Word can tell the reading level of text, typically under the "Grammar" tab.

2.3   Launch and Implementation

Once the product reaches an iteration that test users can endorse, launch and implementation can begin. Ideally, the launch would be a "soft launch," where the product is implemented at specific clinical sites on a trial basis. Clinicians and patients would continue to provide feedback, and the product would be further refined, before its implementation is scaled up to include additional locations [41]. With each iteration, implementation can expand, eventually growing from the local to state or regional level (or beyond) as the team's capacity for growth allows.

Key to a successful implementation is the provision of on-demand technical support. Such support could be offered via email, phone, an online ticket system, and/or site visits [42]. Users must have access to teaching and learning materials to support product adoption as well. These materials can include demonstration and tutorial videos, infographics, explainer text, and/or on-demand webinars. Materials should respect multiple learning styles (auditory, visual, tactile, etc.) and be available in locally appropriate languages [42]. They should account for the fact that, depending on the context/audience, not all end-users may know how to read or open/use multi-media.

In pilot projects, educational materials have included training modules for nursing and medical students, available through project websites. In fact, a unique aspect of the 2TEAM2GO® Model is that project implementations are led in large part by local clinician leaders. Clinicians, including nursing and medical students, typically complete learning exercises through the project website. They then propose locally appropriate implementation strategies and work with the project team to pilot test those strategies.

Products developed under the 2TEAM2GO® model, such as health apps, often collect screening results for large numbers of people. Thus, app data can be valuable to policymakers and public health professionals. By connecting the apps to a data aggregator, the development team can provide decision-makers with near- or real-time insights into the health of local populations. The type of data aggregator an app may require will vary, depending on the size and scope of the project [38, 43]. It can be as simple as creating a form for the application to automatically upload research data to a living Excel sheet on the researcher's computer. As projects grow and more advanced aggregation is needed, a nurse informatician or data scientist can help the team to adopt an appropriate cloud-based data aggregator [38, 44].

A member of the team, ideally a data scientist, would be tasked with managing app data and creating data governance standards in collaboration with stakeholders. Data governance standards must include compliance with all relevant laws and regulations, including the Health Insurance Portability and Accountability Act (HIPAA) [45]. App security and privacy, the de-identification of data, data storage and organization, and rules for data sharing are other data governance issues that must be considered [46].

2.4 Evaluation and Refinement

Evaluation and refinement are central to the 2TEAM2GO® Model. Mechanisms for patient and clinician feedback should be built into each touchpoint with communities. For instance, whenever a technical support call/visit is completed, people should be offered an opportunity to provide anonymous feedback. Formal evaluation work, such as surveys and user interviews, should be completed at agreed-upon benchmark moments as well, such as at 3, 6, and 12 months after implementation.

As with educational materials, feedback mechanisms should be accessible and inclusive, with opportunities to use visual and numeric scales, as well as free-text or spoken responses. Health outcomes data should be combined with user feedback to determine not only how satisfied people are with the application but whether it is measurably impacting their well-being. In addition to app evaluation, the project team should measure the effectiveness of translation and dissemination efforts, such as through assessments of provider and/or patient knowledge.

The team should not only create sharable evaluation reports but also present and discuss their findings at routine strategic meetings. Evaluation meetings should include team leads and key stakeholders, such as representatives from the local community. Each stakeholder group should have opportunities to share evaluation insights, discuss challenges, and contribute to strategies for the next phase of the project.

3 Why Use App and Web-Based Solutions?

If access to basic technologies like the Internet can, arguably, function as a social determinant of health, why create health tools that require access to the Internet, cellphone, and/or computer?

First, it is incumbent upon the project team to build mechanisms into their project and/or acquire funding for the sustainable development of technology infrastructure. In this way, project teams not only stand to impact the issue/condition of focus, but also broader health disparities related to technological barriers to care. In addition, there are several ways in which mobile applications can help to reduce barriers to care—even when there is an up-front investment of time, funds, and/or resources to establish access to the technology. These benefits include:

- **Cost-effectiveness:** The costs of using a mobile app for telehealth tend to be scant in comparison with in-person healthcare service costs. App-based solutions also allow people to avoid the transportation costs and lost wages associated with traveling for in-person care [47]. In the 2TEAM2GO® Model, costs are not passed on to end-users. Instead, project teams rely on mechanisms such as grant funding or sponsorships to support app costs.
- **Accessibility:** Mobile applications can allow patients to coordinate care, use telehealth services, and access health records from anywhere, including rural locations. Apps can offer multiple modes of learning (written, image, interactive, game, etc.) and a user-directed experience, which can solve the often-abrupt sessions they would otherwise have for learning/asking questions in clinical settings [47].
- **Streamlined communication:** Mobile applications can facilitate instant and open communication between patients and providers.

Patient questions do not have to happen within regular business hours, and they are not subject to scheduling delays. App users can share real-time health data, messages, photos, and videos. Remote data sharing allows clinicians to track and alert patients to health risks before people may even realize they are in danger [47, 48].

- **Personal health feedback:** Mobile applications allow patients to track and monitor their health and well-being. Apps can offer insight into subtle health indicators, such as measures of sleep hygiene, and they can show how health indicators relate to other factors (like blood pressure or mood) to reveal cause-and-effect patterns. People can see how their habits impact their well-being and make more informed health decisions [47].

4 Demonstrated Use Cases

Two smartphone applications have been developed within the 2TEAM2GO® Model: Pedia BP® and OH-I-CAN® [49, 50]. Both applications are aimed at increasing community knowledge and access to care. Pedia BP®, which refers to pediatric blood pressure, accurately and efficiently screens for blood pressure conditions in children and teens. OH-I-CAN®, which stands for Oral Health in Communities and Neighborhoods, helps users screen for oral health conditions. In both cases, an app-based approach to screening provides instant results which, in turn, can offer peace of mind and/or next steps for diagnosis and care [49, 50]. One of the authors of this paper served as principal investigator for both applications. The following subsections describe the Pedia BP® and OH-I-CAN® projects in more detail.

4.1 Pedia BP

4.1.1 Overview

Pedia BP is a clinical support tool designed to help clinicians accurately screen for pediatric blood pressure conditions in community settings.

Clinicians download the mobile application, which includes a diagnostic calculator, to their smartphone. When working with a patient, they enter answers to screening criteria (such as weight, height, and age), along with the patient's manual blood pressure reading. The calculator uses an algorithm—formulated based on clinical screening guidelines—to immediately offer an interpretation and recommendation of the pediatric blood pressure measurement [49, 51].

The app is accompanied by educational materials for different stakeholder groups, available on the project's website. Stakeholder groups include children, parents, teachers, and clinicians. In addition, the app continuously uploads anonymous screening data to an Excel-based data aggregator. The team makes aggregator data available, by request, to researchers and policymakers, offering population-level insights into a key indicator of children's health in their communities [49, 51].

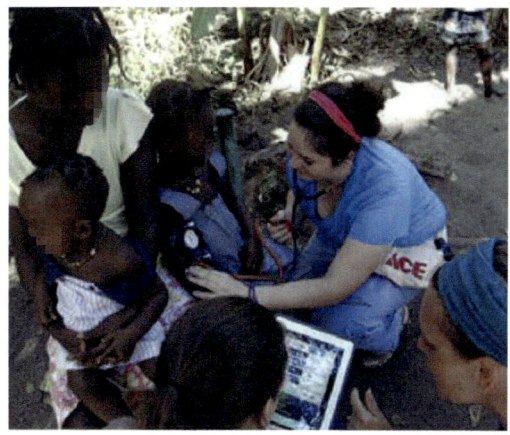

Fig. 2 A mother holds her two children at an Emory Nursing mobile clinic in Haiti. Nursing students work with the mother and children to complete the children's blood pressure readings. One student gathers the readings while speaking with the children and answering questions. The other student enters the readings and other relevant data into the application. Their instructor (pictured in the lower right corner) oversees their work [49]

4.1.2 Launch and Implementation

The Pedia BP® application was initially launched at the local level in South Georgia, USA. It was incorporated into the Family Farmworker Health Program, which provides no-cost healthcare to farmworkers and their families/loved ones in pop-up and community locations in South Georgia [25]. In addition, it was used by the Sheltering Arms Educare Center—an innovative, research-based early learning center—as part of the Georgia Head Start Program. Today, it is available in communities globally, with more than 80,000 users across 50 states and 45 countries. It is being leveraged by patients and clinicians in Turkey, India, Vietnam, Argentina, Brazil, Canada, Ecuador, Netherlands, South Africa, Ethiopia, Spain, and Denmark, to name some.

The project team was able to scale the use of Pedia BP® to the global level thanks in large part to the uniqueness and flexibility of the 2TEAM2GO® implementation model. Namely, before launching the app in any location, nursing, medical, and dental students undergo an orientation program as part of the take2heart initiative [49]. They visit the website associated with Pedia BP®, download the Pedia BP® app, and complete online modules. The students then perform a community assessment to identify culturally appropriate strategies to encourage local adoption of the application. Students, clinicians, and the project team work together with community stakeholders to test and refine the app's implementation in the local context [49]. Figure 2 shows the app in use by nursing students and their instructor at an Emory Nursing mobile clinic in Haiti.

4.1.3 Limitations

The Pedia BP application is continuously evolving. Early iterations of the project have been limited by factors including the app's adherence to the verbiage and parameters of national screening guidelines. Specifically, early versions of the app followed the 2005 and 2017 versions of the American Academy of Pediatrics *Clinical Practice Guidelines for the Screening and Management of High Blood Pressure in Children and Adolescents* [49, 52]. While it is important to adhere to national screening guidelines from a quality-of-care standpoint, the guidelines themselves do not entirely align with certain research practices that the 2TEAM2GO Model encourages.

For instance, the guidelines offer a binary selection for data capture surrounding gender identity (male versus female), as opposed to a spectrum of gender options. They also offer limited race selection categories, such as "African American" only, which does not reflect/is not the same as Black, Afro-Caribbean, Caribbean, and/or Creole identities [53–57]. As another example, the guidelines use the phrase "Hispanic or Latino," which can be limiting in terms of both race and gender inclusivity, depending on local and cultural contexts. Furthermore, the guidelines are based on a systematic search and review for which no exclusion criteria according to clinical setting or the diversity and inclusivity of research practices are named [53–57]. When the guidelines describe differences in blood pressure outcomes according to race, they only mention that risk for hypertension is associated with race. They do not provide essential context or discuss contributing factors. Contributing factors include social determinants of health,[2] structural forms of racism and discrimination,[3] and the chronic stress of interpersonal forms of racism,[4] to name some. Other widely accepted pediatric screening guidelines, such as that offered by the US Preventive Services Task Force (USPSTF) carry similar limitations [58].

The discrepancy between the SDOH-grounded mission of our team and the limitations of national clinical screening guidelines has emerged as an area of strong interest among Pedia BP® teams. The app's Board of Directors is currently planning design thinking workshops to help iterate the next version of the app and website. The workshops will involve a broad array of stakeholders, including community members, researchers, and clinicians. These exercises will focus on ensuring the next iteration is clinically correct, inclusive, and accessible all at once.

The team is discussing updates for optimized accessibility across the website and application. These include systematic checks to confirm all verbiage is clear and complies with ADA standards (as described under the Sect. 2.2). The Board of Directors and project teams are discussing the possibility of offering an automatic/smart-connected blood pressure screening option, in addition to the manual reading/entry option. While manual readings are cheaper and do not require additional technology, smart-connected readings tend to reduce human error. By allowing the app to accommodate both manual and smart-connected readings, it can ensure that the most locally appropriate option is used in each location.

4.1.4   Discussion and Key Take-Aways

By implementing each phase of the Pedia BP project in a locally specific way, the project team can promote alignment among patients, families/caregivers, healthcare providers, students, researchers, and local leaders [49, 51]. They can ensure that the application is not only available in different locations, but that it is accepted, understood, and effectively used. The website, online curricula, audience-specific toolkits, and on-site support are all tactics used to promote access to Pedia BP® [49].

In clinical settings, Pedia BP® has increased the accuracy of blood pressure diagnoses and decreased the time to interpret blood pressure results in children and teens [25]. By saving clinical time, the app can reduce clinical costs; by facilitating blood pressure interpretations, the app can improve the precision of children's care plans. Pedia BP® has been shown to measurably improve awareness of the importance of blood pressure among patients and families/caregivers. Furthermore, the use of Pedia BP® in clinical settings over the past decade suggests there may be a threshold at which body mass index (BMI) starts to influence blood pressure category guidelines and vice versa [59].

In communities, the app has prompted conversations about the importance of assessing children's blood pressure at least once a year. Ideally, annual checks would happen before school starts,

---

[2] I.e., social and environmental factors that put certain groups at increased risk for harm or illness compared to others.

[3] I.e., healthcare processes or systems that favor certain groups more than others based on race, gender, age, income, sexual orientation, or other factors.

[4] I.e., the known trauma and secondary health effects of experiencing racism firsthand.

as part of annual back-to-school forms. When 45th District Congressperson Renee Unterman held office in Georgia, the Pedia BP team provided data and information to support her writing and introduction of a pediatric blood pressure bill. The bill would have required all vital signs to be required on the Georgia Department of Public Health's back-to-school physical examination form (Form 3300). Doing so would have meant every child attending a Georgia school could receive at least one annual blood pressure reading [51]. Because high blood pressure can be an early indicator of several other serious childhood illnesses, including diabetes, this simple measure stood to positively impact numerous childhood health outcomes. Unterman was not reelected in 2021, which has delayed this bill from being considered for a formal vote into law. The Pedia BP team is working to gather and analyze data to reintroduce the bill with current Georgia legislators.

4.2 OH-I-CAN®: Oral Health Screening Tool

4.2.1 Overview

The OH-I-CAN® project is like Pedia BP® in that it is an app-based clinical support tool designed to aid clinicians in community settings. Its focus is on oral health conditions that often go overlooked or untreated due to local barriers to dental care [50]. Specifically, the OH-I-CAN® app combines responses to the Oral Health Impact Profile 14 (OHIP–14), a validated oral health screening questionnaire, with patient images that get uploaded to the app via a camera feature. The clinician works with the person to complete the questionnaire and takes five photos of their mouth [50]. See Figs. 3, 4, 5, and 6 for a screenshot of the in-app photo feature and sample images for upload to the app.

Next, the images are shared and reviewed in real-time, via the app, by a remote team of ear,

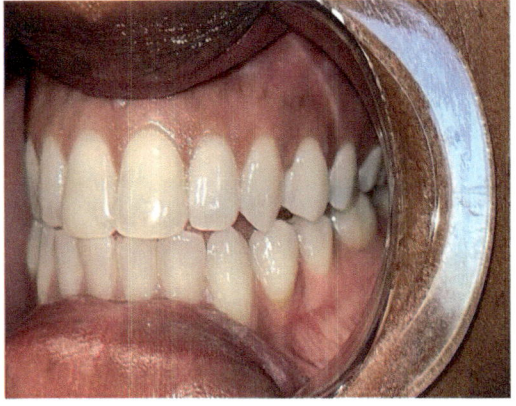

Fig. 3 Photo of a person's oral cavity, taken using the OH-I-CAN® app

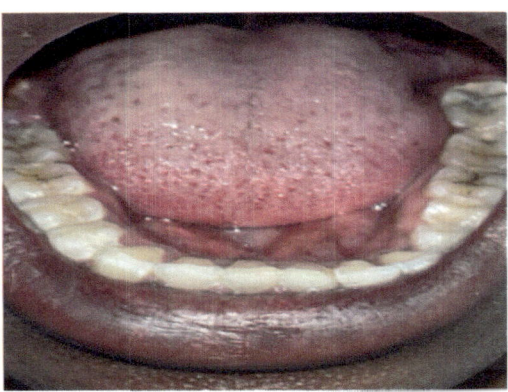

Fig. 4 Photo of a person's oral cavity, taken using the OH-I-CAN® app

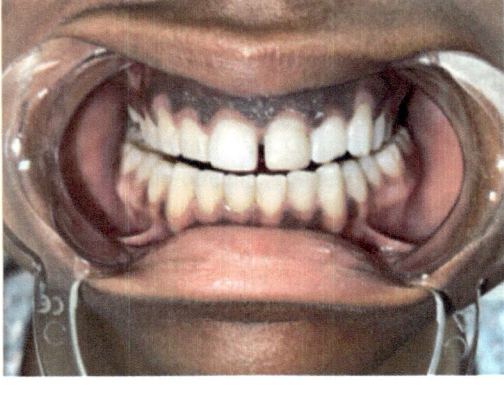

Fig. 5 Photo of a person's oral cavity, taken using the OH-I-CAN® app

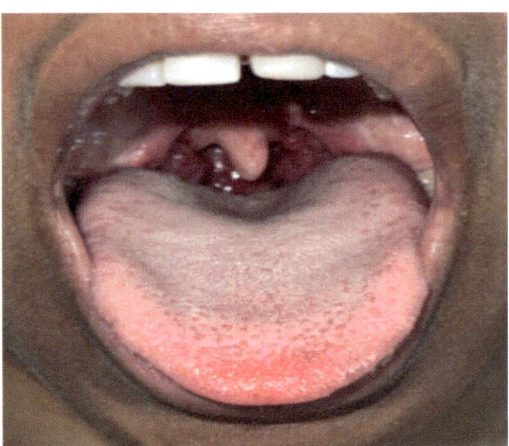

Fig. 6 Photo of a person's oral cavity, taken using the OH-I-CAN® app

nose, and throat (ENT) specialists and dentists. Based on this medical-dental integration review—and the consideration of local factors such as proximity to dental resources—a diagnosis and care plan are offered. The on-site clinician facilitating this process works with the patient to discuss and personalize the care plan further. Patients are not billed for any services provided through the application. Both the photos and responses are kept anonymous and uploaded to a password-protected data aggregator for secondary use by researchers and policymakers [48].

4.2.2 Launch and Implementation

OH-I-CAN® has been tested and implemented in community settings across the state of Georgia. Test sites have included Federally Qualified Health Centers (FQHCs), school-based programs, the Georgia Department of Public Health, clinics for pregnant people and older adults, and nursing, medical, and dental residency programs, to name some. Today it has more than 30,000 users across the state [50].

The OH-I-CAN® team has focused on Georgia for its early iterations because of the state's unique barriers to equitable oral health. As of December 2009, Georgia ranked number 39 out of 50 states for access to dental health services [60]. Among the providers that do practice in the state, many do not accept patients without dental insurance. As a result, dental issues often go

undiagnosed and untreated until discovered by non-dental clinicians during unrelated health services.

Untreated oral health conditions are emblematic of broader health disparities that impact underserved[5] Georgia communities. Oral health can serve as a proxy measure for disparities in several leading causes of morbidity and mortality. Dental plaques contribute to atherosclerosis, which is part of the underlying pathology for conditions like heart disease, stroke, and certain dementias. Untreated dental infections and/or abscesses can lead to infections in the heart. Furthermore, untreated conditions can contribute to preterm birth, diabetes, chronic pain, rheumatoid arthritis, lung infections, intestinal cancer, and mouth cancer [52, 61].

Oral cancer is the eighth leading cause of death in Georgia [62]. The prevalence of oral cancers is concentrated among older adults in Northwest Atlanta, with a median age of 62 years at diagnosis [62]. Several factors converge to increase the risk of mouth cancer within this community: normal changes of aging, the presence of multiple chronic conditions, structural and interpersonal racism, lack of available providers, un- and under-insurance, to name some [62].

The OH-I-CAN application takes an important step toward addressing some of these factors. It provides access to dental health professionals, even if none are locally available—without rendering any personal costs [50, 62]. This is significant because dental diagnostic processes can carry costs and logistical complications. Eliminating costs and steps can help to advance people in the process of accessing and ultimately

---

[5]"Underserved" refers to any geographic area, population, or facility with healthcare needs that exceed the capacity of available healthcare resources or personnel. There are both a great number and great variety of such areas and populations across the US. These include rural, suburban, and urban communities with a spectrum of sociodemographic compositions whose needs for primary care, mental health, and dental services are not being properly met. The Health Resources and Services Administration provides descriptions and examples of many sites captured by the federal "Health Professional Shortage Area" designation list.

receiving dental care. At the very least, the clinician liaising between the patient and the app team can make appropriate referrals for no- or low-cost dental services. The application meets people and communities "where they are" by recognizing that many dental diagnoses in Georgia do not take place in dental offices. It helps non-dental care providers to facilitate correct diagnoses, even if such care falls outside their typical scope of practice [50, 62].

4.2.3 Limitations

Like with Pedia BP®, the OH-I-CAN® app is limited by its reliance on existing screening guidelines. The OHIP-14 Oral Health Impact Profile that informs the app's questions utilizes verbiage that is inconsistent with 2TEAM2GO® practices. This discrepancy has been an ongoing point of discussion among the OH-I-CAN® team. Like the Pedia BP® team, this group is also in the process of holding design thinking workshops to reiterate the application in a way that upholds clinical correctness while accurately representing the experiences of communities.

Another limitation is the fact that the tool only helps to diagnose oral health conditions; it does not offer remote-connected dental care. The OH-I-CAN® team accounts for this to the best of their ability by connecting patients and clinicians with appropriate resources. Partnerships with local providers are multidirectional in that the OH-I-CAN® team both provides knowledge and resources—and receives knowledge and resources in return—from local clinicians. When local clinicians offer system work-arounds or care solutions that would be relevant in other care settings, the OH-I-CAN® team disseminates the information across its network of clinical partners.

Like the Pedia BP® team, the OH-I-CAN® team is engaged in a systematic evaluation for adherence to accessibility best practices. It has taken strides in this regard by offering a Faces Scale to accompany text and/or verbal responses to the oral health questionnaire. The "faces" (emojis) in the scale currently appear in one ethnically ambiguous skin tone, but future iterations will include a broader array of skin tones.

4.2.4 Discussion and Key Take-Aways

The OH-I-CAN® app has been instrumental in revealing oral health disparities at the population level. Those insights have helped to support key policy reforms. App data was written into the Dental Hygiene General Supervision for Preventive Care Bill that passed into law on January 1, 2018. House Bill 154/AP authorizes dental hygienists to perform expanded functions, under general supervision by a dentist, in certain settings [63]. The app team continues to advocate for the ability of advanced practice registered nurses (APRN) to perform certain oral health procedures that could help to close care coverage gaps in many Georgia communities [50, 62].

The OH-I-CAN® aggregator will be made available to support the goals and objectives of Healthy People 2030 [64]. Roll-out efforts for the next app version are slated to include oral health education and the incorporation of development milestone goals into routine pregnancy and early childhood care. Future steps will emphasize head and neck cancer prevention protocols in state outreach programs, clinical settings, and medical and nursing classrooms as well.

5 Conclusion

When it comes to the use of technology in community-centered work, implementation can be thought of as a continuous, shared learning exercise. Nursing students are taught the concept of cultural humility, or the idea that one's understanding of people and communities is never complete—there is always room for self-reflection, and learning is a lifelong endeavor. This is especially true for nurse technologists, who are not only tasked with providing culturally humble care—but with helping communities to benefit from emerging health technologies. This work is nuanced and ever-evolving. There is always room to learn. There are always improvements that can be made to a project or product.

Even technologies needing improvement often play an essential role in connecting people with health services. The 2TEAM2GO® Model, in particular, encourages nurse technologists to focus on areas of community health that are often overlooked. Multidirectional partnerships can ensure these conditions are addressed from the individual to local and state level (and beyond).

At the individual level, app-based technologies can provide a simple, time-efficient way to diagnose health needs and create a care plan. At the population level, the ability to quickly analyze data can help to reveal patterns in care. In this fashion, gaps and trends can be identified. Interventions can be implemented to improve health outcomes, and those interventions can be tracked for further evaluation. With insights into population-level outcomes, community health wins can be tracked, encouraged, and celebrated.

References

1. Brenan M. Nurses retain top ethics rating in U.S., but below 2020 high. Gallup.com. 2023. https://news.gallup.com/poll/467804/nurses-retain-top-ethics-rating-below-2020-high.aspx.
2. Buerhaus P, Hayes R. Leveraging nursing strengths, listening to nursing needs: a keynote paper from the 2022 Emory University business case for nursing summit. Nurs Outlook. 2023;72:101993. https://doi.org/10.1016/j.outlook.2023.101993.
3. Dameron S. A leap of faith: navigating health care innovation with intuition and open-mindedness. Innovation site. 2023. https://www.nursingworld.org/practice-policy/innovation/blog/a-leap-of-faith-navigating-health-care-innovation-with-intuition-and-open-mindedness/.
4. Giuliano K. Nurse-engineer teams: creating the next generation of health care innovation leaders. American Nurses Association Innovation Enterprise; 2023. https://www.nursingworld.org/practice-policy/innovation/blog/nurse-engineer-teams-creating-the-next-generation-of-health-care-innovation-leaders/.
5. National Academies of Sciences, Engineering, and Medicine (NASEM). The future of nursing 2020–2030: charting a path to achieve health equity. 2021. pp. 100–470. https://doi.org/10.17226/25982.
6. Yao R, Zhang W, Evans R, Cao G, Rui T, Shen L. Inequities in health care services caused by the adoption of digital health technologies: scoping review. J Med Internet Res. 2022;24(3):e34144. https://doi.org/10.2196/34144.
7. Lee NT, Makada Henry-Nickie RS, Bartik TJ, Mark Muro JJ, Adie Tomer CG. Why the federal government needs to step up efforts to close the rural broadband divide. Brookings; 2022. http://www.brookings.edu/research/why-the-federal-government-needs-to-step-up-their-efforts-to-close-the-rural-broadband-.
8. US Department of Agriculture (USDA). E-connectivity for all rural Americans is a modern-day necessity. USDA.gov. 2023. https://owl.purdue.edu/owl/research_and_citation/apa_style/apa_formatting_and_style_guide/reference_list_electronic_sources.html.
9. Carlson E, Goss J. The state of the urban/rural digital divide. National Telecommunications and Information Administration; 2020. https://www.ntia.gov/blog/2016/state-urbanrural-digital-divide#:~:text=Overall%2C%20we%20found%20rural%20users,45%20percent%20to%2054%20percent.
10. Vogels EA. Some digital divides persist between rural, urban, and suburban America. Pew Research Center; 2021. https://www.pewresearch.org/short-reads/2021/08/19/some-digital-divides-persist-between-rural-urban-and-suburban-america/
11. Hirko KA, Kerver JM, Ford S, Szafranski C, Beckett J, Kitchen C, Wendling AL. Telehealth in response to the COVID-19 pandemic: implications for rural health disparities. J Am Med Inform Assoc. 2020;27(11):1816–8. https://doi.org/10.1093/jamia/ocaa156.
12. Siek C, Sheon A, Ancker J, Castek J, Callahan B, Siefer A. Digital inclusion as a social determinant of health. Npj Digital Med. 2021, March;4(52):2021. https://doi.org/10.1038/s41746-021-00413-8.
13. Emezue C. Digital or digitally delivered responses to domestic and intimate partner violence during covid-19. JMIR Public Health Surveill. 2020;6(3):e19831. https://doi.org/10.2196/19831.
14. Pesando LM. Safer if connected? Mobile technology and intimate partner violence. Demography. 2022;59(2):653–84. https://doi.org/10.1215/00703370-9774978.
15. Federal Communications Commission. 2020 broadband deployment report. 2020. https://www.fcc.gov/reports-research/reports/broadband-progress-reports/2020-broadband-deployment-report.
16. Kardia. KardiaMobile. 2023. https://store.kardia.com/products/kardiamobile.
17. Zabczyk and Blakely. The effect of connected "Smart" inhalers on medication adherence. Frontiers in Medical Technology 3. 2021; https://doi.org/10.3389/fmedt.2021.657321.
18. ACS. Recent advances in smart contact lenses. American Chemical Society; 2022. https://www.acs.org/pressroom/newsreleases/2022/october/recent-advances-in-smart-contact-lenses.html.
19. Adams HS. Top 10 wearable healthcare devices. Healthcare Digital. 2023. https://healthcare-digital.com/digital-healthcare/top-10-wearable-healthcare-devices.
20. Medilynxsite. MediLynx chosen to participate in NIH study of efficacy of mobile cardiac monitoring

for patients. MediLynx; 2022. https://medilynx.com/news-nih/.

21. GE Healthcare. Vscan, GE Healthcare's newest pocket-sized visualization tool for point-of-care imaging, to support physicians providing medical care for athletes, visitors and trainers at Vancouver 2010 Olympic Winter Games competitions. GE Newsroom; 2010. https://www.gehealthcare.com/about/newsroom/press-releases/vscan-ge-healthcares-newest-pocket-sized-visualization-tool-point-care-imaging-0.

22. Min Wu P, Luo J. Wearable technology applications in healthcare: a literature review. HIMSS; 2021. https://www.himss.org/resources/wearable-technology-applications-healthcare-literature-review.

23. Singh K. You could be wearing the best thing for your health. International Association for Human Resources Information Management; 2023. https://www.ihrim.org/2023/06/you-could-be-wearing-the-best-thing-for-your-health-how-the-inclusion-of-wearable-devices-in-health-plans-could-help-reduce-healthcare-costs/

24. AHQR. Innovative methods in stakeholder engagement: an environmental scan. Agency for Healthcare Quality and Research; 2012. https://effectivehealthcare.ahrq.gov/products/stakeholders-engagement-others/research-2012-1.

25. Bussenius H, Wold JL, Williams BL. Synergy of technology and healthcare: the development of a smartphone application to detect hypertension in children and adolescents. Transl Med. 2013;3(2):116. https://doi.org/10.4172/2161-1025.1000116.

26. Mansour S, Nogues S. Advantages of and barriers to crafting new technology in Healthcare organizations: a qualitative study in the COVID-19 context. Int J Environ Res Public Health. 2022;19(16):9951. https://doi.org/10.3390/ijerph19169951.

27. Crocker L, Johnson BH. Privileged presence: personal stories of connections in health care. Law Bulletin Publishing Company; 2014.

28. Booth RG, Strudwick G, McBride S, O'Connor S, Solano López AL. How the nursing profession should adapt for a digital future. BMJ. 2021; https://doi.org/10.1136/bmj.n1190.

29. Fernandez, Corbie-Smith G, editors. Leading community-based changes in the culture of health in the US—experiences in developing the team and impacting the community. IntechOpen; 2021. https://www.intechopen.com/books/8794.

30. Toney-Butler T, Thayer J. Nursing process. Statpearls: NCBI Bookshelf; 2023. https://www.ncbi.nlm.nih.gov/books/NBK499937/.

31. Coursera. What is agile? And when to use it. 2023. https://www.coursera.org/articles/what-is-agile-a-beginners-guide.

32. Han E. What is design thinking and why is it important? Harvard Business; 2022. https://online.hbs.edu/blog/post/what-is-design-thinking

33. CCPH Board of Directors. Principles of partnership. Community-Campus Partnerships for Health; 2013. https://ccphealth.org/partnering/principles-of-partnering/.

34. Richmond A. Community-campus partnerships for health. Position statement on authentic partnerships. 2019. https://www.ccphealth.org/principles-of-partnership/. Accessed 25 July 2019.

35. Barclay G, Sabina A, Graham G. Population health and technology: placing people first. Am J Public Health. 2014;104(12):2246–7. https://doi.org/10.2105/ajph.2014.302334.

36. Drexel University. Focus groups: a tool for program development and evaluation. Center for Hunger Free Communities; 2015. https://drexel.edu/hunger-free-center/research/briefs-and-reports/focus-groups/

37. Hassan ZA, Schattner P, Mazza D. Doing a pilot study: why is it essential? Malays Family Phys. 2006;1(2–3):70–3.

38. ScienceDirect. Data aggregator: an overview. ScienceDirect Topics; 2013. https://www.sciencedirect.com/topics/computer-science/data-aggregator

39. UNC Greensboro. Why web accessibility is important. Accessibility Resources at UNCG; 2019. https://accessibility.uncg.edu/why-web-accessibility-is-important/.

40. Web Accessibility Initiative (WAI). Introduction to web accessibility. WAI; 2022. https://www.w3.org/WAI/fundamentals/accessibility-intro/.

41. Kothe P. (Host). How to successfully introduce your new product with a soft launch [Audio podcast]. Mastering Medical Device. 2023. https://www.masteringmedicaldevice.com/episodes/soft-launch.

42. MacDonald S. Tech support. why It's crucial to the overall user experience. 2021. https://www.superoffice.com/blog/tech-support/.

43. Sliwa J. Reuse of data from smart medical devices for quality control and evidence-based medicine. In: Pervasive computing. Morgan Kaufmann/Elsevier; 2016. p. 255–97. https://doi.org/10.1016/b978-0-12-803663-1.00009-7.

44. Wheeler A, Winburn M. Application data in the cloud. Cloud Storage Security. 2015:23–55. https://doi.org/10.1016/b978-0-12-802930-5.00002-2.

45. CDC. Health Insurance Portability and Accountability Act of 1996 (HIPAA). Centers for Disease Control and Prevention; 2022. https://www.cdc.gov/phlp/publications/topic/hipaa.html.

46. Dinh-Le C, Chuang R, Chokshi S, Mann D. Wearable health technology and electronic health record integration: scoping review and future directions. JMIR Mhealth Uhealth. 2019;7(9):e12861. https://doi.org/10.2196/12861.

47. Gajarawala SN, Pelkowski JN. Telehealth benefits and barriers. J Nurse Pract. 2021;17(2):218–21. https://doi.org/10.1016/j.nurpra.2020.09.013.

48. Bussenius H. Oral health in communities and neighborhoods. 2022. https://ohican.org/.
49. Bussenius H, Batisky DL, Wold JL, Chalmers S, Williams BL. Pedia BP program: addressing pediatric blood pressure readings using a smartphone application. J Nurse Pract. 2015;11(7):726–9. https://doi.org/10.1016/j.nurpra.2015.04.011.
50. Oral Healthcare in Communities and Neighborhoods Program. Home. OH-I-CAN; 2018. https://ohican.org/.
51. Bussenius H, Zeck AM, Williams B, Haynes-Ferere A. Surveillance of pediatric hypertension using smartphone technology. J Pediatr Health Care. 2018;32(5):e98. https://doi.org/10.1016/j.pedhc.2018.04.003.
52. Bussenius H, Reznik D, Moore C. Building a culture of Oral health care. J Nurse Pract. 2017;13(9):623–7. https://doi.org/10.1016/j.nurpra.2017.07.019.
53. Deutsch MB, Green J, Keatley J, Mayer G, Hastings J, Hall AM, Deutsch MB, Keatley J, Green J, Allison R, Blumer O, Brown S, Cody MK, Fennie K, Hall AM, Hastings J, Mayer GS, Moscoe G, St Claire R, et al. Electronic medical records and the transgender patient: recommendations from the World Professional Association for Transgender Health EMR Working Group. J Am Med Inform Assoc. 2013;20(4):700–3. https://doi.org/10.1136/amiajnl-2012-001472.
54. Kronk CA, Everhart AR, Ashley F, Thompson HM, Schall TE, Goetz TG, Hiatt L, Derrick Z, Queen R, Ram A, Guthman EM, Danforth OM, Lett E, Potter E, Sun SD, Marshall Z, Karnoski R. Transgender data collection in the electronic health record: current concepts and issues. J Am Med Inform Assoc. 2021;29(2):271–84. https://doi.org/10.1093/jamia/ocab136.
55. Nerenz DR, Ulmer C, McFadden B. Race, ethnicity, and language data: standardization for health care quality improvement. National Academies Press; 2009. p. 1–12.
56. Patel K, Lyon ME, Luu HS. Providing inclusive care for transgender patients: capturing sex and gender in the electronic medical record. J Appl Lab Med. 2020;6(1):210–8. https://doi.org/10.1093/jalm/jfaa214.
57. Vega Perez RD, Hayden L, Mesa J, Bickell N, Abner P, Richardson LD, Ngai KM. Improving patient race and ethnicity data capture to address health disparities: a case study from a large urban health system. Cureus. 2022;14(1):e20973. https://doi.org/10.7759/cureus.20973.
58. Flynn JT, Kaelber DC, Baker-Smith CM, Blowey D, Carroll AE, Daniels SR, de Ferranti SD, Dionne JM, Falkner B, Flinn SK, Gidding SS, Goodwin C, Leu MG, Powers ME, Rea C, Samuels J, Simasek M, Thaker VV, Urbina EM. Clinical practice guideline for screening and management of high blood pressure in children and adolescents. Pediatrics. 2017;140(3):e20171904. https://doi.org/10.1542/peds.2017-1904.
59. Bussenius H, Zauche LH. BMI and pediatric hypertension categories. J Nurse Pract. 2021;17(3):299–304. https://doi.org/10.1016/j.nurpra.2020.10.014.
60. Kabore HJ, Smith C, Bernal J, Parker D, Csukas S, Chapple-McGruder T. The burden of oral health in Georgia. Georgia Department of Public Health, Maternal and Child Health, Office of MCH Epidemiology, Georgia Oral Health Program; 2014.
61. Moore CE, Reznik D, Conboy L, Giwa J, Aslam F, Bussenius H, Aidman C, Warren RC. Achieving equity in oral health: a data-driven approach for informing policy changes. J Commun Med Health Educ. 2017;7(2):1–4. https://doi.org/10.4172/2161-0711.1000511.
62. Moore CE, Bussenius H, Reznik D. Oral Health in communities and neighborhoods (OH-I-CAN) pilot project: the burden of poor oral health 2021. https://doi.org/10.5772/intechopen.98456.
63. Cooper S, Hatchett M, Abrams SY, Hawkins L, Henson M. 17 HB 136/AP house Bill 136 (as passed House and Senate)—legis.ga.gov. n.d. https://www.legis.ga.gov/api/legislation/document/20172018/170633.
64. Office of Disease Prevention and Health Promotion (OASH), U.S. Department of Health and Human Services. Healthy People 2030. Oral conditions. 2023. https://health.gov/healthypeople/objectives-and-data/browse-objectives/oral-conditions.

Hope Haynes Bussenius DNP, APRN, FNP-BC, FAANP, FAAN, is an Associate Clinical Professor at the Nell Hodgson Woodruff School of Nursing at Emory University and a tribal member of the Lumbee Tribe of North Carolina. She received her Bachelor of Science in Nursing from the Medical College of Georgia in 1990, her Masters in Nursing from Emory University in 1993, and completed her Doctor of Nursing Practice at Georgia Health Sciences University in 2012. Dr. Bussenius specializes in developing a technology model called the Transformative Technology Evaluation and Assessment Model (2TEAM) and is one of the first nurses to developed an award winning smartphone application with repository, Pedia BP®, and started a non-profit organization, Take2Heart Initiative® for pediatric hypertension, which to date has more than 80,000 downloads in 45 countries.

Rose Hayes RN, BSN, MA, is a nurse and writer. She currently serves as Director of Engagement for Emory Nell Hodgson Woodruff School of Nursing. Hayes uses storytelling and analytics to share nursing knowledge in a way that people will remember and use. Central to her work is the mentorship of students, faculty, and peers in effective storytelling techniques.

Reenvisioning the Social Determinants of Health to Reimagine Population Health Interventions

Catherine M. Waters and Stephanie M. Strozier

The route to achieving equity will not be accomplished through treating everyone equally. It will be achieved by treating everyone justly according to their circumstances.
—Paula Dressel, Race Matters Institute

Reenvisioning the social determinants of health (SDOH) to reimagine population health interventions seems utopian, banal, and a retread of past and extant discourse. We recognize there is not a simple solution or one intervention that addresses population health and its social determinants because people and their socioecological conditions are not monolithic. Rethinking, however, about this dynamic and complex issue and its many nidi can facilitate our understanding of how to move diverse populations along an ever-shifting health continuum toward a healthier society: a nonzero-sum society in which people can achieve their maximum potential for physical, psychological, biological, social, and spiritual health and well-being in a conducive environment, through individual and collective actions.

When people envision the SDOH, they think first of economic and social factors, such as education, income, employment, housing, social networks, and community safety. However, along with the social and economic SDOH, the environmental and lifestyle health behavior SDOH account for 80% of the modifiable variance in health outcomes [1]. Thirty percent of this modifiable or preventable variance is attributable to lifestyle health behaviors, which are strongly correlated with the prevention of chronic diseases, such as cardiovascular disease, type 2 diabetes mellitus, and cancer [2]. Chronic diseases can affect a person's and a population's individual and shared quality of life, activities of daily living, and longevity, respectively.

Sixty percent of adults in the United States have a chronic disease, and Black/African American adults are affected disproportionately by chronic diseases and its risks and sequela of comorbidities [3]. In this chapter, we share our research and experiences collaborating with Black/African American communities, using community-based participatory action research, to promote healthful lifestyle behaviors for the primary prevention of chronic diseases. Specifically, we discuss the Nutrition and Fitness for Life (NuFIT) project, a community-engaged Afrocentric cancer prevention intervention that promoted a physically active lifestyle and healthful nutrition, created and optimized community conditions for the population to engage in healthful behaviors by leveraging the resources of public and private partnerships, enhanced population- and community-level resilience, and

C. M. Waters (✉) · S. M. Strozier
Department of Community Health Systems, School of Nursing, University of California, San Francisco, San Francisco, CA, USA
e-mail: catherine.waters@ucsf.edu;
stephanie.strozier@ucsf.edu

demonstrated sustainability by the community through consortium empowerment and action. NuFIT is an example of our reimagining population health interventions to promote lifestyle health behaviors as a reenvisioning of a dimension of the SDOH to prevent chronic disease development.

1   Contextual Lens

The SDOH or a person's circumstances are shaped by the distribution of power and resources. Health equity and health equality are two interconnected yet opposing concepts that aim to provide fair opportunities for individuals, populations, and communities to achieve optimal health through the impartial distribution of sociopolitical power and healthcare resources [4]. Equity recognizes that individuals have different starting points, which can lead to advantages or disadvantages in all aspects of people's lives, depending on the antecedents, precedents, and consequences of their circumstances or determinants. In principle, health inequities should be preventable, whereas some health inequalities are not preventable because of inheritable differences or presumed volition and control regarding a person's choices.

Equality, unlike equity, is based on fairness and equal opportunity for every person, regardless of a person's starting point [4]. Equality assumes a homogeneous society and a homogeneous environment where individuals, populations, and communities are presumed to have similar circumstances, experiences, outcomes, and access to and utilization of the same resources. We, however, are diverse and unique people from different backgrounds, with different capabilities, needs, reserves, and types and levels of support. While the notion of allocating resources evenly may seem equitable and magnanimous, it can perpetuate the inability to meet people where they are. Furthermore, it can perpetuate the inability to address systemic and structural advantages and disadvantages associated with a population's social determinants or the circumstances that people experience over their life course, often resulting in a cycle of injudicious blame-placing, marginalization, vulnerability, and health disparities.

Cooperative partnerships that promote population health and sustain healthy communities, with an explicit social change or health equity intent, are a guiding principle of community-based or community-engaged participatory action research [5]. The model that underpinned the NuFIT project is an adaptation of the community-based participatory research model [5, 6]. In our adaptation (see Fig. 1), we retain the four domains of the community-based participatory research model: contexts, partnership processes, interventions and research, and outcomes. Additionally, we presume that a community-engaged process that is enhanced by a culturally relevant "village" approach and the resources of public-private partnerships impacts population and community resilience, particularly for communities with strained, low-resourced, or not readily accessible healthcare delivery systems. An egalitarian, community-engaged multisectoral approach can be a bridge to a gap in healthcare or to the ending of a research project, public health program, or demonstration project that is limited in scope, time, and funding.

As educators, scholars, and practitioners working in the public health nursing sphere, the NuFIT intervention was also guided by the principles of public health nursing: population-focused; equity-based; primary prevention; creation of conditions in which populations thrive; collaborations with others; outreach to all who might benefit, not only to those who access and utilize services; optimal use of resources; and evidence-based strategies that enhance the health of the population [7]. Nurses need to reenvision strategies that are comprehensive and encompass both health equality and health equity; advocate for and support social and public health policies; and help to create optimum conditions by reimagining population health interventions that meet people where they are, not solely where we want them to be or how resilient we think they should be [8]. Sometimes, personal responsibility is not enough, and it "takes a village" to solve community health issues and protect community assets through community activism [9].

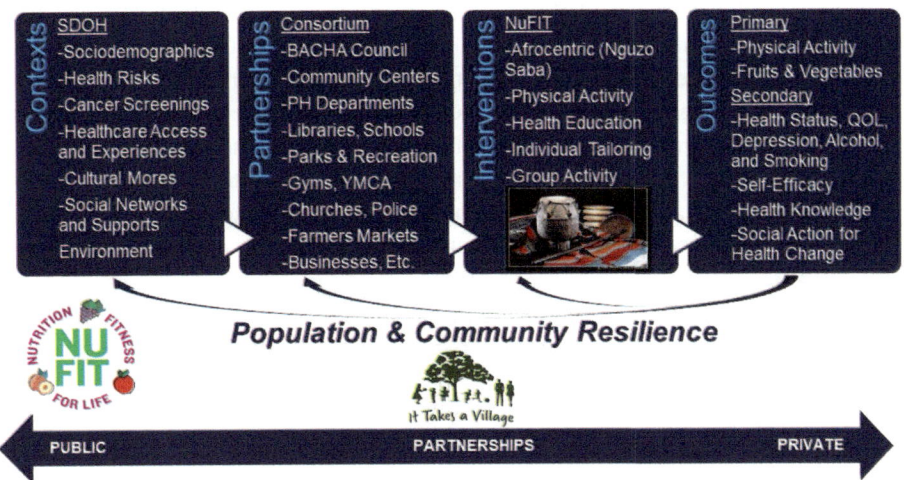

Note. The model that underpinned the NuFIT project is an adaptation of the Community Based

Participatory Research model (Oetzel et al., 2018; Wallerstein et al., 2019;

https://hsc.unm.edu/population-health/research-centers/center-participatory-research/cbpr-

community-engagement/cbpr-model.html).

Fig. 1 NuFIT community-engaged intervention model. *Note.* The model that underpinned the NuFIT project is an adaptation of the community-based participatory research model ([5, 6]; https://hsc.unm.edu/population-health/research-centers/center-participatory-research/cbpr-community-engagement/cbpr-model.html)

2   NuFIT: Nutrition and Fitness for Life Project

The NuFIT project, grounded in sociocultural, socioecological, health equity, and public health nursing perspectives, utilized multiprong approaches and multiple levels of community engagement to promote an active lifestyle and healthful nutrition in Black/African American adults (see Fig. 1). Eating nutritiously and being physically active have been associated with decreased risks for developing certain cancers, many of which are disproportionately represented in the Black/African American population [3, 10].

Funded by the American Cancer Society (RSGT-04-257-01 CPPB), the primary aim of the 5-year NuFIT randomized, controlled community trial was to test the efficacy of an Afrocentric cancer prevention intervention on changes in lifestyle health behaviors, specifically physical activity and dietary fruit and vegetable intake, in a community sample of two groups of Black/African American adults from baseline to 3 months: (a) NuFIT intervention group and (2) delayed NuFIT intervention control group. To promote social justice and access equity in the pursuit and advancement of science and upon recommendation by the community consortium, described later in this chapter, we chose to use a delayed intervention control group instead of a traditional control group to ensure that all control group participants had an opportunity to receive the NuFIT intervention after the 3-month trial period ended. We believe this to be an ethical and morally responsible way to conduct community-based participatory action research. To ensure that participants understood what a research trial is, the community consortium developed a one-page list of frequently asked questions and answers that were vetted and were in response to the community's concerns regarding historical incidents of research misconduct in the Black/African American population.

2.1 NuFIT Team

Consistent with the principles of community-based participatory or community-engaged action research, community representatives were actively engaged in the NuFIT project from conceptualization to dissemination. The multidisciplinary team consisted of the primary author as the project's university partner principal investigator, who specializes in community/public health nursing and has a clinical background in oncology nursing; a university partner coinvestigator, also with a background in community/public health nursing; a community partner coinvestigator, who served additionally as the cancer and cultural nurse consultant; a university partner project director; a university partner community outreach coordinator; a university partner certified fitness trainer; a university partner exercise physiologist consultant; a community partner nutritionist; a community partner health educator; a community partner psychologist; and numerous university graduate student and community partner research assistants.

In recognition of the importance and value of everyone's conceptual contributions, time and effort, all team members were budgeted and paid, including student and community partner research assistants. Too often in the past, community-based participatory research and practice initiatives involved community partners who were considered unpaid volunteers, who should feel privileged to work with university and public health department partners because we were helping their populations and communities. These pseudo-collaborative research and practice initiatives were conducted *on* a population *in* a community, but not *with* the population. The interventions were often designed without the input of the population and without consideration of the SDOH or conditions under which people thrive. Moreover, these partnerships often lacked a common agenda and vision and a foundation of rapport and trust. Yet, *our* uninformed interventions will affect the health of *their* citizenry.

2.2 Community Consortium

Collaborating with a community consortium ensured that the NuFIT project focused on population health issues of local relevance and that the design of the NuFIT intervention and its implementation was reimagined by the population and utilized existing community resources (see Fig. 1). The Bay Area Community Health Advisory Council is the primary author's long-standing community research partner. The Council is comprised of grassroots secular and non-secular stakeholders that work from a health justice perspective with multisectoral entities to create a village united around eliminating health disparities through innovative models of health education and services across the generations and diverse communities [11]. Several NuFIT team members are members of the Council. Along with the Council, the NuFIT community consortium also included other private and public partners: senior and child development centers, public health departments, community clinics, private health practices, public libraries, public schools, parks and recreation facilities, private gyms, YMCA organizations, ecumenical churches, police departments, farmers markets, grocery stores, the small business community, and other stakeholders that operated in and provided services in their communities.

The community consortium created conditions for its residents to live a more physically active and nutritive lifestyle by bolstering their communities' existing built and social environments, SDOH that contribute to 10% of the variance in health outcomes [1]. Some communities reported that the barriers to engaging in regular, leisure-time physical activity and eating healthier are the lack of free or low-cost recreational facilities; community safety related to crime rates; not seeing people being physically active in the community because of the lack of sidewalks, bicycle paths, or interesting things to look at while engaging in exercise; no grocery store in the neighborhood; no transit stop within 10–15 min near home; and unsafe street intersections in the neighborhood. In response to these barriers, the community consortium, for example, worked with the local police departments to provide a police officer to accompany the NuFIT walking groups. The YMCA, private gyms, and parks and recreation programs offered use of their facilities for the NuFIT participants to exercise, and they provided physical space to conduct other NuFIT intervention and research activities, such as classrooms for the health education sessions and kitchens for the cooking demonstrations. Thus, participants did not have to travel outside their communities to engage in healthful lifestyle behaviors.

A businesswoman in one community owned a dance studio. She opened her dance studio to the NuFIT project for exercise classes, and every Saturday, she hosted a farmers market for the NuFIT participants and other community residents. These are a few examples of reimagining population health interventions by reenvisioning the SDOH through community consortium empowerment and action. Moreover, these examples demonstrate that the activities could be sustained by the community upon completion of the NuFIT project at no or low cost to its residents. An additional benefit of these private-public partnerships to the NuFIT project was increased adherence, which minimized participant attrition—an often unavoidable limitation of prospective research studies. To demonstrate reciprocity and goodwill, we hired people from the community, and when possible, we donated the exercise and cooking equipment to the various community organizations upon completion of the NuFIT project.

2.3 The Population and Their Communities

The Black/African American population was the focus of the NuFIT project. Sociodemographic characteristics can provide some context for understanding the starting points of people's lives: the antecedents, precedents, and consequences of their circumstances or SDOH. We presume in our model that individuals are shaped by their backgrounds, experiences, and social networks and relationships (contexts), which impact their health and social outcomes (see Fig. 1). Most participants were middle-aged, on average 45 years old, with a range from 20 to 78 years; were women; were single, not married or partnered; had completed high school or a higher level of education; were employed full-time; and reported a median annual income of $55,000 or higher. The average annual income in the United States is $59,428, and in California, the average annual income is $73,220 [12], indicating an income disparity in this critical SDOH for this Black/African American adult population. As discussed in the community consortium section of this chapter, providing free or low-cost access to recreational facilities and nutrient-rich foods was important to addressing the participants' socioeconomic circumstances.

At the start of the NuFIT project, this Black/African American population was relatively healthy, with some cancer-related health risks: 11% of the participants smoked cigarettes; 41% of them drank alcohol; only 6% of the participants ate the recommended five servings per day of fruits and vegetables; and most participants were sedentary. Tobacco use, excessive alcohol consumption, being sedentary, and low consumption of fruits and vegetables are considered independent, preventable risks for certain cancers [3, 10]. Health behavior-, sedentary-, and diet-related diseases are among the leading causes of death in the United States. Most participants scored low on health knowledge, reported low self-efficacy or confidence to change lifestyle health behaviors, perceived their health to be good or very good, reported fair to good quality of life, did not report depressive symptomatology, had health insurance, engaged in age- and sex-appropriate cancer screenings, described themselves as spiritual, had someone they can depend on, and reported at least one perceived discriminatory healthcare experience.

Most participants lived in single-family residences throughout the Bay Area, which is an urban geographical region in Northern California. The population resided in eight cities in three counties: San Francisco County (city of San Francisco), Alameda County (city of Oakland), and San Mateo County (cities of Daly City, San Mateo, Redwood City, Menlo Park, East Palo Alto, and Livermore). Most recruitment and outreach efforts were concentrated in the city of Oakland, CA. As compared to the other Bay Area cities, Oakland has a larger proportion of the Black/African American population [13]. In addition, these geographical areas were where the community consortium provided services and operated their businesses.

2.4   NuFIT Intervention and Outcomes

The nidus of the community-designed NuFIT intervention was Nguzo Saba, which is a set of Afrocentric ideals based on seven principles: unity (Umoja), self-determination (Kujichagulia), collective work and responsibility (Ujima), cooperative economics (Ujamaa), purpose (Nia), creativity (Kuumba), and faith (Imani) (see Fig. 1). The seven principles are the core of Kwaanza or "first fruits" in Swahili; it is a celebration of family, community, culture, and social justice. Kwaanza was inspired and introduced into the Black/African American culture in 1966 by Maulana Karenga during the civil rights movement in the United States [14]. Despite criticisms about Kwaanza and its creator, we used the seven principles to inspire and guide the NuFIT intervention and to influence the collaborative way we worked with participants, community partners, and each other as a team, with the aim of moving the Black/African American population toward a healthier lifestyle in the context of their everyday

lives. With good health, people can aspire the "pursuit of happiness," a basic idea of the US Declaration of Independence [15].

The 3-month NuFIT intervention consisted of two main components: (a) 1-h group physical activity sessions and 30-min individual physical activity counseling that occurred during weeks 1 through 12 and (b) 1-h group health education and counseling sessions that occurred during weeks 1 through 6. The group sessions were held in the evening, beginning at 6:00 PM with the group health education and counseling session for 1 h, followed by the group physical activity session for 1 h during the first 6 weeks of the NuFIT intervention. For the second 6 weeks, only the 1-h group physical activity sessions were held, and those sessions began at 6:00 PM. Every group session began with a discussion about one of the seven principles of Nguzo Saba and its meaning to the participants' health and general well-being, using a participative group process where participants shared their successes and challenges during the week. Participants could bring their children with them. Paid certified childcare assistants and the university partner community outreach coordinator were onsite to watch and play with the children and to help them with their homework, if needed. Nutritious snacks were also available. Parents were asked if their children had food allergies.

The group health education and counseling sessions were comprised of six modules that focused on promoting healthful lifestyle behaviors: (a) healthful lifestyle choices, (b) cancer prevention, (c) physical activity, (d) weight control, (e) proper nutrition, and (f) cooking demonstration. Each module was facilitated by a NuFIT team member. The community partner health educator and the community partner psychologist were the coleads for the healthful lifestyle choices module. The community partner coinvestigator, also the cancer and cultural consultant, facilitated the cancer prevention module. The university partner certified fitness trainer facilitated the physical activity and weight control modules. The community partner nutritionist facilitated the proper nutrition and cooking demonstration modules. For the cooking demonstrations, the nutritionist asked participants to list their favorite meals. The nutritionist modified the recipes for their favorite meals, teaching the participants how to substitute unhealthful ingredients with more healthful and nutritive ingredients that did not significantly alter the taste of their favorite foods. This approach increased the likelihood that the participants would sustain their health behavioral changes. Upon completion of the NuFIT project, a compilation of these community-inspired recipes was made available to the participants to share with their communities. The nutritionist also showed the participants how to read and interpret the labeling on food products.

The 30-min individual physical activity counseling occurred weekly. During this session, each participant met individually with the community partner certified fitness trainer. Each participant set physical activity goals and reviewed weekly with the fitness trainer the attainment of their goals, discussing their successes and rewards and a plan of action to address their challenges in the following week. In addition to aiding with goal-setting and problem-solving, the fitness trainer provided skills training and demonstration, feedback, and support and encouragement as strategies to increase the self-efficacy or confidence of each participant to engage in regular leisure-time physical activity. The fitness trainer also took into consideration a participant's age and physical functioning level to help tailor a participant's physical activity regimen. For example, if someone used a cane, the fitness trainer designed a plan that included modified exercises that also incorporated the cane, if the participant desired.

While the US federal guidelines for physical activity were used as a metric for research purposes, each person's goal was their metric for their individual physical activity outcome. No comparison was made to the other participants or the federal guidelines during the weekly sessions. The community consortium believed that a better metric would be to pick a percent by which to improve. Instead of setting a goal of 10,000 steps/day or 30 min/day of exercise, a better metric would be, for example, a 5% increase in the number of steps or amount of time engaged in physical activity from the previous week. For the

individual sessions, the fitness trainer met the participant at a mutually agreed upon location, usually the person's residence, a community park, a location in the neighborhood, or at one of the community consortium's sites.

By the end of the 3 months, the NuFIT intervention group participants showed significant increases in the two primary health outcomes: physical activity and dietary intake of fruits and vegetables (see Fig. 1). Consumption of five servings per day of fruits and vegetables increased from 6% to 20% of the population. Participants increased the time they spent walking from 32 to 75 min/day. The median minutes per day that participants were engaged in moderate-intensity physical activity increased from 3 to 42 min. For vigorous-intensity physical activity, the median minutes per day increased from 4 to 31 min. There was no significant change in health status, quality of life, depression, cigarette smoking, or drinking alcohol. Health knowledge and self-efficacy or confidence to change lifestyle health behaviors did increase significantly. During months 4 through 12 of the NuFIT project, participants could choose to attend ongoing group physical activity and health education sessions, which served as a booster to sustain their health behavior changes after their participation in the 3-month NuFIT intervention ended.

3   Celebrations, Lessons Learned, and Forging Onward

Guided by the foundations of community-engaged or community-based participatory action research, health equity, public health nursing, sociocultural mores, and sociological perspectives, a community-designed and reimagined intervention, such as the NuFIT Afrocentric cancer prevention project, that is practical and consistent with the core values of the community and that fits within the context of people's everyday lives can result in beneficial lifestyle health behavior changes, quality of life, and physical, psychological, and spiritual health. With community-level reenvisioning of the SDOH, lifestyle health behavior changes can be sustained, along with increased population and community resilience across the generations. In the long term, hopefully, the risk for developing cancer is minimized, resulting in decreased cancer morbidity- and mortality-related health disparities in the Black/African American population. We must be careful not to assume that populations are monolithic or that a one-size-fits-all intervention, even if it is community-designed and community-driven, will work in other communities, even if the population shares and identifies with the same cultural group.

One key to achieving positive changes in the health of a population is to leverage the resources of a community consortium, comprised of public and private partnerships. The community serves as the catalyst for change. A community consortium can help to create and optimize existing social and environmental conditions in which its residents can realize their full and maximum potential for health, no matter their starting points or reoccurring starting points across their lifespan. Community consortium members understand the unique history, language, religion, social norms, and traditions of the population because they, too, are residents and live, work, play, and socialize in their communities. Furthermore, the sustainability of population-level health interventions by the community can be achieved through the empowerment and action of the community consortium. The reality is that in some communities, there are few social and healthcare safety nets, and those that exist are more illusory than functional. There, however, are not infinite community resources, even with the synergism and cooperation of public and private partnerships.

Community health initiatives, whether the initiatives are status quo, incremental, or revolutionary, take time, effort, human capital, and monetary resources. Community-capacity building is built step-by-step, moving forward, but also at times backward, and concomitantly with economic, social, political, and cultural changes that a community consortium cannot control. Public policy can play a key role to address these challenges.

For public health entities, the availability of more public funding would help not only to strengthen the social and healthcare safety nets but also provide funding to create innovative, health equity focused programs that address the social determinants of population health, which contribute the most to disease morbidity and mortality. Yet only 4.4% of the 4.3 trillion dollar healthcare expenditures in the United States are spent on local, state, and federal government public health activities [16]. For private entities, for- and nonprofit, the availability of more tax exemptions or some other type of noncontroversial financial incentive might encourage more private businesses to engage in activities related to health diplomacy, social democracy, or civic engagement. A model for creating such an incentive is the California's Benefit Program (Senate Bill 697), which requires all private and nonprofit hospitals to "assume a social obligation to provide community benefits in the public interest" in exchange for their tax-exempt status [17].

When populations and communities perceive they have good health and quality of life and are living their best lives, they are more likely to engage in public health and civic activities, such as voting, which can impact public policies about clean air and water, housing, food security, employment, access to public transport systems, education and schools, clinical and quality care, healthcare safety net funding, traffic, crime, etc. All of which have implications for population health and the structural determinants of health: macrolevel factors, such as laws and policies that shape the distribution or maldistribution of the SDOH. Structural determinants are the determinants of the SDOH and thus influence not only population health but also health equity. Public health nurses, partnering with community members who are local experts, can lead and advocate for legislative action and social policy agendas to address and reenvision both the social and structural determinants of health, demonstrating that we specialize in more than documenting problems; we also reimagine and implement solutions for improving the health of populations and communities that have global health implications.

References

1. Magnan S. Social determinants of health 101 for health care: five plus five. National Academy of Medicine's Perspectives; 2017. https://doi.org/10.31478/201710c.
2. National Center for Chronic Disease Prevention and Health Promotion. About chronic diseases. 2022. https://www.cdc.gov/chronicdisease/about/index.htm
3. National Center for Health Statistics. Health, United States, 2020–2021: annual perspective. Hyattsville, MD; 2023. https://doi.org/10.15620/cdc:122044.
4. Gomez CA, Kleinman DV, Pronk N, Wrenn Gordon GL, Ochiai E, Blakey C, Johnson A, Brewer KH. Addressing health equity and social determinants of health through healthy people 2030. J Public Health Manag Pract. 2021;27(6):S249–57. https://doi.org/10.1097/phh.0000000000001297.
5. Wallerstein N, Duran B, Oetzel JG, Minkler M, editors. Community-based participatory research for health: advancing social and health equity. 3rd ed. Jossey-Bass; 2019.
6. Oetzel JG, Wallerstein N, Duran B, Sanchez-Youngman S, Nguyen T, Woo K, Wang J, Schulz A, Kaholokula JK, Israel B, Alegria M. Impact of participatory health research: a test of the community-based participatory research model. Biomed Res Int. 2018;2018:7281405. https://doi.org/10.1155/2018/7281405.
7. American Nurses Association, editor. Public health nursing: scope and standards of practice. 3rd ed. American Nurses Association; 2022.
8. Waters CM. Commentary on "community-based approaches to strengthen cultural competence in nursing education and practice". J Transcult Nurs. 2007;18(1S):66S–7S. https://doi.org/10.1177/1043659606296129.
9. Waters CM. Public health nursing's impact on strengthening community resilience. Am J Public Health. 2022;112(S3):S224–5. https://doi.org/10.2105/AJPH.2022.306873.
10. World Cancer Research Fund/American Institute for Cancer Research. Diet, nutrition, physical activity and cancer: a global perspective. 2018. https://www.wcrf.org/wp-content/uploads/2021/02/Summary-of-Third-Expert-Report-2018.pdf.
11. Bay Area Health Advisory Coalition. Mission and vision. n.d. https://www.bachac.org/mission-visio.n
12. Wong B. Average salary by state. 2023. https://www.forbes.com/advisor/business/average-salary-by-state/#average_salary_by_state_and_occupation_section.
13. Bay Area Census. Cities and Towns. n.d. http://www.bayareacensus.ca.gov/cities/cities.htm.
14. Smithsonian's National Museum of African American History & Culture. Kwaanza First Fruits. n.d. https://nmaahc.si.edu/kwanzaa.
15. National Archives. Declaration of independence: a transcription. n.d. https://www.archives.gov/founding-docs/declaration-transcript.
16. American Medical Association. Trends in health care spending. 2023. https://www.ama-assn.org/about/research/trends-health-care-spending.
17. California's Department of Health Care Access and Information. Hospital Community Benefit Plans. n.d. https://hcai.ca.gov/data-and-reports/cost-transparency/hospital-community-benefit-plans/.

Catherine M. Waters PhD, RN, FAAN, is a Professor, the Sally Bates Endowed Chair in Community Nursing and Health Disparities, and the Associate Dean for Faculty and Academic Affairs in the School of Nursing at the University of California, San Francisco. Appointed by the mayor, Dr. Waters served as a member of the San Francisco Health Commission for 5 years, including 1 year as the Vice President of the Health Commission. Dr. Waters's community-based participatory action research focuses on lifestyle health behaviors as protective mechanisms to prevent chronic disease development, in collaboration with public-private partners and community consortiums. She also has a research interest in end-of-life care planning. Dr. Waters served as a co-editor for the *American Journal of Public Health's* supplement on public health and nursing. She teaches graduate courses on advanced public health nursing and community-based participatory research methods, and previously has taught courses on theory development in nursing, evidence-based program planning, strategic healthcare marketing, behavior theories for nursing research, and interprofessional advanced scholarship in health systems research.

Stephanie M. Strozier MSN, RN, FNP-C, PHCNS-BC, CCRN, is a PhD student in the School of Nursing at the University of California, San Francisco. She was born and raised in Atlanta, Georgia, but relocated to California in 2013 to continue her nursing journey. She earned a Bachelor of Nursing degree from Georgetown University in 2007 and obtained graduate degrees from the University of California, San Francisco, and Yale University in 2017 and 2019, respectively. She has over 15 years of critical care nursing experience.

Fostering Strategic Partnerships to Advance Access to Healthcare Among Georgia's Latino Community

Lalita M. Kaligotla, Jodie L. Guest,
Gilda (Gigi) Pedraza, Pedro Viloria,
Iliana Yamileth Rodriguez, Beth Ann Swan,
and Roxana C. Chicas

> I say this to you as the son of immigrants, knowing that many of you are also immigrants, we must view immigrants as persons - seeing their faces, listening to their stories, trying as best as we can to respond to their situation.
> —Pope Francis, Addressing the United States Joint Sessions of Congress, September 2015

1 Introduction and Overview

There has been exponential growth in the Latino population in Georgia and across much of the Southeast since the late twentieth century. Despite the critical economic and cultural contributions of this population, many Latinos face unique challenges in accessing healthcare due to factors such as cost, language barriers, and immigration status. At present several nonprofit organizations are working to mitigate challenges faced by this historically vulnerable and medically underserved group. In so doing, partnerships between these civil society organizations and universities, particularly those with educational programs in the allied health sciences, are vital. This chapter discusses two such exemplars led by Emory University to advance health equity for the Latino population in the state of Georgia. These partnerships include the collaboration between the Latino Community Fund Georgia (LCF Georgia), the Nell Hodgson Woodruff School of Nursing (NHWSN), and the Emory Farmworker Project (EFP), a robust interprofessional program that provides medical care for the migrant farmworker population in South Georgia. While the partnership between LCF Georgia and NHWSN is an emerging one, the EFP is a well-established and nationally recognized program that continues to make an impact on improving the lives of migrant farmworkers. This chapter provides an overview of these emerging and existing programs and shares best practices and lessons learned for building community coalitions to address health equity with minoritized groups in culturally informed ways.

L. M. Kaligotla · B. A. Swan · R. C. Chicas (✉)
Nell Hodgson Woodruff School of Nursing, Emory University, Atlanta, GA, USA
e-mail: Lalita.kaligotla@emory.edu; beth.ann.swan@emory.edu; rchicas@emory.edu

J. L. Guest
Rollins School of Public Health, Emory University, Atlanta, GA, USA
e-mail: jodie.guest@emory.edu

G. (G.) Pedraza · P. Viloria
Latino Community Fund Georgia, Atlanta, GA, USA
e-mail: gigi@lcfgeorgia.org; pedro@lcfgeorgia.org

I. Y. Rodriguez
The Department of History, College of Art and Sciences, Emory University, Atlanta, GA, USA
e-mail: iliana.yamileth.rodriguez@emory.edu

© The Author(s), under exclusive license to Springer Nature Switzerland AG 2024
J. B. Hamilton, C. E. Moore (eds.), *Transforming Social Determinants to Promote Global Health*,
https://doi.org/10.1007/978-3-031-61160-5_34

2   Latinos in Georgia (History and Growth)

Over the past half a century, the growth of Latinos in the state has been exponential, growing from about 30,000 in the 1970s to over one million as of 2022 constituting 10% of the population and the third largest ethnic group in the state. The establishment of the Latino population in Georgia began in the late 1950s, with small numbers of primarily Cuban and other Spanish-speaking migrants settling in the Metropolitan Atlanta region. By the 1960s and 1970s, Latino laborers migrated in larger numbers to North Georgia, to work in the poultry processing and carpet manufacturing industries, as well as South Georgia, to work primarily in the agricultural sector [1]. The Latino population in Georgia grew rapidly in the 1990s due to unprecedented job growth, partly related to the 1996 Centennial Olympic Games held in Atlanta [2]. The implementation of the H-2A visa program in this era also led to an increase in Latino agricultural workers in the southern part of the state. With new economic and legal possibilities in place, Latinos continued to fill jobs in the booming construction, service, manufacturing, processing, and agricultural industries during this decade. As the Latino population grew, so did their purchasing power. Many local businesses and institutions offering community resources began to tailor their services to the expanding Spanish-speaking population. Furthermore, Latino-owned businesses and Latino-led advocacy organizations were growing to meet the needs of this growing population by the late 1990s.

By the start of the twenty-first century, anti-immigrant rhetoric became hypervisible in Georgia, and the racialized conflation of Latinos with illegality made the population vulnerable to hostility and increased policing. Several Georgia counties implemented section 287(g) of the Immigration and Nationality Act to crack down on undocumented immigrants [3]. Section 287(g) gave local law enforcement the ability to check immigration status and hold individuals suspected of being undocumented until Immigration and Customs Enforcement (ICE) authorities took custody of them. This program adversely impacted Latino communities as even a minor traffic violation by a person without a driver's license could lead to detention and/or deportation [4]. Thus, driving to work, school, and medical appointments was a significant risk for undocumented Latinos in Georgia and mixed-status families. In 2010 undocumented students, primarily Latinos, were met with further barriers to upward mobility as the state Board of Regents implemented a ban on undocumented student admissions to top public universities in the state. Then, in 2011, Georgia House Bill 87 was signed into law to crack down on the employment of undocumented immigrants [5]. It did so by requiring employers to use the federal E-Verify system to check whether employees were eligible to work legally in the United States (USA). Additionally, the law still limits entrepreneurship as a mechanism for undocumented and under-documented communities by requiring legal status in the country before obtaining business licenses and being able to apply for any state or local contracts, effectively reducing avenues for these immigrants to pursue means of securing income for their families.

Despite these anti-immigrant efforts, Latino communities in Georgia continued to flourish and further established a powerful economic presence in the state. Today, the workforces of the manufacturing, poultry processing, and agricultural industries continue to be primarily comprised of Latino workers. Latino-owned businesses and Latino-led institutions dot the state from Dalton to Savannah to Atlanta to Tifton. Georgia is also among the top ten states in terms of the size of the Latino population [6]. At present, the largest national-origin Latino groups in Georgia are Mexicans (57%), Puerto Ricans (10%), South Americans (8%), Guatemalans (6%), and Salvadorans (5%). This diversity of Latino communities in Georgia includes first-, second-, and third-generation Latinos who speak English, Spanish, K'iche', and other languages of the Americas. In short, Latinos contribute to the state's strong and vibrant cultural diversity and social and economic well-being of Georgia.

Although Latinos in general seem to have better health outcomes than non-Hispanic whites, a phenomenon often described as the Hispanic paradox [7], Latinos across the USA and in Georgia experience several adverse social determinants of health. As mentioned previously, Latinos represent over 10% of the state's overall population and as such significantly impact the state's health statistics. However, it is also well documented that racially and ethnically minoritized groups experience health disparities and higher rates of poor health [8]. Given the minoritized status of many members of the Latino community in Georgia, they experience significant health inequities due to barriers to accessing healthcare services. Such challenges include lack of health insurance, monetary costs, language barriers, low health literacy, mistrust in the US healthcare system, and a shortage of culturally competent health providers [8]. These health inequities contribute to members of the Latino community not having regular preventative services, such as vaccinations, health screenings, and annual well-checks, or access to a primary care provider. It is important to note that the diversity of this population means that there are Latinos who are citizens or hold some form of legal status, as well as undocumented Latinos who are among the most vulnerable within the community. Undocumented Latinos and those from mixed-legal status families, therefore, have unique health access needs that must be addressed in appropriate manners. Figure 1 highlights some demographic and health statistics of Latinos in Georgia. To reduce the gap in access to healthcare services within the Latino communities in Georgia, community organizations have formed partnerships with healthcare facilities, academic institutions, public health.

Latinos in Georgia: Demographics & Social Determinants of Health

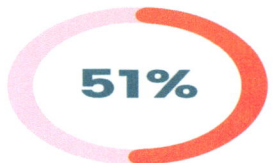

51%

51% Identify as female

- 69% are born in the US
- 69% of undocumented immigrants are Latinos
- 40% of them are foreign born
- Latinos in Georgia have lived in the US for 20 or more years.

Median Age of 26 years
Considered the youngest of all the major racial groups in Georgia

AMONG THOSE WHO SPEAK SPANISH
- 56% report speaking English "very well."
- 20% report speaking English "well."
- 17% report speaking English "not well"
- 8% report speaking English "not at all"
- 38% did not graduate high school

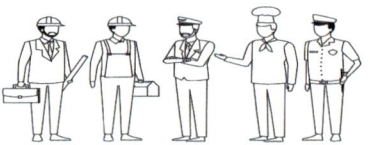

Employed Latinos: Age 16 and over

- 24% work in management, science, business, or arts
- 21% are employed in the service sector
- 14% work in sales and office work
- 22% work in natural resources, construction, or maintenance
- 20% in production, transportation, moving

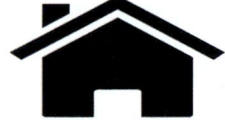

47% of Latinos in Georgia are Homeowners
10% live in overcrowded households

OVER 50% of Latinos in Georgia live in poverty or in low-income conditions

Latino Children's Health
- Infant mortality rate of 5 deaths per 1,000 live births
- Only 72% of children between the ages of 0–35 are immunized.

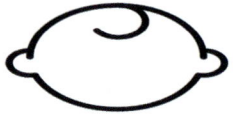

Womens Health
- 29% of Latina women report not seeing a doctor in 12+ months due to cost
- 33% reported not having a doctor or healthcare provider
- 46% of women of reproductive age lack health insurance
- Maternal mortality rate is 18 deaths per 100,000 live births

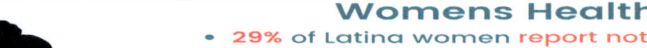

Chronic Health Conditions Among Latinos in Georgia
- 36% are obese
- 6% incidence of diabetes
- 22% incidence of hypertension
- 5% incidence of cardiovascular disease

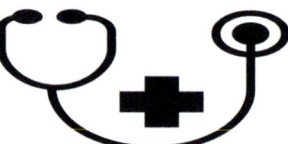

33% of Latinos in Georgia lack health insurance

SOURCES: Please see appendix A for list of sources

Fig. 1 Latinos in Georgia—Demographics and Social Determinants of Health

3   Nonprofits and Civil Society Organizations Advancing Healthcare for Latinos in Georgia

There are several civil society organizations in Georgia that are working to advance healthcare for Latinos in the state. These Latino-led organizations are dedicated to addressing the unique healthcare needs of the Latino community by expanding access to quality healthcare, providing health education, and by advocating for policy changes to positively impact health outcomes among Latinos. Some of these organizations are listed below, along with short descriptions of their mission and work.

1. **Ser Familia:** Incorporated in 2001 as an initiative providing support to couples, the organization has evolved to become the largest consistent provider of parenting, youth, and mental health services for Latinos in their five offices in Gwinnett, Cobb, and Clayton counties regardless of documentation status. Ser Familia is also a state partner on safety net programs enrollment and emergency assistance to the community Georgia.

2. **Latin American Association (LAA—https:// thelaa.org/):** The LAA offers comprehensive social services to the Latino community in Georgia. Founded in 1976 to meet the needs of translation, interpretation, and basic assistance with humble a beginnings when Stratton Frank and Angel Ortiz offered aid from the trunk of a private vehicle, the LAA began as a community service activity led by volunteers and allies to the growing Latino population. Over the decades, the organization has established itself as one of the oldest and largest providers of social service programming in the state. While they offer various programs ranging from youth education to entrepreneurial support, the LAA also organizes health fairs, offers health screenings, and assists individuals and families with obtaining and enrolling for health insurance, language interpretation services, and referrals to health clinics and healthcare providers.

3. **Georgia Association of Latino Elected Officials (GALEO—https://galeo.org/):** GALEO is a nonpartisan, nonprofit organization that is focused on increasing civic participation among Latino communities in Georgia. Founded in 2003 at a time when the community was not as well represented politically in the state, GALEO has focused on expanding and supporting Latino civic engagement and advocacy, including calls to ensure access to health services and reproductive health in the state. GALEO has also supported other local organizations during the pandemic to ensure access to food, and other services are inclusive of the Latino community through language access and cultural competency.

4. **Georgia Latino Alliance for Human Rights (GLAHR—https://glahr.org/):** While GLAHR's primary focus is on immigration and human rights issues, they recognize the importance of healthcare access for the Latino community. Established in 2001 by community activists, GLAHR focuses in particular on the needs of people living with liminal legal statuses. The organization advocates for policies that ensure affordability and access to healthcare including issues of language justice and culturally competent care. GLAHR's work has helped to illuminate the intersections between detention, deportation, and health concerns for Georgia's Latino and immigrant populations.

5. **Latino Community Fund Georgia (LCF Georgia https://lcfgeorgia.org):** Established in 2017, this nonpartisan organization has three pillars driving its work: advancing democracy, protecting, and building communities and expanding economic opportunity. Among its programs, the Health & Wellbeing Program was launched as a response to the pandemic in early 2020 and has evolved into the only free and consistent initiative in the state offering health screenings, preventive education, referrals, and other health-related services like immunizations regardless of documentation status. LCF Georgia has a dedicated staff member at the Mexican Consulate, who also provides services, on a

weekly basis, at other community locations and consulates. The organization also has a team in South Georgia currently being trained in basic health protocols and screenings. LCF Georgia works in collaboration with a number of academic and clinical partners to advance its work and build capacity in communities.

6. **Coalition of Latino Leaders (CLILA https://www.cliladalton.org):** CLILA was established in 2006 in Dalton, Georgia, as a direct service and advocacy organization in response to the lack of engagement from local elected officials. It facilitates academic support, cultural engagement, and civic participation and most recently has launched a health promoters' group providing direct mental health guidance and support to the local community.

7. **Unidos Latino Association (https://www. unidoslatinoassociation.org):** Serving Newton and Rockdale Counties, their work includes partnerships with local groups to organize health fairs to support the local community. They also work with partners across the state to expand access to mental health support to youth across various counties.

8. **Caminar Latino (https://caminarlatino. org):** A nonprofit pioneer in creating safe spaces for each family member to begin their journey toward nonviolence and by centering the Latino experience into social change efforts. They also provide legal and mental health support to participants in their programs.

9. **Feminist Women's Health Center through their Lifting Latina Voices Initiative (https://feministcenter.org):** This is the only nonprofit in Georgia providing comprehensive reproductive health education and services with a sliding scale and language access.

Each of these organizations provides a network of support to the state's Latino community and collaboratively works with each other, policymakers, healthcare institutions and providers, and other stakeholders to address the unique healthcare challenges faced by the Latino population in Georgia. Shared goals among these organizations include expanding access to health-

care services, reducing health disparities, and promoting the overall health and well-being of Latinos in the state. Among these key community organizations is the Latino Community Fund (LCF Georgia). First imagined in 2015, LCF Georgia has grown in reach and capacity over the past few years and supports Latino-led initiatives ranging from healthcare to economic development, and political mobilization. It is to the LCF Georgia and its budding partnerships that we now turn our attention to illustrate the importance of establishing partnerships between community organizations and universities following the COVID-19 pandemic.

4 Partnering to Address Health Challenges Faced by Georgia's Latino Community: The Nell Hodgson Woodruff School of Nursing (NHWSN) and the Latino Community Fund Georgia (LCF Georgia)

One such partnership between a community-based organization serving the needs of Latinos in Georgia and an academic institution is the collaboration between LCF Georgia and the NHWSN at Emory University. LCF Georgia's collaboration with NHWSN spans over 2 years and was born out of the already severe needs of the community that were further exacerbated by the COVID-19 pandemic.

Disparities and inequities in the accessibility and distribution of health services and resources are not new to the Latino community in Georgia, but the pandemic proved that in a crisis, these challenges can have very profound and even fatal consequences. LCF Georgia formally launched its Health and Wellbeing Program in 2021 to mitigate some of these challenges. After a year of coordinating distributions of personal protective equipment (PPE) and food, as well as spearheading Latino and immigrant-centric testing and vaccination initiatives, it was clear that there was a need for more work and for more organizations to advocate for health equity among Georgia's Latino communities. One of the many reasons why COVID-19 disproportionately and so adversely affected the Latino community was because, in many cases, community members suffered from other chronic illnesses, such as diabetes or heart disease, that were previously undiagnosed and/or untreated. LCF Georgia addressed this challenge by launching a health education campaign as well as advocating for increased accessibility, in-language, and in-community, to health services and resources. LCF Georgia became the fiscal sponsor for the Ventanilla de Salud (VDS) program at the Mexican Consulate in 2021. This program served as the only free health educational and preventive program that offered consistent services to the Latino community in Georgia. Through this program and coordination of Spanish-speaking vaccination and testing events in community locations, operations to provide access to healthcare for underserved members of Latino communities were established. Given their mission and focus, LCF Georgia held strengths in community organizing and outreach but needed the medical training and expertise of health professionals. LCF Georgia started their outreach to academic partners like Emory University, Morehouse School of Medicine, and Mercer University in 2020 to collaborate on providing support for COVID-19 mitigation initiatives and for health screenings, referral processes, and education programming. Early in June 2021, LCF Georgia and NHWSN began the process of working together to plan health screenings during Hispanic Heritage Month.

For Hispanic Heritage Month, NHWSN provided over 20 volunteers to support LCF Georgia in providing blood pressure and glucose screenings at three different community health fairs. In addition, Dr. Roxana Chicas hosted health education events via Facebook Live targeted toward the farmworker community on heat exposure and its adverse health effects given this group's heightened risk for heat-related illness.

The collaboration between LCF Georgia and NHWSN during Hispanic Heritage month was successful and the organizations moved forward with implementing a formal Memorandum of Understanding (MOU) in the Summer of 2023 for an ongoing community-based partnership. This MOU established LCF Georgia as a community-based practicum site for Emory nursing courses N315 Population Health: Community & Public Health Nursing and N609 Public Health Nursing Practicum. In both courses, nursing students complete between 45 and 60 practicum hours in a community-based setting focused on the application of public health principles to nursing care of the community/population of focus. During the Summer of 2023, 13 nursing students enrolled in N609 Public Health Nursing Practicum worked with LCF Georgia community health staff to provide over 600 health screenings at the Salvadoran Consulate. Working with LCF Georgia community health workers within a community-based setting allowed nursing students to gain a deeper understanding of how the social determinants of health and environmental health contribute to the health disparities of Salvadorans in Georgia. This collaboration not only provided opportunities for nursing students to apply principals of public health nursing but also allowed students to offer additional health access for members of the Latino community. As such, LCF Georgia became one of the community partners for the Health Resources and Services Administration (HRSA) grant "Toward Health Equity and Literacy: Training for Optimal RN Efficacy in Acute Care" (2HEAL) that was awarded to NHWSON. 2HEAL's goal is to increase the number of undergraduate nursing students in addressing and managing social determinants of health (SDoH) and improve health equity and health literacy for underserved populations in metropolitan Atlanta, Georgia. LCF Georgia, with its in-depth understanding of the various challenges and the SDoH that contribute to Latino health disparities, advises and informs didactic nursing curriculum to strengthen nursing students and the nursing workforce skills and readiness to provide high-quality, culturally sensitive care to address and manage SDoH both in acute care and community health settings.

LCF Georgia is also a community partner for the Fuld Fellowship for Service Learning at NHWSON. This fellowship provides tuition support to students who have a commitment to social responsibility as a component of professional nursing practice. The Fuld Fellow works closely with LCF Georgia's Health and Wellbeing

Program to develop their community health referral process as well as health screenings and health education material.

This community-based partnership has extended to LCF Georgia supporting the Atlanta Region Community Health Workforce Advancement Program (ARCHWAy) at NHWSON to train current and aspiring community health workers supported through a grant from the Health Resources and Services Administration (HRSA). LCF Georgia referred several participants from our member organizations, as well as LCF Georgia navigators to receive training as community health workers. Furthermore, LCF Georgia assists in providing 20 h of simulation experience and is a training site for community health workers to complete 80 h of experiential learning that is grounded in the realities of Latinos in Georgia. The partnership between LCF Georgia and NHWSN continues to grow as we continue to identify community needs and work together to collaboratively addressing them. NHWSN has been a key partner in supporting LCF Georgia's Health and Wellbeing Program outreach at various community health events and health promotion activities.

Collaborating with a nonprofit community organization, such as the Latino Community Fund-Georgia, provides opportunities for academic health institutions to reach the Latino population to provide healthcare services to communities and training in culturally appropriate care to nursing students. The partnership between LCF Georgia and NHWSN continues to grow as we continue to identify community needs and work together to collaboratively addressing them.

NHWSN has been a key partner in supporting LCF Georgia's Health and Wellbeing Program outreach at various community health events and health promotion activities. Collaborating with a nonprofit community organization, such as the Latino Community Fund, Georgia, provides opportunities for academic health institutions to reach the Latino population to provide healthcare

services to communities and training in culturally appropriate care to nursing students. The collaboration between the LCF Georgia and NHWSN is an opportunity for outreach efforts to build trust with communities and the US academic healthcare system to increase access to care and to assist individuals in prevention services and referrals for chronic disease management in Latino underserved communities. These community outreach efforts aim to advance public health, strengthen nursing students' skills in addressing SDoH, and help Latino communities, especially those that are underserved, to achieve health equity. While the partnership between LCF Georgia and NHWSN is relatively recent, established by like-minded stakeholders and volunteers, it joins a long history of related programs that center the needs of Latino community members in Georgia. To illustrate the links between historical and contemporary efforts to address Latino health needs, we now turn our attention to the example of the Emory Farmworker Project, founded in 1996, which continues to work with Latino populations.

5   Addressing the Lack of Access to Health Services in the Latino Agricultural Workers: The Emory Farmworker Project (EFP) Led by Emory University

5.1   History and Overview

The Emory Farmworker Project (EFP), formerly known as South Georgia Farmworker Health Project, provides innovative and culturally appropriate healthcare for the underserved at the juncture of justice and medicine while fostering skills of empathy and the ability to apply medical training in underserved and rural community contexts. In 1996, the Emory University's Physician Assistant (PA) Program created the Emory Farmworker Project (EFP) as a clinical learning opportunity for students interested in migrant healthcare. This program began out of the trunk of a car with one Physician Assistant (PA) faculty member and four PA students. Despite its modest beginnings, the EFP has grown into a logistically complex and community-supported program with vast teaching and care implications and is led by Dr. Jodie Guest at Emory University. The EFP takes place every summer for 1 week each in Bainbridge and Valdosta, two rural communities in Georgia, and one long weekend in the fall in Bainbridge. These cities are home to the largest migrant farmworker populations in Georgia. The vast majority of these individuals (75–80%) have not seen a healthcare provider in the past year, and many have never seen a provider. Most are Latino, primarily from Mexico. Citizenship status is not a consideration for or barrier to care within this program. The EFP is a truly interdisciplinary program and includes the Emory Physical Therapy Program, students and faculty from the Rollins School of Public Health, medical students, nursing students from the Nell Hodgson School of Nursing, Emory medicine residents and fellows, and PharmD residents. At the local level, students from Valdosta State University in the Master of Marriage and Family Therapy Program also participate in the program. Additionally, the program includes local volunteer medical interpreters as language is a significant barrier to care. LCF Georgia and Emory Healthcare recently became important partners in providing translation resources in addition to local community partners in South Georgia.

This is an entirely volunteer faculty-led program and includes members of the PA Program, Department of Family and Preventive Medicine, Department of Pediatrics, Department of Internal Medicine, Department of Emergency Medicine/Toxicology, and the Rollins School of Public Health. Limited dental services are provided in Bainbridge with the Georgia Baptist Dental Van and volunteer dentists from the local communities. The program also provides common pharmaceuticals and care packages with these resources provided through philanthropic donations.

5.2 The Community Served by the EFP

An estimated 4.2 million migrant and seasonal farmworkers (MSFW) work in the USA to plant, cultivate, harvest, and pack fruits, vegetables, and nuts. Although invisible to most people and policymakers, the presence of migrant farm workers in many rural communities throughout the nation is vital as their labor enables the enjoyment of high-quality, low-cost produce all year round. Despite farmworkers' economic and cultural contributions, they continue to be some of the lowest paid, least protected and those with the worst health status among workers in the USA.

Data from the 2012 National Agricultural Workers Survey found that the majority of MSFW do not receive medical care due to cost considerations. The EFP serves MSFW in the Eastern Stream, where there are fewer women and children, have the lowest level of spoken English and the poorest workers with 85% living at less than the federal poverty limit. Most workers send 70% of their weekly incomes to their families in their country of origin. The EFP has received local, regional, and national recognition for innovative and culturally appropriate delivery of healthcare at the juncture of justice and medicine while providing free, healthcare to some of whom may not have survived without the intervention provided by the EFP.

5.3 Partnerships with Local Organizations

EFP collaborates with the local health organizations in Decatur, Lowndes, and Echols counties to determine where care is most needed and engage with their existing protocols to serve the community. Other community partners include churches, local schools operating under the federally funded Migrant Summer School Program, Salvation Army and Goodwill Industries, Southwest Georgia Area Health Education Center, the Georgia Department of Agriculture, the Office of Rural Health, the Farmworker United Foundation, and the Latino Community Fund Georgia.

5.4   EFP Clinics

EFP clinics are held daily in the morning and evening in locations convenient for workers. Morning clinics are offered at different farms and remote field-side areas to provide care prior to the pickers going into the fields while evening clinics are typically at farmworker housing camps or local farmworker clinics. Students bring folding chairs to set up mock exam rooms in vegetable fields, packing plants, and parking lots. Volunteers also commonly bring canopies as the June harvest season in South Georgia brings a heightened risk for heat injuries with the heat index commonly climbing to over 100°.

5.5   EFP as an Innovative Service-Learning Model That Fosters Cultural Change

The EFP is a likeminded group of interprofessional volunteers coming together to provide quality healthcare to those who are severely underserved due to immense barriers to care such as cost, access, language, fear, and the logistics of constantly moving for crop picking. The EFP helps mitigate these barriers by going to the MSFW at their place of work, providing interpreters and access to care. In addition to providing this much-needed medical care, the program works to educate volunteers about the plight of these workers so that they can experience a shared sense of humanity. "Huddles" are used at each clinic to discuss complicated cases and cases that touch and stretch the capacities of student volunteers. Additionally, students witness and reflect upon the high rates of poverty among agricultural workers, differences between H2A and non-H2A workers, varied compensation structures, and severe shortfalls in access to food and other basic necessities.

The EFP assesses student learning outcomes from this program. While most students were enthusiastic about participation in service-learning and had a basic understanding of social determinants of health, the evaluation underscored significant and positive differences in post-participation attitudes and learning. Students who were initially uncertain about the program benefits had a transformed view after participating in the EFP ($p < 0.001$). Additionally, students' desire to participate in service-learning projects increased after participation, as did their sense that the EFP enhanced their learning, and their confidence in participating in these projects with underserved communities ($p = <0.05$ for all). We believe that projects like this are impactful in helping students gain an understanding of SDoH in the context of rural and underserved communities.

5.6   The EFP Improves HealthCare Outcomes for Patients While Improving the Health of the Community and Decreasing Overall HealthCare Costs

Each summer, care and basic pharmaceutical options are provided free of cost to the workers. While the MSFW are eligible to see a clinician for a $25 fee at the local Farmworker Clinic, there remain significant barriers to care such as time out of the fields, lost income, transportation to the clinic, the clinic fee, and inadequate number of available appointments. EFP volunteers come to them and provide needed care at no cost. Last year, 1800 individual patients received care over a 10-day period and close to 21,000 h of free care over the 2 weeks.

5.7   EFP Fosters Leadership Development for Our Students

The EFP has led to many opportunities for students to hone their leadership skills. Due to the program's dependence on fundraising, students lead efforts to raise money to support the EFP through organizing an annual 5K race, including securing corporate sponsorships. Students speak at community events and churches to raise funds and collect clothing and food. During Farmworker

Awareness Week in March, they plan a week of public events to highlight the plight of the MSFW, helping raise awareness among college students, faculty, and staff across campus. Students also have the opportunity to share interesting medical cases with the whole group during huddles.

In 2012, Dr. Guest founded Teen Corp, a program that pairs teens interested in pursuing careers in healthcare with an Emory PA student mentor during the EFP. Teen Corp was the recipient of the Emory Service Award in 2012 and was featured in a national PA journal. A Teen Corp participant was also recognized with the Atlanta Teen Volunteer of the Year Award. The program enables PA students to teach and mentor youth—they lead classes and help Teen Corp mentees present clinical cases. This program has become a wonderful way for senior clinical students to guide younger students on issues of healthcare, compassion, empathy, and justice.

EFP has brought national recognition to the Emory PA Program for collaborating with community partners and clinics to provide care to MSFW. Faculty and students frequently present the work from EFP at Latino Health Conferences, the annual Eastern Stream Migrant Health Conference, and HealthSTAT. Original research articles have been published in peer-reviewed publications including articles on food insecurity published in the Journal of Public Health in 2009, winner of the student research award for JAAPA in 2009, and on heat injuries published in March 2013 in the *American Journal of Preventive Medicine*. These publications include student researchers as authors.

5.8   The EFP Is an Interprofessional Clinical and Educational Partnership with Patients, Families, and Communities

Over the last decade, the EFP has defined and described social and medical issues affecting MSFW. Below are three examples of research conducted in collaboration with the CDC, public health and nutrition students, and local organiza-tions. Low socioeconomic status and a vulnerable position in society increase the risk for food insecurity (the limited or uncertain availability of nutritionally adequate foods), making this an important public health concern for the MSFW population. In 2009, the prevalence of food insecurity was examined in the MSFW served by EFP; 67% of the MSFW were food insecure [9]. The risk was significantly higher in non-H2A workers (risk ratio [RR] = 2.929; 95% confidence interval (CI) = 1.753–4.894); $p < 0.0001$), those without transportation (RR = 5.287; 95% CI = 1.850–5.501; $p < 0.0001$), those without access to a refrigerator and oven (RR = 3.086; 95% CI = 1.121–8.493; $p < 0.0292$), and those with children (RR = 3.190; 95% CI = 1.121–8.493; $p < 0.0001$). These data support the need for policy interventions to protect vulnerable farmworkers. The EFP has worked to improve the food insecurity rates in this population through bian-nual food drives to provide each patient seen during clinics with supplies like cooking oil, corn flour, dried beans, and rice.

Heat-related illnesses (HRI) are a common issue seen at the EFP. In 2011, trained interviewers conducted in-person interviews to determine the risk for heat-related illness. Population intervention models assessed where the greatest potential impact could be made to reduce the prevalence of HRI symptoms. One-third of those seen at the EFP had experienced three or more HRI symptoms in the preceding week [10]. Models showed that the prevalence of HRIs could be reduced by increasing the number of breaks, ensuring breaks are in the shade, increasing access to medical attention, and reducing soda intake [10]. Each of these can be addressed through appropriate training of workers on HRI prevention and dissemination of findings to farm owners to show mitigation of adverse outcomes with modest changes in policies. EFP now distributes bandanas to MSFW printed with HRI reduction techniques and hydration messages in Haitian Creole and Spanish.

MSFW are one of the higher at-risk groups for HIV largely due to the challenging socioeconomic circumstances they face. While the transient nature of their work life hinders the accurate assessment of HIV prevalence, estimates range from 2.6 to 13%. MSFW face typical HIV risk factors such as unprotected sex and IV drug use, all of which are exacerbated by poverty, lack of education, limited access to care, alcohol abuse, high-risk sexual behaviors, social isolation, and inadequate knowledge of risks. In 2015, the program conducted a needs assessment to determine HIV risk awareness, literacy levels, and educational preferences. Low literacy leads to poorer health outcomes. Ninety percent of farmworkers surveyed reported that they read and speak little to no English with the average level of completed education being eighth grade. A low perception of HIV risk, low levels of knowledge regarding transmission methods, and limited testing were found in this population.

While some participants understood the risk of unprotected sex and sex with multiple partners, many others associated risk with promiscuity rather than with the level and consistency of protection used with multiple sex partners. Married and monogamous individuals felt that they did not need condoms or HIV testing to protect themselves from HIV, as they felt protected by the exclusivity of their sexual relations. Moreover, several male participants stated they would doubt their partner's fidelity if the partner requested using condoms. This information was used to design and pilot a culturally sensitive HIV curriculum for MSFW. The content served as a conversational tool between the patient and provider to ensure that training was carried out in a manner conducive to farmworkers' cultural preferences. This pilot has now been adopted as routine care at the EFP. Agriculture is the largest economic driver in Georgia. Many crops need to be picked by hand and these hands belong to farmworkers who have no access to healthcare. Growers desire healthy workers but cannot always provide the infrastructure necessary for ensuring healthcare for their workers.

EFP's long history with the many growers in South Georgia has built trust and recognition of our mutual goal of keeping workers healthy. We strongly promote the belief that a healthier community benefits everyone. By providing free care

to more than 1800 patients each summer, the project has allowed community funds to be spent expanding year-round farmworker clinics, to hire more outreach workers, to purchase fully equipped mobile clinical exam units, and to extend their availability to the entire community.

6   Best Practices and Future Direction

As we reflect upon lessons learned and best practices that can be gleaned from our work on the two exemplars discussed, it seems appropriate to frame them through the acronym, **SALUD GA**. We discuss below the principles exemplified by this acronym and are hopeful, as we continue our work in advocating for health equity for Georgia's burgeoning Latino population, that our collective efforts centered on these principles will continue to move the needle toward greater health equity for the Latino population in our state.

1. **Sensitize communities:** We have learned from our work on both initiatives that education and sensitization are the first steps toward change. As the Latino population in the state has grown and continues to grow in Georgia, they have emerged as an important voice and a political force in the state. Sensitizing businesses, policymakers, and others about the historical challenges and contemporary needs of Latinos in the state is vital to effecting change. With regard to the communities themselves, educating Latinos on preventative care, such as vaccinations, health screenings, and annual well checks, and taking steps to prevent heat-related injuries are all useful ways to ensure the health and well-being of this population. In so doing, we underscore the importance of supporting and collaborating with organizations working on the front lines and at the grassroots to promote wellness in the community. These groups have a deep understanding and are most attuned to the strengths and challenges of communities and often are best equipped to develop culturally appropriate and sustainable solutions.

2. **Address and reduce barriers:** The first step to promoting health with this group that is transferrable to other contexts and to other vulnerable and/or medically underserved groups is to understand the barriers that these individuals and groups face and put in place mechanisms to address them. From both exemplars discussed, we can glean that barriers that many Latino individuals, in particular recent migrants, face include language and literacy issues, mistrust in healthcare systems, a lack of health insurance, and access to care, to name a few. We aimed to address each of these barriers in a variety of creative ways as discussed in this chapter to ensure equitable access to care.

3. **Leverage community coalitions:** A useful lesson that both exemplars offer is the value leveraging and building coalitions. We have learned from our work with LCF Georgia and the more established EFP that partnerships between community-based organizations, institutions of higher education, health systems, religious entities, governmental organizations at the local, state, and federal level, and businesses are vital to advancing health and well-being of individuals and population groups. By working together and recognizing mutually beneficial goals, we are moving the needle on health equity.

4. **Understand and address social determinants of health:** From the perspective of providing enriching educational opportunities for our students and efforts to make a meaningful difference for the communities we serve, it was vital to understand how social determinants of health, such as economic circumstances, living conditions, access to food and appropriate clothing, immigration status, and language barriers can all have an impact on health outcomes and contribute to differences in health equity. Understanding the differential impacts of these factors on individuals and communities is the first step in the journey toward achieving health and well-being for all.

5. **Data-driven decision-making:** We have learned that it is important to measure the impact of the interventions and initiatives we are launching and incorporate the insights from these evaluations for continued program effectiveness and to identify areas of improvement. The EFP has been as effective and as long-standing as it has been because of the willingness to evaluate and address areas of improvement. Given that our partnership with LCF Georgia is relatively new while we have not put in place formal evaluation processes, we have open lines of communication among the partner organizations and with other stakeholders to ensure that we are listening to those whom we are serving and to each other to effect change.

6. **Gain trust and build relationships:** Another useful lesson that this work offers is the importance of establishing relationships with a range of stakeholders and coalescing around common interests. For example, with the EFP, growers want healthy workers but may not always have the infrastructure or resources to ensure adequate healthcare for workers. Working with growers and community advocacy groups and others, we are able to provide healthcare to this vulnerable and medically underserved population. In addition, we have learned that building trust with the Latino community writ large by engaging community members and amplifying community voices is essential to ensure sustainability and justice with this work.

7. **Advocate for policy change:** Ultimately, the purpose of this work is to impact sustainable health outcomes. Therefore, it is imperative to advocate for policy change in several areas, including for affordable healthcare, for language justice, and for culturally competent care. Through the dissemination of our work at local and national forums and by engaging policymakers at all levels, across public and private sectors, and in civil society, we will break down systemic barriers and promote health equity.

By implementing the principles of SALUD GA, we can collectively work toward achieving health equity for Latino populations in our state and across the USA.

Appendix: Sources for Fig. 1

Latinos in Georgia: Demographics and Social Determinants of Health

Ahn T, De Leon H, Dominguez-Villegas R, Zong J, Galdamez M, Oaxaca A, Perez R, Ramos-Vega D, Renteria-Salome L. 15 facts about latino well-being in Georgia. UCLA Latino Policy and Politics; 2022. https://latino.ucla.edu/research/15-facts-latinos-georgia/.

America's Health Rankings. Obesity in Georgia. Explore Obesity in Georgia. 2021. https://www.americashealthrankings.org/explore/measures/Obesity/GA?population=Obesity_LT_25k_C.

America's Health Rankings. Diabetes in Georgia. Explore Diabetes in Georgia. 2021. https://www.americashealthrankings.org/explore/measures/Diabetes/GA.

America's Health Rankings. High blood pressure in Georgia. Explore High Blood Pressure in Georgia. 2021. https://www.americashealthrankings.org/explore/measures/Hypertension/GA?population=hypertension_Hispanic.

America's Health Rankings. Cardiovascular diseases in Georgia. Explore cardiovascular diseases in Georgia. 2021. https://www.americashealthrankings.org/explore/measures/CVD/GA?population=CVD_Hispanic.

Armstrong-Mensah E, Dada D, Bowers A, Muhammad A, Nnoli C. Geographic, health care access, racial discrimination, and socioeconomic determinants of maternal mortality in Georgia, United States. Int J MCH AIDS. 2021;10(2):278–86. https://doi.org/10.21106/ijma.524.

Centers for Disease Control and Prevention. ChildVaxView interactive. Centers for Disease Control and Prevention; 2017. https://www.cdc.gov/vaccines/imz-managers/coverage/childvaxview/data-reports/index.html.

March of Dimes. Mortality and morbidity. March of dimes. 2020. https://www.marchofdimes.org/peristats/data?reg=99&top=6&stop=92&lev=1&slev=4&obj=1&sreg=13.

U.S. Census Bureau. 2021 American Community Survey 1-year public use microdata samples. 2021. https://data.census.gov/all?q=georgia+hispanic+population.

Women's Health. Kaiser Family Foundation. n.d. https://www.kff.org/state-category/womens-health/.

References

1. Murphy A, Blanchard C, Hill J, editors. Latino workers in the contemporary south. Athens: University of Georgia; 2001.
2. Nunez G. Immigration became an economic issue. How Latinos helped Atlanta get Olympic ready. 11 Alive WXIA-TV; 2022. https://www.11alive.com/article/news/community/voices-for-equality/how-latinos-helped-atlanta-get-olympic-ready/85-b94430e3-a8ca-4128-8103-b7b3b04c9c79.
3. Tharpe W. Voluntary immigration enforcement a costly choice for Georgia communities. Georgia Budget & Policy Institute; 2018. https://gbpi.org/voluntary-immigration-enforcement-a-costly-choice-for-georgia-communities/.
4. American Civil Liberties Union Foundation of Georgia. Terror and isolation in cobb: how unchecked police power under 287(g) has torn families apart and threatened public safety. 2009.
5. Baxter T. How Georgia's anti-immigration law could hurt the state's (and the Nation's) economy. Center for American Progress; 2011. https://www.americanprogress.org/article/how-georgias-anti-immigration-law-could-hurt-the-states-and-the-nations-economy/
6. United States Census Bureau. Hispanic heritage month 2022. United States Census Bureau; 2022. https://www.census.gov/newsroom/facts-for-features/2022/hispanic-heritage-month.html.
7. Fernandez J, García-Pérez M, Orozco-Aleman S. Unraveling the Hispanic health paradox. J Econ Perspect. 2023;37(1):145–68. https://doi.org/10.1257/jep.37.1.145.
8. National Academies of Sciences, Engineering, and Medicine; Health and Medicine Division; Board on Population Health and Public Health Practice; Committee on Community-Based Solutions to Promote Health Equity in the United States. In: Baciu A, Negussie Y, Geller A, Weinstein JN, editors. Communities in action: pathways to health equity. National Academies Press; 2017. https://doi.org/10.17226/24624.
9. Hill BG, Moloney AG, Mize T, Himelick T, Guest JL. Prevalence and predictors of food insecurity

in migrant farmworkers in Georgia. Am J Public Health. 2011;101(5):831–3. https://doi.org/10.2105/ajph.2010.199703.

10. Fleischer NL, Tiesman HM, Sumitani J, Mize T, Amarnath KK, Bayakly AR, Murphy MW. Public health impact of heat-related illness among migrant farmworkers. Am J Prev Med. 2013;44(3):199–206. https://doi.org/10.1016/j.amepre.2012.10.020.

Lalita M. Kaligotla PhD, is Professor of the Practice and Senior Director for Leadership and Community Engagement at Emory University's Nell Hodgson Woodruff School of Nursing. Her work is centered on values-based leadership, social innovation, human-centered design, and community-based research. She currently envisions and implements leadership development programming for faculty, staff, and students as well as experiential, and interprofessional, experiences for students. She has a keen interest in addressing inequities in access to healthcare and health outcomes. She also serves as the faculty director for the Fuld Fellowship for Social Responsibility, a scholarship program designed to support high achieving nursing students with a strong commitment to civic engagement and social responsibility.

Jodie L. Guest PhD, MPH, is a Professor and Senior Vice Chair of the Department of Epidemiology at Rollins School of Public Health at Emory University. She is also the Co-Director of the Office of Interprofessional Education and Collaborative Practice, and the Associate Director of Emory PA Program at the School of Medicine. Dr. Guest has a broad background in epidemiology and specific expertise in HIV cohorts and clinical trials and emergency preparedness and has focused her research in racial, sexual, and gender minority populations in HIV care. She has been the recipient of multiple awards at Emory, most recently the 2023 Kenneth Rothman Career Achievement Award from the Society of Epidemiologic Research, the 2022 Distinguished Lifetime Achievement Alumni Award for Rollins School of Public Health, the 2022 and 2020 Rollins School of Public Health Professor of the Year. Dr. Guest is the director of the Emory Farmworker Project, a multidisciplinary program to provide healthcare to thousands of migrant farmworkers each year, and Emory's Outbreak Response Team for COVID-19, working with poultry plant workers, communities in middle Georgia, the Mexican Consulate in Atlanta, and communities with limited access to vaccines and testing due to unstable housing.

Gilda (Gigi) Pedraza is the Executive Director and Founder of the Latino Community Fund (LCF Georgia), a nonprofit organization working to advance people's democracy, protect and build communities, and expand economic opportunities. She is a social entrepreneur with 20 years of experience in both for-profit and nonprofit sectors in the areas of strategy, coalition building, communications, and community engagement.

Pedro Viloria is a Venezuelan-born American immigrant, community advocate, social entrepreneur, and the Health and Wellbeing Program Manager for LCF Georgia. Viloria has coordinated emergency relief during the COVID-19 pandemic in metro-Atlanta and rural Georgia, the 2021 Gainesville Nitrogen Gas Leak, DACA Application Assistance as well as the organization's statewide health equity and advocacy efforts, including access to free glucose, cholesterol, and blood pressure screenings and preventative health workshops.

Iliana Yamileth Rodriguez PhD, is an Assistant Professor of History at Emory University. Rodriguez's research focuses on Latinx history and communities within the US South. Her scholarship examines Latinx histories in relation to culture, race, ethnicity, labor, and migration.

Beth Ann Swan PhD, RN, FNP-C, PHCNS-BC, is a Professor, Clinical Track, Associate Dean and Vice President for Academic Practice Partnerships, Interim Associate Dean for Education, the Charles P. and Peggy Evans Endowed Distinguished Professor in Simulation and Innovation at the Nell Hodgson Woodruff School of Nursing, and Co-Director of the Woodruff Health Sciences Center Interprofessional Education and Clinical Practice Office at Emory University. Throughout her career, Dr. Swan has advocated for engaging consumers in their health care, promoting quality care coordination and safe care transitions, and creating innovative evidence-based practices to improve care.

Roxana C. Chicas PhD, RN, FAAN, is an Assistant Professor at Emory University's Nell Hodgson Woodruff School of Nursing. Dr. Chicas's research is shaping the future of climate and occupational health science, two pressing fields of scientific inquiry. A sought-after scientist with features in Bloomberg News, NPR, and The World, she conducted the first field-based intervention study of methods to reduce core body temperature using real-time biomonitoring equipment among farmworkers in the United States. As a bilingual bicultural nurse scientist, she is committed to conducting research that informs policy to advance environmental justice.

Social Determinants of Health: Strategies for Community Engagement and Practice

Shawana S. Moore, Erica Moore,
Camille Brockett-Walker, and Michael McFarland

1 Health Disparities and Access to Healthcare Services

Health disparities refer to differences in health outcomes and access to healthcare services influenced by social, economic, and environmental factors. These disparities are often associated with social determinants of health, including socioeconomic status, race, ethnicity, education, and access to healthcare. Healthcare providers, specifically advanced practice registered nurses (APRNs), are essential in addressing disparities, with community involvement at the core.

APRNs are a critical component of the modern healthcare ecosystem, providing invaluable services to patients in various healthcare settings. However, healthcare is an ever-evolving system, and in recent years increasing recognition has been given to the impact of social determinants of health (SDOH) on individual and population health outcomes. As the impact of SDOH on healthcare becomes more evident, there is a growing momentum in implementing diversity initiatives within the healthcare workforce. Particularly, enhancing diversity within the APRN workforce has emerged as a crucial approach to improve healthcare service for communities across the United States. Promoting diversity in the APRN workforce aims to better serve and meet the unique needs of diverse communities by addressing the significant disparities in health outcomes among various socioeconomic and demographic groups.

To understand the need for programs to increase diversity within the APRN workforce, it is essential to assess current trends in the field. Data from the American Association of Colleges of Nursing (AACN) indicates that the percentage of non-white APRNs is lower than that of the US population. White APRNs comprise 77.4% of APRN workforce, 6.7% being Hispanic or Latino, 7.9% being Black or African American, and 4.2% being Asian. Similarly, the AACN report showed disparities in male APRN representation, with only 8.2% of APRNs being men. These statistics suggest a need for greater diversity in the APRN workforce to reflect the increasingly diverse populations and meet the needs of the healthcare system.

There is a range of systemic obstacles that hinder the entry of individuals from underrepresented minority groups into the nursing workforce on a scale that accurately represents the overall population. These barriers are primarily fueled by structural racism, which encompasses challenges

S. S. Moore (✉) · E. Moore · C. Brockett-Walker
M. McFarland
Nell Hodgson Woodruff School of Nursing,
Emory University, Atlanta, GA, USA
e-mail: shawana.moore@emory.edu;
Erica.moore@emory.edu;
camille.brockett@emory.edu;
michael.mcFarland@emory.edu

such as limited opportunities for university admission resulting from inadequate funding for primary and secondary schools, long-standing economic policies that perpetuate poverty within minority communities, and unconscious biases in admission procedures (Raghu).

There are numerous identified strategies to enhance the diversity of the APRN workforce. Recruiting underrepresented minority students into nursing programs after high school can contribute to an increased number of students pursuing nursing studies [1]. Scholarships and financial aid should be made available to individuals from diverse backgrounds, reducing the financial burden associated with pursuing advanced nursing degrees. Developing mentoring programs that support and guide aspiring APRNs from diverse backgrounds, providing them with the necessary guidance and encouragement to succeed is key to ensuring diversity in the workforce. Academic support initiatives that aid in retaining and engaging nursing students of color [2]. Additionally, providing academic support through. Mentorship to new faculty along with recruitment and retention of diverse faculty. Lastly, hospitals and healthcare facilities should prioritize diversity in their hiring practices, actively seeking out candidates from different racial, ethnic, and cultural backgrounds. By implementing these strategies, the APRN workforce can become more representative of the diverse populations they serve, leading to improved healthcare outcomes for all.

2 Diversity in the APRN Workforce

Diversity in the APRN workforce is a topic that holds personal significance to us as a minority APRNs invested in enhancing health outcomes, promoting health equity, and minimizing health disparities for marginalized populations. For more than 15 years, we have been honing our skills as APRNs in different specialties. During our time as student nurses and student APRNs, we rarely came across black faculty members or preceptors who reflected our own identities. It was uncommon to encounter another APRN who resembled us throughout our practice. The scarcity of diversity among APRNs not only personally affects us but also raises concerns for patient care, especially for individuals from underrepresented and diverse communities.

Increasing the diversity of providers makes patients more comfortable in seeking out care. According to a study published in JAMA 2020, it is indicated that individuals belonging to minority communities generally prefer healthcare providers who share their racial or ethnic background [3]. When patients have confidence in their providers' ability to comprehend their unique perspectives, relatable and nonjudgmental, they show a higher tendency to book regular checkups, follow prescribed medications diligently, and disclose information more openly and honestly which leads to better health outcomes. While there has been a notable improvement in the diversity and inclusion of APRNs from different racial and ethnic backgrounds, as well as an increase in male representation in the field, there remains considerable progress to be achieved.

Recognizing the importance of fostering a diverse APRN workforce and our understanding of SDOH, the community, including healthcare professionals, community leaders, and individuals impacted by health disparities, plays a crucial role in advocating for transformative change. The literature on health disparities, social determinants of health, and workforce diversity provides insights into the existing inequities and their impact on health outcomes. The overarching goals of addressing social determinants of health and increasing diversity within the APRN workforce may include **promoting equitable access to quality healthcare**, **improving health outcomes**, **reducing health disparities**, **enhancing cultural competence**, and **empowering underrepresented communities**. These goals serve as guiding principles for designing and implementing programs focusing on diversity and inclusion within the APRN workforce, aiming to address social determinants of health and improve health outcomes for all.

3 A Diverse APRN Workforce and Community Engagement

Once we acknowledge the significance of fostering a diverse APRN workforce, how can we effectively collaborate within our communities to introduce programs that promote greater diversity within this profession? The community plays a vital role in addressing social determinants of health and promoting a diverse APRN workforce. Community engagement is crucial in understanding the unique needs and challenges of various populations. It's important to note that the specific community of stakeholders involved may vary based on the geographical location and targeted demographic of the programs aimed at increasing diversity in the APRN workforce. Some of these stakeholders may include practicing APRNs, nursing educators, healthcare administrators, community leaders, and policy makers— all working together for a common purpose of creating opportunities, resources, and support systems to increase diversity within the APRN workforce, with the intention of addressing health disparities and improving health outcomes for underserved populations. By actively involving the community, there is greater potential for meaningful and sustainable change in addressing social determinants of health and promoting diversity among APRNs.

4 Strategies to Diversify the APRN Workforce in Collaboration with Community Stakeholders

By collaborating with the community of stakeholders, we have made significant strides in our efforts to diversify the APRN workforce. We have first started in the area of recruitment and retention of underrepresented nursing faculty. Faculty of color (FOC) in nursing academia are recognized for their contributions in increasing diversity in the nursing workforce, decreasing health disparities, and promoting mentoring for nursing students of color [4]. When students look at faculty, they need to see themselves reflected. This presence provides evidence to students of color that they can succeed in the education arena and become successful health care professionals. With this objective in mind, the Nell Hodgson Woodruff School of Nursing's CRNA program has been purposeful in its efforts to recruit minority CRNAs as faculty. As an illustration of their commitment, they have initiated a recruitment tactic "dating," which involves several steps before formal engagement in academia. This innovative approach allows prospective faculty to shadow current faculty and interact with students, enabling them to gain valuable firsthand experience of the daily dynamics within the academic work environment. During this shadowing experience, they actively participate in simulations to gain hands-on experience and a comprehensive understanding of operational logistics and faculty expectations. Additionally, candidates are invited to contribute as guest lecturers, sharing their expertise and insights with students and the CRNA teaching team. During this phase, transparency is fostered, and a strategic matching process ensures that newer faculty are paired with compatible mentors, ultimately promoting faculty retention. As a result of implementing this approach, the program has successfully expanded its faculty to include several black females, a male, and an alumnus of the program. Through participating in this "dating" process, potential CRNA faculty members from underrepresented backgrounds are able to gain valuable insight into how their presence and unique perspectives can have a positive impact on the quality of education provided. Moreover, this initiative aims to attract minority students to the CRNA profession, thereby contributing to the diversification of the APRN workforce.

Collaboration among stakeholders can also drive policy changes in APRN education that can ultimately impact the diversity of the APRN workforce. Following a thorough review and analysis of data, the Nell Hodgson Woodruff School of Nursing has taken a firm stance by advocating for and successfully removing the GRE requirement for entry into certain APRN programs. This initiative has helped remove a financial barrier for those aspiring to become APRNs and removes the statistical "ism" that the GRE is evidence that an individual has the necessary analytical and critical thinking to be successful in graduate studies. By waiving the GRE requirement, more individuals from economically disadvantaged backgrounds will have the opportunity to apply for APRN programs. This change can potentially increase the number of diverse candidates who aspire to become APRN's. Eliminating the GRE requirement enables programs to attract a wider range of applicants. An APRN workforce that consists of candidates with diverse perspectives and experiences can lead to better patient outcomes.

Lastly, and perhaps most impactful, has been our ability to develop community partnerships with organizations, academic institutions, and healthcare systems to establish pipelines and pathways for individuals from underrepresented backgrounds to enter and succeed in APRN programs. Again, within the DEI department of the SON at Emory University", we have created space for the Fellowship in Nursing Development (FIND) program which is a collaboration between historically black colleges and universities (HBCUs) such as Spelman College, Morehouse College, and Clark Atlanta University and the Nell Hodgson Woodruff School of Nursing. The program aims to allow for an opportunity for underrepresented minorities to experience or expose minorities to different roles of nursing which they may not have the opportunity nor connections to do so on their own, providing support and resources to HBCU students pursuing nursing degrees. The fellowship program offers selected students from Spelman, Morehouse, and Clark Atlanta University finan-cial assistance, mentoring, academic support, and professional development opportunities. These resources are intended to cultivate a strong pipeline of diverse nursing professionals who can contribute to addressing healthcare disparities in marginalized communities. Through FIND, Emory University and the partner HBCUs collaborate to create an environment that supports students' successful completion of nursing degrees. By investing in HBCU students, this program seeks to promote nursing education, professional growth, and leadership by addressing the barriers these students may face due to financial constraints, limited resources, and lack of representation.

Similarly, Emory has programs like the High School to Higher Education Pipeline Program which is a collaborative program developed by two minority faculty members to support and guide high school students from underrepresented backgrounds in their journey to higher education. This is an example of how we reach out to secondary education and address students who may have never identified nursing as a potential career. By nourishing this early stage of the school-to-workforce pipeline, nursing schools can provide the support needed for student from underrepresented backgrounds to thrive in nursing school and beyond. Emory also partners with the CRNA, Leadership Excel and Achievement Program (LEAP), which indirectly promotes APRN workforce diversity through its inclusive approach and commitment to providing opportunities to individuals of diverse backgrounds who are interested in pursuing a career in nursing anesthesia.

The overarching objective of these programs and initiatives is to cultivate a diverse and culturally competent APRN workforce that can effectively address the unique healthcare needs of diverse populations. By increasing diversity within the APRN profession, these initiatives aim to mitigate health disparities, improve patient outcomes, and foster equitable access to healthcare for all individuals, regardless of their socioeconomic status, race, ethnicity, or other social determinants of health.

5 Reflection/Future Directions

Addressing social determinants of health by promoting a diverse APRN workforce comes with its fair share of challenges. One major challenge is overcoming historical disparities and systemic barriers that have limited access to education and opportunities for individuals from underrepresented communities. The lack of diversity within the healthcare workforce itself can make it challenging to attract and retain diverse APRNs. Additionally, cultural competency training and resources are essential to ensure that APRNs can effectively address the specific needs of diverse communities. Building trust and rapport with communities that have been historically marginalized can also be challenging, as it requires active community engagement and ongoing efforts to address the unique social determinants of health in those communities. Despite these challenges, promoting diversity in the APRN workforce is crucial for enhancing healthcare equity and improving outcomes for all populations.

Promoting diversity within the APRN workforce has successfully addressed social determinants of health on various fronts. Firstly, a diverse APRN workforce brings a range of cultural perspectives, experiences, and language skills that allow for more effective and culturally competent care delivery. By understanding different cultural beliefs and practices, APRNs can develop interventions that are more relevant and acceptable to diverse populations. Secondly, a diverse APRN workforce can help reduce health disparities and improve healthcare access for marginalized communities. When individuals see healthcare providers who resemble them, they are more likely to trust and engage in their care. This trust can lead to increased healthcare utilization, better adherence to treatment plans, and, ultimately, improved health outcomes. Furthermore, a diverse APRN workforce can act as role models and mentors for aspiring healthcare professionals from underrepresented backgrounds. Seeing professionals who look like them in leadership positions can inspire future generations to pursue careers in healthcare and diversify the workforce even further. Overall, promoting diversity within the APRN workforce has successfully addressed social determinants of health by fostering cultural competence, reducing health disparities, and inspiring future professionals. However, continued efforts are necessary to ensure equitable opportunities and inclusive environments for all aspiring APRNs.

References

1. Phillips JM, Malone B. Increasing racial/ethnic diversity in nursing to reduce health disparities and achieve health equity. Public Health Rep. 2014;129(Suppl 2):45–50. https://doi.org/10.1177/003335491412 91s209.
2. Barbe T, Kimble LP, Bellury LM, Rubenstein C. Predicting student attrition using social determinants: Implications for a diverse nursing workforce. J Prof Nurs. 2018;34(5):352–6. https://doi.org/10.1016/j.profnurs.2017.12.006.
3. Takeshita J, Wang S, Loren AW, Mitra N, Shults J, Shin DB, Sawinski DL. Association of racial/ethnic and gender concordance between patients and physicians with patient experience ratings. JAMA Netw Open. 2020;3(11):e2024583.
4. Ro K, Sin MK, Villarreal J. Perceptions of support by nursing faculty of color. J Prof Nurs. 2021;37(1):29–33.

Shawana S. Moore , DNP, APRN, WHNP-BC, PNAP, FAAN, is a nationally recognized, board-certified women's health nurse practitioner who specializes in providing women's and gender-related care throughout the lifespan. She has developed a nurse-led mentorship program to support the healthy growth and development of adolescent girls in underserved communities, and she serves on national boards and committees dedicated to women's health care. Her research interests include women's health, environmental/climate and women's health, adolescent female empowerment, well-woman care, contraception, gynecological disorders, telehealth in the women's health care setting, diversity, inclusion, and equity.

Erica Moore , DNP, CRNA, APRN, serves as an Assistant Professor and Assistant Program Director at Emory's Nurse Anesthesia Program. Her research is dedicated to promoting inclusivity and increasing diversity among faculty in the nurse anesthesia profession, with a particular focus on faculty of color. Clinically, she specializes in Trauma and Obstetrics Anesthesia, bringing a wealth of expertise to her academic and clinical roles.

Camille Brockett-Walker , DNP, RN, is an Assistant Professor and the Interim Director of the Adult Gerontology Acute Care Nurse Practitioner program at Emory University. She also maintains a clinical practice as a critical care nurse practitioner. Her research interests include diversity, equity, and inclusion of faculty and students of color in nursing.

Michael McFarland , DNP, AG-ACNP-BC, FNP-BC, is a Senior Clinical Instructor at Emory University NHWSH and serves as a lead faculty member for VANAP-GE and the Atlanta Primary Care Nurse Practitioner Residency program. He is a practicing acute care nurse practitioner in the Division of Hospital Medicine at Emory University Hospital Midtown. He teaches in the Family Nurse Practitioner, Acute Care Nurse Practitioner, Adult Gerontology Nurse Practitioner, and the Master of Nursing (Pre-Licensure) programs at the School of Nursing and lectures in Veteran Affairs Nurse Practitioner Residency Program, which is a partnership between the Atlanta Veteran's Affairs Hospital and Emory NHWSH.

Decolonizing Nursing Education: Promoting Curricula for Community Engagement

Autherine Abiri, Angela Haynes Ferere, Jazzmine Jordan, and Wanjira Kinuthia

1   Introduction

In this chapter, we explore the voices of nurse educators, a Doctor of Nursing Practice student, and a learning designer on their lived experiences with decolonizing nursing education. The authors of this chapter discuss the interconnecting themes of culture, racism, colonialism, and health inequities to arrive at a collective declaration of recommendations to decolonize nursing education.

2   PART 1: Mirror Images by Autherine Abiri

2.1   Denver's Story

It's early in the morning and it's Denver's first day of nursing school. With a mouthful of cereal, she reflects on the moment she initially received the wonderful news of her acceptance into nursing school. Mixed emotions and thoughts race through her mind. Denver's excitement about finally starting nursing school gleams brightly in

her subtle smiles in between her spoonfuls of cereal. Yet, there is a sense of nervousness that runs through her toes as she ponders her potential and ability to represent the first member of her family to go to college. She gently shakes away the doubts, grabs her jacket, and heads out the door to catch the city bus to nursing school. On her way to the bus stop, she sees a small gathering of neighbors in front of her local grocery store. As she gets closer, she sees panic on each face and the atmosphere carries a dense cloud of tension. Denver hears shouts for "help" and as she gets closer, she peers through the crowd. On the ground, there is a man lying there motionless. In that split second as she glances down, her stomach sinks. Time stands still for her, and she wants to move but she's frozen. A little while later, she hears the ambulance arrive. A sense of relief passes through the crowd as they make way for the emergency medical service crew. They begin CPR and the crowd grows as they watch and wait with hope. The man is carried into the ambulance and the crowd begins to slowly dissipate. Denver makes it to nursing school and with a big sigh she takes her seat. Minutes before class start, she thinks to herself how the man had been lying on the ground motionless for what seemed to her like forever.… why didn't anyone try to help him, and no one was prepared or knowledgeable to step in for assistance. The bell rings and class is in session.

A. Abiri (✉) · A. H. Ferere · J. Jordan · W. Kinuthia
Nell Hodgson Woodruff School of Nursing, Emory University, Atlanta, GA, USA
e-mail: Autherine.abiri@emoryhealthcare.org;
angela.haynes-ferere@emory.edu;
Jazzmine.jordan@emory.edu; wkinuth@emory.edu

J. B. Hamilton, C. E. Moore (eds.), *Transforming Social Determinants to Promote Global Health*,
https://doi.org/10.1007/978-3-031-61160-5_36

2.2   Brook's Story

To Brook's surprise she is nervous about the last day of her nursing clinical rotation. In a couple of weeks, she will graduate and officially be a third generation nurse in her family. It had been a lifelong dream for her and now the time had come. She quickly grabs her stethoscope and heads to the elevator of her apartment building. The elevator stops on the eighth floor and a few more residents rush inside before reaching the lobby level. In the lobby, Brook sees a stir of residents gathering around. Immediately, someone shouts "call 911." In the commotion, Brook is shoved to the side, and she sees a woman in gym clothes rush immediately to a man lying on the floor and begins chest compressions. Minutes later, the emergency medical service crew arrives and carries the man to the hospital. Despite the rush of the morning, Brook arrives on time for her clinical rotation on the ICU floor. As she steps into her patient's room, she thinks to herself how familiar he looks. She glances closer and realizes that her patient is the same man from her apartment lobby. She thinks to herself...what would the outcome have been had no one been knowledgeable to respond with CPR.

Health is a state of well-being that is gainfully achieved through the network of community. The attainment of health does not solely rely on isolated and individualistic actions [1]. Moreover, the complex nature of health requires community partnerships. Nursing has its roots embedded deeply in public health and the traditional practice of delivering care to neighborhoods and communities [2]. The history of nursing was established on a model that focuses on community engagement and holistic care. Throughout nursing history, the aim has been to provide health and healing by engaging the community. There is often a preference or bias in healthcare to minimize the preventative measures that regard community health. Most new graduate nurses join the workforce employed in hospital systems versus choosing the traditional roots of nursing in public health. Over the past few decades, nursing education has followed this pattern and has dulled the significance of community engagement by primarily focusing on the practice of acute care within the hospital setting. The problem with emphasizing this new school of thought is that it leaves patients without resources to overcome barriers that meet both medical and social needs. The answer to many health ailments lies within community engagement and mitigating the upstream and downstream effects within society.

In the narratives above, we see the account of two nursing students and their own lived experiences shaped by their communities. In Denver's case, it was apparent that no one in the crowd knew how to perform bystander cardiac pulmonary resuscitation (CPR), whereas with Brook, there was a bystander immediately available and knowledgeable to perform CPR. The factors that contributed to the outcomes in each scenario stem from social determinants of health (SDOH). These are the conditions in the environment and society in which we live and work and how they impact health outcomes [3]. The negative impact of social determinants of health leads to health disparities and inequities as seen in Denver's story. This is an example of why nursing education needs a reform that is designed to highlight and value interventions aimed at promoting community health. To adequately prepare nurses to assess and address social barriers and needs, nursing education must thread social determinants of health throughout pre-licensure and post-licensure curriculum.

Reflecting on my time as a pre-licensure nursing student, I realized not only the need to explore social determinants of health but also to ensure that there is full representation of individuals from diverse backgrounds in the delivery of optimal patient care. Within my nursing program of approximately 100 students, I was one of three students of color. I carried the weight of being this statistic as I attended my nursing classes and clinical rotations. Often, I felt isolated from my classmates as I feared that they and my instructors may not understand my lived experiences as a woman of African descent. It was during my second year in nursing school that one other student of color and I decided to form the Multicultural Student Nursing Organization. At that time, the mission of this inaugural organization was to create a welcoming environment for all nursing students of all backgrounds and to encourage the growth of a diverse nursing workforce. This organization provided a sense of belonging not only for myself but for all students of color. It was in this haven that we as students were able to express our concerns and celebrate our successes. Student associations such as the Multicultural Student Nursing Organization provide an outlet that fosters the development of a diverse nursing workforce and cultivates a culture that values diversity in healthcare.

Now fast forward to my experiences as an Emergency Department Nurse Practitioner, I deliver care to a diverse range of patients that often includes historically underrepresented groups. The accessible nature of the emergency department makes it a central location to serve a diverse range of populations who face social barriers to medical care. For example, social barriers, such as environmental resources, employment, transportation, insurance status, and access to quality food and housing, play a direct role in health and disease outcomes specifically within emergency department patients. Although we tend to consider access to healthcare as a patient experience that only occurs within the hospital walls of a healthcare system, patient outcomes are often dependent upon their social circumstances prior to their arrival at the brick-and-mortar hospital. Frequently, medically underserved and minority populations are left in a plight when it comes to achieving quality health outcomes. In emergency medicine, we observe and experience the intersections of social determinants of health practiced as social emergency medicine (SEM). SEM describes the integration of the social affairs of care into the practice of emergency medicine. SEM sheds light on the necessity of clinicians to take actions that promote health equity for vulnerable populations and the need for an integrated effort that ensures communities are involved. Precious time can be lost with patients if interventions are limited only to the acute care setting. If community partnerships are developed, we can mitigate the upstream factors that influence health disparities.

As a nurse educator, I desire to create a learning environment that promotes ethical nursing practice and social justice in healthcare. Given my own background and experiences as a nurse educator, I have seen the gap in knowledge and clinical practice that exists when integrating social determinants of health into clinical practice. Closing this gap therefore calls for nurse educators to place value on nursing curricula that incorporate experiential learning activities that foster community engagement, thereby allowing nurses in both pre-licensure and post-licensure programs opportunities to develop skills in assessing and addressing SDOH.

Experiential learning activities provide students with opportunities to gain further understanding of didactic coursework rooted in social determinants of health. Examples of experiential learning activities include service-learning opportunities that incorporate social determinants of health and foster community collaboration. The inclusion of service-learning activities in pre-licensure and post-licensure nursing programs allows students the opportunity for full immersion into a community and explore health in the context of social, cultural, environmental, and political concepts. My recommendation for establishing a nursing curriculum that cultivates a future nursing workforce prepared to advance health equity is to endorse requisite service-learning activities that explore elements of social determinants of health and promote community engagement. With experiential learning activities, students take on the role of educating patients within the community setting with knowledge that is beneficial for improving health outcomes.

Relating back to the opening two narratives, one specific example might be to provide students with a service-learning activity tasked with educating community members on how to initiate bystander CPR. Linking this activity with didactic course objectives such as identifying the influence of neighborhood characteristics on health outcomes and discussing barriers to bystander CPR, provides students with a holistic approach to healthcare aimed at mitigating disparities. Offering a structured experiential learning activity built within the curriculum creates an opportunity to change the narrative of nursing education to one that places value on community development and engagement.

In summary, from my lived experiences, recommendations for decolonizing nursing education include:

1. *Placing value on community engagement*
2. *Building a diverse nursing workforce that embraces and celebrates cultural differences*
3. *Requisite experiential learning activities such as service-learning projects that focus on community engagement*

With the implementation of these recommendations, we can work toward achieving a healthcare system liberated from health inequities.

3 PART 2: Who Needs a Red String Anyway? by Angela Haynes Ferere

I felt like I was suffocating as the waves of sweat kept pouring down my face, dripping down my arms, back, and even the ankles around my loose scrub bottoms were clinging to me, soaked with my own moisture. As I glanced around, I could only see waves and waves of faces anxious for me to complete my assessment with the patient in front of me so they could hurry and press closer for a chance to sit in my chair and be seen by the "American." I was hot, exhausted, hungry, and overwhelmed by the desperate moms hoping to have their sick children seen in our mobile clinic. We set up our clinic in the open, under the trees, hopeful for the breeze that rarely rustled the trees. It gave me the chance to keep glancing through the crowds of sick children to triage the most vulnerable and move them to the front of the line.

The day had started before sunup and the 3-h trip over terrible terrain in the back of a beaten up, barely running pickup truck had not improved my mood. It was the sixth day in a row of 14-h clinicals with limited patient resources, never enough providers, too many sick people, little time to rest,

and occasional access to an outdoor latrine. The heat and the mosquitoes were not helping either. Yet each time I looked up to see the pleading, desperate faces of the patiently waiting mothers and fathers, I knew I had to keep going. After all, I chose to keep coming to Haiti to do this very thing month after month and year after year.

I looked over and saw a 3-year-old child riddled with a skin infection and wheezing for air. I moved quickly and brought her and her mother over to my seat. I was frustrated to see that the child was poorly nourished and in such an awful state of health. Both of her ears were oozing with bright, green pus and she was struggling for air. I moved into action quickly. My training kicked in and I went to work. I asked a colleague to help me so we could address the patient's needs more efficiently. I grabbed my scissors and started cutting. I cut the red strings in the child's ears covered in pus and I cut the red string loosely wound around her neck so I could better assess her retractions and breathing workload. As I cut, the mom moaned and several women in the crowd watching gasped. I ignored them and continued caring for the patient. I was oblivious to what I had done, and I was not finished. I looked at the mom and in Creole asked her why she was focused on her child's appearance with the strings rather than finding the healthcare she so desperately needed. I even chastised her for not taking loving care of her child and not feeding her well. Gasp.

I was so focused on stabilizing this young child that I failed to look any deeper than my role as her provider with the knowledge and skills to improve her current health status. I was successful by my standards but had truly violated my patient and her mother by openly rejecting their incredibly powerful spiritual beliefs and dismissing the impacts of relentless poverty. You see, this bone-thin mother had lost everything and was struggling to even feed her child. She herself had lost weight and had been unable to find work because she could not leave her sick child at home. In her despair, she had approached a local healer as a last resort. The local healer had provided the ear strings and the neck string as a symbol of the healing and blessing to protect the child. My irreverent removal of the strings without even asking the patient's mom was such an act of arrogance and cultural dismissal. I had to walk away in shame and gather my thoughts. The mother did not say anything to me, as she was grateful for her child's improving health, but a Haitian interpreter and dear friend in the group pulled me aside to share the consequences of my actions. I had been openly disrespectful of the beliefs and values of those who trusted me to provide their care. I was crushed that I had become so engrossed in my own needs, that I did not even consider the implications of my actions. In that moment, I vowed to do better. I openly apologized in Creole to the patient's mom, and I asked for her forgiveness. I also apologized to the crowd, but that was just the beginning.

I purchased a red band to wear around my watch for the remainder of the trip as a vivid reminder of my experience. I shared my experience with other members of the healthcare team while in Haiti, and I was surprised to find that many did not see any issue with what I had done. They were making excuses for me and defending my actions by reminding me that we were busy and had to work smarter to see everyone, and as foreigners, it would be okay because we could not be expected to know other cultures or include their values in delivering care. Those words made it even harder for me to excuse the actions and not make a real change.

3.1 From Aimless Culture to Intentional Learning

I returned to campus and started exploring the objectives of many of the clinical courses we offered in our distance accelerated BSN (DABSN) program. We moved through the topics of cultural care, but there was no deep dive exploring meaningful ways to increase integration of sensitive topics around social determinants of health. As the program director of the DABSN program, I felt a heavy responsibility to lead change in our cohort of students. The DABSN program is a remote program offered for second-degree students, allowing them to stay in

their home communities for clinical experiences while completing the rigorous one-year program. The program addresses workforce nursing shortage issues by preparing Emory students from all over the country with an emphasis on rural or under-resourced regions. The DABSN program offers an immersive clinical experience through a course titled Vulnerable Populations. This existing course offered the perfect platform for a cultural shift in course delivery. The course description stated that students would explore the health challenges influenced by social, cultural, political, and economic factors but there were no metrics, aligned objectives, or course assignments to fully explore learning about social determinants of health (SDOH). I needed to tell my story and share my lesson. It was not easy to share with my students the lessons learned from my colossal failures. Being vulnerable about my own professional practice shortcomings was not comfortable for me, but when I realized the impact it was having on students, I knew my story had to be included in our shared learning.

3.2 Social Determinants of Health Are Considered Essential

Initially, the focus of the Vulnerable Populations course was on the domains related to person-centered care, such as concepts considering the beliefs of the individual, demonstrating the ability to have difficult conversations, utilizing emotional intelligence in communications, engaging, and demonstrating cultural sensitivity and humility in practice. In 2021, The American Association of Colleges of Nursing released the updated Essentials outlining curriculum expectations for competency at all levels of nursing education (AAACN) and incorporating these updates became a DABSN program priority.

The DABSN faculty recognized integrating social determinants of health (SDOH) in one course in the DABSN program was a good first step, but timely integration of the SDOH pillars in all DABSN courses was necessary, and the planned plan of study update to the new essentials provided the perfect opportunity to integrate change. The faculty focused on adding course objectives with integrated SDOH, evidenced by assignments and unfolding case studies developed for each course. Additionally, each clinical day includes consideration of the influences of one of the four pillars of the social determinants of health. Students and faculty now discuss how social, cultural, environmental, and policy issues inform the health of the patients we care for in all settings in our post-conferences and clinical debriefings.

In the DABSN program, students complete a capstone project as a requirement for graduation. Each student must demonstrate the integration and consideration of the impact of social determinants of health in their intervention. Students also complete care plans and shift reports in clinical with a section for SDOH action. Students completing the clinical immersive experience in either Haiti or South Georgia with farmworkers rely on the course preparation work to complete their population health windshield survey, community assessment, and action plans. Students also rely on the foundational preparation of their courses, including vulnerable populations and population health, to inform their practice for providing care in nontraditional settings. The faculty remain an active part of the cultural transition in our nursing school and were excited to review the content in their courses and explore ways to integrate the content into meaningful learning experiences in the theory and clinical learning settings.

3.3 Lessons Learned from a Red String

As I reflect on an obvious solution, I am reminded that as a nurse, nurse practitioner, educator, and Native American Indian, I did not get it right with my 3-year-old patient in Haiti. Not even close to being right. To someone unfamiliar with the practice of traditional healing arts and the role of spiritual beliefs and reliance on traditional healers, my blunder may seem benign, but that is far from the truth. I am incredibly humbled by the Haitian community that welcomes me into their homes and communities over the past 37 years. Learning this valuable lesson early in my professional practice was life-impactful and changing for me. My goal is to focus on best preparing the next generation of nurses influencing care delivery for individuals, families, and communities with increased expertise and inclusion of social determinants of health in providing care. Maybe they will also wear a red wrist scarf to remain mindful.

4 PART 3: A DNP Student's Journey to Addressing SDOH by Jazzmine Jordan

The day shift nurse approached, eyes rolling and her head shaking from side to side, "Hey good luck with this one, she was a nightmare" she said agitatedly. As I read over the report, I glanced through the patient's history. She was a young woman in her mid-twenties, African American, currently on probation, lack of previous prenatal care, lack of insurance, and unmarried but living with her boyfriend. Her health history indicated she suffered from gestational diabetes and hypertension, and she was being brought into the labor and delivery unit for a diabetic ketoacidosis emergency. Additionally, this was her second pregnancy, but she had no living children, she was 34 weeks (about 8 months) pregnant, and there was a concern for decreased fetal heart tones of her baby. Before entering her room, I gathered my stethoscope, took a deep breath, and I remembered something my mom always told me, "You never know what someone has been through, so treat them with respect, compassion, and a smile… and don't forget to go the extra mile."

4.1 Background and Experience

My name is Jazzmine Jorden. I am a recent graduate of Emory University's Primary Care Pediatric Nurse Practitioner Program. During my tenure at Emory, I attained my Doctor of Nursing

Practice degree with a concentration in Population Health. I chose this track because of my deep passion for public health and the community.

I grew up in a household in the countryside of Georgia, with my mom, who worked as a rural public health nurse; my dad, who served as a phlebotomist and biologist; and my grandmother, who served as a missionary in her church. I am no stranger to the art of serving others through nursing, working in the church, and working in the community. A few core memories I have from childhood are the days I spent traveling with my mom for work. We traveled from house to house, and I watched her care for patients one step at a time. My mom has been a nurse for over 20+ years, and she's never wavered on doing her best to provide the most quality of care to her patients. The smile and joy she had taking care of patients brought me joy and it inspired me to do the same one day. After graduating with my BSN (Bachelor of Science in Nursing) in 2018, I began working as a labor and delivery nurse where I cared for families experiencing the most beautiful moments in life and sometimes the most heartbreaking moments in life. During that time, I learned how impactful social determinants of health can be for each patient and how personalized care can significantly improve patient health outcomes.

4.2 What Are Social Determinants of Health?

Social determinants of health (SDOH) are defined as "the conditions in the environment in which people live, learn, work, play worship, and age that affects a wide range of health, functioning, and quality of life outcomes and risks" [4]. SDOH is divided into five areas: economic stability, i.e., employment, food insecurity, housing instability, poverty; education, i.e. early childhood education and development, language and literacy, high school graduation, and higher education; social and community context, i.e., incarceration, discrimination, and civic participation, health and health care, i.e., access to health care, access to primary care, and health literacy; and finally the neighborhood and built environment,

i.e., access to foods that support health eating habits, crime and violence, quality of housing, and the physical environment that support safe spaces to run and play [4]. Together these determinants can affect anyone in a positive or negative aspect. In my personal experience, the most frequently seen SDOH were access to healthcare and primary care, language and culture, health literacy, access to foods that support healthy eating habits, access to clean water, safe neighborhoods, and clean and open environments for children to play.

One important social determinant to improve the care we provide for our patients is an understanding of cultural influences on language. I specifically recall an interaction with a patient of South Asian descent when I was working as a labor and delivery nurse. At the beginning of the shift, I received a report from the day shift nurse that this patient was "noncompliant" in adhering to the labor plan, and due to a language barrier, "it was impossible to understand her." Throughout my shift that night, I learned that the patient was the gentlest and most compliant patient once she understood the plan of care and her concerns were heard. This mutual understanding between myself and her healthcare provider was possible when we took the time to use language that she could understand and also took the time to understand her. Taking the time to understand patient's concerns and collaborating with the healthcare team to meet the needs of the patient is essential to what we're called to do as nurses. During my interactions with this patient, I was able to develop at trusting relationship and to advocate for her needs to achieve the outcome of a safe and effective delivery—a feat that would not have been possible if I treated the patient as "noncompliant" or "difficult" when I received the initial report from the off-going nurse. Labeling patients with negative descriptors further perpetuate stigma, bias, and discrimination for racialized minority patients. This was the finding of one study that examined the effects of negative descriptors used in the provider notes of the electronic medical record on patient care [5]. The researchers of this study concluded that stigmatizing language may be disproportionately applied to racially minoritized patients and this type of language has the potential to negatively affect the care of the patient among providers and the care delivered by the broader healthcare system [5]. Being more aware of these factors can help to improve the care we deliver to all patients no matter their social or cultural background.

Another social determinant that I have become aware of is related to the family structure of incarcerated patients and their family members. As a nursing student, I have cared for incarcerated patients, patients on probation, and patients with family members who were incarcerated. My beliefs and values as a nurse who respected patients regardless of their social and cultural background allowed me to consider the ways in which an incarceration history can impact the care provided by healthcare professionals. One incident I recall during my time in labor and delivery was that of a recent first-time mother whose husband had been incarcerated since the beginning of the pregnancy. At the end of a successful delivery, this mom opened up to me and shared she wasn't sure she had enough financial resources to care for the newborn once she returned home given the loss of income from her husband who provided their main source of income. She proceeded to ask me to pack extra milk and diapers in her discharge items to ensure she had enough for the newborn when she got home. Once hearing this, I connected the patient with our social services team so they could educate her on proper resources she could access to help her care for her newborn at home. As nurses, we're called to be holistic care providers, which sometimes means going the extra mile to advocate for our patients to have their needs met beyond our care.

4.3 How SDOH Affects Child Health

One thought that has consistently crossed my mind as a labor and delivery nurse was that even if we met every criteria to achieve a seamless delivery of a newborn, those efforts fall short if we don't advocate for our patients to have a warm home to go home to, access to clean water and healthy foods to eat, a safe environment, and access to primary care and healthcare services.

One way to improve our efforts in SDOH and child health advocacy is to educate ourselves on the different resources available to patients and their families [4]. Organizations that assist with providing access to health insurance, social welfare, and food assistance programs do a tremendous job to improve the lives and children and their families. It's important to know about these programs and how to connect patients so that they can have the necessary resources to help them maintain healthy lives. As a student in the pediatric nurse practitioner program, I spent time learning about the importance of access to child health insurance for families. Child health insurance is important to individual quality of life given the finding that expanding health insurance coverage for low-income children increases the rate of high school and college completion [6]. The finding from this study indicates that access to health insurance for children and their families might also result in increased rates of high school completion and decreased rates of dropouts.

Another way to improve advocacy in child health outcomes is to increase our personal knowledge and skills on SDOH [4]. Students of nursing programs and advanced nursing programs have to take on the responsibility of learning about SDOH to improve their own skills. As a PNP student, I requested clinical rotations that included marginalized and underserved communities in order to better understand how to care for individuals and families in those communities. For example, one clinical experience was working in the Migrant Family Farm Workers' program. This program is an H2A Visa government program that provides aid and resources to migrant farmworker families who assist with farming and agricultural work in the United States [6]. In this clinical experience, I was able to assist children of migrant farmworker families obtain their physical exams needed to attend school. Another clinical rotation I had was with the Community of Advanced Practice Nurses'

(CAPN) clinic for nurse practitioners. This clinic is located in Atlanta and designed to provide care for the community's most vulnerable populations. These vulnerable populations served include the Atlanta Children Shelters and the Our House—a nonprofit organization serving children and families experiencing homelessness in the Greater Atlanta Area [7]. These clinical experiences during my tenure at Emory widened my lens and skillset with SDOH to inform the care I am able to provide to these underserved communities. Knowledge and experience in working with the social determinants of health with families who experience diverse social and cultural needs is extremely important to the improvement of child health outcomes.

4.4 Reflection

It is my hope that the dissemination of knowledge and an awareness of social determinants of health will improve the way we care for patients, address their social needs, and improve health outcomes. Achieving this goal requires that we educate ourselves through the integration of SDOH throughout a nursing curriculum. One way this can be achieved is through an examination of programs that already include SDOH curriculum and to find ways to improve and evaluate ways in which students are responding to that curriculum. In my DNP thesis titled "Evaluating the Integration of Social Determinants of Health into a Prelicensure Nursing Curriculum" with the help of Dr. Beth Ann Swan and Dr. Jill Hamilton, I evaluated the integration of SDOH curriculum within the Nell Hodgson Woodruff School of Nursing. I examined the data from course evaluations on student's perceptions to the courses that had a SDOH integrated curriculum and evaluated ways to improve the SDOH curriculum integration. The integrated SDOH curriculum from Emory's School of Nursing is a shining exemplar of the level of in-depth integration we should include across all nursing curriculums across the USA. The integration of SDOH into a nursing curriculum is one way to not only improve our skills and knowledge as nurses, but an additional strategy to improve the lives of children, families, and the communities we care for. A quote by Maya Angelou, author, poet, and civil rights activist says this, "As a nurse we have the opportunity to heal the heart, mind, soul, and body of our patients, their families, and ourselves. They may forget your name, but they will never forget how you made them feel" [4].

5 PART 4: Nursing and Global Health Education in Africa: A Pathway to Equity in Addressing SDOH Through Learning Design by Wanjira Kinuthia

This section explores the intersection of decolonizing health education, learning design, and recognizing social determinants of health (SDOH) in Africa. It highlights the historical context of colonization in healthcare education and how learning design can be employed as a tool for decolonization. Incorporating SDOH within the curriculum examines how nursing and global health education can better prepare students to address healthcare disparities and promote equitable care. In this context, decolonizing nursing education and global health education refer to a comprehensive and transformative process to dismantle historical colonial influences, imperialism, colonial biases, power imbalances, ethnocentrism, and Eurocentric perspectives that have shaped the education structure, content, and practices.

My approach to this narrative seeks to create an inclusive, culturally sensitive, and equitable learning environment that acknowledges the diverse cultural and historical contexts in which healthcare is delivered to prepare students to provide patient-centered and culturally competent care while addressing healthcare disparities and social determinants of health [8, 9]. Having worked as an educator and learning designer across diverse landscapes, from the United States to various African countries, in higher education and healthcare, I have understood education's profound role in shaping societies and healthcare systems.

Creating an equitable educational framework prepares students to engage in global health with humility, cultural competence, and a commitment to social justice. However, the term "global health" is based on assumptions and asymmetries, whereby those from low- and middle-income countries (LMICs) remind us that the concept is a "convenient but artificial construct: developed by high-income countries (HICs) to describe healthcare practiced in LMICs" [8, 10]. This should raise the question about whose perspective global health is being branded and pursued.

Social determinants of health (SDOH) are the conditions in which people are born, grow, live, work, and age and the set of forces and systems shaping the conditions of daily life. SDOH encompasses a wide range of social, economic, and environmental factors that impact an individual's health and well-being, including income, education, employment, housing, access to healthcare, neighborhood environments, and social support networks [11]. Understanding SDOH is critical in public health and healthcare because it influences health outcomes and health disparities, highlighting the need for policies and interventions that address these social and structural determinants to achieve health equity.

Within the African context, broadly, this colonial history impacted nursing education in several ways. The nursing curriculum was developed in line with Western healthcare models and ideologies, often neglecting the existing rich indigenous healing traditions and practices. This omission resulted in an incomplete understanding of the health needs of local communities. The hierarchical structures that characterized colonial rule also influenced the power dynamics within healthcare institutions. This often created inequalities, leaving the local populations marginalized. Additionally, the early development of health education was closely tied to religious missions and field [12]. While these missions played a vital role in healthcare delivery, they also brought Western religious and cultural norms that influenced nursing practice and education, sometimes to the detriment of indigenous traditions.

5.1 The Imperative for Decolonization

Decolonizing health education is a multifaceted and transformative endeavor, and when viewed through the lens of learning design, it becomes a powerful tool for change. In Africa, the imperative for decolonizing nursing and global health education is broadly intertwined with the ongoing efforts to address healthcare disparities. Professional education has generally not kept up with the pace of healthcare challenges. Additionally, the continent needs an effective and efficient health education system to build an adequate, competent, and relevant healthcare workforce to achieve the Sustainable Development Goals [13].

Decolonizing nursing education is essential for fostering cultural sensitivity. It recognizes diverse cultures, traditions, and belief systems and how these influence healthcare practices. By integrating local perspectives, nursing education can create a more culturally sensitive and patient-centered approach to care. Healthcare disparities do persist, with marginalized communities often experiencing poorer health outcomes. Decolonizing nursing education acknowledges the need to address these disparities by preparing healthcare professionals who can understand and effectively respond to the social determinants of health and the unique healthcare challenges in the community [14]. Decolonization of health education aims to create equitable healthcare systems by providing students with a comprehensive experience encompassing local knowledge and practices. This ensures that services are accessible and respectful of the cultural and social context of the communities they serve.

According to Bvumbwe and Mtshali [13], this is in sync with the World Health Organization's framework for the transformative and scale-up of health professions education. Six themes characterize the African education landscape as it relates to nursing education challenges and solutions in Sub-Saharan Africa to inform a model for improving the quality, quantity, and relevance of nursing education at the local level. These are curriculum reforms, professional regulation, transformative teaching strategies, collaboration and partnership, capacity building, infrastructure, and resources. Challenges and solutions in nursing education are common, but significant investment by development partners results in the positive development of nursing education. However, strategic leadership, networking, and partnership to share expertise and best practices remain critical.

5.2   Learning Design as a Catalyst for Change

Learning design in this context can catalyze transformative change by actively promoting decolonization within nursing education. Several vital roles and approaches can be highlighted.

First, instructional designers are tasked with reshaping curricula to include a broader spectrum of cultural and historical perspectives. This entails reevaluating course content, textbooks, and case studies to reflect diverse experiences and healthcare practices. Second, the learning design can promote inclusive pedagogical approaches that acknowledge diverse learning styles and cultural backgrounds [15]. This requires moving beyond a one-size-fits-all model and embracing student-centered strategies. Third, learning designers can harness technology to make education more accessible, especially in underrepresented regions. E-learning platforms, telemedicine, and mobile apps can extend the reach of nursing education, making it a more equitable [14]. Fourth, learning designers can facilitate collaboration among educators, students, and indigenous or marginalized communities to foster cultural competency. This includes developing partnerships with local healthcare practitioners and traditional healers.

5.3   Challenges and Opportunities

Decolonizing health education faces resistance from established norms and traditional power structures. Instructional designers must be prepared to address this resistance with evidence-based arguments and a commitment to change. Additionally, changes in nursing education may

require reform at the policy and accreditation levels, requiring learning designers to collaborate with policymakers to advocate for transformative changes. Finally, learning designers can lead research efforts to measure the impact of decolonization efforts. This includes assessing changes in student outcomes, cultural competence, and healthcare disparities.

5.4   Reflection

As someone who believes in the power of education to shape the future, this section underscores the critical role that learning design can play in dismantling historical colonial influences and fostering cultural sensitivity. In reflecting on the intersection of health education, learning design, and recognizing SDOH, I am struck by the importance of this transformative process. This journey toward decolonization and incorporating SDOH within the curriculum is not merely an academic exercise but a moral imperative and a call to action.

Decolonization should not be seen as a threat to established norms but as an opportunity to develop a more just and equitable healthcare system. It is a chance to bridge the gap between theory and practice, ensuring that healthcare professionals are well-trained, culturally competent, and committed to addressing healthcare disparities. It is not just about revising textbooks or curricula but redefining our values, principles, and the essence of education. The challenges are significant, but the opportunities for transformative change are equally profound. It is a call to create a future where healthcare is provided with humility, cultural competence, and a dedication to social justice.

References

1. Issel LM, Wells R. Health program planning and evaluation: a practical, systematic approach for community health. 4th ed. Jones & Bartlett Learning; 2017.
2. McCauley L. Social determinants of health: call for nursing education reform. In: Hamilton JB, Swan BA, McCauley L, editors. Integrating a

social determinants of health framework into nursing education. Cham: Springer; 2023. https://doi.org/10.1007/978-3-031-21347-2_1.

3. World Health Organization. Social Determinants of Health. 2022. https://www.who.int/health-topics/social-determinants-of-health#tab=tab_1.

4. National Academies of Sciences, Engineering, and Medicine. In: Wakefield MK, Williams DR, Menestrel SL, Flaubert JL, editors. The future of nursing 2020–2030: charting a path to achieve health equity. National Academies Press; 2021. https://doi.org/10.17226/25982.

5. Sun M, Oliwa T, Peek ME, Tung EL. Negative patient descriptors: Documenting racial bias in the electronic health record. Health affairs (Project Hope). 2022;41(2):203–11. https://doi.org/10.1377/hlthaff.2021.01423.

6. Cohodes SR, Grossman DS, Kleiner SA, Lovenheim MF. The effect of child health insurance access on schooling: evidence from public insurance expansions. J Hum Resour. 2016;51(3):727–59. https://doi.org/10.3368/jhr.51.3.1014-6688R1.

7. H-2a Visa Program for Temporary Workers. Farmers.Gov. 2020. https://www.farmers.gov/working-with-us/h2a-visa-program.

8. Our House, Inc. Our house combines with capn clinics. Our House; 2022. https://ourhousega.org/our-house-combines-with-capn-clinics/.

9. Eichbaum QG, Adams LV, Evert J, Ho M-J, Semali IA, van Schalkwyk SC. Decolonizing global health education: rethinking institutional partnerships and approaches. Acad Med. 2021;96(3):329–35.

10. Zappas M, Walton-Moss B, Sanchez C, Hildebrand JA, Kirkland T. The decolonization of nursing education. J Nurse Pract. 2021;17(2):225–9.

11. Salm M, Ali M, Minihane M, Conrad P. Defining global health: findings from a systematic review and thematic analysis of the literature. BMJ Glob Health. 2021;6(6):e005292.

12. WHO. Social determinants of health. World Health Organization; 2008. https://www.who.int/health-topics/social-determinants-of-health#tab=tab_1. Accessed 25 May.

13. Dolamo BL, Olubiyi SK. Nursing education in Africa: South Africa, Nigeria, and Ethiopia experiences. Int J Nurs Midwifery. 2013;5(2):14–21.

14. Bvumbwe T, Mtshali N. Nursing education challenges and solutions in sub Saharan Africa: an integrative review. BMC Nurs. 2018;17(1):1–11.

15. Krouse AM. Instructional design: more important than ever! vol. 54. Thorofare, NJ: SLACK Incorporated; 2015. p. 304–5.

16. Kadioglu M, Tacgin Z, Sahin N. Instructional design and material development progress to eLearning environments: a sample of obstetrical nursing education. Contemporary. Educ Technol. 2020;12(1):ep265.

Autherine Abiri DNP, FNP-C, ENP-C is an Assistant Professor at Nell Hodgson Woodruff School of Nursing. She is a certified family and emergency nurse practitioner. In 2009, Dr. Abiri obtained her Bachelor of Science in Nursing from the University of Wisconsin–Madison. She obtained her Master of Science in Nursing as a family nurse practitioner from Graceland University in 2015. Dr. Abiri graduated with her Doctor of Nursing Practice from Emory University in 2020 where she was recognized with the Nell Hodgson Woodruff School of Nursing Social Responsibility Award for breaking down barriers and creating an environment for diversity, equity, and inclusion. Additionally, Dr. Abiri has served as a national committee member of the American Academy of Emergency Nurse Practitioner's Diversity Equity and Inclusion Committee. With a focus on nursing education, she has served on educational work groups dedicated to integrating social determinants of health within nursing curricula. Dr. Abiri takes a special interest in research that centers on the impact of social determinants of health on patient outcomes and health disparities. She is passionate about providing patient-centered care and implementing processes that promote health equity.

Angela Haynes Ferere DNP, FNP-BC, MPH, is an Associate Clinical Professor and Program Director of the Distance ABSN program at Emory University. In 2022, she was a recipient of the LEAD Program NLN Leadership Institute award. She is a family nurse practitioner with more than 35 years of clinical and nonclinical experience caring for vulnerable populations locally, regionally, and globally. As the Chair of Eternal Hope in Haiti, a not-for-profit organization, she manages healthcare teams in Haiti. She is a Lumbee Indian tribal member and serves on the Emory Native American and Indigenous Studies Initiative.

Jazzmine Jordan DNP, RN, earned her Doctor of Nursing Practice with a concentration in Population Health from the Nell Hodgson Woodruff School of Nursing at Emory University in Atlanta, Georgia in 2023. She earned her Bachelor of Nursing degree from Clayton State University in Morrow, GA in 2018. She has a passion for working with children, adolescents, and families in the pediatric primary care setting and is currently preparing to sit for boards to become a Certified Pediatric Nurse Practitioner. Her research interests include child health advocacy, social determinants of health (SDOH) and health disparities, cultural competency, creative wellness, and nursing education. Her DNP project aimed at evaluating the integration of SDOH into a nursing curriculum. Through her future work and research, she hopes to improve the application of SDOH to pediatric populations to help alleviate health disparities for marginalized and vulnerable communities. In her spare time, she enjoys spending time with close family and friends, engaging in sports (i.e., pickleball), learning new languages, music, traveling, and spiritually serving her church and community. She is a current member of the Alpha Epsilon chapter of Sigma Theta Tau Honor Society and the National Association of Pediatric Nurse Practitioners (NAPNAP).

Wanjira Kinuthia PhD, is involved in teaching, research, curriculum development, and instructional design work in higher education in Africa, the Caribbean, the USA, and the UAE. She also works on learning design health and nursing education programs for international agencies and higher education. Wanjira's research interests are international and comparative education and educational technology policy. Service activities include Editorial Board membership in the International Journal of Education and Development using Information and Communication (IJEDICT) and the e/Merge Africa mentorship program. Research projects include OER, eLearning, and mLearning, where she has edited several books and published many articles. Wanjira received her PhD in Instructional Design and Technology and was an Associate Professor at Georgia State University for many years.

Perceptions of Social Determinants of Health for Emerging Research Scholars

John A. Fuller, Renée Byfield, Seema Das, Jiyoon Jang, Hyein Kim, and Kaprice Welsh

1 An Intersectional Approach to Understanding the Social Determinants of Health Among Sexual and Gender Diverse Populations by John A. Fuller

1.1 Research Interests/ Professional Goals

Due to discrimination and marginalization, sexual and gender diverse (SGD; an inclusive term used to refer to individuals who do not exclusively identify as cisgender and/or heterosexual) populations remain medically underserved and understudied in health behavior research. SGD

Note: The contribution of PhD students Renee Byfield and Kaprice Welsh was partially funded through the National Institutes of Health National Institute of Nursing Research grant number T32NR020778 (PIs: Dr. D. Bruner and Dr. V. Hertzberg) for trainees. The content is solely the responsibility of the authors and does not necessarily represent the official views of the National Institutes of Health.

J. A. Fuller (✉) · R. Byfield · S. Das · J. Jang
H. Kim · K. Welsh
Nell Hodgson Woodruff School of Nursing, Emory University, Atlanta, GA, USA
e-mail: John.fuller@emory.edu;
cecile.renee.byfield@emory.edu;
Seema.das@emory.edu; ji.yoon.jang@emory.edu;
Hyein.Kim@emory.edu;
kaprice.simone.welsh@emory.edu

people experience cancer health disparities, including increased morbidity and mortality, compared to their cisgender-heterosexual counterparts. There are more than one million SGD cancer survivors in the USA [1]. Due to a lack of standardized sexual orientation and gender identity (SOGI) data collection, this number of SGD cancer survivors is likely an underestimate [2].

In 2015, the National Institutes of Health established the Sexual and Gender Minority Research Office (SGMRO), and SGD people were formally designated a health disparity population for research by the National Institute of Minority Health and Health Disparities in 2016. In 2017, the American Society of Clinical Oncology released a position statement on strategies for reducing cancer health disparities among SGD populations. These changes are important since my proposed research will provide an intersectional framework for examining SGD health disparities. I am interested in exploring how intersectional identities (e.g., race/ethnicity, SGD identity, and disability status) interact with systems of oppression (e.g., racism, cis-heterosexism, and ableism) to create barriers in healthcare delivery and cancer survivorship among marginalized populations. To advance health equity for these groups, the representation of public health researchers and their endeavors must reflect the diversity of the communities we serve.

In the spring of 2022, I was admitted to the OSU Comprehensive Cancer Center's Pelotonia

Scholars Program and awarded $12,000 to conduct independent cancer research. My study, entitled "An Intersectional Perspective on Race, Sexual Orientation, and Gender Identity in Cancer Survivorship," was a secondary data analysis of OUT: The National Cancer Survey in collaboration with the National LGBT Cancer Network. Using data from the Out Study, I wrote an undergraduate honors research thesis to examine the association between SGD cancer survivors' social networks and mental health outcomes. During the summer of 2022, I attended my first research conference, the National LGBT Health Conference in Chicago, while completing a research fellowship at Northwestern University.

1.2 Personal Narrative

In the spring of 2019, I graduated high school with an Associate of Arts degree from the University of Akron. When I joined the Ohio State University (OSU) community later that fall, I was a recipient of the Office of Diversity and Inclusion (ODI) Young Scholars Program (YSP) award. The OSU ODI and YSP have played a critical role in my academic development and encouraged my participation in undergraduate research.

As a Black and queer undergraduate researcher from Akron, Ohio, I have a personal connection to my cancer research interests. The fact that cancer has impacted every generation in my family and that we confronted many barriers to my father's care and treatment during my early years in college made me aware that people with few socioeconomic resources, like my father, need advocates. These experiences—my father's terminal illness, my undergraduate coursework, experience on funded quantitative and qualitative research projects, and my teaching, leadership, and additional research experiences—prepared me to undertake new research endeavors that examine the community- and population-level social determinants of health (SDOH) that contribute to health disparities among SGD people at the doctoral level.

1.3 Intersectionality and Social Determinants

Over the course of my first semester in the PhD in Nursing program, I have utilized the rigorous academic structure, extensive research opportunities, and innovative programming at the Nell Hodgson Woodruff School of Nursing to develop my research interest and learn more about the four pillars of SDOH, primarily the social pillar [3].

Despite calls to reduce inequities, cancer health disparities continue to persist among SGD populations, resulting in both poor physical and mental health outcomes [4]. When compared with their cisgender-heterosexual (C/H) counterparts, a growing number of studies have documented increased exposure to cancer risk factors, such as human papillomavirus (HPV) [5], obesity [6], and substance misuse [7]; higher prevalence of cancer types, including breast/chest, cervical, and anal cancers [8]; and greater rates of cancer-related mortality [9] for SGD populations. Additionally, it is a well-established fact that SGD people experience higher levels of mood and anxiety disorders [10, 11], as well as suicidal ideation and behaviors [12, 13] when compared with C/H people. Higher levels of social isolation and weaker social networks have been linked to poorer mental health outcomes among SGD cancer populations [14].

Theory serves as a foundation for the development of knowledge in nursing science and provides meaning, understanding, and context to the practical application of nursing phenomena [15]. The minority stress model offers a conceptual framework to guide understanding of the unique (i.e., not experienced by individuals in the dominant culture), socially constructed (i.e., reinforced by social processes, structures, and institutions), and chronic stressors of SGD populations [16, 17]. Kneale and colleagues [18] developed a logic model to show how experiences of minority stress can lead to weaker social networks, increased social isolation and loneliness, disparate health outcomes, and poorer care experiences, which exacerbate the need for more formal care for older SGD cancer survivors in the United Kingdom. Social support plays a unique role in mitigating stress for sexual and gender-diverse (SGD) populations. With a particular focus on intersectionality and minority stress, my research this semester has landed on understanding the relationship between social support and health outcomes of SGD cancer survivors.

As my research interests have evolved, I have continued to reflect on a quote from Audre Lorde, and I would like my readers to consider the same quote as a reminder that social determinants of health and health outcomes are a result of overlapping, compounded intersectional experiences.

You do not have to be me in order for us to fight alongside each other. I do not have to be you to recognize that our wars are the same.—Audre Lorde

2   From Student to Scholar: A PhD Journey into Obstetric Violence Research Unraveling the Tapestry of Obstetric Violence by Renee Byfield

In the United States, the stark reality persists: Black women face a staggering three to four times higher risk of maternal mortality compared to their White counterparts, irrespective of age, education, or socioeconomic status. In the urgent quest to confront the Black maternal mortality crisis, it becomes evident that the solution to the high maternal mortality rates among Black women extends beyond increasing access to hospital-based care and skilled perinatal clinicians. The provision of quality care demands an unwavering focus on dismantling obstetric violence, a term that encompasses racism, bias, and the disconcerting prevalence of highly medicalized and depersonalized maternal care. This form of care not only constitutes a breach of respect and dignity but also contributes to unsafe childbirth experiences for women and their infants. The pervasiveness of disrespectful and abusive care during facility-based childbirth is an issue that occurs not only in the United States but globally, with a disproportionate impact on Black women, women of color, and those marginalized by poverty or other societal factors [19]. It is within this context that I place myself as a Black woman, a healthcare professional, an advocate, a burgeoning nurse scientist and researcher, and a PhD student.

Embarking on this PhD journey, I am guided by a curiosity in unraveling the intricate components of obstetric violence. In this realm, I am particularly interested in the intersectionality of racism, gender-based violence, and the unequal power dynamics existing within provider-patient relationships. Physical, sexual, and verbal abuse; stigma, racism, and discrimination; failure to meet professional standards of care; poor rapport between women and providers; and health system conditions and constraints are types of disrespectful and abusive care and obstetric violence [20]. This maltreatment has lifelong negative mental and physical health consequences. The problem is multifaceted, comprising healthcare systems where provider behaviors are tainted by bias, a lack of active listening and responsiveness to patient concerns, and other negative actions that collectively contribute to the alarming phenomenon of obstetric violence. This type of maternal violence violates basic obligations in providing care for patients and the basic principles of ethics and human rights. It is preventable, and its eradication can assist in improving maternal mortality rates.

2.1   Navigating the Dynamic Process of Research Refinement

As the semester unfolds, my research questions have been refined to narrow my focus. There has been a shift of my research focus toward evaluating the impact of traumatic birth in terms of the short- and long-term consequences for both mother and infant. The lens through which I view obstetric violence has also expanded to incorporate the broader societal context, with a focus on access to safe healthcare as a social condition that is a pivotal social determinant of health (SDOH) [3]. Within the Emory School of Nursing SDOH

Four Pillar framework [3], the pillar of social conditions plays a role in shaping the experiences associated with obstetric violence. Social conditions include access to financial resources, education, type of occupation, health literacy, access to health care, and social support as a social resource [3]. These social conditions are the result of systemic racism, bias, and disparities in these areas which significantly influence the well-being or lack thereof of individuals [3]. Delving into the intricacies of social conditions, we find that they are influenced by power imbalances and systemic racism, giving rise to a landscape that profoundly impacts survivors of abuse during childbirth [3].

Obstetric violence is marked by a failure to provide access to safe and equitable healthcare, a cornerstone of social conditions. Provider behaviors play a central role in shaping maltreatment in labor, contributing to an environment where the safety of expectant individuals is compromised. This maltreatment is often a culmination of provider actions marked by bias, a lack of individualized cultural responsiveness, and a failure to prioritize effective communication. The biases embedded within healthcare systems can contribute to an environment where individuals, particularly those from marginalized communities, may experience heightened vulnerability and diminished agency during childbirth. Systemic racism within healthcare systems further exacerbates these issues, perpetuating power imbalances that can result in discriminatory practices and suboptimal care. Instances of providers dismissing patient concerns, exhibiting disrespectful attitudes, and engaging in medical interventions without informed consent contribute to an atmosphere where individuals feel disempowered during one of the most vulnerable moments of their lives [20, 21].

Moreover, the medicalization of childbirth, marked by unnecessary interventions and a focus on convenience rather than patient-centered care, underscores the urgent need to reshape provider behavior. To address obstetric violence and ensure access to safe maternity care, provider collaboration is imperative, encompassing empathy and a commitment to dismantling ingrained biases within the healthcare system. Only through a conscientious shift in provider behavior can we aspire to create an environment where every individual experiences childbirth with dignity, respect, and the assurance of their safety at the forefront of care. Health literacy, another dimension of social conditions, becomes a significant factor. Systemic barriers to education and information can impede individuals' ability to understand and advocate for their health needs, potentially exacerbating the impact of obstetric violence. Bridging the gap in health literacy with healthcare advocacy is paramount to empowering survivors with the knowledge and tools necessary to navigate the complex healthcare landscape.

The decision to integrate the social context of maternal care into my research interests stems from a recognition of its crucial role in shaping individuals' experiences within the healthcare system. Access to safe healthcare serves as a linchpin, influencing the quality of care received and the overall well-being of pregnant individuals. For me, this choice is not just academic but deeply personal, rooted in a commitment to addressing the systemic barriers that disproportionately affect populations of certain communities. As I navigate the dynamic process of my research pursuits, the integration of the social pillar as an SDOH enriches my understanding of obstetric violence, paving the way for comprehensive solutions that transcend the confines of individual interactions to address systemic issues at their core.

3 Bridging Disparities in Cardiovascular Care During Pregnancy by Addressing Social Determinates of Health by Seema Das

I am passionate about improving the maternal health outcomes of women specifically focusing on cardiovascular diseases and hypertension in pregnancy. My motivation to work for maternal health came from a decade-long academic and professional experience as a nurse and public health practitioner in Nepal, a low-income country in South Asia. There is huge inequity in maternal health within and between the high-, middle-, and low-income countries. I am keenly interested in addressing this inequity and bridging the gaps in improving maternal health through focusing on hypertension in pregnancy and cardiovascular diseases. I aspire to develop myself as an independent researcher and contribute to improving maternal health. Therefore, a Doctor of Philosophy in Nursing Degree (PhD) at this time is the right next step for me to achieve my professional goal.

I was born and brought up in the eastern part of Nepal. Situated within the Himalayas, Nepal is deeply entwined into a multifaceted cultural tapestry. The Nepalese population is divided into four main castes: Brahmin, Kshatriya, Vaishya, and Shudra; Brahmin is considered the highest caste, and Shudra is the lowest caste [22]. Further, Nepal is divided into 36 subcastes and consists of 125 ethnic groups [23]. This historical and deeply woven caste system is a social structure that has for centuries shaped people's opportunities, lives, and health outcomes and is central to this tapestry. However, discussion of this caste system is a sensitive area and inequities derived from this system are the sensitive areas leading to disparities that need to be approached carefully. In addition to growing up in a socially divisive environment, I am the first generation in my family to complete graduate-level studies and now starting a PhD program in one of the renowned universities in the southeastern USA with support from my parents and brother. However, I come from a society where women are oppressed and discriminated against with regard to education, income, and access to health. Many women my age still do not get the opportunity to pursue a high school education, and the thought of a graduate-level education is far-fetched. I would say growing up, the social determinants of health (SDOH) were a familiar aspect of my life, and I am somewhat familiar with this concept and the ways in which these influences are apparent in societies. However, it was interesting to learn from this course the categorization of SDOH into four pillars: (1) social, (2) environmental, (3) cultural, and (4) policy [3]. This insight offered a systematic framework to comprehend the complex network of factors shaping health outcomes, which are frequently under-discussed. The lectures from knowledgeable instructors from the SDOH course in my PhD program provided a wealth of knowledge on many facets of the SDOH, how they affect health outcomes, and the importance of incorporating these concepts in research studies.

As I was interested in the increased risk of cardiovascular diseases in women with hypertensive disorders in pregnancy, I am finding through reading the literature that hypertensive disorders in pregnancy are more prevalent in Black women [24, 25]. Therefore, the class lectures drew my attention toward the structural and systemic factors influencing this disorder. With my experience in the field of maternal health and experience in maternal health research, this SDOH course inspired me to have a pivotal realization of the critical role of implicit bias as a structural factor that contributes to the increased risk of cardiovascular diseases in women who had hypertensive disorders in pregnancy. However, this is an understudied topic. In my opinion, although this topic is understudied, it is profoundly present almost everywhere in the healthcare system and is considered one of the emerging issues in healthcare. My research aims to shed light on how implicit bias as SDOH contribute to the increased risk of cardiovascular diseases in Black women after hypertensive disorder in pregnancy. My goal is to also illustrate how critical it is to address these often-overlooked social determinants of health for the improvement of maternal health.

4 Addressing the Social Determinants of Health to Mitigate Health Disparities Among Older Adults by Jiyoon Jang

Their numbers are on the rise, while the support struggles to keep pace with their growth.

I have developed a strong scholarly interest in geriatric nursing from my professional and research-related experiences. During my four-

and-a-half years as a nurse in the medical-surgical unit, I frequently cared for older patients with dementia who visited the hospital for surgical treatment. They generally contended that support for patients with dementia was insufficient. Their caregivers were concerned about how to care for the patients after they were discharged. Specifically, they expressed apprehension regarding the potential emergence of further complications in addition to the challenges they were already encountering in their daily care. Even though I knew the discharge instructions for surgery, the scarcity of targeted educational resources for these patients precluded me from informing caregivers about the anticipated difficulties and available assistance. It dawned on me that constant attention and care are critical for people with dementia and their family caregivers. As a result of this experience, I have become motivated to focus my research on the proper care approaches for older adults with dementia and their caregivers in community settings.

Given my clinical background in medical-surgical nursing, my interest in the older population has driven me to work at the Mo-Im Kim Nursing Research Institute in Korea. This Research Institute was established to achieve a healthy aging society by addressing major social concerns, such as dementia, by developing customized therapies and aging-friendly technology. As a research assistant, I was involved in various research using information and communications technology (ICT) that addressed behavioral and psychological symptoms of dementia (BPSD) among community-dwelling older adults with dementia. When I participated in developing an individualized digital care application for managing BPSD, I collected data for evaluating the acceptance of this intervention by participants. Through this project, I became aware of the caregivers' strong demand for effective programs at home. Most caregivers of people with dementia were family members who resided together. They needed interventions to manage care recipients' behavioral and psychological symptoms and alleviate their caregiving burden, which had a profound impact on the families' daily lives and

caregivers' physical and mental health. The caregivers expressed their sincere appreciation for the approaches that supported them in this circumstance. Drawing from these firsthand experiences, I aim to increase my knowledge of ways to facilitate the implementation of beneficial strategies to improve health outcomes for these dementia care dyads. My goal is to ultimately reduce health inequity among this population during my PhD program.

4.1   Above the Seen, in Realms Unseen

In the current academic term, I examined the facilitators and obstacles to social support for older adults with dementia and their caregivers in the community. Initially, my focus centered on individual-level factors, including the cognitive level and severity of behavioral and psychological symptoms of dementia (BPSD) in older adults, the caregiver's attitudes toward social support needs, and the extent of their social network. However, my perspective underwent a substantial change through my engagement in a social determinants of health (SDOH) course, where I explored the four pillars of SDOH (social, environmental, cultural, and policy) [3]. Esteemed researchers provided insights into how each of these four pillars could impact health outcomes and their integration into research through classes. This educational experience significantly enhanced my understanding of the complex connections between SDOH and disparities in health outcomes.

In the four-pillar SDOH structure, I concentrated mainly on the environmental component. The social environment is characterized as the societal context and settings shaped by human influence, encompassing critical social settings associated with health equity, such as housing conditions, the accessibility of affordable transportation, and family composition. For example, a realization occurred recalling a study involving the dementia care dyad, where environmental conditions—among other pillars—played a crucial influence. The family that resided on the third floor encountered challenges due to a steep staircase, leading to a fall occurrence that constrained the older adult's mobility and participation in community programs. The incident brought to light the importance of housing conditions for health outcomes, particularly concerning sedentary behavior and decreased social engagement, which are associated with lower cognitive performance. This recognition prompted me to question whether various studies adequately investigate environmental conditions when examining socioeconomic status (SES) with key variables.

Recognizing the gap, I took the opportunity to broaden my perspective on SDOH, leading to a deeper understanding of issues related to health equity among older adults. This, in turn, facilitated the planning of a comprehensive examination of social determinants of health, focusing on health behaviors, social support, and their changes before and after a dementia diagnosis.

5   Health Equity in Oncological Nursing: Leveraging mHealth and Social Determinants for Underserved Cancer Survivors by Hyein Kim

I am a first-year PhD student and an international student from South Korea. This marks my initial exposure to education in the USA, coinciding with my residence in the USA. My research interest stems from my experience as a staff nurse in the head and neck cancer ward in South Korea, where I encountered many cancer survivors navigating the challenges of diagnosis, treatment, and rehabilitation.

While working as a staff nurse in a head and neck cancer ward in South Korea, I witnessed many cancer survivors who went through a difficult time during diagnosis, treatment, and rehabilitation. Although direct nursing care could help them recover from illness, I realized that scientific evidence did not fully support the patients after their discharge and fundamental

changes in oncological nursing science were needed. This realization forms the basis of my primary research goal: to enhance patient-centered outcomes for cancer survivors through behavioral modification using mobile health (mHealth). I was interested in how mHealth technology contributes to an individual's behavior change for better treatment and rehabilitation during their trajectory with cancer. During my dedication as a graduate research assistant in South Korea, I actively contributed to nursing research involving mHealth for adults at risk of suicide. This involvement included the development of a mobile app utilizing ecological momentary assessment to gauge psychological health in this vulnerable population. I advocate for the incorporation of scientific evidence and user-centered strategies in the development and implementation of mHealth interventions, particularly for at-risk groups like cancer survivors.

Mobile devices have become deeply embedded in our daily lives. Nursing research utilizing mHealth and related technology has contributed to helping people live better in their communities in terms of personalized care, timely communication with medical staff, and tailored symptom management for cancer survivors. I believed that considering current healthcare consumers and the Internet computer technology environment condition, it is important to use these resources and implement those resources in nursing research.

5.1   Current Research Interests

The course taken this semester in my PhD program, "Determinants of Human Health," introduced students to the four pillars of social determinants of health (SDoH) framework: social, cultural, environmental, and policy [3]. Guest speakers elaborated on their research within each pillar, emphasizing the influence of SDoH on the research process. This exposure prompted two key realizations.

Firstly, the importance of considering SDOH as a crucial factor in research became evident. An example was provided by a speaker investigating solutions to problems arising from heat in farmers' working environments and its impact on their health. This highlighted the significance of recognizing the influence of the environment on the health status of diverse communities within our society. Secondly, the course inspired me to incorporate a focus on healthcare access, particularly within the social pillar, into my research. My previous clinical experience and research for adults at risk of suicide in the community did not afford many opportunities to contemplate healthcare access. However, the course prompted me to consider scenarios where individuals, residing in specific geographical areas, might require monthly healthcare visits and how mHealth could facilitate health monitoring in such settings. This addition enriched the social dimension of my research. Each class in the course covered crucial aspects of the four SDOH pillars. For someone accustomed to an environment where SDOH is infrequently utilized in nursing, this class proved invaluable in broadening my understanding of the USA and nursing practices.

A particular focus within the SDOH pillars that I also aim to explore further is the social pillar, encompassing health literacy and access to healthcare. While acknowledging the importance of the culture, environment, and policy pillars, I recognize that, in the context of mHealth, the social pillar provides a link to those in need of resources such as communication methods (e.g., mobile apps) to address their health outcomes. This decision marks a subtle shift in my population of interest, transitioning from a broad focus on "cancer survivors" to a more nuanced consideration of "underserved cancer survivors." Notably, the determination of the medically underserved population (MUP) by the Health Resources and Service Administration relies on several criteria, one of which is the ratio of primary care physicians per 1000 populations. I firmly believe that integrating the "social pillar" into my research interest will yield significant benefits. By intertwining the social pillar with my research topic, I anticipate that individuals in marginalized areas, particularly cancer survivors, will experience enhanced outcomes derived from my research.

6 Is Health Information Technology the Missing Puzzle Piece to Addressing the Social Determinants of Health in the Maternal Health Crises? by Kaprice Welsh

More than 12 years ago, the public health community became aware of the maternal health crises in this country with the release of Amnesty International's Article, Deadly Delivery: The Maternal Health Crises in the USA [26]. It is surprising that since the publishing of this report, we have not made significant improvements in outcomes for Black birthing women. In those years, I worked in public health with maternal and child health policymakers and stakeholders on strategies to address Georgia's maternal morbidity and mortality crises. During that time, I also worked as a midwife within the healthcare system where I saw firsthand some of the ways that Black bodies were not respected. I have witnessed firsthand where their voices were overshadowed by nurses and doctors who felt they knew what was best for them. I could see in their experiences that implicit biases were prevalent. Comments were made in the nurse's station with reference to Black fathers as "baby daddy's" and never the patient's husband, the labeling of Black women as "difficult" when they objected to delivering in certain positions or questioned the language on informed consent documents, and even belittling comments when they objected to their babies receiving vitamin K. These comments all invoked a stereotypical characterization that Black women were difficult. Since my colleagues believed they were treating these patients like "everyone else," they should be grateful for the care that they received. These scenarios of implicit bias played out consistently in labor and delivery wards. Black colleagues who worked in these wards talked about the bias and disrespect that they also witnessed in the care delivered to these women. I was in a unique position to see that there was a disconnect between the care delivered by the healthcare system to improve birth outcomes for Black birthing women and what public health organizations believed was needed to improve these outcomes. The healthcare system looked to implement safety bundles (blueprints) to address some of the top contributors to maternal morbidity and mortality, like hemorrhage and hypertension. However, public health organizations (i.e., American Public Health Association) looked to integrate implicit bias training for healthcare and community health workers to address systemic racism at the system level to improve outcomes for Black women.

As I entered into the Nell Hodgson Woodruff School of Nursing PhD program, I knew that I wanted to focus my work on Black maternal morbidity and mortality. I wanted to focus on policy and system-level changes that could be made to improve the Black birth experience and adverse outcomes. Coming into the program, my research interest was to look at using health information technology tools (HIT) as a strategy to address some of the key drivers of maternal morbidity and mortality during the postpartum period to address the "upstream factors" impacting maternal morbidity and mortality among Back birthing women. I knew that Black women died at two to three times that of White women from cardiovascular diseases. Health information technology (HIT) could potentially be a transformative force for delivering safe healthcare to women across the healthcare spectrum. I believed that leveraging HIT tools to target the underlying drivers of racial disparities at the patient, clinician, healthcare system, and community levels could potentially improve the quality of care throughout the continuum (antepartum, intrapartum, and postpartum) of maternity care. I anticipated that the use of technology like mobile apps, telehealth, and web-based health platforms would permit a timelier triage of potential patient problems and decrease inappropriate emergency room visits or hospital readmissions. This level of patient engagement through technology is grounded in behavioral science principles and allows us to look beyond the "clinical picture." The engagement of patients through technology might also provide insight into how the intersectionality of social

determinants of health (SDOH) conditions is driving racial disparities seen in maternal morbidity and mortality outcomes.

6.1 Conceptualizing the SDOH Framework

During my first semester in the program, I was able to take a class focusing specifically on the social determinants of health. This course has provided a framework that has helped me contextualize how the social determinants of health contribute to the poor outcomes experienced by Black birthing women. In looking back at my initial research interests, I now understand that I will need to look beyond the universality of maternal morbidity and mortality and focus more on the intersectionality of the multiple forms of discrimination that women experience across the Black birth experience that are contributing to the adverse outcomes. In utilizing the SDOH framework addressed in *Integrating a Social Determinants of Health Framework Into Nursing Education* [3], which consists of the four pillars of SDOH—social, cultural, environment, (physical and social), and policy—I can more fully understand how the intersecting forms of social disadvantage and marginalization are linked to the poor health outcomes experienced by Black birthing women. According to the Four-Pillar SDOH Framework, the social conditions are those factors that occur in society due to systemic (structural) racism and imbalances in power, financial resources, education, and occupation that influence wellness or lack thereof [3]. Furthermore, the social conditions, shaped by power imbalances and systemic racism, include access to financial resources, education, type of occupation, health literacy, access to healthcare, and social support as a social resource. The SDOH implications for my research are apparent as social conditions. In looking at the drivers of the healthcare inequities, we cannot ignore the influence that racism/implicit bias, cultural background, social class, and one's social environment (SDOH) have on these maternal outcomes.

6.2   Leveraging HIT in Healthcare to Address SDOH

By leveraging health information technologies, we should be able to mitigate the social conditions that contribute to these disparities by increasing access to care. For example, the ability to provide remote visits for routine prenatal care or postpartum follow-up serves to eliminate barriers to access to healthcare, like inconsistent transportation or childcare issues. When examining why Black women experience such high rates of maternal morbidity and mortality, we must take into account the compounding effects of the SDOH on the Black experience: for example, limited access to consistently affordable healthcare, lack of quality high-earning jobs, lack of adequate housing located in areas in close proximity to high-quality healthcare facilities, institutional racism/implicit bias practices and policies, and the lack of cultural congruent providers. These social and structural inequities are pervasive across this country and cannot be ignored as major contributors to the high maternal morbidity and mortality rates.

Nurses and clinicians can play a pivotal role in utilizing strategies like HIT to enhance patient engagement and improve adherence to clinical guidelines by connecting with moms during the pregnancy and the postpartum period to address their clinical and social needs. Since the COVID-19 pandemic, we have seen a rise in innovation in the healthcare setting, from the implementation of telehealth visits for routine obstetric care, wearable tracking devices, and mobile health technology to remote home blood pressure monitoring programs, all in an effort to enhance clinical care and treatment. It is my hope that the use of HIT to address the intersectionality of women's health and SDOH will help to mitigate unintended consequences and address the persistent racial disparities seen throughout the continuum of maternity care so that Black women can thrive.

References

1. The National LGBT Cancer Network. The national LGBT cancer network. Providence, RI; 2023. https://cancer-network.org/?gclid=EAIaIQobChMIzvSirPzhggMV7TnUAR3WJQHWEAAYASAAEgJTQ_D_BwE.
2. National Academies of Sciences, Engineering, and Medicine. Understanding the well-being of LGBTQI+ populations. Washington, DC: The National Academies Press; 2020. https://doi.org/10.17226/25877.
3. Hamilton JB. Integrating a social determinants of health framework into nursing education. In: Hamilton JB, Swan BA, McCauley L, editors. Integrating a social determinants of health framework into nursing education. Cham: Springer International Publishing; 2023. p. 9–53.
4. Griggs J, Maingi S, Blinder V, Denduluri N, Khorana AA, Norton L, Francisco M, Wollins DS, Rowland JH. American Society of Clinical Oncology position statement: strategies for reducing cancer health disparities among sexual and gender minority populations. J Clin Oncol. 2017;35(19):2203–8. https://doi.org/10.1200/JCO.2016.72.0441.
5. Meites E, Wilkin TJ, Markowitz LE. Review of human papillomavirus (HPV) burden and HPV vaccination for gay, bisexual, and other men who have sex with men and transgender women in the United States. Hum Vaccin Immunother. 2022;18(1):2016007. https://doi.org/10.1080/21645515.2021.2016007.
6. Azagba S, Shan L, Latham K. Overweight and obesity among sexual minority adults in the United States. Int J Environ Res Public Health. 2019;16(10):1828. https://doi.org/10.3390/ijerph16101828.
7. Green KE, Feinstein BA. Substance use in lesbian, gay, and bisexual populations: an update on empirical research and implications for treatment. Psychol Addict Behav J Soc Psychol Addict Behav. 2012;26(2):265–78. https://doi.org/10.1037/a0025424.
8. Quinn GP, Sanchez JA, Sutton SK, Vadaparampil ST, Nguyen GT, Green BL, Kanetsky PA, Schabath MB. Cancer and lesbian, gay, bisexual, transgender/transsexual, and queer/questioning (LGBTQ) populations: cancer and sexual minorities. CA Cancer J Clin. 2015;65(5):384–400. https://doi.org/10.3322/caac.21288.
9. Tamargo CL, Quinn GP, Sanchez JA, Schabath MB. Cancer and the LGBTQ population: quantitative and qualitative results from an oncology providers' survey on knowledge, attitudes, and practice behaviors. J Clin Med. 2017;6(10):93. https://doi.org/10.3390/jcm6100093.

10. Bostwick WB, Boyd CJ, Hughes TL, McCabe SE. Dimensions of sexual orientation and the prevalence of mood and anxiety disorders in the United States. Am J Public Health. 2010;100(3):468–75. https://doi.org/10.2105/AJPH.2008.152942.

11. Nepon J, Belik S-L, Bolton J, Sareen J. The relationship between anxiety disorders and suicide attempts: findings from the National Epidemiologic Survey on alcohol and related conditions. Depress Anxiety. 2010;27(9):791–8. https://doi.org/10.1002/da.20674.

12. King M, Semlyen J, Tai SS, Killaspy H, Osborn D, Popelyuk D, Nazareth I. A systematic review of mental disorder, suicide, and deliberate self harm in lesbian, gay and bisexual people. BMC Psychiatry. 2008;8(1):70. https://doi.org/10.1186/1471-244X-8-70.

13. Kirakosian N, Stanton AM, McKetchnie SM, King D, Dolotina B, O'Cleirigh C, Grasso C, Potter J, Mayer KH, Batchelder AW. Suicidal ideation disparities among transgender and gender diverse compared to cisgender community health patients. J Gen Intern Med. 2023;38:1357. https://doi.org/10.1007/s11606-022-07996-2.

14. Rodriguez-Seijas C, Fields EC, Bottary R, Kark SM, Goldstein MR, Kensinger EA, Payne JD, Cunningham TJ. Comparing the impact of COVID-19-related social distancing on mood and psychiatric indicators in sexual and gender minority (SGM) and non-SGM individuals. Front Psych. 2020;11:590318. https://doi.org/10.3389/fpsyt.2020.590318.

15. Meleis A. Theoretical nursing: development & progress. 5th ed. Philadelphia: Lippincott Williams & Wilkins, Wolters Kluwer; 2012.

16. Meyer IH. Minority stress and mental health in gay men. J Health Soc Behav. 1995;36(1):38–56. https://doi.org/10.2307/2137286.

17. Meyer IH. Prejudice, social stress, and mental health in lesbian, gay, and bisexual populations: conceptual issues and research evidence. Psychol Bull. 2003;129(5):674–97. https://doi.org/10.1037/0033-2909.129.5.674.

18. Kneale D, Henley J, Thomas J, French R. Inequalities in older LGBT people's health and care needs in the United Kingdom: a systematic scoping review. Ageing Soc. 2021;41(3):493–515. https://doi.org/10.1017/S0144686X19001326.

19. World Health Organization. World Health Organization (WHO) statement, the prevention and elimination of disrespect and abuse during facility-based childbirth. WHO/RHR/14.23; 2015.

20. Bohren M, Vogel J, Hunter E, Lutsiv O, Makh S, Souza J, et al. The mistreatment of women during childbirth in health facilities globally: a mixed-methods systematic review. PLoS Med. 2015;12(6):e1001847. https://doi.org/10.1371/journal.pmed.1001847.

21. Vedam S, Stoll K, Taiwo TK, Rubashkin N, Cheyney M, Strauss N, McLemore M, Cadena M, Nethery E, Rushton E, Schummers L, Declercq E, the GVtM-US Steering Council. The giving voice to mothers study: inequity and mistreatment during pregnancy and childbirth in the United States. Reprod Health. 2019;16(77):1–18. https://doi.org/10.1186/s12978-019-0729-2.

22. Caste System in Nepal. Wikipedia 2023. https://en.wikipedia.org/w/index.php?title=Caste_system_in_Nepal&oldid=1182498560.

23. Ethnic Groups in Nepal. Wikipedia. 2023. https://en.wikipedia.org/w/index.php?title=Ethnic_groups_in_Nepal&oldid=1186060522.

24. Burger RJ, Delagrange H, van Valkengoed IGM, de Groot CJM, van den Born B-JH, Gordijn SJ, Ganzevoort W. Hypertensive disorders of pregnancy and cardiovascular disease risk across races and ethnicities: a review. Front Cardiovasc Med. 2022;9:933822. https://doi.org/10.3389/fcvm.2022.933822.

25. Ford ND, Cox S, Ko JY, Ouyang L, Romero L, Colarusso T, Ferre CD, Kroelinger CD, Hayes DK, Barfield WD. Hypertensive disorders in pregnancy and mortality at delivery hospitalization—United States, 2017–2019. Morb Mortal Wkly Rep. 2022;71(17):585.

26. Amnesty International. Deadly delivery: the maternal health care crisis in the USA one year update. New York, NY; 2011. https://www.amnesty.org/en/wp-content/uploads/2021/06/amr510072010en.pdf.

John A. Fuller is a Centennial Scholar, George W. Woodruff Fellow, and doctoral student in the Nell Hodgson Woodruff School of Nursing at Emory University, in addition to being a Building Research Inclusion and Diversity in Graduate Education (BRIDGE) Scholar in the Department of Population Health Sciences at Duke University. Originally from Akron, OH, he is an alumnus of The Ohio State University, where he earned a BS in Human Development and Family Science, magna cum laude, with honors research distinction, a minor in Global Public Health, and a certificate in Health Communication. Daring to end health disparities and achieve health equity for all, his interdisciplinary research training is informed by his interests in examining how social determinants of health influence population-level health outcomes for Black LGBTQ+ cancer survivors. His high-impact, award-winning scholarship is nationally recognized, including support from the National Cancer Institute (NCI) and the National LGBT Cancer Network.

Renée Byfield MS, RN, FNP, C-EFM, is currently a doctoral student at Emory University, Nell Hodgson Woodruff School of Nursing. Ms. Byfield is a professional with diverse experience in obstetric and neonatal care. As a nationally recognized speaker and birth equity coach, she dedicates her efforts to assisting perinatal healthcare teams in developing strategies for achieving birth equity. Her research interest is in obstetric violence and the intersectionality of racism, gender-based violence, and the unequal power dynamics present in provider–patient relationships. Passionate about leveraging data science, Ms. Byfield collaborates with healthcare professionals to raise awareness about the impact of social determinants of health on outcomes and strives to address this human rights issue.

Seema Das is a clinically trained nurse with almost 4 years of research experience in mixed methods study. She completed a Bachelor of Science in Nursing from Nursing Campus Maharajgunj, Institute of Medicine in Nepal, and worked as a clinical nurse in the maternal and child health division at Tribhuvan University Teaching Hospital, Nepal. She graduated with a master's in public health from UiT The Arctic University of Norway. She is keenly interested in addressing the inequity and bridging the gaps to improve maternal health by focusing on hypertension disorder in pregnancy and maternal cardiovascular health.

Jiyoon Jang MSN, RN, is a graduate student at Emory University, Nell Hodgson Woodruff School of Nursing. She has developed a strong scholarly interest in geriatric nursing and has a deep passion for providing age-appropriate, individualized care for older adults. Her background as a registered nurse on a surgical-oncology floor motivated her to focus on effective care approaches for older adults and their caregivers. She expanded her knowledge by participating in gerontological research projects at the Mo-Im Kim Nursing Research Institute in South Korea, which conducts various research projects on aging health science. As a research assistant at this insti-

tute, she witnessed caregivers' high burden of caring for people with dementia and the significant impact on their families' daily lives. Through her doctoral program at Emory University, she hopes to develop strategies for addressing health problems and reducing caregiver burden among older adults with dementia and their caregivers.

Hyein Kim MSN, RN, is a PhD student at Emory University, focusing her expertise on the intricate realm of head and neck cancer research. With bachelor's and master's degrees in nursing from South Korea, she brings a wealth of experience from 3 years of dedicated care for head and neck cancer patients. Her passion lies in revealing the potential implications of mobile health to significantly impact the lives of head and neck cancer patients and survivors while diligently addressing the pervasive health disparities within this community.

Kaprice Welsh CNM, MSN, MPH, is a certified nurse midwife who has worked in women's health care for over 30 years. She holds a Bachelor of Science degree in Nursing from Syracuse University, a Master of Science degree in Nursing, a Certificate in Midwifery, and a Master of Public Health degree from Columbia University. Currently, she is a doctoral student at Emory University's Nell Hodgson Woodruff School of Nursing where she plans to focus her doctoral studies on improving morbidity and mortality for black birthing women.

Transforming Social Determinants of Health: Insights and Future Directions

Jill B. Hamilton, Lalita M. Kaligotla,
Autherine Abiri, Diana Baptiste, Nakia C. Best,
Angie Haynes-Ferere, Jacob K. Kariuki,
Charles E. Moore, and Catherine M. Waters

Social determinants of health (SDOH) conditions can increase or decrease the risk for illness and life expectancy among individuals, populations, communities, and even larger societies. There are a number of recently published books on SDOH; however, none emphasize **global** programs that have been implemented and are being evaluated in marginalized and/or low-resource global communities. Another distinctive feature of this book is the contribution to the evidence on SDOH from not only academic researchers but also clinicians, community partners and stakeholders, and leaders of faith-based institutions. This book addresses the need for scholarly works that include a range of voices—researchers, clinicians, people who work in the community, and leaders of faith-based institutions in various phases of developing, implementing, and evaluating programs that address the well-being, health inequities, and health disparities among marginalized and/or low-resource communities. For ease of reading, we have organized the chapters in this book according to the Nell Hodgson Woodruff Four-Pillar SDOH Framework of social, cultural, environmental (physical and social), and policy conditions.

We anticipate this book will contribute to a diverse perspective on the possibilities of incorporating SDOH into communities and faith-based institutions. Hopefully, long-term outputs will be to inform, inspire, and encourage the novice and senior researcher and clinician, community stakeholder, and faith-based institutional leader to develop, implement, and evaluate the SDOH (cultural, social, environmental, and political conditions) on health and health disparities among marginalized and/or low-resource global communities.

In this book, we were able to include **global** community-based programs that have been implemented. These community-based programs that incorporate the SDOH represent US communities in rural, urban-inner city, southern,

J. B. Hamilton (✉) · L. M. Kaligotla · A. Abiri
A. Haynes-Ferere · J. K. Kariuki
Nell Hodgson Woodruff School of Nursing, Emory University, Atlanta, GA, USA
e-mail: jbhamil@emory.edu;
Lalita.kaligotla@emory.edu; autherine.abiri@emoryhealthcare.org; angela.haynes-ferere@emory.edu; Jacob.kariuki@emory.edu

D. Baptiste
School of Nursing, Johns Hopkins University, Baltimore, MD, USA
e-mail: dbaptis1@jhu.edu

N. C. Best
Sue and Bill Gross School of Nursing, University of California, Irvine, Irvine, CA, USA
e-mail: nbest@hs.uci.edu

C. E. Moore
Emory University School of Medicine, Emory University, Atlanta, GA, USA
e-mail: cemoore@emory.edu

C. M. Waters
School of Nursing, University of California, San Francisco, San Francisco, CA, USA
e-mail: Catherine.waters@ucsf.edu

© The Author(s), under exclusive license to Springer Nature Switzerland AG 2024
J. B. Hamilton, C. E. Moore (eds.), *Transforming Social Determinants to Promote Global Health*,
https://doi.org/10.1007/978-3-031-61160-5_38

northeastern, and western geographical regions as well as international communities, such as Botswana, Ethiopia, Ghana, Kenya, Malawi, Nigeria, and the Grenadines.

Although the Four-Pillar SDOH Framework categorizes the social, cultural, environmental, and policy conditions as concepts that appear distinct from each other, in reality, they are interwoven. In this book, we saw this interwovenness in the work of our contributing authors. In the Four-Pillar SDOH Framework, *the Social Pillar* considers factors that occur in society due to systemic (structural) racism and imbalances in power, financial resources, education, and occupation that influence wellness or lack thereof [1]. For example, within the Social Pillar section, even though the focus of the chapters was on inequities in social conditions, it was also apparent that social conditions also intersect with the cultural and social environmental pillars. This was especially evident in the chapters examining the influences of sociodemographic factors on birth outcome inequalities, where the lead authors from Ethiopia and Botswana brought our attention to the cultural influences that shaped those social factors. Similarly, in the chapter on the SDOH influences on chronic stress and increased risk of heart disease among early midlife African American women, the lead author from the Nell Hodgson Woodruff School of Nursing brought our attention to the interwovenness of social factors, such as wage and wealth inequities that intersect with the social environmental influences from living in impoverished neighborhoods.

The Cultural Pillar considers those customary beliefs, social norms, attitudes, values, and practices shared by a group of people (community or society) in a place and time with regard to health and healthcare [1]. Chapters in this section illustrate community-engaged work related to cultural determinants related to minority health and health disparities in historically underrepresented, racialized, and low-resource communities. Topics within this pillar highlight that SDOH influences can be a source of strength and health-promoting, not merely adverse influences that increase one's risk of disease. For example, faith-based storytelling as a SDOH can promote health,

decrease a person's psychological distress when diagnosed with cancer, and illustrate the historical influence of storytelling for survival in addition to the interwovenness of the religious practice of singing hymns in faith-based institutions. In another chapter, led by an author from the Nell Hodgson Woodruff School of Nursing describes the cultural influence on the increased risk for cardiovascular disease and the need for culturally salient assessment tools and interventions for underserved and high-risk populations in the United States (USA) and Africa.

The Physical Environmental Pillar considers physical, chemical, and biological conditions of the Earth's natural environment that contribute to health inequities and health disparities [1]. Chapters included exemplars of programs implemented to address factors in the physical environment, such as pollution, airborne diseases, and climate change. One lead author from Harvard University describes the process of mapping and modeling an ecological determinant of a vector-borne disease risk from human *African Trypanosomiasis*. In another chapter led by a Spellman University faculty, we learn from the work of an environmental scientist strategies to address environmental injustices and health inequities.

The Social Environmental Pillar considers those conditions influenced by social surroundings and type of relationships (within social settings and institutions) [1]. These chapters included exemplars of programs implemented to address factors in the social environment such increasing access to faith-based institutions and expanding social networks to better access healthcare systems for our aging populations. For example, in the chapter authored by a team at UC Irvine titled "SDOH and school nurse-led interventions: Improving health and education outcomes among school aged children and adolescents," we learn about the importance of nurses in the school environment, where children and adolescents spend a significant amount of time. Schools are opportune settings where school nurses can provide health services that students may not otherwise have access to and help to ensure students have a safe and equitable environment to learn. School nurses are in a unique position to help mitigate the SDOH that impacts students and their families and support them so they may thrive and live healthy lives.

The Policy Pillar considers those guidelines, principles, legislation, and political activities that affect the living conditions conducive to the welfare and quality of life of individuals, populations, communities, and societies [1]. Chapters included in this pillar were written by authors actively involved in policy at the state and national levels, who provided exemplars of programs implemented to address policy specifically in low-resource communities. Ways in which the community should inform policy and ultimately policy should improve the community, particularly as it relates to reenvisioning the SDOH to reimagine population health interventions in mutual collaboration with private and public partnerships.

A particular concept threaded throughout this book revolves around multidisciplinary team-based care, forming the cornerstone for each highlighted approach. The contributions from a diverse group of academic researchers, students, and community members provided a clear lens to the SDOH and community engagement that shifts us apart from an isolated approach of working in silos, particularly within socially vulnerable communities. Moreover, collaborating in teams that include community partners has proven to be an effective strategy, leading to reduced hospitalizations, decreased morbidity, and lower mortality rates, globally. Despite this successful approach, multidisciplinary teams of researchers from diverse disciplines, practitioners, and community partners with expertise in their respective areas may not have regular interactions and may still operate in isolation. The aim is to sustain these transdisciplinary team-based approaches, fostering connections and collaborations within communities while acknowledging the influence of SDOH in crafting effective interventions.

In many chapters in this book, we have witnessed the ways in which authors engaged in a transdisciplinary approach by involving nontraditional healthcare partners, such as community

health workers, local community leaders, and faith-based leaders into the development, implementation, and evaluation of community programs that considered SDOH influences on health disparities and inequities. One example of this transdisciplinary approach was apparent in the chapter that focused on examining digital and health literacy within an inner city among researchers at the Johns Hopkins University School of Nursing. In another chapter titled, *Engaged Scholarship on the Family's Role as a Proximal Health Resource for LGBTQ+ Adolescents*, researchers at the University of Pennsylvania School of Nursing used a transdisciplinary approach that included researchers, students, and community partners. The composition of these transdisciplinary teams extends beyond the boundaries of medicine, public health, and nursing, encompassing collaborative partnerships within the broader community.

While this transdisciplinary approach represents a substantial undertaking, oftentimes spanning multiple settings and requiring substantial resources and funding, it is essential to note that smaller transdisciplinary teams can also thrive within a single setting. This adaptability of a transdisciplinary approach is particularly valuable when integrating community-based outreach and research activities. The specific role of nurses, for example, within these teams may vary depending on their scope of practice, which can differ from one state or country to another. Nevertheless, generally and particularly in the context of community engagement, nurses and other scientists from other disciplines are increasingly encouraged to assume leadership roles, advocate for patients, and foster collaboration among clinicians and community members.

1 The Benefit of Engaging Students

As we have highlighted in this book, engagement with the community is a vital avenue for student education and development. By providing opportunities for community engagement, we enabled students to develop relevant professional, clinical, social, and advocacy skills as well as experiential learning to develop interpersonal skills for professional success. Through engaging with diverse communities and community members, students witnessed firsthand different lived experiences and the differential impacts that these lived experiences had on the health and well-being of individuals, populations, and communities. This form of active learning, in turn, enables students to become better providers of healthcare and more thoughtful and engaged advocates for public health and social justice.

As we have demonstrated through several exemplars featured throughout this book, building sustainable and mutually beneficial relationships with communities is crucial for addressing the SDOH. Collaborating with community partners and community members offers the potential to foster meaningful partnerships, improve health outcomes, and promote health equity for underserved populations and communities. We shared many best practices that we have learned through our own community engagement efforts that we hope will be useful to others engaged in similar work—practitioners, educators, and scholars engaged in community-based work. Below, we highlight in brief a few of these lessons, particularly from the vantage of engaging students in community-based work.

Working Toward a Shared Vision: A lesson that has been reinforced time and again is that alignment with the vision and aspirations of communities is essential for community-engagement work to be effective and just. Students' work with communities that is most efficacious was when they were in active partnership with community members and partner organizations to find a common purpose. We found that helping students see and understand the needs of the communities they serve and the differential impacts of the SDOH contributes to seeking sustainable change.

Focusing on and Facilitating Trust: History is a constant reminder of the importance of building trust and mutuality with communities and their residents. We attempted to highlight this through the many exemplars we have shared in this book. Relationships based on trust and mutual respect are a foundational element of working toward

health equity. Active and respectful engagement with community members, listening to their needs and perspectives with empathy, and involving them in decision-making processes help establish trust and ensures sustainable partnerships. Culturally and linguistically appropriate engagement, along with an asset-based approach, are also important for successful long-term collaborations.

Openness and Honesty of Communications: Open communication, humility, and coordination with those closest to the issues are vital—those most proximal to the issues being tackled are often best equipped to identify solutions. Students are encouraged to communicate frequently with community members for information sharing, feedback, and ongoing support. The students' participation in this book fosters learning opportunities for students and helps build reciprocal networks between academic health centers, civil society organizations, and community members affected by the issues being addressed.

In summary, building collaborations, community, and continuity is crucial to effective and ethical community-engaged pedagogies and ultimately critical to addressing and mitigating the effects of the SDOH. Best practices in community-engaged pedagogies include helping students recognize the importance of building trust, finding a shared vision, and maintaining open communication with community members and community partners. By incorporating these practices, academic health systems, civil society organizations, and government institutions can collectively work toward achieving health equity and improving well-being for all.

2   The Benefit of Engaging a Diverse Group of Authors

We were intentional to include diversity in authors that include type of academic institution, northern and southern global geographic locations, and community partners. It has been especially important to include a diverse group of authors to ensure that the voices of the communities they represent are heard and especially to ensure that negative assumptions about these populations are minimized. Historically, US academic scholars have compared various aspects of the African American/Black lived experiences to those of non-Hispanic Whites without consideration for cultural differences, and these comparisons have resulted in the promotion of negative evaluations, misinformation, and stereotypes of these populations [2, 3]. For example, medical researchers who have considered the experiences of the dominant population of US Whites to African Americans/Blacks have made assumptions that there are biological differences and used these assumptions to justify societal attitudes and beliefs that African Americans/Blacks were an inferior racial group [2, 3]. As early as the late nineteenth and early twentieth centuries, researchers have used findings from these comparison studies to support the notion that African Americans/Blacks were inferior in their anatomy and socially deviant from other members of society [2, 3].

A focus on the SDOH from the lens of authors from diverse populations encourages us to challenge negative assumptions about these populations. The works of diverse scholars in collaboration with individuals in our communities are likely to consider the SDOH influences that affect one's culture or lived experiences. These SDOH influences are likely to extend beyond education and income levels to include factors, such as religious beliefs, work experience, geographic location, healthcare experiences, experiences with segregation and integration, and family structure, to name a few. Consideration of a broader range of SDOH influences from the lens of authors who are also members of their populations is likely to present a more accurate reality of the cultural values and attitudes handed down and adopted from generation to generation [4].

Historically, there has been an imbalance in scientific contributions with most of the data used to inform healthcare decisions being generated by researchers in countries of the global North. Even when studies are conducted in the global South, local investigators are not always involved in the generation and/or dissemination of the data

leading to scholarly parasitism [5, 6] We have embraced authors from the global South who have reached out to us to contribute to this book since we are aware that their contribution promotes mutual learning and an inclusive approach to knowledge creation and dissemination. The contribution from these authors also aims to strengthen research capacity in countries of the global South to accelerate the progress in addressing region-specific challenges related to health disparities. Moreover, the voices of these authors are important to scholars desiring better collaborations to ensure that the implementation of programs is relevant and sustainable to research initiatives in their respective regions. Their voices are also important to promote a better understanding and enhanced ability to navigate the sociocultural contexts in which any community program is conducted.

3 Future Directions

As we conclude this exploration of social determinants to promote global health through the lens of lived experiences, it is essential to contemplate potential future directions that the SDOH might take in the alleviation of health disparities and health inequities. We propose that next steps should include the consistent and widespread integration of the SDOH into clinical care in a variety of settings, such as hospitals, private medical offices, community and primary care clinics, and home health agencies, which we believe is crucial for providing holistic and population-centered healthcare that takes into consideration people's starting points across their life course. Here are a few examples:

- Screening and Assessment Protocols
  - This may involve the use of standardized questionnaires during intake assessments or electronic health record prompts that encourage healthcare providers to inquire about an individual's social circumstances.
  - Screening tools could cover various domains, such as housing stability, food security, employment status, transportation,

and social support. By systematically collecting this information, healthcare providers gain a comprehensive understanding of the social context in which people live, allowing for tailored- and contextual-care plans.

- Training Healthcare Providers in Trauma-Informed Care
  - Recognizing and addressing past trauma as a social determinant can enhance the effectiveness of clinical interventions and improve individual and population health outcomes.
- Care Coordination and Referrals
  - Establishing effective care coordination teams that include social workers, community health workers, and other allied health professionals can help address identified social determinants. These teams can work collaboratively with individuals, their families or significant others, and community organizations or advocacy groups as navigators to develop personalized care plans that consider their SDOH.
  - Referral networks can be created to connect patients and clients with community resources and support services. For instance, if housing instability is identified as a social determinant, a social worker can facilitate connections to local housing assistance programs or community groups and businesses that focus on housing people. This comprehensive approach recognizes that addressing health goes beyond healthcare treatments and includes social and environmental factors.
- Cultural Competency Training for Healthcare Providers
  - Ensuring that healthcare providers are culturally competent and sensitive to the diverse backgrounds of individuals and populations is essential. Training programs can be implemented to educate healthcare professionals on the impact of SDOH outcomes and equip them with the skills to communicate effectively with people from various sociocultural backgrounds.

- Healthcare providers can be trained to ask open-ended questions about patients' social circumstances, fostering a patient/client-provider relationship built on trust. Understanding cultural nuances can also aid in recognizing how social determinants may differ among populations and tailoring care plans accordingly.

Through the incorporation of these strategies, healthcare providers can move beyond traditional clinical models and address the broader determinants that influence the health and social outcomes of individuals, populations, and communities. This socioecologically centered approach acknowledges and responds to the complex interplay between social factors and the health outcomes of individuals and populations that can minimize health inequities and disparities across generations.

References

1. Hamilton JB. Integrating a social determinants of health framework into nursing education. In: Hamilton JB, Swan BA, McCauley L, editors. Integrating a social determinants of health framework into nursing education. Cham: Springer International Publishing; 2023. p. 9–53.
2. Collins PH. Black feminist thought. New York: Routledge, Chapman and Hall, Inc.; 1991.
3. Gamble VN. A legacy of distrust: African Americans and medical research. Am J Prev Med. 1993;9(6 Suppl):35–8. http://www.ncbi.nlm.nih.gov/entrez/query.fcgi?cmd=Retrieve&db=PubMed&dopt=Citation&list_uids=8123285.
4. Hill RB. The strengths of African-American families: twenty-five years later. Baltimore, MD: R & B Publishers; 1997.
5. Rees CA, Ali M, Kisenge R, Ideh RC, Sirna SJ, Britto CD, et al. Where there is no local author: a network bibliometric analysis of authorship parasitism among research conducted in sub-Saharan Africa. BMJ Glob Health. 2021;6(10):e006982. https://doi.org/10.1136/bmjgh-2021-006982.
6. Rees CA, Keating EM, Dearden KA, Haq H, Robison JA, Kazembe PN, et al. Importance of authorship and inappropriate authorship assignment in paediatric research in low- and middle-income countries. Trop Med Int Health. 2019;24(10):1229–42. https://doi.org/10.1111/tmi.13295.

Jill B. Hamilton PhD, MRPL, RN, FAAN, is Professor (tenured) and Senior Faculty Fellow of SDOH and Health Disparities at the Nell Hodgson Woodruff School of Nursing and Affiliate Professor at Candler School of Theology at Emory University in Atlanta, Georgia. Dr. Hamilton earned her BSN, MSN, and PhD in nursing from the University of North Carolina at Chapel Hill, a BS in Accounting from North Carolina Central University, postdoctoral training in the nursing care of older adults at the Oregon Health and Science University, and a Master's in Religion and Public Life at the Candler School of Theology. She previously held faculty positions at Johns Hopkins University and the University of North Carolina at Chapel Hill where she was a tenured Associate Professor. Dr. Hamilton's research interests include social determinants of health, health disparities, and the mental health promoting strategies used among older African American their families in response to life-threatening illness. Dr. Hamilton is Leading Editor of a text with Springer Nature titled *Integrating a Social Determinants of Health Framework into Nursing Education* published in 2023. She has done original research on the effects of storytelling that incorporates Black Sacred Music and scripture on psychological distress among older and younger African Americans. She was a Georgia Cancer Coalition Distinguished Cancer Scholar from 2003 to 2007 and a member of the 2014 Class of the UNC Thorp Faculty Engaged Scholars. Dr. Hamilton is currently a Fellow in the American Academy of Nursing and a Faculty Scholar of the Center for Spirituality, Theology and Health at Duke University. She was the recipient of the 2019 Distinguished Alumni Award from the School of Nursing at the University of North Carolina, the 2011 Oncology Nursing Society (ONS) Publishing's Division Award for Excellence in Writing Qualitative Research and the ONS 2023 Award for Excellence in Cancer Education. Dr. Hamilton was born and raised in the Southern Appalachian region of North Carolina.

Lalita M. Kaligotla PhD, MA, is Professor of the Practice and Senior Director for Leadership and Community Engagement at Emory University's Nell Hodgson Woodruff School of Nursing. Her work is centered on values-based leadership, social innovation, human-centered design, and community-based research. She currently envisions and implements leadership development programming for faculty, staff, and students as well as experiential, and interprofessional, experiences for students. She has a keen interest in addressing inequities in access to healthcare and health outcomes. She also serves as the faculty director for the Fuld Fellowship for Social Responsibility, a scholarship program designed to support high achieving nursing students with a strong commitment to civic engagement and social responsibility.

Autherine Abiri DNP, RN, is an Assistant Professor at Nell Hodgson Woodruff School of Nursing. She is a certified family and emergency nurse practitioner. In 2009, Dr. Abiri obtained her Bachelor of Science in Nursing from the University of Wisconsin–Madison. She obtained her Master of Science in Nursing as a family nurse practitioner from Graceland University in 2015. Dr. Abiri graduated with her Doctor of Nursing Practice from Emory University in 2020 where she was recognized with the Nell Hodgson Woodruff School of Nursing Social Responsibility Award for breaking down barriers and creating an environment for diversity, equity, and inclusion. Additionally, Dr. Abiri has served as a national committee member of the American Academy of Emergency Nurse Practitioner's Diversity Equity and Inclusion Committee. With a focus on nursing education, she has served on educational work groups dedicated to integrating social determinants of health within nursing curricula. Dr. Abiri takes a special interest in research that centers on the impact of social determinants of health on patient outcomes and health disparities. She is passionate about providing patient-centered care and implementing processes that promote health equity.

Diana Baptiste DNP, RN, FAAN, is an Associate Professor at the Johns Hopkins School of Nursing. She is a certified nurse educator whose teaching is grounded in cutting-edge, evidence-based instructional methods with a strong commitment to health equity in education, practice, and research. Her sustained scholarship focuses on cardiovascular health across the care continuum for underserved populations, grounded in responding to social justice issues influencing health outcomes.

Nakia C. Best PhD, RN, is an Assistant Professor in the Sue & Bill Gross School of Nursing at the University of California, Irvine. Dr. Best earned her BSN from Winston Salem State University, MSN in Nursing Education from the University of North Carolina at Greensboro, Post Master's in Applied Health Informatics from Johns Hopkins University, and PhD in Nursing from the University of North Carolina at Chapel Hill. Dr. Best advocates for all students to have daily access to a school nurse. She leverages data to provide valuable insights on how school nurses and the services they provide improve student health and education outcomes.

Angie Haynes-Ferere DNP, RN, is an Associate Clinical Professor and Program Director of the Distance ABSN program at Emory University. In 2022, she was a recipient of the LEAD Program NLN Leadership Institute award. She is a family nurse practitioner with more than 35 years of clinical and nonclinical experience caring for vulnerable populations locally, regionally, and globally. As the Chair of Eternal Hope in Haiti, a not-for-profit organization, she manages healthcare teams in Haiti. She is a Lumbee Indian tribal member and serves on the Emory Native American and Indigenous Studies Initiative.

Jacob K. Kariuki PhD, RN, is a native of Kenya who graduated with a PhD in population health and health policy from UMass Boston in 2016. He was an Assistant Professor at the University of Pittsburgh School of Nursing for 6 years before joining Emory in November

2022. His program of research is focused on prevention of cardiometabolic diseases in high risk and underserved populations, and resource constrained settings.

Charles E. Moore MD, received a Bachelor of Science from Union College and his medical degree from Harvard Medical School. He subsequently completed residency training in Otolaryngology-Head and Neck Surgery and fellowship training in Craniomaxillofacial—Cranial Base, Facial Plastic, and Reconstructive Surgery at the University of Michigan. Dr. Moore is a Professor at Emory University and the Chief of Service in the Department of Otolaryngology—Head and Neck Surgery at Grady Health System. Dr. Moore has a longstanding and profound commitment to the training and development of learners from all backgrounds. His research focus has been in the investigation of factors involved in healthcare disparity with a particular focus on head and neck cancer incidence in medically underserved communities. He is the President and Founder of Health Education, Assessment and Leadership (HEAL), Inc. Through this organization, he strives to educate the community on health issues, assess its needs, and in the process, build leaders from within the community to address those issues. This traveling resource has grown into the Healing Community Center (HCC), one of Atlanta's newest Federally Qualified Healthcare Centers. This center is a free and affordable medical facility with four separate locations, which provide general adult medical care, pediatric medical care, specialty medical care, dental services, as well as mental health services for the uninsured and disadvantaged. The HCC is focused on those who fall in the gap between public funded health care and the privately insured. A primary emphasis is on preventative health, nutrition, and wellness. This center incorporates all of the major Atlanta academic institutions and community organizations in an integrated fashion to provide service-learning experiences while also providing the necessary care to those in need.

Catherine M. Waters PhD, RN, FAAN, is a Professor, the Sally Bates Endowed Chair in Community Nursing and Health Disparities, and the Associate Dean for Faculty and Academic Affairs in the School of Nursing at the University of California, San Francisco. Appointed by the mayor, Dr. Waters served as a member of the San Francisco Health Commission for 5 years, including 1 year as the Vice President of the Health Commission. Dr. Waters's community-based participatory action research focuses on lifestyle health behaviors as protective mechanisms to prevent chronic disease development, in collaboration with public-private partners and community consortiums. She also has a research interest in end-of-life care planning. Dr. Waters served as a co-editor for the *American Journal of Public Health's* supplement on public health and nursing. She teaches graduate courses on advanced public health nursing and community-based participatory research methods, and previously has taught courses on theory development in nursing, evidence-based program planning, strategic healthcare marketing, behavior theories for nursing research, and interprofessional advanced scholarship in health systems research.

Health Informatics

This series is directed to healthcare professionals leading the transformation of healthcare by using information and knowledge. For over 20 years, Health Informatics has offered a broad range of titles: some address specific professions such as nursing, medicine, and health administration; others cover special areas of practice such as trauma and radiology; still other books in the series focus on interdisciplinary issues, such as the computer based patient record, electronic health records, and networked healthcare systems. Editors and authors, eminent experts in their fields, offer their accounts of innovations in health informatics. Increasingly, these accounts go beyond hardware and software to address the role of information in influencing the transformation of healthcare delivery systems around the world. The series also increasingly focuses on the users of the information and systems: the organizational, behavioral, and societal changes that accompany the diffusion of information technology in health services environments.

Developments in healthcare delivery are constant; in recent years, bioinformatics has emerged as a new field in health informatics to support emerging and ongoing developments in molecular biology. At the same time, further evolution of the field of health informatics is reflected in the introduction of concepts at the macro or health systems delivery level with major national initiatives related to electronic health records (EHR), data standards, and public health informatics.

These changes will continue to shape health services in the twenty-first century. By making full and creative use of the technology to tame data and to transform information, Health Informatics will foster the development and use of new knowledge in healthcare.

More information about this series at http://www.springer.com/series/1114

D: 10106023 S: 0001 PT: IX3200-1_i TS: 155x235 Pg: 2/378 BS: 220x251 HW: 3 TW: 13   HB

Kerryn Butler-Henderson
Karen Day • Kathleen Gray
Editors

The Health Information Workforce

Current and Future Developments

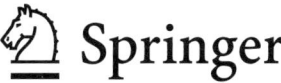
Springer

Editors
Kerryn Butler-Henderson
Digital Health Hub, STEM College
RMIT University
Bundoora
VIC, Australia

Karen Day
School of Population Health
University of Auckland
Auckland, New Zealand

Kathleen Gray
Centre for Digital Transformation of Health
University of Melbourne
Melbourne
VIC, Australia

ISSN 1431-1917   ISSN 2197-3741   (electronic)
Health Informatics
ISBN 978-3-030-81849-4   ISBN 978-3-030-81850-0   (eBook)
https://doi.org/10.1007/978-3-030-81850-0

This Springer imprint is published by the registered company Springer Nature Switzerland AG
The registered company address is: Gewerbestrasse 11, 6330 Cham, Switzerland

Contents

Part I
Introduction

Chapter 1
The Specialised Data, Information, and Knowledge Workforce in Health: Present and Future

Kerryn Butler-Henderson, Karen Day, and Kathleen Gray

Abstract The health information workforce has existed for more than a century yet remains one of the most hidden workforces in health. This workforce supports the planning, delivery, and improvement of healthcare services by analysing, designing, developing, implementing, maintaining, managing, operating, evaluating, or governing health data, information, or knowledge. Lack of awareness about this workforce has flow-on effects: shortages of skilled workers, inadequate skills training opportunities, and ultimately suboptimal health information and communication technology implementation and scaling up. Even in the era of digital health, this essential workforce supporting the safe and efficient management of health and care is a hidden workforce. We call it the HIDDIN workforce. The HIDDIN workforce comprises the practitioners who have key responsibility for the specialised work in Health Informatics, Digital, Data, Information, and kNowledge (HIDDIN). This chapter examines each of these parts of the HIDDIN workforce and defines the framework for this workforce used throughout this book. This chapter also defines the purpose of this book and presents the three conceptual

K. Butler-Henderson (✉)
Digital Health Hub, STEM College, RMIT University, Bundoora, VIC, Australia
e-mail: Kerryn.Butler-Henderson@rmit.edu.au

K. Day
School of Population Health, University of Auckland, Auckland, New Zealand
e-mail: k.day@auckland.ac.nz

K. Gray
Centre for Digital Transformation of Health, University of Melbourne, Melbourne, VIC, Australia
e-mail: kgray@unimelb.edu.au

K. Butler-Henderson et al. (eds.), *The Health Information Workforce*, Health Informatics, https://doi.org/10.1007/978-3-030-81850-0_1

lenses that have been used to frame the structure of this book. This book provides a clearer and more comprehensive view than ever before of the specialised workforce required to manage and govern the health data, information, and knowledge infrastructure now and in the future.

Keywords Health data science · Health informatics · Health information management · Health knowledge management · Health librarianship

Specialising in Data, Information and Knowledge Work in Health

Information is critical in the planning, delivery, and improvement of healthcare services, increasingly so in the twenty-first century era of health big data analytics, digital, and Internet-supported hospitals, artificial intelligence in health, and health self-quantification. Information means many things to many people in the health sector. Broadly, it can be the data of a patient's diagnosis and treatment, such as a fasting blood sugar level. It can be a record of information to inform a prognosis, such as pelvic pain, amenorrhoea, increased CA125 levels, imaging showing an ovarian mass indicating ovarian cancer. It can be the knowledge gained from the outcomes that a healthcare system is achieving, such as the infant mortality rate in place X in decade Y. It can be the wisdom from health messages that are designed to support responsible public health behaviours, such as how to avoid sexually transmitted infections. It can be the summary of evidence from a field of health research, such as what is known about the effects of calcium supplements on osteoarthritis. It can be business intelligence about health care services and how people use them, such as comparative hospital emergency department waiting times, or how rapidly regional governments are rolling out COVID-19 vaccines for people in residential aged care. For the health sector to get full value from health information, the sector needs more than common sense or basic health and information literacy among its professionals; consequently, there is increasing recognition that everyone in the health workforce must acquire basic digital health capabilities. Even so, the need remains for a health workforce group that possesses specialised knowledge and skills, with the capabilities to manage the sophisticated structures, systems, and processes that support and advance everyone's ability to work safely and efficiently with health information.

Who are the health information specialists? What kind of work do they do, where, and when are they needed? Although this work is fundamental, it is hard to see and even harder to understand and define, even for some of the people who do it and certainly for many of the other people who work in the health sector and beyond it. Unlike people in more commonly recognised healthcare roles, these specialists and their employers face challenges in finding one another. Specialised health information workers are not easy to locate in any healthcare organisation, nor is their value to health systems clearly articulated as a component of the overall health workforce (Martín-Sánchez and Gray 2014; Gray et al. 2019). Lack of awareness about this workforce has flow-on effects: shortages of skilled workers, inadequate skills training opportunities, and ultimately suboptimal health information and communication technology implementation and scaling up. Even in the era of digital health, this essential workforce supporting the safe and efficient management of health and care is a hidden workforce. We call it the HIDDIN workforce.

The HIDDIN workforce comprises the practitioners who have key responsibility for the specialised work in *H*ealth *I*nformatics, *D*igital, *D*ata, *I*nformation, and k*N*owledge. Roles in the HIDDIN workforce include functions not only as users of health data, information, or knowledge; rather they are managers, policymakers, clinicians, educators, researchers, and leaders who are tasked with analysing, designing, developing, implementing, maintaining, operating, evaluating, and governing the formats, technologies, systems, and services that mobilise health data, information, and knowledge. Typically, but not exclusively, this may include people who practice, administer, teach, or research in areas such as Biomedical engineering, Biomedical informatics, Biostatistics, Clinical coding, Clinical costings, Clinical documentation improvement, Clinical informatics, Consumer health information services, Digital health infrastructure, eHealth systems, Epidemiology, Health analytics, Health app development, Health artificial intelligence, Health cybersecurity, Health data science, Health informatics, Health information governance, Health information management, Health information systems or services, Health information technology, Health innovation, Health interoperability, Health librarianship, Health simulation, Health technology assessment, Medical research data management, Telehealth platform services, and Translational bioinformatics.

The aim of this book is to make the HIDDIN workforce visible and to explore its place in the health sector. The book begins by setting out the foundations of current knowledge about the HIDDIN workforce—how scholars have described it, how economies have categorised it, how education, professional development and certification have shaped and influenced it. The book continues by giving consideration to some emerging approaches to the work and their implications for this workforce—artificial intelligence and machine learning, consumerism, globalisation, and other leadership challenges. The book also provides a finer-grained analysis of what this workforce contributes to the health sector, in terms of safety and quality, access and equity. The book concludes with case studies of practitioners in the HIDDIN workforce that relate their real-world roles, challenges, changes, and achievements.

Ways of Exploring HIDDIN Work

This book looks at the HIDDIN workforce through three conceptual lenses, as defined in Box 1.1.

Box 1.1 Three conceptual lenses of this book
Identity
    Who is this workforce, and what do they do; what positions do they occupy in the health workforce; what specialised knowledge and skills do they have, and what do they do to acquire these?
Innovation
    What is this workforce doing to advance the ways that its own members practice in response to healthcare changes; what is it doing to transform the ways that other people in the health system gain value from health information?
Impact
    What is the impact of the work done by this workforce, and what criteria can be used to measure or assess its impact; what could be the impact of a more deliberately structured and supported workforce?

The motifs of identity, innovation, and impact (adapted from Bärnighausen and Bloom 2009) frame this book, as applied to specialised work in support of health data, health information, and health knowledge. The three concepts of data, information, and knowledge are fundamental distinctions in the discipline of information science (Zins 2007), and they align with many definitions used in models of this field of work (for example Georgiou 2002). Data, information, and knowledge management work are not easy to define or differentiate, and this is advantageous for our research. This allows us to explore a broad spectrum of people who may identify with this workforce, either exclusively or jointly with another health workforce identity (for example does a chief clinical information officer identify as an information manager, health informatician, as a clinician or as a combination of all three?). This means that we include work which may be called "information technology," but we are not limited to it. Even as data, information, and digital capabilities in health professionals increase, and as the technology changes to automate certain functions, we anticipate that there will be a continuing need for specialised knowledge and skills, even though we cannot be certain who will possess them or review them.

We use the theme of identity to conceptualise the work that is being done by this workforce. We know that this workforce finds it hard to clearly characterise who the people are and what work they do, both within its various professional communities and to external stakeholders. We broadly define work in scope for this book if it meets three criteria: the work is concerned with the management of data, the management of information, and/or the management of knowledge; the work is done in, about, for and/or with health (i.e. by people employed in the system, outsourced workers, government workers, industry, or advocacy groups, and researchers); and the work is done in connection with clinical care, population health, health policy and health research.

Innovation—in terms of what the future holds for what health information work is done, how it is done, and who does it—may be explored using concepts of workforce automation and the digital workforce. The future of work of all kinds, everywhere in the world economy, is expected to change under the influence of the increase in computing power and artificial intelligence and the spread of Internet access and the Internet of Things. (Colbert et al. 2016; OECD 2016; Smith and Page 2016). We can use the theme of innovation to conceptualise the dynamic situation in which the health information workforce finds itself in the era of digital health. The future of the health information workforce may be influenced by intersecting scenarios. Some but not all people in the workforce may keep up with the technical skills required (re-skilling). The work may become the responsibility of another role in the workforce (platform economy). The work may be restructured as some industry sectors shrink and others expand (structural transformation). Human performance of the work may be made obsolete by machines or computer programmes (automation). These considerations apply to the health information workforce as much as they do to all other parts of the health workforce. They allow us to engage with the current workforce and its stakeholders to explore constructive thinking about the work and to plan for inevitable change.

Impact, in the sense of the contribution to the overall operation of the health system of the work done by health information professionals, may be viewed through the lens of health system performance. Many national governments monitor and report the operations of their publicly funded health care systems using performance indicators derived from international frameworks produced by OECD, WHO, and similar agencies (Smith et al. 2012). Typically, a nation's selected indicators are thematically grouped and linked to essential metrics, for example accessibility, appropriateness of care, competence, and capability, comprehensiveness, continuity of care, effectiveness, efficiency, efficient resource allocation, equity, expenditure, and cost, healthy lives, health status, innovation, and capacity to improve integration, patient experience, productivity, technical efficiency, responsiveness, and trust, safety. These aspects of performance can provide a comprehensive, systematic, and contextualised research approach to understanding the impact of the health information workforce in terms of clinical safety and quality of care, the patient or client experience, and service sustainability. We can use the theme of impact to evaluate and improve the work that is done by the health information workforce with a clear view of what we want to achieve for health and care.

The Present Position of HIDDIN Work

Parts of the HIDDIN workforce have been identified and organised formally for well over a century. Consider these milestones: The creation of the Index Medicus in the mid-nineteenth century, the analog-era forerunner of PubMed, led to the establishment of the Medical Library Association in 1898 (Birchette 1973). At a time when clinical notes were written on cards or in large ledgers, medical secretaries began to manage this form of health information and organised themselves into the American Association of Medical Record Librarians in 1928 (Huffman 1947). The International Federation for Information Processing established Technical Committee 4, Health Care and Biomedical Research, and convened the first formal meeting of informaticians in Europe in 1967 (Peterson 2014). With the third and fourth industrial revolutions, health information practitioners have continued to form new associations around new health sector demands. For example a national membership organisation and network "for people working in health information and support … for an improved experience for patients and the public" (https://pifonline.org.uk), and a global community "for health data science and analytics that helps people connect, collaborate, share, learn, and make a meaningful impact on healthcare" (https://www.linkedin.com/company/healthdsa/).

Complex work in new kinds of work environments—sometimes called digital health ecosystems (for example Iyawa et al. 2016)—is being generated by the increasing pace of digital health information technologies in the present century. Managing and governing Internet-connected data, information, and knowledge in the service of healthcare, population health, and biomedical research, popularly called digital health since the 1990s, is critical to achieve higher order health system goals nationally and internationally (Grossmann et al. 2011; World Health Organisation [WHO], 2010a, 2021). This entails broad new strategic planning about how health organisations shift to digitally-enabled ways of operating and how they structure their workforce to do so (Kalra et al. 2016; Topol 2019). One emerging feature of digital health is a more fluid health workforce, less routinised, and more mobile and globalised; this requires major adjustments in how healthcare organisations and health systems are structured, how they support professional learning and development, and how their cultures adapt to digitally enabled ways of working (Accenture 2016). Making these adjustments is an important aspect of managing unforeseen or unintended consequences of digital health initiatives and mitigating risks to their success (Williams 2016).

It is not safe to assume that there are appropriately skilled professional practitioners behind every digital health system's design and operation; instead, the identification and organisation of technologically skilled health information work has gaps and blind spots (French 2014). Despite major investments in digital health systems and high expectations of the benefits that will ensue (Geiger and Gross 2017), there is scant empirical research into the specialised workforce that is needed to manage and govern the associated information infrastructure. Much of the human-centred research in digital health focuses on groups of stakeholders or end users. The considerable research on the technological and economic infrastructure of digital health is mostly silent about the specialised human resources needed to create and maintain it (Baird et al. 2014). This is ironic, to say the least, considering how highly regulated many health professions are.

It is known that many thousands of health information practitioners work in health systems around the world, whether professionally credentialled or self-described. They work as employees, contractors, entrepreneurs, public servants; in public, private, and non-profit organisations in the health sector, in a range of roles that are rapidly being changed and globalised by the networked nature of digital health (Kluge 2017). Up to now, efforts to illuminate their actual and potential contributions to digital health have been scattered. The HIDDIN workforce census is a unique attempt to quantify and qualify the HIDDIN workforce. Originating in Australia (Butler-Henderson et al. 2017), the census was expanded to New Zealand in 2018 (Day and Grainger 2019) and globally in 2021 (Butler-Henderson and Gray 2021). The 2018 Australian HIDDIN census (Butler-Henderson and Gray 2018) confirmed the HIDDIN composition of this workforce and provided insights into the qualifications, credentials, professional memberships, and jobs in this workforce. Results from this census are used below to highlight the differences between each area of HIDDIN. This census is an important tool in the ongoing evaluation of the current and future configuration and development needs of this workforce.

An Overview of HIDDIN Work

Health information work and, as the health sector evolves, digital health work can be seen as a continuum of specialists whose overlapping roles support and advance healthcare through health information, technology, and innovation. Here we offer an overview of the continuum of HIDDIN work.

Health Informatics

*H*ealth *I*nformatics is defined as the theory and practice of health information systems design, development, implementation, and management for the improvement of health outcomes (Friedman 2012). It is the integration of several sciences, including healthcare, computer and information science, business science and cognitive science (Sweeney 2017; Friedman 2012). Health informatics includes the design, development, and implementation of information technologies, analysis of data and information for application in health services, management, and support of information systems and services, and the provision of health services via information and communications technologies, such as video, phone, social media and wearables. Some definitions are specific to an academic field, such as bioinformatics, and others are linked to clinical professions, such as nursing, pharmacy, or medicine (Hübner et al. 2018). Other areas captured above include primary health informatics, population, or public health informatics, health app development, health information systems or services, health information technology, health technology assessment, telehealth platform services, and translational bioinformatics. This diversity of definitions is most likely the result of rapid advances in technology and the diverse adoption of digital and information systems in health services.

An analysis of the health informatics area in the previously referenced Australian health information workforce census reported that most (51.4%) people working in these jobs have done so for less than 10 years, reflecting the relative newness of these jobs in many health organisations (Butler-Henderson et al. 2019a). Furthermore, nearly two-thirds (63.6%) of respondents have been in their current role for less than 5 years, reflecting that most of these jobs are designed as time limited, temporary jobs. The average number of weekly hours worked was 33.5 h, further reflecting the part-time, casualisation of these jobs. A third (31.2%) of respondents undertake another role (i.e. they do not have a dedicated health informatics role), with a quarter (23.9%) reporting they are a registered health practitioners. Less than half (41.5%) of the roles are in a hospital, with roles spread across a wide variety of health settings. The majority of respondents do not hold a formal qualification in health informatics.

Digital Health

The second part of HIDDIN is *D*igital, for digital health. Digital health is "the field of knowledge and practice associated with the development and use of digital technologies to improve health" (WHO 2021). This expands the WHO definition of ehealth to include participatory consumer methods and tools (Kukafka 2019) and a wide range of connected smart devices, such as the Internet of Things, advanced associated sciences and analytics, artificial intelligence, and associated technologies (Jayaraman et al. 2020). Digital health brings the activated and engaged health consumer into the scope of health information workers, as well as leveraging the affordances of automation and advanced technologies. The work roles span all other areas of the HIDDIN continuum, and attract people from backgrounds in enterprise, technology, and education, for example biomedical engineering, digital health infrastructure, health innovation, health interoperability, and health simulation.

Data

Data form the raw materials of the HIDDIN work. Without *D*ata, HIDDIN work would not exist. "Merely using data isn't really what we mean by 'data science'. A data application acquires its value from the data itself, and creates more data as a result. It's not just an application with data; it's a data product. Data science enables the creation of data products." (Loukides 2011). Data scientists analyse data to access actionable insights from information. Data science activities include data gathering, preparation, and exploration, data transformation and representation, computing, data modelling, visualisation and presentation, and the science of data science (Donoho 2017). The data could be "big data," for example large data collection such as routinely collected clinical data, or "little data" e.g. data in EHRs about specific patients. Since data are core to HIDDIN work, they form the foundation of all roles associated with HIDDIN work. Disciplines such as biomedical informatics, population, or public health informatics could be categorised here to the extent that they manage methods and tools for analysing micro or big data to draw meaningful conclusions. Other discipline areas that lead to work in this area include epidemiology and medical research data management, and some specialised mathematical and statistical modelling. Health artificial intelligence and machine learning roles clearly can be located here.

A yet to be published analysis of data roles in the 2018 Australian health information workforce census showed an emerging and evolving field. Most (77.3%) have a formal mathematics or data analytics qualification, but none reported a specific health qualification (which may reflect the small sample included in this census). Like health informatics, the majority (57.0%) have worked in the field for less than 10 years, with 65.1% in their current role for less than 5 years, highlighting the emergence of these jobs in health. Where this area differs from health informatics is that the majority (75.4%) work solely in their data role. Their roles are across health, largely in state or local health departments or for federal government organisations.

Information

Health information is data that has been given context and meaning (Zins 2007), enabling decision-making for clinical, business, and management purposes to support the improvement of health outcomes. In HIDDIN work, *I*nformation processes the raw materials of data to enable the development of meaningful insights. The field of health information ensures "…all stakeholders (providers, consumers, policy-makers, researchers, patients, etc.) have the best data and information available to make informed decisions" (Fenton et al. 2021). One subset of health information professionals, health information managers, are responsible for the creation, analysis, management, and governance of health information (AHIMA 2020; CHIMA 2021; HIMAA 2014). Job roles in health information can include clinical coding, clinical costing, clinical documentation improvement, health cybersecurity, health information governance, and health information managers. Health information management is the only area in HIDDIN recognised in the International Standard Classification of Occupations (International Labour Office 2008), available as a formal tertiary qualification and many roles requiring the qualification. This profession is rapidly changing to include project management, data analyst and statistician influences (Dimick 2012). This area is transforming with a greater focus on information governance (privacy and data protection) and integrity, management of the information lifecycle, and data analytics (Butler-Henderson 2017). Another distinct group within the HIDDIN workforce that historically is identified strongly with health information is health and medical librarians. They develop, store, and make available electronic information resources used by healthcare providers and consumers and HIDDIN workers alike around the globe (Myers 2020). Their expertise has a substantial emphasis on quality assurance of information sources and synthesis of the information to form the evidence base for practice. Their roles are rapidly changing as biomedical publishing and literature search and retrieval are transformed by new technologies. For example the Network of the National Library of Medicine in the USA, and the National Health Service Library and Knowledge Service in the UK aim to provide national and global access to information that enables and supports informed decision-making for health (NNLM 2021; NHS 2021).

An analysis of the subset health information managers in the 2018 Australian health information workforce census (Butler-Henderson et al. 2019b) identified the average length of service in a health information management role was 17.0 years. Over four-fifths (81.4%) of respondents work in just one health information role, with 78.6% in a permanent role. The average weekly hours were 35.6 h, highlighting that most roles are full-time. And most (67.8%) are in a hospital environment, with other settings including state and local health departments and federal government organisations. These roles were more clearly defined by job title than any other area of HIDDIN, with most job titles being health information manager or clinical coder. Three-quarters (77.6%) hold a tertiary qualification in health information management.

Knowledge

Health kNowledge management is the work of systematically distilling value from raw data and tacit knowledge to provide an organised information base for trustworthy health advice, value-based care services, evidence-based clinical practices, learning health organisations, biomedical research impact, health programme evaluations, and other aspects of health systems (Nonaka and von Krogh 2009). Health knowledge management routinises the transformation of both digital data and real-world experiences into explicit, shareable forms of expression that enable a range of people to agree on what is occurring within their remit and to take decisive action on this basis. The central aim of health knowledge management is to keep individuals and communities safe and well; radiating out from this aim, knowledge management is undertaken as part of public health, clinical care, and health administration, research and policy work. Its facets are variously described as knowledge generation, curation, dissemination and translation, and it is essentially methodical work. The tools of the trade include ontologies, standards, guidelines, frameworks, indexes, all designed to give order and structure to cumulative biomedical science and health care knowledge, assure its quality, and make it accessible as appropriate. Health knowledge management is designed into a range of health information and communication technologies: the information architecture of an electronic health record system; the search engine optimisation strategies of a consumer health information website; the forum topics set out in a discussion forum for health professionals; the content included in a clinical decision support system; the form in which a health app enables personal recordkeeping. This field of work is experiencing a resurgence, influenced on the one hand by the COVID-19 data demand and infodemic, and on the other hand by the extraordinary potential of precision medicine and machine learning; overviews are offered by Bowden et al. (2020), Chettipally (2020) and Pereira et al. (2021). The work may not be described as such; the people who do it may come from health administration, health librarianship, health education, biomedical publishing, business information systems, and other disciplines.

An analysis of the health librarian subset of the Australian health information workforce census identified nearly all (94.2%) of respondents are permanent employees, with the average time in the workforce being 21 years (Gilbert et al. 2020). Most respondents only do this role. Over half (58.3%) of respondents are working in a hospital, with other roles in education facilities or state or local health departments. Further, most (79.85%) hold an entry-level (bachelor) qualification in library studies (or similar) or higher, reflecting the need for qualified people in these roles. The average hours worked (28.6 h) is much lower than the average across the HIDDIN workforce (32.6 h), reflecting most roles are part-time.

The Future: A Coherent Framework for HIDDIN Work

Career pathways are not yet clearly defined, although some countries have attempted to develop frameworks to describe the work. There is no specific guideline from the WHO for the health information workforce. The Workload Indicators of Staffing Need (WISN) manual (WHO 2010b) provides a guideline for all health service staffing requirements, but the only reported application of it in the HIDDIN workforce was for health information workforce planning and implementation in Ghana (Ogoe et al. 2018). The more recent WHO (2016) global strategy for human resources for health provides a high-level strategy, yet does not specify the health information workforce. It has been used to create frameworks for specific professions in HIDDIN, such as TIGER (Hübner et al. 2018), but not HIDDIN as a whole. Shah and Mahrin (2021) describe a framework for big data analysts. Mongan et al. (2018) reported the results of a scoping literature review of workforce planning and implementation frameworks for use in strategic planning in Ireland. They indicate that the most commonly used frameworks are the RE-FRAME and PRECEDE-PROCEED frameworks but do not link them to the information workforce. The United Kingdom has produced a set of strategies and frameworks regarding digital health workforce planning, with a focus on health informatics and data science (Liu et al. 2019), and HIMSS has developed a digital health workforce strategy that links workforce to governance and digital health, using principles of governance to frame digital workforce planning (Snowden 2020), but again, neither describe the actual HIDDIN workforce.

The only two frameworks to comprehensively describe the HIDDIN workforce were developed in Australia. Health Workforce Australia (2013) identifies three levels of the workforce. Level 1 consists of the specialist workforce, specifically indicating that specialists who work (usually full time) with health information systems. Level 2 consists of health professionals whose work consists of significant use of information systems in their work. Level 3 consists of all health professionals who contribute, retrieve, use, and reuse information as part of their professional work. Based on the recommendations from Health Workforce Australia for further work to delineate the workforce, the Australian Digital Health Agency (ADHA 2020) describes eight digital profiles, as presented in Box 1.2. The ADHA developed these profiles in consultation with the industry, but these profiles have not been evaluated. The ADHA describes that a job can have multiple digital profiles.

Box 1.2 Australian Digital Health Agency eight digital profiles (ADHA 2020, p.54–55)

1. *Patient, consumer, and carer*: "maintaining health information, protecting the security and privacy of information, and adopting and advocating for new technologies that help manage their health."
2. *Frontline clinical*: "expectations for lifelong learning, adoption of digital technologies, understanding security and privacy, reliable and accurate recordkeeping, ensuring clinical safety with digital technologies, and advocating for consumer use of technology to empower them."
3. *Digital champion*: "a digital teacher and champion locally for a particular technology or system."
4. *Business, administration and clinical support*: "learning, adoption of digital technologies, understanding security and privacy and reliable and accurate recordkeeping."
5. *Leadership and executive*: "leadership of digital transformation and deployment, risk and quality assurance, and understanding sophisticated data analytics to drive better business decisions."
6. *Clinical and technology bridging*: "providing advice during the design and development of new digital technologies and systems, and leveraging clinical networks for user testing and adoption."
7. *Education and research*: "lifelong learning, translational research, evidence-based review, and health reform and innovation. It also addresses expectations relating to education."
8. *Technologist*: "those performing health information technology functions, including cybersecurity, programming, systems maintenance, digital design, interoperability, IT procurement, resilience and continuity planning, health information management and system testing."

The ADHA mapped their digital profiles to the three levels detailed by Health Workforce Australia (p52), identifying profiles 1–3 as aligning with level 3, profiles 4–6 as level 2, and profiles 7–8 as level 1 (the specialist roles). This would suggest only roles that align with the ADHA's description of (7) Education and research and (8) Technologist are HIDDIN roles. Yet the above definitions highlight HIDDIN is more than simply "those performing health information technology functions, including cybersecurity, programming, systems maintenance, digital design, interoperability, IT procurement, resilience and continuity planning, health information management and system testing" (ADHA 2020, p.54–55). So how can we describe these five profile descriptions within the health workforce as a collective group?

Professionalisation of HIDDIN Work

HIDDIN work, as described above, comprises five parts, with many different roles in each. So how do we define what these parts mean to the overall HIDDIN workforce, and what does this mean for professionalisation? Trowler et al. (2012) expanded on the previous work of Becher and Trowler (2001) to define a discipline as (Trowler et al. 2012, p.9):

> Reservoirs of knowledge resources shaping regularised behavioural practices, sets of discourses, ways of thinking, procedures, emotional responses and motivations. These provide structured dispositions for disciplinary practitioners who reshape them in different practice clusters into localised repertoires. While alternative recurrent practices may be in competition within a single discipline, there is common background knowledge about key figures, conflicts and achievements. Disciplines take organisational form, have internal hierarchies and bestow power differentially, conferring advantage and disadvantage.

This definition is appropriate to describe the parts of the HIDDIN workforce; there are discrete knowledge, behaviour, practices, and procedures for each area.

As the digitisation of health increases, the uniqueness between each discipline decreases. This is evident from the HIDDIN definitions outlined above. For example *health informatics* "deals with the storage, retrieval, sharing, and optimal use of data that relates to human health, and it considers how we use this knowledge for problem solving and decision making" (Health Informatics New Zealand 2020). Similarly, *health information management* professionals "create, acquire, analyse and/or manage information to meet the medical, legal, ethical and/or administrative requirements of the health care system" (HIMAA 2014). These two definitions include the same functions, "storage, retrieval, sharing, and optimal use" versus "create, acquire, analyse and/or manage," with the difference being "data" versus "information." Two areas with the same functions at different levels reflects the advancement in digital health: as health move towards the capture of data through information systems as opposed to paper records, this shifts the focus from information brokering to rapid translate of data into actionable knowledge. Digital advances such as data protection, the use of new technologies, innovations such as artificial intelligence and automation of data analysis and management functions will create further overlap across all five areas of HIDDIN. So, whilst it could be argued that each area in HIDDIN is its own discipline, the changing landscape may see these disciplines either merging, transforming, or dissolving over time. Thus, it is possible in the future that HIDDIN itself will become the collective discipline and each of these areas a specialisation.

The different disciplines attract different job titles, recognising that some jobs could be listed in multiple areas and other jobs overlap with one another. The International Standard Classification of Occupations (International Labour Office 2008, p.11) defines a job as "a set of tasks and duties performed, or meant to be performed, by one person, including for an employer or in self employment," with an occupation defined as "a set of jobs whose main tasks and duties are characterised by a high degree of similarity." To have a high level of similarity, there must be a set of practice, processes, and behaviours; in this sense, an occupation can be understood to be a discipline. The above definitions highlight there are specific jobs in each area of HIDDIN that can be found in different health organisations, and therefore the areas in HIDDIN can be defined as occupations. Yet, most of these areas are not defined as occupations in the International Standard Classification of Occupations.

Does this make the HIDDIN workforce a profession? Using the neo-Weberian perspective, a profession "is centred on attaining a particular form of formal legal regulation with registers creating bodies of insiders and excluding outsiders" (Saks 2012, p.4). Whilst several HIDDIN areas require a formal qualification for a job, have a formally structured salary classification linked to that qualification, and have national peak bodies requiring the qualification for membership (excluding outsiders), a register of qualified practitioners is not maintained for any HIDDIN area. There is an emerging trend to link health informatics qualifications to clinical registrations (e.g. in the United States and United Kingdom). Therefore, for HIDDIN to become a profession, it first needs to become a recognised discipline, with a clear body of knowledge underpinned and informed by scholarly research and discourses, and the formalisation of ethical practice and procedures.

These definitions highlight the infancy of the discipline of HIDDIN. The foundation for HIDDIN to be an occupation is present, and this is explored throughout this book through the examination of competencies, education, accreditation, professional development, certification, impact, and jobs. Yet, the only framework in existence, the ADHA digital profiles (2020), does not recognise HIDDIN as a discrete occupational group with its own norms, knowledgebase, and professional code. The emergence of leadership jobs (such as the Chief Information Office, Chief Clinical Information Officer, Chief Medical Information Officer, Chief Nursing Information Officer, Chief Digital Information Officer or the Chief Information Governance Officer) in specialised digital health areas is the start of an occupational structure, from which professionalisation can be achieved.

The Future: Deepening Insights into HIDDIN Work

This book provides a clearer and more comprehensive view than ever before, of the specialised workforce required to manage and govern the health data, information, and knowledge infrastructure now and in the future. It offers a coherent and critical enquiry into a workforce that is essential for healthcare services to function, for care providers to practice at the top of their scope/licence, for researchers to generate significant insights, and for care consumers to be empowered participants in health systems, as digital information and communication technologies transform the health sector. It celebrates and champions those working in the HIDDIN workforce. It informs health sector health executives who need to develop and mobilise this workforce. It is a resource for health workforce planners, professional associations and educators who are responsible for setting and upholding practice and performance standards in this workforce. It sets the stage for forward-looking research and reflective practice to deepen how we understand the specialist knowledge and skills that we rely on in the digital health era.

Acknowledgements   Our Universities, Auckland, Melbourne, RMIT and Tasmania, have encouraged and supported us in writing this book. Associate Professor Rebecca Grainger at the University of Otago was an especially valued collaborator in work that preceded this book. Our colleagues in academia and in the health sector around the world have been generous and genuine in providing chapters and case studies that are unique contributions to describing the HIDDIN workforce. Our reviewers have been invaluable in providing independent peer reviews. Every individual who took the time to complete the health information workforce census in 2018 and 2021 added depth to our collective understanding of this important workforce. Lastly, we wish to acknowledge and pay our respects to the first health information specialists, that is, the traditional owners of the lands on which we all live and work.

References

Accenture. Digital health tech vision. 2016. https://www.accenture.com/au-en/insight-digital-health-liquid-workforce. Accessed 27 May 2021.

AHIMA. Health information 101. 2020. https://www.ahima.org/certification-careers/certifications-overview/career-tools/career-pages/health-information-101/. Accessed 28 May 2021.

Australian Digital Health Agency. National digital health workforce and education roadmap. New South Wales: Australian Government; 2020.

Baird A, Furukawa MF, Rahman B, Schneller ES. Corporate governance and the adoption of health information technology within integrated delivery systems. Health Care Manag Rev. 2014;39(3):234–44.

Bärnighausen T, Bloom DE. Changing research perspectives on the global health workforce (No. w15168). National Bureau of Economic Research; 2009.

Becher T, Trowler P. Academic tribes and territories: intellectual enquiry and the cultures of disciplines (2nd edition). Buckingham: Open University Press/SRHE; 2001.

Birchette KP. The history of medical libraries from 2000 BC to 1900 AD. Bull Medical Library Assoc. 1973;61(3):302.

Bowden DE, Smits SJ, Andrews MA. The challenge of knowledge management in healthcare. In: 13th Annual Conference of the Euromed Academy of Business. 2020. p. 219–30.

Butler-Henderson K. Health information management 2025. What is required to create a sustainable profession in the face of digital transformation? Launceston: University of Tasmania; 2017.

Butler-Henderson K, Gray K. Australia's health information workforce: census summary report 2018. Launceston: University of Tasmania; 2018.

Butler-Henderson K, Gray K. Global HIDDIN workforce census. 2021. https://www.utas.edu.au/health/projects/hiwcensus. Accessed 28 May 2021.

Butler-Henderson K, Gray K, Greenfield D, Low S, Gilbert C, Ritchie A, Trujillo M, Bennett V, Brophy J, Schaper LK. The development of a national census of the health information workforce: expert panel recommendations. Stud Health Technol Inform. 2017;239:8–13.

Butler-Henderson K, Gray K, Pearce C, Ritchie A, Brophy J, Schaper LK, Bennett V, Ryan A. Exploring the health informatics occupational group in the 2018 Australian health information workforce census. Stud Health Technol Informatics. 2019a;266:44–50.

Butler-Henderson K, Gray K, Ritchie A, Ryan A, Brophy J, Pearce C, Schaper LK Bennett V. Health information management in Australia: findings from the 2018 Australian HIW Census. Proceedings of the 36th National Conference of HIMAA & NCCH. 2019b. p. 22–8.

Chettipally UK. Knowledge management in a learning health system. In: Artificial Intelligence: Applications in Healthcare Delivery. Taylor & Francis. 2020. p. 223–30.

CHIMA. Health information overview. 2021. https://www.echima.ca/association/health-information-overview/. Accessed 28 May 2021.

Colbert A, Yee N, George G. The digital workforce and the workplace of the future. Acad Manag J. 2016;59(3):731–9.

Day K, Grainger R. New Zealand's health information workforce: census summary report 2019. Auckland: University of Auckland; 2019. https://hiwcensusnz.blogs.auckland.ac.nz/2019/08/05/2019-summary-report/. Accessed 28 May 2021.

Dimick C. Health information management 2025: Current "health IT revolution" drastically changes HIM in the near future. J AHIMA. 2012;83(8):24–31.

Donoho D. 50 years of data science. J Computat Graphic Stat. 2017;26(4):745–66.

Fenton SH, Butler-Henderson K, Albishi H, Kyabaggu R, Monohur S, Parameswaran Nair D, Paluzie G, Primeau D. IFHIMA workforce white paper. Examining today's HIM profession with recommendations for the future. IFHIMA; 2021. https://ifhima.org/whitepapers/. Accessed 28 May 2021.

French M. Gaps in the gaze: Informatic practice and the work of public health surveillance. Surveill Soc. 2014;12(2):226–43.

Friedman CP. What informatics is and isn't, JAMIA. 2012;20:224–26.

Geiger S, Gross N. Does hype create irreversibilities? Affective circulation and market investments in digital health. Market Theory. 2017;17(4):435–54.

Georgiou A. Data, information and knowledge: the health informatics model and its role in evidence-based medicine. J Eval Clin Pract. 2002;8(2):127–30.

Gilbert C, Gray K, Butler-Henderson K, Ritchie A. Digital health and professional identity in Australian health libraries. Evid Based Libr Inf Pract. 2020;15(1):38–58.

Gray K, Gilbert C, Butler-Henderson K, Day K, Pritchard S. Ghosts in the machine: identifying the digital health information workforce. In: Lau F, et al., editors. Improving usability, safety and patient quality with health information technology. Amsterdam: IOS Press; 2019.

Grossmann C, Powers B, McGinnis JM. Digital infrastructure for the learning health system: the foundation for continuous improvement in health and health care: Workshop series summary. Washington: Institute of Medicine & National Academies Press; 2011.

Health Informatics New Zealand. Infographic: what is HI? 2020. https://www.hinz.org.nz/page/Infograph1. Accessed 15 May 2021.

HIMAA. Definition of the profession. Health Information Management Association of Australia. 2014. https://himaa.org.au/the-professions/. Accessed 25 May 2021.

Health Workforce Australia. Health information workforce report. 2013. https://www.aims.org.au/documents/item/401. Accessed 15 May 2021.

Hübner U, Shaw T, Thye J, Egbert N, de Fatima MH, Chang P, O'Connor S, Day K, Honey M, Blake R, Hovenga E, Skiba D, Ball MJ. Technology informatics guiding education reform–TIGER: an international recommendation framework of core competencies in health informatics for nurses. Methods Inf Med. 2018;57(Suppl 1):e30.

Huffman EK. The medical records librarian: a new career in the medical field. Bios. 1947;18(4):209–15.

International Labour Office. International standard classification of occupations. Switzerland. 2008. https://www.ilo.org/public/english/bureau/stat/isco/. Accessed 28 May 2021.

Iyawa GE, Herselman M, Botha A. Digital health innovation ecosystems: from systematic literature review to conceptual framework. Procedia Comput Sci. 2016;100:244–25.

Jayaraman PP, Forkan AR, Morshed A, Haghighi PD, Kang YB. Healthcare 4.0: a review of frontiers in digital health. Wiley Interdisciplinary Reviews: Data Mining Knowl Discov. 2020;10(2):e1350.

Kalra D, Stroetmann V, Sundgren M, Dupont D, Schlünder I, Thienpont G, Coorevitis P, De Moor G. The European Institute for Innovation through health data. Learn Health Syst. 2016;1(1):e10008.

Kluge EHW. Health information professionals in a global eHealth world: ethical and legal arguments for the international certification and accreditation of health information professionals. Int J Medical Informatics. 2017;97:261–5.

Kukafka R. Digital health consumers on the road to the future. J Medical Internet Res. 2019;21(11):e16359.

Liu D, Milsom R, Calder N, Harry G, Patel P. NHS informatics workforce in England: Phase 1 project report. 2019. https://www.hee.nhs.uk/sites/default/files/documents/Informatics%20Workforce%20Report%202014%20to%202019.pdf. Accessed 28 May 2021.

Loukides M. What is data science? The future belongs to the companies and people that turn data into products. O'Reilly Media: Sebastopol, CA; 2011.

Martin-Sanchez F, Gray K. Recognition of health informatics in Australian standard classifications for research, occupation and education. Stud Health Technol Informatics. 2014;204:92–6.

Mongan D, Farragher L, Long J. Implementation frameworks for use by health workforce planners. Harv Bus Rev. 2018. https://www.hrb.ie/fileadmin/publications_files/Implementation_frameworks_for_use_by_health_workforce_planners_2018.pdf. Accessed 28 May 2021.

Myers B. What we talk about when we talk about medical librarianship: an analysis of Medical Library Association annual meeting abstracts, 2001–2019. J Medical Libr Assoc: JMLA. 2020;108(3):364.

NHS. Knowledge and library services. 2021. https://www.healthcareers.nhs.uk/explore-roles/health-informatics/roles-health-informatics/knowledge-and-library-services. Accessed 28 May 2021.

NNLM. Network of the National Library of Medicine. About NNLM. 2021. https://nnlm.gov/about. Accessed 28 May 2021.

Nonaka I, von Krogh G. Tacit knowledge and knowledge conversion: controversy and advancement in organisational knowledge creation theory. Organ Sci. 2009;20(3):635–52.

OECD. Automation and independent work in a digital economy. 2016. www.oecd.org/employment/emp/Automation-and-independent-work-in-a-digital-economy-2016.pdf. Accessed 28 May 2021.

Ogoe IIA, Asamani JA, Hochheiser H, Douglas GP. Assessing Ghana's eHealth workforce: implications for planning and training. Human Resour Health. 2018;16(1):1–11.

Pereira V, Cooper CL, Chandwani R, Varma A, Tarba SY. Guest editorial: Evaluating and investigating knowledge management practices and ICT in health care: an emerging economies perspective. J Knowl Manag. 2021;25(3):513–24.

Peterson HE. The early history of European Federation of Medical Informatics. Acta Informatica Medica. 2014;22(1):16.

Saks M. Defining a profession: the role of knowledge and expertise. Professions Professionalism. 2012;2(1):1–10.

Shah SMSA, Mahrin MNR. The trend of big data in workforce frameworks and occupational standards towards an educational intelligent economy. J Techn Educ Train. 2021;13(1):176–84.

Smith A, Page D. Public predictions for the future of workforce automation. USA: Pew Research Center; 2016. http://www.pewinternet.org/2016/03/10/public-predictions-for-the-future-of-workforce-automation/. Accessed 28 May 2021.

Smith PC, Anell A, Busse R, Crivelli L, Healy J, Lindahl AK, Westert G, Kene T. Leadership and governance in seven developed health systems. Health Policy. 2012;106(1):37–49.

Snowden A. Digital health: a framework for healthcare transformation. HIMSS. 2020. https://www.gs1ca.org/documents/digital_health-affht.pdf. Accessed 28 May 2021.

Sweeney J. Healthcare informatics. Online J Nurs Informatics (OJNI). 2017;21(1).

Topol E. The Topol review. Preparing the healthcare workforce to deliver the digital future. 2019;1–48.

20   K. Butler-Henderson et al.

Trowler P, Saunders M, Bamber V. Tribes and territories in the 21st century. Rethinking the significance of disciplines in higher education. Milton Keynes: Taylor & Francis Group; 2012.

Williams R. Why is it difficult to achieve e-health systems at scale? Inf Commun Soc. 2016;19(4):540–50.

WHO. Models and tools for health workforce planning and projections. (Human Resources for Health Observer, 3). Geneva: WHO Press; 2010a.

WHO. Workload indicators of staffing need (WISN): a manual (No. WHO/NLM/W76). Geneva: World Health Organization; 2010b.

WHO. Global strategy on human resources for health: workforce 2030. 2016. http://apps.who.int/iris/bitstream/handle/10665/250368/9789241511131-eng.pdf?sequence=1. Accessed 28 May 2021.

WHO. Global strategy on digital health 2020-2025. Geneva: WHO Press; 2021.

Zins C. Conceptual approaches for defining data, information, and knowledge. J Am Soc Inf Sci Technol. 2007;58(4):479–93.

Part II
Identity

Chapter 2
Health Information Work: A Scoping Review

Cecily Gilbert, Kathleen Gray, and Simone Pritchard

Abstract The work of managing health data, health information and health knowledge is fundamental in healthcare systems, as increasingly they are transformed by information and communication technologies. However, this work is not acknowledged or understood as commonly as other kinds of work in healthcare, even though it has been described in scholarly writing for five decades. This chapter is a scoping review of literature from the domains of health sciences, health information technology and health information sciences; bibliometric and thematic analyses explore the responsibilities and the contributions of the health information workforce. 284 publications from 1973 to 2018 outline a wide variety of occupational sub-groups, job titles, work roles and skills. The status and prospects of this kind of work are influenced by: external drivers of role changes; definitions of competency requirements; healthcare professions' needs for general and specialised education regarding new technologies; and fragmented identities within the health information workforce. If specialised professional work is considered essential for healthcare systems to realise the benefits of information and communication technologies, then concerted health workforce planning is needed to consolidate historically disparate health information work practices and to establish a distinctive, accountable workforce that provides the human infrastructure for digital health.

Keywords Competencies · Health workforce · Historical trends · Human resources

C. Gilbert (✉) · K. Gray · S. Pritchard
Centre for Digital Transformation of Health,
The University of Melbourne, Parkville, VIC, Australia
e-mail: cecily.gilbert@unimelb.edu.au; kgray@unimelb.edu.au

23

Introduction

"Historically, the diverse communities working in digital health—including government stakeholders, technologists, clinicians, implementers, network operators, researchers, donors—have lacked a mutually understandable language with which to assess and articulate functionality." (World Health Organization 2018, p. 2). This incoherence is an indicator of the diffuse status of a whole subsection of the health workforce, a multiplicity of people in specialised roles who together are responsible for the systems for capturing and using health data, health information, and health knowledge, and whom we characterise as HIDDIN—referring to their collective specialisations in Health Informatics, Digital, Data, Information and kNowledge management. Their work directly fuels the provision of health services, assures the quality and safety of care and underpins the translation of research into practice. This workforce may have an increasingly important role as the health sector moves toward greater use of digital technologies. Yet precise data about it is difficult to obtain; the work is largely invisible, ill-defined, unregulated and unmonitored (Gray et al. 2019). Further, allusions to it often convey little sense of human agents, creating an abstract impression, of unspecified work done by unspecified workers. The HIDDIN acronym is most apt because this work is so poorly recognised or understood, compared to other areas of work in the health sector.

"Health information" as the description of a specialist work domain emerged in the twentieth century. Individual professions and occupations, such as medical records managers and medical librarians, arose in the early decades of the 1900s, and developed in parallel, rather than intersecting, streams. Further specialisations, in particular health informatics, emerged from the mid-century onward. More recently the field has become very fluid, due in part to technological changes that enhance collaboration between computing or IT staff and those working with health data or health information. A range of professions now claim expertise in health information work, and position titles and career paths also vary greatly. Moreover, in the current era of digital transformation of health, some people in the health information workforce are confronting issues of their relevance and sustainability in the face of possible workforce structuring.

Subsections of the health information workforce have been studied occasionally over the years, for various purposes, in different parts of the world. This chapter takes a holistic approach, inspired by a government workforce planning agency report on the health information workforce (Health Workforce Australia 2013). This chapter is part of a larger research program studying the changing nature and scope of this workforce, starting with a world-first national Health Information Workforce Census in May 2018 (https://www.utas.edu.au/health/projects/hiwcensus), which invited participation by: "…anyone who self-identifies as part of the health information workforce working for/with an organisation that operates in Australia. You are part of the workforce if you work (including volunteer or actively seeking) in a role where the primary function is related to developing, maintaining, or governing the systems for the management of health data, health information, or health knowledge" (Butler-Henderson and Gray 2018a, b).

This chapter addresses the question: How has the concept of "health information work" emerged and developed within writings about the broader workforces in health care, health information technology and health information sciences? The focus is less on abstract ideas of health information work, and more on accounts of how human agency—the capacity of humans to act, and the way that they do act—is manifested in the performance of work with health information, health data, or health knowledge systems. The objectives are to map published descriptions of an instrumental or professional human role in health information work; and to summarise what has been written about the extent, distribution and nature of such work.

Methods

A scoping review methodology was appropriate to this broad research question. Scoping reviews have the goal of "summarising a range of evidence in order to convey the breadth and depth of a field" (Levac et al. 2010, p. 1), for three possible reasons: "…to examine the extent, range and nature of research activities [in a subject]; determine the value of undertaking a full systematic review; or identify research gaps in the extant literature" (Paré et al. 2015, p. 186). The present review has the first and third of these purposes. This review followed the format and stages: (1) identifying the research question; (2) identifying relevant studies; (3) describing study selection criteria; (4) charting the data; (5) collating, summarising and reporting the results (as outlined by Arksey and O'Malley 2005). A completed PRISMA-ScR Checklist for the scoping review (as recommended by Tricco et al. 2018) is not included for reasons of space, however all checklist elements are addressed in the structure of this chapter. The protocol for this review was agreed through consultation with team members in the Health Information Census project. Since scoping reviews were ineligible for registration in the PROSPERO database (Centre for Reviews and Dissemination n.d.), this protocol was published as a preprint (Gray and Gilbert 2019).

To be included in the review, items had to describe or focus on an instrumental or professional human role in health information, health data or health knowledge work. These roles had to be involved in managing health information, health data or health knowledge, in clinical, academic, government or industry settings. Eligible study types included primary research, case studies, reviews, theoretical or analytical studies, policy or planning articles. Editorials, letters and brief items were not included. Descriptions of health information work performed by consumers, patients or carers were not eligible. Non-English items were excluded.

The search was conducted in five online databases: Ovid Medline (1946–June 2017), and associated databases (comprising Ovid Medline Daily, Epub ahead of print, In-process and other non-indexed citations); CINAHL Full Text, searched on 28 March 2018; Embase (Elsevier version) searched on 21 March 2018; Applied Social Sciences Index and Abstracts, searched on 22 March 2018; and Library, Information Science and Technology Abstracts, searched on 27 March 2018. Since the review aimed to trace the evolution and development of the health information workforce, no date restrictions were used.

The search strategies were drafted by an experienced health information practitioner (CG). After a test search in Ovid Medline and discussion with co-researcher (KG), the strategies were refined and translated to the other bibliographic databases. The primary searches were performed by two information professionals (CG and SP) between June 2017 and March 2018. The Medline search strategy can be found in Appendix. In addition, reference lists of relevant items were scanned to identify any further citations. Two grey literature resources—the CORE repository and Google Scholar—were also searched. Two additional criteria were used in screening potential items in these sources: published by a reputable organisation; and contains empirical data about the health information work (i.e. commentary, editorials or opinion items were not eligible). A final search update was conducted in Ovid Medline and CINAHL Full Text to identify any eligible items published up to December 2018. The final span of years searched was 1946–2018.

The search results were exported into the Covidence software (Covidence n.d.) for decisions on selection. The results were de-duplicated in Covidence, then screened by members of the search team. At the outset, both CG and SP reviewed 100 titles and abstracts together, to test consistency of the screening decisions. Following this stage, the two reviewers divided the total set of results and screened allocated items independently. Where judgments disagreed or in the case that items were flagged as "uncertain", these were resolved by consensus. Figure 2.1 shows the flow of items through the retrieval and screening processes. The key reason for exclusion was that the item did not detail the work or the worker in health information activities. A small number were excluded either because the full texts were not in English or they were duplicate reports of a single item. 284 items were judged as eligible for inclusion in this review and appear in the reference list along with all other items cited in this chapter.

Descriptive statistical analysis was used to show bibliometric features such as years of publication, top-ranking subject terms, source journals and prominent authors. Topic analysis was performed by grouping controlled vocabulary items. Deductive thematic analysis was done, based on charting the health information work role characteristics that each item described: identity, responsibilities, functions, knowledge and skills. Open coding was used to identify the main reflections about the work and the workforce that recurred across the dataset.

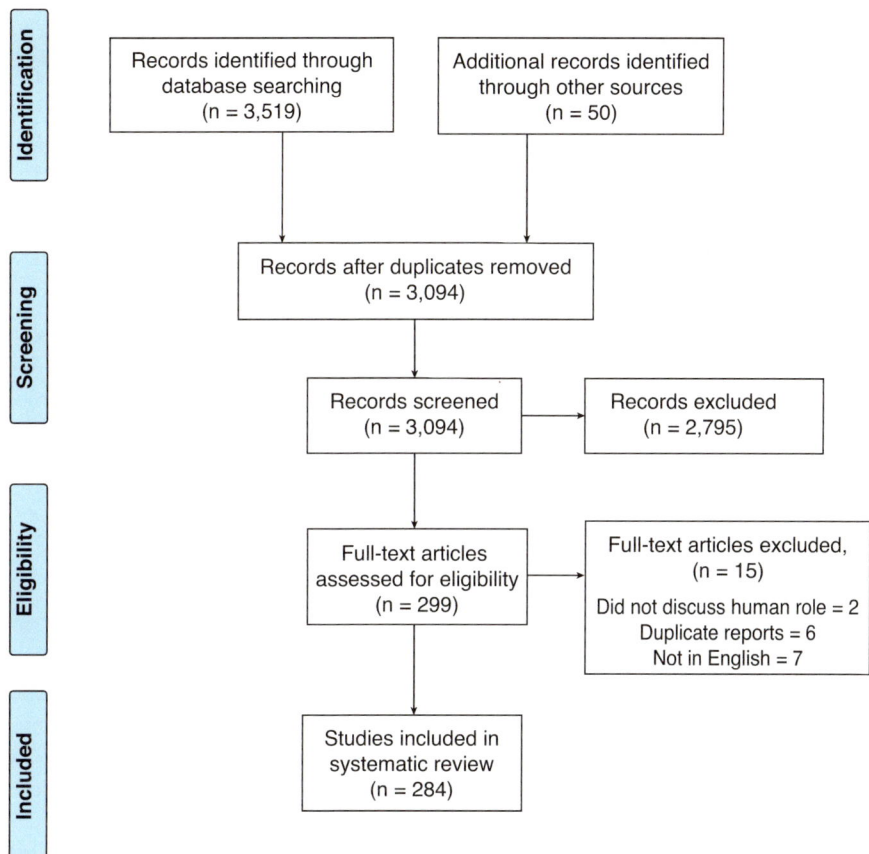

Fig. 2.1 PRISMA Flow diagram

Results

Findings are arranged in four parts: bibliometric analysis (publications over time; publications by author; publication sources); topic analysis (controlled terms used to classify the studies); role analysis (job identities; roles and responsibilities); recurring concerns.

Bibliometric Analysis

Publications explicitly about the health information workforce first appeared in 1973, though the number of items for the first two decades (1973–1990) remained low at 9. However, from 1991 the number of publications steadily increased; for

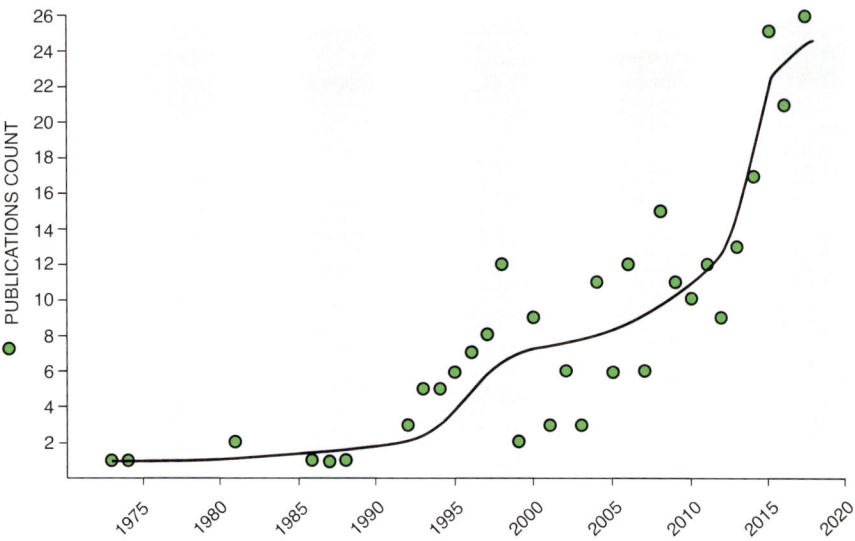

Fig. 2.2 Publications count by year

example, in 1998, 12 items were identified. Substantial growth is evident from the late 1990s onwards, with 60 items (20.9% of the total) appearing in the 1991–2000 decade, 88 items (30.6%) in the 2001–2010 decade, and 127 items (44.7%) since 2011. This was the most productive period, and 2017 with 30 publications (10.6%) was the most productive year. The average annual number of publications (rounded) is 6, or 57 per decade. In contrast, between 2011 and 2015 there were 71 publications, and a further 56 between 2016 and 2018. Figure 2.2 shows the number of retrieved items per publication year.

Most of the included studies reported single cases or primary works; there were only three reviews or overviews of literature. 23 authors appeared as lead authors of more than one publication; in total, these authors contributed 64 items as lead authors (22.5%). Thirty-eight journals or serials published more than one article from the dataset; these are listed in Table 2.1. Titles with two or three articles were from a wide variety of domains: human resources in health, medical decision making, implementation science, information systems education, nursing administration and broader health services administration.

Topic Analysis

Topic analysis was based on analysis of controlled vocabulary. In compiling bibliographic databases such as Medline and CINAHL, a trained indexer assigns subject descriptors from a controlled vocabulary to each newly received article. MeSH (Medical Subject Headings) is the vocabulary used in Medline. Applying the

Table 2.1 Journals which published multiple items in the dataset

No. of items	Journal name and date span of items
26	Studies in Health Technology & Informatics 1996–2017
14	Bulletin of the Medical Library Association 1981–2000
10	International Journal of Medical Informatics 1998–2017
9	AMIA Annual Symposium Proceedings 1999–2008 Journal of the American Medical Informatics Association 1997–2018 Journal of the Medical Library Association 2002–2018 Yearbook of Medical Informatics 1998–2017
8	Health Information & Libraries Journal 2004–2017 Journal of AHIMA 1993–2017
7	Topics in Health Information Management 1992–2002
6	Methods of Information in Medicine 1994–2018
5	Applied Clinical Informatics 2010–2015 Medical Reference Services Quarterly 1998–2013
4	Health Informatics Journal 2000–2017 Health Information Management Journal 2004–2016 Health Libraries Review 1993–2000 Journal of Information Systems Education 2011–2014 Proceedings of Medinfo: World Congress on Medical & Health Informatics 1974–1995
3	Academic Medicine 1995–2017 American Journal of Pharmaceutical Education 2016–2017 BMC Medical Informatics & Decision Making 2009–2016 Journal of Hospital Librarianship 2005–2007 Journal of Nursing Administration 2011–2017 Journal of the Canadian Health Libraries Association 2008–2017 Perspectives in Health Information Management 2012–2013
2	Australian Health Review 2009–2016 Evidence Based Library & Information Practice 2010–2011 Human Resources in Health 2013–2015 Implementation Science 2013–2016 Information Services & Use 2006–2017 Journal of Health Communication 2012 Journal of Healthcare Information Management 2004 Journal of Physical Therapy Education 2004–2010 Journal of Public Health Management & Practice 2015–2016 Journal of the American Society for Information Science 1987–1988 Nursing Administration Quarterly 1997–2007 Online Journal of Public Health Informatics 2012–2014 Telemedicine Journal & E-Health 2012

vocabulary terms enables uniform indexing by subject, rather than relying only on the keywords proposed by the authors. It also links the concepts in the individual record to other records in the database with the same terms, and thus suggests a shared knowledge relationship with those records. Filtering and grouping all the MeSH terms applied this way to the items included in the dataset showed that more than 500 subject descriptors or designated keywords were used. Of these, 32 were applied 10 or more times; these are listed in Table 2.2. They cover domains such as professions (e.g. Medical Informatics, Professional Role), education and curriculum, technological concepts (e.g. Electronic Health Records) and managerial terms (Forecasting, Program Evaluation, Trends). The term Health Personnel—defined in MeSH as "Men and women working in the provision of health services, whether as individual practitioners or employees of health institutions and programs, whether or not professionally trained, and whether or not subject to public regulation"—appears in this group of frequently applied terms, as does one named occupation—Librarians.

The high count for the term "Medical Informatics" can be partly attributed to the gradual evolution of informatics descriptors in the MeSH vocabulary. "Medical Informatics" was introduced in 1987, whereas descriptors for other informatics specialties only became available more than 15 years later: Public Health Informatics

Table 2.2 MeSH subject descriptors assigned to ten or more items in the dataset

No. of items	Subject descriptor
65	Medical Informatics
60	Education
55	Organisation and administration
50	Curriculum
29	Standards
28	Methods
25	Libraries, Medical
22	Professional Competence; Trends
21	Information Services
20	Delivery of Health Care
19	Medical Records, Computerised
18	Surveys and Questionnaires
17	Computer Communication Networks
16	Internet; Professional Role
15	Library Science
14	Information Systems; Statistics and Numerical Data
13	Female; Information Management; Leadership; Librarians; Male
12	Adult; Electronic Health Records; Program Evaluation
11	Health Personnel; Information Storage and Retrieval
10	Education, Medical; Forecasting; Library Services

in 2003, Nursing Informatics and Dental Informatics in 2005, and Consumer Health Informatics in 2018. The broader (parent) term "Informatics" was also introduced in 2005, defined as "The field of information science concerned with the analysis and dissemination of data through the application of computers"; up to 2004, this concept was indexed using the term "Information Systems" (National Library of Medicine 2020).

Role Analysis

The health information occupation identities reported in the publications were grouped into nine broad categories. The "years" shown for each job title in Fig. 2.3 provide an insight into the timeline of the health information work occupations. The occupational groups identified in the earliest years are health information technologists, health information managers (HIMs) and medical or health librarians.

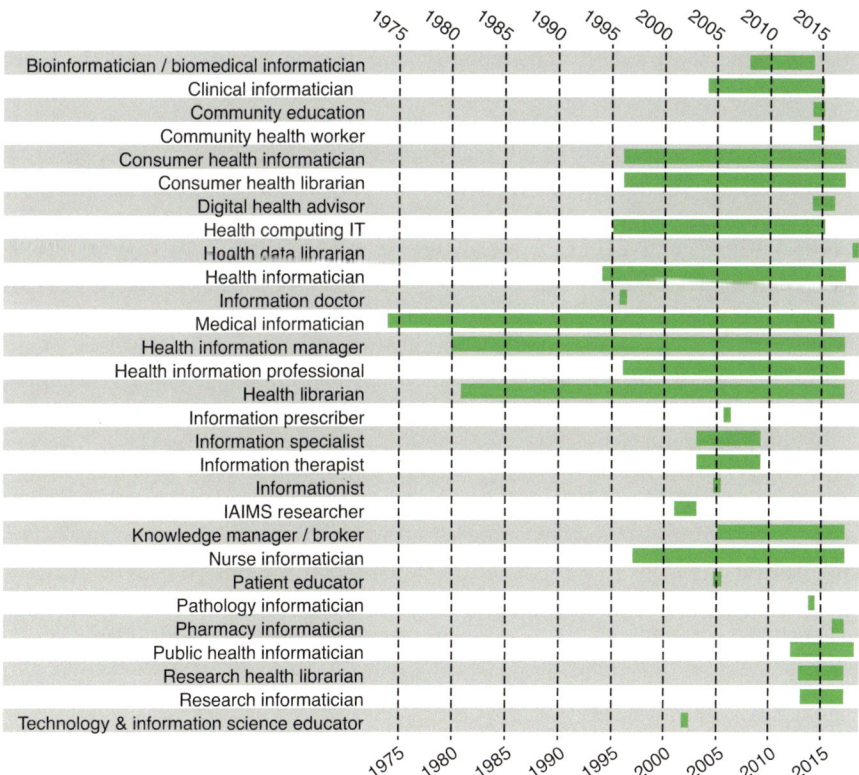

Fig. 2.3 Job titles showing years when used

Reference to clinical participation in this work by medical practitioners also began early and frequently has been linked with advocating informatics education for doctors-in-training (Gonzalo et al. 2017). This trend was followed a decade later, in greater numbers of papers, in the nursing literature. Other occupations, not mentioned often until the twenty-first century, are in the allied health professions (pharmacists and physiotherapists) and in knowledge management. Knowledge work in health has undergone a resurgence, with the recent emergence of knowledge broker and knowledge translator roles, e.g. Glegg and Hoens (2016); Hopkins (2017). A small range of occupations were mentioned only once, such as health administrator, community health worker, researcher and student.

A handful of articles described or advocated for "dual identities" that combined both a health occupation and an information occupation. Examples of these dual identities are: medical practitioner + informatician (Zimmerman et al. 1988), health librarian + informatician (Frisse et al. 1995), nurse + informatician (Bakken et al. 2004) and health information manager + informatician (Bloomrosen and Berner 2017). These illustrate the way that the work of managing information content, information retrieval and information technology in health may form "a tightly woven interdisciplinary braid" (McKnight 2005, p. 13).

More than 60 distinct job titles were used in the publications. A majority matched the titles used in the identity categories listed above, while the less frequent job titles predominantly reflect contemporary or emerging terms. Some of these are creative and intriguing in the way they try to express the scope of work. Examples include decision support manpower and digital information roles (Ash et al. 2015; Dimitrov 2016), community health staff trained in "last-mile" health data collection responsibilities (Bram et al. 2015), a clinician responsible for health data security (Gaunt and Roger-France 1996), information therapist (Mettler and Kemper 2003) and health literacy expert (Vellar et al. 2016). For this analysis the job titles were grouped into 25 categories; Fig. 2.3 displays the job titles matched with their years of usage. Many articles present identity-specific perspectives on the roles, responsibilities, and functions of the nominated profession. The extracts below show examples over the years, for the top four identities: health informatician; health librarian; health information manager; health information technologist.

Health informaticians' perspectives on the work are exemplified here. Greenes and Lorenzi (1998) argued the strategic agenda for health and biomedical informatics work is in incorporating the increasing role of information technology. Sable et al. (2000) identified medical informaticians as interdisciplinary workers who understand clinical medicine, healthcare management and information technology. Kushniruk et al. (2006) observed that informaticians have roles in health services management, development, research and evaluation. McLane and Turley (2011) compared roles of informaticians, project managers and IT professionals in healthcare organisations; speaking from a nursing informatics perspective, they maintained that all three groups ensure the health environment uses IT effectively, with information and knowledge management as core values. Mac McCullough and Goodin (2014) observed that the informatics capacity of staff in local public health departments directly influences how much use is made of the informatics functionality in the health informatics systems. Wholey et al. (2018) asserted that the primary function of public health informatics is to use informatics to improve the health of populations. Khan (2018) gave an example in which informaticians provided "clinical leadership" in the modernisation of the military health system to integrate military-civilian health care delivery. This report also described education of the HI workforce in the U.S. Defense Health Agency. Valenta et al. (2018) described health informatics as an emerging profession with a range of subdisciplines, such as bioinformatics, translational, clinical, public health, consumer health and clinical research informatics.

Health librarians' perspectives: Goffman (1981) advocated for an international health information libraries network and contemplated the personnel, financial and technological requirements for it to be efficient and successful. Bradley (1996) analysed changes in health information and HI work, noting that multiple concepts of information exist, and these depend heavily on different disciplines and professions; this author argued that health librarians' specialty work is relevant to the electronic environment, and professionals in the health library and information science area should redefine and communicate their place in it. Deardorff et al. (2017) described a research project where health librarians tested "authoritative" answers to a real-world corpus of questions submitted by patients and consumers, using the MedlinePlus interface, and saw lessons for evaluating question-answering services and tools. Federer (2018) defined and scoped the knowledge used by librarians specialising in health data librarianship services, and the training and competencies required in these roles.

Health information managers' perspectives: Abdelhak (1980) forecast that the health record practitioner would have an expanded role as a health information specialist. Brunner (1992) argued that medical record professionals need to adapt to the new role of HIMs. Fenton et al. (2017) pointed out that HIM work needs to include roles such as data scientists and data stewards to ensure sound management of data analytics and digital transformation. Butler-Henderson (2017) highlighted updated work practices and educational reform as essential to ensure the on-going inclusion of HIMs in data-driven health systems; this author proposed embedded roles for HIMs in clinical, business, IT and health funder segments of the health industry, and nominated information governance and data management as a strategic focus for this work.

Health Information Technologists' perspectives: Clarke (1997) stated that the information specialist's role was to combine clinical expertise with knowledge of current computer technology with the key tasks being to manage information and health care data. Denham et al. (2013) focused on the work of ensuring health IT safety and argued for the use of proven post-deployment performance assessment of EHR systems in healthcare organisations. Skillman et al. (2015) noted that a trained health IT workforce was required in rural primary care settings, but not likely to be available due to infrastructure weaknesses and workforce barriers. Ammenwerth et al. (2017) described the use of real-world "sub-information systems" for practical exercises in the health information systems curriculum taught in Europe since 2001. Cresswell et al. (2017) argued that expert and experienced health IT personnel were required to optimise the implementation of complex IT systems.

A number of authors gave examples of blended or interdisciplinary roles, such as the following cases in the community and patient education context: Martin et al. (1997) outlined a project involving librarians, primary care and outreach workers, translators and IT staff to deliver health information services and technologies for community AIDS training and education. Oster and Thomas (1998) described teaching "health information internet" classes in a community setting, with providers comprising a medical librarian, a community health activist and a physician with expertise in medical informatics. Greenberg et al. (2004) outlined the roles of consumers, quality experts, search engine experts, researchers, healthcare providers, informatics specialists and others to improve the results of consumers' internet searches for health information. Alamantariotou and Zisi (2010) presented an overview of methods and tools to present health information to consumers, and they noted the interdisciplinary nature of consumer health informatics work. Ndira et al. (2014) described an "information intervention"—a malaria prevention health information package—done in multiple villages by a team of medical students, community health workers and technical experts.

Recurring Concerns

Four main themes preoccupy authors who have written about health information workers, based on an inductive analysis of publications in the dataset: role changes brought about by external drivers; competencies and new curriculum required for specialised information workers to remain relevant; informatics education for the wider health workforce (in undergraduate curricula, and professional development for existing workforce); and cooperation and combined strengths among existing professions and occupations (also for informaticians and HIMs). These themes are unfolded over the years through examples below.

Authors frequently referred to rapid change, external reform and technological innovation as inexorable drivers for change in roles and competencies. Scherrer (2004) reported on new roles adopted by health librarians in the previous decade, and the changing balance of functions performed. This was accompanied by a new job title: academic health information professional. Newly adopted activities included closer faculty liaison, web site design and marketing or promotion using new technologies. Tarver et al. (2013) described how a university health service's clinics used librarians to guide consumers accessing the facility's patient portal, and the MedlinePlus consumer health resource which was contextually linked to it. Baird and Nowak (2014) proposed that primary care practices should extend the concept of "patient portals" by coordinating patients' health data from multiple sources into a digital health information hub, with the added benefit that staff in the practice could provide expert advice and encourage patient engagement. Abdelhak et al. (2016) noted redefined roles for HIM and HI, in the context of a continuous Learning Health system. Butler (2016) suggested that HIM required updated competencies to reflect themes such as informatics, information governance, as well as new academic competencies from AHIMA. Vellar et al. (2016) described an Australian health service's partnership with consumers to address health literacy, aiming to improve the health experience and health outcomes of consumers. Lake (2018) described the librarians' role in offering a consumer medical apps service in a Utah health system. Their expertise was used in digital health technology selection and evaluation to advise both health care professionals and consumers.

With regard to competencies and new curriculum required to remain relevant, in nursing informatics, Bakken et al. (2004) described enhanced informatics competencies and linked this with the broader focus on information technology for safe and effective health care. Further cases are provided by Fetter (2009) citing the TIGER (Technology Informatics Guiding Education Reform) project for the IT competencies needed in the implementation of EHRs, and Yen et al. (2017) who reported the development of a nursing informatics competency assessment aimed at nursing administrators. Murphy and Goossen (2017) described nursing informatics competencies needed for "connected health", highlighting roles including nursing informatics specialists. In health information management, Johns (1995) focused on the leadership qualities that HIM professionals required to manage changes in health care, such as systems thinking and team learning. Butler (2017) outlined skills that HIM professionals needed to practice in the twenty-first century; these included information governance, informatics, data analytics, leadership and project management. Similar competencies were identified by Grzybowski and Orlova (2017), with the addition of soft skills such as ethics, leadership, teamwork and advocacy. Public health informatics education was examined by Joshi and Perin (2012). Their review concluded there was a need for online PHI training programs that could be accessed by professionals worldwide. Drezner et al. (2016) described the skills used by the informatics workforce employed at local public health departments in the USA including: data extraction from information systems, data analytics using statistical programs, GIS systems and website content maintenance. Tremblay et al. (2016) detailed a master's level cross-disciplinary informatics program that added business analysis topics to other skills in health informatics, information systems and data analytics. Several authors highlighted knowledge-based work. Haynes (1998) explained the use of evidence-based informatics, which combines health informatics with best evidence retrieval, summarising, disseminating and applying to improve the transfer of knowledge into health care practice. Haux (2002) described the need for health care professionals well-trained in medical informatics systems to apply medical knowledge resources in patient care. The role of "research informatician lead" was described by Embi et al. (2013), to oversee design, deployment and use of a variety of information resources to advance research and contribute to discoveries and evidence generation.

The concept of a specialist health information workforce exists in relation to a general health workforce, and the distribution of expertise between the two is a perennial balancing act. Zimmerman et al. (1988) discussed the ambiguous and evolving field of "medical informatics", and its place in education and training of health care professionals, in an information-intensive environment. They argued that health care professionals should retain responsibility for medical and patient information; if this is ceded "…they lose control over the quality of care delivered to patients" (p. 139). On this basis, they recommended the introduction of medical informatics training in the curricula for health science professions. The example they cited was the informatics education included in dentistry, nursing and other health professional programs at the University of Maryland at Baltimore. Terry et al. (2008) synthesised lessons from implementing EHR systems in primary care. These included a need to establish the computer literacy of intended users and to address their expectations and willingness to accept the EHR system, in part by use of a leader or champion to assist. Triola et al. (2010) urged the inclusion of core biomedical informatics competencies in medical school curricula, with emphasis on EHR systems, safety and evidence-based care. Ledikwe et al. (2013) described information skills training for health monitoring and evaluation officers in Botswana. The program resulted in improved skills in computer literacy, checking data validity, implementing data quality procedures, using data to support program planning, proposing indicators, and writing monitoring and evaluation reports. Whittaker et al. (2015) documented consensus findings on HIS competencies needed by general health workers, following a consultation process with HIS experts. Their framework enabled improved workforce capability training, particularly in low resource settings. Schleder Goncalves et al. (2015) reported observations on the computing and information literacy of nurses working in hospitals and public health units in southern Brazil. The majority of those surveyed were assessed to have novice-level skills in these areas, despite having some IT exposure in both professional and personal life activities. The authors described educational programs to address these areas in nursing education. Gonzalo et al. (2017) proposed that medical curricula should include health systems science content, to align the education with the needs of the systems currently implemented in health services.

Cooperation and combined strengths among existing professions and occupations have been proposed from many angles. In 2000, a new role, dubbed the informationist, was proposed (Davidoff and Florance 2000). It was envisioned as a knowledge role that would bridge the gap between the findings in published medical literature and applying them in clinical practice. The authors proposed this role would research clinical questions efficiently and effectively using the health information resources and deliver a synopsis to the clinician at the point of care. Davidoff and Florance proposed that the informationist would be educated in both clinical and information science skills. They suggested a multidisciplinary curriculum drawing on input from many, including medical informaticians. They noted "potential turf issues in relation to library science, medical informatics, and clinical medicine" (p. 998). A response from medical informatics came via Hersh (2002, p. 76), who argued that "…individuals do not have to be librarians to become information-ists". This view was based on his belief that medical informatics had "fuzzy bound-aries"; it did not have a common set of skills nor a common curriculum. He agreed that informationist training could be gained through a conventional library science degree complemented by clinical experience. Alternatively, he proposed training in medical informatics would be another pathway to train the informationist. Hersh argued that both fields should "work together to identify the appropriate skills for informationists and ensure that individuals of either training experience can apply and teach them effectively" (p. 79). Perry et al. (2005) offered a similar perspective on the disciplines of medical informatics and health sciences librarianship. They noted that "boundaries are disappearing between the sources and types of, and uses for, health information managed by informaticians and librarians. Definitions of the professional domains of each have been impacted by these changes in informa-tion…Professionals in these disciplines are increasingly functioning collaboratively as 'boundary spanners', uniting technology with health care delivery" (p. 199). Dalrymple and Roderer (2010) noted the expansion of informatics courses in the USA during that decade. Based on their view that health informatics and health information science are converging, they examined education for health information professionals. They argued that "schools of information science have an important role to play…in educating health informationists" (p. 45), alongside the other disci-plines which have established themselves in the informatics sector. Similarly, Gibson et al. (2015) suggested that boundaries between health informatics and health information management were disappearing, in response to changes in health care delivery and information technologies. They concluded with recommendations to strengthen the roles of each profession, and collaboration between them. Bloomrosen and Berner (2017) observed that the discipline of health information management "increasingly is becoming allied with the field of medical and health informatics in that both disciplines have interests in common" (p. 81). They noted that conventional HIM expertise in coding, privacy and security is also essential in contemporary electronic information exchange, and information governance is critical.

Discussion

Two hundred and eighty-four peer-reviewed papers from the past five decades spe-cifically address the question of what people do, in health information work. Synthesis of this body of literature gives a disparate picture: a workforce that is like a large family whose members barely stay in touch, with many different voices, siloed sub-groups, and little appreciation of their interdependence. This characteri-sation is consistent with observations from many quarters, exemplified by the World Health Organization observation that opened this chapter.

The major strength of this study is to go beyond studying or surveying individual workforce segments—just HIMs, or just health librarians, for example—and to show how much irregularity and overlap there is in the definition and expectation of professionalism in this part of the health workforce. The contrast with other areas of the health workforce is plain, as echoed elsewhere, for example in Scott et al. (2018, p. 127): "Data science in healthcare is subject to strong regulatory and ethical controls, minimum educational qualifications, well-established methodologies, mandatory professional accreditation and evidence-based independent scrutiny. By contrast, 'Digital Health' has minimal substantive regulation or ethical foundation, no specified educational requirements, weak methodologies, a contested evidence base and negligible peer scrutiny."

The findings reported here have the potential to affect individual and community views. There is a broader base and longer tradition of knowledge in this kind of work than many current or intending practitioners or employers realise. In the competition for new and emerging roles in the era of digital health, individuals may not be recognised for the knowledge and skills they have, or the scholarly tradition behind them. However, the literature does not show industry or professional associations or health bureaucracies advocating to strengthen recognition of the work. Thus changes that improve this situation for people in this workforce are not certain, unless their collective voice becomes louder and clearer.

Several ways forward are possible. An altogether more collaborative approach to the work may be needed to encompass emerging needs for knowledge and skills, as posited by McKnight (2005). For example, Rajamani et al. (2015) suggest collaborative practice, interprofessional education and health informatics expertise to facilitate a learning health system. Abdelhak et al. (2016, p. S8) proposes "leveraging innovative health data management policies, practices, and developing a collaborative, competent workforce". Alternatively it is possible that one workforce sub-group will outcompete others to become the most distinctive and credible organising force for digital health information work. Another prospect is that a more established group within the health workforce (for example, health service managers) "takes over" the claim to expertise.

This review of the literature is not without limitations. The scoping review process necessarily used very broad search terms, generating a large number of retrieved items in the initial stage of research. Screening the abstracts required a tight focus; articles with scant information were rejected even though they may have made some valid contributions. In a scoping review, quality assessments of the included items are optional (Tricco et al. 2018, item 12); in this review, no quality assessment or critical appraisal was performed. The authors of the current review were unable to include results from databases specific to the engineering and computer science disciplines. The broad search strategies retrieved tens of thousands of items from these resources, which exceeded the team's capacity for screening and selection. In this respect, it has not been possible to conform to the original protocol published in 2019, and this may mean that computer science and information technology aspects that characterise the health information workforce are under-represented in this study. The dataset was limited to English language publications, nevertheless the work originates from many different regions of the world and the findings are widely applicable.

Conclusion

This chapter has mapped the published international literature discussing an instrumental or professional human role in health information work over five decades. This review is unparalleled in its scope and depth; to our knowledge, it offers the most comprehensive overview conducted to date, of scholarly understanding about this segment of the health workforce. The review systematically highlights the human agency in such work and comprises a rich resource for workforce planning. This review illustrates the extent, distribution and nature of the specialised work done by people trained in a variety of disciplines. Their work is described using an assortment of terms for roles and functions, and for the underlying competencies required to discharge these responsibly. It is hard to imagine any other group of specialists in the health workforce that is accountable for such crucial outcomes as health data, information and knowledge are expected to deliver in the twenty-first century, and yet is so diffuse and disjointed. In the era of digital health, an apparently mission-critical part of the health workforce is ill-defined and fragmented.

The review has identified that the absence of a coherent professional identity or a pathway toward professionalisation—including a uniformly defined scope of practice, code of conduct, training and continuing education framework or system of licensing to practice—is a major gap in this part of the health workforce. This gap creates an uneven balance of power between producers and consumers of data, information and knowledge products and services in the health sector. The review has found relatively little empirical research into health information work or the workforce. Isolated project reports exist but do not appear to build toward any major lasting workforce reviews or reforms. Health services research is needed, to analyse how this work contributes to health system performance, and the relative impacts of different approaches to planning and management of the workforce. This review has highlighted the distance that this workforce still needs to travel if its members wish to play visible, vital roles in realising the anticipated benefits of digital information and communication technologies in health. It is a truism that investment in health information and communication technologies is rarely matched with investment in creating a skilled health information workforce. In this case, the investment required is not merely money, but ideas. Innovative thinking is needed, to construct a consolidated identity and community that can be recognised and understood alongside other professions in the health workforce.

Notes This work received funding support from The University of Melbourne. We acknowledge Nadine Ogonek and Patrick Condron for their assistance with elements of the data analysis.

Appendix

Medline search strategy (search performed 14 June 2017)

1. "health information".ab,ti.
2. "healthcare information".ab,ti.
3. "health care information".ab,ti.
4. "health-care information".ab,ti.
5. informatics.ab,ti.
6. management.ab,ti
7. "technolog*".ab,ti
8. (library or libraries).ab,ti.
9. systems.ab,ti.
10. digital.ab,ti.
11. 5 and 6
12. 5 and 7
13. 5 and 8
14. 5 and 9
15. 5 and 10
16. 6 and 7
17. 6 and 8
18. 6 and 9
19. 6 and 10
20. 7 and 8
21. 7 and 9
22. 7 and 10
23. 8 and 9
24. 8 and 10
25. 9 and 10
26. 11 or 12 or 13 or 14 or 15 or 16 or 17 or 18 or 19 or 20 or 21 or 22 or 23 or 24 or 25
27. (work or worker or workers or workforce).ab,ti.
28. (profession or professional or professionals or professions).ab,ti.
29. (role or roles).ab,ti.
30. (staff or staffing).ab,ti.
31. (expert or experts or expertise).ab,ti.
32. (specialist or specialists or specialized or specialised or specialisation* or specialization*).ab,ti.
33. (leader or leaders or leadership).ab,ti.
34. (champion or champions or championing).ab,ti.
35. (manager or managers).ab,ti.
36. ("change agent" or "change agents").ab,ti.
37. 27 or 28 or 29 or 30 or 31 or 32 or 33 or 34 or 35 or 36
38. 1 or 2 or 3 or 4
39. 26 and 38
40. 37 and 39 (1782 items)

Bibliography

Abdelhak M. The expanded role of the health record practitioner: health information specialist. Med Rec News. 1980;51(2):49–52.

Abdelhak M, Ball M, Romero Serrano R, Händel A, Hübner U. Achieving a global learning health system by leveraging innovative health data management policies, practices, and developing a collaborative, competent workforce. Eur J Epidemiol. 2016;31:S8. https://doi.org/10.1007/s10654-016-0183-1.

Abidi SS, Cheah YN, Curran J. A knowledge creation info-structure to acquire and crystallize the tacit knowledge of experts. IEEE Trans Inf Technol Biomed. 2005;9(2):193–204.

Alamantariotou K, Zisi D. Consumer health informatics and interactive visual learning tools for health. Int J Electron Healthc. 2010;5(4):414–24. https://doi.org/10.1504/IJEH.2010.036211.

Alexander S, Frith KH, O'Keefe L, Hennigan MA. Implementation of customized health information technology in diabetes self management programs. Clin Nurse Spec. 2011;25:63–70. https://doi.org/10.1097/NUR.0b013e31820aefd6.

Ali N, Tretiakov A, Whiddett D, Hunter I. Knowledge management systems success in healthcare: leadership matters. Int J Med Inform. 2017;97:331–40. https://doi.org/10.1016/j.ijmedinf.2016.11.004.

American Health Information Management Association. Position Statement. Issue: roles of health information managers and coders in patient-focused care. J AHIMA. 1993;64(10):suppl 2.

American Health Information Management Association. Position statement. Issue: healthcare reform–information systems and the need for computer-based patient records. J AHIMA. 1994;65(1):1st suppl 1-2, following p. 84.

Ammenwerth E, Knaup P, Winter A, Bauer AW, Bott OJ, Gietzelt M, et al. On teaching international courses on health information systems. Lessons learned during 16 years of Frank - van Swieten Lectures on Strategic Information Management in Health Information Systems. Methods Inf Med. 2017;56:e39–48. https://doi.org/10.3414/ME16-01-0124.

Anderson J, Forsythe JM. Abstracts. Medinfo. 1974;1.

Arksey H, O'Malley L. Scoping studies: towards a methodological framework. Int J Soc Res Methodol. 2005;8(1):19–32. https://doi.org/10.1080/1364557032000119616.

Ash JS, Sittig DF, McMullen CK, Wright A, Bunce A, Mohan V, et al. Multiple perspectives on clinical decision support: a qualitative study of fifteen clinical and vendor organizations. BMC Med Inf Decis Mak. 2015;15:35. https://doi.org/10.1186/s12911-015-0156-4.

Assar S, Hickerson L. Exploring information behavior with hierarchical goal decomposition: the case of a web-based consumer-oriented genetics resource. J Hosp Librariansh. 2007;7(2):91–101. https://doi.org/10.1300/J186v07n02_09.

Ayodeji Makinde O, Mami MI, Oweghoro BM, Oyediran KA, Mullen S. Investing in health information management: the right people, in the right place, at the right time. Health Inf Manag J. 2016;45(2):90–6. https://doi.org/10.1177/1833358316639447.

Bachman JA, Panzarine S. Enabling student nurses to use the information superhighway. J Nurs Educ. 1998;37(4):155–61.

Baird A, Nowak S. Why primary care practices should become digital health information hubs for their patients. BMC Fam Pract. 2014;15:190. https://doi.org/10.1186/s12875-014-0190-9.

Bakken S. Informatics for patient safety: a nursing research perspective. Annu Rev Nurs Res. 2006;24:219–54.

Bakken S, Cook SS, Curtis L, Desjardins K, Hyun S, Jenkins M, et al. Promoting patient safety through informatics-based nursing education. Int J Med Inform. 2004;73(7-8):581–9. https://doi.org/10.1016/j.ijmedinf.2004.04.008.

Balloun JL, Stebbins LH, Von Bergen CW. The emerging need for transformational leadership in health information management. Top Health Inf Manag. 1995;15(3):39–46.

Bassi J, Kushniruk AW, Borycki EM. Application of the Technological Pedagogical Content Knowledge framework in integrating an educational EMR into health informatics education. Stud Health Technol Inform. 2013;183:49–53.

Bassinder J, Bali RK, Naguib R. Knowledge management and electronic care records: incorporating social, legal and ethical issues. Stud Health Technol Inform. 2006;121:221–7.

Bayley TJ. Libraries, postgraduate medical education and the management of change. Health Libr Rev. 1993;10(1):3–9.

Bimerew M. Challenges in the use of information technology in processing health information in resource limited settings: a comprehensive systematic review. Afr J Nurs Midwifery. 2015;17:S71–89.

Bloomrosen M, Berner ES. Findings from the 2017 Yearbook section on health information management. Yearb Med Inform. 2017;26:78–83. https://doi.org/10.15265/IY-2017-025.

Bolley HB. Physicians in health care management: 6. Physician *bytes* computer. CMAJ. 1994;150(12):1977–82.

Bomba B, Cooper J, Miller M. Working towards a national health information system in Australia. Medinfo. 1995;8 Pt 2:1633.

Booth A. Bridging the 'Know-do gap': a role for health information professionals? Health Info Libr J. 2011;28(4):331–4. https://doi.org/10.1111/j.1471-1842.2011.00960.x.

Booth A, Carroll C, Papaioannou D, Sutton A, Wong R. Applying findings from a systematic review of workplace-based e-learning: implications for health information professionals. Health Info Libr J. 2009;26(1):4–21. https://doi.org/10.1111/j.1471-1842.2008.00834.x.

Bradley J. The changing face of health information and health information work: a conceptual framework. Bull Med Libr Assoc. 1996;84(1):1–10.

Bradley J, Marshall JG. Using scientific evidence to improve information practice. Health Libr Rev. 1995;12(3):147–57.

Bram JT, Warwick-Clark B, Obeysekare E, Mehta K. Utilization and monetization of healthcare data in developing countries. Big Data. 2015;3(2):59–66. https://doi.org/10.1089/big.2014.0053.

Brander G, Pawliuk C. Research-embedded health librarians as facilitators of a multidisciplinary scoping review. J Can Health Libr Assoc. 2017;38(2):38–43. https://doi.org/10.5596/c17-009.

Breil B, Fritz F, Thiemann V, Dugas M. Multidisciplinary education in medical informatics–a course for medical and informatics students. Stud Health Technol Inform. 2010;160(Pt 1):581–4.

Brennen PW. The medical libraries of Vietnam–a service in transition. Bull Med Libr Assoc. 1992;80(3):294–9.

Brittain JM, Norris AC. Delivery of health informatics education and training. Health Libr Rev. 2000;17(3):117–28.

Brixey JJ. Health informatics competencies, workforce and the DNP: why connect these 'dots'? Stud Health Technol Inform. 2016;225:750–2.

Brunner BK. Health information management in the computer era. Top Health Inf Manag. 1992;13(2):1–8.

Bryant SL, Stewart D, Goswami L. Knowledge for healthcare: the future of health librarianship. Health Info Libr J. 2015;32(3):163–6. https://doi.org/10.1111/hir.12119.

Burrows S, Ginn DS, Love N, Williams TL. A strategy for curriculum integration of information skills instruction. Bull Med Libr Assoc. 1989;77(3):245–51.

Bury R, Martin L, Roberts S. Achieving change through mutual development: supported online learning and the evolving roles of health and information professionals. Health Info Libr J. 2006;23(Suppl 1):22–31. https://doi.org/10.1111/j.1471-1842.2006.00677.x.

Butler M. HIM's Professional SHAKE-UP WAKE-UP. J AHIMA. 2016;87:16–21.

Butler M. Teaching the 'New' HIM. J AHIMA. 2017;88:16–9.

Butler-Henderson K. Health information management 2025. What is required to create a sustainable profession in the face of digital transformation? Launceston, Australia: University of Tasmania; 2017.

Butler-Henderson K, Gray K. Health information workforce census. University of Tasmania. 2018a. http://www.utas.edu.au/business-and-economics/hiwcensus. Accessed 18 Apr 2020.

Butler-Henderson K, Gray K. Australia's health information workforce: census summary report 2018. Launceston: University of Tasmania; 2018b. http://www.utas.edu.au/business-and-economics/hiwcensus. Accessed 18 Apr 2020.

Butler-Henderson K, Gray K, Greenfield D, Low S, Gilbert C, Ritchie A, et al. Development of a national census of the health information workforce: expert panel recommendations. Stud Health Technol Inform. 2017;239:8–13.

Campbell CA. The critical attributes of leadership. Top Health Inf Manag. 1992;13(2):9–19.

Carney TJ, Kong AY. Leveraging health informatics to foster a smart systems response to health disparities and health equity challenges. J Biomed Inform. 2017;68:184–9. https://doi.org/10.1016/j.jbi.2017.02.011.

Caufield-Noll C, Gorman L. Heart-healthy conversations: a librarian-physician partnership to promote disease management and wellness information to cardiology patients. J Consumer Health Internet. 2017;21:148–58. https://doi.org/10.1080/15398285.2017.1309169.

Cellucci LW, Layman EJ, Campbell R, Xiaoming Z. Integrating healthcare ethical issues into IS education. J Inform Syst Educ. 2011;22:215–24.

Centre for Reviews and Dissemination. PROSPERO International prospective register of systematic reviews. Inclusion criteria. CRD, University of York, York. n.d. https://www.crd.york.ac.uk/PROSPERO/#aboutpage. Accessed 18 Apr 2020.

Chen JH, Asch SM. Machine learning and prediction in medicine – beyond the peak of inflated expectations. N Engl J Med. 2017;376(26):2507–9. https://doi.org/10.1056/NEJMp1702071.

Cheng G. The 'market' for medical and health information in transition: the case of the Hong Kong Hospital Authority libraries. Health Libr Rev. 1996;13(2):69–80.

Chi Z, Reichgelt H, Rutherfoord RH, Ju An Wang A. Developing health information technology (HIT) programs and HIT curriculum: the Southern Polytechnic State University experience. J Inform Syst Educ. 2014;25:295–303.

Chonsilapawit T, Rungpragayphan S. Skills and knowledge of informatics, and training needs of hospital pharmacists in Thailand: a self-assessment survey. Int J Med Inform. 2016;94:255–62. https://doi.org/10.1016/j.ijmedinf.2016.08.001.

Chung J, Cho I. The need for academic electronic health record systems in nurse education. Nurse Educ Today. 2017;54:83–8. https://doi.org/10.1016/j.nedt.2017.04.018.

Clarke A. Role and responsibilities of an information specialist. Semin Perioper Nurs. 1997;6(2):81–6.

Cleveland AD. Miles to go before we sleep: education, technology, and the changing paradigms in health information. J Med Libr Assoc. 2011;99(1):61–9. https://doi.org/10.3163/1536-5050.99.1.011.

Collins S, Yen PY, Phillips A, Kennedy MK. Nursing informatics competency assessment for the nurse leader: the Delphi study. J Nurs Adm. 2017;47(4):212–8. https://doi.org/10.1097/NNA.0000000000000467.

Conklin J, Lusk E, Harris M, Stolee P. Knowledge brokers in a knowledge network: the case of Seniors Health Research Transfer Network knowledge brokers. Implement Sci. 2013;8(1):7. https://doi.org/10.1186/1748-5908-8-7.

Connors HR, Weaver C, Warren J, Miller KL. An academic-business partnership for advancing clinical informatics. Nurs Educ Perspect. 2002;23(5):228–33.

Connors H, Warren J, Weaver C. HIT plants SEEDS in healthcare education...Health information technology... Simulated E-hEalth Delivery System. Nurs Adm Q. 2007;31:129–33.

Cooper H. Changing roles of health information managers: an education perspective. Health Inf Manag J. 2009;38:38–42.

Corbett M, Deardorff A, Kovar-Gough I. Emerging data management roles for health librarians in electronic medical records. J Can Health Libr Assoc. 2014;32:55–9. https://doi.org/10.5596/c14-022.

Covidence Systematic Review Software. Veritas Health Innovation, Melbourne, Australia. n.d. https://www.covidence.org/home. Accessed 18 Apr 2020

Cresswell KM, Bates DW, Sheikh A. Ten key considerations for the successful optimization of large-scale health information technology. J Am Med Inform Assoc. 2017;24(1):182–7. https://doi.org/10.1093/jamia/ocw037.

Custis LM, Hawkins SY, Thomason TR. An innovative capstone health care informatics clinical residency: interprofessional team collaboration. Health Inform J. 2017;23(1):69–79. https://doi.org/10.1177/1460458215627188.

D'Alessandro MP, Galvin JR, Erkonen WE, Curry DS, Flanagan JR, D'Alessandro DM, et al. The virtual hospital: an IAIMS integrating continuing education into the work flow. MD Comput. 1996;13(4):323–9.

Dalrymple PW, Roderer NK. Education for health information professionals: perspectives from health informatics in the U.S. Educ Inform. 2010;28(1):45–55.

Davidoff F, Florance V. The informationist: a new health profession? Ann Intern Med. 2000;132(12):996–8. https://doi.org/10.7326/0003-4819-132-12-200006200-00012.

Deardorff A, Masterton K, Roberts K, Kilicoglu H, Demner-Fushman D. A protocol-driven approach to automatically finding authoritative answers to consumer health questions in online resources. J Assoc Inf Sci Technol. 2017;68(7):1724–36. https://doi.org/10.1002/asi.23806.

Demner-Fushman D, Kohli MD, Rosenman MB, Shooshan SE, Rodriguez L, Antani S, et al. Preparing a collection of radiology examinations for distribution and retrieval. J Am Med Inform Assoc. 2016;23(2):304–10. https://doi.org/10.1093/jamia/ocv080.

Denham CR, Classen DC, Swenson SJ, Henderson MJ, Zeltner T, Bates DW. Safe use of electronic health records and health information technology systems: trust but verify. J Patient Saf. 2013;9(4):177–89. https://doi.org/10.1097/PTS.0b013e3182a8c2b2.

Detlefsen EG, Epstein BA, Mickelson P, Detre T. Transforming the present–discovering the future: the University of Pittsburgh's NLM grant on education and training of health sciences librarians. Bull Med Libr Assoc. 1996;84(4):524–33.

Detmer DE. Interprofessional clinical informatics education and practice: essentials for learning healthcare systems worldwide. J Interprof Care. 2017;31(2):187–9. https://doi.org/10.108 0/13561820.2016.1250554.

Devitt N, Murphy J. A survey of the information management and technology training needs of doctors in an acute NHS trust in the United Kingdom. Health Info Libr J. 2004;21(3):164–72. https://doi.org/10.1111/j.1471-1842.2004.00492.x.

DeVore SD, Figlioli K. Lessons premier hospitals learned about implementing electronic health records. Health Aff (Millwood). 2010;29(4):664–7. https://doi.org/10.1377/hlthaff.2010.0250.

DiMarco C, Bray P, Covvey D, Cowan D, DiCiccio V, Hovy E, et al. Authoring and generation of individualised patient education materials. J Inf Technol Healthc. 2008;6:63–71.

Dimitrov DV. Medical internet of things and big data in healthcare. Healthc Inform Res. 2016;22(3):156–63. https://doi.org/10.4258/hir.2016.22.3.156.

Dixon BE, Kaneshiro K. Improving access to HIV and AIDS information resources for patients, caregivers, and clinicians: results from the SHINE Project. Online J Public Health Inform. 2012;4(1). https://doi.org/10.5210/ojphi.v4i1.3849.

Dixon BE, Newlon CM. How do future nursing educators perceive informatics? Advancing the nursing informatics agenda through dialogue. J Prof Nurs. 2010;26(2):82–9. https://doi.org/10.1016/j.profnurs.2009.05.001.

Dixon BE, Kharrazi H, Lehmann HP. Public health and epidemiology informatics: recent research and trends in the United States. Yearb Med Inform. 2015a;24(1):199–206. https://doi.org/10.15265/IY-2015-012.

Dixon BE, McFarlane TD, Dearth S, Grannis SJ, Gibson PJ. Characterizing informatics roles and needs of public health workers: results from the public health workforce interests and needs survey. J Public Health Manag Pract. 2015b;21(Suppl 6):S130–40. https://doi.org/10.1097/PHH.0000000000000304.

Dixon-Lee C, Patena K, Olenik K, Brodnik M. Graduate education bridges the gap between the electronic health record and clinical need. J Healthc Inf Manag. 2004;18(3):19–25.

Dooling JA, Houser SH, Mikaelian R, Smith CP. Transitioning to a data-driven, informatics-oriented department. J AHIMA. 2016;87:58–62.

Dorsey AD, Clements K, Garrie RL, Houser SH, Berner ES. Bridging the gap: a collaborative approach to health information management and informatics education. Appl Clin Inform. 2015;6(2):211–23. https://doi.org/10.4338/ACI-2014-09-RA-0083.

Drawz PE, Archdeacon P, McDonald CJ, Powe NR, Smith KA, Norton J, et al. CKD as a model for improving chronic disease care through electronic health records. Clin J Am Soc Nephrol. 2015;10(8):1488–99. https://doi.org/10.2215/CJN.00940115.

Drezner K, McKeown L, Shah GH. Assessing skills and capacity for informatics: activities most commonly performed by or for local health departments. J Public Health Manag Pract. 2016;22 Suppl 6, Public Health Informatics:S51-S57. https://doi.org/10.1097/PHH.0000000000000459.

Ellis B, Howard J. Clinical governance, education and learning to manage health information. Clin Gov. 2011;16:337–52. https://doi.org/10.1108/14777271111175378.

Embi PJ, Tachinardi U, Lussier Y, Starren J, Silverstein J. Integrating governance of research informatics and health care IT across an enterprise: experiences from the trenches. AMIA Summits Transl Sci Proc. 2013;2013:60–2.

Federer L. Defining data librarianship: a survey of competencies, skills, and training. J Med Libr Assoc. 2018;106(3):294–303. https://doi.org/10.5195/jmla.2018.306.

Feldman SS, Hersh W. Evaluating the AMIA-OHSU 10x10 program to train healthcare professionals in medical informatics. AMIA Annu Symp Proc. 2008:182–6.

Fennessy G. Knowledge management in evidence-based healthcare: issues raised when specialist information services search for the evidence. Health Inform J. 2001;7(1):4–7. https://doi.org/10.1177/146045820100700102.

Fenton SH. Clinical vocabularies and terminologies: impact on the future of health information management. Top Health Inf Manag. 2000;21(2):74–80.

Fenton SH, Gongora-Ferraez MJ, Joost E. Health information technology knowledge and skills needed by HIT employers. Appl Clin Inform. 2012;3(4):448–61. https://doi.org/10.4338/ACI-2012-09-RA-0035.

Fenton SH, Low S, Abrams KJ, Butler-Henderson K. Health information management: changing with time. Yearb Med Inform. 2017;26:72–7. https://doi.org/10.15265/IY-2017-021.

Fernandez-Luque L, Staccini P. All that glitters is not gold: consumer health informatics and education in the era of social media and health apps. Findings from the Yearbook 2016 Section on Consumer Health Informatics. Yearb Med Inform. 2016;25:188–93. https://doi.org/10.15265/IY-2016-045.

Fetter MS. Improving information technology competencies: implications for psychiatric mental health nursing. Issues Ment Health Nurs. 2009;30(1):3–13. https://doi.org/10.1080/01612840802555208.

Forrest M. Learning and teaching retrospective. Health Info Libr J. 2008;25:22–4. https://doi.org/10.1111/j.1471-1842.2008.00799.x.

Forsman RB, Nelson PP. The Academy of Health Information Professionals: a review of the first five years. Bull Med Libr Assoc. 1997;85(4):362–72.

Fox BI, Flynn A, Clauson KA, Seaton TL, Breeden E. An approach for all in pharmacy informatics education. Am J Pharm Educ. 2017;81(2):38. https://doi.org/10.5688/ajpe81238.

Frisse ME, Braude RM, Florance V, Fuller S. Informatics and medical libraries: changing needs and changing roles. Acad Med. 1995;70(1):30–5. https://doi.org/10.1097/00001888-199501000-00010.

Fuller S. Regional health information systems: applying the IAIMS model. J Am Med Inform Assoc. 1997;4(2 Suppl):S47–51.

Gardner RM, Overhage JM, Steen EB, Munger BS, Holmes JH, Williamson JJ, et al. Core content for the subspecialty of clinical informatics. J Am Med Inform Assoc. 2009;16(2):153–7. https://doi.org/10.1197/jamia.M3045.

Gathoni N. Enhancing access to health information in Africa: a librarian's perspective. J Health Commun. 2012;17(Suppl 2):18–22. https://doi.org/10.1080/10810730.2012.666628.

Gaunt N, Roger-France F. Security of the electronic health care record–professional and ethical implications. Stud Health Technol Inform. 1996;27:10–22.

Gibson CJ, Dixon BE, Abrams K. Convergent evolution of health information management and health informatics: a perspective on the future of information professionals in health care. Appl Clin Inform. 2015;6(1):163–84. https://doi.org/10.4338/ACI-2014-09-RA-0077.

Gilmour JA. Reducing disparities in the access and use of Internet health information. A discussion paper. Int J Nurs Stud. 2007;44(7):1270–8. https://doi.org/10.1016/j.ijnurstu.2006.05.007.

Glegg SM, Hoens A. Role domains of knowledge brokering: a model for the health care setting. J Neurol Phys Ther. 2016;40(2):115–23. https://doi.org/10.1097/NPT.0000000000000122.

Gluck JC, Hassig RA, Balogh L, Bandy M, Doyle JD, Kronenfeld MR, et al. Standards for hospital libraries 2002. J Med Libr Assoc. 2002;90(4):465–72.

Goffman W. Theoretical frame of reference for the establishment of an international health information network. Educ Med Salud. 1981;15:467–73.

Gonzalo JD, Dekhtyar M, Starr SR, Borkan J, Brunett P, Fancher T, et al. Health systems science curricula in undergraduate medical education: identifying and defining a potential curricular framework. Acad Med. 2017;92(1):123–31. https://doi.org/10.1097/ACM.0000000000001177.

Grain H, Coote GA. The health informatics professions. Stud Health Technol Inform. 2013;193:169–85.

Gray K. Public health platforms: an emerging informatics approach to health professional learning and development. J Public Health Res. 2016;5(1):665. https://doi.org/10.4081/jphr.2016.665.

Gray K, Gilbert C. Health information work – a scoping review protocol. PeerJ Preprints. 2019;7:e27535v2. https://doi.org/10.7287/peerj.preprints.27535v2.

Gray K, Gilbert C, Butler-Henderson K, Day K, Pritchard S. Ghosts in the machine: identifying the digital health information workforce. Stud Health Technol Inform. 2019;257:146–51. https://doi.org/10.3233/978-1-61499-951-5-146.

Green LA, Potworowski G, Day A, May-Gentile R, Vibbert D, Maki B, et al. Sustaining "meaningful use" of health information technology in low-resource practices. Ann Fam Med. 2015;13(1):17–22. https://doi.org/10.1370/afm.1740.

Greenberg L, D'Andrea G, Lorence D. Setting the public agenda for online health search: a white paper and action agenda. J Med Internet Res. 2004;6(2):e18. https://doi.org/10.2196/jmir.6.2.e18.

Greenes RA. Education in the workplace for the physician: clinical management states as an organizing framework. J Contin Educ Health Prof. 2000;20:219–27.

Greenes RA, Lorenzi NM. Audacious goals for health and biomedical informatics in the new millennium. J Am Med Inform Assoc. 1998;5(5):395–400.

Greyson D, Surette S, Dennett L, Chatterley T. "You're just one of the group when you're embedded": report from a mixed-method investigation of the research-embedded health librarian experience. J Med Libr Assoc. 2013;101(4):287–97. https://doi.org/10.3163/1536-5050.101.4.010.

Grzybowski D, Orlova A. Standards, information governance, informatics–essential components of HIM workforce education. J AHIMA. 2017;88:48–50.

Guangzhi Z, Chi Z, Lei L. Bringing business intelligence to health information technology curriculum. J Inform Syst Educ. 2014;25:317–25.

Haghi N, Shah A, Esposito M, Kothari T, Behiri E. Development of a pathology informatics resident rotation using an inter-departmental training model at a large academic healthcare system. Am J Clin Pathol. 2014;142:A071.

Hammond PA. Immersed in patient care: mission critical decisions for hospital libraries. Against the Grain. 2011;23:22–6.

Hanrahan LP, Foldy S, Barthell EN, Wood S. Medical informatics in population health: building Wisconsin's strategic framework for health information technology. Wis Med J. 2006;105:16–20.

Hardy JL, Lindqvist R, Kristofferzon ML, Dahlberg O. The current status of nursing informatics in undergraduate nursing programs: comparative case studies between Sweden and Australia. Stud Health Technol Inform. 1997;46:132–6.

Harris MR. The librarian's roles in the systematic review process: a case study. J Med Libr Assoc. 2005;93(1):81–7.

Haruna H, Mtoroki M, Gerendasy DD, Detlefsen EG. Health libraries and information services in Tanzania: a strategic assessment. Ann Glob Health. 2016;82(5):912–21.e3. https://doi.org/10.1016/j.aogh.2016.10.003.

Haux R. Health care in the information society: what should be the role of medical informatics? Methods Inf Med. 2002;41(1):31–5.

Haux R. Health information systems – past, present, future. Int J Med Inform. 2006;75(3-4):268–81. https://doi.org/10.1016/j.ijmedinf.2005.08.002.

Haux R. Widening panoramas: current status and future prospects. Health Info Libr J. 2008;25:86–9. https://doi.org/10.1111/j.1471-1842.2008.00814.x.

Haux R, Schmidt D. Master of science program in health information management at Heidelberg/ Heilbronn: a health care oriented approach to medical informatics. Int J Med Inform. 2002;65(1):31–9. https://doi.org/10.1016/s1386-5056(02)00004-7.

Haux R, Leven FJ, Moehr JR, Protti DJ. Health and medical informatics education. Methods Inf Med. 1994;33(3):246–9.

Haux R, Ammenwerth E, Haber A, Hühner-Bloder G, Knaup-Gregori P, Lechleitner G, et al. Medical informatics education needs information system practicums in health care settings: experiences and lessons learned from 32 practicums at four universities in two countries. Methods Inf Med. 2006;45:294–9.

Haynes RB. Using informatics principles and tools to harness research evidence for patient care: evidence-based informatics. Stud Health Technol Inform. 1998;52 Pt 1:Suppl 33-6.

Health Workforce Australia. Health information workforce report: Health Workforce Australia. Report No.: HWA13IAP009. 2013. https://www.aims.org.au/documents/item/401. Accessed 18 Apr 2020.

Hersh W. Medical informatics education: an alternative pathway for training informationists. J Med Libr Assoc. 2002;90(1):76–9.

Hersh W. Who are the informaticians? What we know and should know. J Am Med Inform Assoc. 2006;13:166–70.

Hersh WR. The full spectrum of biomedical informatics education at Oregon Health & Science University. Methods Inf Med. 2007;46(1):80–3.

Hersh W. Health and biomedical informatics: opportunities and challenges for a twenty-first century profession and its education. Yearb Med Inform. 2008a;17:157–64.

Hersh W. Recent trends in biomedical and health informatics education: implications for practice, research, and policy. AMIA Annu Symp Proc. 2008b:1205–6.

Hersh W. A stimulus to define informatics and health information technology. BMC Med Inform Decis Mak. 2009;9:24. https://doi.org/10.1186/1472-6947-9-24.

Hersh W. The health information technology workforce: estimations of demands and a framework for requirements. Appl Clin Inform. 2010a;1(2):197–212. https://doi.org/10.4338/ACI-2009-11-R-0011.

Hersh W. The health informatics workforce: unanswered questions, needed answers. Stud Health Technol Inform. 2010b;151:492–503.

Hersh W, Wright A. What workforce is needed to implement the health information technology agenda? Analysis from the HIMSS analytics database. AMIA Annu Symp Proc. 2008:303–7.

Hincapie AL, Cutler TW, Fingado AR. Incorporating health information technology and pharmacy informatics in a pharmacy professional didactic curriculum – with a team-based learning approach. Am J Pharm Educ. 2016;80(6):107. https://doi.org/10.5688/ajpe806107.

Hoekstra S, Aarts J. A coherent approach to health informatics education: results of the Dutch curriculum project. Stud Health Technol Inform. 2000;57:66–70.

Hopkins E. Knowledge management in healthcare libraries: the current picture. Health Info Libr J. 2017;34(2):103–5. https://doi.org/10.1111/hir.12183.

Houser SH, Morgan D, Clements K, Hart-Hester S. Assessing the planning and implementation strategies for the ICD-10-CM/PCS coding transition in Alabama hospitals. Perspect Health Inf Manag. 2013;10:1a.

Hovenga EJ. Health workforce competencies needed for a digital world. Stud Health Technol Inform. 2013;193:141–68.

Hoyt R, Adler K, Ziesemer B, Palombo G. Evaluating the usability of a free electronic health record for training. Perspect Health Inf Manag. 2013;10:1b.

Huber JT, Swigger K. Preparing health information professionals for the twenty-first century: the Texas Woman's University dual master's degree program. Bull Med Libr Assoc. 2000;88(1):72–4.

Hubner U, Shaw T, Thye J, Egbert N, Marin HF, Chang P, et al. Technology Informatics Guiding Education Reform – TIGER. Methods Inf Med. 2018;57(S01):e30–42. https://doi.org/10.3414/me17-01-0155.

Humphries AW, Kochi JK. Providing consumer health information through institutional collaboration. Bull Med Libr Assoc. 1994;82(1):52–6.

Huston T, Smith J. Surviving and thriving with Vision 2006: information technology in the curriculum. Top Health Inf Manag. 1998;19(2):88–94.

Ingram D. Learning to manage health information – after health informatics. Inform Healthc Aust. 2000;8:35–47.

Johns ML. Issuing the challenge: creating leadership for health information management. Top Health Inf Manag. 1995;15(3):1–8.

Jones WT. A university information and advisory service in occupational health. Ann Occup Hyg. 1973;16:293–6.

Jones CL. Charting a path for health sciences librarians in an integrated information environment. Bull Med Libr Assoc. 1993;81(4):421–5.

Joshi A, Perin DM. Gaps in the existing public health informatics training programs: a challenge to the development of a skilled global workforce. Perspect Health Inf Manag. 2012;9(Fall):1–13.

Kaplan B, Brennan PF. Consumer informatics supporting patients as co-producers of quality. J Am Med Inform Assoc. 2001;8(4):309–16. https://doi.org/10.1136/jamia.2001.0080309.

Khan S. Military health system transformation implications on health information technology modernization. Mil Med. 2018;183:56–9. https://doi.org/10.1093/milmed/usx100.

Kimiafar K, Sheikhtaheri A, Sarbaz M, Hoseini M. Assessing the educational needs of health information management staff of the Mashhad University of Medical Sciences, Iran..."Health Informatics meets eHealth conference," Vienna, Austria, 2017. Stud Health Technol Inform. 2017;236:104–10. https://doi.org/10.3233/978-1-61499-759-7-104.

King SB, Lapidus M. Metropolis revisited: the evolving role of librarians in informatics education for the health professions. J Med Libr Assoc. 2015;103(1):14–8. https://doi.org/10.3163/1536-5050.103.1.003.

King SB, MacDonald K. Metropolis redux: the unique importance of library skills in informatics. J Med Libr Assoc. 2004;92(2):209–17.

Klein MS, Ross F. End-user searching: impetus for an expanding information management and technology role for the hospital librarian. Bull Med Libr Assoc. 1997;85(3):260–8.

Kluge EW. Health information professionals in a global eHealth world: ethical and legal arguments for the international certification and accreditation of health information professionals. Int J Med Inform. 2017;97:261–5. https://doi.org/10.1016/j.ijmedinf.2016.10.020.

Koch S. Meeting the challenges–the role of medical informatics in an ageing society. Stud Health Technol Inform. 2006;124:25–31.

Kushniruk A, Lau F, Borycki E, Protti D. The School of Health Information Science at the University of Victoria: towards an integrative model for health informatics education and research. Yearb Med Inform. 2006;15:159–65.

Lake E. The librarian's role in digital health technology curation and promotion for a health care organization. J Electron Resour Med Libr. 2018;15(2):71–6. https://doi.org/10.1080/15424065.2018.1486261.

Lange LL. Informatics nurse specialist: roles in health care organizations. Nurs Adm Q. 1997;21(3):1–10.

Ledikwe JH, Reason LL, Burnett SM, Busang L, Bodika S, Lebelonyane R, et al. Establishing a health information workforce: innovation for low- and middle-income countries. Hum Resour Health. 2013;11:35. https://doi.org/10.1186/1478-4491-11-35.

Lee A, Moy L, Kruck SE, Rabang J. The doctor is in, but is academia? Re-tooling IT education for a new era in healthcare. J Inform Syst Educ. 2014;25:275–81.

Lei J, Meng Q, Li Y, Liang M, Zheng K. The evolution of medical informatics in China: a retrospective study and lessons learned. Int J Med Inform. 2016;92:8–14. https://doi.org/10.1016/j.ijmedinf.2016.04.011.

Lemmetty K, Kuusela T, Saranto K, Ensio A. Education and training of health information systems–a literature review. Stud Health Technol Inform. 2006;122:176–80.

Levac D, Colquhoun H, O'Brien KK. Scoping studies: advancing the methodology. Implement Sci. 2010;5:69. https://doi.org/10.1186/1748-5908-5-69.

Leven FJ, Knaup P, Schmidt D, Wetter T. Medical informatics at Heidelberg/Heilbronn: status-evaluation-new challenges in a specialised curriculum for medical informatics after thirty years of evolution. Int J Med Inform. 2004;73(2):117–25. https://doi.org/10.1016/j.ijmedinf.2003.11.011.

Leviss J, Kremsdorf R, Mohaideen MF. The CMIO–a new leader for health systems. J Am Med Inform Assoc. 2006;13(5):573–8. https://doi.org/10.1197/jamia.M2097.

Lewis S, Hallam G, Ritchie A, Clark C, Hamill C, Kammermann M, et al. Employers' perspectives on future roles and skills requirements for Australian health librarians. Evid Based Libr Inf Pract. 2011;6(4):57–71.

Lobach DF. Clinical informatics: supporting the use of evidence in practice and relevance to physical therapy education. J Phys Ther Educ. 2004;18:24–34.

Lobach DF, Spell RU, Hales JW, Rabold JS. A Web link management tool for optimizing utilization of distributed knowledge in health care applications. Proc AMIA Symp. 1999:839–43.

Lomas J. The in-between world of knowledge brokering. BMJ. 2007;334(7585):129–32. https://doi.org/10.1136/bmj.39038.593380.AE.

Lorenzi N, Bloomrosen M. Accelerating the deployment of a health information technology and informatics workforce through education, training, research, and evaluation. Stud Health Technol Inform. 2011;170:113–21.

Lun KC, Leong TY, Ong K, Raghavan R, Pung HK. The medical informatics program at the National University of Singapore. Yearb Med Inform. 1998;7(1):85–9.

Mac McCullough J, Goodin K. Patterns and correlates of public health informatics capacity among local health departments: an empirical typology. Online J Public Health Inform. 2014;6(3):e199. https://doi.org/10.5210/ojphi.v6i3.5572.

MacNeill JE, Covvey HD. The development of a model curriculum for applied health informatics. Proc AMIA Symp. 2000:527–31.

Mahoney ME. Transforming health information management through technology. Top Health Inf Manag. 2002;23(1):52–61.

Maloney K, McCray JC. Arizona Health Information Network: the collaborative administration and management of a statewide computing resource for health information. Medinfo. 1995;8(Pt 2):1487–90.

Manifava E, Kolokathi A, Mantas J. Exploring the biomedical and health informatics educational programs in Europe. Stud Health Technol Inform. 2014;202:67–70.

Mantas J. Health and nursing informatics education. Stud Health Technol Inform. 1998a;56:146–52.

Mantas J. Health Informatics Education and Research at the University of Athens. Yearb Med Inform. 1998b;7(1):90–4.

Mantas J. NIGHTINGALE–a new perspective in nursing informatics education in Europe. Stud Health Technol Inform. 1998c;51:102–13.

Margolis A, Vero A, Bessonart L, Barbiel A, Ferla M. Health information systems training for a countrywide implementation in Uruguay. Yearb Med Inform. 2009;18:153–7.

Mars M. Building the capacity to build capacity in e-health in sub-Saharan Africa: the KwaZulu-Natal experience. Telemed J E Health. 2012;18(1):32–7. https://doi.org/10.1089/tmj.2011.0146.

Marshall JG. Linking research to practice: the rise of evidence-based health sciences librarianship. J Med Libr Assoc. 2014;102(1):14–21. https://doi.org/10.3163/1536-5050.102.1.005.

Marshall A. The role of the health information professional. Health Info Libr J. 2017;34(4):293–5. https://doi.org/10.1111/hir.12077.

Martin ER, McDaniels C, Crespo J, Lanier D. Delivering health information services and technologies to urban community health centers: the Chicago AIDS Outreach Project. Bull Med Libr Assoc. 1997;85(4):356–61.

Masic I. Education of medical informatics in Bosnia and Herzegowina. Int J Med Inform. 1998;50(1-3):95–101.

Masic I. Medical informatics between technology, philosophy and science. Med Arh. 2004;58(1 Suppl 2):73–8.

Masys DR. The informatics of health care reform. Bull Med Libr Assoc. 1996;84(1):11–6.

Masys DR. Effects of current and future information technologies on the health care workforce. Health Aff (Millwood). 2002;21(5):33–41. https://doi.org/10.1377/hlthaff.21.5.33.

Matheson NW. A study of the health sciences library: its roles in education for the health sciences. Bull Med Libr Assoc. 1981;69(3):307–10.

Maunder K, Walton K, Williams P, Ferguson M, Beck E, Ayres E, et al. Uptake of nutrition informatics in Australia compared with the USA. Nutr Diet. 2015;72:291–8. https://doi.org/10.1111/1747-0080.12207.

Mayfield MK. Beyond the classroom: self-direction in professional learning. Bull Med Libr Assoc. 1993;81(4):425–32.

McKibbon KA, Eady A, Walker-Dilks CJ. Research, development, and production of information resources and tools. Ref Serv Rev. 2005;33:25–30. https://doi.org/10.1108/00907320410519423.

McKnight M. Librarians, informaticists, informationists, and other information professionals in biomedicine and the health sciences: what do they do? J Hosp Librariansh. 2005;5:13–29.

McLane S, Turley JP. Informaticians: how they may benefit your healthcare organization. J Nurs Adm. 2011;41(1):29–35. https://doi.org/10.1097/NNA.0b013e3181fc19d6.

Meidani Z, Sadoughi F, Ahmadi M, Maleki MR, Zohoor A, Saddik B. National health information infrastructure model: a milestone for health information management education realignment. Telemed J E Health. 2012;18(6):475–83. https://doi.org/10.1089/tmj.2011.0189.

Mettler M, Kemper DW. Information therapy: health education one person at a time. Health Promot Pract. 2003;4(3):214–7. https://doi.org/10.1177/1524839903004003004.

Miller K, Protti D, Wright I, Guerriere M. Innovative informatics education: aligning theory and practice through strategic partnership. Stud Health Technol Inform. 1998;52(Pt 2):752–5.

Mohan V, Abbott P, Acteson S, Berner ES, Devlin C, Hammond WE, et al. Design and evaluation of the ONC health information technology curriculum. J Am Med Inform Assoc. 2014;21(3):509–16. https://doi.org/10.1136/amiajnl-2013-001683.

Moore RA, Berner ES. Comparison of health/medical informatics curricula against multiple sets of professional criteria. AMIA Annu Symp Proc. 2003:942.

Moore RA, Berner ES. Assessing graduate programs for healthcare information management/technology (HIM/T) executives. Int J Med Inform. 2004a;73(2):195–203. https://doi.org/10.1016/j.ijmedinf.2003.12.002.

Moore RA, Berner ES. Comparing health/medical informatics graduate program curricula against two sets of professional criteria. J Healthc Inf Manag. 2004b;18(3):44–50.

Moran BB, Jenkins CG, Friedman CP, Lipscomb CE, Gollop CJ, Moore ME, et al. Preparing tomorrow's health sciences librarians: feasibility and marketing studies. Bull Med Libr Assoc. 1996;84(4):541–8.

Morris M, Boruff JT, Gore GC. Scoping reviews: establishing the role of the librarian. J Med Libr Assoc. 2016;104(4):346–54. https://doi.org/10.3163/1536-5050.104.4.020.

Murphy J. Globalization: implications for health information professionals. Health Info Libr J. 2008;25(1):62–8. https://doi.org/10.1111/j.1471-1842.2007.00761.x.

Murphy J. Health science librarianship's legacy to health informatics. Health Info Libr J. 2010;27(1):75–9. https://doi.org/10.1111/j.1471-1842.2010.00882.x.

Murphy J, Goossen W. Introduction: forecasting informatics competencies for nurses in the future of connected health. Stud Health Technol Inform. 2017;232:1–6. https://doi.org/10.3233/978-1-61499-738-2-1.

National Library of Medicine. MeSH database. Bethesda, Maryland. 2020. https://www.ncbi.nlm.nih.gov/mesh/. Accessed 18 Apr 2020.

Ndira S, Ssebadduka D, Niyonzima N, Sewankambo N, Royall J. Tackling malaria, village by village: a report on a concerted information intervention by medical students and the community in Mifumi, Eastern Uganda. Afr Health Sci. 2014;14(4):882–8. https://doi.org/10.4314/ahs.v14i4.16.

Newbold SK. What practicing nurses need to know about health information technology in order to practice today: continuing education and certification. Stud Health Technol Inform. 2017;232:229–38. https://doi.org/10.3233/978-1-61499-738-2-229.

Newbold SK, Kimmel KC, O'Steen R, Morgan GS. HIMSS Survey results: best practices in implementing nursing/interdisciplinary documentation systems. AMIA Annu Symp Proc. 2008;2008:1067.

Newcomb WL, Lincourt AE, Gersin K, Kercher K, Iannitti D, Kuwada T, et al. Development of a functional, internet-accessible department of surgery outcomes database. Am Surg. 2008;74(6):548–54.

Noh Y. A study comparing public and medical librarians' perceptions of the role and duties of health information-providing librarians. Health Info Libr J. 2015;32(4):300–21. https://doi.org/10.1111/hir.12122.

Norris AC, Brittain JM. Education, training and the development of healthcare informatics...first published in the Proceedings of SHIMR 2000, the Fifth International Symposium on Health Information Management Research, Sheffield, June 2000. Health Inform J. 2000;6:189–95.

Ohno-Machado L. Data science and artificial intelligence to improve clinical practice and research. J Am Med Inform Assoc. 2018;25(10):1273. https://doi.org/10.1093/jamia/ocy136.

Oliver KB, Roderer NK. Working towards the informationist. Health Inform J. 2006;12(1):41–8. https://doi.org/10.1177/1460458206061207.

Oliver KB, Dalrymple P, Lehmann HP, McClellan DA, Robinson KA, Twose C. Bringing evidence to practice: a team approach to teaching skills required for an informationist role in evidence-based clinical and public health practice. J Med Libr Assoc. 2008;96(1):50–7. https://doi.org/10.3163/1536-5050.96.1.50.

Oster NH, Thomas LB. Teaching health information Internet classes in the community: an opportunity for hospital library outreach and collaboration. Med Ref Serv Q. 1998;17(1):69–74.

Palmer RA. Effect of federal programs on health sciences libraries. J Am Soc Inf Sci. 1987;38(1):40–7. https://doi.org/10.1002/(SICI)1097-4571(198701)38:1<40:AID-ASI8>3.0.CO;2-Z.

Pandhi N, Yang WL, Karp Z, Young A, Beasley JW, Kraft S et al. Approaches and challenges to optimising primary care teams' electronic health record usage. Inform Prim Care. 2014;21(3):142–51. https://doi.org/10.14236/jhi.v21i3.57.

Paré G, Trudel M-C, Jaana M, Kitsiou S. Synthesizing information systems knowledge: a typology of literature reviews. Inform Manag. 2015;52(2):183–99. https://doi.org/10.1016/j.im.2014.08.008.

Parry D, Hunter I, Honey M, Holt A, Day K, Kirk R, et al. Building an educated health informatics workforce–the New Zealand experience. Stud Health Technol Inform. 2013a;188:86–90.

Parry D, Hunter I, Honey M, Holt A, Day K, Kirk R, et al. Health informatics community priming in a small nation: the New Zealand experience. Stud Health Technol Inform. 2013b;192:950.

Payne PR, Lussier Y, Foraker RE, Embi PJ. Rethinking the role and impact of health information technology: informatics as an interventional discipline. BMC Med Inform Decis Mak. 2016;16:40. https://doi.org/10.1186/s12911-016-0278-3.

Pentland D, Forsyth K, Maciver D, Walsh M, Murray R, Irvine L. Enabling integrated knowledge acquisition and management in health care teams. Knowl Manage Res Pract. 2014;12(4):362–74. https://doi.org/10.1057/kmrp.2013.13.

Perry GJ, Roderer NK, Assar S. A current perspective on medical informatics and health sciences librarianship. J Med Libr Assoc. 2005;93(2):199–205.

Pienaar ED. The availability of health information in South Africa. Medinfo. 1995;8 Pt 2:1638.

Pittman TJ, Jagodynski KM. Consumer health within an academic medical center state-of-the-art services and technology. J Hosp Librariansh. 2005;5:51–64. https://doi.org/10.1300/J186v05n04_05.

Rajamani S, Westra BL, Monsen KA, LaVenture M, Gatewood LC. Partnership to promote interprofessional education and practice for population and public health informatics: a case study. J Interprof Care. 2015;29(6):555–61. https://doi.org/10.3109/13561820.2015.1029067.

Rao S. The role of libraries in eHealth service delivery in Australia. Aust Libr J. 2009;58:63–72.

Ritchie A. The library's role and challenges in implementing an e-learning strategy: a case study from northern Australia. Health Info Libr J. 2011;28(1):41–9. https://doi.org/10.1111/j.1471-1842.2010.00923.x.

Robertson M, Callen J. The educational needs of health information managers in an electronic environment: what information technology and health informatics skills and knowledge are required? Health Inf Manage J. 2004;32(3):95–101.

Robeson P, Dobbins M, DeCorby K. Life as a knowledge broker in public health. J Can Health Libr Assoc. 2008;29(3):79–82. https://doi.org/10.5596/c08-025.

Rojas CL, Seckman CA. The informatics nurse specialist role in electronic health record usability evaluation. Comput Inform Nurs. 2014;32(5):214–20. https://doi.org/10.1097/CIN.0000000000000042.

Rudman WJ. The effect of education on career advancement patterns of health information professionals. J AHIMA. 1995;66(1):45–8.

Sable JH, Hales JW, Bopp KD. Medical informatics in healthcare organizations: a survey of healthcare information managers. Proc AMIA Symp. 2000:745–8.

Saranto K, Korpela M, Kivinen T. Evaluation of the outcomes of a multi-professional education programme in health informatics. Stud Health Technol Inform. 2001;84(Pt 2):1071–5.

Scherrer CS. Reference librarians' perceptions of the issues they face as academic health information professionals. J Med Libr Assoc. 2004;92(2):226–32.

Schilling L, Dearing JW, Staley P, Harvey P, Fahey L, Kuruppu F. Kaiser Permanente's performance improvement system, Part 4: Creating a learning organization. Jt Comm J Qual Patient Saf. 2011;37(12):532–43. https://doi.org/10.1016/s1553-7250(11)37069-9.

Schleder Goncalves L, Candida Castro T, Fialek S. Computer experience of nurses. Stud Health Technol Inform. 2015;216:1012.

Scott PJ, Dunscombe R, Evans D, Mukherjee M, Wyatt JC. Learning health systems need to bridge the 'two cultures' of clinical informatics and data science. BMJ Health Care Inform. 2018;25(2):126. https://doi.org/10.14236/jhi.v25i2.1062.

Seeley HM, Urquhart C, Hutchinson P, Pickard J. Developing the role of a health information professional in a clinical research setting. Evid Based Libr Inf Pract. 2010;5:47–62.

Shurtz S. Thinking outside the classroom: providing student-centered informatics instruction to first- and second-year medical students. Med Ref Serv Q. 2009;28(3):275–81. https://doi.org/10.1080/02763860903070019.

Sidwell JL. Addressing the health information needs of rural Missouri health care providers: an IAIMS assistant experience. Med Ref Serv Q. 1998;17(1):39–48. https://doi.org/10.1300/J115V17N01_04.

Siegel ER, Logan RA, Harnsberger RL, Cravedi K, Krause JA, Lyon B, et al. Information Rx: evaluation of a new informatics tool for physicians, patients, and libraries. Inf Serv Use. 2006;26(1):1–10. https://doi.org/10.3233/isu-2006-26101.

Skiba DJ. Nursing informatics education: from automation to connected care. Stud Health Technol Inform. 2017;232:9–19. https://doi.org/10.3233/978-1-61499-738-2-9.

Skillman SM, Andrilla CH, Patterson DG, Fenton SH, Ostergard SJ. Health information technology workforce needs of rural primary care practices. J Rural Health. 2015;31(1):58–66. https://doi.org/10.1111/jrh.12081.

Smith SE, Drake LE, Harris J-GB, Watson K, Pohlner PG. Clinical informatics: a workforce priority for 21st century healthcare. Aust Health Rev. 2011;35:130–5. https://doi.org/10.1071/AH10935.

Stearns NS. Tufts academic health information network: concept and scenario. Bull Med Libr Assoc. 1986;74(2):100–3.

Taiwo Adeleke I, Hakeem Lawal A, Adetona Adio R, Adisa Adebisi A. Information technology skills and training needs of health information management professionals in Nigeria: a nationwide study. Health Inf Manag J. 2015;44(1):30–8.

Tan JK. Graduate education in health information systems: having all your eggs in one basket. J Health Adm Educ. 1993;11(1):27–55.

Tarby W, Hogan K. Hospital-based patient information services: a model for collaboration. Bull Med Libr Assoc. 1997;85(2):158–66.

Tarver T, Jones DA, Adams M, Garcia A. The librarian's role in linking patients to their personal health data and contextual information. Med Ref Serv Q. 2013;32(4):459–67. https://doi.org/10.1080/02763869.2013.837730.

Tennant MR, Auten B, Botero CE, Butson LC, Edwards ME, Garcia-Milian R, et al. Changing the face of reference: adapting biomedical and health information services for the classroom, clinic, and beyond. Med Ref Serv Q. 2012;31(3):280–301. https://doi.org/10.1080/0276386 9.2012.698172.

Terry AL, Thorpe CF, Giles G, Brown JB, Harris SB, Reid GJ, et al. Implementing electronic health records: key factors in primary care. Can Fam Physician. 2008;54(5):730–6.

Thomas Gordon L. Inside look. Bridging the HIM present and future. J AHIMA. 2016;87:15.

Tremblay MC, Deckard GJ, Klein R. Health informatics and analytics – building a program to integrate business analytics across clinical and administrative disciplines. J Am Med Inform Assoc. 2016;23(4):824–8. https://doi.org/10.1093/jamia/ocw055.

Tricco AC, Lillie E, Zarin W, O'Brien KK, Colquhoun H, Levac D, et al. PRISMA extension for scoping reviews (PRISMA-ScR): checklist and explanation. Ann Intern Med. 2018;169(7):467–73. https://doi.org/10.7326/m18-0850.

Triola MM, Friedman E, Cimino C, Geyer EM, Wiederhorn J, Mainiero C. Health information technology and the medical school curriculum. Am J Manag Care. 2010;16(12 Suppl HIT):SP54-6.

Ubeyli ED. Medical informatics: a model developed for diabetes education via telemedicine. J Med Syst. 2009;33(2):113–9.

Uneke CJ, Ezeoha AE, Ndukwe CD, Oyibo PG, Onwe F, Aulakh BK. Research priority setting for health policy and health systems strengthening in Nigeria: the policymakers and stakeholders perspective and involvement. Pan Afr Med J. 2013;16:10. https://doi.org/10.11604/pamj.2013.16.10.2318.

Urquhart R, Porter GA, Grunfeld E. Reflections on knowledge brokering within a multidisciplinary research team. J Contin Educ Health Prof. 2011;31(4):283–90. https://doi.org/10.1002/chp.20128.

Valenta AL, Mendola RA, Dieter M, Panko WB. Preparing chief information officers for the clinical information systems environment. Acad Med. 1999;74(5):511–5.

Valenta AL, Berner ES, Boren SA, Deckard GJ, Eldredge C, Fridsma DB, et al. AMIA Board White Paper: AMIA 2017 core competencies for applied health informatics education at the master's degree level. J Am Med Inform Assoc. 2018;25(12):1657–68. https://doi.org/10.1093/jamia/ocy132.

Valerius J, Mohan V, Doctor D, Hersh W. Collaboration leads to enhanced curriculum. Appl Clin Inform. 2015;6(1):200–9. https://doi.org/10.4338/ACI-2014-10-CR-0086.

Van Eerd D, Newman K, DeForge R, Urquhart R, Cornelissen E, Dainty KN. Knowledge brokering for healthy aging: a scoping review of potential approaches. Implement Sci. 2016;11(1):140. https://doi.org/10.1186/s13012-016-0504-5.

Vellar L, Mastroianni F, Lambert K. Embedding health literacy into health systems: a case study of a regional health service. Aust Health Rev. 2016;41(6):621–5. https://doi.org/10.1071/AH16109.

Wales A. Managing knowledge to support the patient journey in NHS Scotland: strategic vision and practical reality. Health Info Libr J. 2005;22(2):83–95. https://doi.org/10.1111/j.1471-18 42.2005.00572.x.

Ward V, House A, Hamer S. Knowledge brokering: the missing link in the evidence to action chain? Evid Policy. 2009;5(3):267–79. https://doi.org/10.1332/174426409X463811.

Westra BL, Delaney CW. Informatics competencies for nursing and healthcare leaders. AMIA Annu Symp Proc. 2008:804–8.

Whetton S, Hazlitt C. Educating the health informatics professional: the impact of an academic program. Stud Health Technol Inform. 2015;214:159–66.

Whitney W, Keselman A, Humphreys B. Libraries and librarians: key partners for progress in health literacy research and practice. Inf Serv Use. 2017;37:85–100. https://doi.org/10.3233/ISU-170821.

Whittaker M, Hodge N, Mares RE, Rodney A. Preparing for the data revolution: identifying minimum health information competencies among the health workforce. Hum Resour Health. 2015;13:17. https://doi.org/10.1186/s12960-015-0002-x.

Wholey DR, LaVenture M, Rajamani S, Kreiger R, Hedberg C, Kenyon C. Developing workforce capacity in public health informatics: core competencies and curriculum design. Front Public Health. 2018;6:124. https://doi.org/10.3389/fpubh.2018.00124.

Wilkinson A, Papaioannou D, Keen C, Booth A. The role of the information specialist in supporting knowledge transfer: a public health information case study. Health Info Libr J. 2009;26(2):118–25. https://doi.org/10.1111/j.1471-1842.2008.00790.x.

Wilkinson SG, Chevan J, Vreeman D. Establishing the centrality of health informatics in physical therapist education: if not now, when? J Phys Ther Educ. 2010;24:10–5.

Williams P, Schaper L. A complex intervention in a complex system: why we must invest now in Australia's health informatics workforce. Pulse+IT magazine. 2013(Apr 1):36–8. https://issuu.com/pulseitmagazine/docs/pulseit_april2013/. Accessed 18 Apr 2020.

Woods SE, Coggan JM. Developing a medical informatics education program to support a statewide health information network. Bull Med Libr Assoc. 1994;82(2):147–52.

World Health Organization. Classification of digital health interventions v1.0: a shared language to describe the uses of digital technology for health. Geneva: World Health Organization, 2018. https://apps.who.int/iris/handle/10665/260480. Accessed 18 Apr 2020.

Yang JY, Yang MQ, Zhu MM, Arabnia HR, Deng Y. Promoting synergistic research and education in genomics and bioinformatics. BMC Genom. 2008;9 Suppl 1:I1. https://doi.org/10.1186/1471-2164-9-S1-I1.

Yarmohammadian MH, Mohebbi N. Review evaluation indicators of health information technology course of master's degree in medical sciences universities based on CIPP Model. J Educ Health Promot. 2015;4:28. https://doi.org/10.4103/2277-9531.154122.

Yen PY, Phillips A, Kennedy MK, Collins S. Nursing informatics competency assessment for the nurse leader: instrument refinement, validation, and psychometric analysis. J Nurs Adm. 2017;47(5):271–7. https://doi.org/10.1097/NNA.0000000000000478.

Yoon S, Shaffer JA, Bakken S. Refining a self-assessment of informatics competency scale using Mokken scaling analysis. J Interprof Care. 2015;29(6):579–86. https://doi.org/10.3109/13561820.2015.1049340.

Zimmerman JL, van Bemmel JH, Rienhoff O. Integrated Academic Information Management Systems (IAIMS). Part III. Implementation of integrated information services. Medical informatics education. J Am Soc Inf Sci. 1988;39(2):138–41. https://doi.org/10.1002/(SICI)1097-4571(198803)39:2<138:AID-ASI14>3.0.CO;2-9.

Chapter 3
The Socio-technical Foundations of Health Information Work

Carey A. Mather and Sue Whetton

Abstract Socio-technical values, principles, and theories are foundational knowledge for health information professionals. These emphasise that people who work with technology are augmented by it, not subordinate to it. Applying them can contribute to more effective design, development, implementation, management, and use of digital health and information systems. This chapter briefly describes the origins and underlying values of the socio-technical approach. It then discusses theories and key concepts. The second section demonstrates the relevance of socio-technical design to the health services in general and health information professionals, in particular. Examples from research and case studies are used to demonstrate how this workforce can apply socio-technical values and principles.

Keywords Design · Socio-technical · Systems theory · Technocentrism · Humanism

Origins, Underlying Values and Principles

Socio-technical thinking is underpinned by humanistic values and principles. A socio-technical system is 'the synergistic combination of humans, machines, environments, work activities and organisational structures and processes that comprise a given enterprise' (Mumford 2006, p.317). This conceptualisation primarily embraces complex systems in which many humans collaborate towards a common

C. A. Mather (✉) · S. Whetton
College of Health and Medicine, University of Tasmania, Launceston, TAS, Australia
e-mail: Carey.Mather@utas.edu.au; Sue.Whetton@utas.edu.au

© The Author(s), under exclusive license to Springer Nature
Switzerland AG 2021
K. Butler-Henderson et al. (eds.), *The Health Information Workforce*,
Health Informatics, https://doi.org/10.1007/978-3-030-81850-0_3

goal. Social refers to individual workers and teams, and needs for coordination, control, and boundary management, while technical includes not only equipment, machines, tools, and technology but also the work organisation.

The term socio-technical was used in the mid-twentieth century by researchers at the Tavistock Institute of Human Relations in London (Whetton 2005). Established in 1946, this Institute applied the social sciences to analysing issues and problems in contemporary society. One focus of their research was industry and commerce. Tavistock researchers expressed concerns about emerging scientific management practices being increasingly adopted in offices and factories in modern industrial society. They argued that these practices were having a de-humanising effect on workers. They felt there was a need to counter this trend, ensuring a more humane, or human-centred, and productive organisation of work in the modern workplace (Whetton 2005). The term socio-technical encapsulated an approach for exploring these workplace issues and trends. Tavistock researchers argued that emerging scientific management practices were prioritising the technical sub-system. They were critical of this trend arguing that the rights and needs of the employee must be given as high a priority as those of the non-human elements of the system. The term socio-technical was intended to emphasise that both the social and technical systems are of equal importance, and that employees are complementary to technology, not subordinate to it. Socio-technical conceptualisations of the system also emphasised that the two sub-systems were interdependent and were impacted by environmental factors (Whetton 2005; Sawyer and Jarrahi 2014; Adaba and Kebebew 2018).

A primary objective of socio-technical researchers was to improve the overall quality of working life through redesigning work practices and workplace technologies. The role of employees was emphasised, with researchers arguing that employees who were to be involved in new systems should be given a voice in the design process of that system. Workers should be encouraged to explore how the new system could improve the quality of their work (Mumford 2006). Sawyer and Jarrahi (2014, p.8) argued this socio-technical approach was, 'a rebellion against the evolution of work-design practices of the time that had adopted an instrumental view of work, workers, and the workforce'. Baxter and Sommerville (2011) further suggested that this implied challenge to existing work practices may impact on the success or otherwise, of attempts to implement socio-technical principles. Mumford (2006), a leader in the field of socio-technical analysis within information systems identified strong uptake of the approach in the 1960s and 1970s, particularly in Britain and Scandinavia. She suggested that application of the principles during this period resulted in improved working practices and agreements between workers and management. However, Mumford found less evidence of the use of socio-technical analyses in the 1980s and 1990s, when the economic focus on streamlining production, downsizing, and cost reduction was less open to discussions of worker conditions and work satisfaction (Mumford 2006).

The initial focus of socio-technical design was on assembly line working conditions, and by the end of the twentieth century it was being applied to a wide range of working environments, including the design of computing and information systems in manufacturing, commerce, and health sectors. In addition, while the initial focus was on employees as end-users, advancements in technology have seen the focus expand to include clients, customers, and consumers as end-users. It is increasingly expected that health services include consumers as co-designers in developing information systems and applications which they may be expected to use. Attempting to implement socio-technical design without acknowledging its humanistic values and principles diminishes planning, development, and implementation of effective, safe, and appropriate health information management systems and applications (Thomassen et al. 2017; Leitch and Warren 2010).

Theories and Concepts for Design and Analysis

Systems theories, which explore and explain systems, their component parts, functions, and goals, are integral to socio-technical thinking. In overview, a system is comprised of a set of elements, either natural or human-made, that are interrelated and interdependent. Systems can include sub-systems, which are themselves systems. For example, a healthcare system may include hospitals, nursing homes, and community centres, which are all sub-systems of it, yet they are each systems in their own right as well. Systems exist to fulfil a purpose which is expressed in terms of goals and objectives. It is possible for a system to have more than one purpose. For example, the purpose of a health information system may be to provide inter-departmental communication for patient treatment, however, it may also be used to aggregate data to facilitate decision-making and research. Individual system components combine to cooperate in achieving goals. Systems theory has long been used by biomedical science as a means of explaining and understanding the entities and processes of healthcare—the physiology of the human body is discussed in terms of skeletal, muscular, or nervous systems and so on. Health information system researchers and practitioners adopt a systems approach to assist in understanding and managing the flow of health information.

General systems theory was first formulated in the 1930s and 1940s within the biological and physical sciences (Whetton 2005). Until this time, the approach to understanding complex organisms such as the human body was to examine individual component parts. Each system within the human body would be isolated and the components examined. This approach is reflected in the structuring of biomedical knowledge, which was typically organised into specialities and sub-specialities. General systems theory focuses on systems as a whole entity, arguing that complex organisms are better understood by studying not only individual components, but also the ways individual parts interact and affect each other (Yurtseven and Buchanan 2013). Since it was first espoused, systems theory has been utilised by many disciplines, including medicine, engineering, sociology, computing, information, and management systems. The approach is based on the premise that individual parts of a system cannot do what the system as a whole can do. Rather, while each individual part may perform particular activities, it is the combination of these parts into a unified whole that makes a system. Once combined, the parts of the system interrelate in a structured way that differs from the activities of individual components. Socio-technical systems theory builds upon general systems theory. Systems theory is part of the specialised knowledge and skills of the HIDDIN workforce. HIDDIN professionals are participants in complex health systems, and much of their work positions them to ensure that the component parts within health systems interact effectively and efficiently.

Socio-technical systems are perceived as comprising social and technical sub-systems with the component parts of each sub-system being interlinked and interacting. The social system comprises the relationships between people, their values and behavioural styles, and formal and informal power structures, while the technical system comprises technology, processes, procedures, and physical arrangements. The term socio-technical emphasises the interrelatedness of these systems and the need to consider them conjointly. It is also necessary to consider the environment within which the socio-technical system is embedded. Interrelatedness of the social and technical sub-systems means that changing the elements in one may affect the other sub-system or the whole system. Therefore, effective implementation of new practices within organisations requires a consideration of both sub-systems and the way they interact. Interactions are thus a key focus in socio-technical systems analysis. The relevance and interaction of both sub-systems is demonstrated in Mather and Cummings (2019), in their digital professionalism model (4E3P) and matrix for assessing organisational readiness of capability of digital technology use by nurses. They highlighted the interconnectedness of the social/human sub-system (engagement, education) and technical sub-system (equipment, electronic access). They found that when any one of these four elements (4Es) of the two sub-systems are hindered, the opportunity for development of digital professionalism by health professionals is at risk. In particular, they noted that even when health professionals are receptive and prepared to use digital health technology, nevertheless if technical factors are unavailable, human or social elements cannot be deployed and capability in digitally professional behaviour cannot develop. Their matrix highlights that recognising interconnectedness between technical and social elements is imperative to enable implementation of technical systems into healthcare environments.

Interactions between the socio-technical system and the external environment within which it is situated are also important to analyse, to achieve effective design and implementation of systems. Thus, the concept of open systems is important (Von Betalanffy 1950; Katz and Kahn 1966). Systems are embedded in wider environments, and separated from these environments by boundaries. Boundaries may be impermeable, denoting a closed system that allows no interaction with the surrounding environment—there are very few closed systems. Rather, most systems are open, having semi-permeable boundaries that allow interaction with their environment. Open systems theory argues that to fully understand the way systems operate, it is necessary to analyse the broader context. The key features of open systems are inputs, processes, and outputs. The system accepts inputs from the environment, processes them in some way, and returns them to the environment. Where a number of systems are arranged as a series, the output of one becomes the input for another. For example, patients enter a hospital (inputs), are treated (processes), and leave the hospital (outputs). Health information systems are generally open systems. The journey of the patient through hospital departments is recorded and documented as an electronic health record within the system. This information can be retrieved as required. It can also be passed across the permeable system boundary and shared with the patient's general practitioner outside the hospital.

Open systems exist in, and interact with, dynamic environments. Open systems need to respond to changes in the external environment if they are to continue to achieve their goals. If open systems cannot adapt, they become non-functional. Therefore, systems are in a constant state of transformation or adjustment to changes in the environment. Contemporary systems increasingly comprise a complex inter-action between humans, technologies, and wider environmental aspects of work systems—not merely the immediate local environments within which the system is located. Socio-technical systems at the local level will be impacted by broader eco-nomic, political, cultural, and technical systems, and vice versa. Today, a socio-technical system that is embedded in one department of a hospital will need to interact with other departments and sections in the hospital. It will also need to interact with the external environment, which may include the hospital's funding bodies and government regulators. This interaction logically extends to the society within which the hospital is located and, in today's increasingly interconnected world, to global health and the global political economy.

Although socio-technical theory and principles have been applied with varying levels of success since the 1940s, there is no consistent, widely adopted method for applying them. An early method was Mumford's Effective Technical and Human Implementation of Computer Systems (ETHICS) which emphasised user participation in the systems design process (Mumford 2006). Initially well accepted, particularly in the United States of America when Mumford worked directly with organisations (Land et al. 1979), the method declined in popularity over several years (Baxter and Sommerville 2011). Other researchers have variously reviewed and developed approaches to socio-technical design, but have concluded that specific details are lacking, about how to implement it in practice (Baxter and Sommerville 2011; Yurtseven and Buchanan 2013; Sittig and Singh 2011; Hughes et al. 2017). Thus, Baxter and Sommerville (2011) suggest that socio-technical system design methods mostly provide advice for sympathetic systems designers rather than detailed notations and a process that should be followed. Similarly, Hughes and colleagues suggest that 'although the socio-technical systems approach to design is well recognised and supported, it is also acknowledged that realising the approach in practice can be challenging' (2017, p.1320). These comments echo Mumford's (2006) observation that 'socio-technical design methods are more akin to philosophies than the types of design methods that are usually associated with systems engineering' (cited by Baxter and Sommerville 2011, p.5).

Theory-Based Analysis of Social and Technical Interchange

Socio-technical principles are reflected in several theories and models that have been applied to analyse work settings: sociomateriality, actor network theory, the technology acceptance model, and the unified theory of acceptance and use of tech-nology are outlined here.

Sociomateriality theorises the complex relationship, or entanglement, between the social and the material that shapes everyday interactions. In health service organisations, 'the social' could refer to the relationships, values and norms, roles, and power structures—like the social sub-system in Tavistock-influenced socio-technical theory. The concept of 'the material' or materiality refers to technology—such as the diagnostic machines, intensive care monitoring systems, electronic records, or mobile communication devices that are used within healthcare organisations. Sociomateriality argues that social practices are intrinsically connected and intertwined with material artefacts and that while they may be theoretically separate, in practice they are inseparable. Technology (material) is designed and developed within the specific values, roles, and practices of organisations (social). A digital clinical information system needs to be consistent with the relationships, values and norms, roles, and power structures of the healthcare environment into which it is introduced; thus, the social influences the material. At the same time, technology is designed with certain capabilities and functions which impose themselves on social practices; while needing to conform to organisational roles and practices (the social), technology (material) shapes what is possible, or expected. For example, digital systems require reports to be typed directly into an electronic data entry form, which may take longer than filling out paper forms, so staff make briefer notes. Over time, staff normalise the expectation that reports should be concise, and when systems are updated, they request that data entry be further modified to ensure even greater conciseness. Sociomateriality allows researchers to study the social and the material simultaneously, and this enriches the evidence about digital work practices and HIDDIN professionals' knowledge base (Leonardi 2013; Orlikowski and Scott 2016; Orlikowski and Baroudi 1991).

Actor Network Theory (ANT) argues that the social and natural worlds exist in constantly shifting networks of relationships. These networks comprise and are constructed through negotiations between human and non-human elements. These elements are referred to as actants. ANT regards non-human actants—objects, ideas, processes, and other relevant factors—as important as human actants, in creating networks. A network forms as actants become closely linked with one another to achieve particular social situations, processes, or outcomes. Thus, in health organisations, technology and human actants merge to create an information system. In doing so, the actants become intertwined, so that it becomes difficult to differentiate a computer program's technical aspects from the influence exerted by the socio-cultural background of the software development team (Cusumano and Selby 1997; Sahay 1997; Callon 1986). From an ANT perspective networks that form are not static and predictable. Interactions that occur cannot be accurately predicted from moment to moment when a digital clinical information system is introduced into a hospital department. Networks evolve as actants interact. ANT theory helps HIDDIN professionals to be aware of active roles of both human and non-human elements in digital health (Cresswell et al. 2010; MacLeod et al. 2019).

The Technology Acceptance Model (TAM) aims to better understand why users accept or reject a given technical system, and how user acceptance can be improved through design of technical systems (Lee et al. 2003). The model posits that an individual's adoption behaviour is directly influenced by his/her attitude towards technology. Two key attitudinal factors are identified. The first is perceived usefulness—the person's expectation that the technical system will enhance their job performance. The second is perceived ease-of-use—the perception of how user-friendly and easy to use a system will be. These two attitudinal factors are connected; users often perceive easy to use systems as more useful. TAM has been critiqued for its emphasis on only two factors (Agarwal and Prasad 1997). The model has been further criticised for its technology focus, as it appears to view user acceptance as depending mostly on the nature of the technology. It is argued that this model ignores the social processes of information systems development and implementation—workflows, roles, and power structures, for instance. It also does not explore cultural and social differences between user groups (clinicians, administrators, patients, clients, or consumers). These criticisms have resulted in revisions, including TAM2 and TAM3. The various forms of the TAM can assist HIDDIN professionals to understand some aspects of how successful the introduction of technology into an organisation has been, and to develop strategies to motivate users to accept the systems.

The Unified Theory of Acceptance and Use of Technology (UTAUT), the outcome of a review of eight other theoretical frameworks, seeks to explain user intention to adopt a technology together with subsequent usage behaviour. Venkatesh et al. (2003) argue that the model developed from this review provides a basic conceptual framework that explains the individual acceptance of information and communication technology. To explore user perceptions and acceptance, UTAUT considers four constructs together with mediating factors: Performance expectancy is the degree to which an individual believes that using the system will help him or her to attain gains in job performance. Effort expectancy is the degree of ease associated with the use of the system. Social influence is the degree to which an individual perceives that important others believe he or she should use the new system. Facilitating conditions refers to the degree to which an individual believes that an organisational and technical infrastructure exists to support use of the system. Social factors considered to potentially influence these factors include gender, age, experience, and voluntariness of use. For example, effort expectancy may be moderated by gender, age, and experience, while social influence may be moderated by gender and age. Various modifications and adaptations of UTAUT have been proposed; some researchers consider it to be accumulation of various research efforts represented in different models and theories, rather than a coherent theory (Ahmed 2014; Venkatesh et al. 2013; Kim et al. 2015; Ayaz and Yanartaş 2020).

Relevance of Socio-technical Principles to Digital Health

Healthcare systems in contemporary society are large and complex, incorporating a mix of community and hospital based public and private services provided for patients, clients, their families, and informal carers, by an array of administrative, clinical, technical, education, and research professionals. They are characterised by multiple networks of communication, governance, and responsibility. Patients typically move within and between departments and services, while clinical and administrative data and information is collected, manipulated, and communicated within and across departmental and service boundaries within healthcare environments. The bulk of this information is of a private and confidential nature, and its collection, storage, and use are subject to legal and ethical guidelines. Technology has become increasingly integral to this collection, management, and dissemination of information. Within the professional staffing component of healthcare systems, there are also producers and consumers of information and services—e.g. clinicians could be considered to 'consume' the outputs provided by educators and researchers. Socio-technical principles are useful to influence or enable decisions ranging from routine administrative processes to obscure clinical diagnoses or decisions about structures or services.

Although there are many success stories, there are many examples of not-so-successful implementation of new health information systems or technologies into workflows. A significant reason for this is a focus on the technology to the detriment of other factors. When information systems were first introduced into healthcare environments, the focus was on technology such as hardware requirements and capabilities, software design and systems development. There was little interest in understanding the organisational and cultural factors already embedded in the organisation (Deluca and Enmark 2000; Venkatesh et al. 2011). It was assumed that information technology would easily slot into health environments and be enthusiastically adopted by end-users, who could include clinicians, management and patients, clients, or consumers. This approach, today described as technocentric, may have worked relatively well for business processes, but not in clinical areas, with a number of consequences: systems not being used as technology designers had intended them to be used; systems being boycotted by health professionals; health professionals using only a limited set of health information system features and functions; and health professionals bypassing or ignoring health information systems features and functions in an effort to complete or conduct healthcare work (Borycki and Kushniruk 2010).

Thus, digital health technologies that are developed to improve workflow do not necessarily do so (Jensen 2015; Westbrook et al. 2011). Socio-technical analyses show a technocentric approach as a significant factor in these less than successful systems implementations. Adaba and Kebebew (2018) noted that up to 90% of information system failures may be attributable to lack of consideration of social and organisational factors in design processes. Unintended consequences and work-arounds occur where there has been insufficient understanding of the impact of socio-technical factors on health information systems or management. While technical issues are an integral element in the development of health information systems, it is necessary to move beyond these to explore organisational and cultural factors—the social sub-system—which interact with the technical system. Information technology systems in healthcare must be able to operate in diverse settings such as hospitals, community health centres, general practice surgeries, and other healthcare environments, and cater to complex and varied information management requirements. Planning an information system means that both information management requirements and the health environment need to be considered. New technologies can disrupt traditional work routines, flows, and relationships. The location of equipment, the need to consult with other health professionals and interact with technology, and the protocols involved may all impact on established work patterns. It follows that a lack of attention to how a new technology will integrate into existing workflows may influence the willingness of health professionals to use it. This may be the case even if health professionals see the benefits of the new technology.

Clinical simulation of workflows has the capacity to reduce opportunity for error or harm before the full implementation of any digital health technologies into healthcare environments (Jensen 2014; Mather et al. 2017a). Clinical simulation are socio-technical methods used to capture how the implementation of new technology can influence established work patterns or create unintended consequences or workarounds. They attempt to uncover the potential for unsafe work practices and highlight deficiencies in effective and efficient deployment of the intended change to the physical and social environment. Clinical simulation can improve quality of care and patient safety by enabling evaluation of digital technologies in context in a controlled environment, prior to implementation in real-world settings. Clinical simulation allows systems designers to explore social environments, analysing user requirements and work practices. The strategy also facilitates stakeholder involvement in the planning and development process. Stakeholders, including anyone involved with seeking or retrieving health data, information, or knowledge, can be involved before, during, and after the clinical simulation. HIDDIN professionals should be involved in the planning and development of the simulation scenarios, observation of the clinical simulation exercises, and debriefing of participants. Additionally, HIDDIN leaders and executives may seek reports of outcomes of clinical simulations to assist with decision-making towards implementation of new products or services.

Workflow studies conducted using ethnography, time and motion studies, and other methods also apply socio-technical principles to capture the complexity of workflows of end-users of technology implementation (Walter et al. 2019). Westbrook et al. (2011) reported from their research into workflows that over time, use of computers to complete tasks increased. This factor is an important consideration when planning to implement any digital health technologies for end-users. Lead time, co-design, and educational preparation of end-users are necessary to ensure social factors which could enhance or reduce acceptance of the new technologies are also understood prior to implementation. Workflow studies have been utilised to investigate the feasibility of introducing digital health technologies, including health education using digital tablet technology into clinical workflows (Driscoll et al. 2019).

A case in point is Baker et al.' (2019) analysis of delivery of a digital tablet to a hospital patient at the point of care, for diabetes education and support. This example demonstrates the importance of considering the nexus of social and technical perspectives in workflow prior to implementation. They found that although current clinical workflows technically enabled the digital health intervention, the social context was such that healthcare providers were not able to spend sufficient time with each patient to instruct them on the technology platform or the content. They concluded that the provision of this support to patients in a general medical ward needed to occur independently from usual care activities. They argued that when there is a lack of alignment between the social and technical aspects of new workflows, consequences may include overload, resistance, or failure of acceptance of the technology (Mather and Cummings 2017). Workarounds can develop which could promote an unsafe environment or potentiate errors. This outcome can be costly in terms of finances, human and physical resources. Additionally, it can be much harder to re-launch a second attempt as a residual lack of acceptance from the initial implementation may remain (Mather 2012). Workarounds highlight the need for the social sub-system to be congruent with the technical sub-system. In this use case there were a number of socio-technical elements that needed to be considered (Mather et al. 2017a). At an individual level the digital and health literacy of the consumer and health professional need to be adequate. At an organisational level access to a digital tablet that has the appropriate software and permissions to connect with the wireless Internet of the healthcare environment needs to be available. At a systems and organisational level there is a need for appropriate governance to enable access and use of the tablet by the consumer and health professional. HIDDIN professionals are responsible for the seemingly easy, high quality, and safe access to the information required by end-users. If privacy, security, or confidentiality are breached or connectivity becomes slow or is unavailable, end-users will notice and as part of risk management processes will let the health service management know. It is during these interruptions to workflows, omissions or failure during the process of enabling end-user access, that end-users become at least minimally aware of the roles and responsibilities that HIDDIN professionals have or should have in their health service.

Relevance of Socio-technical Principles to the HIDDIN Workforce

The rapid growth in the use of digital health technologies has challenged the status quo within healthcare environments at an individual, organisational, and systems level (Huckvale et al. 2019). Using the lens of individual, organisational, and systems highlights opportunities for HIDDIN professionals to promote and apply socio-technical perspectives and augment their own knowledge. National governance structures are overarching components which impact on sub-systems, namely the organisations delivering digital health technologies and providing health services. Within organisations is another sub-system or level comprised of individuals. They are end-users, and are most impacted when socio-technical principles are inadequately considered. Many professionals within health systems may be aware that technology does not always fit smoothly into the environment for which it was intended, however, most may not be able to identify reasons for this quandary. HIDDIN professionals, either through formal training or experiential learning, are competent to address the socio-technical issues that contribute to (in)effective digital health systems. These professionals are able to use their specialised knowledge in promoting digital literacy, advocating for the application of socio-technical principles in the workforce, and contributing to research and knowledge development.

Promoting Digital Health Literacy

Support for a health workforce that can confidently use digital health technologies to deliver health and care is a strategic priority of many governments (e.g. Kennedy and Yaldren 2017; Australian Digital Health Agency 2018). It is essential that consideration be given to the digital health literacy of administrative, clinical, technical, education, and research staff within healthcare environments. If users are inadequately prepared for or engaged in digital health technologies design, development or implementation has potential negative consequences at an individual, organisational, or systems level. However, the needs, motivations, and skills of the various groups within a health service can vary widely.

At systems levels, HIDDIN professionals can advocate that all stakeholder perspectives are considered in decision-making, planning, and implementation of policies, protocols, and programs relating to information management systems and digital health. This work can include contributions to developing effective governance structures. Digital health literacy cannot be promoted if governance structures are not available to support stakeholders. Privacy and security issues become apparent when governance does not keep pace with technological change (Mather et al. 2017b). Additionally, governance structures regarding effective, safe, and appropriate behaviour by health professionals are required to ensure that the public and workers are protected. Enabling the development of digital professionalism is an important aspect of professional identity formation that requires robust governance. Clear direction provided by appropriate governance is necessary for all stakeholders when applying socio-technical values and principles. Use of the socio-technical approach will contribute to reducing the potential for error or harm.

At an organisational level, HIDDIN professionals can liaise with users to ensure unintended consequences and workarounds do not reduce quality and safety for patients (Jensen and Kushniruk 2016). These people can contribute to the development and implementation of usable health applications and systems. While not necessarily software developers themselves, many of them will certainly be involved in the design and/or procurement of systems. This places HIDDIN professionals in a position where they can promote socio-technical values and principles. Doing so during planning or development will assist with ensuring the success of implementation and acceptance of proposed systems. In addition, the concept of digital health literacy is complex as stakeholders develop their own discipline-specific language and perspectives that may not be shared by others; HIDDIN professionals have a role in building mutual understanding throughout organisations, to achieve positive effects on healthcare delivery and outcomes.

At an individual level, HIDDIN professionals can ensure users are adequately guided and supported in being educationally prepared and engaged in accessing and using digital health technologies. They can also promote digital health literacy work with consumers by health professionals. Without the upskilling of society in digital health literacy there will continue to be inequity among end-users, such as those in vulnerable groups (Azzopardi-Muscat and Sorensen 2019; Showell et al. 2017).

Advocating for Users of Technology in Healthcare

At systems and organisational levels, HIDDIN professionals have the opportunity to encourage other potentially influential individuals and groups to respect the views of less dominant stakeholders. Thus, HIDDIN professionals can encourage management to adopt the principle that all intended users of any digital health technologies should be involved at all stages of digital health systems development. This advocacy can challenge narrower thinking about end-user involvement only at the beginning of processes to enable project design or development. Inclusion of all stakeholders over time will enable learning about tasks undertaken and the technical systems that supported them. Developing understanding from multiple perspectives is an integral element of a socio-technical approach. HIDDIN professionals can also advocate for different groups of users. As has previously been noted, the success of many digital health and information system initiatives may depend upon how well diverse perspectives are acknowledged, negotiated, and integrated.

At the individual level, HIDDIN professionals who adopt a socio-technical perspective will be well equipped to challenge technocentric approaches, ensuring that user needs are considered and incorporated into systems design. A socio-technical design perspective could facilitate questions such as: How will the introduction of this system affect stakeholders? How will stakeholders view the introduction of this system? Who will be the main beneficiaries of this application/system? How will this application enable consumers to receive better healthcare? What will the cost be to achieve this aim?

Contributing to Research and Knowledge About Digital Health

Mumford suggested that there should be 'no theory without practice, no practice without research' and notes that 'socio-technical researchers have always tried to test and develop theory' (2006, p.321). Knowledge of socio-technical principles, concepts, and theories is constantly evolving. HIDDIN professionals and researchers can contribute to this growing knowledge base through practice, academic activity, and professional research. Through practical application of socio-technical principles, HIDDIN professionals can informally expand their own knowledge base while demonstrating to colleagues the value of the approach. At a more formal level, HIDDIN professionals can contribute to professional development either as participants to extend their own knowledge, or as leaders to extend the knowledge of other health professionals. HIDDIN professionals have many and varied roles during their careers, which can include research and teaching appointments in higher education institutions where dissemination of new knowledge through academic and professional publications is expected and encouraged. In addition, HIDDIN professionals can collaborate with academics both to contribute to the knowledge base and to disseminate research findings within the workplace and the community.

In summary, HIDDIN professionals are in prime position to show leadership in promoting the humanistic values and principles encompassed within socio-technical approaches, and so to inform health information systems design and implementation for the benefit of all users. Socio-technical approaches enable HIDDIN professionals to explore issues arising from the interaction between information and communication technologies, and the social, professional, and cultural contexts of healthcare. This approach equips HIDDIN professionals to ably recognise and address socio-technical agendas and priorities at many levels in the digital transformation of healthcare systems.

References

Adaba GB, Kebebew Y. Improving a health information system for real-time data entries: an action research project using socio-technical systems theory. Inform Health Social Care. 2018;43(2):159–71.

Agarwal R, Prasad J. The role of innovation characteristics and perceived voluntariness in the acceptance of information technologies. Decis Sci. 1997;28(3):557–82.

Ahmad MI. Unified theory of acceptance and use of technology (UTAUT): a decade of validation and development. Proceedings of the 4th International Conference on ICT in our Lives (ISSN 2314–8942). Egypt: Alexandria University; 2014.

Australian Digital Health Agency. Australia's National Digital Health strategy: safe, seamless and secure: evolving health and care to meet the needs of modern Australia. Australian Government and Australian Digital Health Agency: Sydney; 2018.

Ayaz A, Yanartaş M. An analysis on the unified theory of acceptance and use of technology theory (UTAUT): acceptance of electronic document management system (EDMS). Comput Human Behav Rep. 2020;2:100032.

Azzopardi-Muscat N, Sørensen K. Towards an equitable digital public health era: promoting equity through a health literacy perspective. Eur J Public Health. 2019;29(Suppl 3):13–7.

Baker KM, Magee MF, Smith KM. Understanding nursing workflow for inpatient education delivery: time and motion study. JMIR Nurs. 2019;2(1):e15658.

Baxter G, Sommerville I. Socio-technical systems: from design methods to systems engineering. Interact Comput. 2011;23(1):4–17.

Borycki E, Kushniruk A. Towards an integrative cognitive-socio-technical approach in health informatics: analyzing technology-induced error involving health information systems to improve patient safety. Open Med Inform J. 2010;4:181.

Callon M. The sociology of an actor-network: the case of the electric vehicle. In: Callon M, Law J, Rip A, editors. Mapping the dynamics of science and technology. London: Springer; 1986. p. 19–34.

Cresswell KM, Worth A, Sheikh A. Actor-network theory and its role in understanding the implementation of information technology developments in healthcare. BMC Medical Inform Decis Making. 2010;10(1):1–11.

Cusumano MA, Selby RW. How Microsoft builds software. Commun ACM. 1997;40(6):53–61.

Deluca JM, Enmark R. E-health: the changing model of healthcare. Front Health Serv Manag. 2000;17(1):3.

Driscoll CAH, Gurmu S, Azeem A, El Metwally D. Implementation of smart phones to facilitate in-hospital telephone communication: challenges, successes and lessons from a neonatal intensive care unit. Healthcare; 2019:100331.

Huckvale K, Wang CJ, Majeed A, Car J. Digital health at fifteen: more human (more needed). BMC Med. 2019;17(1):1–4.

Hughes HP, Clegg CW, Bolton LE, Machon LC. Systems scenarios: a tool for facilitating the socio-technical design of work systems. Ergonomics. 2017;60(10):1319–35.

Jensen S. Use of clinical simulation in development of clinical systems. Department of Planning and Development. Denmark: Aalborg University; 2014.

Jensen S. Patient safety and quality of care: how may clinical simulation contribute? Knowl Manag E-Learn. 2015;7(3):412–24.

Jensen S, Kushniruk A. Boundary objects in clinical simulation and design of eHealth. Health Inform J. 2016;22(2):248–64.

Katz D, Kahn RL. The social psychology of organizations. New York: Auflage Wiley; 1966.

Kennedy S, Yaldren J. A look at digital literacy in health and social care. Br J Cardiac Nurs. 2017;12(9):428–32.

Kim S, Lee K-H, Hwang H, Yoo S. Analysis of the factors influencing healthcare professionals' adoption of mobile electronic medical record (EMR) using the unified theory of acceptance and use of technology (UTAUT) in a tertiary hospital. BMC Medical Inform Decis Making. 2015;16(1):1–12.

Land F, Mumford E, Hawgood J. Training the systems analyst for the 1980s: four new design tools to assist the design process. The Information Systems Environment. North Holland; 1979.

Lee Y, Kozar KA, Larsen KR. The technology acceptance model: past, present, and future. Commun Assoc Inf Syst. 2003;12(1):752–80.

Leitch S, Warren MJ. ETHICS: the past, present and future of socio-technical systems design. IFIP International Conference on the History of Computing. 2010:189–97.

Leonardi PM. Theoretical foundations for the study of sociomateriality. Inf Organ. 2013;23(2):59–76.

MacLeod A, Cameron P, Ajjawi R, Kits O, Tummons J. Actor-network theory and ethnography: sociomaterial approaches to researching medical education. Perspect Medical Educ. 2019;8(3):177–86.

Mather C. Case Study: An interdisciplinary evaluation of an e-portfolio: WIL at the University of Tasmania Workready: E-portfolios to support professional placements in Nursing and Construction Management degrees in Australia. Print National: NSW; 2012.

Mather C, Cummings E. Modelling digital knowledge transfer: nurse supervisors transforming learning at point of care to advance nursing practice. Informatics; 2017:12.

Mather CA, Cummings E. Developing and sustaining digital professionalism: a model for assessing readiness of healthcare environments and capability of nurses. BMJ Health Care Inform. 2019;26(1):1–5.

Mather C, Jensen S, Cummings E. Clinical simulation: a protocol for evaluation of mobile technology. Stud Health Technol Inform. 2017a;241:179–84.

Mather CA, Gale F, Cummings EA. Governing mobile technology use for continuing professional development in the Australian nursing profession. BMC Nurs. 2017b;16(1):1–11.

Mumford E. The story of socio-technical design: reflections on its successes, failures and potential. Inf Syst J. 2006;16(4):317–42.

Orlikowski WJ, Baroudi JJ. Studying information technology in organizations: research approaches and assumptions. Inf Syst Res. 1991;2(1):1–28.

Orlikowski WJ, Scott SV. Digital work: a research agenda. A research agenda for management and organization studies. Edward Elgar; 2016.

Sahay S. Implementation of information technology: a time-space perspective. Organ Stud. 1997;18(2):229–60.

Sawyer S, Jarrahi M. Computing handbook: information systems and information technology. Florida: CRC Press; 2014.

Showell C, Cummings E, Turner P. The invisibility of disadvantage: why do we not notice? Stud Health Technol Inform. 2017;235:388–92.

Sittig DF, Singh H. Defining health information technology–related errors: new developments since to err is human. Arch Intern Med. 2011;171(14):1281–4.

Thomassen OJ, Heggen K, Strand R. Applying principles of sociotechnical systems onto working environment research. 2017.

Venkatesh V, Morris MG, Davis GB, Davis FD. User acceptance of information technology: toward a unified view. MIS Q. 2003:425–78.

Venkatesh V, Zhang X, Sykes TA. "Doctors do too little technology": a longitudinal field study of an electronic healthcare system implementation. Inf Syst Res. 2011;22(3):523–46.

Venkatesh V, Brown SA, Bala H. Bridging the qualitative-quantitative divide: guidelines for conducting mixed methods research in information systems. MIS Q. 2013:21–54.

von Bertalanffy L. An outline of general system theory. Br J Philos Sci. 1950;1:134–65.

Walter SR, Dunsmuir WT, Raban MZ, Westbrook JI. Understanding clinical workflow through direct continuous observation: addressing the unique statistical challenges. Cogn Inform. 2019:191–210.

Westbrook JI, Duffield C, Li L, Creswick NJ. How much time do nurses have for patients? A longitudinal study quantifying hospital nurses' patterns of task time distribution and interactions with health professionals. BMC Health Serv Res. 2011;11(1):319.

Whetton S. Health informatics: a socio-technical perspective. South Melbourne: Oxford University Press; 2005.

Yurtseven MK, Buchanan WW. Socio-technical system design: a general systems theory perspective. Proceedings of the International Conference on Engineering and Computer Education- ICECE'2013; 2013.

Chapter 4
Occupational Classifications in the Health Information Disciplines

David T. Marc, Prerna Dua, Susan H. Fenton, Karima Lalani, and Kerryn Butler-Henderson

Abstract If you ask people within the HIDDIN workforce how electronic health records support safe care delivery or how telehealth has shaped service delivery during the time of COVID, there is little dissension. Yet if you ask them what is the umbrella term for the various specialists whose functions relate to managing and governing health data, information, and knowledge, there is little agreement. This chapter explores the HIDDIN workforce as an occupational group. It examines how the workforce is represented in global and national occupation lists. It analyses the way that the workforce is grouped in global job listings. It weighs up role titles versus competencies as an approach to categorise types of work. The chapter concludes by reflecting on the effects of the COVID-19 pandemic and considering workforce development for the future of work.

Keywords Competencies · International Standard Classification of Occupations · Jobs · Roles

D. T. Marc
College of St. Scholastica, Duluth, MN, USA
e-mail: dmarc@css.edu

P. Dua
Louisiana Tech University, Ruston, LA, USA
e-mail: prerna@latech.edu

S. H. Fenton · K. Lalani
The University of Texas Health Science Center at Houston School of Biomedical Informatics, Houston, TX, USA
e-mail: susan.h.fenton@uth.tmc.edu; Karima.Lalani@uth.tmc.edu

K. Butler-Henderson (✉)
Digital Health Hub, College of STEM, RMIT University, Bundoora, VIC, Australia
e-mail: Kerryn.Butler-Henderson@rmit.edu.au

© The Author(s), under exclusive license to Springer Nature Switzerland AG 2021
K. Butler-Henderson et al. (eds.), *The Health Information Workforce*, Health Informatics, https://doi.org/10.1007/978-3-030-81850-0_4

Introduction

The HIDDIN workforce is a dynamically changing workforce, rendering it hard to define workforce boundaries. As countries have moved from paper-based medical records to electronic health records and healthcare-related apps, they have seen a change in operations for planning, management, clinical diagnosis and treatment, disease surveillance, research, and education. However, little attention has been paid to the classification of the workforce required to implement these operations successfully. The American Health Information Management Association is one of many HIDDIN associations asserting the need for professionals to update their skills to manage the transition to digital health (Gibson et al. 2015). Some types of HIDDIN jobs—health information management, for example—require healthcare licensure and specific knowledge and qualifications and are quite formally defined, while others seem barely able to be categorised or described as part of the healthcare industry. As digital health has evolved, overlaps, and synergies have occurred in job roles and occupation titles at the intersection between previously distinct fields of practice in healthcare, information science, and computer science.

Workforce occupational classification systems can be of benefit in organising and ranking similar occupations in groups based on the defined tasks and duties required by certain jobs. These systems enable job placement, employment counselling, and career guidance; using uniform occupational language can effectively match job vacancies and workers (Miller et al. 1980). The classification of occupations helps government agencies and employers to collect and use data on labour market trends and perform comparisons between related occupations. Governments use occupational classifications in the collection and dissemination of statistics from a variety of sources, including population censuses, labour force surveys, household surveys, and employer surveys; these classifications enable occupations to be linked to socioeconomic status, lifestyle (sedentary, physical, or exposed to hazards), and achievement in life (Clougherty et al. 2010). Governments and companies can use classification systems for defining job requirements, identifying educational expectations, reporting industrial accidents, administering workers' compensation, and managing employment-related migration.

How Occupations Are Classified Internationally

To date, over 180 countries have adopted some form of an occupational classification system. Examples include the USA' Standard Occupational Classification System (SOC) (US Bureau of Labor Statistics 2020), the Australian and New Zealand Standard Classification of Occupations (Australian Bureau of Statistics 2020), the South African Standard Classification of Occupations (Africa Check 2001), India's National Classification of Occupation (India's National Career Service 2015), the Classification of Occupations of Costa Rica (Sistema de

Estadistica Nacional 2011), Japan's Standard Occupational Classification System (Japan's Ministry of Internal Affairs and Communications 2009), Germany's Klassifikation der Berufe (FDZ 2013).

In the global economy, a standard to collect and report occupations data has become indispensable. The International Standard Classification of Occupations (ISCO) was first proposed in 1921, created in 1958 by the International Labour Organisation, and has been revised three times since then. ISCO-08 is a four-level hierarchical system that classifies jobs into 10 major, 43 sub-major, 130 minor and 436 unit groups. A title, code number, and definition are associated with each ISCO-08 group. The definition specifies the scope of the group and summarises the main tasks and duties performed in associated occupations. ISCO is the basis for comparisons of occupational statistics between countries and a conceptual model for the development of national occupational classifications (ISCO 2016).

To evaluate global labour trends, the mapping of ISCO-08 to national classifications is essential, although no known ontology specifies how each national classification maps to ISCO-08. One example is the US SOC system, last updated in 2018; the 2018 SOC does not currently include a direct map to ISCO-08; however, the 2010 SOC does, and a 2018 SOC to 2010 SOC crosswalk can be used to map the 2018 SOC to ISCO-08 indirectly. National classification systems that map to ISCO in some way or other are: Australia and New Zealand, Brazil, Bulgaria, Canada, Cape Verde, Costa Rica, Cuba, Czech Republic, Denmark, El Salvador, Germany, India, Indonesia, Israel, Norway, Panama, Paraguay, Philippines, Poland, Portugal, Saudi Arabia, Singapore, South Africa, Spain, Sweden, Switzerland, Thailand, the UK, the USA, Uruguay. Not all national classifications map to ISCO, however, or if a mapping exists, it is not a full crosswalk; the reason for this is that many national classifications offer more specific occupational categories based on their national workforce trends.

Occupational Classification of HIDDIN Work

ISCO-08 has only three categories for HIDDIN occupations: Health Information Technicians (ISCO-08: 3252); Filing and Copying Clerks (ISCO-08: 4415); and Librarians and Related Information Professionals (ISCO-08: 2622). This is a very limited representation of HIDDIN-related occupations. Consequently, many national classifications also lack representation of HIDDIN-related occupations. In the USA in 2014, three peak bodies (the American Health Information Management Association, the American Medical Informatics Association, and the Health Information and Management Systems) jointly recommended changes to the Standard Occupational Classification System Policy Committee, to include additional categories for Health Information Technology occupations in the 2018 SOC update. This resulted in minor modifications—addition of a new occupational category for medical records specialists, modifications to the existing health information technologists to include medical registrars, and expanded career examples including health information analysts and health informatics specialists. However, these changes are not yet reflected in ISCO, and they still do not offer an exhaustive classification of HIDDIN occupations.

The challenge for any occupational classification system is to be able to describe occupations that evolve quickly. All the HIDDIN disciplines are rapidly changing. For instance, the professional tasks, responsibilities, and roles in health information management-related professions have drastically changed in the past 5–10 years: Sandefer et al. (2015), Fenton et al. (2017), and Marc et al. (2019) have found that these professions in the USA anticipate growth in the areas of leadership, data and informatics, and decline in coding work, by 2025. Similar significant changes are occurring in the other HIDDIN disciplines. Continuous change in work focus makes it hard to fully describe and represent the HIDDIN disciplines in occupational classifications, nationally, or internationally.

Categories Derived from Global Job Listings

Occupational trends may suggest categories in the HIDDIN disciplines globally. This is illustrated in an analysis of health informatics and information management recruitment in 64 countries on www.indeed.com during September 2018 (Marc et al. 2019). Using competency areas from the American Health Information Management Association as a guide, 10 terms were applied in search strings to identify relevant job postings. This analysis provided a glimpse into four occupational clusters and differences across countries in the prevalence of job postings with these characteristics.

Most of the jobs in cluster 1 related to health information technology; the terms used were data, engine, software, test, analyst, design, security, system, technology, and solution. The majority of jobs in cluster 2 related to health research and were more clinically focused. Most jobs in cluster 3 were related to health project management and leadership, and the most common terms included sale, market, research, client, business, and project management-related terms. In cluster 4, most of the jobs related to health compliance and included terms such as safety, regulatory, and maintenance.

The analysis also showed a global trend in jobs in the areas of health consumer engagement, health informatics, health information governance, health data analysis, and clinical documentation improvement. The demand for these types of jobs was uneven. The role titles of health consumer engagement and clinical documentation improvement were found in the USA, but they did not often occur in other countries. The title health data analyst was found more frequently in the UK, Canada, Australia, and India than in other countries. Health data analysis jobs were in high demand globally; countries such as the USA, the UK, Canada, Australia, and India each advertised more than 250 positions. Health data analysis jobs were more prevalent in Australia, Canada, India, and the UK, whereas the USA had a high number of consumer engagement, information governance, and clinical documentation improvement jobs.

The job categories derived from this analysis were in keeping with four high-level role types—executive, professional, operational/technical, and supervisory/managerial—identified in a cooperative effort between the USA and the European Union to develop a comprehensive list of health information technology competencies (HITComp 2020).

Categorising Roles or Competencies

Many of the HIDDIN disciplines work together in international organisations, such as the International Medical Informatics Association, the International Federation of Health Information Management Associations, the International Federation of Library Associations Health and Biosciences Libraries Section, and the Institute of Electrical and Electronic Engineering Medicine and Biology Society. Despite these international peak bodies, and the existence of ISCO, differences between countries remain in role titles and functional roles.

Role titles are different in part because the needs of each country's healthcare systems are different. In the USA, the healthcare industry is based on a system of third-party insurance; to date, this has largely meant that providers are paid based on services provided, also known as fee-for-service. The UK, Canada, Australia, New Zealand, and India all have public or nationalised healthcare systems, with many different financing systems. These differences perhaps create a focus less on specific role titles and more on the competencies needed, which may or may not be well-represented by the ISCO or country classifications previously described. Given the diversity of health care systems across the globe, it is also to be expected that roles even within national healthcare settings will be varied. For example in the USA, more nationalised systems and larger integrated health delivery systems may have regional directors or otherwise may manage their health information and data functions centrally, relying on significant specialisation within their health information management department, while small critical access hospitals (less than 25 beds) may employ one or two people who perform all health information-related functions.

This suggests a need to focus on the skills or competencies needed for a specific position and reduce emphasis on occupation classification, at least for the purposes of job placement (Markowitsch and Plaimauer 2009). In response, Austria, Germany, France, Sweden, and the USA have developed taxonomies and databases to document skills and competencies for jobs. Using verbs that describe skills and competencies to be mastered is a standard practice among course designers in competency-based higher education. These same verbs can be used to describe job functions to be performed in the workplace setting. Ideally, this approach helps to align workforce education with labour market demand.

Technology and the skills needed to work with technology are changing at ever-increasing rates. The evolving emphasis on describing skills and competencies, as well as the continuous evolution of job classifications according to skills and competencies needed, are another challenge to the ISCO and national occupational classifications, and related resources. These struggle to keep up with fast-moving technology. Changes in occupational codes can take 4–5 years from proposal to adoption, meaning that the jobs, skills, and competencies proposed are likely to be outdated by the time they are published.

As a result, discussions of the future of work in the digital economy are focused on foundational skills that cross industries, for example "digital building blocks, business enablers, and human skills" (Markow et al. 2018): Within digital building blocks are the skills of managing data, software development, computer programming, analysing data, and digital security and privacy. Business enablers include business processes, project management, digital design, and communicating data. The domain of human skills includes communication, critical thinking, collaboration, analytical skills, and creativity. Analysis of job postings shows high demand for these generic skills in the labour market and also finds that they have higher pay rates than more constrained job titles. An example is the concept of a new "analytics translator" function rather than a role, proposed to be needed across a wide variety of organisations (Henke et al. 2018). The rationale is that, to achieve real impact, organisations looking to hire data scientists so they can utilise advanced analytics and artificial intelligence to improve their decision making and processes also need to hire translators who do not have technical expertise in data science, but rather have domain-specific knowledge, general technical fluency, and project management skills.

HIDDIN role titles may become less and less important as technological change continues to accelerate, whereas skills and competencies will increasingly come into focus. This affects the development of skills and competencies across the globe. For example a common skill might be "interact professionally at all levels of the organisation" or "create effective information visualisations from raw data;" such skills would not need to be role-specific, and a person who possessed them could be employed in multiple roles. The HIDDIN disciplines need to recognise this shift in the future of work and focus on developing skills and competencies that translate across jobs and organisations.

Conclusion

The global digital health market forecast of a compound annual growth rate of 13.4% between 2017 and 2025 (Health Standards 2017) will continue to create opportunities for the specialist HIDDIN workforce. COVID-19 has highlighted not only the importance of information management and governance and how technology can support safe healthcare, but also how important this workforce is to health service management and delivery, at the level of international cooperation. An International Federation of Health Information Management Associations survey (Fernandes et al. 2020) identified the impact of COVID-19 on HIDDIN workforce functions. The rapid transition to electronic capture of information elevated the importance of these roles. Countries where information management uses electronic, digitised, or hybrid record systems, compared to those where the work is still largely paper based, reported higher rates of people in this workforce working remotely and being involved in establishing new systems for information capture and management. This global tragedy accelerated technology adoption, with many of these changes expected to remain or to start further transformation. For example expanded telehealth services are predicted to remain the new normal and to be the catalyst for telehealth for preventative health, consequently requiring new support functions and roles.

What does this mean for occupations in the HIDDIN workforce? Evidence-informed and technology-supported health management and care will continue to reshape specialisations within this workforce. In coming years, many current roles in today's workforce will no longer exist; whilst some will become redundant, others will evolve to meet future needs. The underlying need for this workforce will remain constant, and it ought to be recognised more formally among the health professions in occupation classifications. COVID-19 may be a driver for such change.

Refinement of workforce categories in response to the evidence of global job categories and trends may assist governments and employers to meet future HIDDIN workforce needs in their respective countries. The required competencies continue to evolve rapidly, and the imperative rests on policymakers together with educators to ensure that there is a well-defined workforce able to adapt to technological change and to maintain its relevance.

References

Africa Check. South African Standard Classification of Occupations (SASCO). 2001. https://africacheck.org/wp-content/uploads/2019/05/ghs-2015-occupation-codes.pdf. Accessed 31 Jul 2020.

Australian Bureau of Statistics. Australian and New Zealand Standard Classification of Occupations (ANZSCO). 2020. https://www.abs.gov.au/ANZSCO. Accessed 31 Jul 2020.

Clougherty JE, Souza K, Cullen MR. Work and its role in shaping the social gradient in health. Ann N Y Acad Sci. 2010;1186:102–24.

FDZ. Klassifikation der Berufe (KldB). 2013. http://doku.iab.de/fdz/reporte/2013/MR_08-13_EN.pdf. Accessed 31 Jul 2020.

Fenton SH, Low S, Abrams KJ, Butler-Henderson K. Health information management: changing with time. Yearbook Medical Inform. 2017;26(1):72–7.

Fernandes L, Butler-Henderson K, MacDonald M. The impact of COVID-19 on the work life of HIM professionals: an IFHIMA survey. J AHIMA. 2020. https://journal.ahima.org/the-impact-of-covid-19-on-the-work-life-of-him-professionals-an-ifhima-survey/. Accessed 28 Jul 2020.

Gibson CJ, Abrams K, Crook G. Health information management workforce transformation: new roles, new skills and experiences in Canada. Perspect Health Inf Manag Int Issue. 2015. https://library.ahima.org/doc?oid=301180#.YGQp9z87aUk. Accessed 28 Jul 2020.

Health Standards. Digital health: current state & future growth 2017-2025. 2017. https://health-standards.com/blog/2017/10/25/digital-health-trends-2025/. Accessed 22 Jul 2020.

Henke N, Levine J, McInerney P. You don't have to be a data scientist to fill this must-have analytics role. Harv Bus Rev. 2018. https://hbr.org/2018/02/you-dont-have-to-be-a-data-scientist-to-fill-this-must-have-analytics-role. Accessed 5 Feb 2020.

HITComp. HITComp: Health Information Technology Competencies. 2020. http://hitcomp.org/. Accessed 29 Jun 2020.

India's National Career Service. India's National Classification of Occupation (NCO). 2015. https://www.ncs.gov.in/Documents/National%20Classification%20of%20Occupations%20_Vol%20I-%202015.pdf. Accessed 31 Jul 2020.

ISCO. ISCO-08 Structure, index correspondence with ISCO-88. 2016. https://www.ilo.org/public/english/bureau/stat/isco/isco08/index.htm. Accessed 31 Jul 2020.

Japan's Ministry of Internal Affairs and Communications. Japan's Standard Occupational Classification System. 2009. https://www.soumu.go.jp/english/dgpp_ss/seido/shokgyou/co09-2.htm. Accessed 31 Jul 2020.

Marc D, Butler-Henderson K, Dua P, Lalani K, Fenton SH. Global workforce trends in health informatics & information management. Stud Health Technol Inform. 2019;264:1273–7.

Markow W, Hughes D, Bundy A. The new foundational skills of the digital economy. Developing the professionals of the future. Washington, DC: Burning Glass Technologies. 2018.

Markowitsch J, Plaimauer C. Descriptors for competence: towards an international standard classification for skills and competences. J Eur Indus Train. 2009;33(8/9):817–37.

Miller AR, Treiman DJ, Cain PS, Roos PA. Work, jobs, and occupations: a critical review of the Dictionary of Occupational Titles. Washington, DC: National Academy Press; 1980.

Sandefer R, Marc D, Mancilla D, Hamada D. Survey predicts future HIM workforce shifts: HIM industry estimates the job roles, skills needed in the near future. J AHIMA. 2015;86(7):32–5.

Sistema de Estadistica Nacional. 2011. http://sistemas.inec.cr/sitiosen/sitiosen/Archivos/COCR_2011.pdf. Accessed on 31 Jul 2020.

US Bureau of Labor Statistics: Standard Occupational Classification. 2020. https://www.bls.gov/soc/. Accessed 29 Jun 2020.

Chapter 5
Competencies, Education, and Accreditation of the Health Information Workforce

Ann Ritchie, Gemma Siemensma, Susan H. Fenton, and Kerryn Butler-Henderson

Abstract This chapter looks at the identity of the HIDDIN (Health Informatics, Digital, Data, Information, kNowledge) workforce from the perspective of the competencies that are needed to do these jobs, and the accreditation of formal education and training programmes that confer recognised qualifications for these jobs. We examine definitions and a selection of research articles about how each of the groups has developed and differentiated themselves from others. We also compare the competency sets from a sample of professional associations and industry bodies, noting each group's unique areas of responsibility and overlaps; it appears that information governance is a responsibility common to all groups. Alternative education and training pathways for initial entry and ongoing professional development for the HIDDIN occupations, such as employer-driven on-the-job training and modular certification and micro-credentialing approaches, are emerging as more agile responses to the immediate needs of the workplace, and are challenging traditional post-secondary education structures. This has implica-

A. Ritchie (✉)
Independent Consultant, Melbourne, VIC, Australia

G. Siemensma
Ballarat Health Services, Ballarat, VIC, Australia
e-mail: Gemma.Siemensma@bhs.org.au

S. H. Fenton
The University of Texas Health Science Center at Houston School of Biomedical Informatics, Houston, TX, USA
e-mail: susan.h.fenton@uth.tmc.edu

K. Butler-Henderson
Digital Health Hub, College of STEM, RMIT University, Bundoora, VIC, Australia
e-mail: Kerryn.Butler-Henderson@rmit.edu.au

tions for the identity of these groups as professions. The chapter concludes that a more systematic and coordinated approach to this aspect of strategic workforce development is needed.

Keywords Competencies · Education · Accreditation · Professionalism · Information governance

Introduction

In the past few decades, healthcare managers and employers have witnessed a rise in demand for HIDDIN (Health Informatics, Digital, Data, Information, kNowledge) practitioners with increasingly specialised skill sets and more highly refined scopes of practice. This in turn has brought about a corresponding—although not always well articulated—need for more specialised training in related areas of expertise and competence. In some professions, training courses come with appropriate mechanisms for the individuals who undertake the training to be certified or credentialed, as well as mechanisms for accrediting the training programmes and training providers. Each of the occupational groups who together make up the HIDDIN workforce has recognised competencies and, in some cases, there are competency-based education frameworks against which post-secondary education and training programmes and providers are accredited. Accordingly, this chapter explores the educational structure for the HIDDIN disciplines, with examples where work has already been undertaken in this area.

Competency

In essence, the term "competent" means having expertise, knowing how to do a particular task or activity, and being able to do it. Competencies have been described as:

> integrated sets of Knowledge, Skills and Attributes (KSAs) that are needed to perform tasks in a particular field or circumstance. Competencies are also said to be observable, measurable and able to be taught. Some competency frameworks have basic and advanced levels of practice, and performance measures by which these can be measured.

(Ritchie 2020, p29).

When applied to HIDDIN work and the different occupational groups that make up this workforce, there are a number of competency frameworks that need to be examined. Table 5.1 provides an overview of the ways that competencies are used by different stakeholder groups (where stakeholder is defined as any group that has an interest in their development and use), outlines why they are used (their purpose), and how they are implemented and used. Stakeholders fall into six main groups,

Table 5.1 Health information workforce competencies—their purposes and use by different stakeholder groups

Purpose—why competencies are used?	Stakeholder groups—who uses competencies?					
	Universities and other training organisations	Professional associations/ industry bodies	Health workforce agencies (national)	Employers, e.g. hospitals	Health managers	Health practitioners (individuals)
Education and training (for qualifications, certification)	Curriculum, course development, course accreditation	Regulate and accredit education and training providers; course design and delivery		Recruitment; staff development systems	On-the-job training programmes	
Setting and maintaining standards of practice, safety and quality	Accreditation of education and training providers and courses	Competency frameworks; Continuing Professional Development (CPD); administering certification schemes; credentialing	Oversee and regulate professions and organisations	Training site and work placement accreditation; credentialing	Recruitment; defining scopes of practice; mandatory staff training	Continuing Professional Development (CPD) and specialist certifications
Strategic workforce planning	Education/ research; translation into competency-based curricula	Education/research, funding; translation into competency-based competency frameworks	National health workforce frameworks	Human resource planning; Workplace frameworks	Designing multi-disciplinary teams; team development	
Professional/ workplace/career development and lifelong learning	Teaching staff development	Continuing Professional Development (CPD) programmes and audits	Agency staff development	Staff (workplace) development	Recruitment; job design and position descriptions; team development; performance appraisal/ development	CPD; staff development/ training; career planning; certification, audit/ reflections

each having complementary areas of responsibility and roles: universities and other training organisations, professional associations and industry bodies, health workforce agencies, employers, managers, and health information practitioners themselves. The purposes for which competencies may be used are: education and training; standards, safety, and quality; strategic workforce planning; professional/career/workplace development; and lifelong learning.

In general terms, the work of all the specialist health information groups may be conceptualised as being "responsible for the development, maintenance, and governance of the systems used to manage health data, health information, and health knowledge" (Gilbert et al. 2020, p39). Referring to the centrality of the role of information governance in their mapping of the competencies for the health information professions, The Global Health Workforce Council (2015, p3) state: "The emerging body of knowledge around Information Governance in the healthcare ecosystem anchors the entirety of the health information professions". Figure 5.1 has been adapted from The Global Health Workforce Council (2015, p3) diagram to represent their shared responsibilities for information governance.

Gartner (2020, np) define information governance as:

The specification of decision rights and an accountability framework to ensure appropriate behaviour in the valuation, creation, storage, use, archiving and deletion of information. It includes the processes, roles and policies, standards and metrics that ensure the effective and efficient use of information in enabling an organization to achieve its goals.

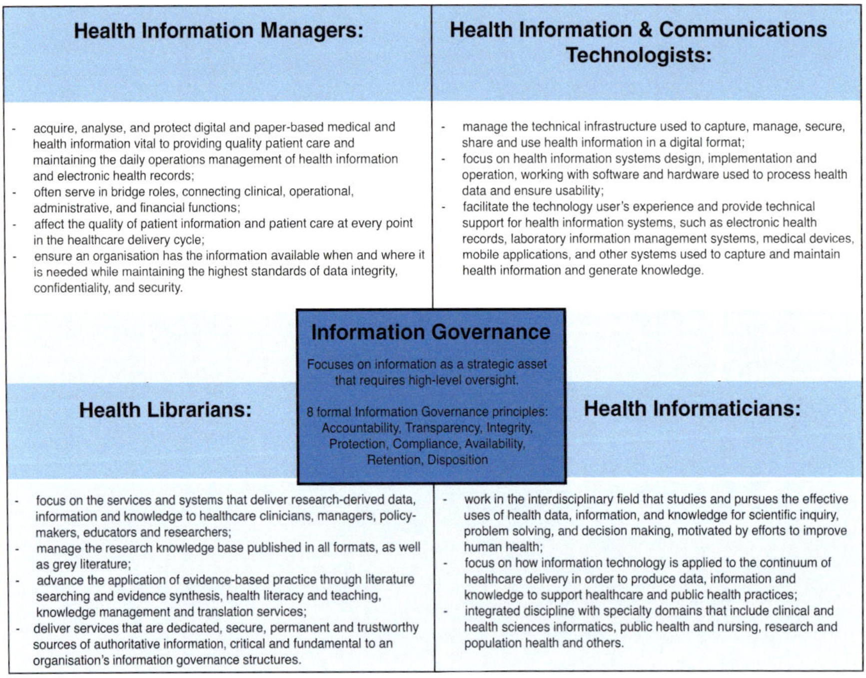

Health Information Managers:

- acquire, analyse, and protect digital and paper-based medical and health information vital to providing quality patient care and maintaining the daily operations management of health information and electronic health records;
- often serve in bridge roles, connecting clinical, operational, administrative, and financial functions;
- affect the quality of patient information and patient care at every point in the healthcare delivery cycle;
- ensure an organisation has the information available when and where it is needed while maintaining the highest standards of data integrity, confidentiality, and security.

Health Information & Communications Technologists:

- manage the technical infrastructure used to capture, manage, secure, share and use health information in a digital format;
- focus on health information systems design, implementation and operation, working with software and hardware used to process health data and ensure usability;
- facilitate the technology user's experience and provide technical support for health information systems, such as electronic health records, laboratory information management systems, medical devices, mobile applications, and other systems used to capture and maintain health information and generate knowledge.

Information Governance

Focuses on information as a strategic asset that requires high-level oversight.

8 formal Information Governance principles: Accountability, Transparency, Integrity, Protection, Compliance, Availability, Retention, Disposition

Health Librarians:

- focus on the services and systems that deliver research-derived data, information and knowledge to healthcare clinicians, managers, policy-makers, educators and researchers;
- manage the research knowledge base published in all formats, as well as grey literature;
- advance the application of evidence-based practice through literature searching and evidence synthesis, health literacy and teaching, knowledge management and translation services;
- deliver services that are dedicated, secure, permanent and trustworthy sources of authoritative information, critical and fundamental to an organisation's information governance structures.

Health Informaticians:

- work in the interdisciplinary field that studies and pursues the effective uses of health data, information, and knowledge for scientific inquiry, problem solving, and decision making, motivated by efforts to improve human health;
- focus on how information technology is applied to the continuum of healthcare delivery in order to produce data, information and knowledge to support healthcare and public health practices;
- integrated discipline with specialty domains that include clinical and health sciences informatics, public health and nursing, research and population health and others.

Fig. 5.1 Responsibilities of the health information professions and information governance

In essence and when applied to the health care sector, information governance is about ensuring the right decisions are made, i.e. decisions that are based on quality-assured information (evidence) derived from two major sources of data and knowledge: patient records and research publications. Each of the health information professions has a role in setting up, maintaining and managing the information systems and processes, and upholding the eight information governance principles: accountability, transparency, integrity, protection, compliance, availability, retention, disposition. Thus, they all have a common interest in getting the right information to the right person at the right time and place and in the right format. And each has a skill set, competencies, roles and responsibilities integral to the complex whole.

The American Health Information Management Association (AHIMA) have defined the ten organisational competencies of information governance for health care: strategic alignment, information governance structure, data governance, enterprise information management, IT governance, analytics, privacy and security safeguards, regulatory and legal, awareness and adherence, and information governance performance (Fenton et al. 2017, p74). Fenton et al. (2017) differentiate between the three levels of governance characterising them as: data governance (process, methods, tools, techniques); IT governance (frameworks, best practices); and information governance (overarching regulations and policies). They state: "data governance is the most basic, rudimentary, level of information governance and if not undertaken properly, the results will substantially affect all other levels of information governance" (p73). They report on the results of a survey of HIMs conducted by AHIMA in 2015, which identified data analytics/mining, informatics, and information governance as the fastest areas of growth in their field. An illustrative example of organisational information governance is seen in the case of hospital librarians. Ritchie et al. (2020) in their study of the contribution of hospital libraries in meeting hospital accreditation standards, state that hospital librarians' expertise and ability to access up-to-date health information and knowledge resources is "integral to an organisation's governance framework… hospital libraries help to ensure that the work of a hospital's employees—clinicians and other health care professionals, managers, administrators, educators, researchers, policy makers—is evidence-based and complies with safety and quality standards".

Understanding the distinctive skill sets (competencies) of the HIDDIN workforce, and recognising their common interest and varying responsibilities in the area of information governance, will help to clarify and make their roles more visible in the digital health care environment.

Competency Frameworks

There are many competency frameworks used by the HIDDIN disciplines. A sample of these is outlined in Table 5.2. Even though these individual disciplines have evolved in relatively separate, specialist streams, there are roles and competencies that are complementary and at times, may have overlapping and/or blurred boundaries. Competency frameworks also vary in the details provided: some specify foundational skills through to advanced skills, while others provide descriptions to indicate the scope of a competency area.

Table 5.2 Health information workforce competency frameworks

Discipline, Name of organisation, and Information source	Number and overview of domains/competencies/quadrants
Health Information Managers (HIM) Health Information Management Association of Australia https://www.himaa.org.au/files/Misc/Docs/HIMAA_HIM_Competency_Standards_Version_3_FNL_June2017.pdf	Domains (9) • Generic professional skills • Health information and records management • Language of healthcare • Healthcare terminologies and classification • Research methods • Health services organisation and delivery • Health information law and ethics • eHealth • Health information services organisation and management
Health Information Managers (HIM) American Health Information Management Association (AHIMA) (2018) https://www.ahima.org/him-curricula/	Domains (6) • Data structure, content, and information governance • Information protection: access, use, disclosure, privacy, and security • Informatics, analytics, and data use • Revenue cycle management • Health law and compliance • Organisational management and leadership
Health Librarianship (HL) Australian Library and Information Association, Health Libraries Australia (2018) https://read.alia.org.au/alia-hla-competencies	Competency areas (8) • The health environment • Reference and research services • Resources • Leadership and management • Digital, ehealth, and technology • Health literacy and teaching • Health research • Professionalism
Health Librarianship (HL) Medical Library Association (2007) https://www.mlanet.org/page/competencies	Competencies (6) • Information services • Information management • Instruction and instructional design • Leadership and management • Evidence-based practice and research • Health Information Professionalism
Health Informatics (HI) Public Health Informatics Institute (2016) https://phii.org/resources/view/9462/applied-public-health-informatics-competency-model	Competencies (8) • Principles and strategy • Standards and interoperability • Project management • Information systems • Communication • Evaluation • Analysis, visualisation, and reporting (VAR) • Policy

Table 5.2   (Continued)

Discipline, Name of organisation, and Information source	Number and overview of domains/competencies/quadrants
Health Informatics (HI) Digital Health Canada (2019) https://digitalhealthcanada.com/wp-content/uploads/2019/12/Competency-Requirements-Exam-Version.pdf	Domains (6) • Information management • Technology ecosystem • Clinical and health sciences • Canadian health system • Healthcare transformation • Project management
Health Information and Communications Technologists (HICT) and Health Informatics (HI) HITCOMP (2015) http://hitcomp.org/competencies/	Quadrants (6) • Operational interactions • Health data interactions • Patient interactions • Administrative interactions • Clinical interactions • Communication interactions
Health Information and Communications Technologists (HICT) and Health Informatics (HI) and Health Information Managers (HIM) Global Health Workforce Council (IFHIMA and AIMA) https://ifhimasitemedia.s3.us-east-2.amazonaws.com/wp-content/uploads/2018/01/20033722/AHIMA-GlobalCurricula_Final_6-30-15.pdf	Domains (29) • Analytics and statistics • Change management • Classification of disease, coding diagnoses, and procedures • Clinical documentation improvement (CDI) • Data management and information governance • Data quality and information integrity • Ethics • Financial management • Health information access, disclosure, and exchange • Health information systems and application design and planning • Health information systems and application development and deployment • Health information systems and application support • Health law, regulation, accreditation, and/or certification • Health record content and documentation • Human resource management • Information and information systems governance • Information protection—data privacy, confidentiality, and security • Information security strategy and management • Organisational management and leadership • Project management • Purchasing and contracting • Quality management • Research design and methods • Risk management • Standards for data content, health information exchange, and interoperability • Strategic planning • Training and development • Work design and process improvement • Healthcare delivery systems

The analysis of the sample sets listed in Table 5.2 shows that although there are differences in each group's primary areas of responsibility, there are similar skills, knowledge, and attributes which could be termed generic competency areas that run through all groups. These include Leadership and Management (variously detailed as financial management, human resource management, project management, change management); Professionalism (ethics, understanding health care environments and contexts, knowledge of legal and regulatory frameworks); Professional and Organisational Development (instruction and instructional design, professional development, training and development). Thus there is some basis for a superficial observation that the disciplines are more alike than different. Further analysis of the competencies related to each groups' areas of focus, however, indicates that there are particular distinguishing features that align with their primary responsibilities, and serve to differentiate each of the specialist groups.

Health Information Management has a key focus on health records and data and exhibits distinguishing features in three main areas: Health information and records management; Healthcare terminologies and classification; Data structure, content, and information governance.

Health Informatics distinguishes itself in three areas focusing on patient information and how technology is applied: Computer science and system design (technology ecosystem); Clinical and health sciences; Healthcare transformation.

Health Information and Communications Technologists distinguishes itself by focusing on the technical infrastructure of health: Health information systems and application; Implementation and operation of systems; Working with software and hardware used to process health data.

Health Librarianship delivers the services and systems for research/evidence-based health care and distinguishes itself through its focus on three areas: Reference and research services; Information resources (in the sense of collection management); Evidence-based practice and research.

Competency-Based Education

Competency-based education is defined as:

> an approach to designing academic programs with a focus on competencies (knowledge, skills and abilities) rather than time spent in a classroom. According to the Competency-Based Education Network (C-BEN): Competency-based education combines an intentional and transparent approach to curricular design with an academic model in which the time it takes to demonstrate competencies varies and the expectations about learning are held constant. Students acquire and demonstrate their knowledge and skills by engaging in learning exercises, activities and experiences that align with clearly defined programmatic outcomes.

(Strategy Labs 2017, p5)

The structure and delivery of formal training varies greatly across the HIDDIN disciplines and between countries. For example, a review of global HIM training (IFHIMA 2021) identified that some countries have been offering training programmes for more than 80 years. The majority of formal training globally is typically through vocational providers and at an educational level below a bachelor or baccalaureate level. Whilst the number of countries offering formal university level training in HIM is increasing, including bachelor (majority) and master (minority) level, this level of required formal training is not recognised globally. No doctorate level training in HIM or clinical classification has been identified. Conversely, digital health and data analytics worldwide are considered relatively new on the educational scene and university programmes are gradually increasing in number and popularity.

There is a paucity of research and evidence to support specialist HIDDIN educational development, compared to research into other areas of health workforce education. One main focus for health informatics and information management education is on the identification of competencies. The US HIM profession conducted a survey to try and identify the roles and skills that are needed for the future (Sandefer et al. 2015), while the US health informatics profession used a more constrained consensus-based approach (Valenta et al. 2018). Interestingly, a survey of both educators and employers conducted in the USA around this time demonstrated a significant difference in the beliefs of these two groups regarding graduates' professional and technical skills, leadership skills, and employability skills (Jackson et al. 2016). There seems to be more research about hybrid education, that is, providing clinical professionals with informatics skills—either interprofessionally (Gray et al. 2015; Whittaker et al. 2015), or in specific clinical disciplines: medicine (Vossen et al. 2020; Jidkov et al. 2019; AMIA 2011; Siribaddana et al. 2019), nursing (Ammenwerth and Hackl 2019), pharmacy (Martin et al. 2019), and the clinical research data management profession (Zozus et al. 2017). Overall, determining the competencies needed to develop hybrid specialists is a work in progress. It is still not unusual to encounter persons working in HIDDIN profession roles who may have no formal training, or who may have done training that was not quality assured or evidence-based.

Healthcare is now witnessing a training evolution beyond competencies to entrustable professional activities (EPAs). According to Cate (2005), EPAs: are part of essential professional work in a given context; must require adequate knowledge, skill, and attitude, generally acquired through training; must lead to recognised output of professional labour. EPAs should be: confined to qualified personnel; independently executable; executable within a time frame; observable and measurable in their process and their outcome, leading to a conclusion ("well done" or "not well done"). EPAs should reflect one or more of the competencies to be acquired. EPAs are a way to transform competencies into practice; EPAs do not describe the learner, but rather describe the work to be done; EPAs often require more than one competency, integrated together (Cate 2013). Finally, for an EPA, it is necessary to determine the needed levels of supervision, including (Cate 2013, p1176): "Observation but no execution, even with direct supervision; Execution with direct, proactive supervision; Execution with reactive supervision, i.e. on request and quickly available; Supervision at a distance and/or post hoc; Supervision provided by the trainee to more junior colleagues". EPAs were initially developed for physicians, though we currently see EPAs for dental (Goodell et al. 2019) and pharmacy (Marshall et al. 2020), along with interest from nursing (Al-Moteri 2020).

Given the continuing integration of more and more information technology into day-to-day clinical practice, the question becomes whether or not the HIDDIN workforce needs to develop entrustable professional activities. For example, how can an organisation determine whether or not the recently developed clinical decision support algorithm has been correctly developed and is acceptable to be implemented for clinical decision-making? How can an organisation determine whether the various reports and dashboards are developed by those with the appropriate training and skill? Currently, the HIDDIN workforce training programmes, especially degree programmes, focus on competencies. While competencies are certainly an improvement over the previous topic-based approach to training the HIDDIN workforce, they may not be adequate in the increasingly digital world. EPAs were introduced to assure patients that they could "trust" their clinicians; so the need to use EPAs is not immediately apparent for the HIDDIN workforce. However, the HIDDIN workforce is increasingly involved in developing information, knowledge, and tools to assist clinicians and consumers to make shared decisions. It is vitally important that all decision-makers have trust in activities performed by the HIDDIN workforce.

For example, "perform exploratory, inferential, predictive, and causal data analysis" is a competency outcome currently in use for an existing master's degree in biomedical informatics. This could translate into an EPA if the component parts are considered. First, to perform these analyses, a trainee would need to understand each type of analysis, including the data needed for each. Second, a trainee would need to understand when it is appropriate to use each type of analysis. Third, a trainee would either need to know how to calculate the analyses manually or how to use various software packages or programs to conduct the analyses. The level of training of the trainee would determine whether or not the trainee could complete this, as would the strictness of the supervisor. Some supervisors might expect the most concise method, while others may not be as stringent, indicating that any method coming to the right conclusion is sufficient. The context, i.e., the type of data and the reason for which the analysis is being completed are important. Finally, if the EPA were to perform exploratory analysis only, the EPA might be simpler, while conducting predictive analyses would be more complex. The supervisor could demonstrate the analyses, progressively giving the trainee more responsibility, until it becomes the responsibility of the trainee to supervise others with less training.

Accreditation

In education, accreditation is a standards-based process that is applied to programmes of study to signify that the provider and the study programme meet the requirements of a profession or industry body. Harrison (2017, p11) explains the role and critical importance of accreditation systems:

> Accreditation in a variety of guises is the norm in a wide range of regulated professions, including architecture, education, engineering, law, medicine and nursing. It serves to validate any academic program for which successful completion is a necessary precondition for entrance

into the profession…. Typically, the accreditation is conducted with reference to standards dictated by the accrediting agency. This is often a body representing the profession itself.

This quality assurance is over and above the generic procedures for accrediting all public post-secondary education providers, so that their degrees are additionally sanctioned by the professions they serve. Although the health information professions are not listed as one of the regulated professions in Harrison's definition, the same logic applies. To qualify to enter and work in their chosen fields, graduates should have baseline levels of knowledge, skills, and attributes, i.e., competencies, as determined by their respective professional associations or industry bodies. Accreditation systems that refer to competencies or standards of professional practice recognise both the education providers and their programmes of study. By attaining a recognised qualification, an individual gains professional status and is deemed entrustable to practice as an appropriately qualified and competent professional; thus accreditation standards provide a measure of quality assurance to employers and the public. An example of the operation of such a system is the Australian Health Practitioner Regulation Agency (AHPRA), which works with national boards of 15 regulated (licensed) clinical health professions; for AHPRA, a health profession accreditation standard means:

> A standard used to assess whether a program of study, and the education provider that provides the program of study, provide persons who complete the program with the knowledge, skills and professional attributes to practise the profession in Australia.

(AHPRA 2020, np)

In the clinical health professions, accreditation of a clinician's professional status serves as a guarantee of public safety and quality care. In contrast, the HIDDIN occupational groups that are the focus of this chapter do not belong to the regulated health professions, and their education and training may not be subject to the same rigorous accreditation systems. In Australia, AHPRA uses the terminology "self-regulating" professions to cover health professional groups such as the HIDDIN workforce. However, given the potential impact of the digital information and systems that they manage—on clinical decision-making and on the lives of patients, the efficiency and accessibility of care, and the policy framework that surrounds clinical care—there is a strong argument that the same rigour and principles should apply across both clinical and HIDDIN professions.

"Academic program accreditation in higher education is both a process and, if a successful process, a mechanism for external quality and integrity validation for education programs" (Feldman et al. 2020, p237). In other words, accreditation is a pathway towards professionalisation of the HIDDIN workforce. Independent bodies are integral to the accreditation process, allowing review from those outside educational facilities. This helps make the system more robust, ensures multiple viewpoints are considered, and offers a higher level of governance and rigour. A multi-disciplinary survey of accrediting organisation members of the US-based Council for Higher Education Accreditation found that, among the 26 of the 85 recognised accrediting organisations (30.5%) that responded, their involvement in competency-based education was minimal, modest, and responsive in nature, partly because most degree programmes are not competency-based (Eaton 2016). The situation for accreditation and competency-based education in the HIDDIN professions is not dissimilar from that described in Eaton's survey.

Of the four disciplines highlighted in this chapter, HIMs appear to be the most regulated, with strong course accreditation reporting lines and frameworks and, together with some health informatics courses, they have demonstrated an intention to follow a competency-based model of education and accreditation. An example is the Health Information Management Association of Australia (HIMAA), the formal accrediting body for all HIM courses in Australia; HIMAA accreditation of HIM degree courses is linked directly to HIMs' eligibility for full graduate membership of HIMAA (2020). Likewise, the Canadian College of Health Information Management (CCHIM) is the national accrediting body for HIM education in Canada. Accreditation with CCHIM confirms that the educational facility is committed to self-assessment and external peer review in meeting or exceeding the standards and to continuously find new ways to enhance the quality of education and training provided (CCHIM 2020). In the United States, the Commission on Accreditation for Health Informatics and Information Management Education (CAHIIM) is an accrediting organisation which has independent authority in all actions pertaining to accreditation of educational programmes in the fields of HIM and HI (Commission on Accreditation for Health Informatics and Information Management Education (CAHIIM 2020)). The International Medical Informatics Association (IMIA) is an international accreditation body that operates separately from universities and local national professional associations. The association's competency-based model is confirmed by the second of IMIA's aims for accreditation of biomedical and health informatics (BMHI) programmes: "To ensure that the level and quality of educational programs offered by academic institutions of various types meet the IMIA recommendations on BMHI competencies" (Jaspers et al. 2017). It is noted that IMIA accreditation provides educational BMHI programmes "with information about whether their curriculum, courses, and student competencies upon graduation meet a global standard". In contrast, Health Information and Communications Technologist and Health Librarianship degree courses are rare—rather, people may undertake training via majors or specialisations within a more generic degree, and be accredited by overarching, generalist industry and professional bodies not specific to health. For instance, the Australian Computer Society (ACS) accredits ICT degrees, and the American Library Association (ALA) accredits librarianship degrees (ACS 2016; ALA 2020).

This brief overview of accreditation and competency-based education has shown this to be an area of weakness for the HIDDIN professions in terms of asserting a health profession identity, although perhaps also it is an opportunity to innovate high quality but more agile forms of education and training than universities typically offer.

Professionalisation

For the health professions in general, and for the HIDDIN workforce in particular, digital health technologies have had disruptive and transformational effects. New and changing models of care are a feature of the clinical digital healthcare environment, and these, in turn, have stimulated demand for increasingly specialised health information professionals who manage health data, information, and knowledge, as well as the technological infrastructure that underpins the delivery of digital services. What is clear is that there is a complex interplay amongst the stakeholder groups who have varied interests, roles, and responsibilities affecting the delivery and outcomes of digital health services. This fluidity has ramifications for the education of the HIDDIN workforce who need to continually learn and adapt to their changing environments.

Although they are not legislated and regulated, there are educational qualifications that confer eligibility for membership of the respective professional associations. But regulatory drivers that are equivalent to regulated professions do not exist—for educational qualifications, continuing professional development or accreditation of education frameworks. Nor are employers legally required to employ credentialed professionals. In addition, the emerging trend towards alternative education pathways that are separate from the traditional post-secondary systems of professional education, carries a risk of deprofessionalisation. We cannot yet be sure that selectively skills-based, modular or "micro" approaches will deliver the competencies required for an individual to develop and practice as a professional. Unfolding in front of our eyes, the uneven approach to train and certify members of the HIDDIN workforce is a social experiment in determining who can be trusted with responsibility and accountability for the digital transformation of health.

Roles and Responsibilities: Specialisation, Convergence, Overlap

This chapter's focus on competencies of the HIDDIN workforce has revealed a shifting terrain with increasing specialisation within the groups, as well as a blurring of boundaries between the groups. Roles and titles have changed, and job descriptions and responsibilities are evolving to fit the requirements of the workplace. In some cases the roles and associated competencies are becoming increasingly specialised and more highly refined, while in other cases, there are areas of overlap. These observations have highlighted two trends which appear to be developing in parallel and independently of each other: Firstly, within particular occupational groups, there is demand for the practitioners to have increasingly specialised and more highly refined skillsets. Secondly, there is a counter trend towards convergence between the groups, demonstrated in the blurring of boundaries, and featuring shared or overlapping areas of competence.

Competencies and Information Governance

Comparing the roles and competencies of the HIDDIN workforce groups has highlighted an important responsibility that is shared across all groups—the area of information governance. All the information professions have a common interest in getting the right information to the right person at the right time and place and in the right format. This is at the core of information governance, which is about account-ability and responsibility for decision-making, and establishing accountability frameworks, systems, and policies, to ensure the right decisions are made (i.e. decisions that are based on high quality information and data) following the correct procedures. The implication of this observation regarding information governance as an area of shared responsibility is that there is a need for a more coordinated and planned approach to workforce development in such a critical area.

Education and Training: Traditional Academic Accredited Model or Alternative Pathways?

Lack of clarity about roles and responsibilities with regard to managing health data, information, and knowledge in the digital workplace can be confusing for employ-ers who may not know who they need to hire to do a particular job, nor how to develop their workforce strategically. It is also confusing for individuals, who may be planning their job progression and career advancement but unclear about where the job opportunities lie or where they can train for these positions.

Employers have tried various approaches to "growing their own" including prod-uct- or vendor-specific training (e.g. using particular Electronic Medical Records systems) and on-the-job workplace learning solutions. These are often product or process-oriented and not designed with broader professional competencies in mind. In its "Workforce and Education Roadmap", the Australian Digital Health Agency (2020, p12) has stated: "Workplace-specific education will play a critical role in driving the new ways of working necessary to achieve the benefits of new technolo-gies". The Agency notes that transformational and situational leadership capabilities will also be required to support the identification and successful delivery of digital health programmes that will cause significant disruption at the enterprise level.

As well as causing disruption in the workplace, lack of clarity about roles and responsibilities for the contemporary HIDDIN workforce is also a significant issue for educators. In general terms, the responses to this issue of "skills deficit" have been uncoordinated and disjointed. A gap in communication between professions, employers, and educators has led to a mismatch between content-based educational courses which focus on learning outcomes, and the competency-based needs of a rapidly developing digital health workplace. Incorporating digital health competen-cies into post-secondary education courses has been cumbersome, and formal accreditation of post-secondary education programmes has not kept pace with industry requirements for a skilled workforce. Alternative education pathways are being forged.

To fill the training and education gaps, industry and professional association-led certification and micro-credentialing initiatives have developed as more immediate responses to the needs of the workplace. Many of the training systems that deliver certification and micro-credentialing are, in fact, based on the various professional groups' competency sets and may be delivered by accredited training providers. Thus although the equivalent rigorous accreditation standards may not be applied to these alternative education pathways, they may have some credibility as standards-based, quality-assured systems. It remains to be seen, however, whether or not there is an ongoing trend in a direction that is outside the traditional academic model of education for the regulated clinical health professions.

Conclusion

This chapter has sought to explore the identity of the HIDDIN workforce from the perspective of their underpinning competencies. It has proposed that understanding their distinctive competencies and recognising their common interest and varying responsibilities in the area of information governance, will help to clarify and make their roles more visible in the broader digital health care environment.

Stakeholder groups who have an interest in the competencies of the HIDDIN workforce comprise: universities and training organisations, professional associations/industry bodies, health workforce agencies, employers, managers, and health information practitioners themselves. Competency-based education pathways are essential if graduates are to be "job-ready" with the requisite skills, knowledge, and attributes that enable them to perform in the workplace, and to maintain standards of professional practice, continually update their knowledge base and improve their skills. It is, therefore, imperative that education providers and employers work together to ensure that their programmes are based on changing workforce needs.

Our analysis has found a paucity of competency-based tertiary education programmes for the HIDDIN professions, which may have led to the apparent mismatch between the content-based education and training programmes offered by education providers and the needs of employers for graduates who are a good fit for the available jobs, as well as programmes for upskilling current employees. Alternative education pathways that may be competency-based include certificates and microcredentials. These are emerging as a more agile response to the needs of the workplace and it remains to be seen if they will replace the more traditional model of academic education, or develop in parallel or in partnership with it.

This chapter suggests that in addition to implications for education and training of the health information workforce, there are higher order issues at stake. If the health field is to address future challenges in digital health and the quality and safety of care, gaps in quality assurance and competency-based accreditation of education for the health information professions need to be addressed. A seriously coordinated and systematic approach to strategic workforce development for the health information professions is needed.

References

Al-Moteri M. Entrustable professional activities in nursing: a concept analysis. Int J Nurs Sci. 2020;7:277–84.

American Health Information Management Association. AHIMA health information management curricula competencies. 2018. https://www.ahima.org/him-curricula/. Accessed 31 Mar 2021.

American Library Association (ALA). ALA accredited programs. 2020. http://www.ala.org/educa-tioncareers/accreditedprograms. Accessed 31 Mar 2021.

AMIA. Becomes a Board-certified medical subspecialty following ABMS Vote. 2011. https://www.amia.org/news-and-publications/press-release/ci-is-subspecialty. Accessed 26 Mar 2021.

Ammenwerth E, Hackl WO. Topics for continuous education in Nursing informatics: results of a survey among 280 Austrian Nurses. Stud Health Technol Inform. 2019;260:162–9.

Australian Computer Society. ACS accreditation of higher education. 2016. https://www.acs.org.au/cpd-education/acs-accreditation-program.html. Accessed 31 Mar 2021.

Australian Digital Health Agency. National digital health workforce and education roadmap. 2020. https://www.digitalhealth.gov.au/healthcare-providers/initiatives-and-programs/workforce-and-education. Accessed 31 Mar 2021.

Australian Health Practitioner Regulation Agency. About AHPRA. 2020. https://www.ahpra.gov.au/About-Ahpra.aspx. Accessed 31 Mar 2021.

Australian Library and Information Association (ALIA). ALIA Health Libraries Australia. 2018. https://read.alia.org.au/alia-hla-competencies. Accessed 31 Mar 2021.

Canadian College of Health Information Management (CCHIM). Program accreditation. 2020. https://www.echima.ca/college/program-accreditation/. Accessed 31 Mar 2021.

Cate OT. Entrustability of professional activities and competency-based training. Med Educ. 2005;39:1176–7.

Cate OT. Nuts and bolts of entrustable professional activities. J Grad Med Educ. 2013;5:157–8.

Commission on Accreditation for Health Informatics and Information Management Education (CAHIIM). Homepage. Chicago: CAHIIM; 2020. Available from: https://www.cahiim.org/.

Digital Health Canada. Competency requirements. 2019. https://digitalhealthcanada.com/wp-content/uploads/2019/12/Competency-Requirements-Exam-Version.pdf. Accessed 31 Mar 2021.

Eaton JS. Accreditation and competency-based education. Competency-based Education. 2016;1:12–6.

Feldman SS, Boren SA, Tesch LH, Valenta AL. Accreditation of health informatics programs. In: Berner ES, editor. Informatics education in healthcare. Switzerland: Springer; 2020.

Fenton SH, Low S, Abrams KJ, Butler-Henderson K. Health information management: changing with time. Yearbook Med Inform. 2017;26(1):72–7.

Gartner. Information governance. 2020. https://www.gartner.com/en/information-technology/glossary/information-governance. Accessed 31 Mar 2021.

Gilbert C, Gray K, Butler-Henderson K, Ritchie A. Digital health and professional identity in Australian health libraries: evidence from the 2018 Australian Health Information Workforce Census. Evid Based Libr Info Pract. 2020;15(1):38–58.

Global Health Workforce Council. Global academic curricula competencies for health information professionals. Chicago: American Health Information Management Association; 2015. https://ifhimasitemedia.s3.us-east-2.amazonaws.com/wp-content/uploads/2018/01/20033722/AHIMA-GlobalCurricula_Final_6-30-15.pdf. Accessed 31 Mar 2021.

Goodell KH, Ticku S, Fazio SB, Riedy CA. Entrustable professional activities in oral health for primary care providers based on a scoping review. J Dent Educ. 2019;83:1370–81.

Gray K, Choo D, Butler-Henderson K, Whetton S, Maeder A. Health informatics and e-health curriculum for clinical health profession degrees. Stud Health Technol Inform. 2015;214:68–73.

Harrison A. Skills, competencies and credentials. Toronto: Higher Education Quality Council of Ontario; 2017. http://www.heqco.ca/SiteCollectionDocuments/Formatted_Skills%20Competencies%20and%20Credentials.pdf. Accessed 31 Mar 2021.

Health Information Management Association of Australia (HIMAA). Accreditation. 2020. https:// himaa.org.au/accreditation/#1584333776893-78843700-02bc. Accessed 31 Mar 2021.

HITCOMP. Health Information Technology Competencies. 2015. http://hitcomp.org/. Accessed 31 Mar 2021.

IFHIMA. IFHIMA workforce white paper. Examining today's HIM profession with recommendations for the future. 2021. https://ifhima.org/. Accessed 13 Apr 2021.

Jackson K, Lower CL, Rudman WJ. Crossroads between workforce and education. Perspectives in Health Information Management. American Health Information Management Association; 2016. http://bok.ahima.org/doc?oid=301567. Accessed 7 Mar 2021.

Jaspers MW, Mantas J, Borycki E, Hasman A. IMIA accreditation of biomedical and health informatics education: current state and future directions. Yearbook Med Inform. 2017:252–6.

Jidkov L, Alexander M, Bark P, Williams JG, Kay J, Taylor P, et al. Health informatics competencies in postgraduate medical education and training in the UK: a mixed methods study. BMJ Open. 2019;9:e025460.

Marshall LL, Kinsey J, Nykamp D, Momary K. Evaluating practice readiness of advanced pharmacy practice experience students using the core Entrustable Professional Activities. AJPE: Am J Pharmaceut Educ. 2020;84(10):7853.

Martin LG, Warholak TL, Hincapie AL, Gallo T, Kjos AL, Task force on informatics AJ. Health informatics competencies for Pharmacists in training. Am J Pharm Educ. 2019;83:6512.

Medical Library Association. Professional competencies. 2007. https://www.mlanet.org/page/competencies. Accessed 31 Mar 2021.

Public Health Informatics Institute. Applied Public Health Informatics Competency Model. 2016. https://phii.org/resources/view/9462/applied-public-health-informatics-competency-model. Accessed 31 Mar 2021.

Ritchie A. ALIA/HLA competencies review 2020: what is a health library and information professional? What do they do and why do they do it? J Health Info Libr Australas. 2020;1(1):28–35. https://www.johila.org/index.php/Johila/article/view/1.

Ritchie A, Gilbert C, Gaca M, Siemensma G, Taylor J. Hospital librarians' contributions to health services' accreditation: an account of the health libraries for the national safety and quality in health services standards (HeLiNS) research project, 2016-18. J Aust Libr Info Assoc. 2020;69(2):215–45.

Sandefer R, Marc D, Mancilla D, Hamada D. Survey predicts future HIM work-force shifts: HIM industry estimates the job roles, skills needed in the near future. J AHIMA. 2015;86:32–5.

Siribaddana P, Hewapathirana R, Jayatilleke AU, Sahay S, Dissanayake VH. Strengthening health systems through informatics capacity development among doctors in low-resource contexts: the Sri Lankan experience. WHO South East Asia J Public Health. 2019;8:87–94.

Strategy Labs. Understanding competency-based education: toolkit. Indianapolis: Lumina Foundation; 2017. https://www.ecs.org/wp-content/uploads/CBE-Toolkit-2017.pdf. Accessed 31 Mar 2021.

Valenta AL, Berner ES, Boren SA, Deckard GJ, Eldredge C, Fridsma DB, Gadd C, Gong Y, Johnson T, Jones J, Manos EL, Phillips KT, Roderer NK, Rosendale D, Turner AM, Tusch G, Williamson JJ, Johnson SB. AMIA Board White Paper: AMIA 2017 core competencies for applied health informatics education at the master's degree level. J Am Med Inform Assoc. 2018;25:1657–68.

Vossen K, Rethans J-J, van Kuijk SMJ, van der Vleuten CP, Kubben PL. Under-standing medical students' attitudes toward learning ehealth: questionnaire study. JMIR Med Educ. 2020;6:e17030.

Whittaker M, Hodge N, Mares RE, Rodney A. Preparing for the data revolution: identifying minimum health information competencies among the health work-force. Human Resour Health. 2015;13:17.

Zozus MN, Lazarov A, Smith LR, Breen TE, Krikorian SL, Zbyszewski PS, et al. Analysis of professional competencies for the clinical research data management profession: implications for training and professional certification. J Am Med Inform Assoc. 2017;24:737–45.

Chapter 6
Professional and Industry Certifications for the Health Information Workforce

Kathleen Gray

Abstract One way to identify individuals in the health information workforce is by the professional and industry certifications they hold. A wide variety of relevant certifications is available outside formal post-secondary education systems. This chapter outlines the major features of these certifications, what aspects of HIDDIN work they highlight, and what body of knowledge they signify. Comparing and contrasting these certifications raises critical considerations for individuals, employers of HIDDIN workers, and certification providers themselves. Analysis suggests that the professional and industry certification business is long on competition and short on quality assurance. This situation undermines the professional standing of a workforce that substantially relies on this means of demonstrating competence to practice.

Keywords Certification · Credential · Examination · Fellowship · Qualification

Introduction

How is it possible to determine which individuals in the health information workforce hold bona fide certification of ability to do work of specific types and levels of complexity? Evidence from the literature and from surveying this workforce points to problems of invisibility and undifferentiation in the way that health information

K. Gray (✉)
Centre for Digital Transformation of Health, University of Melbourne, Melbourne, VIC, Australia
e-mail: kgray@unimelb.edu.au

practitioners work (Gray et al. 2019). Looking at distinguishing features of the specialised Health Informatics, Digital, Data, Information and kNowledge (HIDDIN) workforce around the world, what visibly differentiates a professional from an amateur or an expert from a novice?

A plethora of relevant certifications awarded by professional societies and industry associations are available for individuals to pursue, to identify themselves for this purpose. Earning credentials of this kind is an avenue to workforce differentiation and career progression that has low academic barriers to entry and uncomplicated methods of measuring achievement. Typically, gaining and maintaining this type of credential relies on small, staged quanta of learning, and entails less breadth and depth of learning and assessment than is expected in post-secondary education systems. For this reason, these are sometimes called micro-credentials or micro-certifications (Ellis et al. 2016; NCVER 2018).

This chapter considers the certification of HIDDIN workers in relation to formal post-secondary education, and in the context of certification of practitioners in the related fields of information technology and health care. It reviews an international selection of pertinent certifications awarded by professional societies and industry associations and compares them from both supply and demand perspectives. The overall aim is to make certification options and practices more understandable to current and intending practitioners, employers, and organisations that offer credentialing of practitioners.

Why and How Individuals Are Certified?

In any field of work, if we wish to determine whether an individual has a specialised skill or capability, we rely in part on their own claims, and in part on independent verification of their credentials by a third-party service that provides credible evidence of the person's knowledge, experience, skill, or other eligibility. We attach greater or lesser importance to independent verification, depending on how serious we consider the implications of an individual's competence or the consequences of their incompetence. Society's trust in a professional or industry certification rests not only on a systematic process for certifying individuals and keeping a record of who is and is not certified, but more fundamentally too, on a systematic process for deciding how their competency is framed, that is what knowledge, skills, and attributes they need to demonstrate. The International Standards Organisation standard ISO/IEC 17024 (2012) sets out general requirements for good practice by "bodies offering certification of persons", so that there can be public confidence in certification schemes and understanding of how they relate to each other. The standard also points out that "it is necessary to distinguish between situations where certification schemes for persons are justified and situations where other forms of qualification are more appropriate" and that "alternatives to certification can still be necessary in positions where public services, official or governmental operations are concerned".

Across the HIDDIN workforce, verification of competence to practice may come in the form of a specific qualification awarded by a post-secondary education and training provider, or not. Even if formal educational qualifications are available (not always the case), labour shortages open opportunities to move into this workforce without prior formal education in the field. Historically, many people have entered the HIDDIN workforce opportunistically, becoming skilled by learning on the job or self-taught through personal interest; included among them are some of the most senior and respected figures in HIDDIN communities of practice. Thus, in these communities, there is a persistent tension between academic and industry bona fides of competence (Eckman 2017).

Professional and industry credentialing of individuals in the HIDDIN workforce mirrors a more general social trend to value industry-recognised certificates as a complement or alternative to academic qualifications. Rapidly rising demand for specialised skills, combined with the Internet's facility to support learning interactions and transactions, are driving post-secondary institutions and other organisations to be entrepreneurial in offering credentialing services to individuals who are ambitious to signal their competence to do specific kinds of work (Kato et al. 2020). Among credentialing service providers, terminology, standards, and quality of service are uneven. Thus, there are many nuances to negotiate in HIDDIN workforce credentialing, as shown in an example from the USA: "The terms "certification" and "designation" are usually used interchangeably […]. A professional certification (e.g. PMP, CPHIMS) typically validates that an individual has attained the knowledge and skills necessary for competent practice in a particular profession. A professional designation (e.g. CRNBC, FRCPC) conveys a continuing competency as measured by the issuing national or international professional governing body and as managed by the individual on a regular basis" (Davis 2017). Workforce globalisation and transboundary job markets are a growing consideration for practitioners, employers, and credential providers. However key certification concepts do not translate directly from one country to another because of differences in national systems of education and of healthcare. Therefore, this chapter follows the OECD definition, in which the term "certification" is used to describe recognition by a professional or industry body. This is distinct from a certificate awarded by a post-secondary education institution upon completion of an academic credit-bearing study program (Kato et al. 2020).

Comparisons with Health Care and Information Professions

Where the stakes of individual performance or incompetence are high, society expects high accountability for the management and governance of certification. So, what can we learn from the way that related professions such as healthcare and information technology meet society's expectations of practitioners?

If the HIDDIN workforce aspired to be included among the health professions, the landscape of individuation certification would need to have sharp definition and tight boundaries. Serious attention is paid to the validity and the scope of health practitioner credentials in the interests of safety and quality in healthcare (for example ACSQHC 2015). Standards for registering or licensing individuals to practice are applied through an agency of government (for example, the Australian Health Practitioner Regulation Agency). Though there are many approaches to describing professional competence in those professions, the concept of entrustable professional activity has become a clear way to integrate the type and level of competence of the individual, with the work that needs to be done and the degree of oversight required to do that work legally (Ten Cate et al. 2015). Thus, although a registered doctor/nurse/physiotherapist might undertake some form of certification in nutritional therapy/ultrasound/acupuncture as continuing professional development, that certification alone would not suffice for the individual to practice legally as a registered professional dietitian/medical radiation practitioner/Chinese medicine practitioner.

The HIDDIN workforce has a clear affinity with the information professions, too, for example, De Almeida et al. (2019) found that many health information management professionals are employed in roles such as computer and information research scientists, database administrators, information security analysts, statisticians, and computer occupations. How might HIDDIN certification processes and standards be akin to those professions? Here a different model of trust applies, with a balance very different to the health professions of how individuals acquire competence through learning on, near, or off the job. The peak organisations in the information professions have reached a consensus on certification in major bodies of knowledge (BoK), that is, the prescribed knowledge and skill that an individual must acquire to be certified as a practitioner in a particular area: The Skills Framework for the Information Age (sfia-online.org) lists 40 BoKs that are the internationally accepted definitions of data science, development and operations (DevOps), digital transformation, information and cybersecurity, and software engineering, along with the organisations that curate certification in each field.

By comparison, HIDDIN work rests on a patchwork of curriculum and competency standards that vary greatly around the world, undergo almost no regulation or quality assurance, and are not locatable in a shared framework. Some work in this direction can be seen in a handful of papers over the past two decades: Moore and Berner (2003) compared health informatics graduate program curricula against two sets of professional criteria. Gibson et al. (2015) examined convergence between health informatics and health information management. In 2017, separate papers by Newbold (2017) and by McCormick et al. (2017) itemised certifications relevant to nursing informatics. Nevertheless, there is no universally agreed or observed body of knowledge, or process for demonstrating mastery, to give coherence to the level of competence that an individual has, to do HIDDIN work of defined scope and responsibility.

Certifications for the HIDDIN Workforce

This chapter outlines the terrain of professional and industry certifications for individuals in the HIDDIN workforce. To locate and describe these certifications, firstly search terms were formulated based on the concepts and sources referred to in previous sections of this chapter. Then, searching of the peer-reviewed literature and grey literature 2000–2020 was completed at the end of 2018 (retrieving, for example, McCormick et al. 2017; Zozus et al. 2017), followed by additional Google searching to the end of 2019 (retrieving, for example, Tittel and Kyle 2019). In the first half of 2020, personal communications with professional and industry colleagues helped to refine lists and add details. Excluded were certifications where no information or documentation was openly accessible online, in English, from the primary provider source; a few peer-reviewed sources refer to certifications of this kind (e.g. Gundlapalli et al. 2015; Cummins et al. 2016; Lytle 2017). Also excluded were continuing professional development programs that do not directly award professional or industry certification—examples are the US National Library of Medicine Biomedical Informatics training program (https://www.nlm.nih.gov/bsd/disted/nlm_bmi_training.html) and many massive open online courses (MOOCs) in the HIDDIN domain. Also excluded were certifications by commercial organisations that accredit individuals to work with their products; examples include 3M™ Health Information Systems Certifications (https://www.3m.com/3M/en_US/health-information-systems-us/resources/health-care-academy/certifications/); Intersystems' HealthShare Health Connect HL7 Interface Specialist (https://www.intersystems.com/support-learning/learning-services/certification/healthshare-health-connect-hl7-interface-specialist/); and different types of Epic certification (Sok 2019). Lastly, excluded were not-for-academic-credit certificates offered by institutions that are primarily providers of formal post-secondary education and training; it is noted that growing numbers of universities around the world are engaging in this kind of activity.

Over 50 certifications, offered by over 40 organisations, are summarised in Table 6.1, showing the primary information source, minimum descriptors of high-level knowledge and skill areas, and acronyms widely used to refer to these.

Table 6.1 Professional and industry certifications available to individuals in the HIDDIN workforce

Credential name Credentialing organisation Information source	Outline of knowledge and skills certified
Advanced Analytics for Health Care Strategists Society for Health Care Strategy & Market Development https://www.shsmd.org/education/dgital-badge-certificate-programs	• New and emerging data sets • Changing landscape of inpatient and ambulatory world • Rapid, market-specific strategic decision making • Data visualisation and storytelling
Advanced Health Informatics Certification AHIC; Certified Health Informatics Professional ACHIP American Medical Informatics Association AMIA https://www.amia.org/advanced-health-informatics-certification	• Foundational knowledge • Enhancing health decision-making, processes and outcomes Health information systems Data governance, management and analytics Leadership, professionalism, strategy and transformation

(continued)

Table 6.1 (continued)

Credential name Credentialing organisation Information source	Outline of knowledge and skills certified
Associate/Member/Fellow Faculty of Clinical Informatics https://facultyofclinicalinformatics.org.uk/ how-to-apply	• Experiential exposure to clinical informatics in the workplace • Contributions to advancement of clinical informatics • Leadership • Commitment/engagement
Associate/Fellow of the Australasian Institute of Digital Health AFAIDH/FAIDH (formerly Member/Fellow of the Australasian College of Health Informatics FACHI/MACHI) Australasian Institute of Digital Health AIDH https://digitalhealth.org.au/membership/become-a-fellow-of-the-institute/	• Educational qualifications • Paid and honorary positions • Community achievements • Research and development
Board-Certified Clinical Informatician BC American Board of Preventive Medicine ABPM and American Board of Pathology ABP on behalf of American Board of Medical Specialties ABMS https://www.theabpm.org/become-certified/subspecialties/clinical-informatics/; http://www.abpath.org/index.php/to-become-certified/requirements-for-certification?id=40	• License to practice medicine • Other board certification • Practice experience • References • Graduate degree in informatics
Board-Certified Informatics Nursing Registered Nurse RN-BC American Nurses Credentialing Center ANCC https://www.nursingworld.org/our-certifications/informatics-nurse/	• Foundations of practice—professional practice • Foundations of practice—models and theories • Foundations of practice—rules, regulations, and requirements • System design life cycle—planning and analysis • System design life cycle—designing and building • System design life cycle—implementing and testing • System design life cycle—evaluating, maintaining, and supporting • Data management and health care technology—data standards • Data management and health care technology—data management • Data management and health care technology—data transformation • Data management and health care technology—hardware, software, and peripherals

Table 6.1 (continued)

Credential name Credentialing organisation Information source	Outline of knowledge and skills certified
Certified Associate/Professional in Healthcare Information and Management Systems CAHIMS/CPHIMS Healthcare Information and Management Systems Society HIMSS http://www.himss.org/health-it-certification/cahims; https://www.himss.org/sites/hde/files/CPHIMS%20Handbook%202019.09%20Final.pdf	• General—healthcare environment • General—technology environment • Systems—analysis • Systems—design • Systems—selection, implementation, support, and maintenance • Systems—testing and evaluation • Systems—privacy and security • Administration—leadership • Administration—management
Certified Classification and Coding Specialist CCCS Canadian College of Health Information Management https://www.echima.ca/CCHIM/classification-coding-certification	• Fundamentals • General medicine • Neoplasms • Interventions • Obstetrics and newborns • Iatrogenic disorders, trauma, related conditions • Case scenarios
Certified Clinical Data Manager CCDM Society for Clinical Data Management https://scdm.org/get-certified/	• Project management ... CRF design • Processing lab data … Database updates • SAE reconciliation … Application of randomisation schemes
Certified Clinical Documentation Improvement Specialist CCDIS Canadian College of Health Information Management https://www.echima.ca/CCHIM/CDI	• Anatomy and physiology, clinical pathology, pharmacology, and medical terminology • Clinical coding skills • Documentation improvement • Leadership, communication, and education skills • CDI metrics and analytics
Certified Coding Associate CCA American Health Information Management Association AHIMA https://www.ahima.org/certification/CCA	• Clinical classification systems • Reimbursement methodologies • Health records and data content • Compliance • Information technologies • Confidentiality and privacy
Certified Coding Specialist/-Physician-based CCS/CCS-P American Health Information Management Association AHIMA https://www.ahima.org/certification/CCS; https://www.ahima.org/certification/ccsp	• Clinical documentation • Diagnosis coding • Procedure coding • Reporting requirements for provider-based services • Reporting requirements for inpatient services • Reporting requirements for outpatient services • Data quality management • Health information technology • Privacy, confidentiality, legal, and ethical issues • Compliance

(continued)

Table 6.1 (continued)

Credential name Credentialing organisation Information source	Outline of knowledge and skills certified
Certified Documentation Expert Outpatient CDEO American Association of Professional Coders AAPC https://www.aapc.com/certification/cdeo/	• Purpose of CDI • Provider communication and compliance • Clinical conditions • Diagnosis coding • Documentation requirements • Payment models • Procedure coding • Quality measures
Certified Documentation Improvement Practitioner CDIP American Health Information Management Association AHIMA https://www.ahima.org/certification/cdip	• Clinical coding practice • Leadership • Record review and document clarification • CDI metrics and statistics • Research and education • Compliance
Certified Health Data Analyst CHDA American Health Information Management Association AHIMA https://www.ahima.org/certification/chda	• Business needs assessment • Data acquisition and management • Data analysis • Data interpretation and reporting • Data governance
Certified Health Informatician Australasia CHIA Australasian Institute of Digital Health AIDH http://www.healthinformaticscertification.com/	• Information and communication technology • Health and biomedical science • Information science • Management science • Core principles and methods • Human and social context • Specialisations [to be developed]
Certified Health Informatics Systems Professional CHISP American Society of Health Informatics Managers ASHIM http://www.ashim.com/health-it-certification/	• Health IT • Health care regulations • Computer science • Medical insurance billing • Information and data security • Medical terminology and anatomy • Operational principles in healthcare • Data mining, reports, and queries • Technology in quality of care
Certified in Health Information Management CHIM Canadian College of Health Information Management CCHIM https://www.echima.ca/cchim/certification	• Biomedical sciences • Health care systems in Canada • Information systems and technology • Management • Ethics and practice • Practicum

Table 6.1 (continued)

Credential name Credentialing organisation Information source	Outline of knowledge and skills certified
Certified Health Information Manager/ Practitioner CHIM/CHIP Health Information Management Association of Australia HIMAA https://himaa.org.au/ professional-credentialing/	• Generic professional skills • Health information and records management • Language of medicine • Healthcare terminologies and classification • Research methods • Health services organisation and delivery • Health information law and ethics • eHealth • Health information services organisation and management • Other related qualifications and/or experience
Certified Healthcare Chief Information Officer CHCIO College of Healthcare Information Management Executives CHIME https://chimecentral.org/wp-content/ uploads/2020/01/CHCIO-Brochure-July-2020. pdf	• Organisational vision and strategy • Technology management • Change management • Value assessment and management • Service management • Talent management • Relationship management
Certified Healthcare Information Security Leader CHISL College of Healthcare Information Management Executives CHIME https://chimecentral.org/certification/chisl/	• Policies and solutions • Strategic planning • Situations and responses • Emerging issues, theory, and practice • Risk management • Coordination of operations • Ethical, regulatory, and legal issues • Collaborative business continuity/disaster recovery
Certified in Healthcare Privacy and Security CHPS American Health Information Management Association AHIMA https://www.ahima.org/certification/chps	• Ethical, legal, regulatory issues/environmental assessment • Program management and administration • Information technology/physical and technical safeguards • Investigation, compliance, and enforcement
Certified Healthcare Simulation Educator/ Advanced CHSE/CSHE-A Society for Simulation in Healthcare https://www.ssih.org/Portals/48/Certification/ CHSE_Docs/CHSE%20Handbook.pdf; https:// www.ssih.org/Portals/48/Certification/ CHSE-A_Docs/CHSE-A%20Handbook.pdf	• Professional values and capabilities • Health care and simulation knowledge and principles • Educational principles and activities • Simulation resources and environments • Scholarship and teaching
Certified Healthcare Simulation Operations Specialist CHSOS Society for Simulation in Healthcare https://www.ssih.org/Portals/48/Certification/ CHSOS_Docs/CHSOS%20Handbook.pdf	• Concepts in health care as applied to simulation • Simulation technology operations • Healthcare simulation practices/principles/procedures • Professional role: behaviour and capabilities • Concepts in instructional design as applied to simulation

(continued)

Table 6.1 (continued)

Credential name Credentialing organisation Information source	Outline of knowledge and skills certified
Certified Healthcare Technology Specialist CHTS & subspecialties: -TS, -PW, -IM, -CP, -IS, -TR American Health Information Management Association AHIMA http://www.ahima.org/~/media/AHIMA/Files/Certification/CHTS%20Candidate%20Guide.ashx	[discontinued]
Certified Imaging Informatics Professional CIIP American Board of Imaging Informatics https://www.abii.org/Certification-Overview.aspx	• Procurement • Project management • Operations • Communications • Training and education • Image management • Information technology • Systems management • Clinical engineering • Medical imaging informatics
Certified Inpatient Coder CIC American Academy of Professional Coders AAPC https://www.aapc.com/certification/cic/	• Medical record and healthcare documentation guidelines • Medical terminology, anatomy, and pathophysiology • Inpatient coding • Inpatient payment methodologies • Outpatient payment methodology • Regulatory and payer requirements • Compliance • Coding cases
Certified Outpatient Coder COC Formerly CPC-H American Academy of Professional Coders AAPC https://www.aapc.com/certification/coc/	• Medical terminology • Anatomy • Coding guidelines • Payment methodologies • Compliance • ICD-10-CM • CPT® • HCPCS level II coding • Surgery and modifiers
Certified Physician in BioMedical Informatics CPBMI Korean Society of Medical Informatics KOSMI http://www.cpbmi.or.kr/	[Details unavailable in English]

Table 6.1 (continued)

Credential name Credentialing organisation Information source	Outline of knowledge and skills certified
Certified Professional Coder (CPC) American Academy of Professional Coders AAPC https://www.aapc.com/certification/cpc/	• Surgical procedures performed on the integumentary system • Surgical procedures performed on the musculoskeletal system • Surgical procedures performed on the respiratory system, cardiovascular system, hemic and lymphatic systems, and mediastinum and diaphragm • Surgical procedures performed on the digestive system • Surgical procedures performed on the urinary system, male reproductive system, female reproductive system, and endocrine system • Surgical procedures performed on the nervous system • Evaluation and management • Place of services • Anesthesia • Radiology • Laboratory/pathology • Medicine • Medical terminology • Anatomy • ICD-10-CM/diagnosis • HCPCS Level II • Coding guidelines • Compliance and regulatory
Certified Professional in Electronic Health Records CPEHR Health IT Certification LLC http://www.healthitcertification.com/overview.html	[transferred to HIMSS]
Certified Professional in Health Informatics CPHI American Health Information Management Association AHIMA https://www.ahima.org/education/health-informatics	[discontinued]
Certified Professional Health Specialisation AALIA (CP) Health Librarian or AALIA (CP) Health or ALIATec (CP) Health or ALIA Allied Field (CP) Health Australian Library and Information Association Health Libraries Australia Group ALIA HLA https://membership.alia.org.au/pdinfo/specialisations/health-specialisation	• Health environment • Reference and research services • Resources • Leadership and management • Digital, ehealth, and technology • Health literacy and teaching • Health research • Professionalism

(continued)

Table 6.1 (continued)

Credential name Credentialing organisation Information source	Outline of knowledge and skills certified
Certified Professional in Information Exchange CPHIE Health IT Certification LLC http://www.healthitcertification.com/overview.html	[transferred to HIMSS]
Certified Professional in Healthcare Information and Management Systems–Canada CPHIMS-CA Digital Health Canada https://digitalhealthcanada.com/wp-content/uploads/2019/12/Digital-Health-Canada-Competency-Requirements-Exam-Version-1.pdf	• Information management • Technology ecosystem • Clinical and health services • Canadian health system • Healthcare transformation • Project management
Certified Professional in Healthcare Quality CPHQ National Association for Healthcare Quality—Certification Commission https://nahq.org/wp-content/uploads/attachments/CPHQ_Content_outline_-_effective_01-2018.pdf	• Organisational leadership—structure and integration • Organisational leadership—regulatory, accreditation, and external recognition • Organisational leadership—education, training, and communication • Health data analytics—design and data management • Health data analytics—measurement and analysis • Performance and process improvement—identifying opportunities for improvement • Performance and process improvement—implementation and evaluation • Patient safety—assessment and planning • Patient safety—implementation and evaluation
Certified Professional Medical Auditor CPMA American Association of Professional Coders AAPC https://www.aapc.com/certification/cpma.aspx	• Medical record standards and documentation guidelines • Coding and documentation compliance guidelines • Coding and reimbursement concepts • Scope and statistical sampling methodologies • Medical record auditing abstraction • Category risk analysis and communication
Certified Professional in Operating Rules Administration CPORA Health IT Certification LLC http://www.healthitcertification.com/overview.html	[transferred to HIMSS]

Table 6.1 (continued)

Credential name Credentialing organisation Information source	Outline of knowledge and skills certified
Certified Risk Adjustment Coder CRC American Association of Professional Coders AAPC https://www.aapc.com/certification/crc/	• Compliance • Diagnosis coding • Documentation improvement • Pathophysiology/medical terminology/anatomy • Purpose and use of risk adjustment models • Quality care • Risk adjustment models
Certified Specialist Health Interpreter CSHI National Accreditation Authority for Translators and Interpreters https://www.naati.com.au/become-certified/certification/certified-specialist-health-interpreter/	• Medical terminology • General medical knowledge • Knowledge of health systems • Ethics, culture, and the role of the interpreter • Advanced interactional management • Research and preparation
Certified Terminology Standards Specialist CTSS Canadian Health Information Management Association CHIMA https://www.echima.ca/college/certification/ctss/; https://www.uvic.ca/hsd/hinf/graduate/certificate/HTS-certificate-overview-nov12-2019.pdf	• Health information standards • Controlled terminology standards • Health information exchange standards • Field project in health informatics
Digital Marketing Strategy in Healthcare Society for Health Care Strategy & Market Development SHSMD https://www.shsmd.org/education/digital-badge-certificate-programs	• Building the foundation of a successful contemporary digital marketing program in health care • Telling your story to drive results • Activating your message across the tradigital landscape • Preparing for what is coming next
Fellow of the American Medical Informatics Association FAMIA American Medical Informatics Association AMIA https://www.amia.org/famia	• Education • Certification • Applied informatics experience • Peer recommendation • AMIA membership • AMIA engagement • Future commitments
Fellow of the Health Information Management Association of Australia FHIMAA Health Information Management Association of Australia HIMAA https://himaa.org.au/wp-content/uploads/2019/10/MEMB_HIMAA-MembershipApplicationForm_FellowMember_7March2016.pdf	• Qualifications • CV and references • Service to the organisation • Contribution to the profession • Presentations made/articles published • Level of knowledge and expertise

(continued)

Table 6.1 (continued)

Credential name Credentialing organisation Information source	Outline of knowledge and skills certified
Fellow of the International Academy of Health Sciences Informatics FIAHSI International Medical Informatics Association IMIA https://imia-medinfo.org/wp/iahsi-nomination-process-for-new-fellows/	• Accomplishment • Recognition • Global engagement • CV • Publications
Foundation Certified Healthcare Executive CFCHE College of Healthcare Information Management Executives CHIME https://chimecentral.org/wp-content/uploads/2017/04/CFCHE-Exam-Blueprint.pdf	• Health care vision and strategy • Technical proficiency • Change management • Value commitment • Hospital and healthcare expertise • Relationship building and collaboration
HL7 Clinical Document Architecture Specialist CDA Health Level 7 HL7 http://www.hl7.org/documentcenter/public/training/HL7%20CDA%20Certification%20Study%20Guide.pdf	• CDA overview • CDA document and CDA header • Body choice, section- attributes, participants, relationships, and narrative block entry acts • Entry relationships • Other topics—technical artifacts, document exchange, CDA context
HL7 Fast Healthcare Interoperability Resources FHIR R4 Proficiency Certificate Health Level 7 HL7 http://www.hl7.org/documentcenter/public/training/HL7%20FHIR%20Proficiency%20Study%20Guide.pdf	• FHIR fundamentals • Resource concepts • Exchange mechanisms (includes RESTful API) • Conformance and implementation guidance • Terminology • Representing health care concepts using FHIR resources • Safety and security • FHIR maintenance process • FHIR licensing and IP
HL7 Version 2 Control Specialist V2 Health Level 7 HL7 http://www.hl7.org/documentcenter/public/training/2.8%20Cert%20exam%20study%20tip%20sheet_%20PDF%20Final.pdf	• Conceptual approach of HL7 • HL7 message elements, separators, and lengths 3. • Construction and processing of HL7 messages • Special HL7 protocols 5. • Acknowledgment messages • Message control segments • HL7 data types and their uses • Conformance using message profiles • Other issues
HL7 Version 3 Reference Information Model Specialist V3RIM Health Level 7 HL7 http://www.hl7.org/documentcenter/public/training/RIM%20Version%203%20Study%20Guide.pdf	• Introduction and overview • Foundation subject area diagram • Other subject area diagrams and state transition diagrams • Act, act-relationship, and participation core classes • Entity, role, and role-link core classes • Specialisations of core classes • Data types • Normative structural vocabulary

Table 6.1 (continued)

Credential name Credentialing organisation Information source	Outline of knowledge and skills certified
HealthCare Information Security and Privacy Practitioner HCISPP Information Security Consortium (ISC)[2] https://www.isc2.org/hcispp/default.aspx	• Health care industry • Information governance in healthcare • Information technologies in healthcare • Regulatory and standards environment • Privacy and security in healthcare • Risk management and risk assessment • Third-party risk management
Healthcare IT Technician Computing Technology Industry Association CompTIA https://www.comptia.org/blog/why-comptia-healthcare-it-technician-	[discontinued]
Member/Senior Member/Distinguished Member Academy of Health Information Professionals AHIP https://www.mlanet.org/page/first-time-applicant-member,-senior,-distinguished	• Postgraduate degree that meets competency standards • Full-time professional work experience • Professional accomplishments, continuing education • Professional association participation
Practitioner/Senior Practitioner/Advanced Practitioner/Leading Practitioner Federation for Informatics Professionals in Health and Social Care FEDIP https://uploads-ssl.webflow.com/5af421f1debb da36454953c8/5c5c442fb7e4f65e4e0e2775_fedip-standard.pdf	• Professional competence [9 standards × 4 levels] • Context—patient care and wellbeing • Context—roles within health and care • Context—health and care terminology • Context—health informatics roles and interactions
Registered Health Information Administrator/Technician RHIA/RHIT American Health Information Management Association AHIMA http://www.ahima.org/~/media/AHIMA/Files/Certification/Revised%20Candidate%20Guide%20November%202019.ashx	• Data content, structure, and information governance • Access, disclosure, privacy, and security • Data analytics and use • Revenue cycle management • Compliance • Leadership
Senior Member/Fellow Healthcare Information and Management Systems Society HIMSS https://www.himss.org/membership-participation/member-advancement	• Professional capability • Experience • Leadership • Service • Qualifications • Job description • References

Discussion

The range of professional and industry bodies that provide certification services, and the variety of HIDDIN knowledge and skills that can be certified, attest to a complex specialised workforce, but also a workforce where scopes of practice and levels of expertise are not at all distinct. Points that differentiate these certifications for prospective applicants include: whether eligibility to apply hinges on a prior university degree or prior period of work experience, and how strict that require-ment is; whether there is a written examination, and whether invigilated; whether a more advanced level of certification requires a portfolio of practical work and refer-ees. Key points of difference among providers include: the fee charged for certifica-tion; the duration of certification and the recertification process; whether multiple nested or linked certifications are offered; whether the certifications are jurisdiction-specific or have international recognition. In terms of certification quality and value, most providers cannot readily be seen to address ISO standards for certification of individuals; for example, publicly available descriptions of the body of knowledge often lack details of scope and depth, are undated, and do not explain development processes or identify contributors. It is rare to find scholarly or industry reports with detailed analyses or evaluations of certification programs (such as Gadd et al. 2016).

Some gaps in what is certified are evident here and can be compared with those noted elsewhere. The need for the HIDDIN workforce to be competent to work with genomic data to advance precision healthcare (noted in McCormick et al. 2017) is not yet well addressed. A focus on ethics can be found at the top level in several certifica-tions in the inventory here, contrary to views that certification of HIDDIN work lacks this (such as Kluge et al. 2018). Artificial intelligence is a newly identified area of spe-cialised skill where planning is in early stages, "to credential healthcare professionals and anyone else who seeks a greater understanding of the growing role and use of arti-ficial intelligence, machine learning and deep learning in health care" (ABAIM 2020).

Some inclusions in Table 6.1 are more marginal than others. Including certifica-tions that are emergent (e.g. Advanced Health Informatics Certification) and defunct (e.g. those merged into HIMSS after 2017) makes the point that HIDDIN certifica-tions come and go. Translator and quality manager certifications were deemed to have enough overlap with HIDDIN work to be included, illustrating the potential for scope creep in HIDDIN work. Indistinct language about digital badges as certi-fications was allowed in the case of a marketing certification, to note current interest in digital badging. A certification service run jointly by a professional society (CHIMA) and a university was included, to show a new form of convergence in the certification provider community. Some certifications and providers may have been missed due to a lack of international consensus and coherence in what is offered. There is scope for much further depth in the comparative analysis of certifications, synthesis of their underlying knowledge base, and visualisation of the entire terrain in a way that makes it more accessible to "outsiders". There is also a great need for independent research into certification holders' experiences, employers' evaluation of certified HIDDIN workers, and the efficiency and effectiveness of the varied assessment systems and processes used to certify and recertify individuals.

Conclusions

Analysis of professional and industry credentials provides real-world insights into the body of knowledge and standards of practice of the HIDDIN workforce. The HIDDIN certification landscape is constantly shifting, for two main reasons:

Certification programs are a business activity, where organisations compete to persuade employers and prospective employees to prefer their product or brand. Also, while much HIDDIN work is done within a regional or national healthcare system and its policy and infrastructure, an emerging consequence of digital transformation is a global health services sector that needs a workforce with trans-border expertise.

The certifications listed in this chapter go some way towards answering the questions: What sort of expertise do we need? What guarantees are there that an individual has this expertise? These are fundamental questions for assuring the safety and quality of HIDDIN work that underpins the healthcare sector broadly. However, a more detailed mapping of the certification terrain, and more rationalisation of its features, would help to position the HIDDIN workforce to be seen to have the trustable approaches to self-regulation and self-knowledge that we observe in healthcare and information professions. Rationalisation poses political challenges to the industry and professional associations that presently hold pieces of the puzzle of credentialing health information professionals—accreditation, certification, curriculum standards, competency systems. Undoubtedly improvements on the current situation would be appreciated by health workforce policymakers and employers; HIDDIN workforce education and training providers; and not least, current and prospective practitioners.

References

ABAIM American Board of Artificial Intelligence in Medicine. Press release. 2020. https://www.aithority.com/machine-learning/abaim-aims-to-educate-and-certify-healthcare-professionals-in-ai-and-related-technologies/. Accessed 31 Mar 2021.

ACSQHC Australian Commission on Safety and Quality in Health Care. Credentialing health practitioners and defining their scope of clinical practice: a guide for managers and practitioners. ACSQHC: Sydney; 2015.

Cummins MR, Gundlapalli AV, Murray P, Park HA, Lehmann CU. Nursing informatics certification worldwide: history, pathway, roles, and motivation. IMIA Yearbook. 2016:264–71.

Davis S. Seeking an advanced professional designation. Chapter 20. In: Handbook of continuing professional development for the health IT professional. Boca Raton: CRC Press; 2017.

DeAlmeida DR, Houser SH, Wangia-Anderson V, Fenton SH, Hazelwood A, Barefield AC, Freeman JM, Jones LM, Bakuzonis K, Hamada DL. An exploratory study demonstrating the health information management profession as a STEM discipline. Perspect Health Inf Manag. 2019;16(Summer).

Eckmann J. Earning a certificate to demonstrate competency. Chapter 8. In: Handbook of continuing professional development for the health IT professional. Boca Raton: CRC Press; 2017.

Ellis LE, Nunn SG, Avella JT. Digital badges and micro-credentials: historical overview, motivational aspects, issues, and challenges. In: Foundation of digital badges and micro-credentials. London: Springer; 2016. p. 3–21.

Gadd CS, Williamson JJ, Steen EB, Fridsma DB. Creating advanced health informatics certification. J Am Medical Inform Assoc. 2016;23(4):848–50.

Gibson CJ, Dixon BE, Abrams K. Convergent evolution of health information management and health informatics: a perspective on the future of information professionals in health care. Appl Clin Inform. 2015;6(1):163.

Gray K, Gilbert C, Butler-Henderson K, Day K, Pritchard S. Ghosts in the machine: identifying the digital health information workforce. In: Improving usability, safety and patient outcomes with health information technology. Stud Health Technol Inform. 2019;257:146–51.

Gundlapalli AV, Greaves WW, Kesler D, Murray P, Safran C, Lehmann CU. Clinical informatics board specialty certification for physicians: a global view. In: eHealth-enabled health: Proceedings of the 15th World Congress on Health and Biomedical Informatics. Stud Health Technol Inform. 2015;216:501–5.

ISO International Standards Organisation ISO/IEC 17024:2012. Conformity assessment — General requirements for bodies operating certification of persons. 2012. https://www.iso.org/obp/ui/#iso:std:iso-iec:17024:ed-2:v1:en. Accessed 31 Mar 2021.

Kato S, Galan-Muros V, Weko T. The emergence of alternative credentials. OECD Directorate for Education and Skills. Working Paper 216. 2020. https://www.oecd.org/officialdocuments/publicdisplaydocumentpdf/?cote=EDU/WKP(2020)4&docLanguage=En. Accessed 31 Mar 2021.

Kluge EH, Lacroix P, Ruotsalainen P. Ethics certification of health information professionals. Yearbook Medical Inform. 2018;27(1):37–40.

Lytle KS. Differentiating yourself with a professional certification. Chapter 9. In: Handbook of continuing professional development for the health IT professional. Boca Raton: CRC Press; 2017.

McCormick KA, Gugerty B, Sensmeier J. Comparison of professional informatics-related competencies and certifications. On-Line J Nurs Inform. 2017;21(1).

Moore RA, Berner ES. Comparing health/medical informatics graduate program curricula against two sets of professional criteria. J Healthc Inf Manag JHIM. 2003;18(3):44–50.

NCVER National Centre for Vocational Education Research VOCEDplus. Focus on micro-credentials. 2018. https://www.voced.edu.au/focus-micro-credentials. Accessed 31 Mar 2021.

Newbold SK. What practicing nurses need to know about health information technology in order to practice today: continuing education and certification. In: Forecasting informatics competencies for nurses in the future of connected health. Amsterdam: IOS Press; 2017. p. 229.

Sok S. Different types of Epic modules and highest demand certifications. GlobalHealthIT. 2019. https://www.globalhit.com/different-types-of-epic-modules-and-highest-demand-certifications/. Accessed 31 Mar 2021.

Ten Cate O, Chen HC, Hoff RG, Peters H, Bok H, van der Schaaf M. Curriculum development for the workplace using entrustable professional activities (EPAs): AMEE guide no. 99. Medical Teacher. 2015;37(11):983–1002.

Tittel E, Kyle M. 5 Best healthcare IT certifications 2019. Business News Daily. 2019. https://www.businessnewsdaily.com/10788-healthcare-it-certifications.html. Accessed 31 Mar 2021.

Zozus MN, Lazarov A, Smith LR, Breen TE, Krikorian SL, Zbyszewski PS, Knoll SK, Jendrasek DA, Perrin DC, Zambas DN, Williams TB, Pieper CF. Analysis of professional competencies for the clinical research data management profession: implications for training and professional certification. J Am Medical Inform Assoc JAMIA. 2017;24(4):737–45.

Chapter 7
Professional Learning and Development for the Health Information Workforce

Joseph Crawford and Kerryn Butler-Henderson

Abstract The Health Informatics, Digital, Data, Information, and kNowledge (HIDDIN) workforce is faced with remaining current and relevant in a landscape experiencing rapid change. This chapter provides a holistic learner, employer, and educator perspective to understand the principles of effective professional learning and development. Concepts of evidence-based practice, constructive alignment, and pedagogy are applied to develop a framework for a principles-based assessment of learning environments and activities. Such a framework is needed by learners, to evaluate available professional learning opportunities more critically. Likewise, employers need to evaluate currency and relevance of learning outcomes prior to investing time and resources into professional development programmes. Lastly, providers of professional development can benefit from self-review against a shared set of quality criteria.

Keywords Professional development · Professional learning · Constructive alignment · Professionalism · Educational quality

J. Crawford (✉)
Academic Division, University of Tasmania, Launceston, TAS, Australia
e-mail: Joseph.Crawford@utas.edu.au

K. Butler-Henderson
Digital Health Hub, College of STEM, RMIT University, Bundoora, VIC, Australia
e-mail: Kerryn.Butler-Henderson@rmit.edu.au

© The Author(s), under exclusive license to Springer Nature
Switzerland AG 2021
K. Butler-Henderson et al. (eds.), *The Health Information Workforce*,
Health Informatics, https://doi.org/10.1007/978-3-030-81850-0_7

Introduction

What does it mean, for someone in the Health Informatics, Digital, Data, Information, and kNowledge (HIDDIN) workforce, to stay relevant and remain current in an ever-changing landscape? The way individuals flourish within their personal and professional environments has changed radically in response to many macro-level changes—Web 2.0, the Global Financial Crisis, the dotcom bust, and recently the COVID-19 pandemic (e.g. Crawford et al. 2020). Machine learning and artificial intelligence use was a key factor in responding to COVID-19 (Lalmuanawama et al. 2020). However, as health services everywhere confronted the need for rapid digitisation of information to meet new scientific decision-making, analysis and reporting demands, the pandemic highlighted workforce shortages and gaps that hampered technological transformation and analytics capability (Fernandes et al. 2020). Sudden shifts, such as the pandemic shock, are coupled with the continual and ongoing innovation facing every sector that seeks to be competitive and to improve on current practices.

The impetus of constant social and economic change provides the foundation for myriad professional learning and development opportunities, provided by professional associations, educational institutions, commercial conference and workshop organisers, and digital and print media publishers. However, their professional development offerings may be based more on business than on science; in general, a lack of valid and reliable evidence-based practices plagues the existing professional development scene. Professional competency, skill, and behavioural development often take place in diverse on-the-job and in-service locations without clear evidence for program development (Ramsaroop and Petersen 2020). For example, estimated global spending on training and development exceeded USD370 billion in 2019 (Atd Research 2019), and training and development was found to represent 42.1 work hours per employee in a 2019 industry survey (TrainingMag 2019). Despite the generally growing appetite for professional development, the efficacy of programmes has been challenged by practitioners (Jayaram et al. 2012; Loew and Wentworth 2013; O'Leonard and Loew 2012), academics (Avolio and Hannah 2008; Sung and Choi 2014), and commentators (Glaveski 2019; Pontefract 2019; Vedantam 2008). Many professional development offerings may not result in skill development or behavioural change; however, professional learning is a different story, as we explain shortly, and there are many examples of positive and effective professional learning programmes.

The pandemic aside, the health sector has seen rapid adoption of technology to support more consumer-centred care and service delivery, and to enable better evidence-informed service management and planning. The growth across areas such as artificial intelligence (AI), automation, the Internet of Things (IoT), and analytics is increasing demand for appropriately skilled specialists across the HIDDIN disciplines (Butler-Henderson 2020). Still, the health sector remains highly regulated with regards to biomedical and biopsychosocial scientific knowledge. Therefore, HIDDIN work has to be underpinned by evidence-based practices, professionalism, constructive alignment, and practice-based pedagogy. Many of these elements are commonplace in extensively developed programs (e.g. university qualifications), and have mixed uptake in shorter-form offerings (e.g. conferences, one-day professional workshops) (Percy et al. 2021). Each of these elements is an important link in what it means to remain current from the individual's perspective and the employer's perspective. This chapter unpacks professional learning and development within the HIDDIN workforce, and provides a framework to assess the current professional development environment for this workforce.

What are the ongoing professional development needs for this workforce? Skill development, reading, networking, formal and informal education, gaining visibility, being social, and applying for awards are commonly listed strategies for delivering and supporting professional development (Rees et al. 2018). For practitioners, it is rarely about accessing a discrete professional development opportunity but, rather more often, finding effective professional learning that is efficient for their personal learning goals among the international sea of registered training organisations, private education institutes, peak bodies, and various self-help and professional development offerings. This is often challenged by insufficient digital and ehealth literacy among healthcare professionals (Mather and Cummings 2017), reducing the types of offerings accessible to the workers and learners.

Keeping professionals' skills current and relevant is most pertinent in environments where change is mediated by regular technological innovations (Lorenzi and Riley 2013); healthcare is a key example of the need for continuous professional learning (Manley et al. 2018). This is especially so because entry-to-practice clinical and public health degree programmes do not yet routinely prepare future clinicians to work within a digital health setting; this may be due to lagging degree accreditation standards, or due to a mismatch between theoretical knowledge domains in higher education and practical skills requirements of the healthcare environment (Gray et al. 2014). The same situation also applies to some of the entry-to-practice degrees that exist for the HIDDIN workforce. Thus, to remain current and relevant in a sector being reshaped by external pressures and internal innovations, the HIDDIN workforce requires high-quality opportunities to grow and develop capacity to manage and govern health data, information, and knowledge.

Professional Development and Professional Learning

The evolution of this topic from professional development to professional learning requires explanation and subsequent application to the HIDDIN workforce. Professional development speaks to a defined cycle of individual improvement from identification of needs to learning, application, and reflection on learning (Stewart 2014). In comparison, professional learning speaks to broader concepts including content focus, active learning, coherence, duration, and collective participation (Desimone 2009). The aspirational shift is toward communities of practice to support learning, away from single time-point professional development opportunities (e.g. a one-off conference, or one-off workshop). These broader approaches to professional learning focus on informal learning, personal agency, influencers of learning, and structural influences on learning (Eraut 2012). The individual who engages in professional learning within a professional context likely begins by identifying as an employee, contractor, or consultant with a clear role description, but loosens their identity to participate as a 'learner'; so throughout this chapter, we refer to the person engaging in professional learning or development as a learner.

Many HIDDIN specialists hold a tertiary qualification, which has required them to cultivate generic graduate knowledge, skills, and behaviours, such as critical thinking, responsible collaboration, and formal communication. However, many of these people hold a clinical, business, or information technology or science qualification but have not undertaken training in a specific HIDDIN discipline (Butler-Henderson and Gray 2018). Many report acquiring these skills through on-the-job training; but this can create a mindset that separates the functions of doing from the patterns of knowing (Stange 2010). So, a HIDDIN specialist may understand what to do, without comprehending why this is known to be the way to do it. On-the-job training also tends to create an organisational culture of professional tribalism that can support repeating of existing practice (Ebert et al. 2014), rather than creating a license for individuals to innovate and improve practices to improve healthcare outcomes.

Human resources management (HRM) experts once considered that on-the-job training, with emphasis on single intervention just-in-time skill upgrades, was appropriate for low skill tasks—where the risk to completion of a task without in-depth training is low—and to extend competence in previously developed skill areas (e.g. Acemoglu and Pischke 2003). However, there is some evidence that on-the-job training is ineffective even for these purposes (van der Klink and Streumer 2002), and that employees who have undergone on-the-job training can perpetuate mediocre practices or incorrect norms to their work team. So training and development theory have evolved significantly. The so-called soft HRM seeks to empower employees to continually learn and develop through tailored learning needs analyses of the individual and the organisation. Fulfilling the needs of the individual employee is an important outcome for the organisation (Marescaux et al. 2013). Soft HRM for the HIDDIN workforce, or the cultivation of a high-quality workforce through health sector work environments that are enriched for learning, is not well described.

Evidence-Based Strategies for Professional Learning

The HIDDIN workforce has complex needs for specialised learning, development, and training (Sapci and Sapci 2020). The US Commission on Accreditation for Health Informatics and Information Management Education provides one comprehensive account of foundational knowledge and practice domains of the HIDDIN workforce, including: health information science and technology, human factors and sociotechnical systems, social and behavioural aspects of health, social behavioural and information science and technology applied to health, professionalism, interprofessional collaborative practice, and leadership (Valenta et al. 2018). These domains lend themselves to unique and varied opportunities for professional learning; despite this, there is often a gap between the specific situated needs of the learner, and the types of professional learning that are available.

An integrated framework for evaluating professional learning opportunities will empower individuals in the HIDDIN workforce to transfer knowledge about learning strategies among their immediate co-workers (e.g. informal on-the-job training), and to also expand the knowledge of their wider networks about best practice learning approaches and empirically evaluated learning opportunities. Remaining current with reference to peer-reviewed literature about adult learning strategies (referred to as 'evidence-based learning') will complement and enhance learning on-the-job.

Evidence-based learning is concerned with the relationship between evidence of learning and evidence of its application within practice settings, from the perspective of the learning sciences (Van der Hoof and Doyle 2018). This is quite distinct from professional learning about evidence-based practice, which is concerned with assuring that one learns about best practice in their profession, and is also a highly desirable feature of learning! Some examples of evidence-based professional learning strategies in health are outlined in Table 7.1, recognising the potential transferability of these practices within the HIDDIN learner context.

There is a range of evidence regarding the efficacy of each learning strategy; for example, growth in post-workshop learners' literature use and greater utilisation of evidence-based medicine in supporting inpatient clinical documentation was measured after one hands-on workshop (Sastre et al. 2011). The results of one-off events (e.g. one-day workshops, single classes) are questioned in the literature though (e.g. Mathisen and Bronnick 2009; Taliaferro and Harris 2014); there may be a decaying effect of training outcomes where training is not reinforced, although this is contested (Ashenfelter 1978; Bloom 1984; Gaudine and Saks 2004). The greatest challenge to overcome is the oversupply of single time-point events as an overarching

Table 7.1 Evidence-based strategies for professional learning in health

Professional learning strategies and definitions	References
Case study analysis The presentation of dilemmas to respond to independently or collectively.	Anderson (2004).
Critically appraised topic A focused review of a single article to answer a specific clinical question, with potential for practical clinical reflection.	Capampangan et al. (2010); Ishmach (2004); Sadigh et al. (2012); Shine (2008).
Educational prescription Provision of clinical activities, lectures, and small group discussions for the practitioner to determine the clinical bottom-line.	Ishmach (2004); Straus et al. (2018).
Hands-on workshops A practitioner-led workshop to support literature searching skills.	Sastre et al. (2011).
Journal club Regular meetings among clinicians to share and discuss published journals within their discipline.	Ahmadi et al. (2012); Cramer and Mahoney (2001); Milbrandt and Vincent (2004).
Literature searching Constructing an answerable question and using literature searches to answer it.	Ilic et al. (2012).
Social media sharing Social media reviews of publications post-production, to support ease of information filtering for practitioners.	Topf and Hiremath (2015).

strategy for professional learning. Such professional learning activities likely stem from good intentions, but do not tend to create sustainable long-term growth in the individual. A competing challenge is to systematically measure and interpret the efficacy of other types of learning strategies (Crawford and Kelder 2019)—for example, determining when to evaluate learner and organisational outcomes, regardless of whether pre-post quantitative testing, managerial evaluations, self-reflections, or participant interviews are the tool used for this. Truly effective training programmes may produce short-term declines in quantitative scoring as individuals reflect critically on their skills or, conversely, scores that are inflated as a result of the sense of community and excitement generated by a learning intervention.

Evidence-based learning strategies for the HIDDIN workforce need to be accompanied by convincing evaluation of learning, and an ongoing suite of development opportunities that continually reinforce and build upon initial skills development. This may mean initially intensive programmes with smaller booster activities scaffolded across an annual training and development programme. Opportunities to critically reflect and share findings within a practical context are essential throughout such a cycle. Soft HRM reminds us that it remains important to assure that specific learning activities meet the needs both of the individual learner and of the organisation or organisations where they work (Gaudine and Saks 2004; Hadley et al. 2007).

Current Professional Development Practices

While the need for professional development for digital health capabilities has been reported regularly in recent years in the clinical literature, there is a large gap in the literature with regard to HIDDIN specialist professional development needs. An examination of the literature since 2010 indicates some level of discussion in those disciplines where there are clearer qualification pathways, such as health librarianship and health information management, but less so in all the other HIDDIN discipline areas. This is a critical shortcoming that needs to be addressed as part of a conversation about strengthening professionalisation in this workforce. The literature over the past 10 years largely states the need for continuous professional development in these disciplines, and is not especially current (Abrams and Crook 2011; Blue 2011; Dimitropoulos et al. 2019; Ritchie et al. 2010). Where specific activities are referenced, they are conferences (Jenkins 2015), books (Shepheard 2011), and formal tertiary training (Ritchie et al. 2010). The literature is bereft of empirical evidence about the impact of professional development on this workforce. Interviews with people working in subdisciplines in the HIDDIN workforce identified a lack of incentives and time to incorporate professional learning into their roles, and little support from employers and clients, or recognition from them of the benefits of a workforce that participates in regular professional learning activities (Dimitropoulos et al. 2019).

A 2018 Australian HIDDIN workforce census (Butler-Henderson and Gray 2018) identified that 53.8% (859/1597) of respondents undertook work-based learning (for example, workplace courses, workshops, seminars, journal clubs) during the previous 12 months, 34.3% (548/1597) undertook self-directed learning (reading information online, industry news, podcasts/vodcasts, or blogs), 31.4% (502/1597) participated in a professional activity (for example, events and journal clubs held by peak bodies, reading and contributing to professional journals), and 12.9% (206/1597) participated in formal education and training programmes (short courses, micro-credentials, or tertiary programmes). The majority of professional development activities undertaken by HIDDIN specialists are not aligned clearly with a competency framework, are unregulated and not accredited, and often are not aligned with a formal credentialing programme. As such, professional development for this workforce may be of a lower standard than required, does not always meet industry needs, and may not meet the professional development needs of the individuals. For example, 2020 saw marketing to this workforce of an explosion in short courses about telehealth in response to the COVID-19-driven transition to online services, but with little evidence available on what the professional development needs were or how the offering addressed any quality standards.

When considering engaging with professional learning, it is critical to first understand the need it seeks to fulfil (Marescaux et al. 2013), and subsequently the degree to which the professional learning is likely to achieve that need. For example, one health information systems manager may need technical professional learning to support upskilling in a particular software being added to the hospital they are situated in. Another may require socio-technical development opportunities to enable their ability to influence laggards to engage and support new electronic health records systems usage. During the COVID-19 pandemic, this has been clearly evident with some medical practitioners requiring careful (but quick) onboarding and nudging to enable a move to telehealth and the associated record keeping required. Engaging in critical reflection and evaluation prior to entering the diverse range of learning environments and experiences can support a greater and more relevant skill set developed within the HIDDIN workforce.

Evaluating Before Choosing Professional Learning Options

As an adult learner, it is common to be presented with a series of opportunities to engage in professional development or professional learning. To ascertain the most appropriate opportunities for the individual, it is useful to consider whether an education option aligns with the specific learner context. That is, will the offering support an individual learner's ability to achieve and continuously improve? Table 7.2 presents a series of principles, along with brief questions that a learner can use to assess whether the professional learning activity will be useful for them to pursue.

Table 7.2 speaks to the ongoing balancing act, between the needs of the workforce and the emerging best practice approaches to learning. These are not always perfectly weighted; however, careful consideration to a diverse range of stakeholders will maximise the likelihood that: the learner achieves the personal and professional goals that align to their needs; the educator assures the learner's achievement;

Table 7.2 Principles for evaluating options for future professional learning

Principle definition	Example questions
Evidence-based The relationship between the learning and its basis in evidence, to foster future evidence use in learners.	• Does the learning support future evidence-based practices? • Is the learning based on valid and reliable evidence? • Are the outcomes of the learning measured valid and reliable?
Strategic alignment The alignment between the individual, organisation, sector, and the learnings.	• Has a training needs analysis been conducted prior to learning? • Is there demonstrated connection between the learning and the needs of the individual, organisation, and sector? • Are there opportunities to apply theoretical content to the practical context?
Constructive alignment The demonstrated relationship between intended learning outcomes, assessment, and learning activities.	• Are there clear and transparent intended learning outcomes? • Is there a demonstrated link between learning outcomes and assessment? • Do the learning activities support student success in the assessments, and attainment of the learning outcomes?
Pedagogy The method(s) of teaching	• Is there a clear relationship with the type of pedagogy applied and the context? • Are pedagogies explicitly applied to the learning environment? • Has the educator clearly considered the most appropriate pedagogy?

and the workforce collectively highlights continuous improvement as a result. For example, tertiary education should emphasise constructive alignment and sound pedagogy, but it may not align neatly with the strategies of the organisation preparing to fund their staff to undergo a learning opportunity. Likewise, professional association webinars may support a specific practice-based response to sector-identified needs, yet may lack sufficient time to build a rigorous, aligned, and pedagogically considered professional learning activity.

The learning environment for professional learning requires consideration at every level from the designer to the end user or 'learner'. Each stakeholder will have different needs, however, there is a need to consider explicit components of the learning from each stakeholder's perspective. For example, the individual learner will likely be most concerned with the relationship between their needs and the learning activities, whereas an educator will likely be most concerned with the application of pedagogy and constructive alignment to support learning outcome achievement. These perspectives are not mutually exclusive and may require iterative approaches to incremental improvement beyond initial transformative curriculum development.

Conclusion

This chapter has applied a soft human resource management lens and a learning science lens to the professional development of a current and relevant HIDDIN workforce. The impetus within this research was to support a foundational understanding of the diverse stakeholder views within the professional learning landscape: educator, individual, organisation, and sector. While the educator may bring pedagogy and constructive alignment, the individual may seek rapid learning opportunities that fit within their personal and professional goals. The sector may bring immediate needs and challenges, but may lack the necessary educative expertise and time that the tertiary sector can spend developing postgraduate offerings. This chapter began with an exploration of the challenges to create high-quality valid and reliable learning environments to support learning globally. It considered diverse stakeholder perspectives and evidence-bases. It indicated the relative immaturity of professional learning and development, which is an area of activity that requires maturation to support the emerging professionalism of the HIDDIN workforce. This may be in the form of sector and learning institutional collaboration to build systems and frameworks to support aligned and adaptable professional learning cultures. The chapter also outlined enormous opportunities to improve professional learning opportunities and to improve the contributions of this workforce to essential aspects of health service operations.

References

Abrams K, Crook G. The Canadian Health Information Management Association: health information management in Canada. HIM-Interchange. 2011;1(1):17–21.

Acemoglu D, Pischke JS. Minimum wages and on the job training. Res Labor Econ 2003;22:159–202.

Ahmadi N, McKenzie ME, MacLean A, Brown CJ, Mastracci T, McLeod RS, Evidence-Based Reviews in Surgery Steering Group. Teaching evidence based medicine to surgery residents-is journal club the best format? A systematic review of the literature. J Surgical Educ. 2012;69(1):91–100.

Anderson JG. The role of ethics in information technology decisions: a case-based approach to biomedical informatics education. Int J Med Inform. 2004;73(2):145–50.

Ashenfelter O. Estimating the effect of training programs on earnings. Rev Econ Stat. 1978;63:47–57.

Atd Research. 2019 statee of the industry. 2019. https://www.td.org/research-reports/2019-state-of-the-industry#gsc.tab=0. Accessed 31 Mar 2021.

Avolio BJ, Hannah ST. Developmental readiness: accelerating leader development. Consult Psychol J Pract Res. 2008;60(4):331.

Bloom HS. Estimating the effect of job-training programs, using longitudinal data: Ashenfelter's findings reconsidered. J Hum Resour. 1984;19(4):544–56.

Blue B. Health reform and the health information management profession. HIM-Interchange. 2011;1(1):3–6.

Butler-Henderson K. Health informatics. In: Guyz D, Brown R, Halcomb E, Whitehead D, editors. An introduction to community and primary health care. Cambridge: Cambridge University Press; 2020. p. 206–21.

Butler-Henderson K, Gray K. Australia's Health Information Workforce: Census Summary Report 2018. Launceston: University of Tasmania; 2018.

Capampangan DJ, Wellik KE, Parish JM, Aguilar MI, Snyder CRH, Wingerchuk D, Demaerschalk BM. Is obstructive sleep apnea an independent risk factor for stroke?: a critically appraised topic. Neurologist. 2010;16(4):269–73.

Cramer JS, Mahoney MC. Introducing evidence based medicine to the journal club, using a structured pre and post test: a cohort study. BMC Med Educ. 2001;1(1):6.

Crawford J, Kelder J-A. Do we measure leadership effectively? Articulating and evaluating scale development psychometrics for best practice. Leadersh Q. 2019;30(1):133–44.

Crawford J, Butler-Henderson K, Rudolph J, Malkawi B, Glowatz M, Burton R, Magni P, Lam S. COVID-19: 20 countries' higher education intra-period digital pedagogy responses. J Appl Learn Teach. 2020;3(1):9–28.

Desimone L. Improving impact studies of teachers' professional development: toward better conceptualization and measures. Educ Res. 2009;38(3):181–99.

Dimitropoulos V, Lean N, Butler-Henderson K, Shepheard J. Supporting clinical coders: understanding the challenges. HIM-Interchange. 2019;9(2):4–17.

Ebert L, Hoffman K, Levett-Jones T, Gilligan C. "They have no idea of what we do or what we know": Australian graduates' perceptions of working in a health care team. Nurse Educ Pract. 2014;14(5):544–550

Eraut M. Developing a broader approach to professional learning. In: McKee A, Eraut M, editors. Learning trajectories, innovation and identity for professional development. Dordrecht: Springer; 2012. p. 21–45.

Fernandes L, Butler-Henderson K, MacDonald M. The impact of COVID-19 on the work life of HIM professionals: an IFHIMA survey. J AHIMA. 2020. https://journal.ahima.org/the-impact-of-covid-19-on-the-work-life-of-him-professionals-an-ifhima-survey/. Accessed 31 Mar 2021.

Gaudine AP, Saks AM. A longitudinal quasi-experiment on the effects of posttraining transfer interventions. Hum Resour Dev Q. 2004;15(1):57–76.

Glaveski S. Where companies go wrong with learning and development. Harv Bus Rev. 2019. https://hbr.org/2019/10/where-companies-go-wrong-with-learning-and-development. Accessed 31 Mar 2021.

Gray K, Dattakumar A, Maeder A, Butler-Henderson K, Chenery H. Advancing ehealth education for the clinical health professions. Final report. Australian Government Office for Learning and Teaching. 2014. https://pure.bond.edu.au/ws/portalfiles/portal/26149651/Advancing_Ehealth_Education_for_the_Clinical_Health_Professions_Final_Report_2014.pdf

Hadley JA, Wall D, Khan KS. Learning needs analysis to guide teaching evidence-based medicine: knowledge and beliefs amongst trainees from various specialities. BMC Med Educ. 2007;7(1):1–6.

Ilic D, Tepper K, Misso M. Teaching evidence-based medicine literature searching skills to medical students during the clinical years: a randomized controlled trial. J Med Libr Assoc. 2012;100(3):190.

Ismach RB. Teaching evidence-based medicine to medical students. Acad Emerg Med. 2004;11(12):1283–e6.

Jayaram K, Moffit A, Scott D. Breaking the habit of ineffective professional development for teachers. McKinsey on Society. 2012;1–12. https://www.mckinsey.com/~/media/McKinsey/Industries/Public%20and%20Social%20Sector/Our%20Insights/Breaking%20the%20habit%20of%20ineffective%20professional%20development%20for%20teachers/Breaking_the_habit_of_ineffective_professional_development_for_teachers.pdf. Accessed 31 Mar 2021.

Jenkins R. Professional development through attending conferences: reflections of a health librarian. Health Inf Libr J. 2015;32:156–60.

Lalmuanawma S, Hussain J, Chhakchhuak L. Applications of machine learning and artificial intelligence for Covid-19 (SARS-CoV-2) pandemic: a review. Chaos Solitons Fractals. 2020;139:110059.

Loew L, Wentworth D. Leadership: the state of development programs. Brandon Hall Group: Delray Beach; 2013.

Lorenzi NM, Riley RT. Organizational aspects of health informatics: managing technological change. London: Springer Science & Business Media; 2013.

Manley K, Martin A, Jackson C, Wright T. A realist synthesis of effective continuing professional development (CPD): a case study of healthcare practitioners' CPD. Nurse Educ Today. 2018;69:134–41.

Marescaux E, De Winne S, Sels L. HR practices and HRM outcomes: the role of basic need satisfaction. Pers Rev. 2013;42(1):4–27.

Mather C, Cummings E. Modelling Digital Knowledge Transfer: Nurse Supervisors Transforming Learning at Point of Care to Advance Nursing Practice. Informatics. 2017;4(2):12

Mathisen GE, Bronnick KS. Creative self-efficacy: an intervention study. Int J Educ Res. 2009;48(1):21–9.

Milbrandt EB, Vincent JL. Evidence-based medicine journal club. Crit Care. 2004;8:401.

O'Leonard K, Loew L. Leadership development fact book 2012: benchmarks and trends in US leadership development. Bersin & Associates: Oakland; 2012.

Percy A, Press N, Andrew MB, Pollard V. Reframing theory of, and for, practice in higher education. J Univ Teach Learn Pract. 2021;18(4):1.

Pontefract D. The wasted dollars of corporate training programs. Forbes. 2019. https://www.forbes.com/sites/danpontefract/2019/09/15/the-wasted-dollars-of-corporate-training-programs/?sh=21373fe471f9. Accessed 31 Mar 2021.

Ramsaroop S, Petersen N. Building professional competencies through a service learning 'gallery walk'in primary school teacher education. J Univ Teach Learn Pract. 2020;17(4):3.

Rees CE, Crampton P, Kent F, Brown T, Hood K, Leech M, Newton J, Storr M, Williams B. Understanding students' and clinicians' experiences of informal interprofessional workplace learning: an Australian qualitative study. BMJ Open. 2018;8(4):e021238

Ritchie A, Hallam G, Hamill C, Lewis S, Foti M, O'Connor P, Clark C. Designing a specialist post-graduate qualification and continuing professional development structure for the health librarian workforce of the future. Austral Acad Res Libr. 2010;41(4):276–99.

Sadigh G, Parker R, Kelly AM, Cronin P. How to write a critically appraised topic (CAT). Acad Radiol. 2012;19(7):872–88.

Sapci A, Sapci H. Teaching hands-on informatics skills to future health informaticians: a competency framework proposal and analysis of health care informatics curricula. JMIR Med Inform. 2020;8(1):e15748.

Sastre EA, Denny JC, McCoy JA, McCoy AB, Spickard A III. Teaching evidence-based medicine: impact on students' literature use and inpatient clinical documentation. Med Teach. 2011;33(6):e306–12.

Shepheard J. Industrial relations and human resources: management challenges for Health Information Managers (editorial). Health Inf Manag J. 2011;40(1):4–6.

Shine S. Urinary calculus: IVU vs. CT renal stone? A critically appraised topic. Abdom Imaging. 2008;33(1):41–3.

Stange KC. Ways of knowing, learning, and developing. Ann Fam Med. 2010;8(1):4–10.

Stewart C. Transforming professional development to professional learning. J Adult Educ. 2014;43(1):28–33.

Straus S, Glasziou P, Richardson WS, Haynes RB. Evidence-based medicine: how to practice and teach EBM. 5th ed. New York: Churchill Livingstone; 2018.

Sung SY, Choi JN. Do organizations spend wisely on employees? Effects of training and development investments on learning and innovation in organizations. J Organ Behav. 2014;35(3):393–412.

Taliaferro A, Harris NP. The effects of a one-day workshop on physical educators' self-efficacy toward inclusion of students with autism. Palaestra. 2014;28(3).

Topf JM, Hiremath S. Social media, medicine and the modern journal club. Int Rev Psychiatry. 2015;27(2):147–54.

TrainingMag. 2019 training industry report. TrainingMag. 2019. https://trainingmag.com/sites/default/files/2019_industry_report.pdf. Accessed 31 Mar 2021.

Valenta AL, Berner ES, Boren SA, Deckard GJ, Eldredge C, Fridsma DB, Gadd C, Gong Y, Johnson T, Jones J, Manos EL, Phillips KT, Roderer NK, Rosendale D, Turner AM, Tusch G, Williamson JJ, Johnson SB. AMIA Board White Paper: AMIA 2017 core competencies for applied health informatics education at the master's degree level. J Am Med Inform Assoc. 2018;25(12):1657–68.

van der Klink MR, Streumer JN. Effectiveness of on-the-job training. J Eur Indus Train. 2002;26(2/3/4):196–9.

Van Hoof TJ, Doyle TJ. Learning science as a potential new source of understanding and improvement for continuing education and continuing professional development. Med Teach. 2018;40:880–5.

Vedantam S. Most diversity training ineffective, study finds. Wash Post. 2008;A03.

Part III
Innovation

Chapter 8
Health Workforce Learning in Response to Artificial Intelligence

Sandeep Reddy and Paul Cooper

Abstract In the era of big data and digital technology, artificial intelligence (AI)'s potential and positive implications are becoming prominent. With evidence mounting that AI is performing as well as, or in certain instances better than, clinicians in diagnosis and therapy, it is inevitable the current, and future health workforce will be working with this technology. Yet there is limited or no education or training of healthcare professionals or health information professionals about AI and its appropriate use. We propose an outline for a formal training suite that will inform the health workforce about AI, its types, its application in healthcare and the implications. There are three principal components: computational, translational, and governance; each should be delivered using appropriate pedagogical approaches to enable progressive and productive learning. The current lack of AI training presents a risk when an unprepared health workforce begins using this technology in healthcare settings. This situation has direct implications for the specialist health information workforce.

Keywords Artificial intelligence · Machine learning · Data science · Deep learning · Training

Introduction

We live in an era of big data, and the utility of big datasets for addressing health issues becomes ever more obvious (Puaschunder et al. 2020), but manual processing of large datasets is cumbersome. Fortunately, automated computation of such data via computational reasoning frameworks is one of the most disruptive recent

S. Reddy (✉) · P. Cooper
School of Medicine, Deakin University, Melbourne, VIC, Australia
e-mail: sandeep.reddy@deakin.edu.au; p.cooper@deakin.edu.au

K. Butler-Henderson et al. (eds.), *The Health Information Workforce*,
Health Informatics, https://doi.org/10.1007/978-3-030-81850-0_8

medical services advancements and has drawn clinicians, analysts, and industry experts' attention and efforts (Reddy 2018). Such computational reasoning frameworks mimic human knowledge acquisition by simulating reasoning and self-rectification (Sapci and Sapci 2020). Artificial Intelligence (AI) and distributed computing, which have accelerated the adoption of computer-based reasoning in medicine, have demonstrated the possibility of being more accurate than doctors at predicting or diagnosing some medical conditions, especially in radiology and dermatology (Reddy et al. 2019). Contemporary AI's capacity to advance learning acquisition autonomously separates it from previous generation mechanical or explicit rule-based formulations (Kulkarni et al. 2020). AI can now mirror human knowledge utilising self-learning strategies (Sapci and Sapci 2020). Machine Learning (ML), a subset of AI, permits information gain and forecasting without expressly created rules. Deep Learning (DL) is a subfield of ML utilising a structure of neural networks with feedback loops to obviate the need for express rules. Using DL techniques, computational reasoning frameworks can calculate how to group pictures and appoint names to words in a sentence (semantic naming). Medical imaging analysers, virtual assistants and facial recognition software are some other practical instances of DL. One consequence of DL's approach is the need for enormous amounts of structured and unstructured data to train the system to achieve accurate predictive results; the need for the training data to be unbiased and of high quality adds to this approach's complexity (Puaschunder et al. 2020).

The requirement for digital health specialist expertise in processing extensive high-quality health datasets is therefore twofold: to directly aid clinicians through the combination and analysis of the datasets in new and insightful ways (e.g. to enable early intervention to mitigate disease complications, reduce medical errors and enable keener insights into disease progression and complications); and to provide datasets for training predictive computational reasoning systems that aid clinicians, especially those employing DL techniques. The algorithmic approach of AI and its ability to automate healthcare delivery aspects present unprecedented opportunities for stakeholders (Reddy et al. 2019). Aspects of AI, such as decentralised information curation and more economical processing of data can herald greater affordability and democratisation of healthcare, unlike other technologies. Also, as health data exponentially increases, more training data becomes available for AI, thus increasing clinicians' ability to harness AI for achieving appropriate health outcomes. However, health data managers and clinicians must be properly equipped with the knowledge and skills to realise these opportunities to advance healthcare.

As AI-enabled digital health advances, there will be a net positive benefit for healthcare services and patients, if this technology is used appropriately and safely (Reddy et al. 2019). If not, inequality, discrimination and medical risks may worsen. To support the appropriate use of AI, we need to organise the development of the skills, approaches and performance of the health workforce to become digitally competent and confident (Topol 2019). This means an organised approach to improve digital literacy levels, enable awareness of the competencies required, provide access to education and training, and support technology integration in clinical practice. This is not something any health service can ignore as there is a fundamental shift as to how digital technology is being adopted in healthcare; the COVID-19 pandemic showcased the utility of digital technology adoption in delivering healthcare and how digital systems can be learned and deployed in clinical environments in breath-taking speeds (Keesara et al. 2020). Currently, digital health applications include telemedicine, electronic health records and AI service information sharing and storage platforms, service delivery tools, and decision support, amongst other applications (Topol 2019; Coravos et al. 2019). With expanding telemedicine and AI integration into service delivery, the potential for greater use of remote health monitoring and utilisation of patient feedback in care models is imminent. Although more needs to be done to maximise the benefits of digital systems that include AI computational reasoning frameworks, current digital health knowledge and skills of many health professionals are limited; reasons for this may include unavailability of digital health applications or lack of integration of these applications in routine service delivery (Topol 2019; Alscher and Schmidt 2018), or aptitudinal and attitudinal readiness of the workforce (Department of Health and Ageing 2011). It is the role of clinicians to interpret medical conditions and explain them to the patients (Sapci and Sapci 2020; Wartman and Combs 2019) but the notion that clinicians can be abreast of all the relevant medical and patient information to provide optimal care is a fantasy in the era of overwhelming information sources. One useful path forward is to combine AI computational reasoning systems with human insights (Algorithmic Medicine) to offer combined benefits in processing and digesting huge data sources. It becomes harder and harder for clinicians to be ignorant of AI's technical and functional aspects.

A Framework for Professional Learning

As responsible managers and users of such technologies, the healthcare workforce and health information workforce need to be aware of AI's possibilities in healthcare, and the best-combined capabilities of humans and AI. The workforce needs to understand the characteristics, advantages and limitations of machine learning algorithms, ethical implications, evaluation and audit mechanisms, benchmarking and development of AI models (Sapci and Sapci 2020; Topol 2019; Wartman and Combs 2019). Without such education, clinicians are likely not to adopt AI; where it is implemented, they may make mistakes or have an inability to interpret the algorithms or even be sidelined when deeper integration of AI in service delivery occurs. With such education, clinicians are likely to be confident and capable of seeing the AI as an augmentative process, and thus be more ready to integrate the assistive AI systems into workflows without compromising safety or quality. Three developments are setting the ground for a big shift to integrate AI in healthcare delivery (Topol 2019): the increasing proportion of the population having their genome sequenced, generation of health data that patients can control, and improvements in algorithms' performance to analyse such data. To prepare the health workforce to more effectively and safely participate in the benefits offered by this shift, digital literacy, awareness of the requisite capability, access to education and training, and appropriate skills to utilise technology to improve patient outcomes need to be improved (Topol 2019; Bilimoria et al. 2019). For this to occur, there has to be a multi-level and multi-organisational effort, including investment from authorities and organisations in their workforce and training programs that incorporate the relevant syllabi and assessment structures. So, what should be involved in these training programs?

We know that for safe and appropriate use of data-driven and smart technologies, we require extensive digitisation of patient records, standards for the design and development of these technologies, and evidence-based guidance in the technologies (Puaschunder et al. 2020; Topol 2019; Wyatt and Lin 2002). We also know that to use these technologies in combination with Algorithmic Medicine technologies, the workforce should have the knowledge and skills in data attribution, curation and governance, an understanding of the ethical aspects of the use of patient/healthcare data and the ability to scrutinise digital health technologies for their contextual utility. Further to this, we know for the benefits of AI technology to be harnessed within healthcare there has to be time and willingness amongst the health workforce to adopt the technology, knowledge of the technology amongst the workforce, patient-centred design of the technology and willingness amongst the organisation to fund the adoption of the technology. If we consider all these factors, together with considerations from existing health informatics educational frameworks, and existing AI training courses, an outline for an AI educational package for the health workforce can be designed. AI training courses generally offer computer science, data analytics and algorithm-based platforms in their curriculum to enable students to learn how to interpret AI models and formulate suitable AI strategies, particularly those requiring specialised knowledge; what has to be taken into account for the health workforce are the translational aspects of AI in healthcare, including predictive modelling, clinical AI applications and AI evaluation in healthcare for safety and performance (Reddy 2018). We detail each of these components of an educational package next.

A course on AI targeted at a healthcare workforce should offer students a reasonable understanding of AI model development and deployment and, importantly, of how to ascertain benefits and deficiencies of various models and approaches. To do this, it should cover some aspects of the mathematics, programming and data science behind AI to at least some fundamental competency level. Mathematical concepts that might be considered fundamental include linear algebra, probability, multivariate calculus together with the applied use of these concepts like logical inference, Bayesian networks, Markov models and graph search that underpin the aspects of machine learning. Health data managers and clinicians who work with AI need to be familiar with these topics to understand how AI models are constructed and how they behave in test and real-world environments. Since these topics may be difficult to learn, we propose a pedagogical approach that is experiential, iterative and uses AI techniques to monitor and assist learners. Further to this, we recommend learning at least one of the major programming languages used to build AI models, e.g. Python, R, C++ and Java. Python is the most popular as it has extensive libraries, and a syntax closer to the English language than other programs and is easy to implement (Costa 2020). Learning a programming language also allows learners to interact with data by developing, testing, running, and iterating their code. Data science topics like databases, data query tools, exploratory data analysis, descriptive analysis, regression, classification, network and text analytics, and application programming interfaces are worthwhile to incorporate into the fundamentals. Data fuels AI (particularly DL approaches), and it makes AI relevant in the real world, so to have confidence in applying and managing AI models in healthcare requires some knowledge of the data science concepts of curating and manipulating large datasets in a healthcare context. Visual analysis tools can help in learning about data science.

For AI technology to be adopted in clinical practice and healthcare environments, healthcare professionals need to know how and where AI can be applied. We propose that the healthcare and health information workforce should learn about the main forms of AI currently deployed in healthcare: Machine Learning Analytics (MLA), Computer Vision (CV) and Natural Language Processing (NLP) (Reddy 2021). These AI types are applied in various medical applications such as symptom checkers, real-time transcribers, medical imaging interpreters, clinical decision support systems, robotics, and data mining. MLA is being used in healthcare and by clinicians for diagnosis, prognosis and therapy (Reddy et al. 2019). However, the predominant use is in analysing health data to support healthcare professionals' clinical decisions. These are best exemplified by the non-knowledge-based Clinical Decision Support Systems (CDSS) (Reddy 2018). These CDSS can draw upon complex clinical data and insights from sources like electronic health records and medical guidelines, to direct clinicians in making appropriate medical decisions. MLA also drives CV and NLP (Reddy 2021). CV utilises software to recognise and interpret images and videos, while NLP uses software to interpret human oral and written language. CV is being used for automated interpretation of multiple medical imaging modalities including X-rays, CT, MRI, histopathology and dermatological images, amongst other applications (Reddy 2021). NLP can be used in clinical environments to develop medical chatbots to screen and triage patients, extract clinical concepts from electronic health records and transcribe doctor–patient encounters, as well as for administrative purposes. For AI assistive approaches to be successful in clinical workflow settings, there needs to be a recognition that the human and the AI are part of a combined system; the fact that AI systems are cognitive assistive technologies means that potentially they are much more directly involved in expert guiding or assisting clinician workflows than previous generation healthcare IT systems. Education should emphasise the interactions between healthcare professional, the health information professional and the AI system, as part of learning about what makes implementations successful in clinical settings. For example, the experience of AI applications in radiology has shown that extra emphasis on the AI models' quality assurance is required for methodical use in clinical practice (Vandewinckele et al. 2020).

As the value of AI and its applications in healthcare are recognised by stakeholders, ethical and regulatory aspects and challenges of incorporating AI into existing clinical workflows and systems are coming to the fore (Reddy et al. 2019). There are still very few success stories of AI adoption in actual clinical environments and its operation on prospective data; so far, most of the achievements have been in controlled or simulated settings. Further, where AI has been utilised in healthcare administration type of applications, discriminatory effects particularly against marginalised or vulnerable populations have been found (Reddy et al. 2019). In addition to these concerns, AI applications' autonomous or semi-autonomous nature can present regulatory challenges both at clinical approval and post-approval stages. At the approval stage, regulatory authorities have to consider the privacy of the data being used to develop the AI models and the safety of the AI applications when used in clinical settings. Post approval, there has to be an evaluation mechanism to monitor the efficacy and continued safety of approved AI applications. When errors occur because of approved AI applications, the liability issue needs to be taken into account (Reddy et al. 2020). These issues and their solutions have to be incorporated in the AI education suite, as well as aspects such as trust-building. Schneiderman (2020) has developed guidelines for reliable, safe and trustworthy human-centred AI systems in generic settings; and Cai et al. (2019) have reported that to gain confidence and trust clinicians desired upfront information about basic, global properties of the AI model, including known strengths and limitations, its subjective point-of-view and its overall design objective.

Considering together all three components of AI training customised for a health-oriented workforce—fundamentals, translation, and governance—we recommend these be weighted in the proportions shown in Fig. 8.1. We further recommend that pedagogical approaches be differentiated depending on whether technical aspects or human factor aspects are the focus of learning; all these pedagogical approaches can also be supported by using assistive technologies (pedagogical agents) (Schroder and Adescope 2012).

To support learning the technical elements inherent in the foundational and translational AI topics, we recommend experiential learning approaches such as the use of computer simulations. These have previously been shown to be useful in engineering education, such as the approach proposed by Botelho et al. (2016) which builds on the prior foundational work of Kolb's (1984) experiential learning theory. We recommend this approach because the fundamentals component is essentially technical in nature, thus lends itself to computer simulation modules. Computer

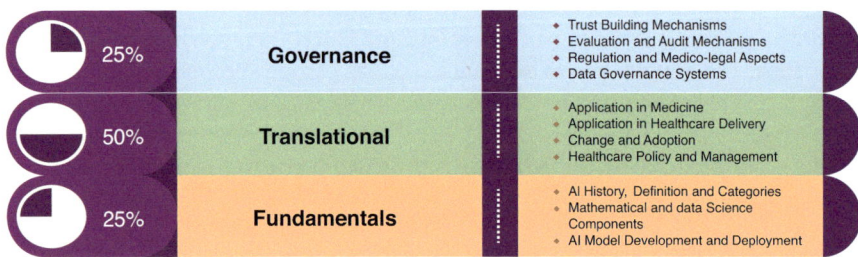

Fig. 8.1 Components of AI in health workforce education and training

simulations would also be appropriate for the translational topics, where the three AI approaches of MLA, CV and DL could be explored and compared in an experimentally rich manner. For example, a variety of software models could be made available to the student to help them understand how a CV model can detect an image through repeat training, and to discover the limitations and benefits of each.

The governance component of our framework and the human factor aspects of the translational and foundational components has inherently strong subjective elements that would be well supported by pedagogies that support frequent learner feedback cycles, such as evaluative feedback, self-regulation and attunement. Evaluative judgement enables learners to make decisions about the quality of work themselves, using practices such as: self-assessment, peer review, feedback as dialogue, rubrics for formative assessment and multiple exemplars with quality indicators (Tai et al. 2018). Feedback approaches for self-regulated learning (Nicol and Macfarlane-Dick 2006) include 'scaffolded feedback', that is, providing incremental hints until a correct answer is self-generated (Finn and Metcalfe 2010). Consideration of ethical and governance aspects of AI would be well suited to responsive attunement techniques where learners and teachers explore issues of importance in syndicate style activities or debates, such as where one group would develop and propose a situation of ethical complexity and another group would tease it out and respond to it.

Discussion

As AI technology's part in digital health becomes increasingly prominent in healthcare delivery, employers, regulatory and professional bodies, and the patient community will expect healthcare professional competency in governance, translation and fundamentals. AI's ability to improve the diagnosis and prognosis of many medical conditions, standardise medical care, decrease the costs of delivering healthcare and reduce medical errors is already evident. AI has the ability to assist healthcare workflows even more when coupled with human involvement, i.e. human in the loop systems (Wang 2019); we already have seen instances where AI, coupled with humans, perform better than AI or humans alone (Lovett 2019). All AI uses in healthcare settings require the stakeholders to understand the technology they are working with, achieved through a structured orientation to the various aspects of AI and its healthcare application.

Innovations in AI in healthcare thus have several direct implications for the specialised health information workforce that is the focus of this book. First, all practitioners in the specialised health information workforce will need to upskill in this field, so that they are prepared for inevitable changes to the roles and functions they presently perform. Following the training approach outlined in this chapter can meet the professional development needs of these practitioners. Additionally, some people in the specialised health information workforce will need to go beyond this training, to develop substantial expertise in AI in healthcare. This will be necessary if they are to remain relevant as advisors and consultants to clinicians, service managers, and policy-makers, about how those groups can work responsibly with computational, translational and governance aspects of AI in healthcare. Finally, a select group within the specialised health information workforce will need to become capable of designing and delivering the type of training described in this chapter, to ensure that professional learning and development is more widely available across the entire health workforce.

As AI evolves, our framework will allow for new technology developments and their healthcare application to be included in curriculum design and delivery. Considering the current situation of limited or no health workforce education about AI and its functions and the imminent possibility of this workforce working with AI directly or indirectly, there is some urgency for educational institutions and healthcare organisations to collaborate to deliver AI-related education not just for the health workforce but also for the larger patient and health consumer community. This wider approach would strengthen awareness of governance needs and challenges in using AI appropriately in healthcare.

References

Alscher MD, Schmidt N. The practice of medicine in the age of information technology. In: eHealth: Making Health Care Smarter. 2018. https://doi.org/10.5772/intechopen.75482.

Bilimoria K, Harish V, McCoy L, Mehta N, Morgado F, Nagaraj S, Wang C, Zheng J. Ontario: Ontario Medical Student Association; 2019. https://omsa.ca/en/position-papers/preparing-medical-students-impact-artificial-intelligence. Accessed 31 Mar 2021.

Botelho WT, Marietto MDGB, Ferreira JCDM, Pimentel EP. Kolb's experiential learning theory and Belhot's learning cycle guiding the use of computer simulation in engineering education: a pedagogical proposal to shift toward an experiential pedagogy. Comput Appl Eng Educ. 2016;24(1):79–88.

Cai CJ, Winter S, Steiner D, Wilcox L, Terry M. "Hello AI": Uncovering the onboarding needs of medical practitioners for human-AI collaborative decision-making. Proc ACM Hum-Comput Interact. 2019;104:1–24. https://doi.org/10.1145/3359206.

Coravos A, Goldsack JC, Karlin DR, Nebeker C, Perakslis E, Zimmerman N, Erb MK. Digital medicine: a primer on measurement. Digit Biomark. 2019;3(2):31–71.

Costa CD. Top programming languages for ai engineers in 2020. Towards data science. 2020. https://towardsdatascience.com/top-programming-languages-for-ai-engineers-in-2020-33a9f16a80b0. Accessed 31 Mar 2021.

Department of Health and Ageing. The eHealth Readiness of Australia's Allied Health Sector. 2011. https://www1.health.gov.au/internet/publications/publishing.nsf/Content/ehealth-readiness-allied-toc. Accessed 31 Mar 2021.

Finn B, Metcalfe J. Scaffolding feedback to maximize long-term error correction. Mem Cognit. 2010;38(7):951–61.

Keesara S, Jonas A, Schulman K. Covid-19 and Health Care's digital revolution. N Engl J Med. 2020;382(23):e82.

Kolb DA. The process of experiential learning: experience as the source of learning and development. Englewood Cliffs, NJ: Prentice-Hall; 1984.

Kulkarni S, Seneviratne N, Baig MS, Khan AHA. Artificial Intelligence in medicine: where are we now? Acad Radiol. 2020;27(1):62–70.

Lovett L. AI in healthcare: not human versus machine, human plus machine. HIMSS. 2019. https://www.mobihealthnews.com/content/ai-healthcare-not-human-versus-machine-human-plus-machine. Accessed 31 Mar 2021.

Nicol DJ, Macfarlane-Dick D. Formative assessment and self-regulated learning: a model and seven principles of good feedback practise. Stud Higher Educ. 2006;31(2):199–218.

Puaschunder J, Mantl J, Plank B. Medicine of the future: the power of artificial intelligence (AI) and big data in healthcare. RAIS J Soc Sci. 2020;4:1–8.

Reddy S. Use of artificial intelligence in healthcare delivery. eHealth – Making health care smarter. 2018. https://doi.org/10.5772/intechopen.74714.

Reddy S. Algorithmic medicine. In: Artificial intelligence: applications in healthcare delivery. London: Routledge; 2021.

Reddy S, Fox J, Purohit MP. Artificial intelligence-enabled healthcare delivery. J R Soc Med. 2019;112(1):22–8.

Reddy S, Allan S, Coghlan S, Cooper P. A governance model for the application of AI in health care. J Am Med Inform Assoc. 2020;27(3):491–7.

Sapci AH, Sapci HA. Artificial intelligence education and tools for medical and health informatics students: systematic review. JMIR Med Educ. 2020;6(1):e19285.

Schneiderman B. Bridging the gap between ethics and practice: guidelines for reliable, safe, and trustworthy human-centered AI Systems. ACM Trans Interact Intell Syst. 2020;10(4):26.

Schroder NL, Adescope OO. A case for the use of pedagogical agents in online learning environments. J Teach Learn Technol. 2012;1(2):43–7.

Tai J, Ajjawi R, Boud D, Dawson P, Panadero E. Developing evaluative judgement: enabling students to make decisions about the quality of work. High Educ. 2018;76:467–81.

Topol E. Preparing the healthcare workforce to deliver the digital future. The Topol Review. An independent report on behalf of the Secretary of State for Health and Social Care. 2019. https://topol.hee.nhs.uk/. Accessed 31 Mar 2021.

Vandewinckele L, Claessens M, Dinkla A, Brouwer C, Crijns W, Verellen D, van Elmpt W. Overview of artificial intelligence-based applications in radiotherapy: recommendations for implementation and quality assurance. Radiother Oncol. 2020;153:55–66.

Wang G. Humans in the loop: the design of interactive AI systems. Human-Centred Artif Intell. 2019. https://hai.stanford.edu/blog/humans-loop-design-interactive-ai-systems. Accessed 31 Mar 2021.

Wartman SA, Combs CD. Reimagining medical education in the age of AI. AMA J Ethics. 2019;21:146–52.

Wyatt JC, Liu JL. Basic concepts in medical informatics. J Epidemiol Community Health. 2002;56(11):808–12.

Chapter 9
The Rise of the Consumer Health Information Specialist

Rachel de Sain

Abstract Healthcare organisations are looking to adopt connected technologies and innovations to empower healthcare consumers with quality information and services to become co-pilots of their own health and wellbeing. This chapter describes the emerging field of the consumer health information specialist (CHIS), their roles, pathways into the profession, places of work and principles of professional practice. It highlights the importance of health, digital and data literacies to ensure that all healthcare consumers can make informed choices for themselves and those they care for. As health technology adoption and adherence by consumers become more and more vital to effective healthcare outcomes, CHIS professionals are increasingly essential in the health workforce to advocate for, create, curate, distribute and analyse quality information and services for all healthcare consumers.

Keywords Consumers · Participatory medicine · Health literacy

Introduction

Consumers want to play an active role in their health and care (Betts and Korenda 2018). This creates a demand for an environment in which health information, tools and services can be personalised for healthcare consumers' own needs. Information should flow seamlessly amongst healthcare professionals and other parties (human or machine) whom the consumer chooses to involve in their care. Thus the consumer's role shifts from passenger to co-pilot (Castle-Clarke and Imison 2016)

R. de Sain (✉)
Codesain, Sydney, NSW, Australia
e-mail: rachel@codesain.com.au

© The Author(s), under exclusive license to Springer Nature
Switzerland AG 2021
K. Butler-Henderson et al. (eds.), *The Health Information Workforce*,
Health Informatics, https://doi.org/10.1007/978-3-030-81850-0_9

continuing to require quality information to guide their decision making while increasingly becoming creators of information themselves.

The term consumer versus patient is debated by many across the health sector (Henderson and Petersen 2002). A healthcare consumer is engaged in preventive and wellness solutions, making decisions about current and future care needs, including being a patient. Patients are a subset of healthcare consumers where there is a consumer-clinician therapeutic relationship. A healthcare consumer is, therefore, an individual who uses the services of a healthcare provider, including patients receiving medical care or treatment.

The health system is increasingly becoming digitised, enabling a greater breadth of information, including from consumers and being used by consumers. This digitsation of information offers transformative opportunities to rethink healthcare delivery models from research to treatment to future policy development (Allen 2020). To leverage the opportunities of this new digital age, health organisations are increasingly looking to professional practitioners who are consumer healthcare information specialists (CHIS) and the unique skills and expertise they bring to support strategic objectives (World Health Organization 2016).

While a clinical audience expects information that is structured and standardised using consistent terminologies and classifications (Seebode et al. 2013), consumers have variable literacy, experiences, access to and needs for information, so they require different formats and styles of information to achieve their health outcomes (Pian et al. 2020). Information management includes policies, procedures, applications and systems to manage the information lifecycle (Boaden and Lockett 1991) but can overlook the activities required to plan, create and curate meaningful, actionable content to engage consumers in health care. Consumers require digital, data and health literacy skills to participate in the digitised health system (Australian Commission on Safety and Quality in Health Care 2013) and improve health outcomes (Hilfiker et al. 2020). This chapter explores the role of consumer health information specialist (CHIS) professionals in providing useful and usable information for health consumers in an increasingly digitised health system that relies on data, information, knowledge and wisdom for improving health outcomes. These CHIS professionals are an important part of the health information workforce.

The Work of Consumer Health Information Specialists

CHIS work spans the domains of data, information and content management. Data management involves creating, obtaining, transforming, sharing, protecting, documenting and preserving data in a binary digital form that is efficient for processing. Information management is the collection, storage, curation, dissemination, archiving and destruction of documents, images, drawings and other sources of processed data. Content management is the set of processes and technologies to support the creation, collection, management and publishing of information in any form or medium. For the purposes of this chapter, these domains are referred to collectively as "information." Working within these domains aligns with a cycle of activities that include planning, creating, curating, distributing and analysing information, with a centralised management, operations and governance function (Fig. 9.1).

A planning stage defines the requirements for information creation. Planning activities may be triggered by a report, a one-off incident, a new clinical system, or a seasonal event. Factors that are analysed for planning purposes include what information sources already exist, the intended audience, governance and approval requirements, publication and distribution and desired outcomes measures. Since the creation of information may require additional expenditure, the commissioning organisation should mandate planning work (in the form of a business case, scoping document or project brief) and approval of a budgeted plan prior to any creation activity. This is particularly relevant if commissioning external services, for example from graphic designers, videographers or marketing agencies. Planning roles may include product manager, project manager, business analyst and technical architect; people in these roles often have specific experience and skills in project management, and organisations may prefer those with additional healthcare experience.

Information creation may involve the acquisition or creation of new information or manipulation of existing content to meet new needs. The high-level information creation requirements developed during the planning phase will require validation

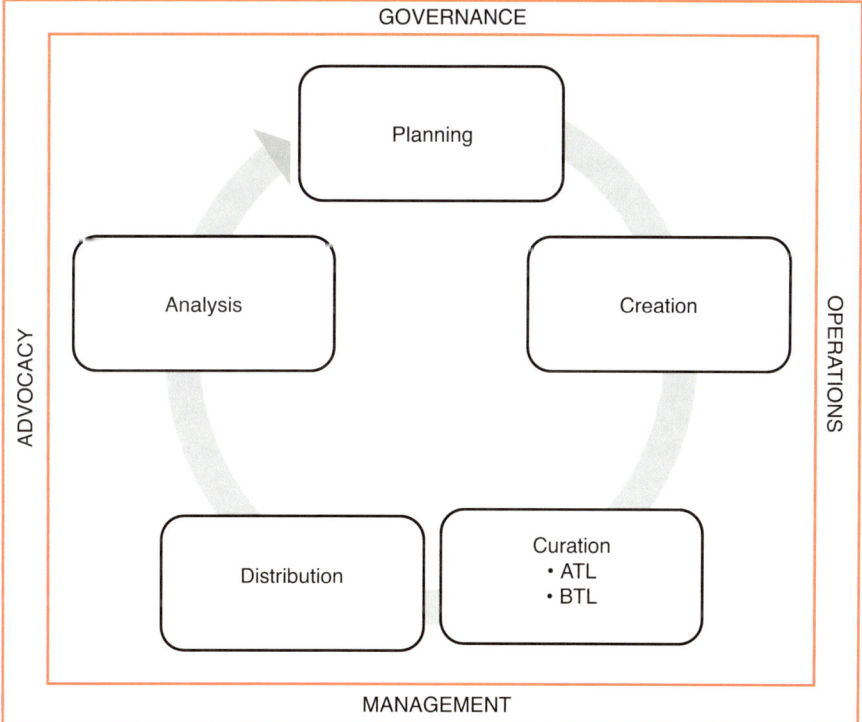

Fig. 9.1 The CHIS work cycle

with end users to understand their needs. Creators use service design principles and design thinking methodologies to co-design solutions with relevant user stakeholders. Creator roles require diverse skills, including copywriting, graphic design, videography and software development. Some organisations may not have permanent staff in these roles and may utilise third-party freelancers, contractors or agencies. Digital professionals are more likely to be working as freelancers within the gig economy (Bergvall-Kareborn and Howcroft 2014), pitching for work on a per-project basis rather than being permanently placed within an organisation. Increasingly organisations are looking to contract creatives with experience in the healthcare sector and a nuanced understanding of its protocols—such as clinical governance of what can be visually portrayed or said within a piece of consumer healthcare information and the impact of non-adherence to clinical quality and safety frameworks.

Once information has been created, it needs to be curated. Information curation consists of above-the-line (ATL) activity and below-the-line (BTL) activity. Marketing and advertising terminology refers to ATL activity as mass media, untargeted communication (e.g. TV or radio) and BTL activity as online or social, often involving targeted communications to specific types of people (Furman 2017). In the context of CHIS, ATL curation activities impact how information is experienced by the end user, how it is seen or presented in a format. ATL curation activities determine the best way to collate multiple pieces of information to deliver a better experience for the healthcare consumer throughout their journey; this work recognises that these consumers access, use and reuse information differently at different stages to meet their perceived needs (Alzougool et al. 2008). Social media has become the primary source of news and information for most people (Shearer and Matsa 2018). Consumers may access health information directly via a social network post, third-party website, navigating from a publisher's website homepage or any number of pathways. Consequently, consumer healthcare information should be modular and responsive, so that it retains its credibility regardless of the access point. ATL curators may work closely with user research, insights and analysis team members and co-design directly with end user consumers to understand their audience's behaviour. BTL curation work is the design, delivery and management of the metadata or descriptive data about the information to be found, shared, reported and managed efficiently. BTL curation roles include health informaticians, data scientists, information managers and health librarians. They are responsible for taxonomies, ontologies and vocabularies that enable information to be categorised, classified and appropriately indexed by various online search engines, websites and content services. BTL curators are responsible for the design, development and ongoing management of information architecture, content modelling, data schemas and overall information models. Many healthcare consumers seeking health information online use a search engine such as Google, Bing or Baidu to begin their search (Tan and Goonawardene 2017; Cocco et al. 2018). As search engine algorithms crawl the metadata to index the information within their catalogue, it is imperative that BTL curation is prioritised, ensuring that consumer healthcare information is easily accessible for all healthcare consumers.

Information distribution requires understanding how the target consumer accesses and interacts with healthcare information that has been created and curated. Digital marketing experts estimated that most Americans some years ago were exposed to around 4000–10,000 ads each day (Simpson 2017), and this "noise" has increased vastly since then. It is challenging—but essential to distribution—to compete successfully against this noise, to ensure that healthcare consumers actually find and engage with the information that a commissioning organisation wishes to provide to them. CHIS distribution roles may exist within a marketing division, depending on the size of an organisation. They are tasked with understanding the best way to distribute the information to reach a target audience or to position the information capture service to elicit the most responses. These types of roles may include search strategists, social media managers, partnership managers. They may also require legal and commercial resources to negotiate distribution, licencing and partnership contracts for making the information available through third-party channels.

The need to analyse the impact and whether information achieves its intended aims is part of the CHIS work cycle. The shift to digital interactions allows for significant insights into health consumer behaviour and an exciting opportunity to rethink the future of healthcare delivery by shifting from a "find and fix" model to a "predict and prevent" system that uses data-driven insights from consumer behaviour to identify and respond to potential health events. The analysis involves business intelligence, web and social media analytics, market research and reporting, as well as customer engagement and research. Analysis closes the loop when it is used in the planning phase of the next project; it guides the development of new requirements and defines what success metrics are used to measure the impact of the new or changed consumer health information.

Management and operations functions are required throughout the work cycle to drive the day-to-day activities, support teamwork and deliver products and services effectively. These skills are transferrable from other industries and often provide an entry point into the field. Management experience in leading diverse teams and overseeing sophisticated, high-turnover online content applications or services is a highly sought-after skill as the volume of work increases for CHIS professionals. Sophisticated skills in assuring data privacy and security are increasingly important, too, as organisations capture and store data about the users of their consumer health information (Managed Healthcare Executive 2019).

Information governance, a vital function of the entire health information workforce, is particularly important for CHIS professionals. Governance includes responsibility for developing the structures and policies that determine how an organisation manages the consumer healthcare information lifecycle. Information governance includes clinical, technical and content governance to ensure the quality of the information, the minimisation of harm from methods of distribution and use, and the engagement of users through adherence to design, usability and accessibility standards. Consumers are beginning to generate and contribute more of their own information either actively through blogs and application interactions or, sometimes passively, through data from wearables and interactions with health systems

(Reinsel et al. 2018). Thus CHIS professionals have ever greater responsibility in that they not only provide the information that they create to consumers; also they are increasingly collecting, storing and managing consumer-generated health information and applications that interact with it. Governance will increasingly need to deal with the legal and ethical implications of how consumer-generated healthcare information is being requested, stored and used. Terms of use and governance policies will require regular updating to maintain transparency with healthcare consumers and meet evolving regulatory requirements.

Consumer health advocates sometimes referred to as ePatients or professional patients, are not typically consumer health information specialists. Some may choose to learn the necessary skills to work in such roles, while others will consult closely with skilled CHIS professionals throughout the work cycle to represent patients' and health consumers' needs. CHIS advocacy work entails support for healthcare consumers to achieve the best overall health outcome for their particular circumstances, considering their specific situation, culture, beliefs and preferences and clinical health needs (Cervantes et al. 2020). CHIS professionals play a vital role to promote health equity and rights, facilitating, promoting and supporting health consumer advocacy, networking and leadership, through engagement, information dissemination and health literacy training.

Pathways into Consumer Health Information Work

Creating and managing quality consumer health information and associated services is a team sport that requires a diverse set of skills and qualities, many of which are transferrable to/from other industries. The number of pathways is as broad as the number of roles associated with this workforce. It is rare within the health sector that specialists can come from such diverse backgrounds. This breadth of experience and knowledge is an asset for organisations tackling the emerging challenges coming from the digital transformation of the sector.

Digitally enabled patients and carers driven by their own experiences may enter the health information workforce as advocates or content creators. They work to help and guide others, sharing their stories via support groups, blogs or dedicated personal websites, or increasingly through patient social networks and online communities like WEGO Health (https://www.wegohealth.com/) and HealthUnlocked (https://healthunlocked.com/). Public and private organisations are embracing the value of this ePatient work, with some creating specific roles for patient experience or outreach, although the majority of such activities are undertaken on a voluntary unpaid basis. Patients and carers may choose to become CHIS professionals by upskilling into the design, product management, strategy and general management roles.

The role of library and information service managers appears to be a natural pathway into CHIS work, given their unique skillset. As health information moved online, many health librarians undertook the BTL curation required to make information searchable and discoverable—by consumers as well as providers of care—through health websites, online catalogues and search engines. Online health information has been a key facilitator for improving, maintaining and recovering health (Hill and Sofra 2018). Library and information service managers may enter the CHIS workforce as BTL curators, remain in those specialised roles as information content managers, and sometimes transition into associated analysis or governance roles.

Since a significant component of CHIS work relies on digital, media and information and communication technology (ICT) professionals, many CHIS professionals begin their careers outside the health sector, which frequently does not have these skills in-house. Healthcare organisations recruit outside of their industry, as they begin to develop digital consumer health information services such as websites, interactive media or mobile apps. Often the first step for digital media and ICT professionals to enter the health sector is to be employed on government-funded projects, either directly or via professional services firms and digital/ICT agencies. Digital, media and ICT professionals may enter the CHIS workforce in any role matching their knowledge domains and skillsets.

Clinicians from all health disciplines may choose to transition into CHIS roles to move away from face-to-face care delivery but continue to apply their skills and expertise to improve patients' outcomes. Clinical professionals may be brought in as advisors or in a clinical governance role within a project, working alongside non-clinical team members to produce consumer healthcare information. Clinical professionals may enter CHIS work as clinical quality assurance advisors or to provide clinical governance of an organisation's consumer information activities. They are detail-oriented and process-driven, skills that make an excellent base for the transition into CHIS planning, creation and curation roles—particularly in user research, user insights and service design.

Others enter CHIS work via public service and peak bodies. Governments from local to state/regional to federal/national are significant funders of population health and hold overall responsibility for their citizens' health and wellbeing. This provides a pathway into CHIS for public sector employees. At all levels of government, population health initiatives require a range of skilled public health professionals who may work on projects that include the development of consumer health information. As well, some government workers have extensive regulatory knowledge and experience as policy analysts about how consumers and their agents trying to procure health and care services must navigate bureaucracies. These public sector professionals may be sought after by healthcare organisations and peak bodies to help them to work more effectively with government agencies on related activities. They are likely to enter CHIS work in management, governance and planning roles.

CHIS professionals may enter the field via post-secondary education programmes or via workplace training. Digital media tertiary qualifications with subjects in public health and social innovation are an excellent starting point for high school leavers wishing to gain a broad understanding of the whole health system whilst becoming qualified in digital media. Also, formal digital health education programmes focusing on clinical informatics, health information technology and healthcare law and management continue to emerge, and these may include aspects of CHIS work. Otherwise, generic degrees—media and communications, marketing, digital media, journalism, visual and graphic design, software engineering and information systems—can be education pathways for digital, media, business and ICT professionals who may find opportunities to develop those skills in a CHIS role. Relevant training targeting consumers may be available from non-governmental organisations and consumer health peak bodies. Some of the skills required to function effectively as a CHIS in a digital age require training in specific computer software, platforms or tools. There may be growing opportunities for traditional education providers in public health and in digital media to co-design specific training for future CHIS professionals.

Where Do Consumer Health Information Specialists Work?

Healthcare consumers interact with every part of the health sector. Therefore, specialists who can design, develop, deliver and manage information to meet their changing needs may work in any part of the system. Healthcare consumers are also increasingly receiving information and making decisions about their health needs in non-clinical environments such as supermarkets, public transport, retail centres and while watching television programmes (Sarasohn-Kahn 2019). While we acknowledge the emergence of these "other" places of work in informing and supporting healthcare consumers, the health sector workplaces are discussed in this chapter.

Healthcare providers from the local family doctor's practice to large hospitals, multinational health insurers and device manufacturers are all increasingly looking to engage CHIS professionals as part of transforming service delivery models and empowering people to become partners in their health and wellbeing. The high volume of interactions these organisations have with healthcare consumers and the rapid pace of change, be it regulatory, clinical or technical, drive the need for CHIS professionals to work within these organisations.

The primary funding sources for public health, government and public sector organisations, will require CHIS professionals to support population health initiatives. Different political structures and funding models for health and care delivery globally create varying organisational structures and responsibilities of CHIS professionals within them. Given the range of work undertaken, there is a need for CHIS professionals in all subsectors that relate to health data, information and knowledge management. These roles may be within a ministry or health department or as part of a specific government agency set up for consumer health needs, population health management or a national health information service—such as Healthdirect in Australia, 1177 in Sweden and NHS Choices in the UK.

CHIS professionals are found working in media organisations. Traditional (newspaper, television and radio) and new (social, online and mobile) media organisations play an essential role in improving a community's health and digital literacy. These organisations may work in partnership with others, particularly health organisations, peak bodies and government agencies, to promote population health initiatives and emergency health information distribution—such as activity to inform citizens about COVID-19. Many countries may also have a legal mandate that any news or content that may cause harm must provide appropriate information and links to support services (Skehan et al. 2020).

Consumer health advocacy plays a vital role in future health reform and ensures an ongoing commitment to improving literacy, influencing policy, and improving the quality of health services for all (Wells 2016). Peak bodies, not-for-profit organisations (NFP) and non-governmental organisations (NGO) represent the interest of healthcare consumers as a whole (e.g. Australia's Consumers Health Forum) or for a specific need such as disease type (e.g. a Cancer Foundation), accessibility (e.g. the Royal Society for the Blind), or socioeconomic factors (e.g. homelessness, rural and remote communities). Similar bodies may operate at a local, national or international level. Healthcare providers and industry organisations such as pharmaceutical companies and insurers are increasingly seeking to work with these groups and the CHIS professionals within them to ensure they provide information and services that meet the needs of the healthcare consumers they serve.

The global healthcare industry reached a value of over $8,000 billion in 2018 (Wood 2019) and is segmented into pharmaceuticals, medical equipment, consumables, medical software and consumer health technology. The consumer health-tech market is a growing area of investment (Consumer Technology Association 2021). Technological advances such as mobile, virtual reality and autonomous vehicles are transforming the healthcare industry by addressing healthcare consumer needs in innovative ways, encouraging new models of engagement to improve prevention and management of various health conditions. CHIS professionals may work in any of these industry segments to support the creation of quality consumer healthcare information. As the health sector transforms into a participatory model, the information created by industry must evolve to be digestible for healthcare consumers and the traditional clinical and business audience. This will, in turn, drive more demand for quality CHIS professionals who understand how to create compelling, engaging content for a diverse audience, including the modern consumer.

Professional services firms, sometimes known as the Big Five (Deloitte, KPMG, Accenture, EY and PWC), are often contracted by government and industry to support strategic business activities, to assess and then implement changes across the healthcare sector. Professional services firms have identified digital transformation as a growth area and have undertaken significant acquisitions of digital media and marketing agencies to provide additional skills to their portfolio of services (Gianatasio 2017). CHIS professionals may work directly as consultants at one of these firms or a subsidiary agency (e.g. Fjord, an interactive agency acquired by Accenture as part of its Accenture interactive services division).

A growing "professional gig economy" of highly skilled independent professionals is flourishing and already changing the shape of the professional services industry (Source Global Research 2018). Independent CHIS consultants are a growing component of the workforce. They support health organisations in coping with short-term spikes in workload, meeting changing regulatory demands, exploring new business opportunities, and researching strategic opportunities. CHIS professionals working as self-employed contractors may work with multiple organisations at the same time or work on short-term projects.

Principles of Professional Practice

There are no formally accepted principles of professional practice in place for CHIS professionals. However, accepted codes of professional practice may be applied to core functions within the speciality, namely those guiding clinical governance, information management, digital media and design. Analysis of existing professional practice principles, codes of ethics and definitions of quality from healthcare, digital media, and information management suggests that the following principles of professional practice may be appropriate for CHIS professionals. Sources included the US Institute of Medicine's six domains of healthcare quality, the Health on the Net (HON) Code, digital media design principles, general principles of information ethics applied to health information and general principles of service design.

1. Consumer-centric—Provide information and services that are respectful, tailored and responsive to an individual's preferences, needs and values. Minimise information entry by pre-populating fields with known information according to privacy rules.
2. Equitable—Ensure that information is accessible, engaging and non-threatening for audiences such as culturally and linguistically diverse groups, First Nation people, LGBTQIA2S+ communities, people with disabilities, other vulnerable or marginalised people.
3. Relevant—Understand the end-to-end consumer experience and how the information provided fits in a broader context of an activity. Present the information or request for information in a suitable, meaningful and contextual manner.
4. Trustable—Understand the responsibility of providing, capturing and managing consumer health information and ensure that it is valid, credible, reliable and safe.
5. Current—Information must be current, up to date and where appropriate, use modern innovative methods for presentation and capture that improve the consumer's access to current information choices.
6. High quality—To facilitate trust and enhance the experience and long-term engagement, information must be professionally produced and consistent using common language and style guides.
7. Digestible—Accessible for all and provided so that consumers can digest the information and process it, as clear, standardised and structured information when shared across different platforms.
8. Actionable—Information should be engaging, practical and directional to support consumers to make informed decisions as to what steps to take next.
9. Beautiful—Information should adhere to design principles to ensure it is engaging and attractive and supports the consumer rather than distracting from the information or task.

Conclusion

Consumer health information specialists play a vital role in shaping the future of the health industry. Professionals who embrace the diversity of skills, experience and knowledge required to deliver the breadth of activities detailed within this chapter will position themselves as leaders and provide quality outcomes for the healthcare consumers, carers, providers and community whom they serve.

Everyone is a healthcare consumer, whether actively seeking treatment or managing a condition as a patient, taking steps to remain healthy or merely existing in the modern digital age. The future healthcare consumer will be in the driving seat of their health outcomes. To interact with this new automated and personalised health landscape, healthcare consumers will require quality consumer health information available in any form they choose; tools to create, manage and share their health information; and the literacies to make informed decisions about the information they consume and the information they choose to share.

These changes provide a transformative opportunity for new forms of work in the health sector to address the rising demand from an ageing population, an increase in non-communicable diseases, and complex care patients, alongside significant regulatory requirements. Improving healthcare can proceed by acknowledging the important role of CHIS professionals within the health information workforce.

References

Allen DS. 2020 Global health care outlook: laying a foundation for the future. 2020. https://www2.deloitte.com. Accessed 22 May 2021.

Alzougool B, Chang S, Gray K. Towards a comprehensive understanding of health information needs. Electr J Health Inform. 2008;3(2):e15.

Australian Commission on Safety and Quality in Health Care. Consumers, the health system and health literacy: consultation paper. 2013. https://www.safetyandquality.gov.au/. Accessed 22 May 2021.

Bergvall-Kareborn B, Howcroft D. Amazon Mechanical Turk and the commodification of labour. New Technol Work Employ. 2014;29(3):213–23.

Betts D, Korenda L. Findings from the Deloitte 2018 health care consumer survey. 2018. https://www2.deloitte.com/. Accessed 22 May 2021.

Boaden R, Lockett G. Information technology, information systems and information management: definition and development. Eur J Inf Syst. 1991;1:23–32.

Castle-Clarke S, Imison C. The digital patient: transforming primary care? Nuffield Trust; 2016. https://www.nuffieldtrust.org.uk/files/2017-06/1497259872_nt-the-digital-patient-web-corrected-p46-.pdf. Accessed 22 May 2021.

Cervantes L, Hasnain-Wynia R, Steiner JF, Chonchol M, Fischer S. Patient navigation: addressing social challenges in dialysis patients. Am J Kidney Dis. 2020;76(1):121–9.

Cocco AM, Zordan R, Taylor DM, Weiland TJ, Dilley SJ, Kant J, Dombagolla M, Hendarto A, Lai F, Hutton J. Dr Google in the ED: searching for online health information by adult emergency department patients. Med J Australia. 2018;209(8):342–7.

Consumer Technology Association. Three investment growth areas in digital health. 2021. https://www.ces.tech/Articles/2021/March/Three-Investment-Growth-Areas-in-Digital-Health.aspx. Accessed 22 May 2021.

Furman J. Everything you need to know about ATL, BTL and TTL advertising. 2017. https://www.business2community.com/marketing/everything-need-know-atl-btl-ttl-advertising-01902793. Accessed 22 May 2021.

Gianatasio D. Global consultancies are buying up agencies and reshaping the brand marketing world. 2017. https://www.adweek.com/brand-marketing/global-consultancies-are-buying-up-agencies-and-reshaping-the-brand-marketing-world/. Accessed 22 May 2021.

Henderson S, Petersen A. Consuming Health: The Commodification of Health Care. London: Routledge; 2002.

Hilfiker SW, Santana S, Freedman M, Harris LM. There's a gap between digital health information and users – let's close it. Stud Health Technol Inform. 2020;269:324–31.

Hill SJ, Sofra TA. How could health information be improved? Recommended actions from the Victorian consultation on health literacy. Australian Health Rev. 2018;42(2):134–9.

Managed Healthcare Executive. The biggest issues facing healthcare today. 2019. https://www.managedhealthcareexecutive.com/view/biggest-issues-facing-healthcare-today. Accessed 22 May 2021.

Pian WJ, Song SJ, Zhang Y. Consumer health information needs: a systematic review of measures. Inf Process Manage. 2020;57(2):11.

Reinsel D, Gantz J, Rydning J. The digitization of the world. From edge to core. International Data Corporation (IDC); 2018. https://www.seagate.com/files/www-content/our-story/trends/files/idc-seagate-dataage-whitepaper.pdf. Accessed 22 May 2021.

Sarasohn-Kahn J. HealthConsuming: from health consumer to health citizen. Phoenxiville, PA: THINK-Health LLC; 2019.

Seebode C, Trautwein M, Ort M, Lehmann JM. A clinical information management platform for semantic exploitation of clinical data. In: Proc. International MultiConference of Engineers and Computer Scientists. 2013. p. 220–2).

Shearer E, Matsa KE. News use across social media platforms. Pew Research Centre. 2018. https://www.journalism.org/2018/09/10/news-use-across-social-media-platforms-2018/. Accessed 22 May 2021.

Simpson J. Finding brand success in the digital world. Forbes. 2017. https://www.forbes.com/sites/forbesagencycouncil/2017/08/25/finding-brand-success-in-the-digital-world/#3228ef4c626e. Accessed 22 May 2021.

Skehan J, Paton E, Tynan R. The uptake of evidence-informed guidelines for reporting suicide into media codes of practice and policies in Australia. Health Promot J Austr. 2020;31(3):482–90.

Source Global Research. The rise of independent professional work & changing demand from European employers. 2018. https://www.odgersconnect.com/fileadmin/uploads/ob/Documents/The_Rise_of_Independent_Professional_Work___Changing_Demand_from_European_Employers.pdf. Accessed 31 Mar 2021.

Tan SSL, Goonawardene N. Internet health information seeking and the patient-physician relationship: a systematic review. J Med Internet Res. 2017;19(1):15.

Wells L. Health workforce: working for consumer-centred care health voices. Consumers Health Forum Australia. 2016. https://healthvoices.org.au/issues/november-2016/health-workforce-working-for-consumer-centred-care/. Accessed 22 May 2021.

Wood L. The $11.9 trillion global healthcare market: key opportunities and strategies (2014-2022). 2019. https://www.businesswire.com/news/home/20190625005862/en/11.9-Trillion-Global-Healthcare-Market-Key-Opportunities. Accessed 22 May 2021.

World Health Organization. Global strategy on human resources for health: workforce 2030. World Health Organization; 2016.

Chapter 10
The Globalisation of Health Information Work

Kathleen Gray

Abstract Globalisation in the health sector challenges conventions about the health workforce, such as where people in this workforce are trained and based geographically, how their work is conducted and regulated for safety and quality and consequently how health information flows. By reviewing scholarly literature on the COVID-19 pandemic, we can see some aspects of the globalisation of health information work, the people doing this work, the innovations they brought to this field of work and the challenges they faced. Three categories in this emergent workforce are described: distinct types of specialists, multidisciplinary coalitions of various kinds of workers, and non-professional Internet users. This review pinpoints some kinds of work that will tend to promote greater globalisation of the HIDDIN workforce and some types of health information challenges that globalisation cannot address without deliberate cooperation at the highest levels in the workforce.

Keywords COVID-19 · Global health · Internet · Public health · Infodemic

Introduction

Globalisation refers to the economic interdependence of countries as a result of heightened international transactions of goods and services, free flow of capital, cross-border migration, and rapid diffusion of new technologies (International Monetary Fund 2002). It is reinforced and intensified by the rise of Internet capacity

K. Gray (✉)
Centre for Digital Transformation of Health, University of Melbourne,
Melbourne, VIC, Australia
e-mail: kgray@unimelb.edu.au

and capabilities that support teleworking and the gig economy (Todoli-Signes 2017), and it affects the health sector. Governments that are signatories to the pertinent United Nations treaties accept that they have a legal obligation to ensure that their citizens have access to timely, acceptable, and affordable health care of appropriate quality and to provide for the underlying determinants of health (World Health Organization 2017). Still, even though we think of health services being the jurisdiction of local and national governments, a combination of market forces and biomedical and technological innovations enables some people to supply and consume health care that is beyond the jurisdiction of specific national governments (Ormond and Toyota 2018). Global economic forces influence cross-border supply, consumption abroad, and the presence or absence of trained personnel and of commercial interests (Smith and Hanefield 2018).

Globalisation of this kind challenges conventions about the health workforce, such as where people in this workforce are trained and based geographically, how their work is conducted and regulated for safety and quality and consequently how health information flows. Some aspects of health care continue to rely on the physical proximity of the patient and the professional, but many other aspects are becoming more possible to accomplish through virtual care (Webster 2020). Similarly, some of the data, information, and knowledge technologies that provide the infrastructure for health care are developed and maintained in and for distinct localities, but digital health is recognised as a global industry (Conor 2020).

What effect does the globalisation of health services have on that section of the health workforce that we call HIDDIN (Health Informatics, Digital, Data, Information and kNowledge management) and, conversely, what influence does the HIDDIN workforce have in the globalisation process? Changes in the world of work driven by the COVID-19 pandemic offer a chance to answer these questions. The pandemic accelerated remote working, disrupted traditional modes of supply and demand and distribution, and also amplified well-known problems such as the digital divide and antisocial uses of the Internet, generally. Information management and information technologies moved to the forefront across social and economic activities, including health care and health research; the ensuing changes to the nature of work—crowdsourcing; process automation; virtual workplaces and teams; the shift to online learning—have the potential to affect the HIDDIN workforce as much as other areas of the health workforce, or perhaps more (Barnes 2020; O'Leary 2020).

The global response to the pandemic had a number of elements that were drivers for new forms of engagement in HIDDIN work. The spread of the virus outpaced localised disease management and triggered renewed attention to World Health Organisation programmes and functions (Tangcharoensathien et al. 2020). Health authorities lost control of public health analysis and reporting standards, as social media placed the power of communication in the hands of anyone who chose to comment publicly (Hou et al. 2020). Thus, the World Health Organisation declared that the pandemic was accompanied by an "infodemic:" "From selling fake coronavirus cures online to a cyberattack on hospitals' critical information systems, criminals are exploiting the COVID-19 crisis, the United Nations has warned, as it also steps up its fight against a proliferation of false information about the virus." (World Health Organization 2020). The idea of an infodemic originated during the SARS epidemic when it was explained thus: "A few facts, mixed with fear, speculation and rumour, amplified and relayed swiftly worldwide by modern information technologies, have affected national and international economies, politics and even security in ways that are utterly disproportionate with the root realities." (Rothkopf 2003).

As the COVID-19 infodemic unfolded in 2020, health information scientists were quick to grasp the information innovations the health sector needed. One area of innovation was managing new volumes of information about sample collection testing and reporting; about critical equipment and drugs in supply chains, and the movements of supply vehicles; about tracking hospital bed and ICU availability; about monitoring patients and people in quarantine (Lal, in Dwivedi et al. 2020). Another area was systems work generated by newly designed COVID-19 apps: managing privacy, crowdsourcing, donating data, tracking cases, and updating models (O'Leary 2020). Another was developing new cost-effective models, frameworks, policies, and applications for delivering healthcare in a post-COVID-19 world (Barnes 2020). Lastly, there was a need to investigate "the centrality of information in the COVID-19 disaster; what constitutes information systems value and success in the context of the COVID-19 pandemic; technology's role in the behavioural, temporal, societal, and organisational aspects of the pandemic; and the negative role of information systems in the COVID-19 pandemic" (Ågerfalk et al. 2020).

The health information work opportunities that arose have been categorised into two dimensions—"fighting against a pandemic" and "adjusting to a new normal"—and six themes—"expanding digital surveillance," "tackling the infodemic," "orchestrating data ecosystems," "adapting information behaviours," "developing the digital workplace," and "maintaining social distancing" (Pan and Zhang 2020). Categorising this globalised work is a start, but it is hard to know who has the expertise to match it. Certainly, no one in any workforce had prior experience of dealing with the combination of an infectious disease demanding such broad and deep decision-making and a digital information ecosystem with so many sources and channels (O'Leary 2020). It is important to those interested in the evolution of the HIDDIN workforce to capture the reality of what the associated health information work entailed and to determine who was doing it.

A Rapid Review of the Literature

This chapter summarises and synthesises globalisation trends in the type of HIDDIN work that the pandemic triggered, the people doing this work, the innovations they brought to this field of work and the challenges they faced. It does this through a rapid review of scholarly literature, with the rationale that "Health care decision makers often need to make decisions in limited timeframes and cannot await the completion of a full evidence review" (Polisena et al. 2015, p.1). Relevant articles were identified by a Google Scholar search in August 2020, "allintitle: COVID-19 information." Removing citation-only items and items with no English language full text yielded 400 papers. Papers were shortlisted first by inspecting titles for words that suggested activities or agents of information management/service/systems/technology. Included were items emphasising activities to do with the source/use/analysis of information and suggesting related work practices (e.g. job*; labo*r; perform*; role*; responsib*; staff*; task*; work*; etc.). Included agents could be healthcare workers, technology workers, administrators, entrepreneurs, patients, and citizens. The next step was to screen the abstracts of included items for references to human actions or agency. Shortlisted items were analysed to find content that mentioned or implied globalisalisation; open coding was used to identify key themes such as inter-country similarities in work, transborder work, worldwide work. If such content was found, further content was sought about details of what the work constituted and details about where, how and by whom the work was done. Final details were extracted about how this reflected changed work practices and what major issues arose in doing the work. This reduced the number of papers to around 100. These were winnowed by: removing multiple papers by the same author (e.g. author SL Pan), including only one representative paper about a topic (e.g. the influence of Twitter), and selecting papers so as to give a perspective from different parts of the world. The resulting 41 (roughly 10% of the items initially retrieved) offer a sample of substantial papers from many different disciplinary forums to illustrate the globalisation of health information work in the first year of the COVID-19 pandemic.

The Globalised Health Information Workforce

Table 10.1 summarises the types of people identified as doing COVID-19 related health information work and the work they did in the papers selected for review. It also summarises innovative elements of this work and challenging aspects of it. Table 10.1 arranges the workforce into three categories. Firstly, distinct types of workers were identified, for example, geographic information systems specialists: librarians; publishers. Some were very specific—proprietors of Facebook; pharmacists in low-income countries; plastic surgery society staff. Secondly, multidisciplinary coalitions of various kinds of workers appeared often. One example was community organisers collaborating with health workers, technology companies, and policy-makers; another example was workers in government agencies collaborating with others in non-government organisations and international news agencies. Finally, a non-professional type of worker emerged strongly from the literature—the health information consumer, the social media influencer, the anonymous Internet user in the crowd.

Table 10.1 Globalised health information workers and their COVID-19 health information work

The workers (Source)	The work: Details	Innovations	Challenges
Distinct identities			
Artificial intelligence researchers (Su et al. 2020)	Retrieving: Combine information extraction with state-of-the-art question answering and query focused multi-document summarisation techniques, selecting and highlighting evidence snippets from existing scientific literature in response to a query	A website for real-time interactions and open code for broader use and refinement	Breaking down a user query and rephrasing complex question sentences into several shorter and simpler queries that convey the same meaning remains a challenge for natural language processing.
Computer scientists (Way et al. 2020)	Translating: Online multi-lingual disease information for scientists and the public, using neural machine translation of English to and from French, Italian, German and Spanish	Minimising the need for translators and interpreters	Automated translation performance can deteriorate without additional training. There is no simple way to do a comparative evaluation of online translation services.
GIS specialists employed by governments (Rezaei et al. 2020)	Mapping: Use of geospatial data technology for systematic collection and representation of details and overview in each disease-affected country	Fast accurate tracking of disease location and spread	The data may not be transparently available to citizens. Mapping alone is insufficient for disease control.
Government agency copywriters (Ojo et al. 2020)	Writing: Making online information readable by the general public, using the SMOG index and US DHHS recommendations for reading levels	Specific attention to readability and comprehension of public health communications	Much public health information on many official websites are not understandable to people without a university education.
Government officials (Baveja et al. 2020)	Valuing: Producing and deploying a government-backed mobile app for citizen contact tracing through ubiquitous, real-time mobile technologies, with clear specifications of roles and responsibilities	An explicit value proposition for citizens to participate voluntarily in information sharing	Official gathering of citizens' personal information poses significant challenges in a free society.

(continued)

Table 10.1 (continued)

The workers (Source)	The work: Details	Innovations	Challenges
Government policy-makers (De Coninck et al. 2020)	Persuading: Ensuring the viability of conventional local news journalism to reach masses by providing incentives for local media outlets to publish reliable information	Journalism infrastructure grants	Business models for "old" media are losing out in competition with global new media.
Health professional society staff (Kearsley and Duffy 2020)	Coordinating: Filtering clinical information quickly and accurately to update clinical guidelines and protocols information in global professional and scientific channels	Professional organisations joining forces to produce a strong united platform with one message	There is a risk that professionals will experience alert fatigue, and important information may be lost in the "noise."
Health sciences librarians (Naeem and Bhatti 2020)	Guiding: Work to identify and collate, also create tools and resources for differentiating fact from false information, and publish these online	New public training and education roles for librarians	There is an increase in stories on social media that at first may appear credible but later prove false.
Journal editors (Song and Karako 2020)	Disseminating: Rapid review and publication of scientific papers, using journals' online advance publication platforms	Papers published simultaneously in English and Chinese to communicate rapidly in the international scientific community	Dissemination of reliable information, including transparent methods of identifying cases, sharing data, unfettered communication, and peer-reviewed research, is hard to do quickly.
Librarians (Ali and Gattti 2020)	Communicating: Creating and disseminating information to the public and to researchers by monitoring emerging resources and tools from publishers and agencies (across South Asia)	Joint responsibility among public, academic, medical, and specialist librarians	Libraries should do more about sharing other useful information, e.g. histories from those who are recovering; advice on lifestyle habits that can reduce the risk of disease.

Table 10.1   (continued)

The workers (Source)	The work: Details	Innovations	Challenges
Media platform proprietors (Wahgre and Seth 2020)	Managing: Influencing quality of information shared on social media platforms by supporting the fact checking and credible journalism; modifying how "explore" sections function or how search results are structured; algorithms for manipulating content to reduce users' interactions with misinformation; new or modified policies about content and user behaviour	New relationships being formed between governments, society, and platforms	Disinformation is overwhelming.
Media professionals (Andreu-Sanchez and Martín-Pascual 2020)	Visualising: using actual or scientific photographs of the virus and avoiding aesthetically retouched illustrations from stock image suppliers	The first electron microscope images SARS-CoV-2, the coronavirus that causes Covid-19, were captured between January and March 2020.	The original, real images are not interesting or informative for most audiences.
Pharmacists (Khatiwada et al. 2020)	Disseminating: providing information, including management approaches, psychological advice, home care and safety, and medical management of chronic comorbid illnesses, in addition to their usual role in providing drug information—both face-to-face in hospitals and central health sites and via teleconferencing and social media sites of drug information centres (in low-income countries)	Upgrading of drug information centres to disease information centres	Centres are understaffed for this work, and some work (e.g. mental health) is not within professional scope.

(continued)

Table 10.1 (continued)

The workers (Source)	The work: Details	Innovations	Challenges
Plastic surgery society staff (Al-Benna 2020)	Standardising: recommending information on websites of these groups in 67 countries, based on comparative review and analysis of content and reference to generic guidelines	The first initiative to evaluate information provided by national plastic surgery society websites	Presently there is little integration and standardisation between websites, governing bodies and plastic surgery societies.
Pseudo-experts encouraged/ employed by government agencies (Sukhankin 2020)	Misinforming: Content creation of falsified data, pseudo-science, and conspiracy theories for social media platforms and state-controlled satellite news media	Amplifying malicious public messages	Propagation of fake news via global social media complicates access to reliable information.
Public health agency staff (Li et al. 2020)	Delivering: using YouTube to deliver timely and accurate information in non-text formats reaching millions of viewers worldwide	Governments engaging with people who use video platforms to find health information	Over one-quarter of the most viewed YouTube videos contained misleading information.
Social media company proprietors, specifically Facebook (Tewfik et al. 2020)	Sharing: Enabling individuals and organisations to publish information, while taking minimal responsibility for content accuracy or quality	Volume and popularity of health misinformation at new levels	There is no easy policy remedy for the preponderance of inaccurate information.
Coalitions			
Artificial intelligence and information retrieval communities (Esteva et al. 2020)	Retrieving: Specialised search tools, using semantic search engines over the scientific literature, developed by teams from 20+ organisations around the world in response to a global research challenge	Combining advanced search technologies, a Wikipedia and PubMed pre-trained question answering system, and other tools for optimal retrieval	Systems that retrieve incorrect results to support frontline healthcare decisions could jeopardise trust and safety.
Authors, editors, peer-reviewers, and journal publishers (Rahimi and Adabi 2020)	Disseminating: Emphasis on COVID-19 related work through open access agreement among 100 academic journals, societies, institutes, and companies	Research and data on COVID-19 publicly available rapidly and widely	Rushed peer review can lead to unethical publishing.

Table 10.1   (continued)

The workers (Source)	The work: Details	Innovations	Challenges
Citizens, platform operators, and researchers (Rodriguez et al. 2020)	Overcoming misinformation: Promoting and sharing a great volume of scientifically-based messages to counter misinformation	Heightened imperative for scientists to increase their use of social media for dissemination	Misinformation has novelty value, leading active social media users to spread it, at the same time as there is long-term lack of investment by mainstream media in science journalism.
Community organisers, health workers, tech companies, and policymakers (Xie et al. 2020)	Combining: Coupling high-tech online and low-tech offline social connectivity services to deliver trustworthy information to older adults, family caregivers, and healthcare providers	Initiatives that take advantage of community organisers who understand the needs of their residents know the local resources available and can move quickly	Increased financial resources are needed for rapid, well-coordinated implementation.
Developers and community leaders of knowledge organisation systems (KOS) (Zeng et al. 2020)	Exchanging: Adapting classification systems, taxonomies, controlled glossaries, thesauri, subject headings, ontologies, and other types of KOS to integrate diverse information sources and targets as a base to support decision-making using semantic technology, data mining and machine learning approaches, graphs, and integration of often Internet based systems	Decentralised standardised search and retrieval systems, interactive maps and charts, repositories and databases	The knowledge and skill to deal with information overload and resolve semantic conflicts are unevenly distributed.
GIS developers and epidemiology researchers (Joao 2020)	Visualising: Dashboard for worldwide pandemic visualisation, drawing upon a data gathering strategy, a commercial GIS tool, and an open online platform	Rapid creation of a global public tool to report and monitor outbreaks as they unfold, with transparent data sources	The tool's output is vulnerable to source errors in data input.

(continued)

Table 10.1 (continued)

The workers (Source)	The work: Details	Innovations	Challenges
Government agencies, media, NGOs, international news sources, and opinion leaders (Fu et al. 2020)	Disclosing: Making information public, using public channels to release Information about cases, medical knowledge, containment policies and compliance	New areas for public policy and administration have arisen due to the scientific and social nature of the disease	Patient privacy and public interest must be balanced and transnational coordination of information disclosure is constrained by anti-globalism geopolitics.
Health care professionals, epidemiologists, and infectious disease experts (Ma et al. 2020)	Communicating: Exercising professional duty to bring evidence-based knowledge to the general public, using new channels such as webinars or online discussion groups	A collective "infodemic patrol" to engage media outlets, scientific agencies, governments	Misinformation is still widespread.
Health information managers and research ethics board members (Robinson 2020)	Governing: Hospital clinical data governance over data supplied to proprietary health databases to reduce risks associated with the assembly and analysis of large health data sets	International clinical dataset as the foundation for COVID-19 research	Disregard data governance can undermine research credibility.
Media professionals and medical librarians (Ashrafi-Rizi and Kazempour 2020)	Categorising: Teaching information literacy and health literacy to citizens so that they differentiate credible information and understand appropriate behaviour in times of crisis	A typology of pandemic information types: valid, comforting, perplexing, mis-, dis-, shocking, contradictory, doubtful (untrusted), progressive, postponed, confidential	To find the best behavioural model for dealing with crises, it is necessary to have knowledge and awareness about information production and dissemination infrastructure and familiarity with information types.
Mobile app proprietors and users (Vanoni et al. 2020)	Volunteering: Using volunteered geographic information collected across many different locations, collated by the developers of a city map mobile phone app, which gathers large amounts of open-source data generated by transport authorities, local transit authorities and individual users, supporting epidemiological analysis	A novel way to evaluate the effectiveness of government restrictions on personal movement	It is a complex matter to determine public interest uses of personal mobile phone data.

Table 10.1 (continued)

The workers (Source)	The work: Details	Innovations	Challenges
Public health agency scientists and technologists (Yu et al. 2020)	Curating: Scientific information about genomics and other precision health tools, through Web portal access into results of database extraction	Information filtering on an important aspect of the disease	Continuous updating of the database is labour intensive, and translational impact is not guaranteed.
Researchers and citizens (Aizawa et al. 2020)	Aggregating: Multi-lingual information aggregation, through a research collaboration that combines crowdsourcing, crawling, machine translation, and a topic classifier	Potential to enrich cross-language sharing of quality information	The complexity of the data processing slows the performance of the system.
Researchers, pharmacists, and allied health professionals (Razonable et al. 2020)	Appraising: Rapid literature reviewing teams with membership, from epidemiology, infection prevention and control, diagnostics, therapeutics, clinical care, and public health with results published at an authoritative medical information website	Multidisciplinary partnership among data analysts and clinical experts	Medical information has increased rapidly and exponentially.
Scientific authors and publishers (Homolak et al. 2020)	Publishing: Adopting open science principles and a mindful approach to data access when publishing research findings and data sets	Submission-to-publication time for most journals reduced tenfold.	It is possible that we are sacrificing the quality of journal content in exchange for speed and reach.
Teachers and parents (Iivari et al. 2020)	Integrating: Incorporating information management and digitalisation topics during the sudden, unexpected digital transformation of children's basic education (Finland and India)	Making visible how significant the field of information management is in supporting and understanding digitalisation, and that through design and digital technology, we can make the world better	Established technology, practices, skills, attitudes, and cultural factors may be barriers to digital transformation.

(continued)

Table 10.1 (continued)

The workers (Source)	The work: Details	Innovations	Challenges
Amorphous workforce			
Community champions among marginalised groups (Schiavo 2020)	Correcting: Dispelling misinformation and false claims about vaccination; building collaborations among clinicians, policy-makers, community leaders, families, academia, and organisations from the public, for profit and non-profit sectors	Improving health and media literacy as well as civic literacy	A great deal of vaccine-related misinformation is spread via social media.
Consumer health information users (Phillips 2020)	Consuming: Choosing information wisely by using health library and information service guidelines and tools	Public participation in the creation of the "vaccine against misinformation"	Misinformation is widespread and readily transmitted.
Crowdsources (Khan Pathan 2020)	Releasing: Providing alternative public access to information about infections, active cases, deaths, critical conditions, infected areas, hospitals, and questioning official information, via crowdsourced contributors to electronic media	New interest in critiquing official versions of events	Even some of the richest and the most developed countries' governments may not be releasing all information to the public.
Health information-seekers (Parshakov et al. 2020)	Searching: Global internet searching using Google search engine	Search intensity depends not only on a nation's disease dynamics, but also on cultural characteristics of that nation	Governmental communication strategies may not address cultural characteristics effectively.
Online opinion leaders (OOL) (Yin et al. 2020)	Propagating: Promoting the development of public opinion on social media platforms, by forwarding/reposting messages accessible to large numbers of followers	Original message communicators understanding of OOL behaviour, so as to design effective communication strategies	Mechanisms are not in place for persuading OOL to shape public understanding of official messages quickly and appropriately.

Table 10.1   (continued)

The workers (Source)	The work: Details	Innovations	Challenges
Prominent commentators (Matthews 2020)	Misinforming: Social media and mainstream media posts, via global online platforms, building up scientifically unfounded criticisms of the national response in a particular country (e.g. in Japan)	Renewing debate about the part played by culture and associated behaviours in reasons for differences among countries	Media attention to cultural differences may mask failures in governance and government responses, and may reinforce stereotypes about cultural behaviours.
Social media influencers (Alqurashi et al. 2020)	Diffusing: Super-spreading of large amounts of information over social media platforms such as Twitter, Instagram, YouTube, Reddit, and Gab.	A global view of Arabic language information dissemination	A focus on the language of content does not necessarily tell us about reliability of information.
Social media users, esp of Twitter (Singh et al. 2020)	Sharing: Tweeting and retweeting disease information in conversations from 217 countries	Possibility to predict global disease outbreak and spread by geotagging conversations	Misinformation is being circulated around the world in more than 30 languages.

HIDDIN Workforce Implications

The force of globalisation, as illustrated by the pandemic, puts pressure on our current understanding of the health information workforce; the health information work and workers described during the pandemic are less conventional and more inclusive than we might expect. This review found that the infodemic that accompanied the pandemic created many vital and stimulating globalised roles and responsibilities for health information workers. However, role titles do not readily convey that specialised health information work is being carried out in those roles, and workers taking on the roles do not always align with existing professions' definitions of who "belongs" in this workforce. From this review, it seems too that many HIDDIN roles remain invisible; particular types of workers not mentioned in the literature here are IT infrastructure managers, data quality managers and informaticians. Descriptions of work of this kind within national boundaries certainly were published, but details of how global work was being done by people in these roles lacked the scholarly profiling that one might expect.

The review highlighted two key features of the globalisation of the HIDDIN workforce. One feature is the emphasis on participation in complex, changing interprofessional workgroups to achieve impact at scale. This is not a field where sole practitioners can succeed, except as consultants to workgroup sponsors and convenors. The other feature is the ascendency of influential efforts by online communities of laypeople, doing roles across a spectrum of health information work. This underlines the importance of formally trained professionals being ready and willing to advise and support this active, worldwide part of the health information workforce.

Familiar terms to describe HIDDIN work appeared in a range of variants: retrieval, curation, integration, and sharing. There were also less conventional ways of describing the work: personalisation, evasion, framing, orchestration, even war. It is dismaying to note that a professional specialisation appears to be emerging to perform work that is agnostic about the scientific quality and benefit of health information content, but skilled at synthesising and distributing (dis)information to serve geopolitical purposes.

This review pinpointed some kinds of work that will inevitably tend to promote greater globalisation of the HIDDIN workforce. Examples include large-scale international data sharing using standards and communication protocols; near real-time scientific information dissemination through open research platforms and new scientific publishing models; rapid multichannel public health information sharing and validation using a considered mix of formal and informal Internet outlets; curation and analysis and representation of data about Internet searching and social media sharing topics.

The lesson of the pandemic is that the professionals conventionally identified with the HIDDIN workforce are meeting some—but not all—of the needs of a globalised health sector. Globalisation brings challenges that HIDDIN workforce professions have not resolved; resolving them is a major a test that may determine whether these professions have a future. The challenges include imperfect and uneven health data collection; multi-lingual scientific information dissemination; incompatible jurisdictional laws and regulations regarding individual data privacy; inconsistent information behaviours of citizens under social and economic stress; commercialisation constraints on the flow of information, e.g. about drug development. Deliberate efforts to overcome these challenges are required at very senior levels in the professions concerned before a formally qualified specialised HIDDIN workforce can be recognised as a serious influence on the way the world works with health information.

Limitations of the rapid review method, considering only the period up to the end of July 2020, mean that it will need expanding and updating to develop a fuller picture. As well, the generic health information search terms may have obscured insights into the globalised workplace for specialised data management and knowledge management workers that the pandemic has created. Another limitation is that studying the context of the pandemic is by no means an exhaustive way to explore the topic of health information workforce globalisation. Further research might reveal transborder work trends driven by a particular multinational corporation's dominance in the health information systems market, or by widespread consumer demand for personal health information technologies such as an app or a wearable, or by an international agency sponsoring a major investment in health information technology infrastructure. Indeed, one or more drivers of this kind may gain momentum from humanity's post-pandemic realisations about our shared health care needs. If so, there are likely to be further worldwide repercussions for HIDDIN workforce skills, supply, demand, and logistics.

References

Ågerfalk PJ, Conboy K, Myers MD. Information systems in the age of pandemics: COVID-19 and beyond. Eur J Inf Syst. 2020;29(3):203–7.

Aizawa A, Bergeron F, Chen J, Cheng F, Hayashi K, Inui K, Ito H, Kawahara D, Kitsuregawa M, Kiyomaru H, Kobayashi M. A system for worldwide COVID-19 information aggregation. arXiv preprint arXiv:2008.01523. 2020. Accessed 28 Jul 2020.

Al-Benna S. Availability of COVID-19 information from National and International Aesthetic Surgery Society websites. Aesthet Plast Surg. 2020;44(3):1043–6. https://doi.org/10.1007/s00266-020-01751-w.

Ali MY, Gatiti P. The COVID-19 (Coronavirus) pandemic: reflections on the roles of librarians and information professionals. Health Inf Libr J. 2020;37(2):158–62.

Alqurashi S, Alashaikh A, Alanazi E. Identifying information superspreaders of COVID-19 from Arabic tweets. Preprints. 2020. https://doi.org/10.20944/preprints202007.0228.v1.

Andreu-Sánchez C, Martín-Pascual MÁ. Fake images of the SARS-CoV-2 coronavirus in the communication of information at the beginning of the first Covid-19 pandemic. El Profesional de la Información. 2020;29(3):e290309.

Ashrafi-Rizi H, Kazempour Z. Information typology in coronavirus (COVID-19) crisis; a commentary. Arch Acad Emerg Med. 2020;8(1):e19.

Barnes SJ. Information management research and practice in the post-COVID-19 world. Int J Inf Manag. 2020:102175.

Baveja A, Kapoor A, Melamed B. Stopping Covid-19: a pandemic-management service value chain approach. Ann Oper Res. 2020:1.

Conor D. Global digital health market size 2019 and 2026 forecast. 2020. https://www.statista.com/statistics/1092869/global-digital-health-market-size-forecast/.

De Coninck D, d'Haenens L, Matthijs K. Forgotten key players in public health: news media as agents of information and persuasion during the COVID-19 pandemic. Public Health. 2020;183:65.

Dwivedi YK, Hughes DL, Coombs C, Constantiou I, Duan Y, Edwards JS, Gupta B, Lal B, Misra S, Prashant P, Raman R. Impact of COVID-19 pandemic on information management research and practice: transforming education, work and life. Int J Inf Manag. 2020:102211.

Esteva A, Kale A, Paulus R, Hashimoto K, Yin W, Radev D, Socher R. Co-search: Covid-19 information retrieval with semantic search, question answering, and abstractive summarization. arXiv preprint arXiv:2006.09595. 2020.

Fu Y, Ma W, Wu J. Fostering voluntary compliance in the COVID-19 pandemic: an analytical framework of information disclosure. Am Rev Public Adm. 2020:0275074020942102.

Homolak J, Kodvanj I, Virag D. Preliminary analysis of COVID-19 academic information patterns: a call for open science in the times of closed borders. Scientometrics. 2020:1–5.

Hou Z, Du F, Zhou X, Jiang H, Martin S, Larson H, Lin L. Cross-country comparison of public awareness, rumors, and behavioral responses to the COVID-19 epidemic: infodemiology study. J Med Internet Res. 2020;22(8):e21143.

Iivari N, Sharma S, Ventä-Olkkonen L. Digital transformation of everyday life–How COVID-19 pandemic transformed the basic education of the young generation and why information management research should care? Int J Inf Manag. 2020:102183.

International Monetary Fund. Globalization: threat or opportunity? 2002. www.imf.org/external/np/exr/ib/2000/041200to.htm. Accessed 31 Mar 2021.

Joao BN. Geographic information systems and COVID-19: The Johns Hopkins University dashboard. 2020. https://doi.org/10.21203/rs.3.rs-15447/v1.

Kearsley R, Duffy CC. The COVID-19 information pandemic: how have we managed the surge? Anaesthesia. 2020.

Khan Pathan AS. Access to information vs blocking of information during COVID-19 pandemic: a governance dilemma in the era of crowdsourcing based on ICT. Int J Comput Appl. 2020;42(6):531–2.

Khatiwada AP, Shakya S, Shrestha S. Paradigm shift of drug information centers during the COVID-19 pandemic. Drugs Therapy Perspect. 2020;36(9):389–95.

Li HO, Bailey A, Huynh D, Chan J. YouTube as a source of information on COVID-19: a pandemic of misinformation? BMJ Glob Health. 2020;5(5):e002604.

Ma X, Vervoort D, Luc JG. When misinformation goes viral: access to evidence-based information in the COVID-19 pandemic. J Glob Health Sci. 2020;2(1).

Matthews J. "Cultural exceptionalism" in the global exchange of (mis) information around Japan's responses to Covid-19. Media Commun. 2020;8(2):448–51.

Naeem SB, Bhatti R. The Covid-19 'infodemic': a new front for information professionals. Health Inf Libr J. 2020;

O'Leary DE. Evolving information systems and technology research issues for COVID-19 and other pandemics. J Organ Comput Electron Commer. 2020:1–8.

Ojo PM, Okeowo TO, Thampy AM, Kabir Z. Readability of selected governmental and popular health organization websites on Covid-19 public health information: a descriptive analysis. medRxiv. 2020.

Ormond M, Toyota M. Transnationalizing the provision of care (Ch.34). In: Routledge handbook of health geography. Abingdon: Routlege; 2018.

Pan SL, Zhang S. From fighting COVID-19 pandemic to tackling sustainable development goals: an opportunity for responsible information systems research. Int J Inf Manag. 2020:102196.

Parshakov P, Permyakova TM, Zavertiaeva M. Health information search during COVID-19: does culture matter? 2020. Available at SSRN 3625158. Accessed 11 Jun 2020.

Phillips K. No, Bananas don't cure HIV, nor will garlic cure COVID-19: searching for, assessing, and consuming health information online. J Consumer Health Internet. 2020;24(2):175–85.

Polisena J, Garritty C, Kamel C, Stevens A, Abou-Setta AM. Rapid review programs to support health care and policy decision making: a descriptive analysis of processes and methods. Syst Rev. 2015;4:26.

Rahimi F, Abadi ATB. Ethical and sensible dissemination of information during the COVID-19 pandemic. Am J Bioeth. 2020:1–3.

Razonable RR, Marshall WF, Stevens RW, Kumar S, Murad MH, Wilson WR. Mayo clinic strategies for COVID-19 rapid appraisal system for COVID-19 medical information. Mayo Clin Proc. 2020.

Rezaei M, Nouri AA, Park GS, Kim DH. Application of geographic information system in monitoring and detecting the COVID-19 outbreak. Iran J Public Health. 2020;49:114–6.

Robinson K. A false promise of COVID-19 'big' health data? Health data integrity and the ethics and realities of Australia's health information management practice. Health Inf Manag J. 2020:1833358320941190.

Rodríguez CP, Carballido BV, Redondo-Sama G, Guo M, Ramis M, Flecha R. False news around COVID-19 circulated less on Sina Weibo than on Twitter. How to overcome false information? Int Multidiscipl J Soc Sci. 2020:1–22.

Rothkopf D. When the buzz bites back. Wash Post. 2003. https://www.washingtonpost.com/archive/opinions/2003/05/11/when-the-buzz-bites-back/bc8cd84f-cab6-4648-bf58-0277261af6cd/. Accessed 31 Mar 2021.

Schiavo R. Vaccine communication in the age of COVID-19: Getting ready for an information war. J Comm Healthc. 2020;2:73–5.

Singh L, Bansal S, Bode L, Budak C, Chi G, Kawintiranon K, Padden C, Vanarsdall R, Vraga E, Wang Y. A first look at COVID-19 information and misinformation sharing on Twitter. arXiv preprint arXiv:2003.13907. 2020. Accessed 31 Mar 2020.

Smith R, Hanefeld J. Globalization, trade, and health economics. In: Oxford research encyclopedia of economics and finance. 2018. https://doi.org/10.1093/acrefore/9780190625979.013.35. Accessed 31 Mar 2020.

Song P, Karako T. COVID-19: Real-time dissemination of scientific information to fight a public health emergency of international concern. Biosci Trends. 2020;14(1):1–2.

Su D, Xu Y, Yu T, Siddique FB, Barezi E, Fung P. CAiRE-COVID: A question answering and query-focused multi-document summarization system for COVID-19 scholarly information management. 2020. https://openreview.net/forum?id=1A83-27cVDW. Accessed 31 Mar 2021.

Sukhankin S. COVID-19 as a tool of information confrontation: Russia's approach. University of Calgary School of Public Policy Publications. 2020;13.

Tangcharoensathien V, Calleja N, Nguyen T, Purnat T, D'Agostino M, Garcia-Saiso S, Landry M, Rashidian A, Hamilton C, AbdAllah A, Ghiga I. Framework for managing the COVID-19 infodemic: methods and results of an online, crowdsourced WHO technical consultation. J Med Internet Res. 2020;22(6):e19659.

Tewfik G, Aziz R, Shulman S, Naftalovich R, Gilels S. Shared content on Facebook often propagates inaccurate or misleading information regarding Covid-19. 2020. https://doi.org/10.21203/rs.3.rs-31047/v1. Accessed 31 Mar 2021.

Todolí-Signes A. The end of the subordinate worker? Collaborative economy, on-demand economy, gig economy, and the crowdworkers' need for protection. Int J Comparative Labour Law Indus Relat (IJCLLIR). 2017;33(2). https://ssrn.com/abstract=2899383. Accessed 31 Mar 2021.

Vanoni M, McKee M, Bonell C, Semenza J, Stuckler D. Using volunteered geographic information to assess mobility in the COVID-19 pandemic context: cross-city time series analysis of 41 cities in 22 countries from March 2nd to 26th 2020. 2020. https://doi.org/10.21203/rs.3.rs-22924/v2. Accessed 31 Mar 2021.

Waghre P, Seth R. Analysing digital platforms' responses to COVID-19 information disorder. Takshashila Institution. 2020. https://takshashila.org.in//. Accessed 31 Mar 2021.

Way A, Haque R, Xie G, Gaspari F, Popović M, Poncelas A. Rapid development of competitive translation engines for access to multilingual COVID-19 information. Informatics. 2020;7(2):19.

Webster P. Virtual health care in the era of COVID-19. Lancet. 2020;395(10231):1180–1.

World Health Organization. Human rights and health. Key facts. 2017. https://www.who.int/en/news-room/fact-sheets/detail/human-rights-and-health. Accessed 31 Mar 2021.

World Health Organization. Department of Global Communications. UN tackles 'infodemic' of misinformation and cybercrime in COVID-19 crisis. 2020. https://www.un.org/en/un-coronavirus-communications-team/un-tackling-%E2%80%98infodemic%E2%80%99-misinformation-and-cybercrime-covid-19. Accessed 31 Mar 2021.

Xie B, Charness N, Fingerman K, Kaye J, Kim MT, Khurshid A. When going digital becomes a necessity: ensuring older adults' needs for information, services, and social inclusion during COVID-19. J Aging Social Policy. 2020:1–1.

Yin F, Xia X, Song N, Zhu L, Wu J. Quantify the role of superspreaders-opinion leaders-on COVID-19 information propagation in the Chinese Sina-microblog. PLoS One. 2020;15(6):e0234023.

Yu W, Gwinn M, Khoury MJ. A new resource for genomics and precision health information and publications on the investigation and control of COVID-19 and other coronaviruses. BioRxiv. 2020.

Zeng ML, Hong Y, Clunis J, He S, Coladangelo LP. Implications of knowledge organization systems for health information exchange and communication during the COVID-19 pandemic. Data Inf Manag. 2020;4(3):148–70.

Part IV
Impact

Chapter 11
Leadership Roles in the Specialist Digital Health Workforce

Tiffany I. Leung, Karen H. Wang, Terika McCall, and Frits van Merode

Abstract Leadership roles in the specialist digital health workforce are incredibly heterogeneous. No one single career pathway suits all aspiring leaders and as society and healthcare become increasingly digitised, the opportunities for new careers grow. Content and methodological expertise form solid foundations for leaders, combined with clear organisational strategy and vision, and the ability to foster work environments for diverse and highly skilled teams to collaborate on innovative projects and programs. This chapter covers foundational principles and important normative considerations for leaders in digital health and provides selected examples.

Keywords Leadership · Diversity · Inclusion · Professional development

Introduction

Health Informatics, Digital, Data, Information and kNowledge (HIDDIN) careers and professional training pathways are highly diverse, leading to a variety of specialised leadership roles. Leadership roles can encompass several scopes which are not mutually exclusive: clinical or non-clinical responsibilities; research across

T. I. Leung (✉) · F. van Merode
Care and Public Health Research Institute/Maastricht University Medical Center+,
Maastricht, The Netherlands
e-mail: t.leung@maastrichtuniversity.nl; f.vanmerode@maastrichtuniversity.nl

K. H. Wang · T. McCall
Center for Medical Informatics, Yale School of Medicine, New Haven, CT, USA
e-mail: karen.wang@yale.edu; terika.mccall@yale.edu

K. Butler-Henderson et al. (eds.), *The Health Information Workforce*,
Health Informatics, https://doi.org/10.1007/978-3-030-81850-0_11

171

basic, translational, and applied health and services or implementation sciences; local, regional, national, and international governmental or non-governmental organisations, which may involve interagency or intersectoral collaborations; entrepreneurial pursuits; and more. This chapter covers foundational principles and important normative considerations for leaders across this workforce. Such principles may be applicable across various career pathways. Leadership profiles and project examples in this chapter are by no means a complete catalogue of possibilities.

To achieve a leadership role, training or hands-on experience is foundational in developing the identity and scope of work for a digital health specialist. Training, for clinicians and non-clinicians, may involve degree-seeking masters-level programs, doctoral programs, or accredited and non-accredited postdoctoral training programs (e.g., Accreditation Council for Graduate Medical Education accredited clinical informatics fellowships for physicians, or National Library of Medicine and other fellowship programs, in the United States of America [USA]). Training program titles in relevant disciplines (e.g., library science, computer science, management science, etc.) may or may not identify health informatics or health analytics explicitly. Formal training programs may not be required; future leaders may instead perform on-the-job work with or without pursuing online learning, acquiring certifications, or working as visiting scholars in academia or interns in industry. However, progressing to a HIDDIN workforce leadership role with a specialised degree or certification is becoming the norm as more customised training programs become available.

Leaders must build on a foundation of expertise, developing a set of advanced skills and competencies that advance their organisation's strategic vision and priorities. In specialist digital health work, common and universal leadership skills draw from multiple disciplines, including organisational management, social sciences and organisational behaviour, organisational professionalism and ethics, and even compassion research and training. Due to the diversity of work and training pathways towards specialist roles in digital health, leaders are vital agents towards achieving the organisation's goals.

Leadership Traits and Skills

In general, effective leaders enable organisational growth, learning, and resilience. Leaders are responsible for engendering organisational professionalism (Egener et al. 2017), which can translate into ensuring a physically and psychologically safe organisation and work environment with a sustainable work culture. This may further include enacting organisational policies that promote diversity, equity, and inclusion in the organisation's workforce to achieve the organisation's mission. The important roles of community and patient partnerships as well as ethical operations and business practice also should be prioritised; this chapter explores these further through a health equity lens on leadership.

Regarding operations and business practices, a well-known paradigm in this field is the learning health system, in which information technologies, standards, and policies are designed in support of healthcare infrastructure that facilitates evidence-based and practice-based healthcare delivery, public health activities, biomedical research, quality improvement, and other population and social services (Friedman et al. 2010). It describes the idea of a virtuous cycle of data-driven practice and evidence-based medicine advancing healthcare (Chambers et al. 2016; Leung and van Merode 2018). To build a learning health system, or lead an organisation that will engage in partnership with others, a leader may need to be especially adept at recognising their unit's needs in terms of operating structures and design.

A leadership role engages in at least one of two functions, strategy making and providing an organising function for their unit or organisation. Strategy making is explored in subsequent sections of this chapter. The organising function, in which the leader is responsible for best matching the design and structure of the unit to achieve its goals within its host organisation, is vital to achieving the unit's goals. For example, organisational design and structures implemented or enforced by leaders may uniquely impact clinical care settings, where logistical and management control can be essential in supporting multiple specialised units or departments providing patient care services. Several units may need their own specialisation with their own logistics devices to meet the needs of different patient populations. However, this can lead to fragmentation and even siloes in healthcare services. At the same time, these units may not be large enough to operate autonomously, for example, because of the use of infrastructure and technology that is connected with other units (e.g., clinical departments or specialties, or functional departments or services such as laboratory or imaging services). Consequently, this requires logistical controls that have a high degree of integration and are capable of taking the specific requirements of each unit into account.

In other words, a leader takes into account not only the entire organisation, but also the resources that it can provide for the differentiated parts to function well and achieve their aims within the whole system. Thus, a leader may need to consider organisational development in system design, with their effort dedicated to the right combination of integration and differentiation. From this perspective, integration is defined as the joint effort of organisational subsystems to affect organisational tasks (Lawrence and Lorsch 1967); and differentiation of organisational units concerns the segmentation of the organisation into subsystems. They perform some of the organisational tasks, but do so in a way that specifically aligns with the task environment (Lawrence and Lorsch 1967). The necessary level of integration is determined by the perceived need for joint decision-making. The degree of differentiation is strongly related to the need for specialisation of subsystems and the specificity of their task environments. Box 11.1 gives an example of when a leader might be called on to balance these organisational structures within a hospital system; this is challenging because organising methods are often very different (van der Ham A et al. 2020). Full integration of healthcare and patient logistics will only be achieved through an effective shared real-time decision-making culture combined with good real-time data provision and physical and digital infrastructures.

> **Box 11.1 MijnIBDCoach: Building a Cross-Disciplinary and Sector Platform**
> Gastroenterologists, in partnership with both academic and non-academic hospitals and a private company, Sananet, developed the MijnIBDCoach, an information technology platform in support of patients with inflammatory bowel disease (IBD), including Crohn's disease and ulcerative colitis (de Jong et al. 2017a). Patients with IBD often are knowledgeable in managing their disease with the right guidance and information. The MijnIBDCoach makes it possible for patients to contribute and transmit data on a daily basis to their clinical care team. As a smartphone or web-based app, instant feedback can be provided to the patient as needed to facilitate self-management. At the same time, a nurse monitors the health status of the patients via a dashboard. If necessary, the patient may be advised to come to the Gastroenterology (GI) clinic and such a visit can be arranged with a very short access time. For example, in a traditional clinical workflow, patients with Crohn's disease have at least one scheduled annual check-up, which is also quite common for other chronic conditions. Diagnostics and surveys of patients' symptoms may be performed, with variable value for the annual visit, as the disease may be quiescent and minimal meaningful information is exchanged between the patient and care team. Additionally, the annual visit appointment can be made weeks or sometimes months in advance, which can contribute to access delays overall for the GI clinics. Furthermore, if disease activity increases and the patient becomes increasingly symptomatic, an intervening visit to the GI clinic would be needed. However, with the development and implementation of MijnIBDCoach, the number of mandatory yet low-value annual visits decreases considerably. The platform allows for collection of patient-reported outcomes and other data from the patient that allow for coordination and completion of on-demand visits on the same or next day, promptly addressing disease instability or changes, without compromising patient care quality (van den Heuvel et al. 2017). Consequently, with digital health leadership, the clinical workflow shifts largely away from routine outpatient clinic appointments to remote monitoring, patient self-management and engagement, and care on demand, with a statistically significant reduction in utilisation of outpatient clinic appointments and a reduction in access time (de Jong et al. 2017b).

Leaders should have a working and updated knowledge of current ethical standards in the field. Especially in digital health, policy changes may significantly impact operations with regard to all data activities and infrastructure (Séroussi et al. 2020). In particular, privacy, confidentiality, and informed consent issues are commonly encountered; however, lack of transparency and explicability of clinical information systems, particularly artificial intelligence and machine learning applications, is ethically problematic (Hübner et al. 2020). Furthermore, the primary and secondary uses and applications of those data are subject to ethical principles, such as the use of information technologies "for good and not evil" (Goodman 2020).

Leaders also have a responsibility to foster an organisational culture conducive for workers to achieve the unit's goals. This may include reducing hierarchy and power distance between employees and their supervisors, and between employees and their coworkers, in order to promote collaboration and reduce unnecessary siloing and competition in the workplace. Enabling interprofessional teamwork may be especially pronounced in digital health work because it involves knowledge work, such as information management, information exchange, and knowledge sharing. Barriers to knowledge sharing and exchange can stymie advancement of the organisation or even the field overall (Lifshitz-Assaf 2018). Another aspect of leadership in work culture is to foster an ethical work climate, in which institutionalised normative systems best match the types of work and communication among workers (Victor and Cullen 1988). Why and how to foster an ethical work climate with special attention to principles of well-being, diversity, equity, and inclusion are discussed next.

Digital Health Leadership for Workforce Well-Being

Digital health leaders are central in influencing those practicing and pursuing HIDDIN careers, as well as shaping the work experiences of those who are end-users of information technologies and digital health tools that are designed or deployed by their organisation. Such influences can be especially vital in sustaining the productivity of diverse HIDDIN professionals. Consequently, promoting workplace well-being warrants special attention to the design of a healthy and sustainable workplace for the digital health experts needed to facilitate the design, deployment, and evaluation of technologies that are equitable, accessible, and as diverse as the populations that they serve.

Despite the rapidly expanding body of literature describing the impact of poorly designed, deployed, or evaluated technologies on clinician burnout—for example, electronic health records—there remains a stark lack of focus on well-being or burnout in the HIDDIN workforce, but we can draw inferences from available data. In market research surveying nurses' experiences using electronic health records (EHR) in 2014, only 15% of the more than 14,000 registered nurses across 40 U.S. states believed that their information technology (IT) department was knowledgeable and receptive to suggestions on improving electronic documentation. Among IT professionals surveyed in the United Kingdom in 2013, two-thirds of IT administrators considered their jobs stressful and 63% of IT staff felt as stressed or more stressed than friends or colleagues, with management the most commonly identified source of stress (35%). In academia, generally, graduate and postgraduate studies are also increasingly recognised as periods of high stress and risk for poor well-being; in one survey of over 6000 graduate students from six continents, more than one-third of respondents sought professional help for depression or anxiety that they attributed to their doctoral studies (Woolston 2019). An example of leadership on digital health specialist work-life concerns and workload sustainability comes from the USA, where addressing the well-being of physician trainees is an accreditation requirement for graduate medical education programs, including clinical informatics subspecialty fellowships.

Leaders should be aware of, even if not engaging specifically in, organisational structures and culture that positively influence employees' well-being and engagement at work. Work engagement is seen as an antidote for burnout and can be promoted through increasing job resources, such as social supports at work, work support (e.g. supportive supervision, team efficiency, access to mentorship and sponsorship, etc.), increased work control such as worker influence over schedule and work planning or pace, and availability of performance feedback (Demerouti et al. 2001). Among clinicians, work engagement is associated with better work ability (Mache et al. 2013), fewer medical errors (Prins et al. 2009), and increased patient-safety-related behaviours and attitudes (Daugherty Biddison et al. 2016), even though better patient care experiences may not be a result (Scheepers et al. 2017). Promoting a culture of psychological safety, in which workers have a perception that there are no negative consequences of taking interpersonal risks, is foundational in enabling idea sharing and interactions (Edmondson and Lei 2014) and important for a productive organisation. However, these constructs have not been systematically studied in digital health workers, highlighting a gap in knowledge about leadership practices to support this workforce, including enhancing their professional development and mitigating attrition and turnover. System-, unit-, and individual level contributors to HIDDIN workers' well-being can also perpetuate workplace inequities and low workforce diversity. To avoid consequences that can be costly to the mission and goals of the unit or organisation, digital health leaders can better prepare to recognise and respond to HIDDIN workers' needs.

Leadership for Diversity, Equity, and Inclusion

Promoting diversity, equity, and inclusion (DEI) and incorporating DEI principles into everyday leadership benefits the HIDDIN workforce and broader society. Leaders in digital health should understand and have competencies in identifying the organisational structures and systems that foster racism, discrimination, and bias, so that they may take corrective actions in order to cultivate the next generation to be a more diverse workforce and to develop informatics tools and methods that do not facilitate inequities (Metzl and Hansen 2014). The aim in embracing such principles is to develop the tools necessary to counteract structural forces, thereby achieving health equity and justice. Leaders can drive healthcare system changes when they carry an awareness of both the structural determinants of health and also best practices in addressing how health inequities negatively affect the health of a population. For example, an equity-sensitive leader would have an understanding of data quality issues, such as data missingness on race or ethnicity or how such data are collected regarding the population their organisation serves, to ensure that services are equitable. Communicating this type of need and knowledge may be necessary to garner executive sponsorship for institutional resources to pursue this aim.

From a system perspective, the learning health system concept does not explicitly include social determinants of health as a component of personalised care (Nwaru et al. 2017). As healthcare systems strive towards the idea of a learning health system, a digital health leader with an understanding of local and regional health inequities could be well-positioned to recognise and incorporate such considerations explicitly into service evolution. Providing healthcare and related services to populations occurs within a complex adaptive system, in which each agent is interdependent and interacts with others, never acting in isolation; changes in one part of the system may influence changes in other parts of the system, intended or not (Waldrop 1993; Plsek and Greenhalgh 2001; Jaaron and Backhouse 2017). Ultimately, a leader in this environment is positioned to foster the needed creativity, learning and adaptability necessary to achieve organisational goals; the present Knowledge Era or Digital Age needs leaders who can address adaptability challenges—rather than technical challenges characteristic of the Industrial Age (Uhl-Bien et al. 2007).

Organisational leadership should design a just, equitable, diverse, and inclusive environment, as part of a larger effort towards organisational professionalism (Leung et al. 2019) and promoting a healthy workplace. Prior studies demonstrate that diversity of workforce fosters innovation and creativity (Phillips et al. 2006). Informational diversity results when people in groups can bring different perspectives, opinions, and information, social diversity in terms of their lived experiences based on societal hierarchies created based on racism, sexism, xenophobia, and other dimensions; such diversity offers unique considerations in group work (Phillips 2014). However, no single occupational category captures specialists in digital health; this is needed in order to provide data for leadership action to lift diversity in the workforce. This complicates further efforts to measure and ensure DEI in leadership.

One study found that between 2017 and 2019, men held leadership positions in 74.7% (71 of 95) of USA academic biomedical informatics programs and 83.3% (35 of 42) of clinical informatics fellowship programs (Griffin et al. 2021). There were no women clinical informatics fellowship program directors in 2018, even though the first such programs had been accredited 4 years earlier (Longhurst et al. 2016). Recently, professional societies are beginning to lead by example, investing in structures to increase DEI. For example, the American Medical Informatics Association (AMIA) developed targeted programs for racial and ethnic minority undergraduate college and university students and women in informatics; deployed a salary survey to begin understanding career and pay gaps; formed a Women in AMIA committee; and convened a Diversity, Equity, and Inclusion task force. A 2017 International Journal of Biomedicine and Healthcare special issue profiled renowned women informaticians towards this aim (Nyänken and Whitehouse 2017).

Digital health leaders can promote DEI through updating institutional policies and practices—for example, hiring practices with an awareness of implicit biases; equitable parental or partner leave policies—or sponsoring DEI task forces or committees to advise on such important considerations. Additionally, sponsoring and mentoring potential leaders is important to sustain diversity in the career pipeline, especially towards influential leadership roles. Leaders as sponsors may publicly support and advocate for protégés in support of their career advancement, recommending them for promotion, connecting them with other leaders, promoting their visibility, and essentially pulling them up the ladder with them (Hewlett 2011; Travis et al. 2013). Gender disparities remain problematic, as do racial, ethnic, and cultural disparities, in perpetuating inequitable access to career advancement opportunities (Hewlett 2011).

Digital health leadership is challenged further to tackle the effects of systemic racism as a key structural determinant of health and its role in creating health disparities, which re-emerged into mainstream dialogue in 2020. This was a result of glaring disparities in COVID-19 morbidity and mortality in Black, Latin, and First Nations populations as compared to White populations in the USA and other countries (Selden and Berdahl 2020; Chowkwanyun and Reed 2020). Also, it arose from the Black Lives Matter campaign fuelled by the violent death of countless Black people at the hands of police or other community members, and the wide acknowledgment of overt and covert racism faced by Black, indigenous, and people of colour (BIPOC) populations daily over generations, to the detriment of their well-being.

Previously unacknowledged bias in clinical medicine, such as predictive algorithms and machine learning (Rajkomar et al. 2018; Vyas et al. 2020), highlight the necessity of ethical, equitable applications of digital health. Structural racism embedded in information systems applications has been described in population access to social services (Eubanks 2018), arrest and incarceration rates (O'Neil 2016), access to and use of digital services like search engines, and even access to broadband internet (Noble 2018). In the last case, lack of access to broadband internet can widen the digital divide for populations who are unable to, for example, access telemedicine services during the COVID-19 pandemic (Rodriguez et al. 2020). Furthermore, data privacy and security as well as digital literacy, or the capabilities that one must develop to live, learn, and work in a digital society (Cooke 2018), remain vital ethical considerations in addressing health inequities (Rivera-Romero et al. 2020).

The importance of structural and social determinants of health and their effects on the well-being of individuals and their communities is increasingly recognised (Daniel et al. 2018; Byhoff et al. 2020). Digital health leadership can sharpen the focus on precision medicine initiatives and data collection efforts to capture social and behavioural determinants of health; both seek to leverage the large volumes of data and develop new data streams to improve individual and population health (Institute of Medicine 2014, 2015). Leaders need to raise awareness in the health sector and wider society that digital health data are critical in contributing to efforts to measure and facilitate individuals' and communities' abilities to intervene on these determinants of health (Veinot et al. 2019). However, considering the volume and sharing of such data, applications of information and computer technologies need to be ethical if they are to offer pathways towards health equity rather than further driving health disparities among patient populations. Thus leaders need to ensure patient engagement through community-based participatory informatics research, patient advisory boards, and citizen science.

Leadership in designing innovative healthcare service delivery options may be one way to help overcome some structural biases in healthcare systems. With high-level knowledge of health policy as well as access to voluminous data on vulnerable populations with poor healthcare access, digital health leaders have the opportunity to achieve a mission of social service. Box 11.2 describes a case of data-driven leadership and innovation, for a traditionally underserved population. In the USA, Medicare insurance coverage is available to all Americans 65 years of age and older and those with a disability; at the State level, Medicaid insurance coverage for low-income individuals is possible, but may vary in terms and services offered due to differences between States' health policies. Many people eligible for either or both insurances (dual eligibility) frequently have higher than average rates of chronic diseases, including mental health disorders, and may live in "health care deserts," where patients have trouble accessing a physician even if they are insured (Porter et al. 2017).

Box 11.2 Oak Street Health: Launching Community Healthcare Service Networks

Oak Street Health is a network of primary health centres in the USA, where a novel care model guides the design of both medical and non-medical services for elderly populations in low-income neighbourhoods. Due to their focus on the vulnerable elderly, they are also entering the social domain (Porter et al. 2017). Integrated health promotion services are offered proactively, whether elders are healthy or have medical conditions that require more management. Healthcare is delivered by a team (doctor, nurse, and care manager) seeing the sickest patients every 3 weeks and those who are healthy, every 3 months. Team nurses also visit patients in the hospital as needed, however prevention plays a prominent role in this care model, especially since the Oak Street Health business model is globally capitated and therefore allocates financial resources towards outpatient services and away from emergency rooms and hospitals. Leaders of this model report a 40% reduction in hospital admissions. Throughout the patient's care continuum, their health data are collected and integrated, as are their patient experience scores. The strength of the model lies in managing the overall coherence of both the patient process and the care system, through integrated data management and funding based on bundled payments. The model is unique in that patient flow to and from the hospital is moderated by primary care networks, and not by the hospital as frequently occurs elsewhere in the USA. Leadership of this innovative model of integrated primary care, constantly driven by digital data applications that directly benefit the community, serves to manage and improve the value-cost ratio of care.

Archetypal Leadership Roles

One quite extensive list of specialist digital health jobs and leadership roles has been published previously (Mack 2016), and the American Health Information Management Association publishes an interactive career map as well (https://my.ahima.org/careermap), however these still underrepresent the breadth of digital health leadership. The diversity of the workforce and the evolution of the domain lend to many possible leadership roles within or bridging different sectors, as well as involving work on a local, regional, national, or international scale. Here, we briefly describe a range of existing roles in and across academic, executive and government sectors, as a way to convey the leadership possibilities.

Academic leadership roles characteristically encompass directing education and research programs, some funded by governmental or institutional resources, some by philanthropic grants and/or industry funders, some by fees from individuals. These leaders are well-positioned to advocate for DEI, to advance science and practice in the field, and to influence the next generations in the workforce. These roles come with expectations that they will provide thought leadership and engage with integrity in defining education and research standards, overseeing accreditation and certification of individuals and organisations. This leadership is often accomplished through service on boards and committees of health agencies and professional societies.

Recognisable executive roles in health services include chief information or informatics officers (CIO), chief technology officers (CTO), and chief digital officers (CDO) all of whom may have varying but overlapping scopes in strategy development and implementation across an enterprise. A health services chief medical informatics officer (CMIO) may be responsible for system-wide information technology applications across clinical settings, including compliance, research, and training. For example, during the COVID-19 pandemic, this role may have overseen rapid implementation of telehealth and remote monitoring capabilities and workflows, as well as rapid development of analytics and decision support tools reflecting best available guidance on the diagnosis and treatment of infected patients. An emerging leadership role in health systems, the chief clinical informatics officer (CCIO) may be similarly responsible for leveraging health information systems, for example, reducing medical errors, promoting evidence-based care, and optimising the effectiveness of electronic documentation while minimising the administrative burden (Sengstack et al. 2016; Kannry et al. 2016). Kannry et al. (2016) offer a concise overview of additional executive roles that draw upon specific clinical disciplines, including chief nursing informatics officer (CNIO), chief pharmacy informatics officer (CPIO), chief dental informatics officer (CDIO), as well as the CMIO role. Another new executive leadership role is the chief research informatics officer (CRIO); the scope of this role most often includes developing and managing infrastructures, such as data warehouses, managing clinical research services, such as those needed for clinical trials, data request services, and research data governance

(Sanchez-Pinto et al. 2017). All these executives may have a significant role in advancing the applications of new information technologies in practice. For example, one such advancement could be establishing an innovation shop or lab, to create a collaboration space for developers, engineers, clinicians and patients, with the capability to disconnect and experiment while developing care processes but at the same time bridge administration and control of technology—a concept called bimodal IT (Mesaglio and Mingay 2014) or two-speed IT (Avedillo et al. 2016; Bossert et al. 2015).

Government leadership roles may overlap with academic and executive leadership roles at times, and people may move in between such roles. During the COVID-19 pandemic, prominent governmental digital health leadership drew from public health institutes and research centres tasked with population health surveillance, including healthcare service utilisation, to guide rapid development of public health policies. Even in non-pandemic periods, leadership of infectious disease surveillance and response, as well as chronic disease surveillance, remains vital to guide policy and budgetary decisions towards population-level health promotion. Formulating and implementing information technology strategies in publicly funded health care services also requires skilled leaders; examples include electronic health record modernisation in primary care or hospitals, health care information systems for military personnel, and community disability and aged care IT systems. In addition to governmental leadership roles, leaders of non-governmental or non-profit organisations also have an important role in convening multiple stakeholders across disciplines and sectors around core values of digital health.

Highly visible health executive leadership roles necessarily exist across all sectors of academia, government and non-governmental agencies, and in the private sector, from small start-ups to large multinational corporations, including public and private health service providers and their suppliers throughout the digital health ecosystem. Leaders in these sectors must be prepared to work together and to work across sectors.

Conclusion

There is no one single pathway for an aspiring digital health leader, and more than likely, such a leader will be positioned in more than one discipline or sector. Also, leaders are likely to face increased demand for a diverse, inclusive, and well-supported HIDDIN workforce. One final consideration in taking on a leadership role or following a leader is to avoid the romanticisation of leadership, or a tendency to view an organisation's successes (or failures) as attributable to a leader (Meindl et al. 1985; Mayo 2017). This chapter has offered several principles that leaders can enact to facilitate positive change in their immediate workplace, in the HIDDIN workforce, and in society.

References

Avedillo JG, Begonha D, Peyracchia A. Two ways to modernize IT systems for the digital era. McKinsey; 2016; Available from: https://www.mckinsey.com/business-functions/mckinsey-digital/our-insights/two-ways-to-modernize-it-systems-for-the-digital-era.

Bossert O, Harrysson M, Roberts R. Organizing for digital acceleration: making a two-speed IT operating model work. McKinsey & Company; 2015. https://www.mckinsey.com/industries/technology-media-and-telecommunications/our-insights/organizing-for-digital-acceleration-making-a-two-speed-it-operating-model-work. Accessed 31 Mar 2021.

Byhoff E, Kangovi S, Berkowitz SA, DeCamp M, Dzeng E, Earnest M, et al. A Society of General Internal Medicine position statement on the Internists' role in social determinants of health. J Gen Intern Med. 2020. https://doi.org/10.1007/s11606-020-05934-8. Accessed 31 Mar 2021.

Chambers DA, Feero WG, Khoury MJ. Convergence of implementation science, precision medicine, and the learning health care system: a new model for Biomedical Research. JAMA. 2016;315:1941–2.

Chowkwanyun M, Reed AL Jr. Racial health disparities and Covid-19 – caution and context. N Engl J Med. 2020;383:201–3.

Cooke C. Library & learning services: digital literacy: what is digital literacy? 2018. https://libguides.aecc.ac.uk/digitalliteracy/introduction. Accessed 26 Aug 2020.

Daniel H, Bornstein SS, Kane GC, Health and Public Policy Committee of the American College of Physicians. Addressing social determinants to improve patient care and promote health equity: an American College of Physicians Position paper. Ann Intern Med. 2018;168:577–8.

Daugherty Biddison EL, Paine L, Murakami P, Herzke C, Weaver SJ. Associations between safety culture and employee engagement over time: a retrospective analysis. BMJ Qual Saf. 2016;25:31–7.

de Jong M, van der Meulen-de Jong A, Romberg-Camps M, Degens J, Becx M, Markus T, et al. Development and feasibility study of a telemedicine tool for all patients with IBD: MyIBDcoach. Inflamm Bowel Dis. 2017a;23:485–93.

de Jong MJ, van der Meulen-de Jong AE, Romberg-Camps MJ, Becx MC, Maljaars JP, Cilissen M, et al. Telemedicine for management of inflammatory bowel disease (myIBDcoach): a pragmatic, multicentre, randomised controlled trial. Lancet. 2017b;390:959–68.

Demerouti E, Bakker AB, Nachreiner F, Schaufeli WB. The job demands-resources model of burnout. J Appl Psychol. 2001;86:499–512.

Edmondson AC, Lei Z. Psychological safety: the history, renaissance, and future of an interpersonal construct. Annu Rev Organ Psychol Organ Behav. 2014;1:23–43.

Egener BE, Mason DJ, McDonald WJ, Okun S, Gaines ME, Fleming DA, et al. The charter on professionalism for health care organizations. Acad Med. 2017;92:1091–9.

Eubanks V. Automating inequality: how high-tech tools profile, police, and punish the poor. St. Martin's Publishing Group; 2018.

Friedman CP, Wong AK, Blumenthal D. Achieving a nationwide learning health system. Sci Transl Med. 2010;2:57cm29.

Goodman KW. Ethics in health informatics. Yearb Med Inform. 2020;29:26–31.

Griffin AC, Leung TI, Tenenbaum JD, Chung AE. Gender representation in U.S. biomedical informatics leadership and recognition. J Am Med Inform Assoc. 2021. https://doi.org/10.1093/jamia/ocaa344.

Hewlett SA. The real benefit of finding a sponsor. Harv Bus Rev. 2011. https://hbr.org/2011/01/the-real-benefit-of-finding-a. Accessed 9 Jul 2020.

Hübner UH, Egbert N, Schulte G. Clinical information systems – seen through the ethics lens. Yearb Med Inform. 2020;29:104–14.

Institute of Medicine. Committee on the Recommended Social and Behavioral Domains and Measures for Electronic Health Records. Capturing social and behavioral domains in electronic health records: Phase 1. Washington: National Academies Press; 2014.

Institute of Medicine. Committee on the Recommended Social and Behavioral Domains and Measures for Electronic Health Records, Board on Population Health and Public Health Practice. Capturing social and behavioral domains in electronic health records: Phase 2. Washington: National Academies Press (US); 2015.

Jaaron AAM, Backhouse CJ. Operationalising "double-loop" learning in service organisations: a systems approach for creating knowledge. Syst Pract Action Res. 2017;30:317–37.

Kannry J, Sengstack P, Thyvalikakath TP, Poikonen J, Middleton B, Payne T, et al. The Chief Clinical Informatics Officer (CCIO): AMIA Task Force Report on CCIO knowledge, education, and skillset requirements. Appl Clin Inform. 2016;7:143–76.

Lawrence PR, Lorsch JW. Differentiation and integration in complex organizations. Adm Sci Q. 1967;1.

Leung TI, van Merode GG. Value-based health care supported by data science. In: Kubben P, Dumontier M, Dekker A, editors. Fundamentals of clinical data science. Cham (CH): Springer; 2018.

Leung TI, Barrett E, Lin TL, Moyer DV. Advancing from perception to reality: How to accelerate and achieve gender equity now. Perspect Med Educ. 2019:317–9.

Lifshitz-Assaf H. Dismantling knowledge boundaries at NASA: the critical role of professional identity in open innovation. Adm Sci Q. 2018;63:746–82.

Longhurst CA, Pageler NM, Palma JP, Finnell JT, Levy BP, Yackel TR, et al. Early experiences of accredited clinical informatics fellowships. J Am Med Inform Assoc. 2016;23:829–34.

Mache S, Danzer G, Klapp BF, Groneberg DA. Surgeons' work ability and performance in surgical care: relations between organisational predictors, work engagement and work ability. Langenbecks Arch Surg. 2013;398:317–25.

Mack J. Healthcare informatics jobs and salaries: what you need to know. 2016. https://onlinedegrees.sandiego.edu/healthcare-informatics-jobs-salary/. Accessed 29 Aug 2020.

Mayo M. If humble people make the best leaders, why do we fall for charismatic narcissists? 2017. https://hbr.org/2017/04/if-humble-people-make-the-best-leaders-why-do-we-fall-for-charismatic-narcissists. Accessed 29 Aug 2021.

Meindl JR, Ehrlich SB, Dukerich JM. The romance of leadership. Adm Sci Q. 1985;78.

Mesaglio M, Mingay S. Bimodal IT: How to be digitally agile without making a mess. Gartner Exec Prog. 2014;55.

Metzl JM, Hansen H. Structural competency: theorizing a new medical engagement with stigma and inequality. Soc Sci Med. 2014;103:126–33.

Noble SU. Algorithms of oppression: how search engines reinforce racism. NYU Press; 2018.

Nwaru BI, Friedman C, Halamka J, Sheikh A. Can learning health systems help organisations deliver personalised care? BMC Med. 2017;15:177.

Nyänken P, Whitehouse D. Int J Biomed Healthc. 2017;5(2):1–60.

O'Neil C. Weapons of math destruction: how big data increases inequality and threatens democracy. UK: Penguin; 2016.

Phillips KW. How diversity makes us smarter. Scientific American. 2014. https://www.scientificamerican.com/article/how-diversity-makes-us-smarter/. Accessed 28 Aug 2020.

Phillips KW, Northcraft GB, Neale MA. Surface-level diversity and decision-making in groups: when does deep-level similarity help? Group process intergroup relations. SAGE. 2006;9:467–82.

Plsek PE, Greenhalgh T. Complexity science: the challenge of complexity in health care. BMJ. 2001;323:625–8.

Porter ME, Lee TH, Alger MA. Oak Street Health: a new model of primary care. Harv Bus Rev. 2017. https://www.hbs.edu/faculty/Pages/item.aspx?num=52357. Accessed 29 Aug 2020.

Prins JT, van der Heijden FMMA, Hoekstra-Weebers JEHM, Bakker AB, van de Wiel HBM, Jacobs B, et al. Burnout, engagement and resident physicians' self-reported errors. Psychol Health Med. 2009;14:654–66.

Rajkomar A, Hardt M, Howell MD, Corrado G, Chin MH. Ensuring fairness in machine learning to advance health equity. Ann Intern Med. 2018;169:866–72.

Rivera-Romero O, Konstantinidis S, Denecke K, Gabarrón E, Petersen C, Househ M, et al. Ethical considerations for participatory health through social media: healthcare workforce and policy maker perspectives. Yearb Med Inform. 2020;29:71–6.

Rodriguez JA, Clark CR, Bates DW. Digital health equity as a necessity in the 21st Century Cures Act Era. JAMA. 2020. https://doi.org/10.1001/jama.2020.7858. Accessed 29 Aug 2020.

Sanchez-Pinto LN, Mosa ASM, Fultz-Hollis K, Tachinardi U, Barnett WK, Embi PJ. The emerging role of the chief research informatics officer in academic health centers. Appl Clin Inform. 2017;8:845–53.

Scheepers RA, Lases LSS, Arah OA, Heineman MJ, Lombarts KMJMH. Job resources, physician work engagement, and patient care experience in an academic medical setting. Acad Med. 2017;92:1472–9.

Selden TM, Berdahl TA. COVID-19 and racial/ethnic disparities in health risk, employment, and household composition. Health Aff. 2020;101377hlthaff202000897.

Sengstack P, Thyvalikakath T, Poikonen J, Middleton B, Payne T, Lehmann C, et al. The Chief Clinical Informatics Officer (CCIO). Appl Clin Inform. 2016:143–176.

Séroussi B, Hollis KF, Soualmia LF. Transparency of health informatics processes as the condition of healthcare professionals' and patients' trust and adoption: the rise of ethical requirements. Yearb Med Inform. 2020;29:7–10.

Travis EL, Doty L, Helitzer DL. Sponsorship: a path to the academic medicine C-suite for women faculty? Acad Med. 2013;88:1414–7.

Uhl-Bien M, Marion R, McKelvey B. Complexity leadership theory: shifting leadership from the industrial age to the knowledge era. Leadersh Q. 2007;18:298–318.

van den Heuvel TRA, Jonkers DM, Jeuring SFG, Romberg-Camps MJL, Oostenbrug LE, Zeegers MP, et al. Cohort Profile: The Inflammatory Bowel Disease South Limburg Cohort (IBDSL). Int J Epidemiol. 2017:e7.

van der Ham A, Van Merode F, Ruwaard D, Van Raak A. Identifying integration and differentiation in a hospital's logistical system: a social network analysis of a case study. 2020. https://doi.org/10.21203/rs.3.rs-22054/v2.

Veinot TC, Ancker JS, Cole-Lewis H, Mynatt ED, Parker AG, Siek KA, et al. Leveling up: on the potential of upstream health informatics interventions to enhance health equity. Med Care. 2019;57(Suppl 6 Suppl 2):S108–14.

Victor B, Cullen JB. The organizational bases of ethical work climates. Adm Sci Q. 1988;101.

Vyas DA, Eisenstein LG, Jones DS. Hidden in plain sight – reconsidering the use of race correction in clinical algorithms. N Engl J Med. 2020.

Waldrop MM. Complexity: the emerging science at the edge of order and chaos. Simon and Schuster; 1993.

Woolston C. PhDs: the tortuous truth. Nature. 2019;575:403–6.

Chapter 12
The Specialist Digital Health Workforce Impact on Access and Equity

Anna G. Shillabeer, Lawrence Sambrooks, and Aydan C. Shillabeer

Abstract HIDDIN (Health Informatics, Digital, Data, Information and kNowledge) work aims to provide ubiquitous healthcare for all: Global healthcare is now data-driven. Health information and support services are accessible 24/7. Wearable devices and smartphones connect people with their health data and enable monitoring by a clinical team for patients at home. Given these tools and technologies and the vast potential they provide for patient access and equity, this chapter asks why so many people still do not have access to a quality healthcare system and why many who do report inequity in treatment and care. Several cases highlight issues with the design and availability of these tools for marginalised and minority groups and lower socio-demographic groups. The chapter argues for a revision to the required skill set for the HIDDIN workforce and a need to bring these professionals out of the silos that they have traditionally worked in and into the communities they aim to serve.

Keywords Marginalised groups · Minority groups · Access · Equity · Socio-economic status

Introduction

Human populations enjoy longer and higher quality lives than at any time in history. The application of evidence-based practices into health in the 1900s facilitated a doubling of a human life span by the end of the twentieth century. However, by the

A. G. Shillabeer (✉) · L. Sambrooks · A. C. Shillabeer
College of Sciences and Engineering, University of Tasmania, Hobart, TAS, Australia
e-mail: anna.shillabeer@utas.edu.au; lawrence.sambrooks@utas.edu.au;
aydan.shillabeer@utas.edu.au

K. Butler-Henderson et al. (eds.), *The Health Information Workforce*,
Health Informatics, https://doi.org/10.1007/978-3-030-81850-0_12

185

beginning of the twenty-first century we had arguably reached the limit of human capacity for such radical progress to be sustained by the work of individuals unaided by new technology. The ability for a healthcare practitioner to adapt, incorporate new knowledge from the rapidly growing big data stores and meet the global drivers for ubiquitous, cross-cultural health care through experimentation and observation in real time has been surpassed. In the twenty-first century reliance on empiricism has faded and digital data is the fundamental tool in healthcare innovation and experimentation. A strong drive to embed technology into clinical practice to continue to realise better diagnostic, treatment and prognostic outcomes has expanded the healthcare toolbox and patient expectations beyond the imagination of previous centuries. Data-driven digital health facilitates rapid responses, decision making, improved and personalised patient care and, with considered implementation, can ensure greater access and equity to high-quality healthcare globally. For these goals to be achieved, we need an enhanced workforce, with cutting-edge technology skills, the ability to build human-centric systems and a global framework for implementation.

The potential for digital health to achieve the stated goals and address community drivers has been evidenced since the beginning of the twenty-first century. In 2005 the World Health Organization (WHO) released resolution WHA58.28 and encouraged all member countries to develop infrastructures and strategies for leveraging the potential of computing technologies to provide 'equitable, affordable and universal access' to quality healthcare (WHO 2020a). This guideline was followed up in 2013 with resolution WHA66.24 which urged members to develop strategies and frameworks to ensure interoperability and a digital health platform underpinned by 'policies and legislative mechanisms linked to an overall national e-health strategy' (WHO 2020a). Two years later, in 2015, the 2030 Agenda was adopted by the UN and aimed to 'bridge the digital divide and to develop knowledge societies' (WHO 2020a). Throughout these resolutions there has been a call for closer collaboration and cooperation between the many stakeholders to achieve the defined goals. In the WHO Thirteenth General Program of Work, 2019–2023 it was stated that the aim was to ensure universal health coverage for a billion currently unserviced people around the world (WHO 2020a). Achieving this would require digital health initiatives to be targeted towards those who currently experience barriers in accessing the current health system structures. It would also require expertise that is not currently available within the domain of traditional clinical health workers or the HIDDIN (Health Informatics, Digital, Data, Information and kNowledge) workforce. As a final guiding statement the WHO Global Strategy on Digital Health defines digital health as 'the field of knowledge and practice associated with the development and use of digital technologies to improve health' and address the social determinants of health (WHO 2019, 2020a, b). The aims should be met through the use of new technologies including artificial intelligence, the Internet of Things, big data analytics and robotics (WHO 2019, 2020a, b). These skills are not commonly found in HIDDIN education degrees (Shillabeer and Anderson 2018). The WHO strategy also outlines four strategic objectives with short-, medium- and long-term goals to provide a standardised global platform from which to effect the implementation of digital health systems and provide a sustainable minimum standard of healthcare for all. Although strategies, frameworks and capabilities are being built, we have not yet reached sufficient global workforce capacity to implement such a broad scale healthcare revolution.

The changing healthcare environment has expanded the expectations of the communities it serves. Current healthcare systems are being driven to deliver personalised health care and preventative health management for complex populations, ensure rapid upscaling and deployment to address emerging health events, and meet local and global community drivers within myriad social, political and financial environments. The WHO has provided a set of overarching principles to guide the development of digital health platforms and systems, but the question that remains is why are we still experiencing global barriers to access and equity in healthcare around the world? This chapter explores some of the challenges that impact access and equity and discusses how the HIDDIN workforce can help to break down the barriers and progress towards a state of universal healthcare for all.

Digital Health as a Facilitator of Access and Equity

Digital health innovation and data dependent technologies present significant benefits for patients. In Australia, a single CSIRO telehealth application was able to provide a 53% reduction in hospital admissions and a 40% reduction in mortality, this is by no means a lone case (Hospital and Healthcare 2020). The demand for a skilled workforce to sustain such benefits is well documented, but the provision of appropriate competencies and capacity has lagged. Primary stakeholders must work together while being mindful of the diverse skill sets and drivers. The HIDDIN workforce often must concentrate on systems to provide back-end data and information to support health services management. Healthcare providers require front-end solutions that provide instant access to accurate patient information, reduce their administrative burden and help develop new treatments and medicines (Australian Digital Health Agency 2017; Deloitte Centre for Health Solutions 2013). Digital health must be a solution for all members of a community, not only those who are technology literate (Azzopardi-Muscat and Sorensen 2019). Meanwhile, members of the community are demanding systems that are user friendly, give them control, ensure that their information is kept confidential and implement digital tools that are safe and secure (Australian Digital Health Agency 2017). The definition of 'user friendly' varies amongst community members, hence developing a digital health solution for a whole community is an almost intractable exercise for HIDDIN workers or healthcare providers without sufficient in-depth understanding of the many sub-communities they are trying to support and serve. This chapter posits that there is an ongoing shortfall in HIDDIN professionals who are suitably trained to facilitate ubiquitous data-driven health care, and this is contributing to persistent inequity in access to healthcare across the globe, especially for disadvantaged populations (Frenk et al. 2010; Kiyumi et al. 2016; Drehobl et al.

2012; Shadmi et al. 2020). We outline the potential impact of the HIDDIN workforce towards ensuring healthcare is available to all and present cases to demonstrate the positive impact that these professionals can have if they are visible and able to engage at the grassroots level.

The (WHO 2011) advocates that all people should have equal opportunity to receive good healthcare and be able to realise their full health potential, without disadvantage. Unfortunately, many social, geographic and political constraints exist to achieving this (WHO 2019; Shadmi et al. 2020; Azzopardi-Muscat and Sorensen 2019; Deloitte Centre for Health Solutions 2013); these constraints form the social determinants of health (SDOH), which are frequently used to measure the potential outcomes of health initiatives and underpin health inequity and disparate access (WHO 2019). Digital health and the workforce that develops and manages it have a significant role to play in reducing this inequity but the real value of this work is yet to be felt.

Health in the general population can be very much enabled by digital tools and technologies, wearable and implantable devices, smartphone apps and digital trackers to name but a very few; their monitoring and feedback functions may trigger health-seeking behaviours, provide digital access to the health system, reduce disparity and increase access and equity (Australasian Telehealth Society 2017). Although the HIDDIN workforce undoubtedly contributes to the design, development and testing of these technologies, this workforce does not generally interact with the population that uses them or directly influence the behaviours that produce health benefits. To reduce the impact of the SDOH, and present opportunities for the HIDDIN workforce to emerge from the shadows, a new professional model is needed, that takes a collaborative approach beyond traditional research and clinical workforce settings to overcome social disparity.

Digital health personal devices, and clinical tools and technologies, often unfortunately exacerbate the potential to increase disparity and inequity for those who are already marginalised. Low socio-demographic or minority cultural groups either may not be able to afford wearable devices or may not have interfaces and information in their native language. Unaffordability excludes such groups from enjoying the potential benefits of information that informs decisions to seek access to healthcare services (Brewer et al. 2020; Azzopardi-Muscat and Sorensen 2019). Given the increasing reliance on and pervasiveness of digital health brought about by the COVID-19 pandemic, it is important to take a broader approach to the design and development of digital interventions. SDOH impede equity already and may be compounded by perceived, or actual, racism and culturally inappropriate digital designs that marginalise those who stand to benefit most (Hardeman et al. 2016). Access and equity in healthcare services are a community problem and are felt hardest by those in marginalised communities (Brewer et al. 2018; Deloitte Centre for Health Solutions 2013). The most significant gains in access and equity can be achieved by addressing the needs of such communities. Digital health should seek to contribute to achieving the WHO Millennium Goals and reducing the SDOH burden. Given the complexities of the populations and environments where digital health is deployed, a visible and capable HIDDIN workforce can have an important impact on community health. Several case studies demonstrate the potential impact of focussing on marginalised communities with the lowest levels of access and equity within the health system. These cases support the position that the digital health developers and champions need to move out of conventional traditional research and clinical settings for their full potential to be realised.

Digital Health Work in US Communities

The American Health System is frequently cited as a health system that fails to serve marginalised communities; these communities may mobilise and create innovative solutions—and research opportunities for digital health workers. One such example is the African-American community in Minnesota which historically experienced a higher incidence of CardioVascular Disease (CVD) than white Americans and almost twice the mortality rate (Minnesota Department of Health 2017). Traditional measures to reduce the problem and create awareness had a low impact, attributed to health services' lack of understanding of community beliefs and social structures leading to a strong community perception of systematic racism and a feeling that the health system tolerated rather than served them (Hardeman et al. 2016). Community improvement initiatives including health were primarily driven through church groups, rather than through health provider organisations or clinicians who were not considered trusted, inclusive entities (Brewer et al. 2018, 2020). Engagement with these marginalised and minority groups by digital health researchers and developers is not common practice and thus perpetuates, and often exacerbates, non-communicable and chronic disease problems in African-American communities (Brewer et al. 2020). Previous research had identified that African-Americans had a similar rate of uptake and ownership of mobile devices as the broader community (around 80%) but were more likely to use smartphones and similar devices to access health information (Ray et al. 2017; Anderson 2015; Pew Research Center 2019). Given the barriers to access described above, reliance on an 'out of clinic' health system is not surprising, but it does call for high-quality information and digital health tools to be available in a form that is easily accessible and applicable to these minority groups.

The 'Fostering African-American Improvement in Total Health' (FAITH!) project was initiated from within the Minnesota community to reduce the CVD burden and facilitate better use of mobile technology as part of a broader community health initiative. The FAITH! premise was to translate community, church-based interventions into a mobile app, so as to have access to information that could be trusted, was relevant to the community and could be used to build and supplement traditional social support mechanisms (Brewer et al. 2020). The project used an approach that included conventional clinical, research and behavioural scientists, some of whom were HIDDIN practitioners, and a range of community partners and church champions, from inception to conclusion. By engaging with community and church leaders, the digital health team developed a bespoke design that incorporated clinical and health education considerations, with messaging framed by biblical and spiritual references and culturally appropriate images and infographics (Brewer et al. 2019a, b). Trial users drawn from the community had a participation rate of 100% and retention rate of 98% and gave the app a high rating for acceptability and satisfaction (Brewer et al. 2018); more importantly, the overall impact on participants' blood pressure, diet and activity was positive (Brewer et al. 2019b). Through subsequent government funding to support clinical integration of the app, the project was also able to influence the target group to access traditional community health centres and services (Brewer et al. 2018). There was a positive impact on equity within and beyond the target population because the general population was able to engage with the app during consultations at participating health centres (Brewer et al. 2020). The multi-level impact was attributed in part to the visibility of HIDDIN practitioners in the community consultations and data gathering processes (Brewer et al. 2018).

Marginalisation and systematic racism are not the only barriers to accessing equitable health care. There are also significant barriers among older people with comorbidities, or who are geographically isolated (Fortuna et al. 2018). Reduced access is an issue in particular locations with significant rural and remote regions where populations have lower socio-demographic characteristics, higher than average age profiles, and often a higher health burden but with low clinical capacity to deliver global best practice in healthcare (Fortuna et al. 2018; Australasian Telehealth Society 2017). An application of digital health in these scenarios is supporting self-management of chronic mental health conditions. As in the previous case study, development of effective and appropriate digital interventions is best facilitated through a collaborative process, for example the 'Peer and Technology Supported Self-Management Training' (PeerTECH) app (Fortuna et al. 2018). This app targets people who have geographic barriers to access, are over 60 years old and have comorbidities which impact on their ability to manage their mental health issues (Fortuna et al. 2019). This cohort was recognised as having lower than average engagement with the health system due to a lack of resources (Fortuna et al. 2019). Peer support was already known to help such groups, so this project focussed on training certified peer specialists to provide outreach support and increase access to mental health services (Brewer et al. 2020). The app took a highly innovative approach, shifting from a medical to a biopsychosocial standpoint. It transformed a traditional mental health management app and moved away from a 'highly medicalized self-management approach' and towards a tool focussed on recovery, social engagement and self-advocacy (Brewer et al. 2020). As with the FAITH! project, there was broad community engagement that sought input from the certified support peers, clinical scientists and the patients themselves. The results could not be achieved at arm's length, and these participants did not have high engagement with the health system so opportunities to collaborate with the usual HIDDIN workforce domain was low. Thus digital health specialists worked within the community to ensure that the app was appropriate for the target user group and that sustained use and acceptance was high. The result was a targeted app that facilitated training for both the patients and their health support peers to enable mental health and comorbidity monitoring and management in their home locations, equitably compared with a clinical setting. The project achieved statistically significant improvements in personal psychiatric and medical management (Brewer et al. 2020).

This US community-based development approach translated internationally, and led to a similar approach in Uttar Pradesh in India (Deloitte Centre for Health Solutions 2013), where again an app was developed through consultation with women, church groups, local government representatives and community health workers. That app was developed as a guide to enable community health workers and health mentors to counsel women on prenatal and postnatal care. Where previous health initiatives had not addressed high maternal and infant mortality rates, this digital health intervention reduced maternal deaths by 16.4% and infant deaths by 5.2% over 10 years (Deloitte Centre for Health Solutions 2013).

Digital Health Work in Australian Communities

Whilst Australia arguably has one of the best health systems in the world, there are still issues with access and equity (Australasian Telehealth Society 2017), and examples where digital health work does not yet serve the community equitably. Australia needs to appropriately expand healthcare services and support to manage an aging population, growing chronic and non-communicable disease rates and the complexities of indigenous health (Australian Government 2011; Australasian Telehealth Society 2017). All of this is underpinned by a need to grow the capacity and capability of the under resourced HIDDIN workforce and develop a strategic and coordinated approach to developing and implementing innovative digital health solutions (Australian Digital Health Agency 2017; Australasian Telehealth Society 2017). The 2017 National Digital Health Strategy (Australian Digital Health Agency 2017) had a focus on the provision of a digital health platform that would enable models of care for supporting the health of rural and remote populations, babies and young children, and the elderly—all very dependent upon non-clinical carers outside of the national health system—and Australia's indigenous communities were also a focus as a hard to reach population. But whilst access to information is integral in this digital health strategy, unfortunately there is no defined focus on addressing equity as the following examples show.

The implementation of a government supported personally controlled health record, My Health Record, (Australian Digital Health Agency 2017; Deloitte Centre for Health Solutions 2013) failed to address how My Health Record would help those who had not engaged with the health system and hence would have a minimal health record. The initiative lacked effective consideration of language and cultural barriers for indigenous people, and a lack of remote area transport impeding access to the clinical health system (Department of Health and Aging 2012). The strategy also intended to reduce medication errors and give prescribing doctors national access to patients' medication records (Australian Digital Health Agency 2017; Deloitte Centre for Health Solutions 2013)—but people must be able to actually access the system to realise those benefits. Insult was added to inequity when the government changed My Health Record from an 'opt in' to an 'opt out' model. The strategy document frequently mentioned 'access' as a benefit, but this referred to access to health information when the underlying issue of access to health care per se was unresolved.

'Care at home' remains a test case for HIDDIN work. 16% of the Australian population live with chronic conditions and many experience issues with poor information flows through their care teams or when being transferred between providers (Australian Bureau of Statistics 2016; Campbell et al. 2017). Information access would seem to be relevant in new telehealth and 'health in the home' initiatives—but many initiatives began unplanned broad scale testing only due to the onset of the COVID-19 pandemic in 2020. Two earlier cases where telehealth implementations have been successful—monitoring chronic health conditions for those in aged care facilities and telehealth facilitated out-patient appointments in three remote towns (Department of Health 2015; Celler et al. 2016)—show the potential of well-informed design and development to improve appointment compliance, reduce hospital admissions and save significant health care system costs. However, evaluation of those cases did not look for, nor find, improvement in access and equity—a missed opportunity to build the evidence-base about the impact of HIDDIN work. In another example, tele-psychiatry has been used as an essential part of Australia's healthcare system to reach geographically distanced communities (O'Connor et al. 2016). This technology became even more essential during COVID-19 to manage the impacts of 'lockdown' measures, which exacerbated already critical levels of mental health problems in rural and remote areas (Meadows et al. 2015). However, effectiveness was impacted by changes in legislation; the initial COVID-19 support package provided by the government mandated that there would be no 'out of pocket' expenses for digital consultations (Shadmi et al. 2020; Hunt 2020), but revisions to legislation led to barriers in accessing cost-free mental health support for all and created inequities for many (Shadmi et al. 2020). Further changes enabling digital consultations at no cost were supported only for those who were defined as 'vulnerable', not for all who needed mental health counselling at that time. Many people who contracted and succumbed to the virus were from designated 'non-vulnerable' groups, and many who had minor symptoms and survived were from groups considered highly vulnerable. The legislative implications of telehealth access, not founded on the evidence-base in the HIDDIN disciplines, served to introduce inequity where it did not previously exist.

Australia experienced a further broadening of the digital divide as a direct consequence of the lockdowns. Those in marginalised and lower socio-demographic groups experienced reduced or no access to digital health tools and technologies due to prohibitions on access to public technology infrastructure. During lockdown, people who could not afford home Internet also could not leave home to access free wi-fi in public spaces such as libraries (Shadmi et al. 2020). This reduced access to social digital health support structures, and in some cases, prevented access to any healthcare services for those in remote areas that were already underserviced (O'Connor et al. 2016; Ward and Agostino 2020). This case, showing that access to the healthcare system during a public health emergency is directly influenced by access to digital technologies in the community, reinforces that building and maintaining a strong grassroots digital health presence is needed to overcome access and equity issues in the future. Similar to the US case studies, for digital health to address access and equity issues in the Australian context, multi-disciplinary teams that integrate peer and community support stakeholders and extended carer networks need to be deployed to reach beyond the mainstream healthcare system (Australasian Telehealth Society 2017; Deloitte Centre for Health Solutions 2013). The economic, geographical, cultural and linguistic needs of the Australian population must become a more fundamental concern in digital health strategy.

Digital Health Work in Responses to COVID-19

The COVID-19 pandemic has been the ultimate case study for the potential of digital health. A range of implementations emerged around the world, and there is a stark contrast in COVID outcomes between countries that have engaged with digital health as part of their management strategy, and those who have not. Countries implementing a two-tier health system response, with one of those tiers based in digital health, have achieved the most positive outcomes. Countries such as Belgium had a first response process utilising digital health systems. Any patient exhibiting symptoms was required to digitally contact their GP who would then triage, and determine if the patient needed to present at a clinic or hospital, or could stay at home (Shadmi et al. 2020). Those who were only mildly symptomatic were advised to remain at home and were provided with a self-management plan that was supplemented with online or phone follow-up until they were considered safe (Shadmi et al. 2020). This freed up clinical care places for those who needed them most. The process also ensured that resources could focus on a rapid response to those who required clinical care, thus enabling access for more patients. Whilst the response in Belgium was underpinned by digital mechanisms, there was still inequity for those not fluent in the national languages (Shadmi et al. 2020). As in most other countries, the first response was for the majority of the population; minorities and marginalised populations were secondary, resulting in higher incidence of COVID-19 in those populations (Shadmi et al. 2020). For them, inability to understand the public health messaging meant greater community and familial transmission, and reduced access to early assessment and treatment. Other countries such as Israel implemented a secondary response mechanism to enable home isolation with digital monitoring, for non-critical cases. These cases were initially triaged in a conventional clinical setting (Shadmi et al. 2020). By implementing an isolation and recovery at home plan, Israel was able to minimise the impact of COVID-19. Although Israel has a comparatively low number of hospital beds per capita (2.2/1000 vs 3.6/100 OECD average), and therefore a reduced capacity to treat cases, it constrained the spread of the virus to relatively low levels (Shadmi et al. 2020; OECD 2020) and is now investigating further tailored measures to protect more vulnerable subpopulations, including those with minimal connectedness to digital platforms (Shadmi et al. 2020). The Israeli Ministry of Health stated that for measures to have a positive impact they must be tailored for the socio-cultural and linguistic needs of each subpopulation; strategies must also include religious and other community leaders and champions at all stages of development and dissemination (Waitzberg et al. 2020).

Although there are many good examples, this discussion must be tempered by examples where digital health and the HIDDIN workforce were not mobilised. In America, the historical minority and marginalised communities, such as the African-American population discussed earlier, experienced even greater disparity and reduced access to healthcare during 2020. Historic inequity issues were exacerbated by a lack of financial, housing and food stability; limited budget for healthcare and Internet connectivity; and reduced access to personal and community technology and community social structures—creating barriers to systems that would otherwise provide connectivity to health services and support (Benfer and Wiley 2020). The African-American population in Chicago recorded over 50% of all cases in the state of Illinois, and the Navaho Nation had more per capita cases than in any other area of the country (Capatides 2020). This almost complete disconnection of some groups of people from any form of healthcare support unquestionably contributed to America having appalling COVID-19 outcomes, with similar stories in other countries, including Brazil and Guatemala (Shadmi et al. 2020). While the inequity could be blamed on the low socio-economic status of the population, there are positive examples from countries with similar socio-demographics such as Armenia. In Armenia, hot lines were set up to provide a first-line response and to provide an outbound call service to directly connect with the population and provide information (WHO 2020b). This was strengthened by public health information announcements on radio and television; mobile phone tracking for contact tracing, and social support mechanisms leveraged to care for the vulnerable and disadvantaged in the community. Armenia did not escape the impact of the pandemic, but it did not see the devastation experienced by the aforementioned countries. Whilst not the cutting edge of digital health technology, this case does highlight the potential for even minimal digital connectedness to have a positive impact on population health access and equity. Digital connectedness is a self-evident crucial factor for any digital health initiative, and even if it is only used to mobilise messaging and education through social media, it can improve wellbeing and save lives in times when no information, or misinformation, can be catastrophic.

Bringing the HIDDIN Workforce Out of the Clinic

A HIDDIN workforce is central to narrowing the digital health information divide, but the cases presented in this chapter suggest that it is not sufficient to simply have a HIDDIN workforce. For that workforce to adequately address community needs and overcome access and equity barriers, they must be in the community, directly working with the marginalised and disadvantaged groups. Providing systems that are culturally, socially and linguistically appropriate is a critical factor in acceptance and adherence; without an understanding of these factors, the HIDDIN workforce cannot possibly meet the requirements of all stakeholders, and their digital health developments will have less impact. The common message from the cases in this chapter is that there is a need for community, patient and clinical engagement in the design and development of digital health solutions most especially where those solutions have an overarching goal to increase access and equity. The call to use digital health to increase access to healthcare suggests that targeted users do not currently engage enough with healthcare practitioners or health-seeking activities. If we accept this, we must also accept that the needs of such potential users cannot inform development that almost exclusively occurs within research and clinical environments governed by national authorities—but this is precisely where the HIDDIN workforce is employed.

Digital health is more than a clinical or health system application and must be contextualised if greater access and equity to healthcare is to be achieved. The social structures and engagement mechanisms must both be understood and be a driving force in digital health initiatives. The workforce must actively and visibly engage otherwise they can never truly realise the true value of their work, even if all stakeholders know they exist. It is incongruous to provide applications to facilitate greater access for those who already access the systems and structures designed to support their health care needs. Relying on a standardised one-size-fits-all digital health development approach is ineffectual, as is relying on practising health professionals to speak authentically for marginalised and disadvantaged communities and cultural groups within their practice catchment.

What this calls for is a broadening of the digital health profession skill set and a redefinition of the workplace boundaries for the HIDDIN workforce. Given the need to change how this workforce functions if access and equity are to be achieved, there needs to be a redefinition of learning and training pathways and outcomes. A broader, more competency-based, vocational education platform would address the education needs of a workforce that requires both lateral pathways and graduate entry; but we note a number of identified issues with equitable and appropriate access to such education opportunities that present barriers for aspiring HIDDIN workers from under-represented social groups (Shillabeer and Anderson 2018).

Some Universities and Colleges now are providing short courses that incorporate micro-credentialing to ensure that the HIDDIN worker can engage with technology, clinicians, terminologies, design and development processes; and also can be mindful of human psychology and behaviour change concepts (Hospital and Healthcare 2020; Shillabeer and Anderson 2018). An example from RMIT in Australia aims to develop graduates who will be 'design thinkers and leaders in health care and social services with the capacity to reimagine and design prototypes of new digitally enabled healthcare services that incorporate good healthcare design principles' (Hospital and Healthcare 2020). Such graduates could have impact at the grassroots level, but only if they work through community engagement in non-traditional settings. Course descriptions suggest that graduates will lead digital health innovations and influence 'transformations within their organisation' (Hospital and Healthcare

2020), even though the greatest demand and potential for impact is outside of structured organisations.

The Australian Digital Health Strategy among its priorities states the need for support for healthcare workers to understand the tools and technologies available. Upskilling is proposed to be provided to all Australian healthcare professionals by 2022 (Australasian Telehealth Society 2017; Australian Institute of Health and Welfare 2006). However, as discussed in this chapter, without specialist training to develop bespoke digital solutions for marginalised and remote communities, equity issues will remain and access to digital health initiatives will be limited. This presents a significant global problem for indigenous and minority populations. Many of these populations have high levels of non-communicable diseases, significant SDOHs; chronic conditions, low literacy, and cultural barriers to engaging with formal health systems (Brewer et al. 2020; Australasian Telehealth Society 2017; Shillabeer 2015; Australian Institute of Health and Welfare 2006; Australian Government 2011; Azzopardi-Muscat and Sorensen 2019). Without a concentrated effort to connect with, understand and include these people, the HIDDIN workforce will have no impact on access and equity. Whilst governments in many countries have detailed strategies to grow their national digital health capacity, this is not yet adequately supported by education for development and management of digital health solutions to address access and equity.

The cases presented in this chapter call for a rethink in how the HIDDIN workforce conceptualises digital health solutions. This work needs to revitalise the principles of altruism, benevolence and personal care upon which healthcare and health research are founded. Patients are people, not diagnoses, and must be considered at the individual and holistic level if health disparities within our communities are to be addressed. This requires a connection with people in their own community, not in unfamiliar and often scary clinical and organisational silos. This can only be possible when our HIDDIN workforce ventures out.

Achieving this dissolution of boundaries will facilitate the provision of a healthcare system that is accessible for all. It will also provide actual, rather than alleged, health equity and not cater only for those who already enjoy the myriad benefits of good health and good healthcare. This is a focus area where the HIDDIN workforce needs to be active and seen—the right people need to be in the right place. As suggested through the case studies presented in this chapter, if digital health is to increase access and equity, we need knowledge and capacity at the grassroots.

Measures implemented around the world in response to COVID-19 have demonstrated that any digital health implementation is better than nothing. However, a generalised approach does not work, and in fact often broadens the access and equity gap. One size simply cannot fit all, and in fact may fit very few. Digital health solutions that aim to increase access and equity need to be developed as part of multi-faceted teams including clinicians, digital health professionals, community leaders and the intended users themselves. Community engagement, cultural and religious beliefs, and innovative implementation science are key mobilisers of outcomes that can reduce or eliminate health disparity. This can take time and requires a much broader skillset and mindset than is usual in the HIDDIN workforce.

Digital health initiatives developed and implemented by a well-skilled and widely visible HIDDIN workforce have the potential to enhance the quality of life of every person on the planet. Longevity is all for naught if it is a life of pain and a constant battle with unmanaged chronic disease.

References

Anderson M. Racial and ethnic differences in how people use mobile technology. 2015. https://www.pewresearch.org/fact-tank/2015/04/30/racial-and-ethnic-differences-in-how-people-use-mobile-technology/. Accessed 17 Jul 2020.

Australasian Telehealth Society. National digital health strategy. Submission 147, Attachment 1. 2017. file:///C:/Users/e105513/AppData/Local/Temp/NBN%20-%20Sub147_attach1.pdf. Accessed 21 Jul 2020.

Australian Bureau of Statistics. Patient experiences in Australia: summary of findings, 2015–2016. 2016. http://www.abs.gov.au/austats/abs@nsf/mf/4839. Accessed 27 Jul 2020.

Australian Digital Health Agency. Safe seamless and secure: evolving heath and care to meet the needs of modern Australia. 2017. https://conversation.digitalhealth.gov.au/sites/default/files/adha-strategy-doc-2ndaug_0_1.pdf. Accessed 21 Jul 2020.

Australian Government. Closing the gap; Prime Ministers Report. 2011. http://www.fahcsia.gov.au/sa/indigenous/pubs/closing_the_gap/2011_ctg_pm_report/Pages/default.aspx. Accessed 25 May 2020.

Australian Institute of Health and Welfare. Australia's health 2006. Canberra: AIHW; 2006. http://www.aihw.gov.au/publications/aus/ah06/ah06.pdf. Accessed 23 Jul 2020.

Azzopardi-Muscat N, Sorensen K. Towards an equitable digital public health era: promoting equity through a health literacy perspective. Eur J Public Health. 2019;29(S3):13–7.

Benfer EA, Wiley LF. Health justice strategies to combat COVID-19: protecting vulnerable communities during a pandemic. Health Aff. 2020. https://doi.org/10.1377/hblog20200319.757883. Accessed 10 Aug 2020.

Brewer LC, Jenkins S, Lackore K, Johnson J, Jones C, Cooper LA, Radecki Breitkopf C, Hayes SN, Patten C. mHealth intervention promoting cardiovascular health among African-Americans: recruitment and baseline characteristics of a pilot study. JMIR Res Protoc. 2018;7(1):31.

Brewer LC, Hayes SN, Caron AR, Derby DA, Breutzman NS, Wicks A, Raman J, Smith CM, Schaepe KS, Sheets RE, Jenkins SM, Lackore KA, Johnson J, Jones C, Radecki Breitkopf C, Cooper LA, Patten CA. Promoting cardiovascular health and wellness among African-Americans: community participatory approach to design an innovative mobile-health intervention. PLoS One. 2019a;14(8):e0218724.

Brewer LC, Hayes SN, Jenkins SM, Lackore KA, Breitkopf CR, Cooper LA, Patten CA. Improving cardiovascular health among African-Americans through mobile health: the FAITH! app pilot study. J Gen Intern Med. 2019b;34(8):1376–8.

Brewer LC, Fortuna KL, Jones C, Walker R, Hayes SN, Patten CA, Cooper LA. Back to the future: achieving health equity through health informatics and digital health. JMIR Mhealth Uhealth. 2020;8(1):e14512.

Campbell B, Stirling C, Cummings E. Continuity matters: examining the 'information gap' in transfer from residential aged care, ambulance t emergency triage in southern Tasmania. Int Emerg Nurs. 2017;32:9–14.

Capatides C. Doctors without borders dispatches team to the Navajo Nation. CBS News. 2020. https://www.cbsnews.com/news/doctors-withoutborders-navajo-nation-coronavirus/. Accessed 15 Aug 2020.

Celler B, Varnfield M, Sparks R, Li J, Surya Nepal S, Jang-Jaccard J, et al. Home monitoring of chronic diseases for aged care. Herston: Australian e-Health Research Centre (AEHRC); 2016.

Deloitte Centre for Health Solutions. Deloitte insights. Digital health technology. Global case studies of healthcare transformation. 2013. www.deloitte.com/centreforhealthsolutions. Accessed 17 Jul 2020.

Department of Health. Evaluation of the PATS-Telehealth Project. Darwin: Northern Territory Government; 2015.

Department of Health and Aging. National Aboriginal and Torres Strait Islander Health Plan 2013-2023. 2012. https://www1.health.gov.au/internet/main/publishing.nsf/content/B92E980680486C3BCA257BF0001BAF01/$File/health-plan.pdf. Accessed 27 Jul 2020.

Drehobl PA, Roush SW, Stoveri BH, Koo D. Public health surveillance workforce of the future. CDC Morbid Mortal Wkly Rep (MMWR). 2012;61(3):25–9.

Fortuna KL, Storm M, Naslund JA, Chow P, Aschbrenner KA, Lohman MC, Bartels SJ. Certified peer specialists and older adults with serious mental illness' perspectives of the impact of a peer-delivered and technology-supported self-management intervention. J Nerv Ment Dis. 2018;206(11):875–81.

Fortuna KL, Ferron J, Pratt SI, Muralidharan A, Aschbrenner KA, Williams AM, Deegan PE, Salzer M. Unmet needs of people with serious mental illness: perspectives from certified peer specialists. Psychiatr Q. 2019;90(3):579–86.

Frenk J, Chen L, Bhutta ZA, Cohen J, Crisp N, Evans T, Fineberg H, Garcia P, Ke Y, Kelley P, Kistnasamy B, Meleis A, Naylor D, Pablos-Mendez A, Reddy S, Scrimshaw S, Sepulveda J, Serwadda D, Zurayk H. Health professionals for a new century: transforming education to strengthen health systems in an interdependent world. Lancet. 2010;376(9756):1923–58.

Hardeman RR, Medina EM, Kozhimannil KB. Structural racism and supporting black lives – the role of health professionals. N Engl J Med. 2016;375(22):2113–5.

Hospital and Healthcare. Digital health micro-credentials to keep workforce up to speed. 2020. http://hospitalhealth.com.au/content/technology/news/digital-health-micro-credentials-to-keep-workforce-up-to-speed-1269548597#ixzz6VK8Bnd2h. Accessed 17 Aug 2020.

Hunt G. Australian government partnership with private health sector secures 30,000 hospital beds and 105,000 nurses and staff, to help fight COVID-19 pandemic. In: Health do. Minister Hunt's media; 2020.

Kiyumi A, Humaid Matar R, Walker S, Tariq A, Fitzgerald G. Health information management professionals [Present circumstances and future expectations]. In: Takahashi O, editor. Proceedings of the 18th IFHIMA International Congress. Japan: International Federation of Health Information Management Association; 2016. p. 518–29.

Meadows GN, Enticott JC, Inder B, Russell GM, Gurr R. Better access to mental health care and the failure of the Medicare principle of universality. Med J Aust. 2015;202(6):297.

Minnesota Department of Health. Cardiovascular health indicator – measure: heart disease death rate. 2017. https://www.health.state.mn.us/diseases/cardiovascular/cardio-dashboard/heart-deathr.html. Accessed 17 Jul 2020.

O'Connor S, Hanlon P, O'Donnell CA, Garcia S, Glanville J, Mair FS. Understanding factors affecting patient and public engagement and recruitment to digital health interventions: a systematic review of qualitative studies. BMC Med Inform Dec. 2016;16(1):120.

OECD. Hospital beds. 2020. https://data.oecd.org/healtheqt/hospital-beds.htm. Accessed 17 Aug 2020.

Pew Research Center. Mobile Fact Sheet. 2019. https://www.pewinternet.org/fact-sheet/mobile/. Accessed 17 Jul 2020.

Ray R, Sewell AA, Gilbert KL, Roberts JD. Missed opportunity? Leveraging mobile technology to reduce racial health disparities. J Health Polit Policy Law. 2017;42(5):901–24.

Shadmi E, Chen Y, Dourado I, Faran-Perach I, Furler J, Hangoma P, Hanvoravongchai P, Obando C, Petrosyan V, Rao KD, Ruano AL, Shi L, de Souza LE, Spitzer-Shohat S, Sturgiss E, Suphanchaimat R, Uribe MV, Willems S. Health equity and COVID-19: global perspectives. Int J Equity Health. 2020;19(1):104.

Shillabeer AG. Health of Vietnam. Singapore: Springer; 2015.

Shillabeer AG, Anderson B. Educating for the next health revolution: are we failing the frontline? In: Proceedings of the Australasian Computer Science Week Multiconference (ACSW '18). Association for Computing Machinery, New York, NY, USA, Article 33, 1–10; 2018.

Waitzberg R, Davidovitch N, Leibner G, Penn N, Brammli-Greenberg S. Israel's response to the COVID-19 pandemic: tailoring measures for vulnerable cultural minority populations. Int J Equity Health. 2020;19(1):71.

Ward J, Agostino J. Coronavirus will devastate Aboriginal communities if we don't act now. The Conversation; 2020.

WHO. mHealth: New horizons for health through mobile technologies. Geneva: World Health Organization; 2011. https://www.who.int/goe/publications/goe_mhealth_web.pdf?ua=1%3E. Accessed 17 Jul 2020.

WHO. Social determinants of health. 2019. https://www.who.int/health-topics/social-determinants-of-health#tab=tab_1. Accessed 17 Jul 2020.

WHO. Draft Global Strategy on digital health 2020–2024. 2020a. https://extranet.who.int/dataform/upload/surveys/183439/files/Draft%20Global%20Strategy%20on%20Digital%20Health.pdf. Accessed 21 Jul 2020.

WHO. COVID-19 health system response monitor. 2020b. https://www.covid19healthsystem.org/countries/armenia/countrypage.aspx. Accessed 10 Aug 2020.

Chapter 13
The Impact on Safety and Quality of Care of the Specialist Digital Health Workforce

Angela Ryan, Brendan Loo Gee, Susan H. Fenton, and Meredith Makeham

Abstract Digital health technologies play a critical role in the safe, effective delivery of care across health systems. The benefits for patients can be significant; however, evidence suggests that poorly designed and implemented technologies can have unintended consequences, with downstream impacts on patient safety and the quality of care provided. Key to the success of these digital health technologies is the specialist digital health workforce, who possess the requisite skills and expertise to manage and govern the safe use of digital health tools and technologies. This chapter explores the specialist digital health workforce and its impact on healthcare safety and quality practices. Following analysis of a set of case studies from US, Australian and other health systems, we highlight the paucity of attention in this important area, and the need for healthcare organisations to acknowledge and promote the specialist skills required to use digital health safely. These cases also highlight the need for further research and evaluation in this area.

Keywords Patient safety · Healthcare quality · Impact · Policy · Risk

A. Ryan (✉)
Australasian Institute of Digital Health, Sydney, NSW, Australia

B. L. Gee
College of Health and Medicine, Australian National University, Canberra, ACT, Australia
e-mail: brendan.loogee@anu.edu.au

S. H. Fenton
The University of Texas Health Science Center at Houston School of Biomedical Informatics, Houston, TX, USA
e-mail: Susan.H.Fenton@uth.tmc.edu

M. Makeham
Faculty of Medicine and Health, University of Sydney, Sydney, NSW, Australia
e-mail: meredith.makeham@sydney.edu.au

© The Author(s), under exclusive license to Springer Nature
Switzerland AG 2021
K. Butler-Henderson et al. (eds.), *The Health Information Workforce*,
Health Informatics, https://doi.org/10.1007/978-3-030-81850-0_13

Introduction

> In complex systems, things happen every day that have never happened before.
>   (Braithwaite 2018).

Digital health technologies play a critical role in the delivery of healthcare across the health system. The digital health strategies of Australia and other nations highlight that the benefits for patients, and the health system more broadly, range from avoided hospital admissions, reductions in adverse medication events and unnecessary duplicate testing, better-informed treatment decisions, and better coordination of care for people with chronic and complex conditions (e.g. Australian Digital Health Agency 2018). However, evidence shows that poorly designed or implemented systems can harm patients and even lead to death (Shortliffe 2010; Ammenwerth et al. 2008; Ash et al. 2004; Coiera et al. 2006). The scale of the problem has grown as digital health has become more ubiquitous. Commonly reported issues in digital health implementations include poorly designed user interfaces that can disrupt clinical workflows, and insufficient training of staff to use health information technology systems during routine care (Kim et al. 2017). For example, a coroner's report found the lack of hospital staff training on the clinical information system was a contributing factor in the death of a 54-year-old patient mistakenly given high doses of opioids (Daly 2018).

The complex adaptive nature of health systems, and the need to acknowledge the impacts of health IT adoption in this context was recognised in a report by the US Institute of Medicine (IOM 2001), following an increasing body of evidence relating to patient injury and death associated with digital health. The report argued that the discipline of safety science needed to be "…better integrated into a health IT-enabled world", and that…. "…safety is the product of the larger sociotechnical system and emerges from the interaction between different parts of this larger system" (IOM 2001). While the authors noted that this was not a new concept, they argued that effort was required across the health system to support this approach. One of the critical factors emerging in this report and the literature has been the under-preparedness of the health workforce to utilise digital health technologies, and the need for training and education programs to ensure a confidently skilled and capable health workforce. The literature also emphasises the critical role of the health informatician in leading the charge, as the specialist who can acknowledge and manage the risks inherent in building and implementing systems into complex adaptive healthcare environments (Kilbridge and Classen 2008; Schneider et al. 2014). This report built on other landmark IOM reports: To Err is Human (IOM 2000) prompted calls to make healthcare safer, estimating that 44,000–98,000 lives are lost in US hospitals every year due to iatrogenesis [in Australia, adverse events in hospitals are estimated to range from 2.9% to 16.6% of admissions, with at least half considered to be preventable (Duckett et al. 2018)]. Crossing the Quality Chasm (IOM 2001) argued for a health system redesign to improve the quality of care. The stimulus to augment the provision of healthcare with widespread implementation of electronic health records (EHRs), followed the introduction of the US Health Information Technology for Economic and Clinical Health Act (HIPAA Journal 2018), resulting in 96% of all nonfederal acute care hospitals possessing certified health IT systems (ONC HIT 2017). In Australia too, governments have prioritised digital health to improve service delivery and health outcomes, as have many healthcare providers, stimulating entrepreneurs and developers to invest in new tools and innovative ways to use data to provide health services (Australian Digital Health Agency 2018). This coalescence of efforts is contributing to the evidence base to support the role of digital technologies in modern clinical practice (Makeham and Ryan 2019). This is also true globally, where digital health is expanding.

Much of this activity did not contemplate the environment into which the technologies were deployed, nor the preparedness of the workforce to utilise them (IOM 2001). Already these technologies are changing profoundly the way healthcare is delivered, having additional impacts on traditional approaches to health occupations, tasks, and leadership functions. A confident and capable health workforce is required to realise the benefits of digital health technologies (Australian Digital Health Agency 2020), that is, health workers who are schooled in the nuances of the digital environment and who can enter the workplace with a degree of digital literacy, regardless of their specific healthcare role. For those who are specialists in digital health, such as informaticians, confidence and capability rely on an in-depth understanding of the component pieces of digital health, such as legal and regulatory requirements, data governance, data quality, and the nexus with patient safety (Ryan 2019). A digitally capable health workforce is still emerging as an area of focus in the health, education, and training sectors; globally, the emphasis is on enhancing digital health technologies rather than improving the capabilities of the workforce to use them effectively and safely. Nevertheless, key works such as Topol (2019) and the Australian Digital Health Agency (2020) highlight the importance of investing in the workforce—fostering a culture of continuous learning, robust governance, leadership, innovation, and the enablers of change (Wachter 2016), and considering the differences across health professional roles and contexts, especially in particular settings where digital inclusion is low (IOM 2001).

Despite the significant investment in digital health technologies, we could find no explicit literature that evaluated the impact of the specialist digital health workforce on patient safety and quality. So, this chapter uses case studies selected to examine workforce education strategies and programs, involving the expertise of digital health specialists, intended to have a positive impact on digital health literacy and patient safety. These give a cross-section of perspectives on the potential for digital health impacts on patient safety and healthcare quality: responding to a pandemic; building a cohesive workforce; managing risk; increasing transparency; operating a virtual clinic; and sharing knowledge globally. Table 13.1 provides a summary of the case studies.

Table 13.1 Case studies of workforce development for safety and quality of digital healthcare

Author (Year) Education program or strategy	Goal of program or strategy How was the case study implemented?
Annis et al. (2020) Virtual health rotation at the University of Minnesota	To improve the *use* of remote monitoring solutions. − Using existing medical resources from multiple local programs to rapidly establish a virtual health rotation. − Collaboration among clinicians, academia, and industry as being instrumental to its success. − Limitations include inefficient manual processes, and limited customisation capabilities.
Australian Digital Health Agency (2020) Workforce and Education Roadmap	To inform policy for education and training for *digital health specialists*, and to aid in the development of curricula and resources for the health workforce. − Led by the Australian Digital Health Agency, and supported by leading health informaticians, the Roadmap was co-developed with all Australian jurisdictions, including the Commonwealth, and States and Territories, university and education providers, clinical and consumer peaks, researchers and industry, and healthcare providers and consumers. − The Roadmap defined a set of digital role profiles that articulate the digital health capability requirements for the health workforce in Australia.
Bellringer et al. (2017) In-house specialist training for senior therapists and advanced clinical practitioners.	To provide staff with skills to *use* digital health technologies. − The Brighton and Sussex University Hospital Trust in the United Kingdom established new roles for senior therapists and advanced clinical practitioners who received specialist training in-house, in the area of digital technologies, imaging, and acute injury management.
Global Digital Health Partnership (2018) Learning Networks (Network-based Learning Health Systems)	To provide a policy for education and training for *digital health specialists*. − The Global Digital Health Partnership (GDHP) was established by the Australian government, in concert with international governments and territories, government agencies, and the WHO. − The specialist digital health workforce from participating countries is organised across five different workstreams, with a number of white papers developed and published in collaboration.
Greenhalgh et al. (2020) Article disseminated via BMJ on the 25 March 2020.	To improve *use* of telehealth. − Tool was developed from previous research findings and official guidance. − Doctors responded to a straw poll with advice.
OpenNotes (2010) Sharing of clinician notes.	To provide patients with skill to *use* digital health. − The OpenNotes system was designed by experts at the Beth Israel Deaconess Medical Center, a teaching hospital of Harvard Medical School in Boston, and located in the Division of General Medicine. − The study involved 105 primary care doctors and 20,000 of their patients.

Table 13.1 (continued)

Author (Year) Education program or strategy	Goal of program or strategy How was the case study implemented?
Queensland Digital Academy (CSDS 2019) Certification, basic computer training, leadership and governance training, university partnerships, grand rounds, and just-in-time training.	To provide staff with digital health specialists skills, and training opportunities to build confidence in *using* digital health technologies. – The QDA is led by a specialist digital health workforce and operates within the Clinical Skills Development Service on the Herston Campus of Metro North Hospital and Health Service, in Brisbane. – Learning opportunities are maximised through a centrally coordinated hub and spoke model.
Reeves et al. (2020) Online self-guided learning videos on virtual patient care in conjunction with "boots-on-the-ground" resources provided onboarding assistance to clinical areas enabling rapid deployment of telemedicine visits.	To improve *use* of telemedicine. – Implementation of the telemedicine system was led by the Chief Medical Information Officer and Associate Chief Medical Officer. – Training material was broadcast and communicated on the telemedicine platform which provided scripted triaging, electronic check-in, standard ordering and documentation, secure messaging and real-time data analytics, and specific metrics to key organisational leaders in real time.
Singh et al. (2013) A set of Safety Assurance Factors for EHR Resilience (SAFER) guides that was published by the ONC.	To provide staff with skills to *use* EHRs in routine care to improve patient safety. – Guides published by experts who have published widely on the topic of digital health and are internationally recognised health informaticians. – The guides were originally conceived using rigorous iterative methodologies that sourced material on unintended consequences of EHR implementation.
Sittig et al. (2018, 2020) Implementation of the Safety Assurance Factors for EHR Resilience (SAFER) guides in Australia and the United States.	To provide staff with skills to *use* EHRs in routine care to improve patient safety. – Healthcare organisations in Australia and the United States self-assessed their adherence to 140 recommendations contained across the SAFER guides.
Wright et al. (2015) Sharing of clinician notes via a patient-facing web portal	To provide patients with skill to *use* digital health. – Patients were invited to examine their records for perceived errors and mistakes.

Responding to a Pandemic

Following the declaration of a global pandemic in March 2020 (WHO 2020), tele-health became according to some, a 20-year overnight success (Dyer 2020; Warraich 2020), as the only mechanism in many parts of the world by which to deliver health-care without exacerbating disease spread; "all the red tape [had] suddenly been cut" (Webster 2020). Numerous resources were made available online worldwide to support health services as they struggled to respond to the immediate need to consult with patients via telephone or video.

For example, the United Kingdom saw sweeping developments in the use of telehealth; a research project that had been tracking the use of video conferencing in Scotland for the previous 6 months described a 1000% increase in use in 2 weeks. Greenhalgh, a noted expert in the evaluation and use of digital health technologies, and colleagues (2020) developed a remote assessment tool to aid clinicians in treating new diseases such as COVID-19. The telehealth aspects of the assessment tool were developed at speed and crafted from published and unpublished research findings and official guidance. Due to the paucity of evidence on how to assess breathlessness over the phone, a straw poll was used to elicit (mostly) doctors' expert advice. This was a case of marshalling and disseminating key learnings about how to use digital health technologies effectively in a crisis.

Reeves et al. (2020) described a US digital health implementation in response to the COVID-19 outbreak, that saw over 300 health employees trained in telemedicine and approximately 1000 video visits scheduled, within 72 hours of the executive proclamation of a national emergency. This was enhanced by a pre-existing telemedicine infrastructure and associated specialist digital health workforce in situ. Online self-guided learning videos on virtual patient care in conjunction with "boots-on-the-ground" resources provided onboarding assistance to clinical areas, enabling rapid deployment of telemedicine visits and real-time responsiveness to the evolving situation. There were challenges, including the need to frequently adjust the system build, the voluminous stream of information and communication being broadcast, and the necessity to continue to provide safe high-quality healthcare to non-COVID-19 patients. This case offers lessons for the rapid deployment and translation of digital health expertise.

Annis et al. (2020) describe a remote patient monitoring solution for patients with COVID-19 symptoms that provided healthcare to them while minimising virus exposure and in-patient admissions. The study also examined the impact of an existing rapid technology deployment platform that was repurposed as a remote monitoring solution, staffed by medical students and residents from multiple local programs through the timely establishment of a virtual healthcare rotation program at the University of Minnesota. The authors highlighted the "significant learning opportunities (in virtual health) for medical resources which may have otherwise been sidelined". The virtual healthcare rotation program was an approach to ensure patients heard a consistent narrative about the care they were receiving, especially given the dynamic and evolving nature of treatment guidance. 2,255 patients reported a 74% satisfaction rating, and patients described a sense of safety overall.

Building a Cohesive Workforce

Two Australian examples illustrate healthcare system approaches to define and shape the digital health workforce, as part of acknowledging the impact of digital health tools and technologies on patient safety and quality of care. In 2020, the

Australian Digital Health Agency's National Digital Health Workforce & Education Roadmap established eight digital role profiles as a mechanism to guide individuals and organisations in understanding their needs, roles, and responsibilities for the design, development, implementation, adoption, evaluation, and monitoring of digital health technologies. Further, these digital profiles were intended to aid the development of health workforce curricula and resources for the education and training sector, and specifically for developing specialist digital health expertise. The Clinical and Technology Bridging digital profile, for example, includes the functions of Clinical Designer and Specification Advisor; Clinical Information Analyser; Risk and Governance Enforcer; Digital Change Champion; User Tester; Problem Solver; Health Reformer and Innovator; and Quality Controller. The elements of this profile have been tested with this specific cohort for their relevance and applicability, as have the other seven profiles.

The Queensland Digital Academy (QDA) is a cross-organisational collaboration working in partnership with multiple agencies, established in 2019. The Academy is addressing the burgeoning need for digital literacy and capability within the State of Queensland's health workforce in order to assure and improve patient safety. Multiple locations across the State provide staff with education and training opportunities in digital healthcare, literacy, and leadership capability and capacity to help support digital transformation, with many achievements in a short time: The Academy has provided access through sponsorship to the Certified Health Informatician Australasia (CHIA) certification (2021), with additional learning support. It has provided access to basic computer training through a computer fundamentals course and touch-typing practice to ensure no one is left behind in the digital environment. It has provided digital onboarding sessions and electronic medical record introductory sessions to grow the digital capability of key leadership and governance group members. It has led to the development of university partnerships to design undergraduate and postgraduate curricula. It has provided monthly Digital Health Grand Rounds, an opportunity to showcase insights and engage academics, clinical informaticians, and the broader health workforce. It has provided just-in-time training, leveraging technology to provide training directly to clinicians when needed.

Managing Risk

A landmark study compared the effects of two commercial electronic prescribing systems on two Australian hospitals' inpatients, examining effects on reducing prescribing error rates and on introducing new errors (Westbrook et al. 2012). Both hospitals experienced statistically significant reductions in prescribing error rates, including a reduction in serious errors. Both hospitals also demonstrated system-related errors, which the study noted required ongoing monitoring to detect and address through redesign and user training. While the study did not comment specifically on the makeup of the workforce involved to introduce the two systems, it did note that clinicians' greatest concern regarding systems introduction was their impact on workflows. The study highlighted the complexity of introducing such systems, particularly across an organisation, and the number of work process and cultural factors that must be considered, noting that organisations should commit to resourcing for the long term. It also emphasised the requirement for ongoing surveillance and refinement to ensure the systems are optimised for safer practice.

Safety guides have appeared in response to the rapid implementation of EHRs in the United States—from the ONC HIT (2018) and earlier, from Sittig et al. (2014). The SAFER guides are in three broad categories: Foundational guides, Infrastructure guides, and Clinical Process guides. Recommendations within the guides are organised into three broad domains: "safe health IT" (45 recommendations), 'using health IT safely' (80 recommendations), and "monitoring health IT" (15 recommendations). The guides were designed to assess risk and eliminate or minimise the unintended consequences that arise from the implementation of EHRs into complex adaptive health systems. The guides also introduce the importance of the development and ongoing promotion of a safety culture across organisations, to identify and mitigate risks to patient safety (Ryan 2019). Risk assessments across eight different healthcare organisations spanning the United States and Australia, examining their adherence to the SAFER guides, found that only 25 of the 140 SAFER recommendations (18%) had been fully implemented, with adherence higher for the "safe health IT" domain (82.1%) vs "using health IT safely" (72.5%) and "monitoring health IT" (67.3%). The authors concluded that despite the availability of the guides, governments need to prioritise policy initiatives to ensure greater awareness of best practice guidelines and embed them as part of EHR implementations (Sittig et al. 2018).

Similarly, a paper by Sittig et al. (2020) describe an approach to support healthcare organisations, researchers, funders, and policymakers to better contemplate and address digital health-related patient safety. The paper articulates areas of emphasis across the digital health lifecycle, providing a set of challenges to apply to every implementation to ensure patient safety. The challenges take a stepped approach and are described through nine different stages, across three themes. Design and Development challenges include Developing models, methods, and tools to enable risk assessment; Developing standard user interface design features and functions; Ensuring the safety of software in an interfaced, network-enabled clinical environment; and Implementing a method for unambiguous patient identification. Implementation and Use challenges include Developing and implementing decision support which improves safety; and Identifying practices to safely manage IT system transitions. Monitoring, Evaluation, and Optimization challenges include Developing real-time methods to enable automated surveillance and monitoring of system performance and safety; Establishing the cultural and legal framework/safe harbor to allow sharing information about hazards and adverse events; and Developing models and methods for consumers/patients to improve Health IT safety. Using a systems-based approach, risks can be minimised and EHR design optimised to drive healthcare safety and quality improvements.

Improving Transparency

OpenNotes (2010) is an "international movement committed to spreading the availability of open visit notes and studying the effects", with a mission to provide patients, families, and caregivers with open access to their clinicians' notes. OpenNotes was first conceived in 2010 following the launch of an exploratory study (Walker et al. 2011) examining the impact of sharing clinician notes with patients. Results from this study showed that patients felt more in control of their health as a result of the exposure. Since this initial study, the movement has grown to represent more than 40 million patients across the United States and Canada. A study by Wright et al. (2015) found greater adherence to medication regimes following exposure to primary care physician notes via a patient-facing web portal. The authors conducted a retrospective comparative analysis of 2417 patients aged 18 years or above. They found adherence rates of 79.7% among patients using antihypertensive medications versus 75.3% in a control group who did not have access to their notes; even though there was little difference among patients using antihyperlipidemic medications. The authors concluded that patient exposure to notes might be associated with positive behaviour change, particularly as records become more transparent over time. However, a report by Bell et al. (2020) found that patients perceived errors within their notes to be associated with important safety and quality implications. Among 29,656 patients invited to examine their records for perceived errors, 20% of the cohort reported a perceived mistake. Based on the findings, Bell et al. have concluded that note transparency may be associated with greater patient engagement in safety along with improved accuracy within their records, although further research is necessary to expand the evidence base. This study illustrates the potentially overlooked role of patients and consumers in the work of digital health safety and quality.

Operating a Virtual Clinic

Bellringer et al. (2017) described the establishment of specialised in-house training for a virtual fracture clinic for acute fractures and soft tissue injuries at a hospital in the United Kingdom. Patients presenting in the Emergency Department with an ankle fracture were X-rayed and assessed, and then discharged when surgical intervention was not required. Patients were followed up post discharge with a telephone call, replacing the need to attend a clinic in person. Telephone calls were guided by the use of a consistent guideline, which articulated the treatment protocol. Education and training requirements were minimal due to the use of the protocol and the involvement of experienced staff. This study examined the safety and effectiveness of this intervention. In particular, the study found that the model was able to deliver safe care with no evidence of serious complications and delivered significant savings to the Clinical Commissioning Group. Similar studies in Australia have replicated these findings, demonstrating patient satisfaction with the quality of care: avoiding unnecessary travel, needing fewer outpatient appointments, experiencing shorter wait times for first orthopaedic contact, and being managed locally by primary care providers (Cross 2019).

Sharing Knowledge Globally

In 2018, the Global Digital Health Partnership was established to bring together a network of countries to collaborate on best practices and to share evidence and learnings of digital health implementations. The vision of the partnership is to guide policy on the delivery of digital health services to drive improvements in patient safety and quality of care (GDHP 2020). Similar network-based learning health systems (or learning networks) have been established over the last 13 years (Britto et al. 2018), recognising the value of exchanging knowledge internationally among digital health specialists. Participant countries are organised across five different work streams, identified as key areas where there are shared challenges, covering clinical and consumer engagement, evidence and evaluation, policy environments, interoperability, and cybersecurity, with a number of white papers developed and published in collaboration. Further work will be required to determine the impact of these white papers on local country policies.

Discussion and Conclusions

The case studies in this chapter examine different workforce development strategies and programs focused on improving digital health safety and quality, either directly through designing and implementing technology interventions or indirectly through improving the digital health literacy of the broader health workforce. The methods used to achieve these goals include the rapid dissemination of academic articles, online self-guided videos, virtual health rotations, certification programs, leadership and governance training, university partnerships, grand rounds, just-in-time training, guideline formulation, clinician note sharing, and learning networks. There is little consistency in their approach, and the accounts provided by researchers and policy-makers offer only fragments of insight into the role of digital health specialists in their execution.

The explosion of online resources to support pandemic-driven use of telehealth has left many clinicians searching for standardised, reliable, and consistent guidelines. This is a prime example of an opportunity for digital health specialists to create and curate, in a centralised location, standardised programs and guidelines to support telehealth use at least at a national level. Such initiatives would be effective and efficient and would enable digital health specialists to monitor and evaluate the impact of their work on healthcare safety and quality.

Many of the case studies did not include a patient safety framework, such as that described by Sittig et al. (2014), that contemplates the environment in which a digital health system is implemented. The implementation of patient safety frameworks should be considered at the outset and led and managed by digital health specialists working in concert with the broader health workforce. These frameworks can be applied across any healthcare environment—from primary and community care environments to hospital and health service environments. The aim should be to assign responsibility to digital health specialists, to maintain control of the intervention over different environments and hence minimising the risk for any adverse events.

There is a need to place a greater emphasis on the complex adaptive nature of the health system as an underpinning tenet, and the overarching principles of patient safety and quality as the necessary outcomes. Further, there is limited application of ongoing monitoring and surveillance to detect and respond to issues that arise, leading to the likelihood of unintended consequences – consequences that the technologies have been put in place to avoid. The specialist digital health workforce has a growing role to play in the design, development, deployment and ongoing monitoring of these technologies and there is an opportunity for health leaders across the system to respond to this need and invest further in the education and training of this important workforce.

The majority of the case studies showed training programs targeting the wider health workforce to utilise digital health tools safely. There has not been a concomitant investment in the training of the specialist digital health workforce, nor widespread recognition of the important role of the digital health specialist. There are a number of federally funded programs in the United States, including the National Library of Medicine (NLM 2021) fellowship program for pre- and postdoctoral trainees and those funded by the Agency for Healthcare Research and Quality (AHRQ 2021) regarding the dissemination of best practices around HIT, which support the emerging digital health specialist workforce. Alongside these are small-scale fellowship programs in the United Kingdom (Faculty of Clinical Informatics 2021) and Australia and New Zealand (Australasian Institute of Digital Health 2021). Overall, greater investment in a confident and capable workforce could assist governments and health services to scale digital health projects and proofs of concept. We need to know more about the impact of digital health specialists' work on safety and quality outcomes, and also about the impact of their efforts to train the health workforce to utilise digital health tools.

Novel approaches are essential to move beyond traditional models of developing the specialist digital health workforce. Multi-actor collaborations at a global level, among governments, healthcare organisations, clinicians, consumers, and resources are critical to implementing strategies and programs to build the digital health workforce and digital health specialist workforce effectively. Learning networks (Britto et al. 2018)—aligning participating healthcare agencies with a common goal, transparency of outcome measures, and collaborative shared resources for cooperative learning and co-production of ideas and knowledge at scale—could support the digital health specialist workforce to address and improve overall patient safety and health outcomes.

It is clear that much more research into the specialist digital health workforce is required to understand its actual effectiveness and potential for impact with respect to patient safety and healthcare quality.

References

Agarwal S, LeFevre AE, Lee J, L'Engle K, Mehl G, Sinha C, WHO mHealth Technical Evidence Review Group. Guidelines for reporting of health interventions using mobile phones: mobile health (mHealth) evidence reporting and assessment (mERA) checklist. BMJ. 2016;352:i1174.

AHRQ Agency for Healthcare Research and Quality. Funding announcements. 2021. http://www.ahrq.gov/funding/fund-opps/index.html. Accessed 8 Feb 2021.

Ammenwerth E, Schnell-Inderst P, Machan C, Siebert U. The effect of electronic prescribing on medication errors and adverse drug events: a systematic review. J Am Med Inform Assoc. 2008;15(5):585–600.

Annis T, Pleasants S, Hultman G, Lindemann E, Thompson JA, Billecke S, Badlani S, Melton GB. Rapid implementation of a COVID-19 remote patient monitoring program. J Am Med Inform Assoc. 2020;27(8):1326–30.

Ash JS, Berg M, Coiera E. Some unintended consequences of information technology in health care: the nature of patient care information system-related errors. J Am Med Inform Assoc. 2004;11(2):104–12.

Australasian Institute of Digital Health. Certified Health Informatician Australasia. 2021. https://www.healthinformaticscertification.com/. Accessed 31 Mar 2021.

Australasian Institute of Digital Health. Fellowship by training program. 2021. https://digital-health.org.au/fellowship-by-training-program/. Accessed 31 Mar 2021.

Australian Digital Health Agency. Seamless and secure: evolving health and care to meet the needs of modern Australia, Australia's National Digital Health Strategy. 2018. https://www.digitalhealth.gov.au/sites/default/files/2020-11/Australia%27s%20National%20Digital%20Health%20Strategy%20-%20Safe%2C%20seamless%20and%20secure.pdf. Accessed 31 Mar 2021.

Australian Digital Health Agency. The national digital health workforce & education roadmap. 2020. https://www.digitalhealth.gov.au/sites/default/files/2020-11/Workforce_and_Education-Roadmap.pdf. Accessed 31 Mar 2021.

Bell SK, Delbanco T, Elmore JG, Fitzgerald PS, Fossa A, Harcourt K, Leveille SG, Payne TH, Stametz RA, Walker J, DesRoches CM. Frequency and types of patient-reported errors in electronic health record ambulatory care notes. JAMA Netw Open. 2020;3(6):e205867.

Bellringer SF, Brogan K, Cassidy L, Gibbs J. Standardised virtual fracture clinic management of radiographically stable Weber B ankle fractures is safe, cost effective and reproducible. Injury. 2017;48(7):1670–3.

Bergmo TS. How to measure costs and benefits of eHealth interventions: an overview of methods and frameworks. J Med Internet Res. 2015;17(11):e254.

Braithwaite J. Refashioning the quality agenda over the next decade. In: Health Quality Transformation. 2018.

Britto MT, Fuller SC, Kaplan HC, Kotagal U, Lannon C, Margolis PA, Muething SE, Schoettker PJ, Seid M. Using a network organizational architecture to support the development of Learning Healthcare Systems. BMJ Qual Saf. 2018;27:937–46.

Coiera E, Westbrook J, Wyatt J. The safety and quality of decision support systems. Yearb Med Inform. 2006:20–5.

Cross E. The safety and efficacy of a virtual fracture clinic in a major Australian tertiary trauma hospital. 2019. https://www.thermh.org.au/health-professionals/clinical-services/orthopaedic-surgery/virtual-fracture-clinic. Accessed 31 Mar 2021.

CSDS Clinical Skills Development Service. CSDS welcomes the Queensland Digital Academy. 2019. https://csds.qld.edu.au/blog/csds-welcomes-the-queensland-digital-academy/. Accessed 31 Mar 2021.

Daly N. Medical staff lacked 'critical thinking' in accidental overdose of Paul Lau, coroner finds. ABC News (online). 2018. https://www.abc.net.au/news/2018-03-29/medical-staff-lacked-critical-thinking-overdose-man-says-coroner/9600076. Accessed 31 Mar 2021.

Duckett S, Jorm C, Danks L, Moran G. All complications should count: using our data to make hospitals safer. Grattan Inst. 2018. https://grattan.edu.au/wp-content/uploads/2018/02/897-All-complications-should-count.pdf. Accessed 31 Mar 2021.

Dyer J. Telehealth in the time of COVID-19: a 20-year overnight success. Infect Control Today. 2020;24(5). https://www.infectioncontroltoday.com/covid-19/telehealth-time-covid-19-20-year-overnight-success. Accessed 14 Feb 2021.

Faculty of Clinical Informatics. Competency framework for clinical informaticians. 2021. https://facultyofclinicalinformatics.org.uk/core-competencies. Accessed 31 Mar 2021.

GHDP Global Digital Health Partnership. White papers. 2020. https://gdhp.org/home/index/white-paper-2020. Accessed 31 Mar 2021.

Greenhalgh T, Koh GCH, Car J. Covid-19: a remote assessment in primary care. BMJ. 2020;368:m1182.

HIPAA Journal. What is the HITECH Act? 2018. https://www.hipaajournal.com/what-is-the-hitech-act/. Accessed 14 Feb 2021.

IOM Institute of Medicine. Committee on quality of health care in America. To err is human: building a safer health system. In: Kohn LT, Corrigan JM, Donaldson MS, editors. 2000. https://pubmed.ncbi.nlm.nih.gov/25077248/. Accessed 31 Mar 2021.

IOM. Committee on quality of health care in America. Crossing the quality chasm: a new health system for the 21st century. 2001. PMID: 25057539. https://pubmed.ncbi.nlm.nih.gov/25057539/. Accessed 31 Mar 2021.

IOM Institute of Medicine. Committee on quality of health care in America. Crossing the quality chasm: a new health system for the 21st century. 2001. PMID: 25057539. https://pubmed.ncbi.nlm.nih.gov/25057539/. Accessed 31 Mar 2021.

Kilbridge PM, Classen DC. The informatics opportunities at the intersection of patient safety and clinical informatics. J Am Med Inform Assoc. 2008;15(4):397–407.

Kim MO, Coiera E, Magrabi F. Problems with health information technology and their effects on care delivery and patient outcomes: a systematic review. J Am Med Inform Assoc. 2017;24(2):246–50.

Makeham MA, Ryan A. Sharing information safely and securely: the foundation of a modern health care system. Med J Aust. 2019;210(Suppl 6):S3–4.

NLM National Library of Medicine. Extramural grant programs [product, program, and project descriptions]. Grants and funding; U.S. National Library of Medicine. 2021. https://www.nlm.nih.gov/ep/Grants.html. Accessed 8 Feb 2021.

ONC HIT. Health IT dashboard, 2017, percent of hospitals, by type, that possess certified health IT. 2017. https://dashboard.healthit.gov/quickstats/quickstats.php. Accessed 14 Feb 2021.

ONC HIT. SAFER guides. 2018. https://www.healthit.gov/topic/safety/safer-guides. Accessed 14 Feb 2021.

OpenNotes. About. 2010. https://www.opennotes.org/about/. Accessed 14 Feb 2021.

OpenNotes. More than 40 million patients can access their clinicians' visit notes via secure portals at 200 health systems. 2018. https://www.opennotes.org/news/more-than-40-million-patients-can-access-their-clinicians-visit-notes-via-secure-portals-at-200-health-systems/. Accessed 14 Feb 2021.

Reeves JJ, Hollandsworth HM, Torriani FJ, Taplitz R, Abeles S, Tai-Seale M, Millen M, Clay BJ, Longhurst CA. Rapid response to COVID-19: health informatics support for outbreak management in an academic health system. J Am Med Inform Assoc. 2020;27(6):853–9.

Ryan A. To investigate methods to reduce patient harm through national digital health safety governance. Churchill Fellowship Report. 2019. https://www.churchilltrust.com.au/fellows/detail/4293/Angela+Ryan. Accessed 31 Mar 2021.

Schneider EC, Ridgely MS, Meeker D, Hunter LE, Khodyakov D, Rudin RS. Promoting patient safety through effective health information technology risk management. Rand Health Q. 2014;4(3):7.

Shortliffe EH. AMIA testimony to HIT policy committee adoption/certification workgroup. 2010. https://www.amia.org/sites/default/files/files_2/Shortliffe-HIT-policy-testimony-feb2010.pdf. Accessed 14 Feb 2021.

Singh H, Ash JS, Sittig DF. Safety Assurance Factors for Electronic Health Record Resilience (SAFER): study protocol. BMC Med Inform Decis Mak. 2013;13:46.

Sittig DF, Ash JS, Singh H. The SAFER guides: empowering organizations to improve the safety and effectiveness of electronic health records. Am J Manag Care. 2014;20(5):418–23.

Sittig DF, Salimi M, Aiyagari R, Banas C, Clay B, Gibson KA, Goel A, Hines R, Longhurst CA, Mishra V, Sirajuddin AM, Satterly T, Singh H. Adherence to recommended electronic health record safety practices across eight health care organizations. J Am Med Inform Assoc. 2018;25(7):913–8.

Sittig DF, Wright A, Coiera E, Magrabi F, Ratwani R, Bates DW, Singh H. Current challenges in health information technology–related patient safety. Health Inform J. 2020:181–9.

Topol E. The Topol review, preparing the healthcare workforce to deliver the digital future, An independent report on behalf of the Secretary of State for Health and Social Care February. 2019. https://topol.hee.nhs.uk/wp-content/uploads/HEE-Topol-Review-2019.pdf. Accessed 8 Feb 2021.

Wachter RM. Making IT work: harnessing the power of health information technology to improve care in England. Report of the National Advisory Group on health information technology in England. 2016. https://assets.publishing.service.gov.uk/government/uploads/system/uploads/attachment_data/file/550866/Wachter_Review_Accessible.pdf. Accessed 8 Feb 2021.

Walker J, Leveille SG, Ngo L, Vodicka E, Darer JD, Dhanireddy S, Elmore JG, Feldman HJ, Lichtenfeld MJ, Oster N, Ralston JD, Ross SE, Delbanco T. Inviting patients to read their doctors' notes: patients and doctors look ahead: patient and physician surveys. Ann Intern Med. 2011;155(12):811–9.

Warraich HJ. As a doctor, I use telemedicine. With the coronavirus threat, it could revolutionize healthcare. Los Angeles Times (online). 2020. https://www.latimes.com/opinion/story/2020-03-17/op-ed-as-a-doctor-i-use-telemedicine-with-the-coronavirus-threat-it-could-revolutionize-healthcare. Accessed 14 Feb 2021.

Webster P. Virtual health care in the era of COVID-19. Lancet. 2020;395(10231):1180–1.

Westbrook JI, Reckmann M, Li L, Runciman WB, Burke R, Lo C, Baysari MT, Braithwaite J, Day RO. Effects of two commercial electronic prescribing systems on prescribing error rates in hospital in-patients: a before and after study. PLoS Med. 2012;9(1):e1001164.

WHO. WHO timeline – COVID-19. 2020. https://www.who.int/news-room/detail/27-04-2020-who-timeline%2D%2D-covid-19. Accessed 14 Feb 2021.

Wright E, Darer J, Tang X, Thompson J, Tusing L, Fossa A, Delbanco T, Ngo L, Walker J. Sharing physician notes through an electronic portal is associated with improved medication adherence: quasi-experimental study. J Med Internet Res. 2015;17(10):e226.

Part V
Case Studies

Chapter 14
Working as a CIO in Healthcare

Meredith Makeham, Angela Ryan, Richard Taggart, Clair Sullivan, Peter Sprivulis, and Keith McNeil

Abstract Healthcare Chief Information Officers (CIOs), through their stewardship of technology, have become key players in the healthcare innovation agenda. However, the introduction of technology is much more than just a technical task; it involves new ways of working, networking and organising globally. These changes require the expertise and guidance of professionals with health informatics knowledge, combined with management and leadership skills (particularly in the context of change), as well as clinical experience and an understanding of the demands faced by frontline clinicians in healthcare services and settings. This chapter provides historical context for the development of these roles, their key attributes, challenges and next steps for the healthcare CIO of the future.

M. Makeham (✉)
Faculty of Medicine and Health, University of Sydney, Sydney, NSW, Australia
e-mail: meredith.makeham@sydney.edu.au

A. Ryan
Australasian Institute of Digital Health, Sydney, NSW, Australia

R. Taggart
Sydney Local Health District, Sydney, NSW, Australia
e-mail: Richard.Taggart@health.nsw.gov.au

C. Sullivan
Metro North Hospital and Health Service, Brisbane, QLD, Australia
e-mail: Clair.Sullivan@health.qld.gov.au

P. Sprivulis
Western Australia Department of Health, Perth, WA, Australia
e-mail: peter.sprivulis@health.wa.gov.au

K. McNeil
Queensland Health, Brisbane, QLD, Australia
e-mail: Keith.McNeil@health.qld.gov.au

© The Author(s), under exclusive license to Springer Nature
Switzerland AG 2021
K. Butler-Henderson et al. (eds.), *The Health Information Workforce*,
Health Informatics, https://doi.org/10.1007/978-3-030-81850-0_14

217

Keywords Case study · Chief information officer · Chief clinical information officer · Chief digital health officer · Leadership

Introduction

Healthcare planners and governments across the globe are involved in efforts to stimulate innovation and reform health systems to enhance the delivery of safe, effective and quality care 'to patients'. Digital information and communication technologies (ICT) have become essential; today there are almost no parts of healthcare systems anywhere in the world that do not rely on any form of ICT (WHO 2020). Increasingly, technology underpins the continuum—the supply chain, medical research, people management, operations, finance and billing, patient diagnosis, treatment, monitoring, and handover of care. Health services are being technology-enabled to address consumer demands and expectations, provide relevant, appropriate and useful real-time information to clinical practitioners, and enhance the management and monitoring of healthcare delivery performance. Whether it is the deployment of mobile phones to monitor pregnant mothers in Sub-Saharan Africa (Holst et al. 2020), or the implementation of a comprehensive electronic medicines system in hospitals across New South Wales, Australia (eHealth NSW 2019), the momentum of technology adoption has transformed the industry, and demonstrated improved quality, safety and efficiency of patient care (ACSQHC 2018). Governments and healthcare providers are cognisant of these opportunities but must balance up them up against available resources and possible risks. For every successful ICT implementation, there are countless examples of failure; however, these are often difficult to learn from, tending to be reported less frequently in the literature. ICT also presents new risks to health organisations such as cybersecurity and technology-related adverse events (Sujan et al. 2020). International collaborations such as the Global Digital Health Partnership are emerging to guide reform initiatives in the best use of evidence-based technologies (Global Digital Health Partnership 2020). Industry organisations have created maturity models (HIMSS 2020), best practice guidance, communities of practice (Australian Institute of Digital Health 2020) and training programs to help health organisations navigate the complexities involved in healthcare ICT.

Emergence of the CIO

Chief Information Officers (CIOs) have become critical players in the healthcare innovation agenda, through stewardship of the technology. The introduction of ICT is much more than just a technical task; it involves new ways of working, networking and organising globally. These changes require the expertise and guidance of professionals with health informatics knowledge, combined with management and leadership skills, clinical experience and an understanding of the demands faced by frontline clinicians in healthcare services and settings. Specialisations within health-care ICT leadership and CIO roles have emerged in response to the requirements for senior roles within the Health Informatics, Digital, Data, Information and kNowl-edge (HIDDIN) workforce. By way of background, although healthcare organisa-tions had been establishing information management and technology functions since the 1970s, it was not until the mid-1990s that the CIO's role was commonly found on the organisation charts of leading healthcare providers (Glasser 1993). In the early years, the CIO's role was very technology-centric, responsible for estab-lishing telephone and network infrastructure, email systems and necessary comput-ing hardware (Sullivan and Miliard 2018). By the 2000s, health providers worldwide were beginning to identify the benefits that health information technology could make to the safety, efficiency and quality of care.

In Australia, both public and private providers were making large investments into electronic medical records (EMRs) and several States and Territories commit-ted significant funding to roll out programs. By the early 2010s, EMRs and other clinical information systems were becoming ubiquitous in Australia. CIOs became key to delivering these transformational technologies within government health departments and health provider organisations. The role moved from 'back of house' IT support, to become an essential strategic role within the business. Increasingly CIOs were required to have a deep understanding of healthcare and the delivery and management of technology operations. As more systems were imple-mented and new features added, the IT department needed to grow to keep these systems running, updated and secure, and to provide around-the-clock support to clinical and administrative staff users.

Related healthcare CIO roles became more commonplace in healthcare, as demand increased for organisational leaders who could merge the traditional skills of a health CIO with deep clinical expertise and experience. Some original CIOs had this skill set, but it was not denoted in their position title. As the importance of dual qualifications increased, roles emerged with titles such as Chief Clinical Information Officer (CCIO), Chief Medical Information Officer (CMIO), Chief Nursing Information Officer (CNIO), and more recently, Chief Digital Health Officer (CDHO). These professionals were expected to have qualifications or in-depth knowledge and experience relevant to informatics, combined with either broad clinical expertise or qualifications in a specified clinical discipline. In many healthcare organisations the traditional technology focussed CIO role continues today, combined with a range of healthcare C'X'IO. In larger healthcare organisa-tions, their partnership plays a vital role in delivering digital health services to front-line clinicians and healthcare consumers, as well as balancing the technical and non-technical aspects of change.

For example, in Australia the National Digital Health Strategy provides a plan and a vision of safer and better-connected healthcare, supported by digital health technology (Australian Digital Health Agency 2019); the application of this strat-egy in the late 2010s required CIOs to coordinate and lead the approach in many organisations (Eden et al. 2020). These organisations also became increasingly interested in emerging technologies such as clinical mobility, voice assistants and artificial intelligence, to name but a few, and needed healthcare CIOs to stay current with the latest trends and opportunities created by these tools. In the 2020s, the healthcare CIO specialist must often balance maintaining the operation of complex clinical environments and providing line management to large departments of IT professionals. They must manage the expectations of healthcare professionals whilst controlling costs and delivering business innovation (Kark 2017). Their frontline healthcare delivery experiences and qualifications provide an important skillset to deliver these functions in a way that best incorporates the needs and expectations of patients and frontline clinical staff. It also helps them lead co-design processes with technologists, clinicians and healthcare consumers to develop and implement new digital health technologies and services for their organisations.

An Australian case study is that of Clair Sullivan. She started her career intending to become an endocrinologist, completing her training and a research doctorate in the UK. After 2 years as a consultant endocrinologist in a metropolitan academic tertiary hospital in Australia, she became the Director of Physician Training. This provided initial experience in system management. Following this role, she was promoted to Deputy Chair of Medicine. When the health system embarked on a digital transformation with an initial implementation of an integrated electronic medical record, she became the Clinical Lead for the AUD70 million project. She then moved to a State-wide role as the Medical Director of the EMR governance team. Her next role was as Chief Digital Health Officer for Australia's largest hospital and healthcare service. Throughout this time, she maintained a portfolio of academic activity, continuing to publish, research, and supervise PhD students. She also undertook governance roles, serving on several national advisory boards. She has remained a practising clinician throughout this career trajectory.

Key Functions of CIOs

CIO roles are unique leadership positions in healthcare. They have an extensive remit to transform the health systems in which they work. They must combine their knowledge of the health system with technology expertise and business acumen. To achieve success, people in these roles should have organisational knowledge and skills across strategy and vision, cybersecurity and privacy, and many domains of management: people; services; relationships; vendors; finances; technology; projects and portfolios. The healthcare CIO needs to work in alignment with their Chief Executive Officer and others in the organisation's senior leadership team, on the business goals of the organisation and the role technology will play in achieving them. Although protecting patient confidentiality and data security is a shared organisational responsibility, the CIO is often the most senior executive accountable for protecting information systems—they must be abreast of the threats facing the health industry and be proactive in averting them.

The ability of the CIO to lead a team and relate to others is one of the most important of all the domains. They must inspire their department, partners and key stakeholders to understand the opportunity that technology offers their business and overcome the inevitable challenges that arise. They must build a high-performing team through recruitment, talent management and professional development, manage the performance of their team, and deal with human resource issues as they arise. A key to their success is their knowledge of and experience with change management principles, since the effective implementation of any large-scale digital project is at its heart, a change management process involving all the people affected by the change. An essential part of the role is maintaining relationships both internal and external to the organisation, across both technology and healthcare stakeholders. From the Emergency Department to the fracture clinic up to the finance office, the CIO role must be responsive regarding the technology tools others in the organisation need to achieve their goals.

The CIO must lead their teams to plan, build and deploy a complex set of ICT services, such as monitoring, maintaining and supporting production systems and managing incidents as they arise. They must also outsource some service provision, by interacting with a range of providers from hardware and software vendors to consultancies and resource agencies. They must navigate complicated procurement and contractual issues, and ensure that the deliverables provide value for money and achieve their stated outcomes. Information technology can add significant value to an organisation, but it can come at a substantial cost, so the CIO is likely to be responsible for a multi-million-dollar budget, and balance how to invest this in maintaining operations, upgrading systems and delivering innovative solutions.

Although not required to be deep technical experts, the CIO must have a thorough understanding of technology, and how it should be governed and managed. They must continue to develop, maintain and manage the infrastructure and applications upon which their organisation depends. They must stay current with emerging technologies, understand their organisation's needs and have a strategy that enables interoperability between systems. These roles will often be relied on to oversee cybersecurity systems, policies and procedures that are based on working knowledge of both the technical and behavioural aspects of cybersecurity. Especially in the wake of COVID-19, many healthcare organisations have a comprehensive digital transformation program underway, from EMRs to telehealth and everything in between. Effective program and project management are essential to ensure that these initiatives are delivered within the time, quality and cost parameters acceptable to their organisation. The CIO must therefore balance the portfolio of initiatives underway within the organisation, based on available resources and ability to deliver.

Becoming a CIO

Many healthcare CIOs start from a health professional background, and then either through experience or by seeking post-graduate qualifications in IT, they develop their interest in health informatics and subsequently pursue careers in this specialised field. Many choose to undertake professional or industry certifications; some more senior executives undertake Master's degrees, for example, in information management or business administration.

CIOs and senior health technology executives have generally followed a more traditional technology career path. These professionals often hold a computer science or informatics-based undergraduate degree before entering the health industry. Then, either through further education or experience, they develop their knowledge of the healthcare industry. At the time of writing, the authors know of only one specific formal pathway to becoming a CIO—through the College of Healthcare Information Management Executives (CHIME 2020), a US-based non-profit organisation that offers a certification program open to international applicants. In addition or alternatively, many CIOs have obtained Fellowship with a professional or industry association, for example in health services management, health information management or health informatics.

Challenges and Directions for CIO Roles

Healthcare CIOs are interpreters of information technology for their organisations and clinical colleagues. A principal barrier they face is the lack of digital health literacy in the management ranks of most health organisations and indeed, the clinical community. Being able to successfully answer an email on an iPhone or use common applications in a desktop environment may give people a sense that they understand the complexities of enabling digital health capabilities far more than they do. This makes the role of a CIO more challenging, as they balance the principles of co-design, engagement and feasibility. Demonstration rather than description is by far the best means of breaking through this barrier. An opportunistic approach is often required, such as taking opportunities to act as an interpreter while simultaneously increasing the digital literacy of management tiers. Active promotion of digital literacy in the clinical and management workforce is required for the successful engagement and implementation of new digital tools and services in a healthcare organisation. The investment required for workforce digital capacity and capability uplift varies between settings and is under-resourced in some.

Progressing the role of CIOs in healthcare involves them in exercising leadership beyond their immediate roles, and working across the health sector broadly. They need to contribute to efforts that can support digital health specialist capacity building. They need to participate actively in the formulation and advancement of national digital health strategies and policies.

References

ACSQHC. Impact of digital health on the safety and quality of healthcare. Australian Commission on Safety and Quality in Health Care, 2018. https://www.safetyandquality.gov.au/sites/default/files/migrated/Report-The-Impact-of-Digital-Health-on-Safety-and-Quality-of-Healthcar.... pdf. Accessed 15 May 2021.

Australian Digital Health Agency. Safe, seamless and secure: evolving health and care to meet the needs of modern Australia – Australia's National Digital Health Strategy. 2019. https://www.digitalhealth.gov.au/about-us/national-digital-health-strategy-and-framework-for-action. Accessed 15 May 2021.

Australian Institute of Digital Health. Communities of practice. 2020. https://digitalhealth.org.au/communities-of-practice/. Accessed 15 May 2021.

College of Healthcare Information Management Executives. About. 2020. https://chimecentral.org/. Accessed 15 May 2021.

Eden R, Burton-Jones A, Ballantine C, Staib A, Sullivan C. The transformation of Australia's first large digital hospital: a teaching case. In: Proceedings of the 41st International Conference on Information Systems (ICIS 2020). Association for Information Systems; 2020.

eHealth NSW. Milestone for electronic medication management roll-out. NSW Health. 2019. https://www.ehealth.nsw.gov.au/features/milestone-for-electronic-medication-management-roll-out. Accessed 15 May 2021.

Glasser JP. The role of the Chief Information Officer in the health care organization in the 1990s. Top Health Inf Manag. 1993;13(3):62–8.

Global Digital Health Partnership. About the global digital health partnership: our vision. 2020. https://www.gdhp.org/our-vision. Accessed 15 May 2021.

HIMSS. Adoption model for analytics maturity. 2020. https://www.himssanalytics.org/amam. Accessed 15 May 2021.

Holst C, Sukums F, Radovanovic D, Ngowi B, Noll J, Winkler AS. Sub-Saharan Africa-the new breeding ground for global digital health. Lancet Digit Health. 2020;2(4):e160–e162.

Kark K. The CIO balancing act: operations and business innovation. Harv Bus Rev. 2017. https://hbr.org/webinar/2017/09/the-cio-balancing-act-operations-and-business-innovation. Accessed 15 May 2021.

Sujan M, Scott P, Cresswell K. Digital health and patient safety: technology is not a magic wand. Health Inform J. 2020;2295–2299.

Sullivan T, Miliard M. Meet the modern healthcare CIO: a business leader that is casting off their traditional IT role, in Healthcare IT News. 2018.

World Health Organization. Global strategy on digital health 2020-2025. 2020. https://www.who.int/docs/default-source/documents/gs4dhdaa2a9f352b0445bafbc79ca799dce4d.pdf?sfvrsn=f112ede5_42. Accessed 15 May 2021.

Chapter 15
Working as a Health Cybersecurity Specialist

Patricia A. H. Williams, Simon Cowley, Christopher Bolan, Ken Fowle, and Richard Staynings

Abstract The need for cybersecurity expertise in the health workforce is rapidly growing as security compromises and attacks on hospitals and government departments accelerate at an alarming rate. Healthcare presents a rich and unique environment to protect, requiring an informed perspective on how to protect it. The challenges of applying cybersecurity protections in healthcare, the pace of technical change, the complexity of regulation and the potential for patient safety impact means healthcare needs specialised skills in cybersecurity. The characterisation of this specialty, together with five case studies, describes its vital importance and the variety of careers in this area.

Keywords Case study · Cybersecurity · Data breach · Incident response · Risk management

P. A. H. Williams (✉)
Flinders University, Adelaide, SA, Australia
e-mail: trish.williams@flinders.edu.au

S. Cowley
Department of Health, Melbourne, VIC, Australia
e-mail: Simon.Cowley@health.vic.gov.au

C. Bolan
St John of God Healthcare, Perth, WA, Australia
e-mail: chris@seamlessintelligence.com.au

K. Fowle
Child and Adolescent Health Service, Perth, WA, Australia
e-mail: Kenneth.Fowle@health.wa.gov.au

R. Staynings
Cylera, New York, NY, USA
e-mail: richard.staynings@cylera.com

225

Introduction

Australia faces a shortage of job-ready cybersecurity professionals, and the demand will increase to 16,600 additional professionals by 2026 (AustCyber 2020). This is a microcosm of the situation around the world where a 2020 study found that organisations could use over 3 million additional workers, that is, nearly double the existing workforce ((ISC)^2, 2020b). This shortage is a significant challenge for all industries; however, the healthcare sector has specific reasons to take this challenge seriously. Healthcare has become a high-profile target because of the breadth and amount of personal and sensitive information recorded. Healthcare has an ethical and regulatory obligation to society to keep patients' information confidential and maintain their privacy because of the damage to reputation, identity and safety that can ensue from medical data breaches. Real-time access to patient histories, monitoring equipment data and medical device data is important, for example in emergency care; but threats to real-time access have increased, with disruptive ransomware attacks impacting critical healthcare delivery (Ronquillo et al. 2018; Chernyshev et al. 2018).

The issues in cybersecurity will only increase for healthcare and are driven by the integration of systems, our necessity to share patient information, and the move to new models of patient-centred care (Coventry and Branley 2018; Williams et al. 2020). For instance, the increased use of telehealth and adoption of virtual care, accelerated by the COVID-19 pandemic, means the inherent vulnerability of connectivity becomes a broader problem for healthcare organisations (Langer 2020). Further, the shift to patient empowerment and demand for greater access to information (CSIRO 2018) are driving change in the expectations of digital technology users and the experiences they desire. Coupled with wireless medical devices, the Internet-of-Things (IoT), mobile data sharing and health apps, the growing complexity of the healthcare environment demands increased protection as the cyber-physical boundaries are integrated into our information systems (Williams and Woodward 2015; Webb and Dayal 2017; Altawy and Youssef 2016). It is widely acknowledged that security and privacy measures have not been able to keep up with such technology.

The cybersecurity specialist role is at the centre of healthcare's information infrastructure, to protect the information, systems and the infrastructure itself. The potential threats, whilst not unique to healthcare, include social engineering, insider misuse, malware, unsecured mobile devices, connected devices, unrestricted access, inadequate disposal of retired hardware and systems, and unintentional mistakes. This chapter does not detail the generic cybersecurity skills, nor the litany of cybersecurity breaches in healthcare. Instead, it highlights what makes cybersecurity in healthcare an advanced specialisation. Then it provides five case studies of how cybersecurity specialists characterise their work and the specific skills they need to have for this work.

The Challenge of Being a Healthcare Cybersecurity Specialist

Cybersecurity in healthcare is complicated. The reasons are fourfold. Firstly, security is not the core business of healthcare. We often rely on healthcare workers to adapt to the security procedures and the information systems developed to manage information securely; however, this can be problematic in the healthcare environment. Healthcare workers' primary task is the delivery of quality healthcare to patients, and therefore we cannot arbitrarily change their clinical processes to adapt to the demands of information technology (IT) and cybersecurity. Better integration of cybersecurity is required, so that it is woven seamlessly into clinical workflow (Garg et al. 2018; Williams 2008). Education of non-security personnel in cybersecurity risks is also needed.

Secondly, the pace of change, development and adoption of new technologies outpaces our ability to secure these technologies from an end-to-end systems perspective. For instance, the rise in the availability of IoT devices for healthcare, a technology that already has significant security concerns, will require knowledge of application programming interface (API) security, IoT security frameworks, integration risks and safe deployment management (Williams and McCauley 2016). The detection of physical signals and their translation into vast amounts of data that can be recorded and analysed requires oversight and understanding of the nature of these devices, in particular where this data is life critical (Mohapatro and Snigdh 2020). Also, health and wellness apps connected to health systems, proliferating in, and useful to, patient care are not well regulated.

Thirdly, the lack of cybersecurity expertise is an issue, and cybersecurity skills are not the same as IT skills. Whilst IT staff play an important role in developing, implementing, and managing the technical aspects of patient health information systems and infrastructure, they generally do not have specialised skills in cybersecurity. In an environment with multiple networks, diverse health software systems, legacy systems, medical devices, together with the associated risks that integration of these systems poses, a comprehensive understanding of their operation is vitally important. Further, the threats to sensitive patient information and device data, and the availability, integrity and protection of these data, must be well understood in the context of their use in healthcare; the consequences for patient safety can be significant and life-threatening (Ross 2017).

Lastly, a unique brand of complexity arises from the inter-related demands of legislation, regulation, data protection standards, breach notification rules, and expanded approaches to using data in healthcare; the increasing connectivity and digitisation of health technologies continue to create new vulnerabilities (Therapeutic Goods Administration 2019).

A cybersecurity specialist is not just another IT person. There are numerous roles within the cybersecurity discipline, including cybersecurity analyst, operations, regulatory compliance, testing and architecture functions, each with its own specialised skill set (Australian Signals Directorate 2020). Frameworks such as the Workforce Framework for Cybersecurity (NICE Framework) (Petersen et al. 2020) detail the skills a cybersecurity specialist requires. In addition to the broad, fundamental, and necessary cybersecurity skills of information security governance, threat and risk assessment, operational security management, incident management, investigation and digital forensics, health cybersecurity specialists need the following skills. They need to understand the sensitive nature of health data and the associated privacy concerns, including how to meet regulatory requirements. Also, they need an in-depth knowledge of the complexity of the attack surface (the totality of ways that an IT system can be attacked) and how this interacts with the healthcare environment. They must understand how cybersecurity impacts patient safety and how to protect systems where attacks could result directly in adverse events and physical harm—for example, medical devices such as ventilators, incubators and pacemakers. They must have the knowledge to take responsibility for the safety and security of the complex healthcare ecosystem, not just the individual information systems, separate medical devices or sections of infrastructure. They need advanced knowledge of the risks related to artificial intelligence (AI) and machine learning algorithms. The healthcare cybersecurity specialist must not only understand but also communicate their contribution to the overall operation of healthcare facilities and health system performance; because awareness about cybersecurity amongst healthcare workers is low, the cybersecurity professional has a significant role to play to advocate for a cybersecurity culture and best practice ((ISC)², 2020a).

Simon Cowley, Department of Health, Australia

As Principal Cybersecurity Officer with the State of Victoria's Department of Health, Digital Health Branch, I work with public health services on assurance activities, initiatives to uplift cybersecurity maturity and cyber incident response. The position of Principal Cybersecurity Officer involves engagement with health services across the Victorian public health sector. I assist with assurance activities, such as assessments to monitor the progress of health services implementing controls based on the NIST Cybersecurity Framework. These assessments often lead to initiatives such as implementing tools and technologies to assist health services to improve cybersecurity capabilities; I am involved in project design and project management. I also participate in cyber incident response and collaborate closely with an Incident Response Team and trusted partners in this work.

Cybersecurity is a recent career change. I have a Bachelor of Science in Biomedical Sciences and electronics engineering qualifications from my previous career as a biomedical engineer for over 15 years in the public health service, with my last position at The Royal Melbourne Hospital. Prior to this, I worked in the industrial control sector, installing, and maintaining control systems used in manufacturing, petrochemical and food industries. My career progression from a biomedical engineer into healthcare cybersecurity had a natural flow. As a biomedical engineer working in a large health service, I was exposed on a daily basis to the operational challenges of network-connected medical devices. I worked collaboratively with key stakeholders (medical device manufacturers, IT professionals, facility managers, project managers) to ensure medical IT systems were safe and resilient. To equip me to confront these challenges, I drew on my experience from the industrial control sector and pursued further training in IT networking to understand the concepts and 'language' of IT. I observed that as medical device technology advanced, it became more digitised and interconnected. This increased system complexity also increased the cybersecurity risk through hardware and software vulnerabilities and increased exposure to network and internet-based threats. This risk to the safety of medical devices was emerging and unlike other risks to medical devices, it had a dynamic threat landscape. At The Royal Melbourne Hospital, I worked collaboratively with IT on secure medical IT network architectures, and practical cybersecurity controls for medical devices, adapted from best practices used in the industrial control sector. This work led to several biomedical engineering conference presentations on medical IT and cybersecurity, growing a further interest to move towards a career in healthcare cybersecurity.

I concluded that it was necessary to pursue industry recognised training in cybersecurity to assist with this new career path, and therefore completed my first cybersecurity certification whilst working as a biomedical engineer. I hold an ISACA CSX Certification in Cybersecurity Fundamentals, and I am currently pursuing ethical hacking and cyber incident management training. It is essential to have a fundamental knowledge of patient care workflow, health technologies and health ICT systems used in health services. This background assists with the understanding of the practicalities of applying cybersecurity controls and technologies within the health sector. The completion of industry-recognised cybersecurity training/certifications is also beneficial. This training assists in building specific skill sets, such as penetration testing, cyber incident response and digital forensics.

Inspiration comes from the knowledge that my work is instrumental in improving the safety and resilience of health technology and ICT systems within the public health sector. Cybersecurity is a challenging profession, primarily due to an ever-changing threat landscape. It requires regular analysis of threat intelligence and sharing actionable information with health services. This activity is rewarding, knowing that this is one of many preventative activities protecting hospitals from cyber incidents. The profession also provides an opportunity to apply my knowledge and experience from other fields throughout my career to real-world challenges, such as medical device security. Globally, there is a shortage of cybersecurity professionals across many industries, including healthcare. The healthcare sector is also particularly exposed to cybersecurity risk, due to low maturity and investment in security, along with vast repositories of protected health information, a commodity highly sought-after by threat actors. There have also been numerous cyber incidents globally within the healthcare sector, resulting in the disruption of clinical services, exposure of protected health information and extortion of health services/individuals. I foresee the demand for healthcare cybersecurity professionals will continue to grow well into the future, driven by the increased digitisation of healthcare technologies and health ICT systems. The healthcare sector is well placed to build these professions from within, augmenting the experience of existing health professionals, similar to my experience.

Christopher Bolan, St John of God Healthcare, Australia

I started my IT journey with a Bachelor of Science in Computer Science followed by Honours in Software Engineering, and this was eventually followed by a PhD in cybersecurity. I have also completed several industry certifications (e.g. CISA) and training on specific cyber technologies. I started my IT career as a programmer within the WA Government which grew into a project lead role. From there, I became a University Lecturer in both Australia and the United Kingdom whilst simultaneously keeping my hand in the industry as an IT Security consultant. When the time came to leave academia, I took up the position as the National IT Security, Risk & Audit manager for the prominent ANZ hardware retailer Bunnings. After several years, my career moved back to service provision, undertaking a role with Kinetic IT to establish their Security Operation Centre and lead the development of their Cybersecurity services. In 2017, I accepted the challenge to build an internal cyber capability for St John of God Healthcare, in Perth, Western Australia where I am now Group Manager, Digital Security. For someone like myself who has moved between industry verticals, the continuously evolving challenges of cybersecurity generally are coupled with the need to gain understanding rapidly of a large amount of healthcare-specific knowledge. Healthcare does offer some interesting challenges, such as in infection control, medical technologies and legacy systems, that require you to adapt your thinking.

Healthcare is a people-focused industry that looks after those at their most vulnerable, and being able to use my skills to support the people in St John of God Healthcare, is a way to make a significant impact on all those within our care. My current role reports both to the senior executive and the Board and focuses on uplifting and ensuring security across the organisation. The role of cybersecurity specialists is undoubtedly becoming more critical within healthcare as each new technology and system increases the risk associated with a significant breach or attack. There are already suggestions that cyber incidents have had direct impacts on patient outcomes, and as these become more publicised the focus on cybersecurity's role will be more prominent. I believe this will be driven in part by a push for more significant cybersecurity regulation and Board accountability.

Ken Fowle, Child and Adolescent Health Service, Australia

I am the Director of Procurement and Contract Management, Child and Adolescent Health Service, Perth Western Australia. My education and training include a Bachelor of Business (Information Processing) from the Western Australian College of Advanced Education; a Doctor of Philosophy from the University of Nottingham, UK; and various short industry training programs. My previous work experience includes project and contract manager, investigator, academic and computer professional, and I have managed a range of multifaceted teams and led significantly sized and complex projects. I have undertaken complex procurement, contract and ICT project management activities on behalf of the Child and Adolescent Health Service, the WA Department of Health, the Department of Mines and Petroleum, and Edith Cowan University.

The public service does not cater to specialists. There are Network people, Programmers, Project Leaders, and other ICT professionals who have good general knowledge in their area but no specialist knowledge of cybersecurity. Progression and maintaining permanency are difficult as the public service has restricted staffing numbers. Therefore, it is easier and beneficial for ICT departments to outsource this specialist area as these positions command higher salaries (something the public service cannot afford). My challenge was that once you remove yourself from ICT, the ICT community does not necessarily recognise your ICT skills and knowledge, they see you as the client and not as a resource who has been on "both sides of the fence".

I moved from ICT to Director of Procurement and Contract Manager and to undertake large-scale ICT work in my current role. The ICT knowledge was very beneficial in working with ICT people in developing specifications, evaluating ICT responses and managing the ICT contracts. When I was working in cybersecurity, what inspired me was looking at the issues (investigating), looking for a solution (researching) and seeing the outcome (realising the solution).

The skills and knowledge that I think are needed, and are unique, for a health cybersecurity specialist are fivefold. Excellent communication is one—you need to explain the technical in simplified terms to enable your clients to understand the issue/concerns/solution. Relationship building is another—you want to continue the journey with your clients and if needed an external provider, with trust/honesty and knowing that your clients have confidence that you can or know someone who can. Hands-on technical skill, not just theoretical knowledge, is important. You need to be inquisitive—ask why did that happen and how did that happen? Doing research to keep up to date as to what is happening in the security area and providing an effective, comprehensive solution is the final thing I would emphasise. Currently establishing stable and fast networks and keeping all hardware up to date seems to be a priority as not all health services are operating on the same technology; however, as more information is transferred from hard copy to the digital platforms, there will be a greater emphasis on data security.

Richard Staynings, Cylera, USA

My job is Chief Security Strategist at Cylera—a leading innovator in biomedical and healthcare Internet of Things cybersecurity—in New York, USA. Like many people today working in cybersecurity, I entered the field in a rather indirect way.

My undergraduate degree was in Government and Public Policy, followed by post-graduate diplomas in Business and Public Administration. Still, a career in the Civil Service was not one that I aspired to. Instead, I began my working career in IT in the City of London, gathering business and systems requirements for high-volume, transaction processing trading systems for a merchant bank. Information technology fascinated me and had done so for many years. I was the very first student on my liberal arts degree to type out his dissertation on his computer, and the bug stuck with me. How could IT not be the future of business and society I rightly assumed?

Leaving London some years later, I headed down-under to work on the Western Australia Gas Pipeline. Here, I was exposed to SCADA systems to control LPG flow rates, temperatures, and pressures—and more than a few snakes in the Western Desert. Trying to secure these simple systems proved to be a significant challenge. When my part of the project was completed, I headed to Hong Kong and found work deploying networks and IT systems, while training customers on proper computer usage. Following this, I headed to the USA and joined a Big-Six accounting firm as a Consultant. There I first worked in IT infrastructure management and systems development, where I led a team that developed one of the first identity and access management (IAM) systems. Assigned to various clients, over the years, I moved between information technology and Information Security projects, later known as "Cybersecurity". I ended up leading security for the US Rocky Mountain region. Along the way, I gained a Master's in Cybersecurity Management and Policy and multiple certificates in Cybersecurity Risk Management and related fields.

Growing up in the United Kingdom, my father worked in the British National Health Service, so I was exposed to healthcare terminology and healthcare practices from an early age. My familiarity with the industry has led to working as a consultant on many security assessments and healthcare customer audits. I quickly became an expert in healthcare security risk and compliance, gaining a solid understanding of the nuances of healthcare security and privacy, and consequently leading a national consulting practice in healthcare security on behalf of a large company in the space. This consultancy led to a position as the global cybersecurity leader for healthcare life sciences, for a major IT vendor, as well as several corporate executive roles leading security and IT, and ultimately to my current role at Cylera.

Cybersecurity was still an emerging discipline when I entered the field, so like many of my peers, we had to learn as we went along. Security frameworks like BS7799 later became ISO 27001, and the NIST CSF evolved, and the various healthcare compliance requirements changed frequently. Working with international life sciences organisations and supporting an extensive global list of healthcare delivery organisations exposed me to numerous national and supranational security and privacy requirements—GDPR, Caldicott, HIPAA, Joint Commission, APA and PDPA are just some of these. However, the major challenge in healthcare is not about compliance; the challenge is about patient safety and providing holistic security. Healthcare security is so much more than a compliance checklist today. If you are secure, you are usually compliant, but not the other way around. This is a lesson that some health systems and governments have yet to learn, unfortunately.

My primary role today is advising CISOs and other security leaders on what they need to consider as threats and risks change. I also spend a lot of time educating and briefing their managers on cybersecurity risk concerns and remediation strategies. I am no longer focused on day-to-day operational security concerns but instead focus on providing the people in the driver's seat with a lot of the information they need to be successful. I also share my research with peers, presenting at healthcare and security conferences. I teach master's degree-level courses in cybersecurity and healthcare IT to the next generation of cybersecurity leaders.

Unlike an attack against a bank, where funds are insured against theft, in healthcare, you cannot provide insurance against increased patient morbidity and mortality. There are real implications when critical life-sustaining systems are held to ransom while needed to diagnose, treat, monitor, and manage the sick, the elderly and infirm. Perhaps that is why I feel drawn to work in this space and to bring the weight of my knowledge and experience to bear. Healthcare is an area in which I can make a significant difference, and not just for myself but for the greater good of society.

There are many ways to enter the profession of cybersecurity, laterally from various IT areas, from risk management, from engineering and with a background in IT audit and compliance. Also, there are academic, and vocational certification programs focused on the multiple disciplines in cybersecurity, at undergraduate and post-graduate levels, that equip students with the necessary skills to be successful. However, most important of all is experience and aptitude. As a cybersecurity professional, you need to continually think outside of the box and deal with the challenges of being knocked off your feet yet be able to get back up straight away.

With demand for cybersecurity professionals far exceeding supply, those willing and capable of working in this space will never be unemployed for long. Tens of thousands are entering the discipline each year globally, but it is not enough. We need more, many times more, people to defend against rising attacks. It is a broadening profession with almost unlimited opportunities for specialisation and advancement. In healthcare it is a vital and necessary role, to protect patients and the hospitals and clinics we all need throughout our lives. A career in healthcare cybersecurity requires more than just an aptitude with different technologies. It requires an understanding and appreciation of the business of providing care, and of the risks that that healthcare provider organisations are facing.

Trish Williams, Flinders University, Australia

I am the Cisco Chair and Professor of Digital Health Systems at Flinders University in Adelaide, South Australia. My education includes a Bachelor of Science (with Honours) in Mathematics and Computing, a Master of Science in Computer Science and a PhD in Medical Information Security. I am a Certified Health Informatician Australasia; I hold a Graduate Certificate in Tertiary Teaching; and I was a certified Unix Administrator. My entire working life has been in computing and security in healthcare. Coming from a medical family and growing up in the UK, I started as an Analyst/Programmer in the UK at Update Software, then moved to Australia to join Amfac/Medrecord to write clinical software and worked as the Customer Service Manager and Systems Consultant. After 15 years in the industry, I decided that passing on my knowledge was essential, joining academia in 2000. Commencing as Lecturer, I was promoted over the intervening years, becoming Associate Professor in 2013 and Associate Dean in 2015, at Edith Cowan University in Perth. In 2016, I took up the position of Cisco Chair and Professor of Digital Health Systems, Director of Flinders Digital Health Research Centre (Co-Director until 2021) and Director of Cisco-Flinders Digital Health Design Lab at Flinders University in Adelaide. I also hold the position of College of Science and Engineering, Research Section Head for Data and Information Science.

Most obviously, I faced the challenge of being a female in male-dominated professions, and this applied equally to computer science in the 1980s and 1990s, as it did to cybersecurity in the 2000s and still does today. For me, this was not necessarily a negative but highlighted the reality that you need to focus without losing your feminine identity, and that you do not need to display male behaviour to succeed in cybersecurity. I had the opportunity to move from highly technical roles to management and leadership positions because of my ability to communicate effectively and understanding the broader perspective of the challenges healthcare faces. Despite the technical aspects of cybersecurity, there is an equally crucial human side to the profession. I believe that my communication abilities as well as my technical skills, allow me to bring different and complementary perspectives to cybersecurity.

My current role includes many diverse activities related to cybersecurity in healthcare, and leadership within the university sector. My research activities include the application of cybersecurity in a practical manner and integrating this into healthcare workflow, and the impact of cybersecurity on patient safety. This work is about improving healthcare through digital infrastructure, including how to provide better experiences for patients and clinicians. I am heavily involved in developing international standards in healthcare cybersecurity and patient safety through HL7 and ISO. I am excited by the ability to make a difference in a sector that so needs it! Healthcare's focus is on patient care, and as a profession, cybersecurity needs to help by understanding this working environment and adapting cybersecurity practice to work within this environment. The challenges of doing this with skill and compassion inspire me.

In addition to superior cybersecurity skills, a cybersecurity specialist in healthcare needs to have a pragmatic perspective on how to protect the healthcare information environment and how to support the organisation, clinicians, administration and patients. Possessing a good understanding of, and empathy with, how the healthcare operates, and be responsive to the needs of this setting and the people working within it, is critical. The skills required will always include technical cybersecurity and risk management skills. However, as digital health disrupts healthcare and new technologies emerge, this will drive changes in how healthcare is provided. Virtual care is one such example, where care supported by technology and information sharing is taken out of the hospital and primary care practices, and often delivered in the home or perhaps an aged care facility. The increased use of healthcare technologies, outside the confines of an organisation, such as a hospital, results in a broader and less controlled digital footprint that needs protection. The use of the Internet of Medical Things, remote monitoring, health apps and other data sources will require new perspectives on how to protect data, networks, and communications, end-to-end, outside of the traditional controllable perimeter. This means the cybersecurity specialist will need to be knowledgeable and adaptable, and take a systems perspective to protections encompassing the technology, people and processes involved.

Conclusion

The dynamic nature of healthcare makes it vital to stay up to date on new and emerging technologies that will transform healthcare. Artificial intelligence and machine learning will become commonplace, and there will always be new health software, apps, and connected devices. Increasingly, patients will use the Internet of Medical Things and personalised monitoring devices, and bring these into healthcare delivery environments. These innovations will certainly stretch, if not eliminate, traditional network boundaries and organisational cyber-perimeters. Future healthcare delivery scenarios that incorporate more virtual care will require advanced knowledge of API integration, interconnected cross-platform systems, secure data transfer and storage, integration into electronic health records, and secure communications.

There is not yet a specific job title of healthcare cybersecurity specialist, nor explicit training for such a specialisation. Yet many cybersecurity specialists, such as those in these case studies, demonstrate the advanced knowledge and skills required to pursue this career. Healthcare is different from other sectors. It is critically reliant on national and international information infrastructure, and poor cybersecurity can lead to harm to human lives. The quantity, criticality and importance of the data held by healthcare providers and organisations, and the impact that breaches can have on individuals, mean that cybersecurity is now an essential component of management and governance across the whole of healthcare. Balancing digital health operations with appropriate protections is a complex task that requires specific skills and knowledge—it needs healthcare cybersecurity specialists.

References

(ISC)². Not all life savers wear white coats. 2020a. https://www.isc2.org/-/media/ISC2/Landing-Pages/2020/HCISPP-B2C-White-Paper/MAR-HCISPP-Not-All-Life-Savers-B2C-Whitepaper.ashx?la=en&hash=4487C2B81A8E6228E5DEC05DB34A7AD4EBBA3B90. Accessed 15 May 2021.
(ISC)². Cybersecurity experts stand up to a pandemic: (ISC)² Cybersecurity workforce study. 2020b. https://www.isc2.org/Research/Workforce-Study# Accessed 15 May 2021.

Altawy R, Youssef AM. Security tradeoffs in cyber physical systems: a case study survey on implantable medical devices. IEEE Access. 2016;4:959–79.

AustCyber. SCP – Chapter 3 – Accelerating and sustaining growth. In: Australia's Cyber Security: Sector Competitiveness Plan [Internet]. Canberra: Australian Cyber Security Growth Network; 2020. https://www.austcyber.com/resources/sector-competitiveness-plan/chapter3. Accessed 15 May 2021.

Australian Signals Directorate. ASD cyber skills framework. 2020. https://www.cyber.gov.au/acsc/view-all-content/publications/asd-cyber-skills-framework. Accessed 15 May 2021.

Chernyshev M, Zeadally S, Baig Z. Healthcare data breaches: implications for digital forensic readiness. J Med Syst. 2018;43(1):7.

Coventry L, Branley D. Cybersecurity in healthcare: a narrative review of trends, threats and ways forward. Maturitas. 2018;113:48–52.

CSIRO. Cyber security: A roadmap to enable growth opportunities in Australia. CSIRO Futures. 2018. https://www.csiro.au/en/Do-business/Futures/Reports/Future-Industries/Cyber-Security. Accessed 15 May 2021.

Garg S, Williams NL, Ip A, Dicker AP. Clinical integration of digital solutions in health care: an overview of the current landscape of digital technologies in cancer care. JCO Clin Cancer Inform. 2018;2:1–9.

Langer J. Mitigating health care's cybersecurity risks in the era of hyperconnectivity. Med Econ. 2020;97(10):43–5.

Mohapatro M, Snigdh I. Security in IoT healthcare. In: IoT security paradigms and applications: research and practices. Milton: Taylor & Francis Group; 2020. p. 237–60.

Petersen R, Santos D, Smith MC, Wetzel KA, Witte G. Workforce framework for cybersecurity (NICE Framework). 2020. https://nvlpubs.nist.gov/nistpubs/SpecialPublications/NIST.SP.800-181r1.pdf. Accessed 15 May 2021.

Ronquillo JG, Erik Winterholler J, Cwikla K, Szymanski R, Levy C. Health IT, hacking, and cybersecurity: national trends in data breaches of protected health information. JAMIA Open. 2018;1(1):15–9.

Ross J. Cybersecurity: a real threat to patient safety. J PeriAnesth Nurs. 2017;32(4):370–2.

Therapeutic Goods Administration. Medical device cyber security guidance for industry. 2019. https://www.tga.gov.au/sites/default/files/medical-device-cyber-security-guidance-industry.pdf. Accessed 15 May 2021.

Webb T, Dayal S. Building the wall: addressing cybersecurity risks in medical devices in the U.S.A. and Australia. Comput Law Secur Rev. 2017;33(4):559–63.

Williams PAH. When trust defies common security sense. Health Inform J. 2008;14(3):211–21.

Williams PAH, McCauley V. Always connected: the security challenges of the healthcare internet of things. IEEE World Forum in Internet of Things. Reston, VA: IEEE; 2016. p. 30–5.

Williams PAH, Woodward A. Cybersecurity vulnerabilities in medical devices. Medical Devices Evid Res. 2015;8:305–16.

Williams PAH, Perimal-Lewis L, Mudd G, Gunasekara G. Reimagining a better healthcare system through virtual care [White Paper]. 2020. https://www.cisco.com/c/dam/en_us/solutions/industries/resources/healthcare/reimagining-better-healthcare-system-through-virtual-care.pdf. Accessed 15 May 2021.

Chapter 16
Working as a Health Data Scientist

Natasha Donnolley, Lachlan Rudd, Oisin Fitzgerald, and Miranda Davies-Tuck

Abstract The health data scientist is a relatively new specialty within the HIDDIN workforce. In this chapter we profile four very different people working in this critical role: a Research Project Manager, a Director for Data and Analytics, a Statistician and an Epidemiologist. While their job titles and journeys to become a health data scientist differ significantly, the case studies presented in this chapter demonstrate the one thing that they all have in common—harnessing the power of health data to address real-world problems.

Keywords Case study · Health data scientist · Big data · Data analytics · Epidemiology

N. Donnolley (✉)
National Perinatal Epidemiology and Statistics Unit, UNSW, Sydney, NSW, Australia
e-mail: n.donnolley@unsw.edu.au

L. Rudd
eHealth New South Wales, Sydney, NSW, Australia
e-mail: lachlan.rudd@health.nsw.gov.au

O. Fitzgerald
Centre for Big Data Research in Health, UNSW, Sydney, NSW, Australia
e-mail: o.fitzgerald@unsw.edu.au

M. Davies-Tuck
The Ritchie Centre, Hudson Institute of Medical Research, Clayton, VIC, Australia
e-mail: miranda.davies@hudson.org.au

Introduction

The increasing amount of real-world data—often known as "big data"—being generated through our health and welfare systems creates opportunities and careers never imagined before. If the COVID-19 pandemic highlighted just one thing, it was the need for real-time, real-world health data and specialists who know how to make use of it. Health data scientists have a lot in common with other specialists in the HIDDIN workforce (that is, Health Informatics, Digital, Data, Information and KNowledge experts) and often the roles overlap—epidemiologist, biostatistician, data analyst, data engineer, health information manager. An effective research team will involve collaboration between all these roles (Goldstein et al. 2020). However, one specialist—health data scientist—often brings together aspects of all these roles into one (Goldstein et al. 2020). According to Granville (2014) what sets them apart is the way they work with data: "DAD (Discover/Access/Distill)". Data scientists are involved across the whole life cycle of data—they identify what data can be sourced or needs to be created, they identify how to access those data, and then they extract and distill information and knowledge in an applied manner. They often have the domain knowledge that a statistician may not have, the computer programming that an epidemiologist may not have, the communication skills that an engineer may not have, and bring together different aspects of all those roles in order to address real-world, real-time questions. They are an essential part of the HIDDIN workforce that work with "big data". Although this field was virtually non-existent 20 years ago, things are changing rapidly, particularly with the burgeoning availability and use of "big data". Now it is not only a recognised career, as well there are university degrees specifically to teach the skills needed. Several exist in the USA and the UK, for example, and the Master of Science in Health Data Science run by the Centre for Big Data Research in Health at the University of New South Wales is the first postgraduate program in Australia to focus entirely on this discipline. As can be seen from the four case studies presented in this chapter, many people working in this relatively new specialty area may not necessarily go by the title of "Health Data Scientist", but that is what their role encompasses. The case studies aim to showcase how the profession has evolved over the past two decades, how the paths to become a health data scientist are so varied, and some examples of the diverse work they undertake. Their titles are all very different, but the one thing they have in common is using their knowledge, experience and skills working with health data to address real-world health problems.

Natasha Donnolley, University of New South Wales, Australia

Like many people who work in this area, I did not make a conscious decision to become a health data scientist. It took me several other careers and a personal tragedy before I ended up where I am, and even so, it still happened somewhat by accident. Having had a varied career since leaving school (including an unfinished science degree, a brief brush with politics and a series of jobs that had a health and later IT focus), I found myself out of the full-time workforce after having four children, and a need to retrain from my last career as an international IT consultant. Following the term stillbirth of my second child, I had become involved in consumer advocacy in maternity care. I knew I wanted to do something that could capitalise on my experience and networks in that area and make use of my background in IT and health. That is when I discovered the Bachelor of Science in Health Information Management then offered by distance education at Curtin University in Western Australia. I had never heard of Health Information Managers or clinical coding. I still was not entirely sure what I wanted to do with my future career, but I knew I wanted to work in research, and this degree seemed to combine my health and IT backgrounds perfectly. The BSc (HIM) was a great platform to develop the skills and knowledge I needed to work with health information and health data. Along with a foundation in anatomy and physiology, it gave me the knowledge and skills in nosology and clinical coding to work with the large routinely collected datasets generated by the Australian health system, and a basic level of biostatistics and epidemiology to get me started.

I started a new career working in perinatal research at the National Perinatal Epidemiology and Statistics Unit (NPESU), at the University of New South Wales, in the last semester of my degree. I managed to combine the content knowledge I had developed over the previous 8 years as a maternity consumer advocate, with my experience in health and IT, with the health data science skills I had developed through my degree, and roll them all into the perfect role. Not only did my HIM degree prepare me for the role, it also gave me the grounding I needed later to undertake a PhD in the area. Even after commencing at the NPESU, I did not consciously think of myself as a health data scientist. When I started in 2011, it still was not a role or title that was used, yet there are many of us in the university sector who would identify as one. My titles have varied between Project Officer, Project Manager, Research Assistant and currently Research Project Manager. But essentially, I am a Health Data Scientist. All my projects revolve around creating, using, analysing and understanding health data—specifically related to mothers and babies—and increasingly utilising "big data".

The focus of my work at the NPESU initially was on data development. Using the skills I had developed during my degree in clinical classification, combined with my knowledge of maternity services, I developed the world-first Maternity Care Classification System (MaCCS) for the Australian Commonwealth government. The MaCCS is now being rolled out in all Australian maternity services to classify their models of maternity care as well as being used in the UK to evaluate components of the National Health Service Better Births policy. In addition to undertaking data development, I have worked with routinely collected national datasets, data collected through surveys, electronic medical records, focus groups and interviews, designed governance systems to manage "big data" platforms, and analysed and interpreted data. Everything I do revolves around health-related data and the "real-world" application of those data. For me, this work came from a very personal place—trying to understand why my own daughter died; trying to understand and improve the lives of pregnant and birthing women and their babies; and trying to prevent other families from experiencing the same unnecessary tragic loss that I experienced. I am not a doctor in a white coat, but I can make a contribution with health data science.

Lachlan Rudd, eHealth New South Wales, Australia

Like many people in this sector, I took quite a round-about route to become a health data scientist. I completed my undergraduate Bachelor of Business at the Queensland University of Technology (QUT), majoring in Finance and Mandarin language. In my second and third year of that degree, I also worked with an innovative ICT start-up company led by a business mentor I had met during networking in my first year of study. I came in on the ground floor when the company was just a three-person garage start-up. I flew from Brisbane to Sydney to work 4 days per week and tried to condense my undergraduate coursework in Brisbane into a Friday. In the final year of my undergrad, the company moved to New Zealand to scale up development. I had an opportunity to defer completion of my degree and gain management experience, however, after a couple of weeks in New Zealand and much consideration, I decided to focus on finishing university first. At that stage, I had completed all subjects required for my finance major but still needed to complete six subjects in a minor. QUT had an international exchange program to learn Chinese, which I took advantage of. As I finished up my undergraduate degree in Shandong Province, China, my father and I decided to form a company together in the mining and infrastructure investment sector. I would base myself in China, focusing on Chinese government loans and provincial State-Owned Enterprise investors. My father looked at investment opportunities in Australasia that met the criteria of China's regulators. After 5 years in China, I thought I'd take a break back in Australia and study mathematics, something I'd heavily considered out of high school, but feared to do as the career path was less clear. Two years later, I graduated with a graduate certificate and diploma of applied mathematics (statistics), followed by a Masters. I supported myself in between with a lead business development role, helping an ICT security penetration testing company expand into the Queensland market.

Upon graduation, jobs in the applied mathematics space were highly competitive. My previous experience in China did not readily translate to the Australian market. I had spent 10 months in the final year of my Masters searching for opportunities without success. Unsuccessful in Australia, I was offered a private equity role in Shanghai, China. However, in my first 2 weeks there, an offer at CSIRO Canberra came through, so I returned to Australia to accept it. I spent several years at CSIRO building stochastic models for a behavioural economics team. We worked on a wide variety of projects predominately in the health, education, employment, auction design and strategic foresight domains. Following my time at CSIRO, I took a management job at Quantium, one of the first Australian private sector consultancies to focus on big data and advanced analytics. I spent just over 2 years there, leading several large international projects. I led teams of developers, data scientists, consultants and testers. Although none of the projects was health-based, my worked involved data analytics, cutting-edge machine learning and big data visual insight tools. All skills and experience that helped prepare me for my future work in health data science.

Fast forward to today: I am now Director of Data and Analytics in eHealth NSW, the ICT services provider to the New South Wales Health Department. I have oversight of all data, analytics and research activity within eHealth NSW. I have been able to take the breadth of my experience and focus it on leveraging data and advanced analytics to drive value for NSW Health patients, clinicians and the system more broadly. Knowing I can make a meaningful difference, positively impacting patient experiences, motivates me to succeed. I see the future of data science focusing less on the development of complex and accurate forecasting techniques and more on how data can be made actionable. Analysing data in a dark room, and producing endless executive dashboards, lacking clearly actionable insights, will be a thing of the past. Data scientists will collaborate more with operational roles to truly understand where automation and prediction can be best applied to improve decision-making and maximise efficiency.

Oisin Fitzgerald, University of New South Wales, Australia

My journey to health data science has taken me across the globe—from my home in Ireland studying a Bachelor of Science in Sports Science and Health to my new home in Sydney where I am currently completing my PhD at the University of New South Wales (UNSW). My first exposure to "big data" was during my honours project in sports biomechanics at Dublin City University, Ireland. I was very interested in the computational and signal processing aspects of the project and considered doing some postgraduate study in computing. Later I became more interested in how data could be used for decision-making, deciding to study statistics to further that interest. I enrolled in a Master of Statistics and Operations Research at RMIT University in Melbourne. I can distinctly remember a "light-bulb" moment where, despite being overwhelmed and lost in the equations, I experienced a level of satisfaction I had not gotten from previous study. Before finishing the degree, I left for Sydney, essentially doing the equivalent of a graduate diploma, and continued studying a Master of Statistics at UNSW. The two courses had different focuses which I found very beneficial. At RMIT, there was a strong applied focus, on written and presented communication of results, including practice team consulting projects with real data which were very enjoyable and remarkably similar to workplace experiences. In contrast, UNSW had a more mathematical focus, on model derivations and fundamental thinking about data. This combination of experiences and courses was great as the mathematical approach gives an understanding that generalises well but learning how to communicate statistical results and make reports is an excellent job-ready skill.

Like many students during university, I worked a variety of jobs. One summer, I worked as a research assistant during a PhD project on walkability which involved surveying households across Dublin, Ireland. I later did a similar job when studying in Melbourne, where I performed surveys for local councils. These seemingly unrelated jobs gave me a fascinating insight into the importance of the data collection process. Bias due to unrepresentative or poorly analysed datasets are two concerns in data science, and both these roles emphasised just how much work needs to go into well-designed research. While studying at UNSW, I began working as a Data Manager at the National Perinatal Epidemiology and Statistics Unit there, primarily working on the Australian and New Zealand Assisted Reproduction Database. This is a registry of all in-vitro fertilisation (IVF) cycles undertaken in Australia and New Zealand. The role involved a significant amount of reporting which resulted in developing my programming skills, learning about reproducibility, automation and building tools for making data cleaning and reporting easier. This was the real beginning of my work as a health data scientist as the role evolved into more of a statistician and data analyst, working on applied projects such as the detection of underperforming IVF clinics and developing IVF prediction models. The detection of underperforming IVF clinics was a particularly interesting challenge that taught me the importance of considering how the data was generated, and how this relates to actual clinical practice, the "map-territory" concept.

I am currently doing a PhD at the Centre for Big Data Research in Health (UNSW Sydney) and working part-time. My PhD focuses on how to better use electronic medical records (EMRs) for personalised medicine—can EMRs inform clinical decisions about subgroups of patients? EMRs are very much a focus in health data science now, and an impressive data source as they are quite detailed, allowing for reasonably unconfounded analyses in some settings and modelling of the many decisions during a course of care. However, this detail is not without its challenges, with a lot of data cleaning and a general lack of interpretability of models that suitably account for the temporal and complex data generating process.

I see a lot of changes for data science in the future, particularly around improving access to data while maintaining privacy. There has been a focus on software and empirical approaches to secure privacy-preserving data analytics in recent years, along with several advances in theoretical data science (e.g. homomorphic encryption), that makes me hopeful this will become an important toolset for data scientists. On the one hand, we have arguably intrusive use of our personal data by some companies, combined on the other hand with the general difficulty of access to healthcare data for research purposes (by both public and private institutions). I am hopeful we can move to a more principled approach to privacy-preserving analysis and data sharing that will ultimately benefit healthcare-focused research and technology. Lastly, I hope to see more practical applications of health data science. There are ethical issues that data scientists must understand about their work not existing in a vacuum. Taking a more methodological focus increases understanding of the importance of causality in data science. Data science is not about optimising the area under the receiver operating characteristic curve (AUROC) but improving decisions in real life. Students and practitioners need to learn and think about how data is created, and the biases and decisions that go into that process. Causal thinking about the data can make this clear and is an important skill for a data scientist.

Miranda Davies-Tuck, Hudson Institute of Medical Research, Melbourne

I have probably had a more traditional pathway to becoming a health data scientist than some. I completed an undergraduate degree in Biomedical Sciences with Honours. My undergraduate degree gave me a broad base in both basic and medical sciences. I then undertook a PhD at the School of Public Health and Preventive Medicine within the Department of Epidemiology and Biostatistics, at Monash University in Melbourne. My PhD focussed on non-communicable diseases epidemiology, and I was involved in several prospective cohort studies identifying modifiable factors for osteoarthritis development and disease progression. As part of my PhD, I also undertook coursework in epidemiology, biostatistics and research methodology. My PhD supervisors were both academic clinicians with strong collaborations with epidemiologists and biostatisticians. This provided many opportunities for me to learn new methods to analyse data and the importance of the clinical question being front and centre. During my PhD, I also had opportunities to be involved in teaching epidemiology, biostatistics and research methods and to work on large cohort studies and clinical trials where students were able to gain experience in fieldwork and data collection. These opportunities showed me many facets of clinical data science, including the challenges around recruitment and measurement.

It was through my personal experiences with maternity care when I was having my children that my interest in maternal and perinatal research began. After 5 years at the School of Public Health, I moved to the Ritchie Centre, Victoria's leading perinatal research centre. I extended my training by undertaking further coursework in biostatistics, and it was here that my exposure to large, routinely reported datasets began. My previous background had involved the recruitment, measurement and collection of data directly from individuals, rather than through accessing databases of clinical information or mandatory reported public health data. During my earlier work, my datasets may have had 300 or so participants, and now I had access to data on tens- and even hundreds-of thousands of women and babies. This created exciting opportunities to examine rare outcomes and overcame many of the sampling challenges I experienced undertaking prospective studies, as the entire population was captured. Perinatal datasets, however, have their specific challenges that I had to learn. There can be non-independence in the dataset as women may have multiple babies over the periods studied, and it is not always possible to identify them. There may be differences and or errors in how fields are reported, and sometimes the things you want are not captured. From an analysis point of view, it is imperative to carefully consider how to build models and how to present data, given the sheer number of fields available.

My current work aims to address inequities in maternal and perinatal health; this includes inequities in access and care, and inequities in outcomes. My program of work spans laboratory-based discovery research embedded within prospective cohort studies, clinical trials, implementation science and health policy, working in partnership with academics, clinicians, health services and government. The opportunity that data science has to bridge these gaps is enormous; things can be observed at a population level in epidemiological studies, we can then take this back to the laboratory or undertake more detailed prospective studies and to understand the mechanisms. From there, we can then trial interventions or implement changes to practice. Coming full circle, large population-based datasets can then be used again to see whether these changes are effective. We also now have the ability to link datasets, so the life course impacts of different exposures and treatments can be observed. I see health data science and knowing how to analyse data as being the key to all aspects of medical research and the field of science that will drive future research, treatments and policy.

Conclusion

These case studies highlight the diverse backgrounds, qualifications and work environments of health data scientists working in the field today. Health data scientists fill a variety of functions and roles within the health system in Australia and in other countries around the world: from Miranda's more traditional epidemiology-based role, to the age of big data analytics in Lachlan's role, and the use of data-rich electronic medical records that form the basis of Oisin's PhD study. Despite their very different settings, the people profiled in this chapter are all part of one of the top emerging career fields. For all their differences, what ties them together is that the work they undertake has real-world application and impact; it combines the traditional areas of epidemiology and biostatistics with innovative cutting-edge computer science and machine-learning methodologies; and it involves the full life-cycle of health data. As their careers and skills have evolved, so too have their identities as health data scientists.

"Big data" is the way of the future in health data science; with access to "real-world" data changing the way we view population-based health research and a greater focus on machine learning to find connections in data that may have been missed using more traditional research methods. Along with these changes comes the need for more formal career pathways and qualifications to prepare the health data science workforce of the future. Although Lachlan, Miranda, Oisin and Natasha have demonstrated how related qualifications and roles in epidemiology, statistics and health information management prepared them for their current roles as health data scientists, as this field matures we are beginning to see the emergence of new degrees and qualifications designed specifically for health data science. Along with maturity comes growing appreciation of the complexity and responsibility of the work of health data scientists: In the words of a prescient paper, their work spans re-use of clinical data for second order usages; design of artefacts and infrastructures; politics of creating and using data; algorithmic authority of information infrastructures in healthcare, and effects on the exercise of expertise and discretion of healthcare professions; new forms of healthcare data work, including new occupations; data-driven accountability and management in healthcare (Bossen et al. 2016).

References

Bossen C, Pine K, Elllingsen G, Cabitza F. Data-work in healthcare: the new work ecologies of healthcare infrastructures. In: Proceedings of the 19th ACM Conference on Computer Supported Cooperative Work and Social Computing Companion. 2016. p. 509–14.
Goldstein ND, LeVasseur M, McClure LA. On the convergence of epidemiology, biostatistics, and data science. Harv Data Sci Rev. [Internet]. 2020;2(2). https://hdsr.mitpress.mit.edu/pub/twqhhlhr.
Granville V. Developing analytic talent: becoming a data scientist. 1st ed. Somerset: WILEY; 2014.

Chapter 17
Working as a Health AI Specialist

Angela C. Davies, Alan Davies, Anthony Wilson, Haroon Saeed, Catherine Pringle, Iliada Eleftheriou, and Paul A. Bromiley

Abstract Artificial intelligence and the sub-field of machine learning offer the potential to deliver data-driven healthcare solutions that can improve patient care and increase efficiency in healthcare services. Despite this, the methods and models are new and complicated, to those who work in healthcare. This chapter explores the implementation of such solutions in healthcare settings, through five real-world case studies of experts applying this technology in a variety of clinical settings and at different stages of implementation. These cases highlight the challenges and opportunities posed by implementing artificial intelligence and data-driven solutions, and the lessons learnt from colleagues pioneering its adoption in the healthcare sector.

Keywords Case study · Artificial intelligence · Machine learning · Clinical informatics · Predictive algorithms

A. C. Davies (✉) · A. Davies · P. A. Bromiley
School of Health Sciences, The University of Manchester, Manchester, UK
e-mail: Angela.davies@manchester.ac.uk; alan.davies-2@manchester.ac.uk;
Paul.a.bromiley@manchester.ac.uk

A. Wilson
Manchester University Hospitals NHS Foundation Trust, Manchester, UK
e-mail: Anthony.wilson@mft.nhs.uk

H. Saeed · C. Pringle
Royal Manchester Children's Hospital, Manchester, UK
e-mail: hsaeed@doctors.org.uk; cjpringle@doctors.org.uk

I. Eleftheriou
The Christie NHS Foundation Trust, Manchester, Manchester, UK
e-mail: Iliada.Eleftheriou@manchester.ac.uk

K. Butler-Henderson et al. (eds.), *The Health Information Workforce*,
Health Informatics, https://doi.org/10.1007/978-3-030-81850-0_17

247

Introduction

Artificial intelligence (AI) has been applied to digital transformation in healthcare services with the aim of deriving value from the volume of available digital data that is being gathered. AI is concerned with mimicking human activities related to cognition and problem solving. A sub-field of AI, machine learning (ML) allows us to generate mathematical models from "training data" that can be applied to new, hitherto unseen data in order to identify patterns and make predictions. There are four key considerations when embedding AI in healthcare: the digitisation of patient records; professional development, which includes staff being able to appraise data-driven technologies; the evidence base about AI technology; and the ethical and regulatory issues surrounding using AI in clinical settings (Topol 2019a). Ethical considerations are especially important given that some ML algorithms (especially deep neural networks) have been described as "black boxes", where it is unclear how output is obtained (Topol 2019b), rendering clinical decisions based on such methods questionable from an ethical-legal perspective. Also an algorithm may obtain very high accuracy scores among other metrics but have little clinical utility if it fails to improve clinical outcomes (Topol 2019b). These caveats have led to the publication of advice relating to the transparency, human oversight and evaluation of such methods when they are applied to healthcare (for example, the European Commission, United States Food and Drug Administration (US FDA) and United Kingdom (UK) Government) (US FDA 2019; European Commission 2020; Department of Health and Social Care 2020). Areas of healthcare like medical imaging have seen a growth in interest in line with increases in computational performance (Wernick et al. 2010), and ML has been applied to other areas such as cardiac conditions detectable on electrocardiograms (Alfaras et al. 2019) and mental health conditions (Triffin and Paton 2018). This chapter explores five case studies based in the National Health Service (NHS) in the UK, covering a range of projects at different stages of development, all using or aiming to use AI in healthcare settings: initial feasibility work to introduce ML models for chemotherapy screening in a hospital pharmacy department; two paediatrics proofs-of-concept for ML applications, in rare children's tumours and congenital hearing loss; promoting quality improvements in an intensive care unit; and automating vertebral fracture detection and reporting. In each case study, the project lead was interviewed by author Alan Davies or Angela Davies.

Case Study 1: Feasibility of ML for Chemotherapy Screening

The project lead, Iliada Eleftheriou is an academic consultant at The Christie NHS Foundation Trust (a leading centre for cancer care in England) and a lecturer in healthcare sciences at The University of Manchester. She has a background in

Computer Science (a PhD) and IT business management. Her expertise lies in mapping data landscapes in large-scale organisations for the identification of challenges and costs related to the movement and flow of data in digital transformation projects. This project looks at the feasibility of embedding ML models into clinical pathways in the chemotherapy screening process. When thought to be of benefit, chemotherapy is prescribed to cancer patients, in a regimen to prolong the patient's life, for curative purposes or for palliative purposes. A regimen defines the types of drugs used, duration, dose and frequency (Feather et al. 2020). Pharmacists validate the regimen prescribed by a consultant (called chemotherapy screening) to ensure there are no contraindications with any other medications the patient may have been prescribed. There are well-defined criteria, baselines and protocols for screening; around 90% of screenings find no further action required. However, the number of screenings is estimated to increase by 5–7% each year, thus increasing clinical workload and the need for additional capacity. ML approaches have the potential to automate parts of this process, to decrease the time pharmacists must spend on screening and at the same time to scale up the volume of screening.

Introducing a new AI model within an already complex infrastructure comes with a myriad of challenges. These challenges are not merely technical in nature but often stem from the variety of organisational structures or human processes involved in the patient and clinical pathways (Eleftheriou et al. 2016b). Technical difficulties arise when sharing or integrating information from the diverse data sources involved. Other challenges stem from the social aspects of the organisation, its people, policies, processes and governance. For example, we find people being reluctant to change their current processes to use the new system in place, or user requirements are not met because of conflicting organisational policies and governance issues (Eleftheriou et al. 2016a). So Iliada's project used a mix of methods and tools to assess feasibility: focus groups and observation sessions with pharmacists were undertaken in order to understand the current workflows and processes. The Landscape, Organisations, Actors and Data (LOAD) model (Fig. 17.1) was used to organise and structure findings. A data journey model was used to map the current data landscape and existing data movements to identify challenges and potential risks. A new data landscape was proposed to reduce risks and costs of embedding ML models in the workflows.

The data to be used for the ML project are in both structured and unstructured forms, including unstructured data in scanned text and documents and hand-written notes. Data are stored and captured in several systems and require significant manual curation. The data landscape refers to the infrastructure within the Trust where the data reside; the storage locations of the data (both digital and physical) as well as where the data come from, where it goes and who accesses it. Data journey modelling can be utilised to map the movement of data around the systems in the organisation, to find areas of increased risk or areas that could be improved. This can model the human, technical and organisational challenges in data flow (Eleftheriou et al. 2016a, 2018).

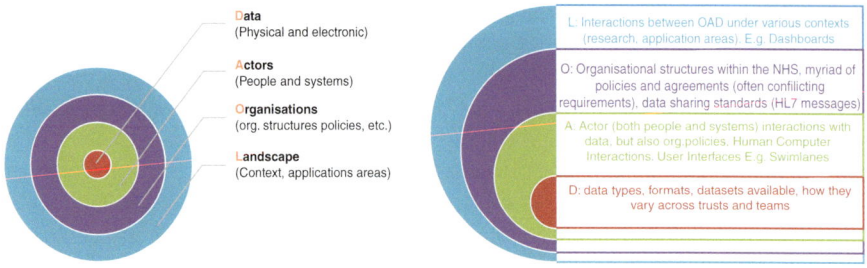

Fig. 17.1 LOAD dimensions and factors affecting the adoption of new AI models

In Iliada's words: "We're analysing the pathway associated with the Trastuzumab, a monoclonal antibody used to treat breast cancer. We're particularly focusing on this drug, as prescribed for early breast cancer, because the clinical guidelines involved in this drug are simpler with a very well-defined, straightforward protocol (National Institute for Health and Care Excellence 2002). Other drug protocols are more complicated, so we wanted an easy example to start our analysis. In order to map the current data landscape, we're not only analysing the data itself, we're also analysing the processes needed to capture the required data and which data to collect and store in the systems. We had to look into how this information is being used, how the information is being transformed, the various actors involved, the people along the patient pathway that would have to interact with the information, as well as the systems that will store and use the information."

From this analysis, the primary challenges to feasibility have been found to be: processing large volumes of unstructured data; dealing with missing information; identifying the correct document and determining its position in the timeline; determining data provenance. Many clinical datasets have missing values (Köse et al. 2020), but discounting missing data during analysis can reduce statistical power (Enders 2010). Many ML algorithms are adversely affected by missing data and decision-making using such methods (support vector machines, principal component analysis, random forests and neural networks) would be inadvisable (Köse et al. 2020). Observation sessions with pharmacists going through several screening processes found that most of the time of a pharmacist's workflow is taken to trace the right documents in the system, trying to identify the timeline of events that happened for a particular patient, in order to identify the missing values.

Human factors and the mode of engagement with stakeholders are critical, although some may think that automation is a straightforward process—we have a protocol, we create an ML tool, we embed it into the workflow, and we hope for the best. Doing feasibility analysis early on will flag up any warning signs, identify the socio-technical factors and potential costs and risks that might arise throughout the project, try to anticipate the human and organisational elements; it is equally important to keep analysing and identifying upcoming factors throughout the life cycle of the project. The acceptability of the solution is as important as achieving good quality outcomes from the tools developed. A challenging part of the work is simply finding time to work with busy clinicians and pharmacists, to illustrate the benefits for their everyday routines and encourage their questions—but it is crucial for them to be invested in the project. Some may fear AI replacing human jobs, so part of the feasibility analysis ensures appropriate communication that such tools are designed to support end-users, not to replace them, and to work alongside the essential human element of healthcare.

The project team involves many different disciplines, trying to break the boundaries between academia and healthcare, academia and industry and governmental bodies, to work on this clinical problem: pharmacists, the head of the pharmacy department, the analytics team, the data warehouse team, machine learning experts, and the business intelligence team and directors and managers. Having to analyse the social aspects of the project—for example, the people involved, the governance of bringing the data into that form where it can be used—is complicated and takes time, but the lessons learned are very important to create the right foundation for developing the right AI model. For example, one of the biggest challenges originally was having access to the data and processes involved; this was overcome by relatively quickly setting up contracts for honorary appointments, with the organisation providing the data. This brought the data scientists to the data instead of trying to move the data to the data scientists, and created a new way to collaborate.

The project makes use of the Agile software development methodology (Agile Alliance 2020) that focuses on iterative development. Agile is often also considered a mindset rather than just a methodology, and the way that we have tried to establish effective practices and ways of working within the team, is by following the Agile mindset. So, we emphasise a set of values within the team, for example, including respecting each other, collaboration within the team and continuous improvement. We have learning cycles, we take pride in ownership, focus on delivering value and, most importantly, the ability to adapt to change.

The impact of the feasibility work is difficult to measure during the first stage of a larger project, but this phase concludes with a report summarising the data journey models (Eleftheriou et al. 2018) and feeding into the next phase, where a team will produce the ML tool/algorithm that will be embedded within the patient pathway. The technical aspect of the project—the maths behind it, the data, transforming the data into a form where you can use it and train your AI models—is the easy part, in Iliada's experience.

Case Study 2: Predicting Outcomes in Children's Brain Tumours

Catherine Pringle is a neurosurgery trainee based at the Royal Manchester Children's Hospital and also a PhD student at The University of Manchester. Catherine works in an extremely emotive area of medicine, children's brain tumours, aiming to provide more personalised outcome predictions and recurrence and relapse profiles. As a study cohort, they are quite a challenging group to deal with, and it is a heterogeneous diagnostic field. As more is being discovered regarding these tumours from a molecular and biological point of view, observations indicate that they fall into more and more diverse sub-groups. Children's brain tumours are the second most common childhood malignancy and the leading cause of cancer-related death in children (Shih and Koeller 2018), however the overall numbers are very small, compared to adult colon or breast cancers. This creates a high dimensional data field, with relatively small numbers of study patients, but with a lot of deep information about each individual patient. Firstly, Catherine and colleagues are looking to harness the information generated from advanced multiparametric magnetic resonance imaging (MRI) of brain tumours, but then to combine it with the full data set held for these patients. Using this large retrospective data set they hope to identify more accurate and precise survival trends within these patient groups than detected by traditional methods such as Kaplan Meier survival analysis (Rich et al. 2010). Repeated patient imaging has associated patient-centred risks of repeated general anaesthetics and impacts on anxiety and quality of life (Cravero et al. 2009), and more precise and individualised survival outcomes could streamline its use.

Current predictive models for childhood brain tumours use tumour diagnostic type data and possibly surgical resection data, however, Catherine's work is one of the first projects aiming to incorporate whole patient data to make predictive models. This involves collecting large amounts of structured and unstructured data from tumours in the posterior fossa in the cerebellum of children (the most commonly occurring tumour location). Additional data may include histological data and biological diagnoses, which are identifying a lot more discrete tumour types. This kind of data can be used to support imaging data, historically CT imaging or more advanced MRI imaging. In addition to diagnostic data, there is also a large amount of demographic data such as presenting signs and symptoms, how long patients had symptoms before they presented, the surgical techniques used and whether any surgical adjuncts were used during the procedure, and also oncological treatment such as chemotherapy or radiotherapy. Relapse and recurrence data too are being captured, including when, how long after initial presentation, surgery, any other treatments and whether at the same site or distant sites.

The data are heterogeneous: from newborns to 18-year-olds; located in a variety of notes, scan reports and histological data; many are paper-based but some are held within a partial electronic system within the hospital. Catherine's patients can come from a large catchment area, meaning that some of their imaging is done at other hospitals and they attend clinics in other hospitals, so their data may be held elsewhere. Decentralised storage makes accessing imaging data and scan reports challenging, and could lead to gaps in the data sets. Imaging data files are large so moving them between hospitals would be challenging, but fortunately the focus of Catherine's work is on specific findings already known from imaging that has been done. Magnetic resonance imaging as a technique is evolving every few years, meaning that more recent scans may have more detailed imaging in comparison with earlier scans, which could affect outcome predictions (Villanueva-Meyer et al.

2017). Additionally the content in scan reports can vary, sometimes simply providing a disease assessment and not always describing the scan features in sufficient detail.

Progress toward undertaking machine learning is in its early stages: following data collection, the data will be split into trial and test sets, thereby creating a set of data not previously used during the study, ready to trial with any potential successful techniques. The trial set is going to raise the question of statistical overfitting, and whether increasing our data set size can overcome that problem. Ethical approval covers two external NHS sites, so if the study set is too small, there is access to additional cases to build up the trial set and to create a completely unseen test set.

In terms of human factors, Catherine's project is supervised by a small but highly qualified academic team, including clinical professors in paediatric neurosurgery, paediatric neuro-oncology and paediatric neuroradiology, whom she works with on a daily basis, so their shared language already is familiar and routinely used in such teams. Her project also involves working with a professor of data science and will grow to incorporate further data science based academic collaborations.

Case Study 3: Precision Medicine for Congenital Hearing Loss

Haroon Saeed is a specialist trainee in ear nose and throat (ENT) surgery, currently employed by Manchester University NHS Foundation Trust and also a PhD student based at The University of Manchester. Haroon's project involves assessing a group of children who have a congenital and progressive hearing loss condition, called enlarged vestibular aqueduct (EVA) syndrome, caused by an enlargement of one of the bones in the inner ear known as the vestibular aqueduct (Belenky et al. 1993). This condition causes progressive hearing loss and ultimately it leads children to be profoundly deaf by adolescence. Haroon is able to rehabilitate children's hearing by implanting a hearing aid device, known as a cochlear implant, and audiologists are able to provide hearing aids to them. The issue for these children and their parents is that it is very difficult to predict when their child's hearing loss is likely to worsen, how fast, which ear it will be affected the most, and importantly when to do cochlear implantation surgery. Haroon's work aims to improve precision medicine in EVA syndrome, first by discovering the prognostic features or clinical biomarkers that relate to worsening hearing and then by using these to build a prognostic model or decision support tool. The aim for a newly diagnosed patient is to predict the severity and degree of their hearing loss, and plan appropriately for their surgery or hearing aid implementation. This will ensure that the team provides the right treatment to the right patient at the right time and will streamline the correct hearing surveillance and audiological testing.

In data science terms, Haroon and colleagues are using different methodologies to approach this research—one approach is based on established inferential statistics and the other is exploring the role of ML. They have data about a large number of patients from cochlear implant centres in Manchester and London. Haroon's project is using retrospective unstructured data, collected from approximately 450 patients' ears, across three different NHS sites. Each site has different electronic patient record systems, ways of coding their data and different scanning machines. The data collection for this project has been informed by the current prognostic literature for this disorder and includes: genetic variant data, features in the inner ear from the radiological scan, demographic features (age and sex) and hearing loss data (Aimoni et al. 2017). These prognostic biomarkers are a mixture of quantitative and qualitative data. An important consideration when collecting the radiological data will be to ensure that the measurements and features selected are reproducible. It is vital that reproducible measures are used to form the building blocks of a clinical prediction model to ensure that it is both generalisable and transferable across healthcare settings. The data are being collected in a bespoke cloud database platform, which means pseudo-anonymised data can be uploaded remotely, from different sites, ensuring that the data are collected in a unified way.

In terms of human factors, Haroon has brought together an interdisciplinary team with complementary expertise, including an ENT surgeon specialising in working with children with this condition, a professor of genetics, a neuroradiologist, an academic with expertise in data science and also another academic with experience in inferential statistics. Haroon has had to invest time in developing his knowledge and understanding of the respective areas of expertise; in doing so, he has developed a shared language and knowledge base for the team to use to discuss the project.

Ethics and Governance in Cases 2 and 3

Catherine's project is a retrospective study requiring ethical approval to access and work with data from her own hospital and two external sites but in this small disease cohort even pseudo-anonymised data have the potential to identify a patient. The system for ethical approval through the Integrated Research Application System (IRAS) within the NHS assumes randomised controlled studies involving very large cohort sizes. It is not set up to deal with projects that are applying ML techniques to investigate much smaller patient cohorts, using retrospective data (Grist et al. 2020). Generally ethics committee members lack understanding of ML and this can result in rejections or issues being raised during review, even though the studies are based on safe and appropriate approaches. Similarly, funding bodies might not always see the applicability of ML approaches to healthcare data, perhaps deeming that this is not sufficiently big enough data to be used to make predictive models. There may also be debate over whether the tool or model is a medical device, which would then need approval by appropriate regulatory bodies such as the US FDA (2019) or UK MHRA (Rowley et al. 2019).

The studies described by both Catherine and Haroon aim to produce an academic model rather than an externally validated clinical prediction model. It can be extremely time-consuming to get the correct ethical approval and informatics governance in place and to set up contracts and data processing agreements for these kinds of multi-site retrospective studies. A longer term issue even after a study is approved is to build clinician trust and confidence in accepting electronically generated outcomes, therefore successful implementation depends on robust evaluation and clinical governance of ML approaches. This can be difficult to achieve, as demonstrated in these cases, where the data have never been assembled and interrogated in a similar way before.

Training the Humans, in Cases 2 and 3

Haroon had no previous experience in machine learning or programming, and it is unusual for a clinician to have these skill sets. As more concrete examples come through from landmark studies that illustrate real benefits to patients (Hildebrand et al. 2009; Taylor et al. 2013), Catherine and Haroon agreed that these sorts of cases should be integrated into the undergraduate medical curriculum. They also thought that ML or data science should be included within the medical curriculum. At an introductory level medical students have the option of undertaking 6- to 12-week clinical or research based modules, which they suggested could be based on an underlying artificial intelligence methodology. Medical students with a strong interest in ML and data science could intercalate a Bachelor's or Master's degree into their medical degree. In terms of postgraduate opportunities for specialist training in this area clinicians could contribute to audit or quality improvement projects, which are more of a taster-level introduction to ML approaches. In terms of more formal postgraduate training in the UK, AI could be taken up through some of the limited numbers of highly competitive clinical training posts, called academic foundation posts, with designated research time. Once in a clinical post, carving time out to do research can be challenging. Both Haroon and Catherine were successful in applying for independent charitable funding to support this, but they also do intense out-of-hours clinical work to make time for their research. Health Education England's Topol Fellowship programme (NHS Health Education England 2019) is another avenue for healthcare professionals to dedicate time to data science driven projects.

Impact in Cases 2 and 3

Both Catherine and Haroon were asked what the impact of their projects had been to date. Haroon: "When you are within your speciality as a trainee, that is your world essentially, and you're not aware of all these other things that are going on around you. One of the added benefits of this project is actually eye-opening, in terms of what expertise there is within the university and, indeed, within our other specialities within our NHS Trust. So I'd say those two are impacts, and the culmination of that has been a collaborative paper." Catherine: "We've looked at a rare children's tumour group and we think we've found a radiological phenotype for separating it into two tumours, one of which you can operate on, and, theoretically have a big impact on survival. The other still unfortunately has a dismal outcome, but they are two completely discrete tumour groups and when you apply these levels of filters of the advanced imaging, you can separate them out and decide which one should have surgery and which should not. This reinforces the role for using these advanced metric scans to characterise small rare tumour groups and, even though it's not something big from a health economics point of view, you can actually make a big impact to a child's survival." Haroon has published a literature search investigating potential prognostic markers for his project in a very high impact journal, disseminating his research and hopefully influencing others in their fields in the future (Saeed et al. 2020).

Conclusions Regarding Cases 2 and 3

Although Catherine and Haroon's projects are quite different in their clinical focus, they are both proof-of-concept projects to determine if AI approaches can help to discover prognostic markers within the retrospective study groups and so both raise similar workforce issues. Data collection for these kinds of prognostic studies concerning heterogeneous data is laborious and time-consuming but requires clinical expertise and domain knowledge to enable assessment of the quality of the data to see if it is suitable to be used for ML algorithms. Data need to be collected in an agile manner; databases for the collection of this sort of complex data need to quickly adapt to capture the richness of the data, particularly with techniques such as MRI which are developing all the time. When data are captured from very diverse systems and reporting structures, manual curation and data entry may lead to introduced errors, which could flaw the starting data sets. A secondary benefit of a detailed analysis of retrospective data is that it can also be used to find important patterns in the data, which have not been previously possible as the data have not been held in one single place, this may help to drive quality improvement projects. Education about ML and how we can use it on health data to improve patient outcomes needs to be much more accessible—among the healthcare workforce, among important gatekeepers such as ethics committees, and among community stakeholders such as future patients. Within hospitals there is a need for a translator role, that is, clinicians who understand the data in detail know the questions that the data can answer and are conversant with the kinds of ML to apply. Placing people in such roles would make it much easier to have conversations in collaborative teams with experts in ML and data science, to drive healthcare projects forward.

Case Study 4: Building a Learning System in the Intensive Care Unit

Anthony Wilson is a consultant in anaesthesia and critical care medicine at Manchester University Hospitals NHS Foundation Trust. He is the clinical lead for healthcare informatics in the Department of Adult Critical Care and works in the Intensive Care Unit (ICU). Within the adult ICU where Anthony works there are a number of healthcare databases that record vital signs and details of interventions that doctors and nurses carry out with the patients. Anthony's project aims to bring together all those data, link them and start to apply ML techniques to the data set to promote quality improvements for patient care. Anthony aspires to "mimic" MIMIC III (Medical Information Mart for Intensive Care), a landmark US project that created an open access single database with integrated de-identified clinical data of patients admitted to a tertiary care hospital (Johnson et al. 2016), or emulate other initiatives of this kind such as the Paediatric Intensive Care (PIC) database developed by a tertiary hospital in China, freely accessible under the terms of a data access agreement (Zeng et al. 2020).

Bringing all the data together is not a simple matter. In the ICU patients are monitored in more detail and more frequently than anywhere else in the hospital. For the entirety of their stay, each patient is connected to a continuous vital-signs monitor, recording their heart rate and blood pressure, and also closely observed by a critical care nurse stationed at the end of their bed. Unfortunately, patient data are sequestered in many data silos and not easy to access in one central database. One of these is the ICU Electronic Patient Record (EPR); it contains approximately 10 million records, including electronic free-text notes written by doctors and nurses about the patients they're caring for, and structured forms that doctors and nurses use to enter specific care events such as admission and discharge data. It also collates information such as vital-signs data pulled directly from monitors and ventilators and, from other hospital departments, blood, X-ray and microbiology results. In addition the EPR contains quantitative data that the nurses measure and record and enter manually, such as volume of urine, or blood exiting from a drain. The hospital also has an ICU outcomes database covering key patient parameters and critical care outcomes, where data are entered retrospectively by data clerks. Some information also is drawn from a national audit project that supports comparisons among ICUs. Data are not always used to advantage; one example is that the patient vital-signs monitor outputs a lot of data such as heart rates and oxygen saturations as waveforms, complex and useful data that currently are discarded after 72 hours. Another example is that when a patient leaves the ICU, their still largely paper-based notes are scanned into the EPR as a PDF file, an unstructured document that makes it difficult to automate extraction of information.

The benefit for patients is personalised local healthcare, which Anthony calls "evidence-based medicine 2.0", because it is an advance on how doctors now practice evidence-based medicine and use trials and apply trials in their specific patient circumstance. What ML enables is to personalise the care that patients receive down to the individual level and the local level as well; clinicians will be able to look through the data and understand what they've done for ICU patients in Manchester and how that has worked. So, they can say to a patient: "bearing in mind all this evidence that's already come from our intensive care unit and with our patient population, this is what we think will work best for you". ML also enables clinicians to improve the amount of harm-free care that they give. To minimise the chance of iatrogenic injury constant vigilance is required, but no human being is able to provide this level of vigilance, and no ICU doctor is able to look at all the available data all the time. According to Anthony, "So much of intensive care is about doing simple things well; it is not actually that difficult to provide organ support and look after a patient intensively, it just needs to be done systematically and well all the time." A quality improvement project underway across the entire NHS called "Getting it Right First Time" has a large focus on anaesthesia (Getting It Right First Time 2020). Anthony believes the data that he is collecting can be used to provide individualised performance feedback to clinicians about patients they have treated and whether a patient deteriorated following discharge (similar to the system implemented for measuring the outcomes for surgeons in the NHS). "So one of the things that we're doing with the data at the moment is a little extubation project. Patients go on a mechanical ventilator with an endotracheal tube, not having an anaesthetic, and then at some point in time when they get better we take them off the ventilator. You have to choose the right time to take the breathing tube out, and one of the markers of performance is how many patients need to go back on the breathing machine within 48 hours. That's really based on a decision about whether or not this is the right time to take the tube out or not. [Staff in the ICU] are really interested to see how we do as a unit and how they all perform individually."

Getting access to the data, which is held in a Structured Query Language (SQL) database, was initially difficult as local informatics teams are not used to clinicians requesting this kind of access, Anthony and a colleague approached this by teaching themselves to programme in SQL, enabling access to the data needed. The database is complex as it holds data from four different ICUs in the hospital, each of which set up their own data structure. The database from Philips is based on SNOMED CT (Systematized Nomenclature of Medicine Clinical Terms) (Bodenreider et al. 2018) and has all of the SNOMED codes built into it. However, each ICU team decided to make their own structure within the existing SNOMED structure as each team had specific requirements, meaning that mining the data for the right clinical term was very complicated. In addition, as clinicians in the ICU weren't able to visualise the data in its rawest form they couldn't advise the informaticians over the best way to address the database. The key step forward was when Anthony and his colleague were given access to the SQL database, in order to query it and work through the structure, and mine the database much more effectively. Access to the database still needs to be very controlled, ensuring that hospital laptops and VPN access are used if accessing the database from off-site. Mutual trust and deeper understanding of the SNOMED codes used allowed them to work together with the informatics team to build a dashboard with a graphical user interface to display patients' ventilatory parameters during the COVID-19 pandemic.

The importance of developing a culture of mutual trust was exemplified in another project focused on outcomes from ICU patients with COVID-19. In this example clinical colleagues appeared reticent to undertake any statistics or propose models themselves, however Anthony would like to see a much more proactive approach—clinicians taking the lead with more of the data analysis in the future, working collaboratively with statisticians to refine the models. He aspires to promote a two-way dialogue regarding what could be achieved with the data, arguing that if some of the data cleansing and structuring can be undertaken by clinicians with experience in that clinical area then it will reduce input and time needed from the data scientists. In terms of the broader team Anthony describes that it is important to have support from the Chief Informatics Officer (CIO) or equivalent informatics lead in the hospital. In his hospital they are not only the data controller but also somebody who can act as a figurehead and be an advocate for data science in the ICU. Having the support of the Medical Director is also important in taking any data science projects forward in the ICU. Anthony's ICU now has a member of the hospital informatics team embedded within the ICU, who has been integral to setting up the databases and now is particularly invested in the unit's data science projects and keen to see the outcomes from using the collected data. The collaborative team within the ICU also consists of an ICU registrar, contract software and database engineers and research software engineers collaborating from the academic side, all working to create an API linked to a server to collect the waveform data. As yet there are no data scientists or statisticians collaborating on the project, but the focus to date has been on assembling and curating the data to see what is feasible, before the main clinical research questions are defined.

In terms of ethics and governance within this project, Anthony has found it challenging to find out exactly what is permissible with the data he is collecting, and hard to find expert governance advice from somebody with a strong understanding of ML approaches. There is a need to widen the pool of colleagues who can act as decision makers for information governance, enabling better use of the data that the hospital is collecting and improved guidance on how to pseudo-anonymise data for use in these sorts of studies. His view was that the hospital has a duty to undertake health-related research, and that this should be the main aim of any such work with the priority being to ensure that individual patient anonymity is retained. Much of Anthony's work will lead to service improvements; simply having all the data located in one place will save huge amounts of staff time during audit and quality projects, typically undertaken by junior doctors attempting to collate disparate and distributed datasets. Describing himself as a "positive disrupter", he argues that the time saved could be used to change attitudes and effect more immediate changes in performance, through constant monitoring using dashboards for example. His aim is to see patterns and new things in the data that perhaps would not have been possible previously whilst all the data were distributed; using ML approaches to make predictions from the data would be beyond the primary reason for collection because such manipulation and interrogation of the data means that the project is defined as research and therefore requires ethical approval.

Anthony describes mistrust of ML, elaborating that although colleagues may know that these approaches exist they may not understand what they can do or how they might relate to existing statistical techniques. Best practice in scientific computing advises working in small steps and obtaining frequent feedback from end-users, working in an agile manner, responsive to changing demands (Wilson et al. 2014). For Anthony's projects one of his main concerns relates to the end-user interface where any final tools will be deployed, as this will influence adoption by clinical colleagues. He suggests adoption is most likely to be supported if implemented within a device that was easily accessible at the time needed. The type of interface and choice of device for deployment might vary considerably depending on the part of the care pathway it was being used to support. For example, there would be some tools that would be beneficial at the bedside for direct patient care; others during ward-round events where Anthony might be leading overall direction of care decisions with a team of junior doctors; still others in critical care and management events which might provide direction on quality of care for the entire unit. The requirements and the questions that each of these scenarios would ask of the data vary considerably. Anthony's view is that it is likely to be in the more senior management events where any kind of decision-making tool would have the most likelihood of adoption and success. Regarding integration of decision-making tools, Anthony comments: "How you put that interface into people's hands in the hospital is a concern for anything that I do with machine learning or whatever it might be in any data-driven project. The set tools that people use to interact with data and hospital patients, like the Philips database system—the front end of that is the monitor for the ventilator. [It is unsatisfactory that] these are all manufactured pieces of equipment where I can't interact with the source code at all, I can't do anything about that; so anything that I produce is going to sit on some random computer screen, or it's going to be separate from the work streams that people use routinely."

In terms of training, Anthony has built up his expertise in AI in healthcare informally. Prior to becoming a doctor Anthony completed a physics degree which has helped him with the maths and statistical knowledge needed to understand ML. He has also accessed informal training through online freely accessible courses such as Massive Online Open Courses (MOOCs) and also open community resources to support programmers, such as Stack Overflow (https://stackoverflow.com/). Like other UK doctors, he has a limited budget towards his own training and development; in the future, he would like to use this to develop his knowledge through more formal training in high quality data science courses. He, like Catherine and Haroon, feels the need to strengthen the data science taught in the medical curriculum, including data cleansing, structuring and interpretation and argues that too much of the curriculum focuses on interpreting tests and confidence intervals, rather than focusing on the data, and what is possible from analysing it. He also supports much earlier immersion in data science as a trainee doctor, such as options to do intercalating degrees within your fifth year of study. Following completion of a medical degree there is the option to undertake an academic foundation training programme, which could incorporate a 4 month data-driven research project; however, this would need champions and supervisors among consultants with experience of these kinds of projects. The next level up would then be clinical fellowships where clinicians would be able to pursue dedicated master's degrees to develop data science expertise.

Conclusions:

- Collaborative relationships between informatics teams and clinicians where the barriers are less distinct develops a mutual understanding and trust of what is achievable and what each party can bring to a data-driven project.
- To improve outcomes for patients, we need more clinical colleagues with expertise in the governance of data-driven projects, who understand what is possible and facilitate discussions with research ethics and governance bodies.
- The data that is routinely collected within a critical care unit is complex, rich and large, and can be used to drive data-driven clinical decision support and improve the quality of care. The choice of interface and route of deployment for any such tool needs to involve the end-user to ensure adoption.
- Training in data science should follow the pathway of training for a clinician, being embedded within research opportunities within the medical degree through to data-intensive research projects during registrar training, supported by clinical champions with data science expertise.

Case Study 5: Automating Vertebral Fracture Detection and Reporting

Paul A. Bromiley is a lecturer in Health Data Sciences at The University of Manchester, where he works on the development of computer-aided diagnostics for medical imaging, with a focus on musculoskeletal radiology. Paul's project involves the development of a system for the opportunistic detection of vertebral fractures on computed tomography (CT) images. These images are requested for other clinical reasons, but often image the spine and so provide the opportunity to detect vertebral fractures. Vertebral fracture detection is important because these fractures are often the earliest clinical manifestation of osteoporosis (Gonnelli et al. 2013); the earlier a patient can be diagnosed, the earlier they can be treated, so improving current diagnostic rates will in turn have a positive impact on healthcare quality and cost. Paul says: "Vertebral fractures should be reported by the radiologist as an incidental finding, but we know from clinical practice that those vertebral fractures are quite rarely reported. The Royal College of Radiologists' national audit in 2019 (Howlett et al. 2020) found that on average, only 26.4% of the vertebral fractures visualised incidentally in CT images were accurately reported and 2.6% of the patients were referred on for proper management." One of the issues affecting diagnostic rates is the shortfall of available radiologists in the country; it isn't just a matter of asking radiologists to spend more time processing images and reporting vertebral fractures;

there simply are not enough of them. This is where the idea of using ML and computer-aided diagnostic systems comes into Paul's project.

Clinical image data are often presented in the DICOM (Digital Imaging and Communications in Medicine) format. These images have an extensive header which contains information regarding the patient, including, weight, height and sex, some of which provide information on fracture risk. They also, however, contain personal identifiable information such as the patient's name, address, referring physician and NHS number, which need to be anonymised. Despite the DICOM format being a standard, it is often poorly adhered to. There is a DICOM dictionary which is used to provide information on what should be included; each entry has a tag number, and these are all even numbers. The DICOM format allows individual manufacturers to add non-standard, odd-numbered tags to include additional information, which can include a field containing patient information, also requiring removal to prevent identification. In this case study the quality of the data itself is fairly high as it is used for diagnostic purposes. However radiographic artefacts and the presence of extraneous items like cardiac pacemakers/defibrillators, stents, shunts, surgical clips and other medical devices can obscure bony edges.

For data analysis, the team has developed several bespoke software packages, most of which are open source or licensed to users, e.g. TINA (Schunke et al. 2012) and VXL (University of Manchester 2020), to identify landmark points in images. Landmark detection has been used for tasks like facial recognition, where facial landmarks like the eyes, nose and mouth can be detected. The team Paul works in has been developing algorithms for 25 years and aims to develop an algorithm that can annotate landmark points on structures in a given image. These points should be identifiable across all the images in a given image class. Aside from developing their own algorithms, the team also use "off the shelf" solutions, for example various Python libraries for results processing and producing graphics. The team often combine methods (e.g. TINA, VXL and Python) for the purpose of rapid prototyping. When identifying landmark points, it is important to try to identify commonality. For spinal image annotation, points are marked on the edges of the vertebrae. This allows the development of a shape model. By annotating landmark points across a number of individuals with variation in shape, the covariances of the points can be determined to produce a model with parameters that can be varied to fit a given image. Image intensity can also be included, producing an appearance model. The most recent version of this approach uses a random forest to model the image intensities around each landmark point, together with a shape model describing the whole set of points. The shape model acts as a constraint during fitting of the individual intensity models, helping to guide them to the correct locations in the image (Lindner et al. 2015). The team has had considerable success with using that particular kind of model in a whole range of different image types, for example, various different musculoskeletal imaging problems, in the spine, the hip and the knee.

When it comes to training data, humans are required to mark up the images to define these landmarks, annotating points in training data. This involves potentially marking up thousands of points in hundreds of images, each image taking about typically 30–40 min. For Paul's project, external contractors in the form of retired radiographers from the Manchester Royal Infirmary were used. The contractors had all worked in the bone health unit and had undergone training in this area.

Ethics and governance in this project respect all seven key requirements of the European Commission's report on ethical guidelines for trustworthy AI (European Commission 2020). However Paul argues that in a medical context, human agency and oversight is of particular relevance. This includes having a human "in the loop", demonstrated here by having a trained radiologist as part of the loop. The algorithm generates the clinical reports that would be reviewed and, if necessary, corrected by the radiologist, prior to return to the hospital. Aside from the standard issues of applying for ethical approval to access clinical data and the need to anonymise the data, deeper ethical and philosophical issues have arisen around how to handle hitherto undiagnosed conditions detected through the course of the project. Since the data are anonymised, there is no easy way to feed such diagnoses back to inform (and potentially treat) a patient. The dilemma, thus, is whether or not the team should maintain a pseudo-anonymisation system that, if required, could enable the re-identification of patients by the clinical facing part of the system. The main drawback of this kind of system is increased risk of identification of patients by staff unauthorised to do so. The eventual compromise was to anonymise everything. In Paul's words: "we argued this back and forwards for years, I'm very unhappy with that system, particularly in the case of osteoporosis where we're talking about images that we know will be under-diagnosed in clinical practice, that's the whole point. We know we've got diagnoses of people that, when those scans were taken, those fractures were missed. I think there are ethical risks on both sides of the equation there. So, ultimately the solution is probably a technological one." Paul considers that such technological solutions could allow the patient to be identified by the clinical team if a previously undiagnosed condition is detected.

This project involved an academic group from the University, clinical partners and also a commercial partner, Optasia Medical (https://www.optasiamedical.com/). Clinical partners are necessary for several reasons including access to the data and their clinical knowledge, specifically relating to what the intended solution should look like and its clinical utility. This partnership has helped to overcome certain issues, especially around the longer term support and maintenance of such solutions. Paul highlights that the kind of approach applied to developing open-source software in other domains doesn't translate well into the clinical arena. In clinical medicine the solutions require specialised knowledge and expertise and regulatory approval as well as long-term maintenance of the software. Working with commercial companies can bring different expertise to such projects. They are often familiar with setting up and running customer support services that extend over time and have different funding models that can support such services. Companies can also assist in managing scaling of projects. Paul identifies that there is a significant difference between supporting a single hospital site and nationwide service, which could rapidly increase image processing demands from a few thousand images to millions, and he stresses the importance of sourcing expertise about high tech, rapid expansion types of companies from the people who work in that area and who are familiar with ways that you mitigate the kinds of commercial risks involved. Paul talks about the importance of a tight-knit, close team, who are all committed to getting the formal contracts complete and out of the way as soon as possible so the project can succeed. Paul talks about the value of leadership in place of management, with a mix of people with different skills all invested towards a single mutually understood goal. Working with medical charities (Royal Osteoporosis Society) and organisations (Bone Research Academy), especially for generating grant proposals, is useful, and carrying out public and patient involvement and consultation throughout the course of the project.

The work carried out by the team in this area has already had a positive direct impact on patient outcomes. By working with Fracture Liaison Services (FLS), it has provided a direct route to feedback information about patients so they could be treated. The FLS model was pioneered in Glasgow (Scotland) and has emerged as the most effective service model for the management of osteoporosis (McLellan et al. 2003). Around 2000 people were reported to the FLS that otherwise would have remained undiagnosed, which potentially has saved the lives across the next 5 years of somewhere between 10 and 30 people who would have died from a hip fracture that now has been avoided by early diagnosis. One of the trials Paul's team was involved with in London influenced an NHS Trust to put in place a system similar to cancer reporting, to ensure that all patients with fractures were referred to the bone health team—a permanent improvement in health services for around 360,000 people in that Trust's catchment (Rajak et al. 2019).

Paul has a background in physics and astrophysics. He taught himself C programming during his PhD and then undertook on-the-job training in computer vision when he started at Manchester, but received no real formal training in computer vision or data science. Paul recommends a solid foundation in statistics and maths for this type of work, otherwise: "It's relatively easy to take a bunch of data, put it in your model and look at the response [...] it won't be a particularly useful solution because you haven't got any of the expertise to know what you are doing, how it is working, whether it's working properly, whether there are particular things you could enforce invariances in to make it much more accurate. All of this is basically statistics… the science of analysing things where you've got a stochastic element, where there's noise in the data."

Paul commented on the sort of training that might be of use to clinicians approaching this subject, considering the level of understanding and application required. Like Haroon, he cited the Topol Fellowships (NHS Health Education England 2019) as a good opportunity for selected clinicians to specialise in AI. For the majority though, given that they already have very extensive training, adding more requirements to this already considerable workload may lead to burnout (Dauphinee 2020). They need to be in a position, not necessarily where they can program AI systems or train a convolutional neural network to solve a problem, but where they have enough knowledge to be able to understand what those systems are doing, what they mean and how to use the results from them. Paul suggested that clinicians do not necessarily need to understand the intricate inner workings of ML processes in order to make effective use of their output. The key for clinicians is to understand and interpret the output with some understanding of how reliable it is. Clinicians must recognise the models' limitations and vulnerabilities as well as their potential applications. Adversarial ML can be used to fool models, and show that sometimes just changing a few pixels in an image is enough to change the output of an ML model, even though such a change is imperceptible to a human viewing the image.

Conclusions and Recommendations

The use of patient data either retrospectively or prospectively is central to the success of any ML-based clinical decision approach. Patients need to understand how their data might be used and why it might aid improvements in health and treatment for other patients, and patients must be consented appropriately. This is more complicated when it concerns the data of children and adolescents, and needs some careful public and patient involvement. Active dialogue and involvement with patients and the public can be facilitated by those who work in and with appropriate patient support and advocacy groups, such as the UK organisation "Understanding Patient Data" (Wellcome Trust Ltd. 2020). Largely, many patients are very positive with respect to wanting to share their data, but they want close regulation of how it will be used and by whom; perceptions that ML approaches might replace clinicians may be a negative factor, or alternatively may be welcomed by the public (Wong et al. 2019).

Mistrust of ML approaches is not unique to patients—many clinicians and senior stakeholders in hospitals remain sceptical. Therefore clinicians, whilst not necessarily needing to become experts in the field, must be equipped with sufficient knowledge to rigorously question and appraise any potential approaches that are being considered in their hospital. Health AI experts need to assist their healthcare co-workers and colleagues to understand the richness of their data, its complexity and what is and is not achievable when considering ML approaches.

The use of patient data to inform ML approaches in healthcare must be undertaken within ethical and governance guidelines and frameworks for research and practice; these are still developing and therefore not always fit-for-purpose. It is incumbent upon the collective community working in this area to actively define and refine appropriate uses of AI in healthcare, and work together closely with regulators to minimise risks and barriers.

AI has not yet reached the point where it is capable of fully replicating human performance in complex data analysis tasks, so its clinical utility relies on incorporating AI into existing workflows, rather than replacing them. Human oversight is essential. Clinicians need to be able to interpret the results that algorithms produce. Those who develop algorithms must ensure that they are not "black boxes".

Data-driven ML projects require a collaborative team approach, garnering interdisciplinary skills and domain-specific knowledge. Team members must develop a culture of trust, be willing to develop themselves and others, and work towards developing a shared common language. A collaborative team working on this kind of project is likely to be most successful with the support of a senior champion or stakeholder, such as a Chief Clinical Information Officer, who is well-versed in these kinds of approaches and can act as an advocate in strategic planning and management meetings.

References

Agile Alliance. What is Agile software development? Agil. 101. What is Agil. 2020. https://www.agilealliance.org/agile101/. Accessed 25 Jan 2021.

Aimoni C, Ciorba A, Cerritelli L, Ceruti S, Skarżyński PH, Hatzopoulos S. Enlarged vestibular aqueduct: audiological and genetical features in children and adolescents. Int J Pediatr Otorhinolaryngol. 2017;101:254–8.

Alfaras M, Soriano MC, Ortín S. A fast machine learning model for ECG-based heartbeat classification and arrhythmia detection. Front Phys. 2019;7:1–11.

Belenky W, Madgy D, Leider J, Becker C, Hotaling A. The enlarged vestibular aqueduct syndrome (EVA syndrome). Ear Nose Throat J. 1993;72:746–51.

Bodenreider O, Cornet R, Vreeman DJ. Recent developments in clinical terminologies – SNOMED CT, LOINC, and RxNorm. Yearb Med Inform. 2018;27:129–39.

Cravero JP, Beach ML, Blike GT, Gallagher SM, Hertzog JH, Pediatric Sedation Research Consortium. The incidence and nature of adverse events during pediatric sedation/anesthesia with propofol for procedures outside the operating room: a report from the Pediatric Sedation Research Consortium. Anesth Analg. 2009;108(3):795–804.

Dauphinee WD. Building a core competency assessment program for all stakeholders: the design and building of sailing ships can inform core competency frameworks. Adv Heal Sci Educ. 2020;25:189–93.

Department of Health and Social Care. GOV.UK. In: Code conduct data-driven health care technology. 2020. https://www.gov.uk/government/publications/code-of-conduct-for-data-driven-health-and-care-technology/initial-code-of-conduct-for-data-driven-health-and-care-technology. Accessed 15 Sep 2020.

Eleftheriou I, Embury S, Brass A. Data journey modelling: predicting risk for IT developments. In: Pract. Enterp. Model. Skövde, Sweden: Springer Link; 2016a. p. 72–86.

Eleftheriou I, Embury SM, Moden R, Dobinson P, Brass A. Data journeys: identifying social and technical barriers to data movement in large, complex organisations. Tech Report, Sch Comput Sci. 2016b.

Eleftheriou I, Embury SM, Moden R, Dobinson P, Brass A. Data journeys: identifying social and technical barriers to data movement in large, complex organisations. J Biomed Inform. 2018;78:102–22.

Enders C. Applied missing data analysis. New York: Guildford Publications; 2010.

European Commission. Shaping Europe's digital future. In: Ethics Guide. Trust. AI. 2020. https://ec.europa.eu/digital-single-market/en/news/ethics-guidelines-trustworthy-ai. Accessed 16 Sep 2020.

Feather A, Randall D, Waterhouse M. Kumar and Clark's Clinical Medicine. 10th ed. Elsevier; 2020.

Getting It Right First Time. Getting it right first time. In: Anaesth. Perioper. Med. 2020. https://gettingitrightfirsttime.co.uk/medical-specialties/anaesthesia-perioperative-medicine/#. Accessed 22 Sep 2020.

Gonnelli S, Caffarelli C, Maggi S, et al. itail.pdf. Osteoporos Int. 2013;24:1151–9.

Grist JT, Withey S, MacPherson L, et al. Distinguishing between paediatric brain tumour types using multi-parametric magnetic resonance imaging and machine learning: a multi-site study. NeuroImage Clin. 2020;25:102172.

Hildebrand MS, DeLuca AP, Taylor KR, Hoskinson DP, Hur IA, Tack D, McMordie SJ, Huygen PLM, Casavant TL, Smith RJH. A contemporary review of Audio Gene audio profiling: a machine-based candidate gene prediction tool for autosomal dominant nonsyndromic hearing loss. Laryngoscope. 2009;119:2211–5.

Howlett DC, Drinkwater KJ, Mahmood N, Illes J, Griffin J, Javaid K. Radiology reporting of osteoporotic vertebral fragility fractures on computed tomography studies: results of a UK national audit. Eur Radiol. 2020;30:4713–23.

Johnson AEW, Pollard TJ, Shen L, Lehman LH, Feng M, Ghassemi M, Moody B, Szolovits P, Anthony Celi L, Mark RG. MIMIC-III, a freely accessible critical care database. Sci Data. 2016;3:160035.

Köse T, Özgür S, Coşgun E, Keskinoğlu A, Keskinoğlu P. Effect of missing data imputation on deep learning prediction performance for vesicoureteral reflux and recurrent urinary tract infection clinical study. Biomed Res Int. 2020:1895076.

Lindner C, Bromiley PA, Ionita MC, Cootes TF. Robust and accurate shape model matching using random forest regression-voting. IEEE Trans Pattern Anal Mach Intell. 2015;37:1862–74.

McLellan AR, Gallacher SJ, Fraser M, McQuillian C. The fracture liaison service: success of a program for the evaluation and management of patients with osteoporotic fracture. Osteoporos Int. 2003;14:1028–34.

National Institute for Health and Care Excellence. Guidance on the use of trastuzumab for the treatment of advanced breast cancer. 2002;24.

NHS Health Education England. Topol digital fellowships. In: About Topol Digit. Fellowsh. Program. 2019. https://topol.hee.nhs.uk/digital-fellowships/. Accessed 14 Sep 2020.

Rajak R, Patel K, Lawless R, Staal J, Holmes A. Incidental capture of vertebral fragility fractures (VFFs) from CT imaging in a large district general hospital in London. Rheumatology. 2019;58:kez108.073.

Rich JT, Neely JG, Paniello RC, Voelker CC, Nussenbaum B, Wang EW. A practical guide to understanding Kaplan-Meier curves. Otolaryngol Head Neck Surg. 2010;143(3):331–6.

Rowley A, Turpin R, Walton S. The emergence of artificial intelligence and machine learning algorithms in healthcare: recommendations to support governance and regulation. BSI Gr. 2019:1–18.

Saeed H, Kenth J, Black G, Saeed S, Stivaros S, Bruce I. Hearing loss in Enlarged vestibular aqueduct: a prognostic factor systematic review of the literature. Otol Neurotol Off Publ Am Otol Soc Am Neurotol Soc [and] Eur Acad Otol Neurotol 2020.

Schunke AC, Bromiley PA, Tautz D, Thacker NA. TINA manual landmarking tool: software for the precise digitization of 3D landmarks. 2012.

Shih RY, Koeller KK. Embryonal tumors of the central nervous system: from the radiologic pathology archives. RadioGraphics. 2018;38:525–41.

Taylor KR, DeLuca AP, Shearer AE, et al. AudioGene: Predicting hearing loss genotypes from phenotypes to guide genetic screening. Hum Mutat. 2013;34:539–45.

The University of Manchester. UoMqVXL: University of Manchester's Qt libraries for VXL. 2020. http://uomqvxl.sourceforge.net/. Accessed 16 Sep 2020.

Tiffin PA, Paton LW. Rise of the machines? Machine learning approaches and mental health: opportunities and challenges. Br J Psychiatry. 2018;213:509–10.

Topol E. The Topol review: preparing the healthcare workforce to deliver the digital future. London: 2019a.

Topol EJ. High-performance medicine: the convergence of human and artificial intelligence. Nat Med. 2019b;25:44–56.

US FDA. Proposed regulatory framework for modifications to artificial intelligence/machine learning (AI/ML) based software as a medical device (SaMD). 2019.

Villanueva-Meyer JE, Mabray MC, Cha S. Current clinical brain tumor imaging. Neurosurgery. 2017;81:397–415.

Wellcome Trust Ltd. Understanding patient data. In: Putt. people Cent. Decis. about patient data. 2020. https://understandingpatientdata.org.uk/. Accessed 16 Sep 2020.

Wernick M, Yang Y, Brankov J, Yourganov G, Strother S. Machine learning in medical imaging. IEEE Signal Process Mag. 2010;27:25–38.

Wilson G, Aruliah DA, Brown CT, et al. Best practices for scientific computing. PLoS Biol. 2014;12:1–7.

Wong SH, Al-Hasani H, Alam Z, Alam A. Artificial intelligence in radiology: how will we be affected? Eur Radiol. 2019;29:141–3.

Zeng X, Yu G, Lu Y, Tan L, Wu X, Shi S, Duan H, Shu Q, Li H. PIC, a paediatric-specific intensive care database. Sci Data. 2020;7:14.

Chapter 18
Working as a Health Information Manager

Trixie Kemp, Lorraine Fernandes, Cameron Barnes, Deneice Marshall, Mandy Burns, Sabu Karakka Mandapam, Gemala Hatta, Oknam Kim, and Kerryn Butler-Henderson

T. Kemp (✉)
College of Health and Medicine, University of Tasmania, Burnie, TAS, Australia
e-mail: trixie.kemp@utas.edu.au

L. Fernandes
Fernandes Healthcare Insights, Bigfork, MT, USA
e-mail: lorraine@fhci.biz

C. Barnes
Cabrini Health, Malvern, VIC, Australia
e-mail: cbarnes@cabrini.com.au

D. Marshall
Barbados Community College, Bridgetown, St. Michael, Barbados
e-mail: deneice.marshall@bcc.edu.bb

M. Burns
Manchester University NHS Foundation Trust, Manchester, Greater Manchester, UK
e-mail: Mandy.Burns@MFT.nhs.uk

S. K. Mandapam
MCHP, Manipal Academy of Higher Education, Manipal, Karnataka, India
e-mail: sabu.km@manipal.edu

G. Hatta
University of Indonesia and Repati Indonesia University, Jakarta, Indonesia

O. Kim
Sungkyunkwan University, Suwon, Republic of Korea

K. Butler-Henderson
Digital Health Hub, College of STEM, RMIT University, Bundoora, VIC, Australia
e-mail: Kerryn.Butler-Henderson@rmit.edu.au

© The Author(s), under exclusive license to Springer Nature   269
Switzerland AG 2021
K. Butler-Henderson et al. (eds.), *The Health Information Workforce*,
Health Informatics, https://doi.org/10.1007/978-3-030-81850-0_18

Abstract Health Information Management (HIM) professionals have knowledge and skills in health record management, clinical coding and classification, information management, human resource management, and healthcare processes. HIM professionals take responsible roles in data integrity, information governance, and health informatics, at the same time as they continue to modernise the fundamentals of HIM. This occupation has a range of options that allow people to work within a health-related field while not being on the frontline providing direct care. There are opportunities to work in healthcare, academia, research, health IT, and anywhere that uses health data, across the globe. Case studies from leaders in the field tell stories of personal growth, education, camaraderie, and contributions to health systems that impact lives globally.

Keywords Case study · Health information management · Clinical documentation · Information governance · Data governance

Introduction

The work of documentation to support the safe delivery of health care has evolved over thousands of years (Kemp et al. 2021). Today, the Health Information Management (HIM) professional "plans, develops, implements and manages health information services, such as patient information systems, and clinical and administrative data, to meet the medical, legal, ethical and administrative requirements of health care delivery" (HIMAA 2016). HIM professionals may work in any organisation which requires the creation, management, governance, analysis, or destruction of health information. They may manage the paper health record, develop and implement the electronic health record, classify and analyse health information, or protect and safeguard health data entrusted to the organisation. Further, they may implement and manage the technology to collect health data, and distil, analyse, and report health information to inform health decisions. Professionalisation of this work has increased over time. Positions of medical record librarian were created in hospitals (Watson 2013) and in the first half of the twentieth century professional bodies formed in the USA (AHIMA 2020), Canada (CHIMA 2019), UK (Abdelhak 2016), and Australia (HIMAA 2016). Formal vocational qualifications started to emerge around the same time. The International Federation of Health Record Organisations (IFHRO) was formed in 1968 (IFHIMA 2020) and established official relations with the World Health Organization in 1970. As their roles evolved to have greater responsibility, medical record librarians became medical record administrators (~1970s) then health information managers (~1990s). Bachelor qualifications emerged in the 1980s in countries where the role had become a recognised profession. In 1987 HIM was included in the International Classification of Occupations. IFHRO changed its name to the International Federation of Health Information Management Associations (IFHIMA) in 2010. The following case studies highlight the diversity of HIM roles across all health system areas, and the importance of the HIM professional in supporting safe health delivery and management.

Lorraine Fernandes, Fernandes Healthcare Insights, USA

My career has been a wandering path of education and experience in different roles as I have worked in many aspects of the health industry, both domestically and internationally. I started as a medical record clerk in a 20-bed hospital in rural South Dakota, in the middle of the USA.

My formal health information education has been at the technical and baccalaureate levels. During the first decade of my career, I worked in teaching hospitals and small community hospitals. I managed 10–50 staff in areas including traditional HIM departments, trauma and cancer registries, and ancillary departments including risk management, discharge planning, and utilisation review. These management roles prepared me for opportunities in large and small technology companies where I served as a healthcare subject matter expert developing or executing corporate strategy, or directly interacting with customers. Additionally, at various points in my career, I have worked as a management consultant, and more recently as a data governance consultant.

At the beginning of my career, I did not appreciate the importance of the two fields I would cross: health information management and health informatics. But I have learned the value of data, from managing clinical registries such as trauma and cancer and being responsible for reporting data to meet local, state, and federal requirements. I witnessed the shortcomings when data in the applications and systems could not easily be exported and used or understood for broader purposes. I have become a believer in the critical need for accurate, trusted data. This need creates many roles, such as privacy or compliance officer, data steward, data analyst, for HIM professionals.

A couple of years ago, I read The Fourth Industrial Revolution by Klaus Schwab (2016), which discussed the need for a multi-stakeholder approach in using data and new technologies and advocated for a comprehensive, global view of how technology is reshaping our world economically, socially, and culturally. HIM professionals can play leadership roles in the new multi-stakeholder era as organisations define their information and data governance practices. Schwab (2016) summarised the tension between the past and the future, which the HIM profession certainly sees: "decision-makers are too often caught in traditional, linear (and non-disruptive) thinking or are too absorbed by immediate concerns to think strategically about the forces of disruption and innovation shaping our future".

Throughout my career volunteerism has played a crucial role in expanding my personal and professional horizons. I have enjoyed roles as Board member and President of the California Health Information Association and served on national workgroups and committees. Since 2013 I have served IFHIMA through being the Editor of Global News, website coordinator, Board member, and President 2019–2022.

Cameron Barnes, Cabrini Health, Australia

Despite a privileged school setting, there was not an abundance of career advice in my final year of secondary school. My application for several courses failed leaving my only option for tertiary education, a humble number five on my wish list, a Bachelor of Applied Science in Medical Record Administration. My mother had suggested it as the course prerequisites included biology, typing 60 words per minute (thankfully not required), and only the 11th form maths I had completed the previous year. I commenced the course in 1986 and promptly failed most of the first-year subjects; I was forced to present myself to the "Committee to Review Unsatisfactory Progress" and plead my case to continue. Thankfully, they recognised my unfulfilled potential and allowed me to complete my first year. I subsequently passed the remaining 2 years and was set to embrace my Medical Record Administrator's career, after a 9-month break to explore Western Europe.

On return to Australia, I applied for a position at St Vincent's Public Hospital in Melbourne. I was 23, with no experience but of course pretty sure that I knew everything I needed to know about managing 15 staff all older than me, acute coding, the Freedom of Information Act, submitting data to the Department of Health and many other duties. I stumbled through my first few years with help from my manager, peers, and the staff themselves who took pity on me as a young and foolish boy whose heart was in the right place. It was an excellent grounding, and I learnt a lot in 7 years at St Vincent's, knowledge that I still refer to today. I became involved in our professional association (now the Health Information Management Association of Australia) at this time, an involvement which I continue 30 years later.

During my tenure at St Vincent's two co-workers and I established an independent coding contracting business that kept 15 casual staff busy, and us busy too most weekends for a couple of years. Our increasing success and workload eventually meant we had to either move into this full time or sell up. We sold up.

After becoming Deputy Manager at St Vincent's, I was approached to do a role at The Royal Children's and Women's Hospitals, managing 70 staff and a budget that made my eyes water. I accepted this role with glee and subsequently failed impressively in the first 12 months. Working across two big campuses meant I was never in the place I needed to be, and the staff were not impressed. The decision was made to base me solely at "The Children's", and I set about my department manager tasks. This role included more strategic work, interaction with executive, planning the building of a brand-new hospital and department, a patient administration system implementation, and planning for a scanned medical record solution. I also went to Vietnam for a period as an advisor for Royal Children's Hospital International. During this time, I completed my Masters in Health Administration, and I did surprisingly well because the study seemed so relevant to my day-to-day work.

I worked at 'The Children's' for 12 years until I was approached by Cabrini Hospital, a private hospital with around 700 beds and five sites, to take on a new role that included a departmental cultural transformation. I am now the Director, Health Information Services and Information Governance. My position's information governance aspect came about due to the increasing realisation of the need for good quality data to inform business decision making. It is a perfect role for a HIM professional as we generally have an eye for detail, like to solve problems, and understand the interface between administrative and clinical work. We are also used to data reporting and know that "data" is not always "information". During my 10 years at Cabrini, I have also instigated some ground-breaking projects including secure messaging, data integrity software, and e-referrals.

My ongoing interest and desire to "be part of the solution" meant I became involved with the IFHRO (now IFHIMA) as the Australian representative. I also presented papers internationally. I have been able to travel extensively nationally and internationally as part of my profession and make friends and colleagues throughout the world. As an elder statesman of the profession now, I still love to solve problems, make work more efficient, and mentor HIM staff.

Deneice Marshall, Barbados Community College, Barbados

My career in HIM started 17 years ago. I never imagined I would have the opportunity to serve my country, the region, and my profession as IFHIMA Director for the Americas 2019–2022, or become the Founding President of the Barbados Health Information Management Association. Further, I could not have envisioned being appointed HIM Coordinator at my country's only community college. In this role, I administer and provide leadership in the day-to-day operations of the HIM education programme. My responsibilities also include developing, implementing, and delivering an updated HIM curriculum. Besides my educational responsibilities, I have conducted HIM consultancies as a Pan American Health Organization (PAHO) Temporary Advisor for several regional Ministries of Health in the Caribbean.

My unpredictable journey started in 2003 at the Barbados Community College. Initially, I wanted to pursue a degree in environmental sciences; however, the programme was fully subscribed. The alternative options were minimal, and HIM was the only option that intrigued me at the time; little did I know that it would become my profession and my passion today.

At that time, the HIM curriculum combined the disciplines of medical records management, basic information technology, health care, and the traditional principles and practices of acquiring, analysing, and protecting health information. Upon completing the programme's theoretical components, I embarked on a 3-month directed practice training period at the local hospital, a polyclinic, and a health insurance company. This work-based learning allowed me to connect the dots, to acquire a genuine appreciation and understanding for the concepts taught and the importance of the HIM profession. Many people equated this profession with the simple filing of records; however, my academic programme and directed practice exposed me to a much broader and more detailed view.

After completing my associate degree, my first job was as a medical records clerk at the local hospital for a short period; I worked primarily in the appointment and library section. I subsequently accepted a job offer from the insurance company where I had completed a part of my directed practice, working as a healthcare administrative assistant. My duties included researching and managing health claims inquiries, advising customers on claim-filing procedures and the status of health claims cases and insurance policies, coding clients' claims using International Classification of Disease version 9 Clinical Modification (ICD-9-CM) and Current Procedural Terminology (CPT) and adjusting clients' requests for reimbursement.

I began to think more deeply about how my profession impacted the community's life and health. I started to reflect on how a lack of knowledge about the value added by my chosen profession could stifle its growth. Moreover, I became curious about how other parts of the world were using HIM to better manage patient care. Further study and professional development were warranted. My HIM education continued at Tennessee State University, where I completed a Bachelor of Science in HIM with a minor in General Business in 2009. I subsequently earned my American Health Information Management Association (AHIMA) Registered Health Information Administrator certification in 2010. While studying in the United States, I capitalised on opportunities to work at both acute and long-term care settings as a HIM Consultant. I worked primarily on clinical coding projects, Joint Commission accreditation, and quality improvement initiatives.

My research and exposure to international conferences and other forums showed me a whole new world. The use of health data and new technologies to manage patient information was more extensive, with closer links acknowledged between HIM and patient care outcomes. Inexorably, my educational journey continued; in 2014, I completed my joint Master of Science from the College of St Scholastica in Duluth, Minnesota, in HIM and Information Technology Leadership. My published research thesis focused on HIM and information technology education challenges in developing countries (Marshall 2014).

In 1978 the Associate of Applied Science degree in HIM programme formerly known as the Medical Records Technology programme was established at the Barbados Community College. This programme has evolved to integrate health information technology, current trends in HIM, and various continuing education courses in health informatics, coding, and classification of health data (Barbados Community College 2020). The Medical Records Management/HIM profession in Barbados has a cadre of trained HIM professionals working across various health institutions locally, regionally, and internationally. Employment opportunities on the island are mainly at acute, ambulatory, and behavioural health facilities in the public and private sectors. However, on the island, there is still a lack of awareness of the value of the HIM professional, or of the importance of their roles and responsibilities, especially in regard to the integration of information communication and technology (ICT) and electronic health records in health care delivery. We are still recognised by traditional role names such as chief medical records officer, medical records officer, medical records supervisor, and medical records clerk, designations that are no longer aligned with global benchmarks and tend to undervalue the work. The Barbados Health Information Management Association is working to bring awareness and enact reform of the HIM profession.

Mandy Burns, Manchester University, UK

My education journey to becoming a HIM professional included Institute of Health Records and Information Management (IHRIM) Foundation Qualification, IHRIM Certificate Qualification, IHRIM Diploma Qualification, IHRIM Certificate of Technical Competence Assessor Certificate, Certificate in Post 16 Education, and a variety of training and courses including a National Vocation Qualification (NVQ) through the City and Guilds of London Institute, local courses such as anatomy and physiology, along with attending numerous conferences and congresses.

I started my career as a secretary for a therapy service in a small district general hospital, taking minutes, organising appointments, typing, and other administration work. I then moved to work at a large teaching hospital as a secretary/reception manager with the district therapy services; while there I started training therapists and administrative staff on the hospital patient administration system (PAS). This opportunity provided me with the knowledge for my next role as the Training Coordinator, Medical Records, training new staff on all areas within the department including library, reception, booking, referrals, templates, call centre, bed bureau, clinical coding, ward clerks, secretaries, waiting list, and preoperative staff. I delivered the mandatory training and undertook the NVQ training and assessments. I progressed to a large teaching hospital as Medical Records Manager, where I managed staff across two sites delivering all the services just listed. I also became Master Trainer for the newly implemented PAS; I provided train the trainer sessions and direct teaching sessions. My responsibilities included coordinating the clinic template and outpatient appointment migration across systems and staffing the Go-Live helpline for a month. I had key responsibility for sections of the Information Governance Toolkit, which is mandatory for all National Health Service organisations to complete and reach acceptable levels.

My next role was Admin, Records, Child Health, Data Quality, and Information Governance Manager for a Community Trust. I was responsible for supporting all community services within these functions over a large and diverse population. No services had previously existed for records or data quality in this organisation. I established and delivered them, ensuring compliance with all legal requirements. Here my responsibilities also included vital sections of the Information Governance Toolkit. The Trust went through various mergers and transformations as part of National Transforming Community Services work, which involved many changes in records, information governance, and data quality.

Next I went to a Paediatric Hospital as Patient Services Manager, with responsibility for records, transcription, booking, admissions, and reception and becoming lead for Outpatient Global Digital Exemplar (GDE) work. I made decisions and informed direction for the organisation as it moved towards the Healthcare Information and Management Systems Society (HIMSS) Level 7. I am currently the Informatics Head of Patient Services for the second largest NHS Trust in England, where I manage records and coding services. I work with both teams to support daily management and the organisation's single electronic patient record programme, i.e. merging nine hospital systems and records. During COVID, I worked alongside the Director of Technology in establishing the local Nightingale Hospital. I was responsible for establishing and agreeing on the documentation requirements for the unit and all administration services.

In addition to my employment, I have been the CEO of IHIRM for the last 6 years and served on the Board of the Federation for Informatics Professionals (FEDIP). I also set and mark papers within IHRIM's Informatics suite of exams and am part of the Education Board for the Institute. I am the United Kingdom IFHIMA representative.

Sabu Karakka Mandapam, Manipal Academy of Higher Education, India

The HIM profession's prospects in India were not clear when I joined the Medical Documentation Master's programme in 1996. The curriculum and training mainly focused on medical records and management (MRM) in a traditional hospital setting. My professional career started in 2000 as an Administrator—Medical Records in a private medical college hospital. The role's primary responsibilities were to assemble a multitude of patient clinical information for various administrative decisions at the Medical Director level. It was a great learning experience, as my activities were different from my education and training. In 2000, I joined as a lecturer with my current organisation and started teaching medical terminology, disease classification systems, and basic MRM subjects to Master students. In 2003, I was entrusted with the responsibility of managing the department. I have utilised the initial period of my career to strengthen my HIM academic competencies mainly through the self-learning. In 2006, I earned the first Doctor of Philosophy degree awarded to a HIM professional in India.

My progression to Associate Professor and Head of the department has allowed me to persuade the university to establish the first full-fledged HIM programme of global curriculum standards in India. As a senior faculty member and administrator, my key responsibilities included teaching, guiding student projects, research activities, streamlining curriculum, creating awareness about the HIM profession, exploring international collaborations, and strengthening the academic processes as per regulatory requirements. During this phase, the department built up the value of

HIM professionals among many corporate hospitals through guided student projects, which increased demand for HIM trainees in the market. I also initiated the preliminary work for a Master level Health Informatics programme during this period. In 2012, I was promoted to Professor of HIM. I was assigned additional administrative responsibility as Associate Dean of the institution to oversee several health professional departments' academic and non-academic functions.

My exposure to many national and international conferences worldwide has enabled me to learn and integrate evolving HIM concepts in my profession. My first ever participation in an IFHIMA international congress in Canada in 2013 gave me a professional breakthrough by establishing connections with many international experts from academia, industry, and professional bodies. This network helped me associate with several global councils and continued collaboration with various HIM professional bodies worldwide to strengthen the HIM workforce and training competencies. As a member of a national taskforce formed by the Government of India, I have influenced the national committee to gain approval for a model curriculum for HIM education and HIM as a professional title for the first time in India. More institutions and universities must start formal education and training programmes in the HIM domain, as the existing volume of HIM graduates is insufficient to meet the demand for qualified and trained HIM professionals. India needs a large workforce of trained HIM professionals to efficiently integrate newer technologies and manage health information at multiple levels in its evolving healthcare system.

Gemala Hatta, University of Indonesia and Repati Indonesia University

Starting in 1976, upon my graduation from Medical Record Administration (MRA) School in Sydney, I joined the Ministry of Health (MOH) of Indonesia. A new chapter of progress towards a medical record system had commenced. In 1978 the Minister of Health signed the first organogram for Indonesia's hospitals (SK 134/1978), known as MOH Decree 134/1978. For the first time, a medical records section in the hospital had a place, i.e. under the secretariat. This was a critical recognition and the beginning of medical records in Indonesia's hospital organisation. In 1977 I asked MOH's Directorate General of Disease Prevention and Control to design medical record systems and MRA short training courses for the MoH in Indonesia. From 1980 to 1989 Jakarta Municipality Health Department established a Medical Record Working Group Committee which I chaired. We published the first medical record serial publication (MR News) and distributed copies of 29 quarterly editions to 100 hospitals. We also delivered a regular 1-day training session per month and provided medical record training courses for 2 months for each group of trainees (once or twice a year), training more than a thousand hospital medical record staff from many provinces this way. In 1989 the first MRA school's 3-year programme was opened; I designed the curriculum based on the MRA School in Sydney but with some local adjustments. Even though there has been significant work undertaken to progress medical record administration towards the HIM era in Indonesia, even with 70 schools now teaching HIM, there is still a way to go. We need to supply a HIM workforce for a country covering three time zones with more than 2000 hospitals and 17,000 health centres that provide services to 267 million people across 17,000 islands. By building on lessons learned from other nations, and by involving myself in numerous public policy and education initiatives related to professional practice, I have been able to help Indonesia step towards excellence.

Oknam Kim, Sungkyunkwan University, Republic of Korea

My HIM career began in 1976 at Yonsei University Severance Hospital in Seoul after completing the Severance Hospital Institution Registered Record Administration (RRA) Training Course. The concept of medical record management began at Severance Hospital in 1962 when a Canadian missionary established unit numbering, disease classification, and a patient index system. Also, Severance Hospital had established and operated the only specialised curriculum for medical record librarians (Severance Hospital Institution RRA Training Course) since 1965 and produced about two or three RRAs every year. Fewer than 20 RRAs were employed in the medical record department when I completed my training.

In 1977, the Korea Medical Records Association (KMRA) was approved by the Ministry of Health and Welfare as a legal entity—in 2018, the association's name was changed to the Korea Health Information Management Association (KHIMA). From 1978 to 1983, KMRA operated a private qualification screening course in medical record libraries for Certification as Accredited Record Technician (ART) and Registered Records Administrator (RRA). Despite my short career, I had the opportunity to participate as an educator, teaching ART trainees medical terminology, disease classification, and hospital statistics every weekend for several years. RRAs who graduated from Severance Training Institution voluntarily participated in KRMA-led ART education and led the curriculum to organise medical record management as a speciality. From the beginning, KMRA had promoted the legislation of a medical record librarian licence system as a top priority, and I devoted myself to this project as a lead member. A review of the Medical Service Technologies, etc., Act in 1983 led to the establishment of the Medical Record Librarian Licence System.

With the introduction of the national licence system, regular HIM curriculum for colleges and universities was opened to enhance professionalism, and record librarians were included in the government-managed medical personnel. There was a shortage of professional education about medical information management theory and practice, so I worked as an administrator of a medical record department at a hospital and continued to teach medical information management at a university. To meet university faculty requirements, I obtained master's and doctoral degrees in health information management. Now I have worked as an administrator in several university hospital medical records departments for 30 years and taught health information management at colleges and universities.

My life as a HIM is made meaningful by volunteer activities. From the beginning of KMRA/KHIMA, I participated as an executive member prominent in advocating for the medical record librarian license system. I served as President and the Director of the Research Institute; most memorably as KMRA President I organised the 15th IFHRO Assembly in Seoul in May 2007. Currently I am working as a member of the Korean National Standards Committee for the International Organization for Standardization's Technical Committee on health informatics (ISO/TC 215). Korea urgently needs to establish standards for interoperability of health information; therefore, I plan to contribute to the development of health information interoperability standards during the rest of my lifelong HIM activities.

Conclusion

These case studies have shown similarities and differences in the HIM profession across the world. Each demonstrates the personal growth of the individuals from entry-level positions, working their way up to leadership positions in a range of roles that demonstrate the profession's breadth of knowledge and skill. Their careers include managing health information services in health care facilities, consultancy, projects, legislation and standards development, education curriculum, and working directly with the professional associations that represent HIM.

Each person featured in this chapter received formal education at the start of their career, but that was only the start of their lifelong learning and growth in the field. Many have taught or mentored other HIM professionals and established education pathways for HIM students and graduates. Each of these HIM leaders embraced opportunities to further their skills and knowledge, with several working towards or completing a PhD. Some of these careers have unfolded under strict regulation and support of the HIM profession; others occurred while working towards recognition as a HIM professional, rather than as a medical records clerk or administrator of the past.

A few of the case studies show HIM professionals in senior information governance roles. They provide examples of work in developing strategy and standards to manage health information. There is also recognition of the synergies among health information management and health informatics and data management and high-quality information for decision making. Amid rapid growth of data with the implementation and expansion of digital health, the HIM workforce is well placed due to their qualifications and training (Butler-Henderson 2017).

Challenges for the HIM profession have been discussed also. The domain is relatively unknown in some countries. There is difficulty in keeping up with the demand for a qualified HIM workforce to support the needs of millions of people across various geographic landscapes. Each country has its own professional education and regulation system, with varying degrees of engagement or support from governing bodies. The introduction of the International Classification of Diseases 11th edition (ICD-11) poses the big imminent challenge of educating future HIMs and preparing the existing workforce to transition from existing versions and modifications of ICD (Fenton et al. 2017).

But the most significant point to emerge from these cases is the passion and commitment of HIM professionals to improve citizens' lives, make healthcare safe, and drive the growth of HIM as a profession.

References

Abdelhak MH. Health information: management of a strategy resource 5th edition. Elsevier Saunders: Missouri; 2016.

AHIMA. AHIMA who we are web. AHIMA; 2020. https://www.ahima.org/who-we-are/about-us/history/.

Barbados Community College. Overview of health information management web. Barbados Community College; 2020. http://www.bcc.edu.bb/Divisions/HealthSciences/HealthInformationManagement.aspx.

Butler-Henderson K. Health information management 2025: 'What is required to create a sustainable profession in the face of digital transformation?'. Launceston: University of Tasmania; 2017. Contract No.: ISBN 978-1-82695-88-3.

CHIMA. The history of the Canadian Health Information Management Association. Canadian Health Information Management Association; 2019. https://www.echima.ca/uploaded/pdf/CHIMA_History.pdf. Accessed 28 Jun 2019.

Fenton SH, Low S, Abrams KJ, Butler-Henderson K. Health information management: changing with time. Yearb Med Inform. 2017;26(1):72–7.

HIMAA. About HIMAA. Health Information Management Association of Australia; 2016. http://www.himaa2.org.au/index.php?q=node/41.

HIMAA. About HIMAA. Health Information Management Association of Australia; 2016. http://www.himaa2.org.au/index.php?q=node/41.

IFHIMA. IFHIMA about us web. International Federation of Health Information Management Associations; 2020. https://ifhima.org/about-us-2/.

Kemp T, Butler-Henderson K, Allen P, Ayton JE. Evolution of the health record as a communication tool to support patient safety. In: Chisita C, Enakrire R, Durodolu O, Tsabedze V, editors. Handbook of research on records and information management strategies for enhanced knowledge coordination. Hershey, PA: IGI Global; 2021. p. 127–155.

Marshall DL. A guide for restructuring and transforming health information management education in Barbados and other developing countries [M.S.]. Ann Arbor: The College of St. Scholastica; 2014.

Schwab K. The fourth industrial revolution. Geneva: World Economic Forum; 2016.

Watson PJ. The first fifty years 1949-1999 Medical Record Librarian to Health Information Manager. Kingswood, Australia: Health Information Management Association of Australia; 2013.

Chapter 19
Working as a Health Librarian

Ann Ritchie, Sarah Hayman, Aoife Lawton, Gemma Siemensma, Helen Baxter, Meena Gupta, and Blair Kelly

Abstract Health librarians were one of the first health information specialist groups to organise as a professional association, dating back to the late nineteenth century and the early days of organising the medical literature. The late twentieth century saw the introduction of many digital health information products and services and the transformation of health librarianship's models of service delivery. Six case studies in this chapter apply a practitioner's lens to the transition that has taken place over the last 30 years. They highlight the impact of several major influences, in particular, evidence-based medicine, health literacy and digital health or e-health. Their careers illustrate a range of educational pathways to becoming a health librarian and the variety of roles and settings in which they work. Their motivations provide

A. Ritchie (✉)
Independent Consultant, Melbourne, VIC, Australia

S. Hayman
Barwon Health, Geelong, VIC, Australia

A. Lawton
National Health Service, Dublin, Ireland
e-mail: aoife.lawton@hse.ie

G. Siemensma
Ballarat Health Services, Ballarat, VIC, Australia
e-mail: gemma.siemensma@bhs.org.au

H. Baxter
Austin Health, Melbourne, VIC, Australia

M. Gupta
Australian Catholic University, Melbourne, VIC, Australia
e-mail: meena.gupta@acu.edu.au

B. Kelly
Deakin University, Geelong, VIC, Australia
e-mail: blair.kelly@deakin.edu.au

© The Author(s), under exclusive license to Springer Nature
Switzerland AG 2021
K. Butler-Henderson et al. (eds.), *The Health Information Workforce*,
Health Informatics, https://doi.org/10.1007/978-3-030-81850-0_19

281

insights into an evolving future for this professional group. The conclusion summarises the impact of health librarians in terms of their organisational roles in knowledge management and information governance, and their value to society in advancing equitable access to high-quality evidence-based information.

Keywords Case study · Evidence-based healthcare · Governance · Health librarians · Health literacy

Introduction

In responding to the question "what is a health librarian?" it is tempting to reply: "any librarian who works in a health organisation". But as with any simple answer to a complex question, this does not tell the whole story; it belies the intricacies, specialist nature, knowledge and advanced skill set required to practise competently as a health librarian (Ritchie 2020), and may, in fact, be misleading. Health library and information specialists work in various types of organisations and a number work outside of traditional libraries (Kammermann 2016). Anecdotal evidence suggests that there may be a growing number of health librarians working online and remotely, and a couple of the case studies in this chapter illustrate this tendency towards remote work. Most health librarians do, however, work in hospitals, community care and social care organisations, meeting the needs of clinicians who deliver direct care and services to individual patients and defined communities (Kammermann 2016). Others are located in government health departments and agencies that operate at population and policy levels; and still, another group is located in academic health organisations, including universities and institutes that have teaching and research remits. Some health librarians work in specialist health information roles in commercial organisations, such as pharmaceutical, biomedical and publishing companies. The common characteristic for all the health librarians who work in these various types of organisations is the set of competencies that define the scope of their professional practice (ALIA HLA 2018). Depending on their organisational context and the focus of their roles (generally reflected in their position title), they may specialise in particular areas. The six case studies in this chapter sample the different organisational contexts and various types of health librarian roles.

Before delving into the case studies, however, it is instructive to give some perspective on the development of this relatively small but dynamic profession by examining briefly some of the main factors that have influenced the development of health librarianship in the recent past. As with all service professions, health librarianship has been exposed to the disruptive influence of digital technologies that have transformed many traditional models of in-person service delivery. The past three decades have witnessed the evolution of health library and information services from largely physical, face-to-face interactions and print-based transactions, to online, remote and electronic modes of delivery. The US Medical Library Association was established in 1898 at the time when Index Medicus, the forerunner of the US National Library of Medicine's PubMed database, was the ever-growing, bulky and voluminous, paper-based tool used for finding the evidence located in the published literature. In the transition to the digital health world, health librarians have proved to be responsive, adaptable and collaborative, often early adopters and experimenters with new technologies. They have transferred the principles of their professional practice in information and knowledge management to the digital products and services of the e-health world. For example, health librarians no longer deal with just books and journals—there is an ever-expanding range of electronic resource formats, products and bundles of offerings from publishers. Developing library collections is no longer as simple as buying a resource once from a known publisher, owning it forever, lending it to whomever you choose—there are intricate permutations on licencing and purchasing models for different conditions and rights of access, available from an array of suppliers. Working collaboratively across departments, professional groups and organisations, health librarians have used digital technologies to deliver services beyond the boundaries of a physical library; for example, online and real-time reference and research consultations with national and international reach; embedded librarians (also known as "informationists") working in multidisciplinary clinical, research and teaching teams.

Health librarians have been on the front foot in creating innovative digital solutions to problems stemming from the limitations imposed by print-based, physical service delivery models. They realised quickly the advantages of electronic technologies for improving equity of access, making information available regardless of time and place. At the same time, health librarians recognised that the digital divide has exacerbated the "information rich/information poor" divergence. They have driven digital literacy and information literacy training programs that have reached out to health consumers, as well as to practicing and trainee medical, nursing and allied health professionals.

Health librarians have been champions of the evidence-based practice (EBP) model of clinical decision-making. In this model, the current best available evidence (most often supplied through the specialised health reference services of librarians) is combined with health professionals' expertise, knowledge and understanding of their individual patients, and the values, preferences and informed consent of the patients themselves. Health librarians very quickly recognised the connection between EBP, consumer health literacy and patients' ability to find, understand and apply good quality information in their choices about their treatment (Schardt 2011). Hospital librarians have taken their support for EBP and health literacy one step further through their assistance in developing and implementing organisational literacy strategies. Recent research shows how their consumer health literacy initiatives support hospital accreditation requirements and objectives—patient engagement, health literacy and patient empowerment—and thus patients' ability to give their truly informed consent (Ritchie et al. 2020).

All has not run smoothly for health librarians in the transition to digital models of delivering health library services. One of the biggest risks in moving to a digital world has been the problem of invisibility of both the information resources and the health librarians who are delivering the services. While the aim has been to create seamless and joined-up services, the unintended consequence has often been that the professional expertise that makes it all happen has been taken for granted. Digital health means more than simply delivering health services online. The clinicians delivering consultations are the face of telemedicine, but there are many health information professionals behind the technology—collectively they are the human infrastructure who bring it all together. The ability of clinical health professionals and health policy-makers to apply the principles of good governance and evidence-based decision-making is dependent on the specialist health librarians who manage the information that is the stuff of decision-making. They ensure that the right information (the best available evidence) is delivered in the right place (whether physical or online), at the right time (at point-of-need), to the right person, so that evidence-based decisions can be made. This chapter contains six case studies of health librarians working in three sectors—hospitals, universities and government health departments. They illustrate some of the challenges they have encountered along the way and touch on their ideas and visions for the future of health librarians in the digital health world.

Sarah Hayman, Barwon Health, Australia

I gained a Bachelor of Arts from The University of Adelaide with majors in English, Old and Middle English and Philosophy in 1977, and a Graduate Diploma of Librarianship from the University of New South Wales (1979). I have worked almost always in special (research) libraries, in education and health. My first job was running a small research library for the Australian Wool Corporation. I followed that with 2 years in the central cataloguing department of NSW TAFE, where I received a thorough grounding in cataloguing rules; it gave me an excellent grasp of the principles of structured information, which I believe to be essential for understanding information retrieval. My main job after that was for the National Centre for Vocational Education Research, where I managed a team responsible for producing the then VOCED research database. We moved from a disc-based and physically mailed-out database to the excitement of developing a web-based bibliographic research database. It was one of the earliest to be linked to an online thesaurus, and we achieved UNESCO endorsement for the database as a vital underpinning for research in that field worldwide. This job instilled my passion for excellence and for meeting the needs of information users; our work supported and enabled research, practice and policy-making, with the ultimate beneficiaries being those engaged in vocational education, and especially the students. (Now, in health, I see a similar ultimate aim of meeting the needs of the patients.)

After a brief stint in health libraries, I moved to education.au, a leading government-funded education technology company. Here I built on my more formal understanding of information provision to incorporate growing concepts of the opening up of user access and user evaluation via web 2.0 philosophies and mechanisms such as crowd-sourcing and user tagging. It gave me a new understanding of different ways of determining quality while maintaining the need to support practice with evidence of the highest quality. I had the opportunity to write and publish papers and present at conferences. Still, my most cited paper is one on taxonomy-directed folksonomies—how to maximise benefit from user knowledge and formal taxonomies combined. Through these jobs I was developing my passion for supporting practice and research with evidence, using my own technical knowledge, experience and understanding of user needs and approaches.

I then had an opportunity to move back into the health world with a position in the CareSearch palliative care project, at Flinders University, to work in the highly specialised and fascinating field of search filter development. I loved the mix of technical and intellectual challenges along with the chance it gave to me to develop my own searching skills and to support work in the valuable field of palliative care. Working in an academic environment gave me the opportunity to write and publish in peer-reviewed journals. In 2017 I moved to my current job at Barwon Health where I am a research librarian, undertaking literature searches for hospital staff—for research, clinical and protocol development purposes—and I do the entire job remotely from my home in Adelaide! Meanwhile, alongside my formal employment, I always took every opportunity for involvement in wider professional work through committees, conferences, working groups, etc. This can seem tedious at times but I have met some wonderful colleagues and learned a huge amount from them. Indirectly it is through these contacts that I found my way into my present role.

In this role, I search a range of health and other databases for evidence that answers questions that come from clinical, research and administrative staff. These questions are hugely varied and I get excited each time I open a new one—I love the technical and even sometimes creative challenge of finding the best possible information, of being as sure as I can that I have not missed any vital reference, and of fitting what I find to what the user wants. They may want a comprehensive search (recently I have done searches for five systematic reviews) or they may want only a few key recent references, and there is an art to selecting those. I also love the feeling of learning new information each time I do a search; I often do not retain it beyond the end of the search, and I certainly could not begin to work as a clinician, but I find health knowledge fascinating. Most importantly, I love knowing that I am part of the cohort of people contributing to health outcomes for patients. Health is an area that touches every single person, and it is a privilege to work in it.

The remote nature of the work I do is less remarkable than formerly, after the time of the COVID-19 lockdowns. In this period the world has woken up to the importance of having the highest quality medical evidence delivered quickly, which is the heart of our job as health librarians. Librarians do need to adapt and respond to the changing world, as we always have done. Our role is one of navigating information and facilitating user access to it. In the health world, this means customising what we do to fit the needs of our users. We can provide tools and training for those who want to do their own searches, for those who want all the searches and acquisition of the information done for them, and for those at all points in between. We fit in that space between the users and the information and we can teach them how to find, identify and evaluate evidence. I believe we need to say "yes" to all opportunities to be involved in the transition to digital health. This may mean that we are moving further into research roles, learning more about technological approaches and embedding ourselves into research and clinical teams. I think we may be required in future to go beyond basic literature searches to undertaking more synthesis of evidence—and this may require the development of different more research-aligned skills. I have always found health librarians to be extraordinarily passionate, skilled and dedicated and I believe we are well capable of moving into these areas.

Aoife Lawton, National Health Service Executive Librarian, Ireland

My personal journey to become the first national health service librarian in Ireland was a mix of serendipity and silent determination. I am not sure that anyone answers the question "what would you like to be when you grow up?" with the response "a librarian"! It is a path that I consciously chose at a certain point in my life when it seemed like a job I would like to try out. I did not know much about it at the time and ended up enjoying it.

My education is a primary honour's degree in European Studies from Trinity College Dublin which places an emphasis on languages, culture, politics and the history of ideas. It was a good grounding in critical thinking skills which translate well to the work environment regardless of the profession. I was offered my first job with the IBM corporation, after my final exams, at the same the time as I was offered a place on a Master of Arts course in journalism. I came to an early career crossroad with an important decision to make; regular income held a lot of appeal as a recent graduate so I accepted the job with IBM and reasoned that I could always return to journalism at a later stage. I was thrust into a world of computers and corporate culture at IBM which gave me solid training and foundational knowledge of hardware, software, teamwork and customer service which benefits me to this day. In a conversation with a work colleague about the future and where we saw our careers going, she suggested to me that I might like to pursue a career in librarianship. She had worked in an architectural library and it had been her happiest job with the greatest job satisfaction. I got a place on a Higher Diploma in Library and Information Studies at University College Dublin (UCD) and gained experience in a public library as a library assistant. Fast forward a few years, I gained international experience with a library management system supplier and got a Master's in Library and Information Studies from UCD while working full-time. I held other roles including a brief period as a sole trader selling school library management systems, as a librarian in a specialist nursing library, and eventually as a systems librarian with the National Health Service. Despite other opportunities, I held this job for almost 14 years. Working in the health service is a great way to keep your work interesting and your skills up-to-date because it is a challenging environment and an area where information is continually changing and needed.

I got the job of National Health Service librarian at the end of 2016, a position I hold today. This role is brand new and with no predecessors, I get to walk in my own shoes, set out a new path, inspire others to hopefully follow it and lay foundations for librarians and paraprofessionals for a solid future in the health service. This position inspires me because I see the difference that library staff makes to patient care and the potential that we have as an integrated service going forward. This is a leadership role and it requires strategic planning, positioning and management of resources and people. There is a staff of 53 with a mix of librarians, library assistants, senior library assistants and library managers; they are geographically dispersed with approximately 30 libraries located primarily in hospitals throughout the country. This separation has meant that virtual teams and digital communication are the primary way of working, with their own unique challenges. I set the direction of travel for the library service and work at positioning the library in a busy and changing organisation so that it is responsive to the needs of the health workforce and its service is aligned with the strategic objectives and values of the organisation. Ensuring that the library team has adequate and suitable resources and competencies to do the job to the best of their ability is a key function of the role. I enjoy many aspects of the job, from planning annual staff engagement days, to participating in five-nation knowledge exchanges with counterparts in England, Scotland, Northern Ireland and Wales. Working in partnership with others in the health sector is key to getting things done. In the area of innovation for example we have introduced an "Energy Pod" as a rest facility for clinical staff at one of our hospital libraries. This has been a big success, attracting new clients into the library and affording an opportunity to promote library services at the same time. Reporting performance indicators that make sense to stakeholders is very important. Integrating library services with the broader infrastructure of the health service is also key to sustainability and growth.

Reflecting on the transition to digital health, the skills required by the health librarian will continue to be specialised. The traditional skills of critical thinking, logical reasoning, collating information and making it easily accessible to busy clinicians will all remain important, while seeking innovative ways to deliver and filter information, for example, using artificial intelligence and big data may become more mainstream. The specialist health librarian will need to keep ICT skills up-to-date to make the best contribution to the health system. The COVID-19 global pandemic has highlighted the value of advanced searching and research skills that health librarian specialists have across the world. As long as platforms like PubMed, Cochrane Library, Embase, medRxiv and bioRxiv continue to exist, these searching skills will be in high demand. Evidence searching, synthesis, summaries and reviews are all knowledge products that health librarians provide; this is a niche but respected area. We save the health service time and money by carrying out these searches expertly; we stamp out "fake news" and stand up for truth. Evidence-based librarianship will hold its own, although the future will see more integration of our services with complementary departments, e.g., Research & Evidence, ICT. We are a well-organised profession and our national and international professional associations do the hard work of continually updating competencies to future proof our skills.

Gemma Siemensma, Ballarat Health Services, Australia

My journey to health libraries came in a rambling way when I was 21. As a child and adolescent, I adored reading and really had no grand plans for my future but after secondary school, chose to undertake the TAFE qualification for Library Technician because I loved to read (such a cliché)! During this time, I worked at a public library. My partner lived a few hours away and when I finished TAFE, a job for a Library Technician came up in the hospital library near his hometown, Ballarat. Thus began my career in health libraries. I knew very little about health libraries but was enthusiastic. I had an inspiring boss who encouraged me to study for a Bachelor's degree in Librarianship via distance education. I completed this and went on to study my Master's in Librarianship and then my MBA. Working in health libraries has allowed me to gain an understanding of all the different functions library staff undertake. As I worked my way up, I undertook tasks including article requests, document delivery, literature searches, alerting services, implementing online systems, complex research queries and cataloguing. Now in the Library Manager position, I get to enjoy budgeting, planning, inspiring my team and aligning health librarian expertise with the goals of the organisation. This is coupled with professional development opportunities which help me hone my skills, gain new knowledge and implement changing practices.

I am motivated by the people within my workplace. Clinicians do an incredible job of caring for those in need and I think the interprofessional collaboration between clinicians and health librarians creates a continuous improvement ethos. In a hospital, the ultimate goals relate to patient care and population health, and the scope and focus of hospital libraries' activities are defined by reference to these primary areas of responsibility. This includes providing access to the best available evidence, and provision of professional information services delivered by trained and credentialed information professionals. The information we provide modifies current clinical practice, diagnosis and medication choices. It is an empowering role, knowing that the information we make available improves clinical outcomes.

I have been involved with my professional library association for almost 20 years. I am a big believer that you get out more than you put in. I am currently the Convenor of Health Libraries Australia. This voluntary role has opened up collegial networks, amazing opportunities and friendships. I have worked on projects I never thought I would have been capable of, have been pushed to undertake challenging tasks, and grown as an individual and as a librarian. I get to work with colleagues across the country who are helping to shape health libraries in Australia and advocate and influence our professional landscape. In turn, these opportunities have opened up other avenues within my organisation and allowed me to dream big and strategically place the library in new and emerging situations. My library offers services to other health organisations within our region as none have a library or librarian onsite. This makes equity of access to information a possibility for my whole region. Statistics show that those in rural and regional areas have poorer health outcomes but we know that evidence-based information can bridge this divide. Getting the right information, to the right people, at the right time is one of the reasons I love working as a health librarian. One of my passions is equality. Smaller services should not be disadvantaged because they do not have resources or access to much-needed information. Filling this evidence gap allows the health system to work as a whole, with better outcomes for individuals and organisations.

As we have moved into the digital health realm, technology has enabled health librarians to make information seamlessly available; as technology develops, I think more avenues will open up and we will see more information in more places. One of the challenges for health librarians is to ensure clinicians and consumers are accessing reliable and accurate information—health literacy is a growing area as we grapple with information overload. Another huge shift in the coming years for health librarians is in open access publishing; this is evolving rapidly and as mediators of information our roles and systems need to change and develop. Also, as technology advances, systems need to be interoperable rather than the current piecemeal and disjointed experience. The evolution of digital health brings new ways to get information to people; this, in turn, leads to better clinical outcomes which is what everyone working in health is striving for.

Helen Baxter, Austin Health, Australia

I work as the Clinical Librarian at Austin Health, a major teaching hospital in Melbourne, Australia. Like many librarians this was not my first career; my initial university studies were in nursing followed by several years working in the health care system as a Registered Nurse. I returned to university, undertaking postgraduate study in Library and Information Management. I was keen to combine these two qualifications and therefore actively pursued health librarianship opportunities. I was initially employed as a member of the Health Library team at Austin Health, working at its rehabilitation campus, then later at the main hospital campus. During this time, it became clear to me that a health librarian's role does not need to be defined or constrained by the physical library space. In 2014, a new Chief Librarian at Austin Health envisaged a new role for a Clinical Librarian and I was given the opportunity to build and shape this outward-facing role for the organisation.

As a Clinical Librarian, my goal is ensuring the timely provision of evidence at the point of care, or as learning opportunities arise, for all clinicians. I am passionate about contributing to research evidence that can be translated into clinical practice that ultimately improves the quality and safety of patient care. The clinical knowledge gained by studying and working as a nurse is a considerable advantage to my role today. Information is often required quickly by clinicians and being able to rapidly decipher the medical literature aids in effective searching to find relevant evidence. My role is visible to hospital staff via my participation in clinical meetings, grand rounds, journal clubs and education sessions, and it carries a broad range of responsibilities. The Library is a pivotal contributor to the organisation's research outputs, and in this sphere, I design complex search strategies, provide comprehensive advice for complex topics, and as a result, have contributed as a co-author on several systematic and scoping reviews.

As Clinical Librarian I lead the development and delivery of tailored education and training to promote the culture of evidence-based practice across all levels of the organisation. In collaboration with the Library team, I contribute to the planning, coordination and delivery of interdisciplinary research courses; prepare synthesised evidence briefs for the hospital executive; contribute to the development of our library website; and actively keep the team abreast of best practice literature searching methods to support the convergence of new technologies and clinical decisions. I am conscious of how a Clinical Librarian's expertise can contribute to the decisions of care teams and research groups. With an enormous variety of clinical questions arising in the hospital setting, and clinicians keen to ensure that the care they deliver aligns with best practice recommendations, there is little time for sitting still! Being part of a process that ultimately improves patient care is what drives my passion for the job: playing a pivotal role in supporting an evidence-based practice model to enable practitioners at the coalface to know how to access the latest evidence in their specialty, critically consider and apply it.

Professional health librarians face a rapidly evolving work environment. The burgeoning of internet-based health information means that both digital information literacy and health literacy are critical. In the future of evidence-based healthcare, health librarians have a role in ensuring evidence underpins the adoption of new digital health technologies, particularly clinical decision-support systems. In the research realm, data management and the interoperability of technologies are emerging areas of focus—this will require expanding the health librarian's skills further to meet the challenges associated with the digital transformation of healthcare information systems and information management. We will need to adapt as software automating the management of large evidence reviews becomes ubiquitous, and as "living documents" become mainstream. Our ability to work across health disciplines and contribute a broad knowledge perspective of the local healthcare environment remains an important asset and enables us to tailor large amounts of evidence to an immediate clinically relevant context.

Meena Gupta, Australian Catholic University, Australia

I am an early career health liaison librarian in an academic setting. The three pillars of an academic institution, namely teaching, learning and research, underpin my primary mission. Goal setting and being agile in researching and using educational opportunities have been central to perform my liaison tasks better. I have a Bachelor's degree in Business Information and Knowledge Management along with a Master of Business (Information Technology). Both courses helped me understand information needs, information-seeking behaviour, and the value of credible knowledge sources to enable informed decision-making processes in personal and professional endeavours. Whilst working, I wanted to learn more about teaching in adult learning environments, with a Certificate IV in Workplace Training & Assessment. There is no formula when choosing the qualifications befitting a health librarian. However, given the opportunity to become one, I identified a skills and knowledge gap so I enrolled in 2019 in a micro-credential on Digital Health Information Services offered by the University of Melbourne and Australian Library and Information Association Health Libraries Australia (ALIA HLA). The course was aligned with the ALIA HLA (2018) competencies framework and gave me confidence in health information work. I also volunteer as a member of the ALIA HLA Executive Committee and in that way actively contribute towards professional development opportunities for myself and others.

I always wanted to be a librarian from a young age—an information detective! The knowledge and skills obtained from my education informed my choice to pursue a career in academic librarianship. I began in a liaison position at Australia's Deakin University as Science, Engineering & Built Environment Liaison Librarian; then at Australian Catholic University (ACU) as Senior Librarian in Business; now continuing as a Senior Librarian in Health (Nursing, Midwifery and Paramedicine). I deliver flexible access to information resources, providing services that partner with academics and researchers to achieve their goals of furthering knowledge and education. I liaise with other health librarian colleagues, academic e-learning advisors and students to determine their data and information needs, and I enable them to do independent research locating, summarising and synthesising evidence tailored to meet their needs. I provide outreach services such as videoconferencing, scaffolded information literacy classes, understanding relevant tools within specialist health databases, providing research metric services to enhance academic researcher profiles. I can identify gaps in where information users search for information and present the information via learning management platforms or reports. Previous positions in marketing, law firm libraries and market research helped me appreciate how I could help people understand the importance of informed decision-making in a digital environment, with expert knowledge of what, where, how and when information was needed. Being an academic librarian/health information specialist is an opportunity to contribute to researcher and student success. Enabling users to find and use information ethically within a professional capacity, engaging in real-world research, and demonstrating ways to access information are only the tip of the iceberg. Integral parts of my role include being able to show people how to use the information and think critically about health information systems, use decision-making tools, processes and strategies to enable evidence-based practice. My personal motto has always been "providing quality information services with a smile"; it offers ways to engage in daily acts of kindness in a sensitive and volatile work environment.

The future of the health librarian is now, with increased access points for health information and health-related data. Therefore, we must continue to work on finding (e.g. delivering tailored information literacy and resource literacy), on using (e.g. understanding systematic searching, on informing the development of systematic reviews and academic curriculum development) and on disseminating information (e.g. research impact reports). Future health librarians may use and adapt technology such as virtual and augmented reality to inform critical decision-making around health professional practice; these kinds of innovations may keep them central in the health professionals team.

Blair Kelly, Deakin University, Australia

I came to librarianship as a career change, seeking a profession that helped others, solved problems and performed a social good; librarianship met these criteria. I began by enrolling in a library technician degree and in the ensuing move from the classroom to employment found library work to be greatly satisfying. My first library job was at the University of Western Australia, followed by a longer period working at the University of Notre Dame Australia. Here I worked in a number of positions, from library assistant to technician to senior library technician, eventually moving into the roles of liaison librarian and university copyright coordinator. Being in a small library there was an expectation that daily duties covered a wide range of tasks and in hindsight, this was an excellent experience for my move into health librarianship as a Reference Librarian at Barwon Health, another small library environment. My initial challenge was shifting from an education-focused mindset to one which focused on providing a service while including elements of education where appropriate; I was used to teaching people to search the literature, not searching the literature on their behalf. In my current role as Medical Librarian at Deakin University, I am grateful for my time working in healthcare service. An understanding of the Victorian public health system and clinician life is something I now regularly use to connect the experiences of the student to their post-graduation professional life.

As Medical Librarian I am part of the Deakin University Library's Faculty of Health team, with an emphasis on its School of Medicine. The Library plays an important part in supporting digital literacy and this gives focus to my interactions with the School. These involve working with teachers, students and researchers. These interactions may happen in person, including instances where I am teaching students in physical classrooms, or online, commonly in the form of slide presentations or through the creation of learning resources such as library resource guides and information pages. The aim is to provide learning experiences that are aligned, and where possible integrated, with curriculum, and this relies on me maintaining close relationships with teaching staff. Collection development is part of my role which supports teaching, learning and research. This includes value analysis for purchases or subscriptions and decisions on how the Library budget could best be spent. Here I work closely with colleagues in the Library's Collections, Copyright and Licensing department to identify resources for inclusion or removal from the collection, keeping in mind the teaching and research needs of the School, as well as the university's broader areas of focus, with the aim of providing a solid return on investment. Finally, my role includes leadership activities. In the Library's Health Team, I assist the Team Manager to build capacity among team members. I also assist the Campus Manager with actions related to the campus library building and team. My role has also presented me with opportunities to conduct my own research; dissemination of this research via journals and conferences is another area where I provide leadership by example. This role is exciting and dynamic; every day is different, there is always something new to learn, and while the learning and the work are never done, things are never boring. It is rewarding to come to work with intelligent and creative people—library staff, academics and students—and to play a part in the development of future health professionals and the success of health research.

Looking to the future, research support is an area where health librarians will see rising demand for their skills and, in some organisations, have the opportunity to step into areas of unmet need. Today's deluge of research publications, and the accompanying feedback loop of an increased push for practitioners and researchers to publish, mean that skills with the activities in the research cycle will be valued, including teaching and/or direct application of advanced literature search skills, including using text mining and artificial intelligence/machine learning to speed up comprehensive literature reviews. Another area will be research data management best practices, to support research integrity, transparency and replicability. Expertise in methods for demonstrating research impact beyond citation counts will be increasingly valuable as competition for research funding increases. Lastly understanding and working with open science principles, including open access options for dissemination, will be valued. Advocating for the importance of the above skills, and developing relationships in order to produce and promote reliable, replicable processes, will continue to underpin the work of the specialist health librarian.

Conclusion

The case studies in this chapter convey a pragmatic approach combined with a principled vision and a passion for helping people. They demonstrate health librarians' distinctive discipline knowledge and technical skills in managing health information to deliver highly valued services to clients at the coalface of health care delivery, education and research. They provide examples of the range of education and employment pathways that can lead an individual to a career in the specialist area of health librarianship. They highlight health librarians' advanced competencies and expertise in literature searching and knowledge of health research information sources beyond the generic librarians' skills base. They also highlight some of the national and international collaborative professional networks and systems that facilitate resource sharing and seamless access to information for all those who work in the health world.

Health librarians' stories have highlighted transformative changes that have occurred over the past decades in the ways that health library services are delivered, particularly in relation to the impact of evidence-based medicine, health literacy and digital health. As well as delivering information services, health librarians have been at the forefront of teaching others the information and digital literacy skills associated with evidence-based practice. Collectively the case studies serve to illustrate health librarians' knowledge management and information governance functions and roles in their organisations. On a societal level, health librarians have been champions and enablers of equitable access to high-quality health information.

References

ALIA HLA. ALIA HLA competencies. 2018. https://www.alia.org.au/sites/default/files/HLA%20 Competencies_0.pdf. Accessed 1 Jun 2020.

Kammermann M. The census of Australian health libraries and health librarians working outside the traditional library setting: the final report. ALIA. 2016. https://www.alia.org.au/sites/ default/files/CENSUS%20of%20Aus%20Hlth%20Libs%202012-14_Final%20Report_2016. pdf. Accessed 1 Jun 2020.

Ritchie A. ALIA/HLA competencies review 2018: What is a health library and information professional? What do they do and why do they do it? JoHILA. 2020;1:28–35.

Ritchie A, Siemensma G, Gilbert C, Gaca M, Taylor J. Hospital librarians' contributions to health services' accreditation: an account of the Health Libraries for the National Safety and Quality in Health Services Standards (HeLiNS) research project, 2016-18. JALIA. 2020;69(2):215–45.

Schardt C. Health information literacy meets evidence-based practice. J Med Libr Assoc. 2011;99:1–2.

Chapter 20
Working as a Health Research Information Specialist

Ann Ritchie, Steve McDonald, Suzanne Lewis, Cecily Gilbert, Terena Solomons, Kristan Kang, and Mari-Elisa Kuusniemi

Abstract Working with health research information is an evolving and specialised area of health data, information, and knowledge management. The individuals who perform these roles have been characterised as being an emerging third tribe, sitting between and complementing the research work of scientists and administrators. Their specialist information management work facilitates the research process, intersecting at many points and stages in the research lifecycle. A thorough knowledge of scientific research methods as well as information and knowledge management competencies are essential. The six research information specialist case

A. Ritchie (✉)
Independent Consultant, Melbourne, VIC, Australia

S. McDonald
Cochrane Australia, Melbourne, VIC, Australia
e-mail: steve.mcdonald@monash.edu

S. Lewis
Central Coast Local Health District, Gosford, NSW, Australia
e-mail: Suzanne.Lewis@health.nsw.gov.au

C. Gilbert
Centre for Digital Transformation of Health, The University of Melbourne,
Parkville, VIC, Australia
e-mail: cecily.gilbert@unimelb.edu.au

T. Solomons
Western Australian Group for Evidence-Informed Healthcare Practice, Perth, WA, Australia
e-mail: t.solomons@curtin.edu.au

K. Kang
Australian Research Data Commons, Canberra, ACT, Australia
e-mail: kristan.kang@ardc.edu.au

M.-E. Kuusniemi
Research Services, Helsinki University Library, Helsinki, Finland
e-mail: mari.elisa.kuusniemi@helsinki.fi

K. Butler-Henderson et al. (eds.), *The Health Information Workforce*,
Health Informatics, https://doi.org/10.1007/978-3-030-81850-0_20

studies described in this chapter have been selected to demonstrate the variety of the roles, types of work, and skillsets that are required.

Keywords Case study · Evidence-based healthcare · Health research lifecycle · Knowledge translation · Research data management

Introduction

This chapter contains six case studies that create a composite picture of how and where the work of health information research specialists has an impact on the different stages in the health research lifecycle.

During the early research scoping stages, conducting a literature search helps to identify and refine a research question and find the evidence on a particular topic; searching the literature begins to reveal what is already known as well as alerting the researcher to potential gaps in the current evidence base. Research information specialists have unique skills in literature searching and devising and implementing search strategies according to established and robust protocols, which ensure replicability. They are skilled in managing the resultant reference lists, and identifying abstracts and full text articles for appraisal, evidence syntheses, and the creation of the various types of reviews. Artificial Intelligence (AI) and machine learning tools are already assisting in the task of sifting through extraordinary numbers of abstracts, selecting articles for further scrutiny, and critical appraisal before synthesising in reviews of various sorts. Designing and executing a comprehensive literature search forms the basis of a solid systematic review; literature searches for systematic reviews are, in themselves substantial pieces of research often taking around 6 months to complete.

In the planning stages of the research lifecycle, decisions affecting research records and data management need to be addressed, usually through the production of research data management plans. This is a growing area of specialisation that calls for a range of skills, with the study data needing to be actively managed during the project and for years after the research has been completed. Also in the planning stages, the literature searching services of research information specialists contribute to the production of research protocols, research grant proposals, and ethics submissions.

How to translate research knowledge into practice is a problem that has preoccupied many researchers, practitioners, and policy-makers. Research information and knowledge management specialists bring an evidence-based healthcare philosophy to a multidisciplinary review team. Their expertise is critical in the scholarly communications and publication stages, when choices about how to disseminate results and the most effective publication channels are important.

An open science model allows freedom of access to the research literature (via open access publishing models) and re-use of health research data (by adherence to the FAIR—Findable, Accessible, Interoperable, Re-usable—principles).

The integration of research-derived knowledge obtained from the published literature with real-world data from accessible datasets produces what has been termed "living" evidence—applicable to individual health care decision-making as well as the creation and ongoing review of health policies and guidelines. The exciting possibility of continuous evidence surveillance is created when barriers to access (such as paywalls and restrictions on re-use of data) are removed.

Steve McDonald, Cochrane Australia, Australia

Studying social and political science was my ringside seat in momentous times— during the fall of communism in Eastern Europe and the demise of Thatcherism in Britain. A few years later, faced with economic realities, my interest in revolutionary politics gave way to the more refined pursuit of indexing and classification. To be fair, by the mid-1990s, library and information science was on the verge of its own revolution, sparked by the arrival of the internet. Medicine, too, was a profession in the throes of radical change: evidence-based medicine was shiny and new (and viewed with suspicion by many) and the Cochrane Collaboration (formed in 1993) quickly became the vanguard of the evidence movement, coalescing around a formidable group of pioneers and iconoclasts. This was the environment I stepped into as a naïve information science graduate 25 years ago in Oxford. They were genuinely exciting times; to be a health information specialist as evidence synthesis took off, was to feel that you were helping to right a long-standing wrong.

My career has been spent on the frontline of evidence synthesis—doing, supporting, teaching, advocating, and researching. The focus of those early years was to find the evidence to feed into systematic reviews. In the absence of adequate indexing, we scoured Medline (and later Embase) for reports of trials, screening tens of thousands of abstracts and working with the National Library of Medicine to re-tag records. I supervised volunteers who would spend hours in libraries searching journals by hand to find trials that either pre-dated databases or were so poorly reported they were unlikely ever to be retrieved. The Cochrane trials register is the ongoing legacy of that early effort. Knowledge and skills acquired during those formative years with Cochrane in the United Kingdom—around search strategy development and design, research methods, and supporting systematic reviews—have evolved and, happily, are once again central to my roles and responsibilities. I have been the resident health information specialist at Cochrane Australia for 20 years, contributing to commissioned evidence syntheses, getting involved in research, and teaching search methods to systematic reviewers. However, only in the last few years have I returned to my information science roots, having previously managed international research projects with our Cochrane partners in the region and served as a board member for Cochrane internationally.

Although evidence-based medicine is now so mainstream it is a more historical than contemporary movement, the impetus to see that decisions about health and health care are informed by reliable evidence remains personally highly motivating.

Alongside this is a desire to improve the efficiency of evidence synthesis by improving timeliness and reducing duplication of effort. The health information specialist's role in supporting traditional systematic reviews is not radically different from that of yesteryear—the expert searcher's value is well-recognised in the field of evidence synthesis—but we need to continually acquire diverse skills and techniques that reflect new technologies and approaches. Some of these new technologies, such as machine learning and text mining, bear directly on how we design search strategies and facilitate the assessment of study eligibility. New approaches to evidence synthesis, such as living systematic reviews and guidelines, are becoming more commonplace and more feasible because of these new technologies—a trend that accelerated during the COVID-19 pandemic. My involvement in some of the early pioneering work around living evidence has led me to PhD studies in which I am evaluating how continuous evidence surveillance and the use of machine learning classifiers can improve the efficiency and feasibility of living reviews and guidelines. These are interesting times in evidence synthesis. While fully computable evidence syntheses, in which structured data are derived from different sources, are not a reality yet, it is also true that the days of relying on a single study publication from a bibliographic database as the sole source of evidence are disappearing. We recognise that studies have lifecycles and shed data and information along the way that are critical to the reliability of evidence synthesis (via protocols, study registers, data repositories, publications, and open science platforms). As health information specialists, we have skills in searching, data storage and data linking, but we must be prepared to embrace new technologies, hone our skills, and consider how we position ourselves in the changing landscape of evidence synthesis.

Suzanne Lewis, NSW Central Coast Local Health District, Australia

I came to health librarianship via a Bachelor of Arts and PhD in English literature, followed by a Graduate Diploma in Library and Information Science. I became a health librarian almost by default as I was successful in the first job I applied for after graduation. The fact that I am still a health librarian more than 20 years later is a reflection of how much I enjoy my role, and the opportunities I have been afforded by my employer and via my engagement with the professional community of health sciences librarians in Australia and internationally.

During the first few years of my career learning the foundations of health librarianship, I became aware of the evidence-based practice philosophy and framework as it applied to both health and librarianship. I completed one of the early online courses in evidence-based librarianship offered by the University of Sheffield School of Health and Related Research and made available to Australian librarians via the Australian Library and Information Association (ALIA). Together with several enthusiastic colleagues, I began applying evidence-based principles to workplace projects, and disseminating the results via several publications in the Evidence-Based Library and Information Practice journal. I became an evidence summary writer for the journal, which involved critiquing a recent research publication in the library and information science (LIS) field. I progressed to reviewing evidence summaries and peer reviewing original research for publication.

As I became more confident with critical appraisal of LIS research, I wanted to be able to apply those skills to the health and biomedical research I dealt with every day on behalf of clinicians. I could search the biomedical literature and was confident in selecting the most relevant literature from the results, but was aware of my uncertainty around the concepts of methodological rigour and quality of published research. What were these randomized controlled trials, cohort studies, and meta-analyses that health professionals talked about? I completed a Graduate Certificate in Epidemiology, which enabled me to teach critical appraisal skills in addition to literature searching skills, and also to talk to clinicians about clinical research. Having an understanding of clinical research methodology, including the best research design to answer different types of clinical questions, is a valuable foundation for advanced skills in searching the biomedical literature.

In 2011, I was asked to be a tutor at the first Australian Evidence-Based Practice Librarians' Institute (AEBPLI), a residential workshop for health librarians on the principles of evidence-based practice, research methodology, and critical appraisal. Working in a team of Australian and US-based health librarians was a game-changer for me. The intensive preparation for teaching at the Institute, plus mentoring from the highly experienced US-based tutors, consolidated my knowledge. However, the learning is not all one-way; the format of the Institute encourages knowledge sharing among tutors and students in the programmed sessions and via informal networking. I have returned as a tutor and co-convenor of the Institute every year it has been held since 2011.

Another teaching opportunity arose when the Australian Library and Information Association Health Libraries Australia (ALIA HLA) group developed and delivered an online subject in health librarianship in partnership with the Queensland University of Technology (Health Librarianship Essentials) and later with the University of Melbourne (Digital Health Information Services). I led the development and teaching of an Evidence-Based Practice module each time this course ran.

These four initiatives—early adoption of evidence-based library and information practice, a Graduate Certificate in Epidemiology, the AEBPLI, and the online specialist health librarianship/digital health information subject—have allowed me to achieve three ALIA HLA competencies (ALIA HLA 2018): health literacy, curricular design and instruction, and teaching the information skills associated with evidence-based practice; health research and the application of health research methodologies; and health information professionalism. Like most of my colleagues, I spent the early years of my health librarian career achieving competence in delivering reference and information services (a separate HLA competency), including completing a course in medical terminology and building skills in searching the biomedical and nursing bibliographic databases. More recently, I led a project to build a validated search filter for retrieval of integrated care literature in PubMed. This gave me the opportunity to further develop my knowledge of bibliometrics, Medical Subject Headings (MeSH), and search syntax. Moreover, the process of building a tool that is of direct benefit to clinicians and researchers. Working with an expert advisory group gave me invaluable insights into researchers, clinicians, and health service planners and their priorities and how they approach information in a digital world.

Over the last 20 years, improvements in online search platforms and discovery tools, and increased access to digital information resources, mean that most clinicians are able to find the information they need to ensure their routine clinical decision-making is based on reliable evidence. The role of the health research information specialist has changed from research gatekeeper to a more nuanced role perhaps best described as a research information facilitator. Such a role includes searching for evidence on the complex, multi-faceted, wicked questions that arise from clinical practice and health service planning; appraisal and summary of evidence in the form of evidence checks or rapid reviews; creation and testing of tools such as validated search filters that provide fast-track access to published research; teaching health literacy skills in context; and facilitating knowledge translation from research to practice. I think it is this last facet of the role that inspires me most—being part of the process that translates evidence into clinical practice that directly benefits patients. As healthcare organisations make the transition to digital health, the discipline of health research information specialists will continue to work at the evidence/clinical practice interface, continually adapting to new technology but retaining the role of facilitator.

Cecily Gilbert, University of Melbourne, Australia

Since 2012, I have worked as a health information specialist and research assistant in the Centre for Digital Transformation of Health (CDTH) at the University of Melbourne. But my working life began in libraries, and most of it has been in health; I count myself lucky to have experienced the huge transition in information management, which has occurred in the course of my career.

After matriculation in 1970, I did a 3-year diploma of librarianship at RMIT University in Melbourne. We were introduced to principles and practice in reference service, cataloguing and classification, systems analysis, and library administration; in 1990 I upgraded this qualification to a library and information science degree. Between 1974 and 1978, I held librarian positions in higher education and science, maintaining and searching large card catalogues, and using printed subject indexes for reference queries. My first taste of health work was as a librarian at Melbourne's Queen Victoria Medical Centre between 1978 and 1984. In this period, I accessed remote databases using an acoustic coupler to connect a dumb terminal to the phone line, to send literature search commands and to receive the results. I returned to university library reference work in 1987, then moved back to a hospital librarian position 10 years later. By 1997, web access was possible in hospitals, PubMed provided free MEDLINE access, and gradually other databases transitioned to online services. These technological developments fully enabled end-users to search their own questions: a dramatic change that also altered my role in teaching and information provision. The Cochrane Collaboration, which had emerged in 1993, promoted systematic reviews to examine the evidence on healthcare questions; as a result, my literature searching was transformed by the levels-of-evidence paradigm.

In 2004, I undertook a 12-week placement at Monash Health Centre for Clinical Effectiveness (CCE), which conducts tailored syntheses of health information sources, in response to clinicians' enquiries, and fosters evidence-informed practice. I was supervised by an experienced information specialist, participated in syntheses on two detailed topics, became familiar with health technology assessment resources, and honed my skills in critical appraisal. I gained greater confidence and a broader view of information specialist work, which fits my current role at CDTH. I am embedded in the health informatician research team, providing customised information services and research assistance to between 10 and 15 researchers in various roles including practitioners, clinicians, researchers, and educators. My tasks include: literature searching; analysing, summarising, and scoping information sources; preparing quick environmental scans; obtaining, extracting, managing, and analysing data; teaching postgraduate students; research data management; writing and proofreading; and preparing ethics and funding applications. These activities are in line with four of the seven competency areas for Australian health library and information professionals (ALIA HLA 2018): health reference and research services and delivering best practice information services; management of health knowledge and information resources in a variety of formats; the digital and ehealth context, and the technology and systems used to manage data, information and knowledge resources in the delivery of library and information services; health research and the application of health research methodologies.

While many of the duties are similar to those performed by health librarians in a library, there are differences. The key variation is my ongoing link with a defined group of informaticians: it is a huge advantage to be attached to a specialist group, to gain a deeper knowledge of the body of relevant information resources, as well as the research projects and interests. It allows me to anticipate some information needs, and to draw on conceptual sources that apply in this field. I am challenged by involvement in new tasks (such as supporting the weekly presentation of a fully online subject on digital health resources, and becoming competent with visualisation tools). I have three main observations about the health research information specialist in the digital health future. First, more widespread research use of health datasets of many kinds will require the information specialist to keep abreast of such sources and where to locate them, effectively extending their "knowing where to find" capability to non-bibliographic repositories. Second, the shift to translational research—translating research findings into evidence-based practice and policy—means that time-poor clinicians and researchers will require and value literature reviews that synthesise current knowledge and lessons from existing research. There is an imperative from government to gain maximum benefit from its research investment, and health research information specialists with the capability to synthesise and assess sources will need to be ready for this. Third, health research information specialists should claim a place in the frameworks for learning health systems (LHS), which integrate real-world data and evidence in a health system to improve outcomes. The LHS literature is replete with references to digital knowledge objects "curated and managed in digital libraries…and made available to users" (Guise et al. 2018: 2237), but lack any mention of digital health librarians, whose skills in filtering, summarising, and organising information would be highly relevant. Finally, as a general point, the health research information specialist workforce does not have the level of diversity that is evident in the general population; we have an obligation to redress this.

Terena Solomons, Western Australian Group of Evidence-Informed Healthcare Practice, Australia

With my father a surgeon and mother a nurse, it was by osmosis that I picked up medical terminology over dinner table conversations whilst growing up. Since 2013, I have worked as a health research information specialist and as a research librarian for the Western Australian Group for Evidence Informed Healthcare Practice (WAGEIHP), a Joanna Briggs Institute (JBI) collaboration centre.

I completed a Bachelor of Arts majoring in History and Geography from James Cook University in Townsville, Queensland, Australia. I wanted a profession that allowed me to travel and work overseas without having to re-qualify. Librarianship offered this and I studied the Graduate Diploma of Library Science at the Queensland University of Technology. I worked in higher education and special libraries in Australia and the United Kingdom before my first foray into health libraries, a 6-month contract in the Health Science team at Curtin University Library in 1999 in Perth, Western Australia (WA). I ran information literacy workshops focusing on the main health databases and worked on a project evaluating their platforms. For 17 years I managed Hollywood Private Hospital Library, overseeing the change from print to digital collections. The service I enjoyed most was searching the literature for busy doctors, nurses, allied health, and corporate staff.

With ALIA HLA support, in 2002 I attended the Evidence Based Clinical Practice Workshop in Adelaide, along with two other WA health librarians with whom I ran Evidence Based Practice (EBP) workshops for WA librarians. This experience gave me a good understanding of EBP and was the catalyst for working with the Clinical Pathways Co-ordinator at Hollywood Hospital in finding evidence to support clinical pathways and the clinical practice manual. Serendipitously, discussions over a cup of coffee with school mums led me to my role with WAGEIHP, based at the School of Nursing, Midwifery, and Paramedicine at Curtin University. I met a paediatric nurse who had conducted a systematic review as part of her Masters of Nursing degree and had been approached to write evidence summaries for the JBI. The thought of searching databases, however, was daunting for her. We began a job-share—I would find the evidence and she would synthesise it.

I am now embedded within research teams at WAGEIHP, where I began 7 years ago searching for studies relating to wound care. The focus of the initial evidence summaries was on low resource countries' use of naturally available wound products like banana leaves, potato peels, acetic acid, turmeric, and coconut products. To get up to speed with wound management practices and to understand the fundamentals of wound healing I undertook Wound Care Australia's online learning modules. My childhood years of flicking through my father's surgical textbooks prepared me for seeing photos of some horrible wounds. My self-education to acquire a wound care vocabulary was important for identifying keywords and indexed terms and developing comprehensive search strategies to identify relevant studies. I learnt many interesting facts in my research and one article I will always remember about the use of coconut products for wound healing was "Skull trepanation in the Bismarck Archipelago"; coconut juice was used to irrigate the wound from trepanation (the process of drilling a hole in the skull) and it was also used to wash the hands of the surgeon (Watters 2007).

Since 2015, I have been involved with research teams undertaking systematic and scoping reviews. Tasks include preliminary environmental scans; conducting searches across all databases and grey literature; establishing shared EndNote or Mendeley libraries and de-duplicating results; exporting results to Rayyan for the team to screen, finding full text articles, PRISMA flowchart and writing the search methodology section for the protocol and review. I also critique search strategies for postgraduate students planning to submit manuscripts to JBI.

I enjoy working with researchers at the start of a project when they are working out their protocol. I like scoping the literature and using text mining tools like MeSH on Demand, PubMed Reminer, and Yale MeSH analyser to develop the Concept Table (sometimes referred to as Logic Grid, Matrix) to capture all keywords and indexed terms.

Extensive literature searching as a hospital librarian gave me the initial skills and experience for this role. Since then I have gained knowledge and developed skills in the following ways: reading JBI, Cochrane and Campbell Collaboration reviewer manuals and professional literature related to evidence synthesis; participating in the Expert Searchers listserv and following information specialists on Twitter; co-chairing the JBI Information Science Methods Group; attending HLA professional development events (particularly advanced searching workshops led by Julie Glanville and Carol Lefebvre); and the continuing education workshops at EAHIL (European Association for Health Information and Libraries). Learning about new sources of evidence and new software tools like Rayyan, DistillerSR, EndNote sharing, and Mendeley for managing results is what excites me (or horrifies me when it does not work as expected!).

In the digital health future, the tsunami of systematic and other types of reviews offers fantastic opportunities for health research information specialists to make a valuable contribution to review teams. Finding the evidence is a crucial step in the process, and there is further scope for information specialists to improve practice by peer-reviewing search strategies for systematic and scoping reviews (Grossetta Nardini et al. 2019). From my experience, there is demand for health research information specialist skills that are not always explicit; often word-of-mouth recommendations have led to me being involved in reviews. Artificial intelligence applications will assist in managing large amounts of data for evidence synthesis in the future, but they are unlikely to take over the role of the health research information specialist. This work will always need human input and checking.

Kristan Kang, Australian Research Data Commons, Australia

Inspired (embarrassingly enough) by FBI Agent Dana Scully from the TV show "The X-Files", I started a Bachelor of Science degree fascinated by the idea of using evidence to solve complex problems. I majored in psychology/neuroscience, completed an Honours research project on brain activity in attention deficit hyperactivity disorder (ADHD), and then continued to a PhD project, which aimed to understand the neural mechanisms underlying consciousness. I was part of a group effort to collect large amounts of information on brain function and human behaviour that was divided up among many different projects. Many of the business processes to support this effort were being made up along the way, and my project became deprioritised as time went on; I completed my degree but the experience was not pleasant. My research was limited by the practicalities of obtaining good data in a timely fashion, and my introduction to doing science as a profession was less than ideal. After 6 years as a trainee researcher, I was turned off being a career academic, but I had no idea what I did want.

Eventually, I accepted a research support role with a dementia research group that needed someone to manage their large data collection and data sharing activities. Initially, I was not sure it was the right fit for me. I understood the science they were doing, but my role as data manager required me to learn a whole new set of skills on the job: technical knowledge of databases and applications, data storage and security, as well as a range of general business skills like strategic prioritisation, relationship building, and project management. As the group evolved into a research centre, I gained additional experience in research governance, ethics, and privacy and contract law. I never had formal training in these things apart from the occasional half-day staff development sessions offered by the university, but through trial and error, I learnt how they worked in practice and how they influenced the productivity of research. In essence, I transitioned from knowing the science to knowing the business of science, and I was promoted to the role of research manager as a result. Despite my earlier reservations about moving from science to research support, I ended up contributing directly and indirectly to hundreds of research projects. I had a pivotal behind-the-scenes role, and while I was not receiving personal academic accolades, my colleagues appreciated my contribution and frequently acknowledged that our group's achievements relied (at least in part) on the work I did.

When the opportunity arose to move to a national eResearch infrastructure organisation as their health and medical data specialist, I was excited by the prospect but nervous; eResearch entails the use of information technology to support existing and new forms of research, and this role would draw on knowledge and skills that I had built up informally. Moving from the coalface of research to a national infrastructure role felt like a big leap, but my research experience got me the job. There are many principles and policies around eResearch and open science, but effectively translating these into research practice can be problematic. Those who know only the theory can struggle to understand why researchers are hesitant or simply unable to implement it in daily practice. Understanding the science, the data, and the realities of being a scientist might not be essential for all research support roles, but the more experience you have with these things, the better you can translate between the differing contexts of infrastructure and science in a meaningful and impactful way.

The research sector has evolved well beyond the two original tribes of scientists and administrators. The problems with decreased financial support combined with an increased focus on research translation and public benefit means that research as a sector has had to figure out how to operate more efficiently and productively, particularly through digital transformation of traditional processes. The emergence of a third tribe, research support specialists who have a combination of technical and professional skills and research experience, is essential to the evolution of the sector. This is something I know not only in theory, but from nearly two decades of personal experience in both being a researcher and supporting other researchers. The power of evidence-based decision-making is what drew me to science, as did the desire to improve our knowledge of the world and consequently the quality of our lives. However, I have learnt that simply trying to do good science is not enough to produce these outcomes; scientific research is an information-intensive industry like many others, and must function as such.

Mari Elisa Kuusniemi, Helsinki University Library, Finland

First, I studied science/organic chemistry. I specialised in bioinformatics. In my master's thesis, I used bioinformatics methods to predict protein structure for a research group working on drug chemistry. Bioinformatics is a classic example of data science. I have a Master's degree in Information Science. I specialised in networks and other electronic resources. As a part of this master's program, I studied computer science at bachelor level. I have also studied educational sciences, but I have not finished the last course of the program; I have used the skills and knowledge a lot, but have not needed the certificate.

I got my first position in a library in Finland's National Public Health Institute. I worked as an information specialist in a small information services unit. The main customers were medical researchers and national health administration staff. I worked with an experienced information specialist from whom I learned most of the important skills needed for research services. I learned the rules of academic research, academic merit, and funding. I developed skills in information retrieval, bibliometrics, communication, and marketing. I also learned project management when working in various projects with research groups and the health administration. My last big project was about interoperability of electronic health services. I was responsible for creating data models, ontologies, and terminologies ensuring semantic interoperability.

After 8 years, I got a job in the medical library of the University of Helsinki. I worked as an information specialist in the library of the medical faculty, which also serves the University Hospital (mainly nurses and physicians). Part of my role was to develop data management services. Research data management was a new thing at the time. Starting from scratch, in 2012–2013, I organised in-house training and, together with my colleagues (Kuusniemi et al. 2014), started the library's first data management services, including developing basic guidance and training for doctoral students. Gradually we built up a data management team in the library and started networking with other services around research data management in the university. I worked for a while as a team leader. At the same time, we got national funding for a project where we developed the national requirements for data management plans (DMP), launched a national instance of a DMP tool (the software is DMPonline), and built up a network of data management planning experts. I was the project manager of the DMP project 2015–2017. During 2015, I got an opportunity to work as a visiting scholar in a hospital library at Geelong, Australia for 3 months. The visit gave me the opportunity to reflect on the importance of research librarians in a hospital setting, while also launching new services and working in a new environment.

Continuing in my university career, I worked in a data management infrastructure project developing services for all disciplines. I worked as data librarian in data management services, with various tasks including training, consultancy, and marketing. However, the medical field has been the one I feel most at home with, because of my health background. Nowadays, I work mainly in national and international projects and working groups around research data management. At the university, I work primarily with policy-level issues. The main topics are data management planning, research data documentation and metadata (FAIR—Findable, Accessible, Interoperable, Re-usable), data curation and developing new professional skills in research data in libraries. Research data have huge value as information sources in fast moving disciplines. When dealing with current hot topics there is no time to wait until an article is published. Openly available data make global cooperation possible. The potential of open data has not yet been reached, and this area will grow fast in the future. Although it is challenging, I love being part of the movement towards a true digital era.

In the transition to digital health, as a specialised health research information professional, I see the need for specialising even further. New professions will be needed and will develop at least in the bigger libraries and research institutes. Traditional skills around networking and cooperation will be even more important in the future, when we need to bridge the gaps that separate the needs of researchers from all different disciplines. Forms of information are changing along with publication channels; health research information specialists need to be part of that transformation too. The US National Library of Medicine sees the library as an important player in medicine and data science (Fridsma 2015) and I hope that other medical libraries join this movement.

Conclusion

There is no single professional degree or certificate that qualifies an individual to practise as a health research information specialist. The roles go by different names: information service manager, library manager, research assistant, research librarian, evidence researcher, research data specialist, and information specialist. As one case study author commented: "The research sector has evolved well beyond the two original tribes of scientists and administrators". This third tribe, of health research information specialists, is emerging as an essential part of the research team. The case studies in this chapter have shown various pathways, qualifications, and experiences, that can lead to becoming a health research information specialist. The practitioners who work in this field operate in different capacities and levels, and are employed by different types of organisations. Their work permeates and facilitates the research lifecycle. Whatever the area of health research—clinical, medical, pharmaceutical, bioinformatics, or evidence research—the common element demonstrated in the case studies is that they all have an interest and a passion for research-based knowledge and the potential for knowledge to be used to good effect.

References

Australian Library and Information Association/Health Libraries Australia. ALIA HLA competencies. 2018. https://www.alia.org.au/sites/default/files/HLA%20Competencies_0.pdf. Accessed 1 Jun 2020.

Fridsma DB. A new vision for the National Library of Medicine. J Am Med Inform Assoc. 2015;22:1111.

Grossetta Nardini HK, Batten J, Funaro MC, Garcia-Milian R, Nyhan K, Spak JM, et al. Librarians as methodological peer reviewers for systematic reviews: results of an online survey. Res Integr Peer Rev. 2019;4:23.

Guise JM, Savitz LA, Friedman CP. Mind the gap: putting evidence into practice in the era of learning health systems. J Gen Intern Med. 2018;33(12):2237–9.

Kuusniemi ME, Heino T, Larmo K. How to get started with research data management training services for the academic library? Helsinki University Library. 2014. http://old.iss.it/binary/eahi/cont/76_Mari_Elisa_Kuusniemi_Full_text.pdf. Accessed 12 May 2020.

Watters DA. Skull trepanation in the Bismarck archipelago. P N G Med J. 2007;50(1–2):20–4.

Chapter 21
Working as an Allied Health Informatician

**Mark Merolli, Kirsty Maunder, Dawn Choo, Khye Davey,
and Yasmine Probst**

Abstract Allied health professionals are fast recognising the need to adopt digital health technologies in their service delivery models. Reasons driving this need include greater digitisation of healthcare systems, such as electronic medical records, and pressures on healthcare systems to rapidly deploy digital models of care, such as telehealth consultations. Despite a growing need to support the digital allied health workforce, there has been much volatility in formal educational opportunities, career development pathways, and leadership roles. The future of allied health informatics faces challenges, including its heterogeneity of professions, siloed tools and technologies, and ongoing issues surrounding change management, for example. However, striving to increase the profile and provide support for the advancement of digital health and informatics amongst this group of professions will help foster success; success in terms of improved patient outcomes, health system performance, and job satisfaction (to name a few). With greater attention to educating the emerging and existing workforce, mapping career progression, and lobbying for leadership opportunities, we envisage that a clearer profile of the digital allied health information workforce will emerge.

Keywords Case study · Allied health · Dietitians · Physiotherapists · Competencies

M. Merolli (✉) · D. Choo
Centre for Digital Transformation of Health, The University of Melbourne, Parkville, VIC, Australia
e-mail: merollim@unimelb.edu.au; dawn.choo@unimelb.edu.au

K. Maunder · Y. Probst
School of Medicine, University of Wollongong, Wollongong, NSW, Australia
e-mail: kmaunder@uow.edu.au; yasmine@uow.edu.au

K. Davey
East Metropolitan Health Service, Perth, WA, Australia

K. Butler-Henderson et al. (eds.), *The Health Information Workforce*, Health Informatics, https://doi.org/10.1007/978-3-030-81850-0_21

Introduction

Allied health professionals (AHPs) are a diverse mix of health practitioners who are trained in complementary clinical disciplines outside of medicine and nursing. Examples include, but are not limited to: audiologists, dietitians, occupational therapists, optometrists, physiotherapists, psychologists, speech pathologists, and social workers. AHPs can be found in varying roles (i.e. clinician, educator, researcher, policymaker), across a range of healthcare settings (i.e. acute or tertiary public and private hospitals, aged care facilities, private practice, community and in-home care), and in colleges and universities, industry, and consulting. It is fast becoming recognised that there is a need for AHPs to embrace digital health—including electronic medical records (EMR), telehealth, mobile applications, online resources, analytics dashboards and/or ubiquitous care—for (1) the ability to capture patient data in a more complete, systematic, accurate, and efficient manner to improve healthcare recording accuracy; (2) adapting and mobilising digital models of care in light of unprecedented challenges to healthcare (e.g. pandemics); (3) evaluating and improving the quality and safety of care; and (4) collecting and using health data to support the transformation of care, research and/or funding decisions. There are also ever-increasing patient expectations about digital empowerment and a more observable focus on the continuum of care from the hospital/clinic to the home/community environment (NHS 2019; Philip 2015; Maunder et al. 2018; Greenhalgh et al. 2020).

The digital health workforce across the varied allied health disciplines needs to include technologically informed and competent clinicians with diverse specialised clinical skills and also AHPs in information and communication technology (ICT) specialist roles. The types of digital health and clinical informatics competencies which different healthcare professionals must possess have been proposed over the years and mapped, with relevance to the allied health workforce (Coiera 2013; Gray et al. 2015; Fridsma 2018, 2019; Butler-Henderson et al. 2020). Such workforce development is an initiative with global support, for example in international scientific forums (Maunder et al. 2018; Houston et al. 2018), in UK National Health Service policy documents (NHS 2017, 2018, 2019). Key underpinning themes are (NHS 2019): being digitally ready (strategic, leadership, digital literacy, and governance), being digitally mature (effective use, interoperable, and transformative), and being data-enabled (safety and quality, outcome-driven, and sustainable).

Despite a clear argument for the role which AHPs play in the delivery, planning, and coordinating of healthcare, designated leadership roles in digital health continue to elude these professions. While clearly defined roles exist for Chief Medical and Nursing Information Officers (i.e. CMIO/CNIO), support and understanding for the leadership role that AHPs can play in senior executive health teams (has lagged in Australia and internationally; only a handful of Chief Allied Health Information Officer (CAHIO) positions exist. Author Maunder, has worked to promote the importance of such leadership in dietetics (Maunder et al. 2019), and the Australasian Institute of Digital Health (AIDH) has produced a whitepaper calling for greater visibility and a future for the role of CAHIO in 2019 (HISA 2019).

Collectively the authors of this chapter represent experiences across the disciplines of physiotherapy, dietetics, and speech pathology. Our careers span several settings, including but not limited to private/public hospitals, private practice, community-based, and aged care, industry (IT vendor solutions), consulting, academia, and research. Further, we are actively engaged members of the digital allied health community, keenly involved in digital health initiatives around the world; we have chaired national and international committees in clinical informatics and been actively involved in annual scientific conferences as presenters, chairpersons, and reviewers to advocate for the engagement of allied health professionals in this discipline. Using a pseudo-collaborative autoethnographic approach (Chang 2016), we have individually reflected upon our career journeys, impact, and progression through allied health informatics, meeting afterwards and reflecting iteratively to distil our experiences of working in this sub-community of the HIDDIN (Health Informatics, Digital, Data, Information, and Knowledge) workforce.

Here we present the result of analysing our collective career narratives (Benoot and Bilsen 2016) as four major themes (see Table 21.1 for a full list of themes and sub-themes), drawing on thematic analysis in qualitative research (Anderson 2007): preparing for a career in allied health and AHI; building knowledge and skills in digital health; the unique attributes of the digital AHI workforce; predictions for the future of the allied health information workforce. Taking this further, we have also identified particular themes that are inherently related to our professional training as an AHP and those seen to be purely related to informatics. It is at this intersection of informatics and AHP that we see the unique attributes of an allied health informatician. Our themes are accompanied by short excerpts or quotes from our individual narratives. To further contextualise this chapter, Table 21.2 offers two case studies that depict sample career paths in digital allied health informatics.

Table 21.1 Allied health informatician career themes and sub-themes summary

Themes	Sub-themes
1. Educational background	1.1 Interest in the sciences 1.2 Desire to help people 1.3 Big picture thinking 1.4 Pursuing further education and credentialing in informatics
2. Career history	2.1 Careers paralleling advances in digital health 2.2 Experience with digital health quality improvement and service redesign projects
3. Unique attributes of the digital allied health informatician	3.1 Personal advancement and life-long learning 3.2 Analytical curiosity
4. A future view of the allied health informatics workforce	4.1 Opportunity to advance and transform practice supported by digital health technologies 4.2 Essential role of the allied health professional (leadership and engagement) in digital health 4.3 Change management 4.4 Maintaining a patient-centred focus

In the educational backgrounds of AHPs who move into the field of digital health, there are consistent threads. One is interested in the sciences. AHPs curiosity about the STEM disciplines (science, technology, engineering, mathematics) goes as far back as high school, especially biology, chemistry, physics, and psychology, with some also interested then in information-communication technology (ICT) and information systems. "Science and technology have been constant gravity wells." (Author KD).

Another such thread is desire to help people. We collectively identified a common theme that spurred all of us to pursue our careers, the interpersonal nature of being a practicing AHP. This was sometimes augmented by an AHP having prior experience with receiving healthcare treatment or with sharing in the health journey of a loved one.

At the intersection of health informatics and AHPs are "big picture" thinkers, a macro-level view of health and wellbeing. We all agreed that positive change requires an appreciation for the role of the patient in their own care (participatory health) and across their continuum of care and a willingness to embrace evidence-based practice grounded in sound research. "Insights…about the performance of health systems…helped me to recognise the value of big picture thinking in advancing health beyond one-to-one clinical care." (Author DC).

While much of AHPs' journey into digital health is work-based or experiential, we found that people interested in this area will take it upon themselves to pursue further education opportunities related to digital health and informatics—continuing professional development modules, graduate coursework, doctoral studies. "I pursued my PhD… This was a way for me to combine my knowledge of clinical healthcare, with an interest and foundational knowledge of ICT from my earlier years." (Author MM) In the absence of a formal clinical informatics training pathway, some proceed to gain credentials such as the Certified Health Informatician Australasia (CHIA) or international equivalents; some apply to have their years of experience and education recognised in Fellowship status in a professional college in Health Informatics (MM, KM and YP are Founding Fellows of the Australasian Institute of Digital Health). "…There were no academic or formal education channels to prepare me for my work in this field." (Author KM).

The career development of AHPs who move into the field of digital health parallels the advances in digital health and involves project-based experiences. A common theme in our personal journeys in AHI is our evolution alongside that of digital health. We have noted a paradigm shift from traditional patriarchal healthcare structures towards participatory healthcare, in part driven by increasing ubiquitous computing and digital connectedness (i.e. Internet and online information availability, rising prevalence of smartphones, mobile health and remote monitoring). For those of us in the vanguard, digital health practice meant being early adopters and willing to embrace innovation to support how we work; for those only just entering the digital workforce now, it means an opportunity to drive forward cutting edge AHP practice utilising advances in ICT.

In career journeys in allied health, AHPs past and present may recall personal involvement with service- or quality-improvement projects. Whether working in a

Table 21.2 Two case studies of careers in digital allied health informatics

	Case study #1	Case study #2
Domain	Physiotherapist clinician; clinical lead for EMR implementation; large metropolitan hospital	Dietitian; clinical background, now in academic role
Education background and preparation for allied (digital) health	– Interest in science and technology growing up – Undergraduate studies in marine and biological sciences – Pursued degree in physiotherapy to capture the opportunity to combine interest in life sciences with communication and people skills, critical thinking, and ability to add value to people's lives	– Graduated as a Dietitian – Six tertiary degrees; bachelor degree, two graduate certificates, two masters degrees, PhD
Work history: role(s), why it is interesting, the how/what of building knowledge and skills in their area	– Career in public tertiary and rehabilitation hospitals – Started career in paper-based clinical records systems; technology was siloed and scarcely used, for results look-up and email – Worked in various clinical teams over the years as technology outside of the hospital rapidly evolved; web-based clinical applications slowly began to emerge, allowing better access to patient information and requests, plus it created the opportunity for digitally literate clinicians to start innovating and improving systems – Expansion of role into clinical quality improvement projects (continued use of clinical skills and learning new skills; i.e. project management, problem-solving, system-level thinking, clinical workflows, process mapping, data analysis, human-factors) – Developed into role as an allied health educator; teaching a range of allied health professionals about clinical information systems and health ICT – Eventual role as clinical lead in an EMR implementation, a newly created role	– While working as a dietitian and doing doctoral research, I wanted to challenge the key premise about how dietitians worked; this led to upskilling in informatics – Research focused on informatics in dietetics to bridge the gap between clinical care and information science/ICT) – Career experience in hospitals, primary care, the food industry, consulting, and universities – Long research career in clinical and translational studies – Very few informaticians working in the nutrition field (unique skillset in clinical healthcare and informatics provided a pivotal bridge between both areas) – Created a virtual centre for nutrition informatics research – Also experience as a patient (lived experience and merging of personal and professional research interests) – Keen interest and observations of how health professionals document their notes; spurred desire to trial digital systems, data capture forms, and electronic documentation in own practice – Much of early journey was self-directed; including forming collaborative networks with like-minded professionals – Own journey paralleled advancement of digital technology into allied health systems

(continued)

Table 21.2 (continued)

Domain	Case study #1 Physiotherapist clinician; clinical lead for EMR implementation; large metropolitan hospital	Case study #2 Dietitian; clinical background, now in academic role
Future of allied health informatics: where do you see the discipline going in the future?	– A real opportunity to take more leading roles in informatics and digital health, particularly in hospitals. Driving factors behind this include; many of us work in interprofessional teams with a good understanding of the roles and skills different professions bring, expertise in person-centred care, and career paths for allied health are generally more constrained; giving rise to branching out and expanding scope.	– Informatics will not hinder, but rather improve efficiencies within the various professions to allow us to use our health training and communication skills more effectively – Expect to see health informatics become more ingrained in practice from the beginning of the professional career journey – The time frame of these cycles of acceptance will begin to decrease; in part due to the parallel changes occurring within society (i.e. with our patients/clients)
Other thoughts	– For a long time, digital health and informatics for allied health professionals has been challenging to get involved in (partly workplace and/or network dependent) – Career paths for allied health professionals in informatics have not been clear – The digital health community would be well advised to bring greater attention to this area to allied health professionals – The allied health workforce is an untapped resource in digital health	– We should continue to challenge ourselves and take the next step – Early fear was transformed to passion and a need to advocate for something I continue to feel very strongly about

public hospital system, community care setting or private practice, because of our intimate knowledge of the patient journey, care planning and coordination, AHPs are frequently called upon to take leading roles in major projects to transform practice such as EMR implementations, development of portals and dashboards, telehealth service redesign. "While the electronic systems worked, in some cases the fall back of paper methods were still heavily ingrained in the hospital environment." (Author YP). We are able to pinpoint systems or processes that are fragmented or working inefficiently and are able to accurately identify areas for improvement, e.g. "ability to prioritise at risk patients accurately was dependent on subjective and often inaccurate information." (Author KM). As a result of our roles in major projects, we are often well-placed to demonstrate the benefit of digital tools and services and act as a conduit between clinical colleagues, ICT teams, and senior executives in helping to ensure major digital health projects are a success. "These skills honed along my career have allowed me to add value to multiple clinical change programs and projects." (Author KD).

The digital allied health informatician has unique attributes, the first of which is personal advancement. AHPs share an intellectual curiosity for progress and self-determination; this includes a personal desire to excel. We identified an "Aha moment," when AHPs discover and pursue digital health and informatics as an area of fascination, historically down a path less trodden. "I found that we were speaking two different languages which at times slowed progress... my focus was to learn the 'language' of informatics." (Author YP) It runs through to a desire to stay ahead of technological advancements that can improve care outcomes and clinical efficiencies (e.g. telehealth solutions and remote monitoring for improved access to care). We have pursued greenfield opportunities beyond the realm of traditional allied health practices whilst balancing a diverse portfolio of work in the clinic, research, teaching, health system administration and industry.

Analytical curiosity occurs in conjunction with this desire to embrace solutions at the cutting edge of practice, AHPs are by nature analytically curious about how to support evidence-based practice. AHPs may naturally gravitate towards the digital health informatics sciences because of the innate ability of technologies to support intelligence gathering and processing remotely, which is frequently in the scope of work of an AHP. For example we want to use analytics techniques and the growing field of artificial intelligence on big data that is collected away from the clinic to inform patient progress and care plans. "...continue to leverage technologies...to inform patient progress and clinical metrics outside of the traditional clinical environment and how technology can assist to analyse big data to predict patient outcomes" (Author MM).

The future for the Allied Health Informatics workforce is influential and important. The benefits of incorporating informatics and digital initiatives into usual care practices continue to compound and resonate across the allied health disciplines to improve the efficiencies in the way that we currently work. Access to electronic patient data, for example has enabled AHPs to tap into data analytics capabilities for prioritising caseloads, managing workflow, reviewing intervention outcomes as well as to allow for clinical audits to be conducted rapidly to inform service improvements. AHPs have a key role in influencing the integration of digital health and ensuring that the utility and delivery of system support standards and terminologies align with our professional practice. Furthermore, there is a need to ensure that the AHP workforce is sufficiently equipped to best utilise the electronic solutions that are available or drive the development of electronic solutions to support best practice. "Allied health has a key role to play in the integration of eHealth, ensuring the delivery of these systems support standards and terminologies to their professional practice" (Author KM).

In teaching and training future clinicians, we observe that student willingness to engage with artificial intelligence, sensor, mobile, and even ubiquitous methods of assessment has been high. There is a shared view that the transformation of care practices supported by digital health technologies could be further bolstered by the infusion of digital health curricula into standard clinical teaching.

We can see an essential leadership and engagement role for allied health professionals in digital health. There is a well-known ceiling effect for conventional career trajectories for AHPs practicing within their specialised clinical field. This could be the impetus in the future for experienced AHPs—given our exposure to working in interprofessional teams and our common understanding of the roles and skills which different care providers bring to the clinical management of patients—to take leadership opportunities in furthering the digitisation of health within the wider arena of the healthcare system. AHPs can lead all the way from the design and development of digital and informatics solutions through to the generation of research evidence to support implementation in clinical practice.

Our observations about change management suggest that the evolution of the digital health informatics workforce within allied health has arguably occurred as cycles of acceptance rather than a linear progression towards our current state. The adoption of technology in healthcare was initially met with resistance and could be attributed to a fear of the unknown or fear of losing jobs to technology. We have found that the number of early adopters has tended to increase with the diffusion of knowledge and information about digital technology use amongst the clinical community; this, in turn, has activated a growing sense of urgency to integrate informatics into practice. The momentum of these cycles of acceptance has continued to build over the years, ultimately leading to the formal recognition of health informatics as a discipline in its own right. "Acceptance generally appears to be driven by urgency while the number of early adopter groups were evidently increasing in number and size." (Author YP). There is an expectation that these cycles of acceptance and change might occur more rapidly throughout healthcare as AHPs acclimatise to the complementary role that digital health technology has in standard clinical practice. In addition to technological acceptance, we recognise that life-long learning can ensure a smoother transition as new ways of working continue to arise with new technological innovations and new digital information flows. Thus not only is there a need to assimilate digital health and informatics within standard university curricula to prepare the future health informatics workforce but as well as it is a priority to continue to provide professional development initiatives for AHPs in the current workforce, "to the point that we essentially stop referring to the 'digital' in 'health'." (Author MM).

Maintaining a patient-centred focus in the fast-evolving age of digital technology accompanies the growing expectation that individuals will engage with and manage their own health with information technologies across a range of mediums and scenarios. AHPs are generally invested in the life course of individuals and hence need to be adaptable in different digital environments across the continuum of care and over the patient journey. From our perspective as healthcare providers, however, it is folly for technology to overshadow the clinician-patient interaction or to allow it to diminish the patient experience. Patient-centred care, being respectful of an individual's preferences, needs, and values, has been instilled in AHPs as a cornerstone of practice. In the participatory health paradigm, the clinician strives to uphold patients as the focus of healthcare by engaging with them as equal partners in the process of shared decision-making towards managing their own health. The growing shift towards participatory health also provides an avenue for patients to influence the design of digital tools and solutions; we see that these, in turn, could strengthen patient engagement with their own care as well as improve the patient experience. "Basic premise of care for the patient should always remain at the cornerstone of our interactions." (Author YP).

Implications and Recommendations

The themes uncovered and discussed in this chapter (education steps, career pathways, unique attributes, and future perspectives) speak to the existing and future allied health workforce and provide them with a compass to navigate their careers in an increasingly digitised world.

The field of allied health poses challenges due to its heterogeneity while at the same time it affords unique opportunities to drive the digital information workforce forward. The advancement of the digital allied health informatics workforce is driven from the desire for the digital enablement of better data collection and synthesis to improve health care and reporting. Success will require addressing the substantial data and information silos created across the various allied health disciplines, as well as greater attention to interoperability challenges created by multiple discrete connected devices and systems. This workforce can bring about change from the push to provide evidence of outcomes to support funding of healthcare and to incorporate digital into models of care to improve access and empower clients to engage in their own care.

Coordinated and concerted efforts need to go into advancing both the formal and informal channels for education in digital health information for allied health professionals. Also required is attention to the development of formal career pathways that included leadership roles for AHPs in digital health information. For this work to progress, further research needs to be undertaken to understand better and manage resistance to change in this space.

Developing and harnessing a digital allied health information workforce will deliver benefits for clients in improved health outcomes, satisfaction with care, participatory health, and safety of care. It will deliver benefits for allied health practitioners regarding better access to data, data quality improvements, workflow efficiencies, career, and leadership opportunities. A stronger allied health information workforce is a stronger basis for sound evidence for health funding, and sound health system performance, and a culture of innovation in care.

References

Anderson R. Thematic Content Analysis (TCA): descriptive presentation of qualitative data. Institute of Transpersonal Psychology: Palo Alto, CA; 2007.

Benoot C, Bilsen J. An auto-ethnographic study of the disembodied experience of a novice researcher doing qualitative cancer research. Qual Health Res. 2016;26(4):482–9.

Butler-Henderson K, Dalton L, Probst Y, Maunder K, Merolli M. A meta-synthesis of competency standards suggest allied health are not preparing for a digital health future. Int J Med Inform. 2020;144:104296.

Chang H. Autoethnography in health research: growing pains? Qual Health Res. 2016;26(4):443–51.

Coiera E. Why e-health is so hard. Med J Australia. 2013;198(4):178–9.

Fridsma DB. Health informatics: a required skill for 21st century clinicians. BMJ (Clinical research ed). 2018;362:k3043.

Fridsma DB. Strengthening our profession by defining clinical and health informatics practice. J Am Med Inform Assoc: JAMIA. 2019;26(7):585.

Gray K, Choo D, Butler-Henderson K, Whetton S, Maeder A. Health informatics and e-health curriculum for clinical health profession degrees. Stud Health Technol Inform. 2015;214:68–73.

Greenhalgh T, Wherton J, Shaw S, Morrison C. Video consultations for COVID-19. BMJ (Clinical research ed). 2020;368:m998.

Health Informatics Society of Australia (HISA). Allied health professionals: the untapped potential in digital health – Position Statement. Melbourne; 2019.

Houston ML, Yu AP, Martin DA, Probst DY. Defining and developing a generic framework for monitoring data quality in clinical research. AMIA Annu Symp Proc. 2018;2018:1300–9.

Maunder K, Walton K, Williams P, Ferguson M, Beck E. A framework for eHealth readiness of dietitians. Int J Med Inform. 2018;115:43–52.

Maunder K, Walton K, Williams P, Ferguson M, Beck E. Strategic leadership will be essential for dietitian eHealth readiness: a qualitative study exploring dietitian perspectives of eHealth readiness. Nutr Diet. 2019;76(4):373–81.

NHS. Allied health professions into action: using Allied Health Professionals to transform health, care and wellbeing. England: NHS; 2017.

NHS. Clinical informatics and digital delivery in health and care: a career framework for nurses and allied health professionals. England: NHS; 2018.

NHS. A digital framework for allied health professionals. England: NHS; 2019.

Philip K. Allied health: untapped potential in the Australian health system. Aust Health Rev. 2015;39(3):244–7.

Chapter 22
Working as a Medical Informatician

Daniel Capurro, Rebecca Grainger, and Daniel Luna

Abstract Medical professionals frequently have to forge their own paths to achieve proficiency and learn the core components of clinical informatics, understood as the "application of informatics and information technology to deliver healthcare services" [American Medical Informatics Association (Clinical informatics. 2021. https://www.amia.org/applications-informatics/clinical-informatics)]. In this chapter, we present the personal stories of three medical doctors, from different parts of the world, and what motivated, guided, and inspired their journey. Several common themes emerge. The first is self-directed learning, strong mentorship, and the need for the on-going building of communities of practices to share experiences and knowledge. Secondly, there is strong desire to formalise learning during our careers, and we found different ways to achieve this. Finally, health informatics is more about health, clinicians, healthcare and patients and less about informatics, and clinical informatics sits at the core of clinical care. Although the routes and timing of these journeys varied, resonating throughout is a deep desire to impact patients' lives and improve the ways we provide healthcare.

Keywords Case study · Clinical informatics · Chief Medical Information Officer · Mentorship · Community of practice

D. Capurro (✉)
University of Melbourne, Melbourne, Australia
e-mail: dcapurro@unimelb.edu.au

R. Grainger
University of Otago, Wellington, New Zealand
e-mail: rebecca.grainger@otago.ac.nz

D. Luna
Hospital Italiano de Buenos Aires, Buenos Aires, Argentina
e-mail: daniel.luna@hospitalitaliano.org.ar

K. Butler-Henderson et al. (eds.), *The Health Information Workforce*, Health Informatics, https://doi.org/10.1007/978-3-030-81850-0_22

Daniel Luna: Hospital Italiano, Buenos Aires

I am currently the Chief Information Officer (CIO) of a private hospital in Buenos Aires, Argentina. Hospital Italiano de Buenos Aires (HIBA) is a non-profit medical academic centre established in 1853. It has a network of 2 hospitals with 750 beds, 41 operating rooms, 800 home care beds, 25 outpatient clinics and 150 associated private practices located in Buenos Aires City and its suburban area. Since 1998, HIBA has been running an internally developed health information system, which encompasses both clinical and administrative data. Recently, we achieved the Health and Information Management System Society (HIMSS) Electronic Medical Record Adoption Model (EMRAM) certification at Level 7, the highest level possible.

When I was 17, my father suggested that there were no physicians in the family, so I decided to become a doctor. I went to Buenos Aires University. During my time in medical school I held different jobs, including in a public library, as an electrical technician, even as a DJ in a famous discotheque, which I loved. Having two or three jobs allowed me to be completely independent of my parents, which was pretty exciting at the time. I always thought that I would have certainly found passion in many other activities too.

After graduating from university, I decided to become a practising clinician. Someone recommended me to train at HIBA; I have been there ever since. I have worked as a clinician for more than 20 years and, as a primary care physician, I have had more than 900 patients under my care. In daily practice, I could experience first-hand the doctor's information needs in the decision-making process. I also realised that data integration for public health was a complex fundamental essential requirement.

During my internal medicine residency, we were required to prepare training resources for our colleagues. Usually, I could use slide presentations as graphic resources, but I felt that this was not enough. For me, one of the biggest challenges was how to treat diabetic ketoacidosis. At that time, I created a spread sheet containing formulas for the standardised and systematic treatment of these patients. That was my first contact with informatics tools. It was also during my residence when I was asked to join a team of local researchers. That is when I met Doctor Fernán Quiros, a real mentor, who has had the most significant professional influence on me. Among the many projects we were engaged in, the most complex one was addressing the need for an electronic medical record. I thought of this as a personal challenge. After evaluating different commercial products worldwide, we proposed an in-house-development project.

It was then when I started to study the field of medical informatics on my own. I often searched for articles related to implementation experiences, participated in conferences, and began publishing scientific papers on the topic. I spent many summer vacations reading the proceedings of the American Medical Informatics Association (AMIA) Annual Symposium while at the beach. We began to slowly design an electronic health record based on our daily work. While working as a clinician, I would think of possible functionalities, and I would ask the system engineer to develop them. I became a tester and a bug reporter. In this way, I actively participated in the iterative cycle of software development.

After years of working for free and teaching myself about medical informatics, the Department of Health Informatics was finally established at HIBA in 2000. I was responsible for leading the development and implementation of the institution-wide Clinical Information System and served as Chief Medical Information Officer for 10 years. We created and coordinated the Medical Informatics Residency at HIBA to train clinicians in the discipline. To date, it is the only one of its kind in Latin America. Soon, I realised that I needed formal training, as I was missing the latest knowledge—on security and infrastructure issues for example. I began a master's degree and a PhD. This was a significant challenge since, at that time I was married, and we had three children. I completed a Master of Science in Engineering of Information Systems at Universidad Tecnológica Nacional in 2016. The following year I obtained my PhD in Informatics Engineering at the Technological Institute of Buenos Aires. At that time, I became a HIMSS Certified Professional in Health Information Management Systems, and in 2020 I was named an Independent Researcher of the National Scientific and Technical Research Council (CONICET) of Argentina.

As a Chief Information Officer my constant challenge is to nurture an innovative, high-performance team of professionals who can develop local and regional leadership. I consider that a big part of that has been achieved.

Today, after 20 years of working in the health informatics department, 10 years as a CIO, and visiting 38 different countries around the world because of my professional activities, there are two key lessons I have learned. First, health informatics is not only about computers, monitors or mobile devices. It involves information systems: information workflow in health organisations, and information needs of both healthcare providers and patients. Devices may change over time, but the information system will always exist and always be the necessary foundation. Second, health informatics is not different to any other clinical specialty; it is an opportunity to change a patient's life. In this case, the discipline has allowed me to change hundreds and maybe thousands of patients' lives at the same time.

Rebecca Grainger: Hutt Hospital and University of Otago, New Zealand

My formal journey in health informatics started with an informal conversation in a corridor. I was known by my clinical rheumatology colleagues in a New Zealand public hospital and academic colleagues at a university as an early adopter of technology. Our patients and other stakeholders were increasingly wondering why the "health system" did not adopt more flexible and user-friendly ways of interacting— mobile technology and web-based. One lunchtime a colleague asked me "Rebecca, you are into technology, would an app be useful in patient-led management of rheumatoid arthritis?" I was intrigued by the idea but being "into technology" did not extend much past Twitter, Evernote and a few useful apps on my phone. I had no formal, or even informal, training or education in anything that seemed remotely related to the emerging field of digital health. This suddenly seemed untenable in a world where digital was the direction of travel for all business and social aspects of life. Thus began a new direction in my career—into health informatics. Now, 5 years later, much of my research focuses on aspects of health informatics and I contribute to the local information and communications infrastructure development in my hospital.

After that conversation I looked for every opportunity to learn and upskill in health informatics. Knowing myself and theories of adult learning, I found communities of practice where I could learn with and from others. Joining Health Informatics New Zealand and attending every seminar, workshop and conference provided insights into the current status of, challenges to, and trends in the digital health landscape in New Zealand. This also provided some base knowledge in the principles and practice of health informatics as a discipline. However, I was aware my knowledge was patchy. The health informatics competencies framework developed for the Certified Health Informatics Australasia (CHIA) (2013) certification provided me a comprehensive and regionally relevant resource to understand the knowledge and skills necessary for competent practice. My undergraduate and postgraduate medical education had already provided ample training in relevant aspects of scientific skills, health science and human and social factors but little in aspects of health informatics, information and communication technology, information science or management science. I, therefore, directed my learning to these areas, using recommended readings from the CHIA certification and any in-person or online learning that I could access. This included completing several MOOCs—massive online open courses—from top international institutions. This organic and self-directed learning may not be ideal, and I would recommend that others explore formal tertiary offerings in health informatics, however with significant work and family commitments, formal studies were not an option for me. After my knowledge increased, I registered for the CHIA certification and successfully passed the rigorous examination. Using the CHIA competencies, I established an on-going professional development plan in health informatics which meant I was able to recertify after 3 years. My research activities, mainly focusing on technology in supporting self-management in chronic conditions and medical education, keep my knowledge up to date, along with reading key health informatics journals regularly and attending regional health informatics conferences. A key motivator of my health informatics research theme is to provide increased knowledge about how technology can enhance and improve health outcomes, without assuming that a product will always be the answer. A key theme of my research has been a focus on the people and processes around the product—these are often overlooked. It has been possible to apply research skills developed in biomedical and health sciences to health informatics, however research methods are sometimes less well defined and challenges, such as the ethical considerations of research in social media, abound.

My clinical work has been influenced by my health informatics journey too. For health professionals in 2020, the use of information and communication technology is an everyday part of clinical care. Within my clinical service, I have contributed to the development of information, communication and technology (ICT) tools for management of team processes and patient care. Within my District Health Board (providers of government-funded health and disability services for a local population in New Zealand) I contribute to committees which address practical and governance aspects of ICT developments. I have found that the multidisciplinary nature of these committees continues to enhance my understanding of how interdependent different parts of the health system are, which is highly evident when focusing on shared electronic tools, patient care and staff workflows.

Most recently, my clinical, academic and health informatics roles and skills provided a unique and meaningful way to contribute to the global response to COVID-19. In early March 2020, one of my online communities of practice, the Rheumatology community on Twitter, identified that the COVID-19 pandemic was likely to have a particular impact on the patients we serve. This potentially included increased vulnerability to infection with or outcomes from COVID-19, and reduced access to pharmacological treatments, which were being disrupted by a rush to use hydroxychloroquine for COVID-19. This Twitter community responded by forming a virtual team collaborating online, the COVID-19 Global Rheumatology Alliance, who rapidly developed a global disease registry and an international patient registry, facilitated via social media. This international initiative leveraged knowledge and skills across all six competency streams of health informatics, showing that in 2020 health informatics is really just about health.

Daniel Capurro: University of Melbourne

As happens with many clinical informaticists, I stumbled upon this career through chance; the path has been winding and mentorship has been fundamental in understanding a field that was still defining itself.

I trained as a medical doctor (MD) in Chile, where medical education is a 7-year program that includes clinical internships. Halfway through my training—in 1998—I met a senior clinician who, after a quick chat, suggested I read Learning Clinical Reasoning, a book by a former Chief Editor of the New England Journal of Medicine (Kassirer and Kopelman 1991). Being able to understand the diagnostic process explicitly, and quantify how each symptom, physical finding, and laboratory test could contribute to structured reasoning about the probabilities of disease, was transformational. Immediately, it became apparent that we, clinicians, were making clinical decisions with uncertain information; we were using data about what we remember, about what we had experienced in the past, subject to our individual biases. There had to be a better way. Those were the early days of the Internet, Amazon was already around, and I ordered a copy of Ted Shortliffe's Medical Informatics (1991).

After graduating with my MD, it was time to decide my next steps, but there weren't many people to ask about medical informatics (as we called the field back then). It was hard then, as it is still today, to explain what a health informatician is or does; a few academics suggested talking to the School of Medicine's webmaster; that conversation didn't go very far. My interest in quantitative decision-making pushed me towards Evidence-Based Medicine (EBM) where I learned how health informatics, the biomedical literature, and—overall—the whole problem of knowledge translation are deeply connected. With a significant proportion of our time as clinicians spent searching, organising and generating information, healthcare has become an information discipline.

I finally decided to complete my medical training in internal medicine, where the spectrum of clinical decision-making would be fully expressed, and I would obtain a broad perspective on how clinical care really worked. During the residency years, I met lifelong mentors from whom I learned about patient care and rigorous decision-making. My understanding of health informatics was still peripheral. With no training programs in Chile, I moved to the USA, supported by a Fulbright Fellowship and the Chilean Ministry of Education. I enrolled in a PhD in Biomedical and Health Informatics at the University of Washington. The PhD years were spent learning about the shortcomings of clinical informatics and the need for sound methods to improve our ability to reuse routinely collected clinical data for secondary purposes such as quality improvement and research.

After the PhD, I returned to Chile and began working at a university healthcare network consisting of two hospitals (approximately 600 beds) and 11 outpatient clinics. I became an advisor to the clinician who was leading the implementation of a new electronic medical record. Shortly, I was asked to step in as the network's first Chief Medical Information Officer. Only then I realised how much I did not know about clinical informatics.

Juggling my research on digital phenotyping in parallel, I became forcefully exposed to concepts I never learned during my medical training nor the PhD. Project management, change management, clinician engagement, software quality assurance, stress tests, development environments, contract management, 24/7 on-call duties and so on. I found some comfort in reading "All systems down", an article describing a major system crash that happened at Beth Israel Deaconess, in Boston, back in 2002 (Berinato 2003). If you work in clinical informatics and haven't read it, you should. But even more relevant than all the IT stuff I learned during those years, the most significant learning came from working with nurses. None of them had a formal education in clinical informatics—they had all learned a lot by doing—but they all had a deep understanding of clinical workflow, patient-centred care, and the clinical risks of incorporating technologies into clinical care. Just as nurses' perception of a patient's gravity can be a powerful predictor of adverse events (Romero-Brufau et al. 2019), I experienced first-hand their ability to detect risks imposed by new technologies. It was a humbling and productive period, certainly not pain-free. We were able to create the Clinical Informatics Unit and make it part of the organisational chart and slowly started to incorporate clinical informatics into crucial decision-making processes inside the organisation. Together we learned about the perils and consequences of embarking on implementing a new electronic medical record when it is not an explicit part of the strategy. Before spending so much energy and resources, clinical organisations must ensure that it perfectly aligns with its mission, vision and values. Return on investment is not a useful metric to assess such an endeavour.

I spent almost 4 years as CMIO before moving to Australia to pursue a full-time involvement in health informatics research. During those years, I had the privilege of working with colleagues in other Chilean universities and, with them, founded the National Centre for Health Information Systems. I recently joined the University of Melbourne School of Computing and Information Systems; I believe I am the only medical doctor among the academic staff of that School. I feel that the impostor syndrome has reached new heights as a result of me being among people who know so much about things of which I know so little. On the other hand, I believe that my combined 15 years of clinical experience and the time I spent as CMIO helps provide a different perspective and understanding to those who conduct research in digital health.

There is still a long way to go. I still struggle to explain what I do to people unfamiliar with health informatics, but it feels like we are now at a turning point. The COVID-19 epidemic forced everyone, including patients, to rethink the way we seek and deliver healthcare. Health data analytics and predictive models are in the news daily. It is time to embrace that healthcare is an information discipline and health informatics is at its core.

References

American Medical Informatics Association. Clinical informatics. 2021. https://www.amia.org/applications-informatics/clinical-informatics. Accessed 17 Feb 2021.

Berinato S. All systems down. Computerworld. 2003. https://www.computerworld.com/article/2581420/all-systems-down.html. Accessed 29 Jul 2020.

CHIA. Health informatics competencies framework. 2013. https://www.healthinformaticscertification.com/wp-content/uploads/2016/02/CHIA-competencies-Framework_FINAL.pdf. Accessed 28 Jul 2020.

Kassirer JP, Kopelman RI. Learning clinical reasoning. Baltimore: Williams & Wilkins; 1991.

Romero-Brufau S, Gaines K, Nicolas CT, Johnson MG, Hickman J, Huddleston JM. The fifth vital sign? Nurse worry predicts inpatient deterioration within 24 hours. JAMIA Open. 2019;2:465–70.

Chapter 23
Working as a Nursing and Midwifery Informatician

Karen Day, Sally Britnell, Lisa Livingstone, Abin Chacko, and Karen Blake

Abstract Information is integral to the work of nurses and midwives, as they gather, analyse and use data to perform clinical activities, keep private information confidential, and support the healing of those for whom they care. Evidence-based care is fundamental to their practice, and information management is part of their training, to varying degrees. Once they have completed their training, some nurses and midwives augment their professional profile and become information specialists. Nurses and midwives are the largest component of the clinical workforce, so possibly nursing and midwifery information specialists are the largest invisible subgroup in the health information specialist workforce. In this chapter we explore the history of nursing and midwifery informatics, how it has been incorporated in training, and what nurses are doing now. Five narratives from practitioners in Australasian health care systems describe their identity, the impact of their work (now and yet to

K. Day (✉)
School of Population Health, University of Auckland, Auckland, New Zealand
e-mail: k.day@auckland.ac.nz

S. Britnell
Nursing Department, School of Clinical Sciences, Auckland University of Technology, Auckland, New Zealand
e-mail: sally.britnell@aut.ac.nz

L. Livingstone
Nelson Marlborough District Health Board, Nelson, New Zealand
e-mail: Lisa.Livingstone@nmdhb.govt.nz

A. Chacko
Waitemata District Health Board, Auckland, New Zealand
e-mail: Abin.Chacko@waitload.dhb.govt.nz

K. Blake
Office of the CCIO, healthAlliance NZ Ltd, Auckland, New Zealand
e-mail: karen.blake@healthalliance.co.nz

© The Author(s), under exclusive license to Springer Nature Switzerland AG 2021
K. Butler-Henderson et al. (eds.), *The Health Information Workforce*, Health Informatics, https://doi.org/10.1007/978-3-030-81850-0_23

be seen) and their role in creating and implementing innovations to improve the care they and their colleagues deliver.

Keywords Case study · Nursing · Midwifery · Clinical informatics · Nursing informatics

Introduction

Nursing and midwifery take on many forms, but this field is essentially about care, advocacy and assisting people through life and health transitions (Meleis et al. 2000). A great deal of this caring relies on a broad range of skills and activities that are based on co-ordination with other clinicians (from the multidisciplinary team), safe processes that enhance health outcomes, and reliable and trustworthy information systems to support the information needs of those both providing and consuming nursing and midwifery services (Nursing Council of New Zealand 2017). The nursing workforce accounts for 59% of the total health professional workforce globally (World Health organization 2020). If nursing is the largest group of the health workforce, then nursing and midwifery informaticians are the most invisible subgroup amongst the Health Informatics, Digital, Data Information and kNowledge (HIDDIN) specialist workforce. This is despite the fact that nursing informatics competencies have been clearly documented over the years (Hübner et al. 2018), especially since the inception of Technology Informatics Guiding Education Reform (TIGER) in 2004. Florence Nightingale, a statistician, a trained nurse, and famous for her work in the Crimean War, is the first known nursing information specialist (Brixey et al. 2020). Her own claim that her work with data would not become the norm in nursing for another 150 years was prescient. The earliest signs of digital nursing informatics as a specialisation appeared in the late 1960s when electronic health records were just beginning to emerge from the medico-legal records of clinicians (Honey et al. 2020). Paradoxically, the development of information systems in the nursing and midwifery workplace has been slower than for medicine. Nursing information needs are in some ways different from, and in other ways similar to, those of other clinicians, e.g. laboratory results are shared by the whole interdisciplinary healthcare team, but nurses need nursing-specific data (e.g. to calculate patient acuity in order to map nursing resources appropriately), the automation of certain activities (e.g. vital signs measurements), and support for evidence-based nursing care. A survey during the 2020 International Year of the Nurse and the Midwife documents dynamic changes in nursing information specialist roles in the development, implementation, and optimisation of electronic medical/health records, nursing clinical documentation, point-of-care clinical decision support, and computerised practitioner order entry (HIMSS 2020). The case studies in this chapter describe the career journeys of five nursing information specialists in New Zealand and Australia. They outline how their early nursing or midwifery identities were expanded or defined by information specialisation, and what they were able to achieve in terms of impact and innovation.

Sally Britnell, Auckland University of Technology, New Zealand

The theme that runs through my narrative is improving patient care by doing a 'defrag'. All my life I have been known as someone curious who strived to help others to be the best that they could be. After doing a post-secondary overseas experience year and completing a Diploma in Recreation Management, I started my journey to becoming a registered nurse as a mature student in 1994. I completed my degree at a time when nursing informatics was just beginning to emerge, but as a new graduate nurse, my focus was on learning to become a nurse, which meant that innovation and incorporation of informatics did not appear on my radar immediately.

I was privileged to marry a man who was a researcher and developer in a successful software company, which reignited my passion for data and technology. I coupled this with my keen interest in improving what we do through streamlining processes and I was always tinkering with things that made my job as a registered nurse more effective and agile. What I ran up against in the healthcare system was a series of solutions that solved parts of problems, but these were not united, and although this tendency has improved, the siloed approach is still evident in practice today. At that time, the nursing workforce in New Zealand was not using health data or technology on an everyday basis to improve patient care.

In the late 1990s, I worked as a Practice Nurse in a low socioeconomic status area. The immunisation statistics at the practice showed that 6.6% of eligible children were immunised. It seemed hard to believe that the families of the remaining 93.4% of children chose not to immunise. The MS-DOS-based computer system used at the time included a recall system via printing letters and making phone calls. I found that patient data was missing or incorrect in many places, coupled with many households having low health literacy and no access to a phone, which made follow-up challenging. It was this experience that showed me the importance of accurate data in providing optimal healthcare. I made it my mission to collect accurate data and implement strategies such as spending time in the waiting room talking with families and getting to know their challenges, thus allowing more open communication, all the while updating patient records using the information I found out, which led to an immunisation rate of over 60% after 1 year.

These challenges prompted me to study Computer Science at the University of Auckland while working part-time as a practice nurse. Although I didn't finish a formal qualification at this time, I learned what was possible. I used my new skills to develop software for tracking medical staff for a volunteer organisation and other smaller projects. These included assisting with an Installfest (an event where experienced users help others install a computer operating system) for the Engineering Department at the University of Auckland, speaking at a conference (giving an introduction to Linux and promoting Linux at a Computerworld event) and assisting in running a Quake Server (an online multi-player game) at an Armageddon Expo.

In 2004 while working as a registered nurse in a large District Health Board (DHB) in Auckland I again ran into siloed systems and a culture of very controlled use of technology. For example, nurses across a department were not allowed email addresses or a computer login of their own; instead, they shared a department login to look up patient information, lab results, and X-rays. A DHB could not digitally share much information, such as X-rays, blood results, and patient alerts, making patient care fragmented on a national level. It was at this point that I began to question why the systems and technology were not fit for purpose. I knew what was possible using data and technology but was unable to implement this in the role I had. I tried to discover why processes and systems were siloed and whether it was the healthcare system, or the DHB, or the advancement of technology, that was making integration impossible. I changed roles to become an infection control nurse specialist, where I enjoyed and valued the use of data to improve patient care.

In 2011 I moved into academia, allowing me to research, educate future nurses, and ultimately change and streamline their practice. I gained a Master of Health Science including a thesis, completing many small projects along the way in nursing informatics and online learning. I became known for innovation and investigating emerging technologies and became a part of the health informatics community in New Zealand and internationally. In 2015 I began my PhD in Computing and Mathematics, where I could finally combine my nursing knowledge and passion for streamlining processes using technology. My PhD project modelled the New Zealand Health Survey data and used this in the design and development of a mobile application for clinical decision making in paediatric resuscitation (MOH NZ 2020; Britnell 2020).

My informatics journey continues through doing research, inspiring future nurses, and working in a team developing informatics guidelines and resources to support nursing informatics in New Zealand. It has taken 25 years to reach an expert position where I can pass on my passions, curiosity, innovation, technology, and nursing to improve patient care. I plan to continue challenging the status quo to allow us to work smarter in providing healthcare for New Zealanders.

Lisa Livingstone, Nelson Marlborough District Health Board, New Zealand

Advocating for clinician-friendly information systems is the theme of my narrative. Nursing is in my blood, the 'family business', although I fought the call for a long time. After being accepted into training and turning it down in 1990 I finally graduated in 2002. By this time, I had been very successful in my chosen career of hospitality and I suddenly went from expert to novice overnight.

Curiosity has been a strong theme in my nursing career to date; I always questioned why and was never satisfied with the answer, 'Because that's how it is done'.

My constant need to see improvements in healthcare, along with a strong management background, led to my career move into nursing management in 2008. This was where my interest in processes and informatics really began. I could see that clinical staff were struggling to achieve outcomes, not due to clinical abilities, but rather because the information systems they were using to collect data were not set up in a way that supported them. In theory the systems were in place to improve patient flow and support the clinical team to identify barriers, but in fact the systems themselves were the barriers. I worked on these systems, being involved in clinical projects and looking at ways we could work with the technology provided to support and guide the work being done. I never once thought about the fact that I was becoming involved in health informatics; I am not sure whether I even knew then that it was a field in which I possibly could work.

Over the next 10 years I developed my nursing career, moving around a number of organisations, always questioning how the clinical informatics systems that we were using worked for the clinician: Were we capturing the right data at the right time and then presenting this to the right people? One organisation where I worked was building a new hospital that aimed to be paperless. I left the organisation before the hospital opened; when I later visited with their newly appointed Chief Nursing Informatics Officer I learned that they did not move into the building paperless, but they were paper-light. We both reflected on the challenges of enabling enough clinical voices to be heard, to ensure change that works for clinicians—but not so many voices that you end up trying to 'boil the ocean' and never see any change.

In 2018 I moved to where I now work full time in clinical informatics within a large DHB. Initially I was seconded for 12 months to be the clinical lead on a project to implement an electronic observation and assessment system. I finally had an opportunity to work with vendors and clinicians on making sure that the system worked for the clinician not the other way around. I learnt so much during that first 12 months and at the end of the project, with the system successfully introduced into the DHB, I accepted a permanent role within the informatics team. My role is ever evolving which in itself has challenges at times. I am a project manager, sometimes a clinical advocate, and often an interpreter between the clinical and informatics teams. My role is at a strategic level looking at opportunities and working others to set the organisation's health informatics direction; it also entails working alongside clinicians to bring ideas to life in the organisation.

What has not changed in my purpose, and in fact has been cemented, is the need for health informatics to be data driven, patient driven, and clinician-friendly. Too often I have seen clinical applications that silo information, and in turn create silos within clinical teams, and thus create patient safety issues. Another barrier I see within many organisations is the impact of low digital literacy on clinicians' engagement with the informatics team. Having experienced going from expert to novice several times in my life, I know that unless you approach change with curiosity and willingness you create barriers to learning. I believe that my work has brought down some of these barriers and given clinical teams and informatics teams a better way to communicate with each other. There is still a long way to go, but we are now at least on the same page and talking.

Abin Chacko, Waitemata District Health Board, New Zealand

The theme of my career is walking the floor with digital implementations. In 2009 I migrated from India to New Zealand as a registered nurse. The main difference I noticed in my new ward at a New Zealand metropolitan hospital was the presence of an electronic medication dispensing system called Pyxis. There were a few computers available in the ward, and as a nurse, I accessed the computers in the ward only when required, e.g., to review blood results and radiology reports. The desktop computers were usually occupied by doctors reviewing results or completing discharge summaries.

Soon after I arrived, we received the exciting news that the DHB was introducing an electronic workload management system where you could predict a patient's acuity, analyse the requirement of nursing hours, and document shift notes electronically for handover. Before that, the nursing shift handover was a manual process where you waited for your turn to scribble down notes against your patient's name on a piece of paper, so that the coordinators could hand over to the incoming shift. The time-consuming handover process involved referring to these notes and ran the risk of missing essential things that may not have been written down on the piece of paper. The new technology was exciting, and I took the opportunity to be a super-user, providing support to new users as part of the implementation team. Post-implementation, I noticed a dramatic change in our clinical work: electronic prescribing, smart messaging, electronic bedside patient monitoring and other aspects of care were poured into the nursing workflow. During this time, I completed a Master's degree in nursing, with a project focus on the nursing leadership role in managing chronic post-surgical pain and incorporating electronic solutions in assessing a patient's pain.

In 2017, I took a role as a clinical coach in a project team managing the implementation of an electronic bedside patient monitoring system where nurses can record vital signs and most of their nursing assessments electronically. I was a bit nervous during the initial days as the workspace was entirely different from what I was used to, and I started hearing new technical terminologies. Many times, it felt like this was not for me; I could not see myself enjoying work away from caring at the patient's bedside. Going back to the floor of the ward in a different role was not initially comfortable, but the move eventually helped me to listen and understand many things which I had never imagined that my nursing colleagues felt about digital changes. Most nurses felt very optimistic about the digital changes but, at the same time, some nurses shared their concerns in terms of computer skills, time management, and increasing complexity in the nursing workload. I realised that I needed to learn more about leadership and coaching to be more efficient in my role, so I completed a UK National Health Service online leadership course as well as other leadership training locally. The organisation where I work was very supportive and provided training for clinical leaders managing clinical workflow changes. I took the opportunity to be in the first cohort of a Digital Academy for clinical leaders run by the DHB.

I stepped up to a clinical nurse specialist role from the clinical coach role in late 2019. I enjoy meeting various clinical experts, understanding their needs and work-flow and assisting them with a digital solution wherever possible. It is a great plea-sure consulting about the clinical needs with a vendor so that they can translate it into a technical functionality. I believe change management is still a great challenge, but I can lead change effectively by listening to end-users, by supporting, directing and guiding them regularly, and by responding to their queries.

I am very optimistic about the digital future of nursing. Being a nurse is a highly rewarding job where you receive an opportunity to touch many lives, and ultimately, we want to provide safer care to patients. Digital solutions have the potential to enhance a nurse's decision making and the nursing care process in order to provide better patient care, faster and smarter. Chasing after clinical notes, time-consuming searches for relevant data, one-way pager communication and duplicated documen-tation—among other things—will soon be history in many hospitals. Digital solu-tions will enable nurses to enjoy improved access to health records, more coordinated and streamlined care planning, the ability to schedule assessments with automated reminders, and effective communication with the healthcare team. However the nursing profession, including those in teaching, policy-making and clinical practice, faces a massive responsibility to prepare the current and future nursing workforce to use technology effectively. With the increasing use of technology in nursing care, strategies to maintain patient privacy and to reduce the risk of negative impact on nurses' critical thinking abilities and patient outcomes are paramount. Constant monitoring and robust research are required to assess the impact of digital solutions on nursing practice and patient outcomes.

Karen Blake, healthAlliance NZ Ltd, New Zealand

'Learning and leading, leading and learning' is the story of how I approach my work. When I first trained as a direct-entry midwife (that is, becoming a creden-tialed midwife without first becoming a nurse) in the late 1990s in New Zealand the career options seemed threefold—work as a clinical midwife, work in management, or work in education—and during my 20 years as a practicing midwife I have done all those things. I have practised clinically in New Zealand and in Australia, from maternal foetal medicine in large tertiary hospitals to water births and home births in the community. I was the first direct-entry midwife in Australia to become a Director of Nursing and Midwifery, managing a sub-acute and day surgery facility. I am passionate about education, working both as a clinical educator and university lecturer. I have also discovered new career options as a senior policy advisor in Australian state government, learning to understand the machinery of government and the development and implementation of policy.

An enterprise Electronic Medical Record (EMR) project first propelled me into clinical informatics. I had worked as a clinical super-user of an EMR, had done project management and service redesign, and was generally known as someone who was 'good with computers'. During a coffee break with the Executive Director of Nursing and Midwifery at the Melbourne hospital where I worked, I was asked to apply for a newly created role to support this EMR project: Chief Nursing and Midwifery Information Officer (CNMIO). I tried to appear knowledgeable, enthusiastic and excited about the opportunity; however, the first thing I did after going back to my office was to Google, 'What is a CNMIO?' and (because I was curious), 'What does a CNMIO earn?'. I wholeheartedly embraced this opportunity and experience, finding my feet relatively quickly and working with the newly appointed Chief Medical Information Officer (CMIO) to create a team of clinical subject matter experts. I loved working alongside the EMR project team too, and learning all about a large EMR implementation. This role became a strong foundation to build the next steps in my career in clinical informatics.

Following a move back to New Zealand—having already accumulated a wealth of qualifications from health care leadership to project management, data standards, complex obstetrics and informatics—I embarked on more postgraduate study in health informatics. I also took on a new role at healthAlliance, a shared service provider that provides the Information and Communications Technology (ICT) services for the four northern region DHBs. As Head of Clinical Informatics, I work to ensure that everything we provide and implement meets the requirements of the clinicians working across the region and the patients they care for. In order to do the breadth or work required, I have collaborated with the Chief Clinical Information Officer (CCIO) to build a team of specialist informaticians, including nursing, midwifery, pharmacy, and medicine. I believe that in order to fully understand health and how best to develop and implement ICT, we need the collective wisdom of a multidisciplinary team with a wide range of clinical experience underpinned by a theoretical knowledge base.

What continues to resonate with me and forms a large part of my approach to my work as a clinical informatician is being able to learn and critically evaluate new information, and bring that into my work, becoming a more effective advisor with every opportunity. I have an in-depth understanding about the healthcare system and the impacts of technology on clinical staff, patients and consumers, and health operations. I also am able to learn about technology, processes and systems—distributed denial of service attacks, and containerisation to support a cloud migration strategy, and application programming interface gateways, and identity and access management. It is this on going quest for learning that contributes to success in my role and makes my work so rewarding.

Karen Day, University of Auckland, New Zealand

Changing how we work is the theme of my narrative. It was 1980 and I was training for my Diploma in General Nursing and Midwifery. In the half-kilometre-long building that was the new Johannesburg Hospital, we sat before computers and learned how to search for patients, complete the midnight report, and admit, transfer and discharge patients electronically. It was exciting and scary in the belly of this immense 2000 bed hospital, where we had to walk through the 'tunnel' and past the mortuary to get to the computer department. My dream was to influence how health care was organised, managed and delivered on a national level, so I went on to complete a Bachelor of Arts, majoring in public health nursing and health service management. By then I was nursing in a small urban hospital rehabilitation unit for people recovering from brain injuries and spinal cord injuries and associated complications. There were no computers. When the Nursing Process was introduced to standardise care, in the late 1980s, I felt overwhelmed by the documentation and I wondered how a computer could support this work.

By 1995 I was half way through my Master of Arts, using data on 100,000 members of a medical insurance scheme to apply a managed care intervention in an effort to create a market advantage for my employer. My nursing skills, coupled with latterly acquired insurance underwriting skills, were leveraged to manage a prescription benefit for people with long-term health issues. Fourteen per cent of the membership base had long-term health issues, and we applied a managed care structure and rules to their use of the benefit. This was the basis of my Master's thesis. A year later this work became the reason for a start-up insurance scheme in a gold mining house west of Johannesburg, to employ me to establish its claims and managed care divisions. When the pre-selected information system failed, we recruited a software company to co-design and develop a bespoke claims system that included managed care processes. As the claims data grew in the information system, I analysed the practice profiles of the services and clinicians such as general practitioners (GPs) to detect variance in clinical care and resource use. I had no idea that the work I was doing was informatics.

By the time I arrived in New Zealand in 1999 I was comfortable at the computer, and had other skills such as data analysis in spread sheets, information system design and implementation, data driven staff management skills, and the ability to use routinely collected claims data to assess the quality of care delivered by clinicians in primary and secondary care. My first job in New Zealand was to build a decision support system for prescribing in software designed for use by primary care clinicians—although I did not understand what I was doing until years later, in these terms. At the time I was called a 'knowledge advisor' and asked to source information about medications available in New Zealand and set up a system to support GPs as they wrote prescriptions.

When I moved on and joined a project team as a change manager in a large urban District Health Board in Auckland, it felt like this was the kind of work I wanted to do for the rest of my life, this blend of nursing, midwifery, information systems, innovation and bringing about changes to improve how we do health care. The Chief Information Officer recommended that I enrol in a PhD in information systems. Once again, my studies were based on my job, inextricably blended into the work I was doing through action research. At that point I discovered that I was doing health informatics and it became part of my identity.

With a PhD I became an academic—learning, teaching, and researching health informatics. As a supervisor of research students, I relate to clinicians, their environment and the learning they do that will enrich their roles. My experience in hosting hackathons, leading and teaching postgraduate and undergraduate informatics, conducting research in telehealth, consumer informatics, evaluation of information systems, and change management, have left their mark on me. I deeply identify with health informatics as seen in my teaching and workforce research—it means a lot to me to influence the next generation of the HIDDIN workforce, and to have far-reaching positive impacts on the way people do their jobs.

Discussion and Conclusion

Our original identities as nurses and midwives have been enriched with understanding how the whole health system works. We are successors of Florence Nightingale, in this respect; 200 years after her birth we are as baffled as she was by the institutional and processual silos that interfere with clinical workflow, continuity of care and quality of care. All of us have extended our clinical roles to reach into the possibilities associated with digital health. To varying degrees, we learnt something about clinical informatics in our basic training and augmented that with information specialist learning to solve problems and advocate for change—to ensure that clinical information systems meet nurses' and midwives' needs as well as those of other clinicians. We are prepared to keep advocating for change through leadership and support for those who need to learn and adapt to new digital health ways of working.

The impact of informatics was dramatic in Nightingale's time, when she developed visualisations of patient data for the first time in history so that funders and administrators were able to see at a glance the effects of hygiene, appropriate staff training and management, and environmental conditions on the morbidity and mortality of hospital patients. We take this for granted now and we have the advantage of digital data management and associated informatics initiatives. Innovation is at our fingertips, as described by Sally and Karen Day. We become the bridges between information systems designers and implementers, and the clinicians who use those systems, as described by Lisa, Sally and Karen Blake. We are the voice of leadership to advocate for improved clinical care, as described by Lisa, Karen Blake and Karen Day. And because we are nurses and midwives, we provide support for those who need our help, whether as our patients or as our colleagues who are learning new ways of working, as described by Abin. All of us solve problems that require our information specialist skills, which lie in the sweet spot between what it means to be a nurse and/or midwife and to be an information specialist. Like Nightingale, we may not see the full impact of our work in our lifetime, but we work to ensure that one day we will no longer be the most invisible subgroup of the HIDDIN workforce.

References

Britnell S. Weight estimation without waiting: design, development and testing of a mobile application to measure the length and estimate the weight of New Zealand children for advanced paediatric resuscitation. Auckland University of Technology; 2020.

Brixey J, Salyer P, Simmons D. Nightingale power: the advent of nursing informatics. Nurs Manage. 2020;51(7):51–3.

HIMSS. Nursing informatics workforce survey. 2020. https://www.himss.org/sites/hde/files/media/file/2020/05/15/himss_nursinginformaticssurvey2020_v4.pdf. Accessed 15 May 2021.

Honey M, Collins E, Britnell S. Education into policy: embedding health informatics to prepare future nurses – New Zealand case study. JMIR Nursing. 2020;3(1):e16186.

Hübner U, Shaw T, Thye J, Egbert N, de Fatima MH, Chang P, et al. Technology Informatics Guiding Education Reform–TIGER. Meth Inf Med. 2018;57(S01):e30–42.

Meleis AI, Sawyer LM, Im E-O, Messias DKH, Schumacher K. Experiencing transitions: an emerging middle-range theory. Adv Nurs Sci. 2000;23(1):12–28.

MOH NZ. New Zealand Health Survey. Wellington: Ministry of Health New Zealand; 2020. https://www.health.govt.nz/nz-health-statistics/national-collections-and-surveys/surveys/new-zealand-health-survey. Accessed 22 Oct 2020.

Nursing Council of New Zealand. Trends in the New Zealand Nursing workforce: 2012–2016. Wellington; 2017.

World Health Organization. State of the World's Nursing Report. 2020. https://www.who.int/publications/i/item/9789240003279. Accessed 15 May 2021.

Chapter 24
Working as a Public Health Informatician

Karen Day, Robyn Whittaker, Vicki Bennett, Vanessa Selak, and Brian Stokes

Abstract Public health realises its potential when information specialisation is part of the job of protecting and improving the health of populations. With the benefit of information specialisation, practitioners are able to tap into evidence, leverage the value that data adds and improve services at individual, local, regional, national and global levels. This chapter contains four narratives of careers of public health information specialists in which they describe their career journeys, the innovations they have spearheaded, and the impact of their work on the health of populations. We then relate their narratives to identity, impact and innovation to illustrate how diverse career pathways converge on public health information specialisation, enable innovation and define far-reaching impacts.

Keywords Case study · Public health · Population health · Global health · Community health

K. Day (✉) · V. Selak
School of Population Health, University of Auckland, Auckland, New Zealand
e-mail: k.day@auckland.ac.nz; v.selak@auckland.ac.nz

R. Whittaker
Institute for Innovation and Improvement, Waitemata District Health Board,
Auckland, New Zealand
e-mail: robyn.whittaker@waitematadhb.govt.nz

V. Bennett
Metadata and METeOR Unit, Australian Institute of Health and Welfare,
Canberra, ACT, Australia
e-mail: vicki.bennett@aihw.gov.au

B. Stokes
Menzies Institute for Medical Research, University of Tasmania, Hobart, TAS, Australia
e-mail: brian.stokes@utas.edu.au

339

Introduction

Public health focuses on the community. The community has many faces, e.g. local communities, populations and nations. Within each of these communities, public health practitioners work to prevent illness, promote health and address health issues from a population and infrastructure perspective that results in improved health outcomes simultaneously for individuals and groups of people. Public health typically involves monitoring, diagnosing and investigating health issues in communities; informing and educating people about health issues and identifying ways for them to access services that are out of their reach; mobilising communities and developing policies to address health issues that affect communities and policing policies and regulations; evaluating the impact of public health policies and implementations; researching insights and innovations to take public health to the next level, and assuring an appropriately qualified and skilled workforce to provide public health services for individuals and communities (Magnuson and Dixon 2020). The information needs of public health practitioners include statistics, guidelines, research, government reports and finding data (Barr-Walker 2017). Electronic data collections, such as immunisation registers, are a valued source for public health. Creating, maintaining and making best use of these databases requires public health information specialists.

The inclusion of digital health and information science in public health is a small step, since public health work so obviously relies on information management. Public health informatics is defined as 'the systematic application of information, computer science and technology in areas of public health, including surveillance, prevention, preparedness, and health promotion' (Aziz 2017: 78). The context and scope of public health informatics is as broad as it is wide. Its identity lies within this scope; with a focus on illness prevention and health promotion that ranges from interventions that affect the environment to interventions aimed at individuals within their communities. This reach benefits from digital technologies and associated innovations that take public health interventions into the homes of individuals. The impact of such a reach is woven into everyday lives, e.g. by targeting a population (such as people with diabetes) on their mobile phones with a diabetes monitoring and management program via texts (Dobson et al. 2018). The digital and information challenges faced by the public health workforce stem from new health issues too, such as the COVID-19 pandemic. This poses opportunities for the public health workforce to reposition itself (Meng 2020). The ability to create large databases raises opportunities to create innovative public health interventions, but to make the most of the data, the workforce requires new skills in big data analytics and the use of artificial intelligence in making sense of the data. However, many public health databases remain manual or based on localised use of Excel spread sheets—thus are not readily connected with other useful databases, e.g. a cancer registry separated from electronic health records. The pandemic juxtaposed the lack of inter-regional laboratory data sharing to manage epidemics with the need to share data globally with other countries and with the World Health Organisation. The public health workforce must expand its information skills to address new and old problems. This chapter examines the careers of four people who have done so.

Robyn Whittaker, Waitemata District Health Board, New Zealand

Mobilising public health has been a key theme in my career. I am a public health physician—a doctor specialised in public health, population health, epidemiology, health impact assessment and health services planning. My first placements as a trainee were in health informatics—in regional health services planning and then in a hospital assessing clinical indicators. I went on to do more traditional public health service roles but returned to digital health initially through an academic role. I was employed at the University of Auckland to help with the dissemination and implementation of the first health intervention delivered solely by text messages, proven effective in a randomised controlled trial (Rodgers et al. 2005). This started my interest in using mobile communications to deliver healthy behaviour change and self-management support programmes directly to people. The mobile phone was fast becoming ubiquitous and outstripping any previous technology in terms of the speed of global spread and penetration into vulnerable communities. New Zealand was at the forefront of mobile health (mHealth) research and development, cementing my role and the topic of my PhD. This has led to a body of mHealth interventions, co-designed with communities and clinicians, tested in real-world randomised trials, and several implemented in practice across a variety of contexts and countries (Whittaker et al. 2012a–c).

My international networks in mHealth were given a huge boost through a Harkness Fellowship in Healthcare Policy and Practice and 12 months working in the US federal health system (Whittaker et al. 2012a). Upon return to New Zealand, I took up a role at Waitematā District Health Board while continuing my academic career. This role led to a strategic programme of work in digitising the hospital system and implementing innovations in the health service as part of establishing an Institute for Innovation and Improvement. My interest in making cool things happen has led to dabbling in a variety of different specific fields including mHealth, health IT, telehealth, wearables, big data and AI. I think that the public health perspective brings big picture thinking and the population perspective to all this work. Conversely, I think an interest in informatics and digital brings an openness to new ways of doing things to the public health sector.

Learning from others and particularly other countries has always been a large part of my work. I enjoy working internationally, on mHealth trials and implementations, as well as with the World Health Organization (WHO) as part of their Digital Health Technical Advisory Group and 'Be Healthy Be Mobile' global initiative (WHO 2020). Recently I have been involved in developing an in-house course for clinicians with an interest in digital, causing me to reflect on the paths my colleagues have taken to get to the roles they now occupy. These pathways are varied and were not often planned in advance—mine certainly wasn't. Those who have taken circuitous routes to digital health often have a breadth of experience and passion for improvement in general that adds substantially to what they bring. A clinical background or deep experience of the health sector is invaluable, and works well alongside the fresh perspective and new approaches brought by those completing health informatics and related courses.

Vicki Bennett, Australian Institute of Health and Welfare, Australia

My career has taken me from Health Information Management (HIM) to population health. When I finished high school, I started an accounting degree, but quickly worked out that I had too much personality for that! So, I enrolled in a Bachelor of Applied Science (HIM) at the University of Sydney. Not only was the varied content intellectually appealing, but I was told that there were lots of jobs available, including part-time. I knew that I wanted to have a family, so work flexibility was important. I was pregnant when I finished my degree, so the ensuing years included lots of part-time and contract roles including working as a data manager in a cancer unit (arguably my first foray as a Public Health Information Manager (PHIM), teaching IT units in the HIM degree program, and developing a database for the first set of Australian Clinical Coding Standards. Then, with two toddlers in tow, I moved to a village in the catchment region of the national capital, Canberra; over the next 5 years, I worked at Yass Hospital 1 day a week looking after all things health information- and data-related, and had another two children. During this time, I also continued to stay strongly committed to my professional identity as a HIM and often self-funded my attendance at professional development events. I then moved into Canberra and I worked at a private hospital as the Administration Manager; I led the implementation of a new patient information system managing a team of 40 staff, and completed a Master of Science (Health Informatics) at the University of Sydney.

I was offered the opportunity to work as a HIM for 2 months on an Australian aid funded program in Vanuatu, due to a relationship between my hospital and one there. My CEO asked if I wanted to go, following up with 'but you probably can't because you have four kids'; notwithstanding, living and working in Vanuatu turned into an experience for my whole family, and was the true beginning of my appreciation of public health information and the vital role it plays in improving health outcomes. When I returned, I took on a position as the Manager of the Health Information Section at Medicare Australia, responsible for a team who provided publicly subsidised medical and pharmaceutical services data (MBS and PBS) to internal and external requestors. This was a new and interesting area involving the use of national health data to inform health policy, planning and research, including the establishment of a number of important major cohort studies. My heart was still in the Pacific Islands, so over the next few years I developed a health data dictionary and national health indicators for Tonga, then became the national HIM for the Ministry of Health in Fiji, again moving my whole family there. When I returned, I started work at the Australian Institute of Health and Welfare (AIHW) where I have held a range of roles managing national health and welfare data assets and developing national health indicators, including running the My Health Record Data Unit, the Expenditure and Workforce Unit, and now the Metadata and Classifications Unit.

In 2009, I took on the role of Project Manager of the Health Information Systems Knowledge Hub for Health at the School of Population Health at the University of Queensland. I worked extensively with the WHO and other international agencies and made ten international trips for work in 2010. I have since returned to work at the AIHW where I am able to continue to work in an area that allows me to fulfil my passion for public health and for using evidence to inform decision making in health continues. As well I remain committed to Pacific Island nations—I am now the official advisor to the Pacific Health Information Network Board. I could not be happier with the career I have had and I hope to continue to make a positive impact on public health outcomes for many years to come.

Vanessa Selak, University of Auckland, New Zealand

Using routinely collected electronic data to support improvements in health service quality has increasingly fascinated me during my career, as clinician and a health researcher. I completed training in medicine in 1998, specialist training in public health medicine in 2007, and a PhD in cardiovascular epidemiology in 2015. I have 20 years' experience working within the health sector, in roles spanning clinical medicine, planning, funding and quality improvement. In my most recent health sector role, in quality improvement, my job was to work with clinical directors of hospital specialty departments to help them to develop clinical quality indicators that could be reported on automatically and displayed in near real-time on specialty-specific dashboards using routinely collected electronic data. A critical aspect of the role was in being able to effectively translate between clinicians and their clinical priorities, and the analysts and the available electronic data.

A particularly fruitful collaboration emerged when working with a rheumatologist who wanted to develop an indicator of the proportion of patients with rheumatoid arthritis who were receiving disease-modifying anti-rheumatic drugs (DMARDs). Rheumatoid arthritis is primarily managed by rheumatologists in the outpatient department in the hospital, and medication is dispensed in community pharmacies. While we could identify all patients attending rheumatology outpatient clinics (and could determine whether this was for a first or subsequent specialist assessment) and all the medications that had been dispensed in the community (including DMARDs), we had no way of knowing which of the rheumatology patients had rheumatoid arthritis without manually looking up the records of each patient. This was because, although coding of clinical diagnoses is undertaken routinely for admissions (by administrators), it is not done for outpatient appointments at that hospital. There was no funding to support extension of coding of clinical diagnoses by administrators to include outpatient appointments, so the rheumatologist and I, supported by a quality improvement team, developed and implemented a sustainable system for integrating the coding of clinical diagnoses within the existing workflow of the rheumatologists for all outpatient clinic appointments. Initially we modified an existing paper-based process but were then able to progress to an electronic system. Not only was the rheumatologist able to receive automated reporting on the proportion of rheumatology patients receiving a DMARD, but for the first time they were able to automatically generate reports of their patient population by clinical diagnosis.

Since completing my PhD, which was based on data from randomised controlled trials, my research has increasingly focused on observational methods which use routinely collected electronic data. Undertaking such research is extremely attractive for a public health physician in New Zealand, for a number of reasons. We have a unique national health identifier (NHI), which enables us with ethics approval to link data for individuals across different data sets. As researchers we don't need to know who these individuals are, just that their data are linked, so we are able to maximise the privacy of included individuals by using encrypted, rather than live, NHIs. Our Ministry of Health collates and maintains a comprehensive selection of national datasets, including for mortality, hospitalisation, primary health organisation enrolment, community dispensing and laboratory test requests. Using these data collections, we are able to create national (or subnational) cohorts of health-contact populations. This means that research can be conducted at a truly population level at a manageable cost because data collection leverages existing data sources. We are currently restricted primarily to structured data, but efforts are underway to unpack the potential of unstructured data (such as from specialist letters and hospital discharge summaries) using methods such as natural language processing. Combining unstructured with structured data will increase our ability to identify and characterise clinically relevant cohorts of people from a population perspective, for example in order to assess the extent to which evidence-based interventions are being implemented for these cohorts. Further, we are also able to characterise these clinical cohorts according to important demographic factors such as ethnicity and socioeconomic status, which will increasingly enable us to assess the equity of the implementation of such interventions.

Brian Stokes, University of Tasmania, Australia

The undeniable value of data in public health is the theme running throughout my working life. I have always worked with data in differing forms. Earlier in my career, I worked in public sector tourism as a technology specialist with responsibility for data management and reporting. With a primary interest in using data to evidence and inform government and public policy, I completed a Bachelor of Arts degree with majors in political science and public policy, and with a focus on the emerging role of information technology in supporting data management. With the emergence of digital health in the early 2000s, I found myself drawn to the enormous opportunities presented through the growing use of technologies in the healthcare sector.

After a period working in central government in policy and project roles, in 2006 I joined the Mental Health and State-wide Services areas of the Tasmanian Department of Health, with responsibility for technology, data and information management. In this demanding but rewarding role, I found myself drawn to strategies centred on improving data quality to support state and national reporting across the mental health and alcohol and drug sectors. A key area of my responsibility was providing data annually to the Australian Institute of Health and Welfare across multiple national minimum datasets. At that time, data was collected manually by clinicians across acute inpatient, ambulatory and residential settings with unit record data coded manually according to the International Classification of Diseases (ICD) system and entered into a standalone database. The timeliness, accuracy, completeness and overall quality of data was considered low and presented problems at multiple levels. Nationally, when compared to other jurisdictions, certain key performance indicators suggested Tasmania was underperforming. Locally, with incomplete data and significant delays in coding of patient episodes of care, the absence of high quality data made resource and service planning challenging—especially when developing policy specific to requests for increased funding and service expansion, from consumers, carers, staff and the broader mental health and alcohol and drug sector.

For the past 9 years, I have been employed as Manager of the Tasmanian Cancer Registry (TCR) and the Tasmanian Data Linkage Unit (TDLU) of the Menzies Institute for Medical Research, University of Tasmania. In the former, data is collected specific to the incidence and mortality of malignant neoplasms in Tasmania. Cancer registration is required by law under the Public Health Act Tasmania 1997, with data used in a multiplicity of ways including those of previous roles—to inform policy direction, strategic planning and service provision. Data is coded centrally by TCR staff according to the ICD Version 3.1 classification system and reported at State and local levels. In the TDLU, a range of health and related datasets, collected and classified according to agreed standards, are used to support de-identified, Human Research Ethics Committee approved, whole of population research in Tasmania and Australia-wide. Today, as when I commenced working with health data earlier in my career, my unwavering focus remains on the collection, availability, reporting and quality of healthcare data and the innovative use of technology and systems that underpin timely data collection and reporting.

Discussion and Conclusion

Few people wake up in the morning and say, 'Today I want to start a career as a public health information specialist' and follow that up with an inquiry into the training they would need to complete or an appropriate career path to enter. Public health informatics is a logical progression from public health (Aziz 2017), but there is no equivalent to public health icon John Snow, to inspire future public health information specialists—this is still in the stage of 'becoming' an identifiable role. The identities of public health information specialists derive from an associated identity: as a public health physician, a health information manager or a public health policy maker and implementer, all with an interest in how information technologies influence the impact of public health. They have converged on the public health information specialisation from different trajectories, rather than identifying with it at the beginning of their career.

While Robyn took what some would say is a traditional journey as a public health physician and career path into policy, Brian started with policy. Vanessa flipped clinical reliance on randomised controlled trials, to explore routinely collected data as a means to improve the quality of care of a population of patients with rheumatoid arthritis. In contrast to Robyn's and Vanessa's journeys, Vicki was first an HIM and then became a public health information specialist.

In different ways their work has had an impact on the health of their communities (local, regional, national and beyond) demonstrating the breadth and depth of public health and the potential of information specialisation. Both Vicki and Robyn describe working within the global community of the World Health Organisation, to contribute to public health outside their own countries.

All our case study authors have been innovative, though not limited to information technology innovation. All have used the evidence derived from information systems to design and implement novel solutions to new and old problems. Innovative thinking and design are at the heart of solving the problems faced by public health information specialists; here, we have shown solutions in the form of an mHealth intervention, a data dictionary, a cancer registry and a creative use for routinely collected patient data. Increasingly, people in these roles need to know their way around the associated information systems, build and use evidence, and influence the health of populations, in ways that make sense and scale up in digitally enabled health systems.

References

Aziz HA. A review of the role of public health informatics in healthcare. J Taibah Univ Med Sci. 2017;12(1):78–81.

Barr-Walker J. Evidence-based information needs of public health workers: a systematized review. J Med Libr Assoc: JMLA. 2017;105(1):69.

Dobson R, Whittaker R, Jiang Y, Maddison R, Shepherd M, McNamara C, et al. Effectiveness of text message based, diabetes self management support programme (SMS4BG): two arm, parallel randomised controlled trial. BMJ. 2018;361:k1959.

Magnuson J, Dixon BE. Public health informatics: an introduction. In: Public health informatics and information systems. Springer; 2020. p. 3–16.

Meng X-L. COVID-19: a massive stress test with many unexpected opportunities (for data science). Harv Data Sci Rev. 2020.

Rodgers A, Corbett T, Bramley D, Riddell T, Wills M, Lin RB, Jones M. Do u smoke after txt? Results of a randomised trial of smoking cessation using mobile phone text messaging. Tobacco Control. 2005;14(4):255–61.

Whittaker R, Matoff-Stepp S, Kendrick J, Jordan E, Stange P, Cash A, et al. Text4baby: development and implementation of a National Text Messaging Health Information Service. Am J Public Health. 2012a;102(12):2207–13.

Whittaker R, McRobbie H, Bullen C, Borland R, Rodgers A, Gu Y. Mobile phone-based interventions for smoking cessation. Cochrane Database of Systematic Reviews. 2012b;(11 Art No.: CD006611).

Whittaker R, Merry SN, Stasiak K, McDowell H, Shepherd M, Dorey E, et al. MEMO–a mobile phone depression prevention intervention for adolescents: development process and post-program findings on acceptability from a randomised controlled trial. J Med Internet Res. 2012c;14(1):e13.

WHO. Addressing mobile health. WHO; 2020. https://www.who.int/activities/Addressing-mobile-health. Accessed 16 Oct 2020.

Chapter 25
Journeys into Becoming a Digital Health Specialist

Urooj R. Khan, Leanna Woods, Gerardo Luis C. Dimaguila, Mohamed Khalifa, Elizabeth Schoff, Greig Russell, and Saswata Ray

Abstract Digital health specialists are by definition a pluralistic heterogeneous professional group; their career pathways are neither straight nor smooth. This chapter contains seven narratives of professionals, their journeys into becoming digital health specialists, their aspirations, and their career prospects. These narratives speak of identity, impact, and innovation and illustrate how diverse career pathways out of clinical and technological careers have converged to define roles in digital health. These narratives have important implications for how this specialised workforce needs to be trained, identified, and retained, to meet the growing needs of digital health in patient care, health system planning, and policy making.

Keywords Case study · Doctoral degree · Fellowship · Training · Mentorship

U. R. Khan (✉)
La Trobe University, Bundoora, VIC, Australia
e-mail: u.razakhan@latrobe.edu.au

L. Woods
The University of Queensland, Brisbane, QLD, Australia
e-mail: lee.woods@uq.edu.au

G. L. C. Dimaguila
Murdoch Children's Research Institute, Parkville, VIC, Australia
e-mail: gerardoluis.dimaguil@mcri.edu.au

M. Khalifa
Macquarie University, Sydney, NSW, Australia
e-mail: Mohamed.khalifa@mq.edu.au

E. Schoff · S. Ray
University of Auckland, Auckland, New Zealand
e-mail: liz@pleioneconsulting.com; saswata.ray@auckland.ac.nz

G. Russell
Massey University, Palmerston North, New Zealand
e-mail: greig.russell@russellhealth.org

© The Author(s), under exclusive license to Springer Nature
Switzerland AG 2021
K. Butler-Henderson et al. (eds.), *The Health Information Workforce*,
Health Informatics, https://doi.org/10.1007/978-3-030-81850-0_25

349

Introduction

The potential of digital technologies to benefit healthcare has been evident in recent years, but implementation has encountered challenges at various levels; the effort required to deliver on significant digital health investments is often underestimated and the workforce required is often invisible (Gray et al. 2019). Technology is not a panacea, and theories of technology adoption put the focus on workflow, process, task-fitness, and other user-related factors that indicate the cultural shift needed to use technologies effectively in complex and sensitive healthcare environments (Raza Khan et al. 2019). Such use of digital technologies requires a multidisciplinary approach (Smith et al. 2011), specifically the development of a specialist workforce that understands both the technical and clinical aspects of a digital health program (Parry et al. 2013; Whetton 2005). Digital health specialists are critical in the digital transformation of health (Butler-Henderson and Gray 2019), in two key roles: creating and managing clinical information from raw patient data and delivering it to the point of care; and acting as the bridge between the work cultures of clinical and technical teams across the health organisation. Technical, clinical, and other communities within the broad health environment often resemble tribes, looking within to define who they are to themselves and others (Mannion and Davies 2018). But digital health specialists exist to enable the binding and integrating of health workforce tribes. Some of them choose to keep one foot in their tribe of origin, and one foot in a self-defined digital health tribe (Dave et al. 2008), and maybe this is why they are hard to perceive distinctly. Some reports indicate that the current specialist workforce is ageing and consequently the future productivity of the health sector is at risk (Butler-Henderson and Gray 2018); the COVID-19 pandemic resulted in rapid adoption of virtual care and other related digital health technologies, indicating a rising need for such specialised professionals (Sarbadhikari et al. 2020). However digital health specialist career structures are unclear—how someone lands into this space, gains professional recognition, finds pathways forward. Building capacity—through workforce planning, developing specialist qualifications, training programs, and career pathways—is essential to satisfy the growing demand for such roles (Butler-Henderson et al. 2020). This chapter explores the stories of seven clinical and technology professionals to trace common threads in their profiles, their motivations and trajectory in becoming digital health specialists, and to relate their reflections to the concepts of workforce identity, impact, and innovation.

Urooj Raza Khan: "I wanted my health records anywhere anytime."

Sometimes a moment can change your life aims. It was such a moment for me in August 2012, lying in the operating theatre, nearly unconscious after going through immense pain from a ruptured ectopic pregnancy, thinking that I am in a technology era in a developed country that has a world-class health system… there must be a way to inform these clinicians, when I can't speak, about my chronic illness, sensitivities and its effects on me….before I could think anything else, I was asleep. The background to this incident is that I relocated from the city to the countryside in 2012 and was trying to transfer my health records from a general practice in Melbourne to a new one in regional Victoria; after the initial consultation with my new GP, I kept my next check-ups on hold for some time, thinking I would follow up once my health records were transferred. Thus I came out of hospital frustrated, sad, and angry, wondering how it is possible in today's world that I am unable to inform clinicians about my condition in an emergency or how can take so long to transfer GP records? My career as a technologist with 12 years of experience in IT business systems implementation and management of various electronic record systems, eGovernment and eCommerce solutions, made it impossible for me to comprehend the situation in the health sector. Dealing with post-natal depression, I was encouraged to use my disappointment and energy positively, so I started investigating any technological solutions that could ease health records transfer among clinicians and enable health record accessibility by clinicians when one is unable to speak. My mantra was "there has to be a better way!".

I learnt there was such a solution, which could store my health records and make them accessible to clinicians and myself easily, Australia's Personally Controlled Electronic Health Record (PCEHR). I conducted a Master of Science research project investigating PCEHR adoption in regional Victoria and realised its teething issues. Not satisfied with my findings, I pursued doctoral research about MyHealthRecord (the new name for PCEHR) adoption in general practices. I started with curiosity, thinking I was exploring technology issues. Soon I learnt that there were process- and people-related socio-technical challenges, limited provisions for change management and cultural shift, significantly delaying system adoption. I investigated the problems with ten general practices and developed a framework for improving the integration of the MyHealthRecord system into their workflow.

After one of my industry supervisors directed me to the field of health informatics, I was accepted in a fellowship training program that extended my professional development into digital health. During my associated work placement, I was involved in planning and initiating various innovative digital health projects. I discovered the real-world challenges of fragmented health data and its silos. I also learnt not only that digital health is surrounded by numerous challenges related to data, technology, organisations and people, but also that technology implementation is handled very differently by various disciplines. Even when people are motivated to progress in digital health with all good intentions, their journey is protracted as they learn new dimensions of each other's knowledge and communication conventions.

To date, I am unable to find a satisfactory answer to the question, why is it so difficult to have our health records accessible anytime, anywhere? The legacy of my own hospital emergency episode now seems like a lifetime reminder; it has given me a purpose to do more so that no one else should have to go through what I have suffered. It leads me on to explore my opportunities to make an impact in digital health through projects, education and research: in 2020, I joined La Trobe

University as a senior lecturer. In this role, I am involved to coordinate, develop, and teach postgraduate courses in digital health. I am also leading a community of practice to mentor students and interns who are conducting various virtual care related industry research projects (in collaboration with Australia's Digital Health Cooperative Research Centre). I feel this is my calling now, to make a difference and make a contribution to a better healthcare system. I believe my journey entails much more learning about digital health, and many further opportunities to find answers. Bring it on!

Leanna (Lee) Woods: "Administration should not absorb one third of my time as a nurse."

It was 2 o'clock in the morning at the nurses' station, when I realised something was dramatically inefficient with the way healthcare was delivered. With 8 years of clinical practice behind me, I had seen advances in biomedical science—so how could it be that I was writing my new patient's admission weight, with pen on paper, four times, across the various admission documents? Tired and frustrated, I placed multiple admission paperwork pages for a single patient end-to-end on the floor, lay down alongside these, and measured their length, amused at its relation to my own. Administration would absorb some 30% of my time as a nurse, pulling me away from the bedside where my patients lay afraid, confused or in pain. I made the decision to get qualified, be heard and make a difference on a larger scale than six patients I cared for in a single shift. I knew it was time to make my contribution to the digital transformation of healthcare.

Six years later, I have a two post graduate certificates, a research honours degree and Doctor of Philosophy which span the fields of clinical nursing, research, and digital health. My doctorate investigated clinician-led innovation, mobile health, and patient empowerment. Following this I undertook the requirements of the Fellowship by Training program with the Australasian Institute of Digital Health, affording me the opportunity to complete coursework in digital health topics and learn from experts across industry, health, and research. The highlight was contributing to national policy development in a 12-month work placement with a federal government department.

Digital health offers powerful ways to connect information to people when and where it is needed, to keep the patient at the centre of their health. Unless digital health is used to its full potential, there is a missed opportunity to better health outcomes both at an individual and population level. Nurses are innovative, adaptable, and committed to people, yet the data we generate, correct, and use is stored in paper records in vaults under hospitals. As the largest workforce in health, nurses advocate for safe, quality patient care across a great number of settings, however nursing leadership in senior positions in the health, education and government sector is less than proportionate to the numbers in the workforce. I now have a seat at the table to make positive change, because of the pre- and post-nominals I have earned and the professional network I am developing.

My becoming a specialist has been based on my mission to focus on the humans behind the technology, to enable the realisation of digital health technologies in practice. My pursuit of learning and impact has continued with my return to academic research, in collaboration with a State health system, to advance the connection of patient information across the healthcare journey. Digital health specialists are fearless optimists from a variety of backgrounds working on the same goal but from different angles.

Gerardo Luis (Ikee) Dimaguila: "…passionate about patient empowerment and bridging healthcare gaps through technological innovation."

When I finished my bachelor's degree in Computer Science in the Philippines, I didn't know what to do next. I loved my degree, but I didn't want to work as a full-time programmer. I was driven by curiosity and the desire to contribute positively, and in the university, I spent a significant amount of time constantly finding ways to be involved in volunteering activities and community organisations. I was fortunate to be accepted as the consultant and designer of a project to develop the first national registry of child neurological diseases. In my role, I had to understand and implement data documentation and reporting using the ICD-10 standard. I was not even aware of any health standard at the time! I had to learn about the standard so we could integrate it into the database. I also had my first taste of digital health challenges, such as how some terminologies used by neurology practices may not be directly mappable to the ICD codes; and how data collection processes and resources available at different clinics across the country could vary. Through successive consultations, my team established processes for nationwide neurological data collection and management, and a feedback loop so varying terminologies could be flagged, and consensus reached. My first dip into digital health was a relative success, but I felt that there were many things I could have done better—but I was not sure what, or how.

Serendipitously, a new Master of IT degree with a health specialisation launched at the University of Melbourne around the same time as the registry project ended. I enrolled in this degree and secured an Australian government Endeavour scholarship. I learned that the challenges I had encountered in designing and developing the registry were quite common, and that digital health frameworks, principles, and methods could have guided me then. I became passionate about patient empowerment and bridging healthcare gaps through technological innovation and digital health expertise, and I researched and published an evaluation of the possible challenges facing mobile health technologies in under-resourced settings. To merge my digital health interests, I decided to pursue a PhD in digital health. I developed a novel framework enabling people to report their health effects and outcomes, when they use the data that they generate from engaging with health information technologies, and I disseminated my research through six publications in high-quality journals.

In digital health one does not have to look far to find meaningful work. In our State's vaccine safety service, I work closely with clinicians and epidemiologists so data and information guide government policies on Covid vaccine roll outs. I also hope to learn and look for ways to bridge healthcare access gaps, especially in under-resourced settings, through critical and thoughtful use of digital health design and evaluation frameworks and principles. I am excited to be in a field that continually challenges its practitioners and experts to ask: What can I do best, and better; where are my skills needed now and in the future?

Mohamed Khalifa: "I could add greater value in population health through informatics, as compared to treating individual patients."

My childhood was spent closely connected to computers, however, I studied medicine and graduated in 2001 as a medical doctor. Based on the slowness and inefficiency of healthcare processes that I experienced shortly thereafter, I decided to use my computer skills to improve the clinical outcomes of patients. I believed technology could save time and provide more accurate results. In 2002 I had the opportunity to implement a health information system to run the oncology medical centre where I worked, which resulted in improvements in our services to patients.

This experience changed my mindset: I realised that I could add a greater value in population health through informatics, as compared to treating individual patients. I took a full-time job as a medical IT consultant, developing and implementing health information systems. For my professional development in this field, I studied healthcare management at the American University in Cairo. It brought me an opportunity to teaching health informatics to doctors. I continued my studies from 2009 to 2012 in a Master of Science in Health Informatics at the University of Edinburgh, and I became a member of the Royal College of Surgeons of Edinburgh. I also became a HIMSS Certified Professional in Healthcare Information & Management Systems.

In 2012, I moved to a major tertiary care hospital to lead the Health Informatics and Performance Improvement departments. Over 5 years, I led diverse teams of healthcare and IT professionals to use health informatics in improving patient safety, effectiveness, efficiency, and timeliness of healthcare services. I worked on reducing waiting times, improving productivity, streamlining discharge processes, and reducing unnecessary lab tests. I also worked on reducing avoidable hospital admissions and frequent non-urgent emergency visits. I developed key performance indicators, operational dashboards, and strategic scorecards to improve services. I published over 30 papers documenting my projects and sharing my experience with colleagues worldwide.

I moved to Australia in 2017, as a distinguished talent permanent resident, and joined the PhD in Health Innovation at Macquarie University, after I had been awarded a Commonwealth government funded PhD scholarship. I developed an evidence-based framework for grading and assessment of clinical predictive tools—the GRASP framework. In 2018, I was granted my first innovation patent from IP Australia for my framework. In 2020, my core published PhD paper was selected by the International Medical Informatics Association as best paper worldwide in medical informatics, and appeared in the IMIA 2020 Yearbook.

Over 20 years I have developed a global career as a consultant and director in health informatics, business intelligence, and digital health, and I have engaged from three main perspectives: business development and implementation, professional hospital operation and utilisation, and academic research and training. Going forward, I am interested in investing in my skills, knowledge, and experience to contribute to the continuing digital transformation of the Australian healthcare system.

Greig Russell: "The daylight is slowly creeping in."

Describing myself as a health informaticist and getting the newly created sole full-time role in my hospital felt akin to telling people something socially stigmatising about myself. My friends said they had known all along but did not want to say anything. I was instantly demoted to a second-class citizen in the professional pecking order in the hospital, but I was happy! Paying my way through medical school as a software developer for actuarial software might have given some clues. My honours thesis was in health informatics, rebadged of course. Still, once I became a doctor, everyone let me put my sordid IT past behind me and start again: my mother was so proud of her son the real doctor.

So my double life started, working as a clinician by day, and at night using health information to improve clinical outcomes. This study evolved into studying extramurally at the local university, but always on the quiet. Many colleagues looked the other way, though a few were incredibly supportive. Slowly my health informatics skillset grew, in computer science, statistics, clinical coding and classification systems, as well as health systems theory. I moved from solving a specific problem through ad hoc learning to the broader joined-up knowledge base, one course, one book, one video at a time, with lots of mistakes and many blind alleys.

Slowly, various doors started to open as I worked on shared problems with new colleagues, particularly from the local university. The statisticians and philosophers in particular welcomed me into the most fascinating and exhilarating conversations of my life. Transactional medicine was getting in the way of my secret academic life; my desire grew to use health informatics to contribute to population health outcomes and optimisation of health system management to support clinicians. However, when I seized the chance for my dream job, as a health informaticist, this triggered new challenges. In my mind, I am still a clinician, but I just use different tools and have a population health focus; the snag is that there is no recognised health informatics speciality in medicine. Growing as a practitioner is no problem, thanks to the internet, Amazon and the fantastic Rstats community around the world, but getting this learning recognised as clinical activity is not straightforward. I have included my health informatics study into my clinical speciality continuing medical education system, and hoped for the best, and so far everyone has looked the other way, and it has worked out—but a vehicle for professional recognition is badly needed. I quickly discovered that my academic knowledge and practical experience were not the reason I was hired for my dream job, nor are these valued greatly in the digital health business culture of personalities and events—I have a presence in that world though still not a much of a voice. I hope and believe that a new day is dawning, however slowly, on professional recognition and respect for the role of the health informaticist.

Elizabeth (Liz) Schoff: "Technology has changed, but people are still key to leveraging its value."

My journey into the world of health informatics started from a completely unrelated life situation and I had no idea where it would lead me. I'm a techie—not the geeky kind, but instead the people kind. I love working with people who are having trouble understanding when technology can help and how. I'm also the first person to wave a banner when technology is not the answer. My journey into health informatics started while I supported my mother in her final years. As we travelled from doctor to doctor, I would listen to her recount her medical history to each newly acquired specialist, gently correcting and prompting her when she left out major medical events or conditions, or confused dates and people. I tried to help by creating (what I now know!) her medical record—a spread sheet of her medications and medication history and a chronological (e.g. longitudinal) health record.

Fast forward a couple of years, I had relocated from California to New Zealand, and was looking for a job that would allow me to stay. Because of my technology and management skills, I landed a job heading Northern Region Professional Services at the healthcare software vendor, Orion Health. During my interviews, I leaned on my personal experience creating my mother's medical record. Working at Orion Health and with the Northern Region healthcare providers, I realised I had fallen into a world that fit me—people who wanted to help people, but who didn't have the right fit, or sometimes any fit, for the technology that would make a difference. This was an opportunity to build into systems, the constant need to balance people, process and technology—a three-legged stool that would surely topple if one leg grew too long.

I needed more training. I signed up for a Master of Science degree at the University of Auckland's School of Population Health, focusing on health informatics. I was often the only techie in classes of nurses, doctors, and researchers. Listening to the discussions of those who had come from the clinical world really broadened my empathy for the challenges that technology has brought to healthcare. I wanted more involvement. I joined Health Informatics New Zealand (HINZ), then joined the Executive Committee, and moved into a lead role to restructure the HINZ organisation. This time, I was working to balance the perspectives of clinical, academic, and commercial stakeholders; again, it was all about the balance.

Through all this, I have continued to work in hospitals and healthcare related entities. Technology has changed, as has our cultural acceptance of technology, but people are still key to leveraging its value. Now I focus on cybersecurity, where we look at how people, process, and technology work together to keep our electronic health information under our own control, secure and private, as it should be.

Saswata (Sas) Ray: "Some beautiful paths can't be discovered without getting lost." (Erol Ozan)

I certainly don't want to get lost on my career path, but I feel this quote has something to do with my career decisions, maybe something to do with my subconscious performing silent tricks on my conscious, before my conscious being typed a search into Google, 'digital health'.

I was in Mumbai, India, working for the number one healthcare service provider in the country. I had worked in clinical operations, medical writing, pharmacovigilance, and clinical research data management over a span of 8 years. Life was sorted out almost perfectly, but I felt a push from inside to do something that was not written in a 'protocol' and that would allow me to leave a digital footprint (by writing a thesis). Thus I landed in Aotearoa, New Zealand, to do a PhD at the University of Auckland. My PhD is exploring how social media may influence food decisions for young adults. The urge to find a research topic outside clinical research grew after I wrote a review paper on social media and clinical research. As a professional I was attracted to research that had the potential to influence our daily lives in health related ways, and I became fascinated with the power of the virtual world to affect us in so many ways. I am excited that my PhD topic is the first national study of its kind at this point, and this helps me to keep going.

Moving on from clinical trials to embark on a new path was not an easy choice, but when I made the decision, I banked on my skills being transferable in an informatics role. Working in all domains of clinical research had given me a positive mindset about being able to traverse new domains, to rise to a challenge and to shift from one stream of healthcare research to another. In addition I imagined the fun and satisfaction in contributing to a project that could improve patient outcomes. As I gain more exposure to the field of health informatics I am feeling more confident to meet other professionals and have conversations about fascinating topics, and I am getting to know more about different roles and requirements. Given an opportunity, I would like to work as a clinical business analyst who knows what happens in the clinical field and is able to translate the needs to a software developer.

Discussion and Conclusion

The case studies in this chapter tell of passionate professionals with various information sciences and health sciences backgrounds and pivotal life and work experiences. Urooj, Liz, and Ikee worked through multiple roles in the technology industry whereas Khalifa, Lee, Greig, and Sas worked in clinical positions. They observed and experienced problems in patient care, health records inaccessibility and fragmentation, technology adoption resistance, and systems inefficiencies. They realised how digital technologies can help the healthcare industry deal with these challenges and became determined to explore how to contribute to improve efficiency, effectiveness, and safety of health technology design, development, and evaluation. A personal drive sustained the momentum in each of them, as they proceeded through the indeterminate nature of the digital health profession. Their stories illustrate the lack of a formal pathway to enter and advance in the field. Greig and Liz were able to find their way into digital health through years of work experience. Others followed PhD pathways, and some undertook a fellowship training program as well. All navigated different routes to come to identify themselves as digital health specialists. Coming through such individualised experiences has made them resilient; in them, the digital health workforce has dedicated emotionally intelligent real-world problem solvers, likely to have significant impact through work in academia, in applied research, and in the digital health industry. They will view challenges through diverse lenses and develop multidisciplinary solutions using outside-the-box thinking and evidence-based approaches. Each one brings something unique to the evolution of the health care system.

The healthcare industry is often tribal (Dave et al. 2008), and such a culture can be the source of harm and conflict, but it is also possible that culture can be a source of remedy, as can technology. Health information ideally is a force multiplier, reducing the stress on staff and improving both patient experiences and clinical outcomes. Digital health specialists are a pluralistic heterogeneous professional group that builds information and communication bridges between the technical and the clinical tribes. Their work is translational and holistic; more than merely having expertise in dual disciplines, the whole of their skillset is greater than the sum of the parts, and they can make key contributions once they find their voice and assert their ability. Imagine how much more powerful these individuals' contributions could be if they had a firm base of professional recognition from which to build! In concluding, this chapter shares their experiences to frame a call for the health sector: to raise awareness of the exciting possibilities to work as a digital health specialist; to provide high-quality specialist learning and training options; to encourage consistent specialist identification and affiliation; and to formally recognise the value of this specialist workforce. Innovations in these aspects of workforce culture will widen and deepen understanding of the need for change in healthcare and of the positive transformation that is possible through digital health.

References

Butler-Henderson K, Gray K. Australia's Health Information Workforce: Census Summary Report. Launceston, Australia: University of Tasmania; 2018.

Butler-Henderson K, Gray K. A Glimpse at the Australian Health Information Workforce: findings from the First Australian Census. Stud Health Technol Inform. 2019;264:1145–9.

Butler-Henderson K, Gray K, Day K, Grainger R, editors. Defining the Health Information Technology discipline: results from the 2018 Australian and New Zealand censuses. Proceedings of the Australasian Computer Science Week Multiconference. 2020.

Dave L, John K, Halee F-W. Tribal leadership. Aurora: HR.COM; 2008. 4 p

Gray K, Gilbert C, Butler-Henderson K, Day K, Pritchard S. Ghosts in the machine: identifying the digital health information workforce. Stud Health Technol Inform. 2019;257:146–51.

Mannion R, Davies H. Understanding organisational culture for healthcare quality improvement. BMJ. 2018;363:k4907.

Parry D, Hunter I, Honey M, Holt A, Day K, Kirk R, Cullen R. Building an educated health informatics workforce–the New Zealand experience. In: Grain H, Schaper L, editors. Health informatics: digital health service delivery-the future is now!: Selected Papers from the 21st Australian National Health Informatics Conference (HIC 2013). IOS Press; 2013.

Raza Khan U, Zia T, Perera K, Pearce C. User acceptance of MyHealthRecord system in general practices. Int J Cyber-Physical Syst IJCPS. 2019;1(1).

Sarbadhikari SN, Pradhan KBJS, Work Ha. The need for developing technology-enabled, safe, and ethical workforce for healthcare delivery. 2020.

Smith SE, Drake LE, Harris J-GB, Watson K, Pohlner PG. Clinical informatics: a workforce priority for 21st century healthcare. JAHR. 2011;35(2):130–5.

Whetton S, editor. Health informatics workforce skills: technology is king, time for a consort? HINZ: Proceedings. 2005.

Index

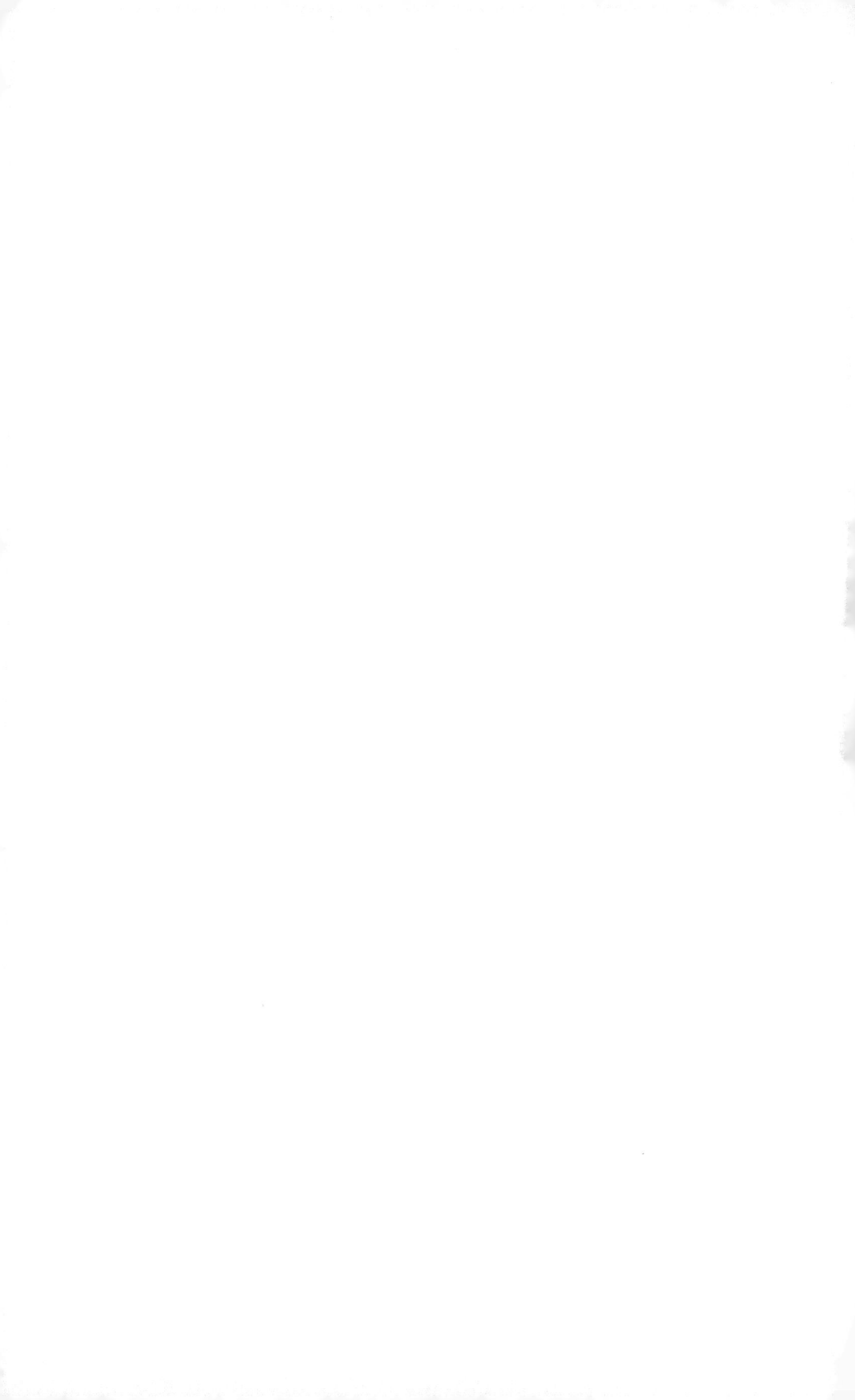